S0-BPY-000

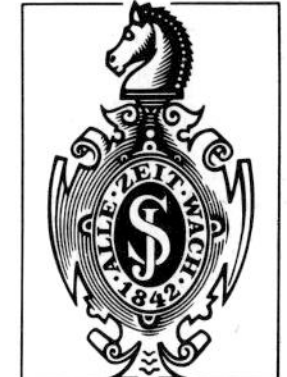

Julien L. Van Lancker

Molecular and Cellular Mechanisms in Disease

2

Cell Death · Blood Lipids and Arteriosclerosis · Radiation Injury · Inflammation Immunopathology · Regeneration and Wound Healing · Cancer

With 145 Figures

Springer-Verlag
Berlin Heidelberg New York 1976

Professor JULIEN L. VAN LANCKER, M.D., Department of Pathology, U.C.L.A. School of Medicine, Los Angeles, California 90024/U.S.A.

ISBN 3-540-06932-1 Springer-Verlag Berlin Heidelberg New York
ISBN 0-387-06932-1 Springer-Verlag New York Heidelberg Berlin

Library of Congress Cataloging in Publication Data. Van Lancker, Julien L. 1924– Molecular and cellular mechanisms in disease. Includes bibliographical references and indexes. 1. Pathology, Molecular. 2. Pathology, Cellular. I. Title. [DNLM: 1. Pathology. 2. Molecular biology. QZ4 V259m] RB27.V33 611′.0181 76-4844

Printed in Germany.

Typesetting, printing, and bookbinding by Universitätsdruckerei H. Stürtz AG, Würzburg

Contents · Volume 2

Chapter 10. Cellular Death and Degeneration 604

Introduction 607
Cell Death in Biology 607
Necrosis 608
Role of Hydrolases in Cell Death 620
The Point of No Return 627
The Role of Trypsin in Cell Death 630
Intracellular Macromolecular Deposits 635
Liver Injuries in Humans 641
Extracellular Accumulation of Degenerative Macromolecules 655
Elementary Lesions of the Nervous System 661
References 673

Chapter 11. Blood Lipids in Arteriosclerosis and Hyperlipidemia 676

Atherosclerosis 679
Morphology of the Arteries 679
Biochemistry 679
Arterial Regeneration 680
Elementary Lesions in Atherosclerosis 681
Fat Metabolism and Atherosclerosis 685
Cholesterol Metabolism 692
Pathogenesis of Arteriosclerosis 697
Consequences of Atherosclerosis 705
Working Hypothesis on the Pathogenesis of Arteriosclerosis 709
Hyperlipidemia 710
Conclusion 711
References 713

Chapter 12. Radiation 715

Physical Phases of Biological Effects of UV and X-Irradiation 717
Biological Effects of UV Irradiation 724
Biological Effects of Ionizing Radiation 733
Radiation Carcinogenesis 740
Biochemical Effects of Ionizing Irradiation 746
Conclusion 757
References 758

Chapter 13. Inflammation 763

History 765
Inflammatory Process as a Whole 765
Vascular Reaction to Inflammation 766
Kinins—Structure and Metabolism 771
Kinins in Disease 774
Prostaglandins 775
Cellular Changes in Inflammation 778
Gross and Histological Appearance of Inflammation 792
References 799

Chapter 14. Immunopathology 803

Introduction 805
Antigens 805
Antibodies 805
Antigen Determinants 808
Theories on Antigen-Antibody Contact 810
Activation of Complement 813
Blood Levels of Antibodies 816
Antibody Synthesis 817
The Cellular Aspects of Immunity 820
Mode of Action of Humoral Antibodies 832
Cell-Mediated Hypersensitivity, Tuberculin Reactions, and Graft Rejection 837
Blood Groups 840
Histocompatibility 845
Immunological Disease 854
References 887

Chapter 15. Regeneration, Hypertrophy, and Wound Healing 893

Regeneration 895
Wound Healing 920
References 939

Chapter 16. Cancer 943

Introduction 947
Benign and Malignant Tumors 947
Cancer and Heredity 955
Hormones and Cancer 959
Carcinogens, Their Metabolism and Mode of Action 970
Viruses and Cancer Viruses 996
Viral Replication 1019
Transformation 1022
Metabolic Pathways in the Cancer Cell 1027
Metabolic Regulation and the Malignant State 1041
Regulation of Gene Expression and Differentiation 1052

The Cell Membrane and the Malignant State 1065
Metabolic Regulation in Minimal Deviation Hepatomas 1081
Invasion, Metastasis, and Host Reactions 1088
Tumor-Host Relationships 1096
Miscellaneous Alterations in Cancer Patients 1097
Cancer Immunity 1098
References 1105

Subject Index · Volumes 1 and 2

Contents · Volume 1

Chapter 1. Cellular Sources of Energy 1

Bioenergetic Pathways 8
References 68

Chapter 2. Determination of Cellular Specificity 71

The Nucleus 73
The Chromosomes 84
Protein Synthesis 106
Elaboration of Polypeptide Chains 123
Operon Theory 130
The Endoplasmic Reticulum 133
Microbodies-Peroxisomes 137
References 137

Chapter 3. Inborn Errors of Metabolism 143

Hereditary Disease 145
Therapy for Inborn Errors of Metabolism 232
Chromosomal Anomalies 233
References 241

Chapter 4. Malnutrition 245

General Malnutrition 247
Protein Deficiency 253
Vitamin Deficiency 266
Malnutrition Due to Disease 318
Obesity 325
References 327

Chapter 5. Calcium and Phosphorus Metabolism 331

Importance of Calcium 333
Sources of Calcium 333
Calcium Absorption 333
Serum Calcium 333
Ossification and Bone Metabolism 334
Rickets 341
Parathyroid Glands 346
Pseudohypoparathyroidism 354
Osteoporosis 355
Calcitonin-Thyrocalcitonin 356

Pathological Calcification 358
References 359

Chapter 6. Iron and Bile Pigment Metabolism 363
Iron Metabolism 363
Iron Metabolism and the Red Cell 366
Control of Iron Metabolism 373
The Biological Role of Iron and Other Metals 375
Siderosis, Hemosiderosis, and Hemochromatosis 379
Iron Deficiency 383
Bile Pigments: Metabolism and Jaundice 385
References 394

Chapter 7. Blood Coagulation 397
Introduction 399
The Coagulation Theory 399
Interference with Blood-Coagulating Factors 406
The Role of Platelets in Blood Coagulation 409
Vascular Factors in Blood Coagulation 413
Fibrinolysis 413
Thrombi and Emboli 415
Conclusion 421
References 421

Chapter 8. Hormones 423
Diseases of the Hypophysis 425
Diseases of the Thyroid 439
The Adrenal Cortex: Function and Diseases 458
Sex Hormones 479
Diabetes of Pancreatic Origin. The Mode of Action of Insulin, and Hypoglycemia 495
Common Denominators in Hormone Action: Receptors and Second Messengers 527
References 534

Chapter 9. Alterations of Body Fluids and Electrolyte Metabolism 537
Anatomy of the Kidney 539
Sodium Metabolism 551
Potassium Metabolism 567
Chloride Metabolism 570
Acids and Bases 570
Edema 582
Urea Metabolism and Uremia 585
Lithiasis 592
References 602

Subject Index · Volumes 1 and 2

Chapter 10

Cellular Death and Degeneration

Introduction 607

Cell Death in Biology 607

Necrosis 608

Microscopy of Cellular Death 609
Dynamic Changes in Necrocytosis 611
Biochemistry and Ultrastructure of Cell Death 613
Cellular Death, DNA Synthesis, Transcription, and Translation 613
Cellular Death and Source of Energy 616
Cellular Death and Membrane Lesions 617

Role of Hydrolases in Cell Death 620

Role of Lysosomes in Cell Physiology and Cell Pathology 620
Pinocytic Theory

Hydrolases in Autolysis 621
Hydrolases and Necrobiosis 622
Hydrolases in Experimental and Pathological Necrosis 623
Biochemical and Ultrastructural Correlation of the Lysosomal Concept 624

The "Point of No Return" 627

Relationship between Spontaneous and Provoked Cellular Death 629

The Role of Trypsin in Cell Death 630

Pancreatitis 630
α_1-Antitrypsin Deficiency
Conclusions and Comments on Cell Death

Intracellular Macromolecular Deposits 635

Liver Steatosis 635
Light Microscopy and Ultrastructure
Effects of Carbon Tetrachloride on Liver—Metabolic Alteration
Primary Molecular Injury of Carbon Tetrachloride
Some Other Forms of Steatosis
Steatosis in Tissues Other Than Liver

Liver Injuries in Humans 641

Effects of Alcohol and Alcoholism 641
Alcohol Metabolism
Catalase and Alcohol Oxidation
Alcohol and Diet
Acute Behavioral Effects
Metabolic Alterations Caused by Ethanol
Acute Effects on Liver
Electron Microscopic Alterations in Alcoholism
Chronic Effects on Liver
Gross Findings
Alcohol and Drugs
Deterioration

Acute Viral Hepatitis 650
Epidemiology
Clinical Manifestation
Drug Hepatitis
Chronic Hepatitis
Experimental Viral Hepatitis
Mushroom Toxins 654
Reye's Syndrome 654
Extracellular Accumulation of Degenerative Macromolecules 655
Amyloidosis 655
Classification
Pathological Anatomy
Pathogenesis
Experimental Production and Spontaneous Incidents
Amyloid Fibrils
Hyalinization and Fibrinoid Necrosis 660
Elementary Lesions of the Nervous System 661
The Nerve Cell and Its Appendages 661
Types of Nerve Cell Injury 662
Nonconductive Elements 663
Demyelinization 668
Axon Degeneration
Allergic Encephalitis
Multiple Sclerosis 669
Factors Influencing the Incidence of Multiple Sclerosis
Pathology of Multiple Sclerosis
Amyotrophic Lateral Sclerosis
Conclusion
References 673

Introduction

Generations of pathologists have devoted their efforts to studying the chemistry of necrotic and degenerated tissues. Such material constitutes a source of abundant normal and abnormal cellular components. In addition, chemical identification of cellular products that are quantitatively or qualitatively abnormal is often of diagnostic value. An adequate understanding of the sequence of biochemical events that lead to cellular death or degeneration hopefully will help to prevent irreversible damage and to restore normalcy.

Nevertheless, it is impossible to describe all forms of cellular degeneration in detailed biochemical terms. This chapter provides a classical description of the various forms of necrosis and cellular degeneration, followed by an outline of some biochemical and ultrastructural information acquired during the last decennia.

Classically, the life of the cell has three stages: mitosis, differentiation, and elimination. The dominant events during cellular division are replication of the DNA molecules and chromosomes, and redistribution of the genetic material between two identical nuclei. Although the nucleus is important in differentiation, many of the manifestations of that process occur in the cytoplasm where differentiation is expressed by a specific mosaic of enzymes, substrates, and products inserted within a specific structural arrangement. Depending upon the cell type, some of these biochemical components are quite conspicuous. For example, the liver manufactures large amounts of albumin. Some cells of the epithelia of the gastrointestinal and respiratory tracts specialize in secreting mucus; others, like the cells of the thyroid gland, synthesize large quantities of specific hormones.

Cellular populations are categorized three ways with respect to a life span. Some have a relatively short life span; for example, the epithelial cells lining body cavities go through a cycle during which the superficial layers are regularly eliminated by desquamation, and are continuously replaced by the cells proliferating in the basal layers. A second type of cell has a longer life span. In parenchymal tissue, like the liver, cellular turnover also occurs, but the elimination is less conspicuous and probably results from a discrete form of physiological autolysis. The neural cells of the brain illustrate the third cell type, those with a long life span. The neural cells do not divide from adulthood until bodily death.

Ideally, this normal pattern of cellular development should continue uninterrupted; unfortunately, it is frequently altered by mistakes of nature and man, leading to disease. Whenever the normal processes of replication of the genetic material, differentiation, or the natural turnover of the cell are interfered with, cell biochemistry and morphology are altered. Often these changes are of little consequence for the entire organism. The development of a wart or the appearance of a pigmented area may constitute a minor cosmetic disadvantage, not endangering life; however, even discrete changes in the life of the cell cycle may lead to dramatic pathological manifestations, such as mongolism, Parkinson's disease, cancer, and myocardial infarcts. Thus, in warts, as in adenocarcinoma; in a pimple, as in appendicitis; in baldness, as in Fallot's tetralogy, it is the cell that constitutes the target for injury. For these reasons, an adequate understanding of the injury at the cellular level is fundamental to an appropriate understanding of all forms of disease. It should be kept in mind, however, that many products of cellular origin are extracellular, such as collagen and nervous fibers. Disease, although cellular at the origin, often ultimately manifests itself by altering the extracellular structures.

Cell Death in Biology

Almost nothing is known of the factors that control the life cycle of mammalian cells. Although the cellular life span is normally rigorously timed for a given cell type, it can be modified by injurious agents. Normally a cell that divides in the crypt of the intestinal epithelium is transformed after a day and a half into a mucus-laden cell, which is ultimately shed by exfoliation into the intestinal lumen. The life span of the cell is extended to 5 days after irradiation of the gastrointestinal tract. Whether the increased life span of the superficial cell results from an attempt to compensate for the block of mitosis in the crypt cell remains to be seen. In any event, the crypt cell seems to communicate with the superficial cell. The information received by the superficial cell tells it when it must die. Chemical mediators could well be involved in transferring the information. Yet we cannot even begin to suspect what type of molecules are involved. Needless to say, the site of action of such natural chemical transmitters within the receptive cells is unknown. The intracellular receptor could be: (1) the nucleus or cytoplasmic machinery involved in protein synthesis; (2) one or more steps of the aerobic or anaerobic bioenergetic pathway; (3) the activities of catabolic pathways; or (4) the cell membrane. In any event, normal cellular death is important in embryogenesis and in the maintenance of the histological equilibrium.

Under physiological condition, cells die by dissolution and ultradifferentiation. Cellular dissolution resembles autolysis, which will be discussed in detail later. During ultradifferentiation, the cell progressively loses its mosaic of bioenergetic and biosynthetic pathways and devotes all its potential to elaborating a specific substance—hemoglobin, keratin, or mucus. Cellular dissolution and ultradifferentiation may mechanistically not be very different.

Except for the fact that cell death is an essential feature of the development of embryos, little is known of the mechanism triggering programmed cellular death in the fetus or in the growing and mature mammalian organism. For example, in human embryos the separation of fingers, toes, and lips results from the death of connecting cells. Yet, if these cells are transplanted at other sites in an early embryo, they will live [146].

The mechanism of death of a red cell is particularly interesting; the mammalian red cell is typical of this highly specialized career. The undifferentiated mother cell has a varied and complex metabolic life. The hemocytoblast synthesizes DNA, RNA, enzymes, and protein. It produces ATP with fully developed Krebs cycles, glycolytic pathways, and hexose monophosphate shunts. As the cell matures and becomes an erythrocyte, it progressively loses its nucleus; its cytoplasmic basophilia and, consequently, its cytoplasmic machinery for protein synthesis; and its mitochondria and aerobic pathway.

An interesting mechanism has been proposed for red cell enucleation. After they mature, the enucleated red cells are thought to leave the bone marrow by passing through the endothelium of capillaries. During this process, the nucleus is squeezed out of the red cell because the flexible cytoplasm can adjust to the size of the pores but the nucleus cannot.

In the reticulocyte stage, the red cell has only a remnant of the genome: a stable messenger RNA needed for hemoglobin biosynthesis. At the end of the process, the cell is a bag surrounded by a membrane filled with hemoglobin, retaining a few enzymes needed to maintain its energy requirements. Among these enzymes are glucose-6-phosphate dehydrogenase and pyruvic kinase. When the activites of these enzymes are also reduced the cell dies, possibly because glutathione can no longer be reduced. Glutathione oxidation is probably responsible for membrane instability.

Red cell death, and possibly all cellular death, can be thought of as special forms of cellular differentiation. The process involves maintaining restricted pathways and destroying all other pathways. But what triggers the destruction of specific pathways, and what determines the selection of the surviving pathways? The destruction could result from massive repression of biosynthetic pathways by some factor in blood and progressive elimination of preexisting material by the normal catabolic pathway. The restrictive cellular death could also result from the activation of catabolic pathways. Finally, a combination of a block of biosynthesis and activation of catabolic pathways could also be responsible for the death of the red cell.

Whatever the triggering mechanism may be, it must be selective and affect some pathways and not others. Thus, when part of the red cell is destroyed, another part goes on to make specific proteins. What barrier separates these two zones—one destined to die, the other destined to make a single protein?

Necrosis

The term necrosis comes from the Greek word *νεκρος*, which means the dead, death, and dead body. Pathologists use it in a very restricted sense, referring to a localized process resulting in the death of a group of cells. (The term necrobiosis is used to describe a slow process of death resembling atrophy.) A necrotic process could involve only one or very few cells. In general, such events are so inconspicuous that they are not detected by the pathologist. In a few cases, however, the cell type is of such functional importance that the destruction of a few cells causes considerable physiological impairment. An example of this is the cells of the anterior horns of the spinal cord in acute poliomyelitis. More often the term necrosis refers to a rather massive destruction of the cells, and therefore necrosis is acute in nature (see Fig. 10-1). Some major causes of necrosis are trauma, toxins (bacterial, antimetabolites, etc.), and vascular occlusion.

Obviously, every organ in the body is subject to necrosis, but some organs are affected preferentially because they are more accessible to trauma, because the life of the cells of the organ depends on the presence of enzymes or other biochemical compounds particularly sensitive to specific toxins, or because the vascular tree that nourishes that organ, for some mechanical or metabolic reason, is prone to occlusion.

Since necrosis is an acute process leading to the simultaneous death of a large number of cells, it is recognizable macroscopically. The gross appearance is naturally a function of the agent responsible for necrosis and of the organ involved. In this respect, various gross appearances of necrosis can be described. Pathologists have described an incredible variety of necrotic forms in detail, but these various types can be grouped into two major categories, and the difference between these two categories resides in the ability of part or all of the material in the necrotic tissue to be hydrolyzed.

In some types of necrosis, the necrotic agent does not inhibit all hydrolytic enzymes and does not produce indigestible products. The necrotic mass is rapidly liquified under the influence of the hydrolytic enzymes that are normally present in tissue or are brought into the necrotic territory by migrating leukocytes. This type of necrosis is called liquefaction necrosis. But, under some circumstances, part or all of the necrotic tissue is not readily hydrolyzed, and the necrotic tissue appears as a dry plaque at the surface of the skin, as a massive core within parenchymal tissues, or as a thick membrane covering the mucosa. This occurs when an injurious agent, such as electrocoagulation or formaldehyde, precipitates all proteins at once, including the hydrolytic enzymes. It also results when a terminal vasculature is blocked so suddenly that cellular death is quickly followed by dehydration, preventing hydrolysis. Such necrosis is observed in some forms of gangrene (dry gangrene), or when the dead cellular elements are trapped in thick membranes of unvascularized fibrin (as is the case in diphtheria).

Sometimes, however, bacteria produce the indigestible material, which then accumulates. The caseous material in tuberculosis and the rubbery material found in the syphilitic gumma are examples of this.

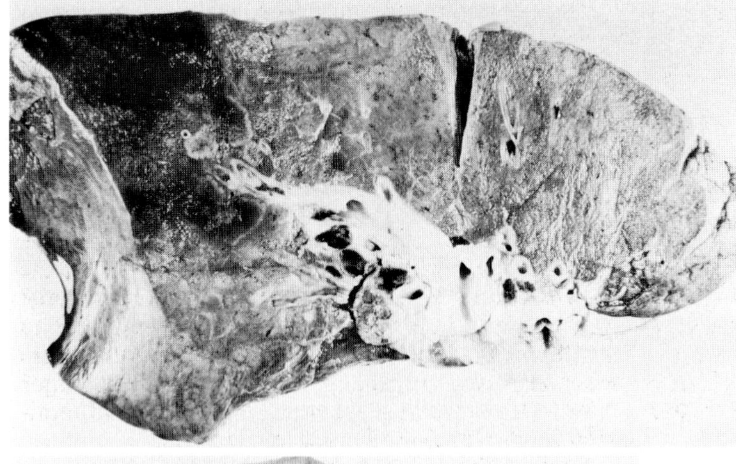

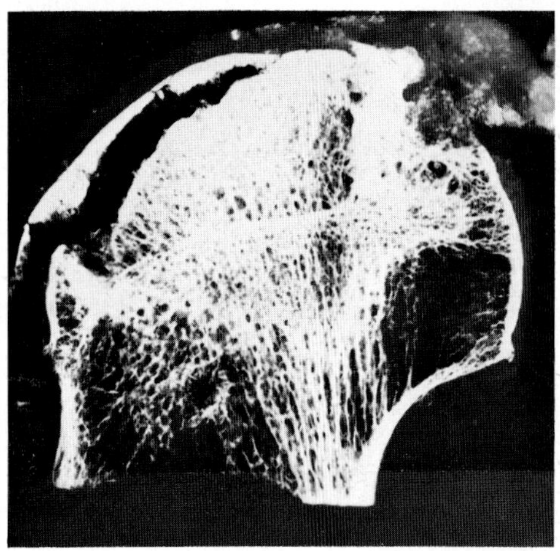

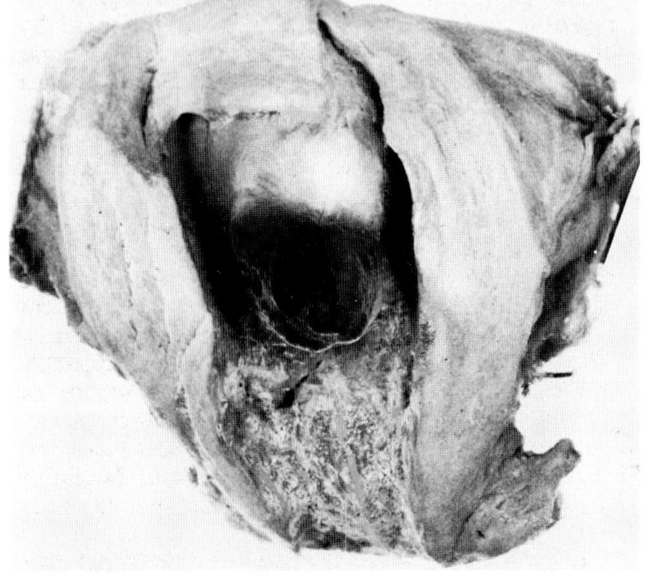

Fig. 10-1. Gross appearance of various forms of necrosis due to vascular obstruction. Infarct of lung *(top left)*, uterus *(bottom)*, and vascular necrosis of bone *(top right)*

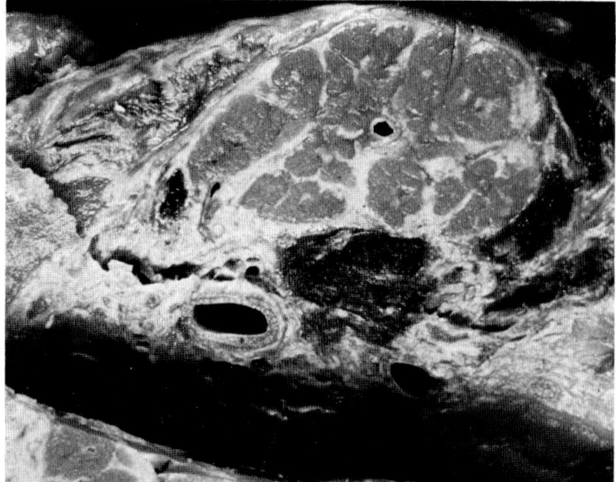

Fig. 10-2. Areas of fat necrosis in the pancreas (perpendicular section). The normal pancreas (dark gray) is streaked with white areas of fat necrosis, resulting from the digestion of extracellular lipids

All other forms of necrosis are modifications of these two main types. Fat necrosis (see Fig. 10-2), for example, is a limited form of liquefaction—hydrolysis affects only the fat deposits. Triglyceride splits into fatty acids and glycerol when the medium becomes sufficiently alkaline, and the fatty acids are precipitated in the form of soaps while the glycerol is lost in the circulation. Such necrosis occurs in pancreatic disease associated with the release of pancreatic lipase into the circulation or the surrounding medium. Putrefaction is an accelerated form of hydrolysis in which bacteria participate in digesting the tissues.

Microscopy of Cellular Death

The microscopic changes that accompany the gross alterations due to necrosis include the changes that take place within the necrotic cell and the reaction of the surrounding tissue. The reaction of the surrounding tissues to the dead cells is discussed in detail

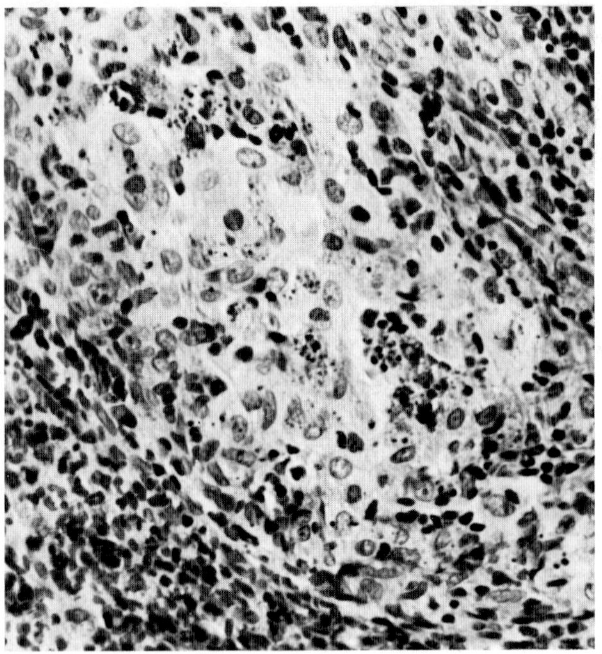

Fig. 10-3. Pyknosis, karyolysis and karyorrhexis of nuclei of spleen lymphocytes after exposure to radiation

in the chapter on inflammation. Suffice it to point out that these reactions are of two types: reabsorption of the dead tissue by granulation tissue, and encapsulation of the dead tissue by connective tissue with or without calcification.

Perhaps the simplest way to observe the cellular alterations that take place during cellular death is to observe those changes during ischemic death or autolysis.

Autolysis is a form of spontaneous cellular death that occurs in excised organs or in all organs after death. Autolysis is important because it can be studied experimentally and probably reflects some basic events of cellular death uncomplicated by vascular or cellular interference. The changes visible under the light microscope affect both the cytoplasm and the nucleus. Soon after death, the cell membranes, which at the onset may be accentuated, disappear. The cells swell and their cytoplasm loses its granular structure, becoming homogeneously eosinophilic. The nucleus may progressively lose its chromatin and resemble an empty vacuole (karyolysis—see Figs. 10-3 and 10-4), its chromatin may clump to form a single black core (pyknosis—see Figs. 10-5 and 10-6), or it may fragment, leaving chromatin debris throughout the cytoplasm

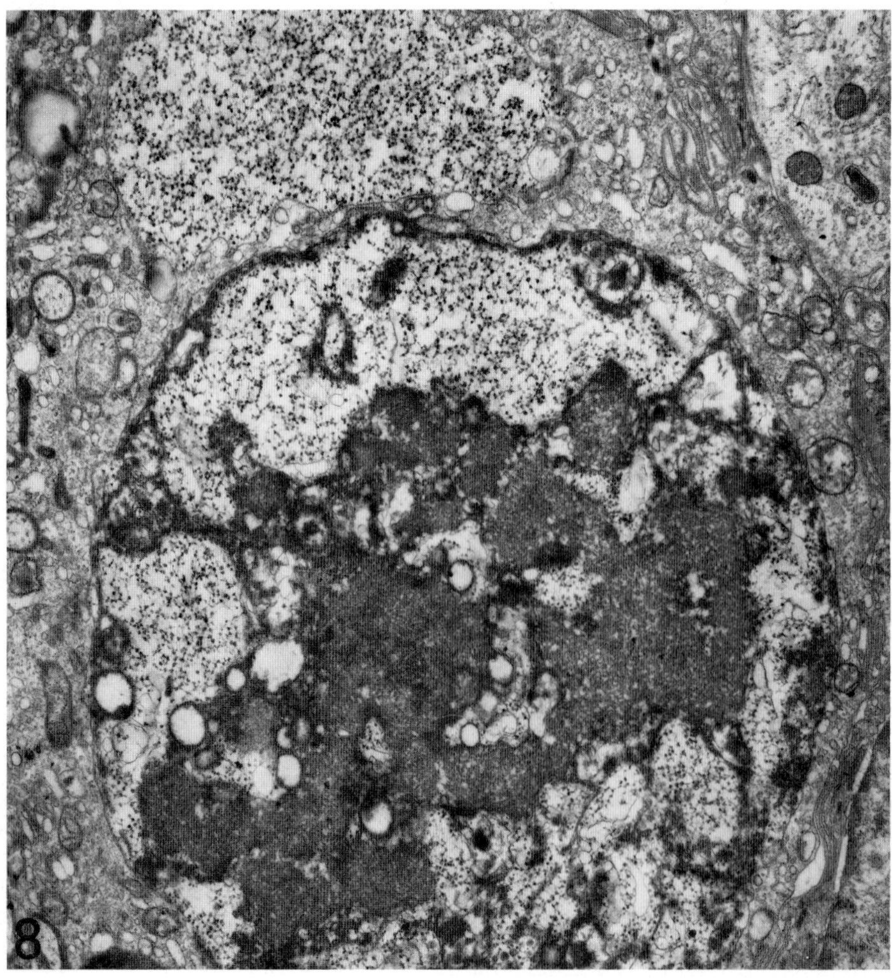

Fig. 10-4. Karyolysis of a hepatic cell in a case of infectious hepatitis. Note the dissolution of the chromatin, which appears as confluent aggregates of coarsely granular material without a membranous envelope ($\times$ 9,000; from Zamboni)

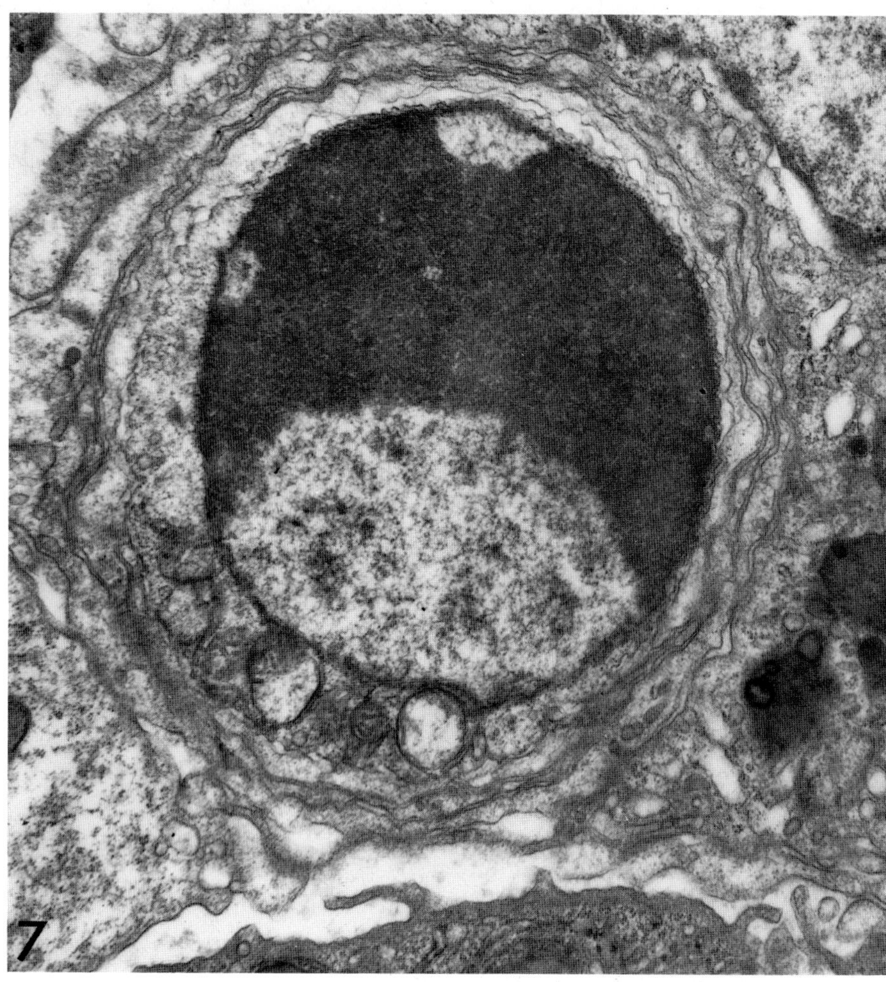

Fig. 10-5. Pyknosis of nucleus in a hepatic lymphocyte of a patient with infectious hepatitis (× 13,500; from Zamboni)

(karyorrhexis). When such morphological signs are present, the cells are dead.

We know little of the biochemical mechanisms responsible for the development of pyknosis and karyorrhexis. Presumably they result from the action of specific endonucleases, exonucleases, and phosphatases. The changes in the staining properties of the DNA in dying cells are likely to be related to the availability of phosphorus residues to the basic dyes. In the early stages of cellular death, the release of proteins and the breakdown of the polynucleotides to smaller nucleotides yield more phosphorus residues capable of reacting with the hematoxylin; in the later stages, as the phosphatases remove the phosphorus, the staining properties disappear.

Dynamic Changes in Necrocytosis

Pathologists become accustomed to observing injured cells on fixed material. But the development of the cell cycle should not be described in terms of the successive projection of a number of color slides. The cell cycle is a dynamic deployment of complexly interrelated movements and modifications of the membrane, intracellular organelles, and nucleus. Even when the cell is injured and finally dies, its agony is associated with dramatic dynamic changes.

Bessis and his associates [1-3] have described the dynamic changes that occur early after cellular injury. Dying leukocytes and fibroblasts were examined by microcinematography. One or more pseudopods form and the consistency of the cytoplasm changes before obvious signs of cellular death take place. When more than one pseudopod is formed, various morphological effects are described: the star-shaped pseudopod, the spinwheel effect, the scarflike pseudopod, etc. The viscosity of the cytoplasm may be either increased or decreased. When liquefaction occurs, the movement of the organelles is accelerated. Conversely, when gelation occurs, the movement of the organelles is slowed down. The early changes are followed by autolysis of the cytoplasm, and karyorrhexis, karyolysis, or pyknosis of the nucleus. The dead cell may then be phagocytized by neighboring cells. According to Bessis, the phagocytizing cells are attracted by chemotactism. However, the possibility that movements toward the dead cells occur at random has not been completely excluded. The changes in permeability are responsible

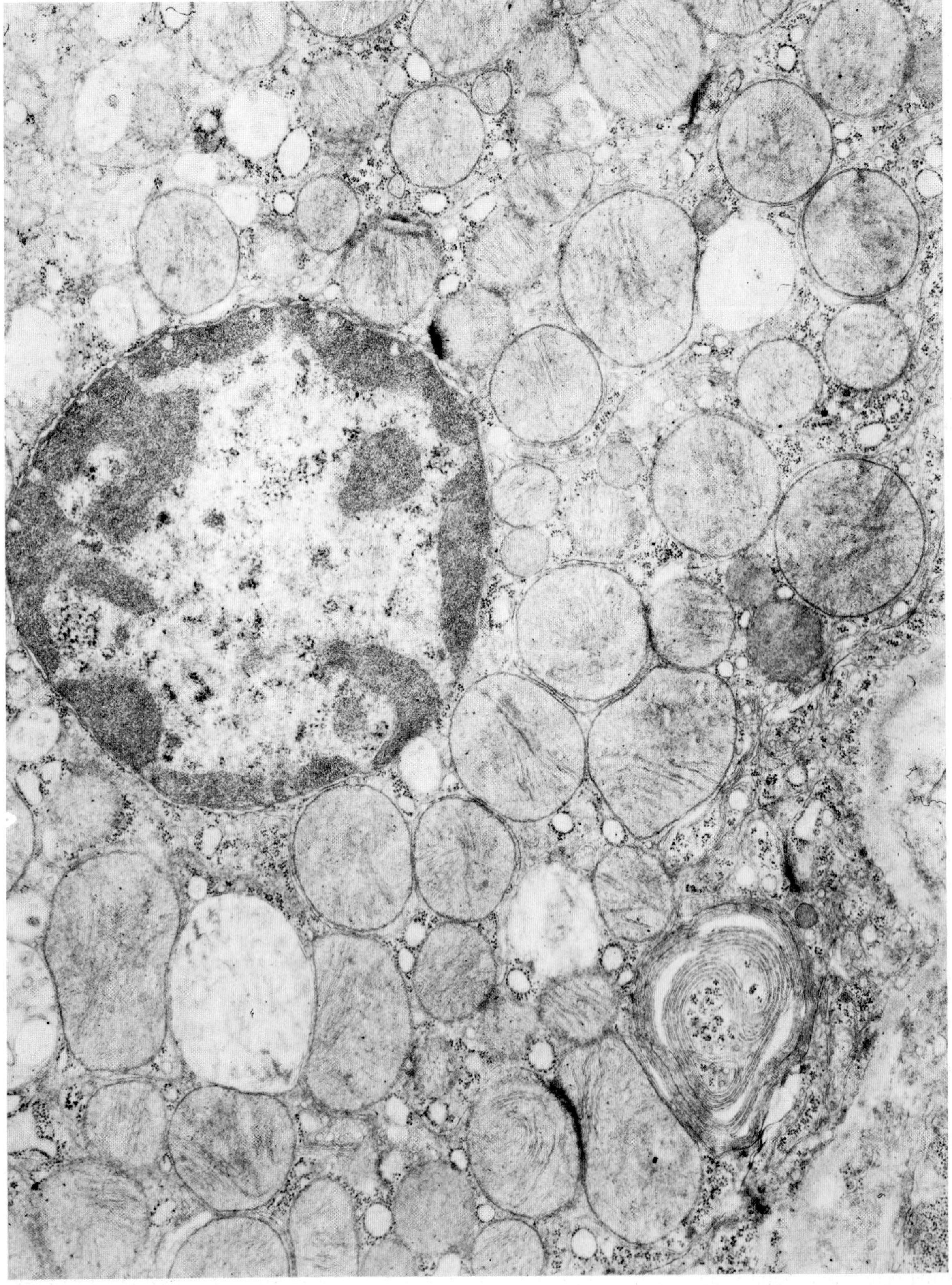

Fig. 10-6. Proximal convoluted tubule cell of a rat kidney after 4 hours of autolysis, showing the pyknotic type of cell death. At the base of the cell *(lower right)*, a concentric proliferation of the plasma membranes encloses portions of cytoplasm. The mitochondria have fragmented into spherical forms. Several light cytoplasmic bodies probably represent lysosomes. The nucleus shows considerable chromatin margination. Electron micrograph, ×20,000. [From Latta, Osvaldo, Jackson, and Cook, Lab. Invest., **14**, 635 (1965)]

for cellular swelling and possibly for the formation of superficial and intracellular vacuoles.

These cinematographic studies provide a new dimension in the study of cellular death, but they have not revealed which cellular structure is the primary target of the injurious agent. In blood cells killed by antibodies, the primary changes seem to involve the cell membrane. In lupus erythematosus, Bessis claims that death results from alteration of the nucleus as a result of the uptake of specific antinuclear antibodies. It remains to be established whether the antibody can be brought to the nucleus in a living cell. Bessis thinks that this can be accomplished by pinocytosis.

Streptolysin is believed to rupture the granules of the polymorphonuclears and kill the cell by releasing the granular content into the cell sap. Again, it is not clear whether the primary injury of streptolysin involves the cell membrane. The effect of streptolysin is instantaneous; therefore, it seems to modify the permeability of the intracellular membranes as well as that of the cell membrane.

Even living cells can be engulfed by other cells; in fact, in tissue culture, lymphocytes have been seen entering and leaving cells. The Hodgkin-Sternberg cell (also called the Reed-Sternberg cell) often phagocytizes whole lymphocytes, and in hemochromatosis the reticuloendothelial cells phagocytize intact red cells. The acinar cells of the pancreas have been seen to contain red cells and leukocytes. Moreover, the engulfment of intact cells by other cells is not restricted to pathological conditions. The most typical physiological example of an intact cell being engulfed by another cell is the penetration of the spermatozoan into the ovum.

Little is known of the mechanism that brings cells together—one to be engulfed, the other to engulf. It has been proposed that cellular death modifies the electrostatic charges at the surface, eliminating the natural electrostatic repulsion exerted between two cells. These changes in the electrostatic charges would then make the cell "sticky." This theory meets with many objections: what happens when live cells are ingested? How can it be that both nonsticky cells, such as red cells, and sticky cells, such as the polymorphonuclears, have the same electrophoretic mobility? This point will be further discussed in the chapter on metastasis.

Biochemistry and Ultrastructure of Cell Death

It is naturally important to identify the point of no return in the time elapsing between the application of the injurious agent and the moment of death. Indeed, all morphological and biochemical changes occurring before that point should be reversible, and it should be possible to restore the tissues to normal with appropriate therapy. For these reasons, considerable effort has been devoted to elucidating the early ultrastructural and biochemical changes occurring during necrosis.

Although the cause of cellular death is not always clear, a number of biochemical events have been associated with cellular death. They include: (1) interference with macromolecular synthesis (DNA synthesis, RNA transcription, and protein synthesis); (2) interference with the bioenergetic pathways; (3) release of hydrolytic enzymes; and (4) alterations of the plasma membrane.

Cellular Death, DNA Synthesis, Transcription, and Translation

Interference with DNA synthesis has long been known to be associated with cellular death. Interference with DNA synthesis may result from direct damage to the DNA molecule, from interference with enzymes involved in the last steps of DNA synthesis, from substrate deprivation, and from interference with mitosis. An example of interference with DNA synthesis resulting from damage to DNA will be described in detail in the section devoted to ultraviolet and ionizing radiation.

Typical of a block of DNA synthesis resulting from interference with enzymes is the block of nucleotide reductase by cytosine arabinoside or hydroxyurea. However, these compounds do not cause cellular death in all tissues exposed to them. For example, if hydroxyurea is injected in animals after partial hepatectomy, it interferes with DNA synthesis in the regenerating liver temporarily, but the liver recovers and the cell lives. In contrast, after administration of these substances, DNA synthesis is interrupted in growing cells of the intestinal mucosa, the bone marrow, and the lymphocytes; extensive necrosis of these cells follows. Nucleotide reductase can also be blocked in tissue culture by adding excess thymidine. The thymidine is converted to the triphosphate nucleotide, which exerts an allosteric inhibition of the nucleotide reductase.

Block of DNA synthesis by substrate depletion has been demonstrated in bacteria that depend on thymine for survival. The exclusion of thymine from the culture medium blocks DNA synthesis and leads to cellular death.

Compounds like colchicine and vinblastine block cell division in mitosis, and cell division and DNA synthesis are interrupted as long as the block is maintained. Again, cells derived from tissues that do not normally grow unless stimulated (like liver) do not die after the administration of this antimitotic agent, but rapidly growing cells show a block in metaphase and the cytoplasm is rapidly degraded. All these examples illustrate that when DNA synthesis is blocked, cells that normally grow rapidly die, whereas cells that grow slowly survive unless very large doses are given. The reasons for these differences in the response to the block in DNA synthesis are not known.

A number of chemical compounds interfere with transcription of DNA into messenger RNA. Cells from various tissues exhibit different degrees of sensitivity to these substances, but probably no cell survives the administration of agents blocking transcription if the dose is large enough or repeated frequently enough.

Actinomycin D (see Fig. 10-7) penetrates permeable cell membranes and traverses the cytoplasm in unknown ways to reach the nucleus, where the molecule intercalates between DNA strands. The intercalation leads to conformational changes, which in turn are believed to interfere with the binding of RNA polymerase along the double-stranded DNA and consequently with transcription of template.

It has been known for a long time that deoxyguanosine residues are essential for the binding of actinomycin D to DNA. Two major mechanisms have been proposed: direct binding between the guanosine residues and the chromophore of actinomycin D and intercalation of the phenoxazone ring system between the base pairs of the DNA helix, as is the case for aminoacridine. The second possibility does not, however, take into account the specificity of the binding to guanine. Sobell has recently cocrystallized actinomycin D with its binding site, the deoxyguanosine, and studied the crystals by X-ray crystallography and concluded that the phenoxazone ring system intercalates between the base pair nucleotide sequence dG and dC. The peptide subunit lies in the narrow groove of the DNA helix and interacts through hydrogen bonding with the deoxyguanosine residues on the opposite chain [101].

Intercalation of the bulky actinomycin molecule in between the DNA strands distorts the winding of the double helix, and consequently interferes with the binding of RNA polymerase to the double-stranded DNA molecules and transcription of templates. If a few molecules of actinomycin bind to DNA, only the transcription of the larger templates (mRNA) is interfered with, and the small templates (rRNA and tRNA) continue to be transcribed. If the concentration of actinomycin added to the medium is great, more actinomycin molecules bind to the DNA molecules, and transcription of all templates is prevented. Despite the uniformity of the primary insult in permeable cells, the manifestations of the injury in the affected cells vary considerably.

Such a difference in sensitivity has been demonstrated in cultured cells. For example, when actinomycin is added to the cells in culture during the period of logarithmic growth in amounts that block 85% of RNA synthesis, depending upon the types of cells used, three kinds of damage can be described: acute cell death, delayed interphase death, and premitotic or reproductive death. These differences in response could result from varied interferences with the action of actinomycin. These interferences may alter the binding of actinomycin to DNA, or they may trigger one or more of the steps of a cascade of insults that links the primary molecular injury to functional, biochemical, or structural pathology.

Some factors that modify the expression of the primary insult in terms of cellular pathology are: (1) differences in site and mode of binding (It is known that the presence of histones modifies the tightness of the binding and the amounts of actinomycin that binds to DNA. For example, much less actinomycin binds to DNA included in chromatin than to native DNA.); (2) the life span of existing indispensable templates; (3) the ability to restore template transcription through initiation processes; and (4) the ability to repair DNA with a specific repair enzyme.

Mitomycins and porfiromycin are closely related antibiotics produced by several species of Streptomyces. The basic component is mitosan which can be further expanded by adding various side chains: R^1, R^2, R^3 (see Table 10-1).

Table 10-1. Structure of mitomycins and porfiromycins

	R^1	R^2	R^3
Mitomycin A	H	CH_3	H_3CO
N-Methyl-mitomycin A	CH_3	CH_3	H_3CO
Mitomycin B	CH_3	H	H_3CO
Mitomycin C	H	CH_3	H_2N
Porfiromycin (N-Methyl-mitomycin C)	CH_3	CH_3	H_2N
7-Hydroxy-porfiromycin	CH_3	CH_3	HO

Mitomycin is a good example of a bifunctional alkylating agent. When mitomycin or porfiromycin is administered *in vivo*, it binds covalently with complementary strands, thus forming interstrand cross-links. High contents of guanine and cytosine in the DNA sequence favor cross-linking. Cross-linking blocks DNA synthesis, interferes with DNA transcription, and in some unknown fashion causes cellular death.

Direct exposure of DNA to mitomycin *in vitro* does not yield cross-links because the antibiotic must first be reduced and lose its tertiary methoxy group to yield an aromatic indole system before it can effectively bind to DNA [4].

Rifamycins [5] are antibiotics found among the fermentation products of *Streptomyces mediterranei*. These antibiotics specifically inhibit bacterial and viral RNA polymerase. Chemically, rifamycin consists of a naphthoquinonic chromophore and a long aliphatic side chain with one end attached to the nitrogen in position 2 and the other attached to the oxygen in position 12 of the chromophore. Thus, the aliphatic chain forms a crescent, each end of which is attached to one side of the chromophore like the handle of a basket. The model is rifamycin B, the formula of which is given in Fig. 10-7.

Although most rifamycin derivatives are inactive on mammalian polymerases, a 3-formyl rifamycin SV:O-n-octyloxime has been prepared which inhibits RNA polymerases of rat liver, calf thymus and lymphocytes. In both bacteria and mammalian cells rifamycin derivatives bind to DNA dependent RNA polymerase, thereby preventing the attachment to the DNA template and interfering with initiation [102].

One could argue that cellular lesions that follow D-galactosamine intoxication result from UDP hexose or UTP depletion. Keppler [103] seems to have settled

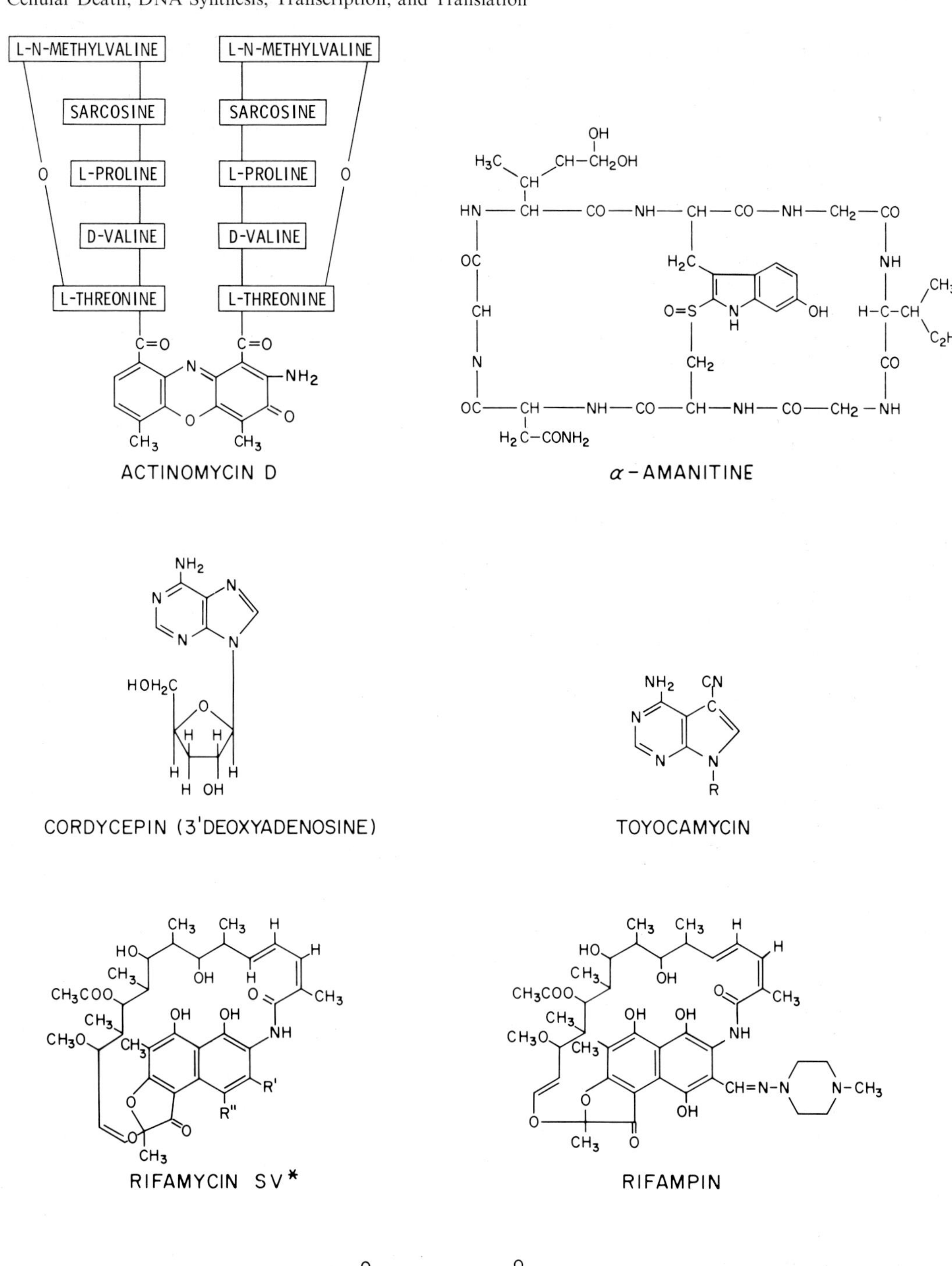

Fig. 10-7. Some agents blocking transcription

the matter by using ascites cells which contain no detectable amounts of UDP hexoses. In these cells UTP deprivation results in complete growth inhibition and loss of transplantation ability and ultimately cell death. The administration of uridine restores all cell functions.

A large number of substances interfere by one or another mechanism with the translation of the polypeptide chain. Most of these agents are primarily effective on bacteria. A partial list of such compounds and their sites of action in the sequence of steps of translation are given in Table 10-2. At least two of these compounds—cycloheximide and puromycin—are effective in mammalian cells and under some circumstances cause cellular death.

Table 10-2. Some inhibitors of translation

Inhibitor	Site of action
Streptomycin Tetracycline[a] (low concentration) Edeine	Inhibits chain elongation by blocking the binding of amino acyl tRNA to the A site of the ribosome
Neomycin Kanamycin Tetracycline	Binds to 30 S subunit at several sites and inhibits peptide bond formation
Spectinomycin	Interferes with messenger RNA: 30 S subunit interaction occurs during translocation
Pactamycin	Inhibits initiation by interfering with the attachment of initiator tRNA to the initiation complex
Puromycin	Competes with amino acyl tRNA for the 50 S binding site
Amicetin	Inhibits transpeptidation
Chloramphenicol	Inhibits binding of mRNA to RNA to 50 S unit
Cycloheximide	Inhibits peptide elongation

[a] Low concentration of tetracycline inhibits polysome formation; in contrast, high concentration yields longer polysomal chains, probably because the antibiotic interferes with termination as well.

Tannic acid, a component of many foodstuffs, causes disaggregation of polysomes, as well as interference with protein synthesis. The endoplasmic reticulum is modified so that the membranes are denuded and the ribosomes are free. Areas of focal cytoplasmic degradation have not been observed [164].

Agents that interfere with RNA synthesis—either by blocking transcription, inhibiting RNA polymerase, or even interfering with translation (e.g., ethionine)—often cause nucleolar damage. The nucleolar morphological alterations vary somewhat with the molecular structure and the dose of the injurious agents administered. However, it is impossible to decide whether the nucleolar alterations constitute an unspecific response to a block in RNA synthesis, or whether they are varied and highly specific manifestations of injuries. In any event, the prototype of such nucleolar injuries is the sequence that develops after actinomycin D administration: the nucleolus decreases in size, nucleolar components are redistributed, and opaque alternating with translucent zones appear.

Three stages can be distinguished in the development of the nucleolar alteration—the formation of microspherules, the segregation of the nucleolar components, and disintegration. Soon after actinomycin is administered, small, dense spherules composed of a central fibrillar mass and small granules appear at the periphery of the nucleolonema. In the second stage, the nucleolar components are segregated into three distinct zones: fibrillar, granular, and a dense opaque area. In the final stage, the opaque mass and the granules disappear, leaving a nucleolonema filled with fibrils.

Ethionine also induces a fragmentation of the nucleoli, but the lesion can be reverted by adenine administration. Restoration of intact nucleoli does not seem to require protein synthesis since cycloheximide administration does not prevent reconstruction. However, the doses of cycloheximide administered block only 40–45% of protein synthesis. Therefore, it cannot be excluded that small amounts of protein are synthesized, some of which are indispensable to nucleolar reconstruction.

Early after the onset of ischemia in rats, protein synthesis is impaired and polyribosomes are degraded yielding free ribosomes with a low affinity for the membranes of the endoplasmic reticulum [105]. Available evidence suggests that this does not result from degradation of messenger RNA, but rather from an inability of the ribosomes to be recycled on the messenger RNA strands. These events are reversible provided that the ischemia is not extended too long. The experiments of Vogt and Farber exclude the possibility that drops in ATP are responsible for the block of protein synthesis. It would therefore appear that a defect either involves the ribosome or factors involved in induction or termination of protein synthesis [41].

Cellular Death and Source of Energy

A simple way of investigating cellular death is to observe the events that develop during autolysis. For these reasons, autolysis has been investigated in several laboratories. Most of these investigations are concerned with the early changes in the bioenergetic pathway, or with the release of hydrolytic enzymes from their granular support.

Judah and his associates [6, 7] have concentrated their efforts on studying the changes in energy metabolism occurring in fragments of tissue undergoing autolysis. They found that the oxidation of all substrates (except succinate) of the Krebs cycle is reduced 30 minutes after the onset of autolysis. This, they think, results from the inability of the cell, or possibly the mitochondria, to retain NAD because adding NAD to the system restored oxidation. But the restoration was incomplete; therefore, the reduced oxidation of the Krebs cycle substrates cannot result only from coenzyme loss.

The coupling of oxidation to phosphorylation is completely blocked in perfused tissues 30 minutes after the onset of autolysis. However, if glucose is added to the perfusate coupling is maintained, but only to a certain degree. Glucose perfusion probably acts by providing the system with a source of ATP through anaerobic glycolysis. Judah's experiment thus suggests that the first manifestation of injury is a loss of ATP. Indeed, the main source of ATP—the Krebs cycle—is out of order since there is no oxygen in the system, and glycolysis—an anaerobic process—soon exhausts preexisting glucose or that generated at the expense of glycogen. In contrast, if glucose is perfused into the system, ATP production is prolonged. In the absence of ATP, all synthetic processes probably stop, and the membrane's structural integrity cannot be maintained possibly because some of the structural elements have a very rapid turnover. Furthermore, the permeability of the cellular organelles is modified; this has been well demonstrated for the mitochondria, which swell with aging but can be made to contract again by the addition of ATP. Mitochondrial swelling leads to the distension of the cristae modifying the relationship between the mitochondrial enzymes and their substrate. Coenzymes like NADP or even enzymes may be lost in the process.

Without ATP, no new cellular components are synthesized; therefore, the concentration of all structural compounds or catalytic proteins with a high turnover decreases. Unless vital structural elements are replaced, the delicate enzyme mosaic of the dying cytoplasm is disrupted. Even when an enzyme is normally involved in anabolism, the conditions in the dying cytoplasm may shift the equilibrium in favor of hydrolysis. The turnover of the hydrolases must be much slower than that of the average proteins because using puromycin the overall rate of protein synthesis can be reduced without interfering with the total acid phosphatase and β-glucuronidase activities. Thus, the hydrolase concentration seems to be an inevitable consequence of cellular death. In conclusion, although the first event in ischemic necrosis or autolysis may be a decrease in the ATP concentration because of lack of substrate, the critical alteration seems to be a distortion of the delicate equilibrium between cellular anabolic and catabolic pathways.

Deprivation of the cell from bioenergetic substrates is not likely to be the only mechanism by which the equilibrium can be distorted. Direct alteration of important biosynthetic pathways could lead to a similar imbalance. For example, in some cases, X-irradiation interferes with the biosynthesis of newly made mRNA and thereby deprives the cytoplasm of new template needed to replace the exhausted stock. This could then well result in focal cytoplasmic or cell-wide imbalance between anabolic and catabolic pathways. Some antimetabolites (actinomycin) and some toxins may also kill the cell by similar mechanisms.

Alterations of cell membrane permeability could distort the distribution of intracellular components, consequently depriving biosynthetic or bioenergetic pathways of needed substrates or introducing within the cell inhibitors of these pathways. For example, Judah and McLean have proposed that cellular death might be triggered by changes in the membrane permeability that lead to calcium mobilization. The membrane's calcium loss would in turn permit excessive sodium entry and potassium loss. As a result, the cell must accelerate sodium pumping, so ATP reserves are soon exhausted. When the intracellular ATP drops to excessively low values, the mitochondrial changes described above take place and death follows. The alteration in membrane permeability may finally lead to sodium and calcium accumulation inside the damaged cell.

The studies of Trump and Bulger [8–10] on the isolated flounder tubules treated with cyanide provide experimental support for the theory expounded by Judah and his associates.

Time-lapse cinematography indicates that two stages of swelling occur when a cell's electron transport chain has been blocked. The first stage is a moderate form of swelling associated with water intake. Na^+ intake is likely to be responsible for the swelling. Lack of ATP due to mitochondrial damage causes ineffective performance of the sodium pump, which probably is responsible for the increased sodium flux. This stage is reversible, but if it is not reversed it explodes into massive swelling with Na^+ and Ca^{++} and extracellular fluid intake. The second phase of the swelling resembles changes produced by direct damage to the plasma membrane.

Electron microscopic studies of the system revealed early swelling and densification of the mitochondrial matrix associated with reduction of histochemical ATPase in the membrane. Other changes include reversible clumping of the nuclear chromatin similar to that observed in ischemia or hypoxia. The "dense bodies" do not burst even after irreversible swelling of the cells, indicating that hydrolase release cannot be responsible for triggering cellular death.

Cellular Death and Membrane Lesions

At a first approximation, examination of the cell membrane under the light or electron microscope may leave the observer with the impression of a static envelope that prevents the extrusion of cytoplasm in the environmental milieu and the intrusion of foreign material. In reality, as we shall see in more detail in Chapter 16, the functions of the cell membrane are numerous; they include ion transport, cell communication, cell locomotion, and phagocytosis, among others.

Injurious agents must either bind to the cell membrane or traverse the membrane to reach their target in the cell. There can be no doubt that many agents traverse the cell membrane without causing any permanent damage to the membrane and kill the cell by interfering with other vital functions.

The structure of the cell membrane will be described in more detail in Chapter 16. The membrane is a mosaic composed of structural and functional units. Injurious agents may either bind to a structural unit and cause severe leakage that may or may not be repaired or they may inhibit one of the functional units such as the sodium pump.

Examples of agents that are believed to cause primarily membrane damage are hyposmolarity, antigen-antibody reactions, phalloidine, and inhibitors of the sodium pump. The effects of sodium pump inhibitors have already been discussed.

Osmotic shock, which has been studied best with the red cell, can be caused slowly, for example by dialysis, or rapidly by plunging the red cells in a hypotonic solution. Three stages can be distinguished: the prelytic events, osmocytolysis, and hemoglobin exit. The most important alteration in the prelytic stage is the loss of potassium with entry of sodium and water, leading to progressive swelling of the cell. The causes for the potassium loss are not known, but it is certainly not linked to loss of cholesterol, phospholipids, or proteins because those events occur later (24 to 48 hours after incubation). In the rapid hemolytic process, the red cells swell and acquire a spherical shape a minute before lysis. Approximately 10 seconds before lysis, membrane defects can be observed in the shocked red cells. They appear as holes of 2 A to 1 μmm in diameter. The holes have a tendency to occur in clusters. If lysis occurs slowly, hemoglobin oozes out of the cell in all directions, but if it occurs rapidly, the hemoglobin is ejected usually at one point of the red cell membrane. The membrane lesion is not irreversible, in fact the membrane heals within 25 to 50 seconds of incubation in hypotonic solutions buffered with phosphate, but not in hypotonic solutions buffered with Tris. As a result of this restoration, ferritin that was able to enter the red cell ghost during the lytic period is unable to do so after repair.

However, in spite of the morphological sealing, the membrane continues to be leaky to ions for rather long periods of time and it is only after further incubation (up to 1 or 2 hours) that tight sealing of the membrane occurs.

The erythrocyte can also be lysed by the action of detergents such as Filipin or saponins. Those substances combine with cholesterol and form rings which are visible under standard electron micrographs. Freeze etching reveals that pits (which do not penetrate through the entire membrane) are formed in the case of Filipin, while holes that perforate the membrane develop in the case of saponins.

When sheep erythrocytes are incubated with sheep erythrocyte antibodies and complement, the reaction between antigen, antibody, and complement culminates in a lytic process that ultimately leads to hemolysis. Three morphological observations have been made at the surface of the erythrocyte subjected to immune lysis: (1) Formation of rings (90 to 235 A in diameter) at the extracellular surface of the erythrocyte membrane. The rings are not depressions because their center is level with the plane of the membrane. (2) The aggregation of globules in the cleave-etched plane of the membrane suggesting a rearrangement of the protein component of the erythrocyte membrane. A correlation between the aggregation of globules and ring formation has been suggested. (3) The formation of small holes identical to those seen in osmotic hemolysis.

On the basis of these findings Seemen has proposed a sequence of steps for membrane lysis in the erythrocyte which involves the binding of antibody to antigen, the reaction with complement, the prelytic loss of potassium with cellular swelling, hemolysis and ultimately the resealing of the cell membrane.

We have already seen in some cases and we will see later in other cases that drugs cause hemolysis of the red cell because of an enzyme defect like that of glucose-6-phosphate dehydrogenase, the presence of abnormal hemoglobins, or through immunological mechanisms. The molecular events that lead to the cellular lysis caused by drugs are not clear, but it is believed that the drugs cause the prelytic loss of potassium and intrusion of sodium and water with further osmotic swelling and disruption of the cell. It has been claimed, but not confirmed, that drug injury requires ATP.

Even less is known about modes of cellular death where a direct attack on the membrane is likely to occur. Examples are the killing of the target cell by sensitized lymphocytes, or that of leukocytes by platelets, or of EDTA-treated blood in patients with Behçet's disease. In each case it is believed that the contact between the killer and the victim causes a tangential sheer force to be exerted by the killer on the target cell membrane. The sheer results in prelytic loss of potassium [106].

Although neither the electron microscopic details nor the biochemical alterations are known, it is possible that similar biochemical mechanisms obtain in the cellular death caused by ischemia in myocardial tissues. When the circumflex branch of the left coronary artery is occluded for 40 minutes, relaxation of the occlusion after that length of time will not prevent cellular damage. Yet, during the period of occlusion there are no changes in the electrolyte composition of the ischemic muscle. Reperfusion of the artery after 40 minutes rapidly increases potassium leakage with concomitant increases in water, sodium chloride, and calcium intake. Intracellular vacuoles appear and mitochondria swell. Dense bodies of calcium accumulate in the mitochondria. No significant changes in the lysosomes are seen. Whether the cellular swelling can be explained by the formation of holes in the membranes as is the case in erythrocytes remains to be established [107, 108].

Thus, during the ischemic period anabolic events are slowed down, if not completely stopped, and catabolic processes cause alterations of the macromolecular structure of the cell membrane leading to leakage of potassium and penetration of water, sodium, etc. The macromolecular alterations could result from the inability to replace a molecular component with a very high turnover, or from the denaturation of a molecule highly sensitive to ischemic conditions. An example of membrane damage caused by molecular denaturation of the membrane is provided in the case of the aging red cell.

As will be discussed later (Chapter 16), SDS-polyacrylamide gel electrophoresis of red cell membranes yields a number of proteins: a surface protein with a molecular weight of 90,000 to 110,000 daltons that can be attacked by trypsin, a protein with a subunit mass of 33,000 to 35,000 daltons which is known to be a D-glyceraldehyde-3-phosphate NAD oxidoreductase, and a high-protein subunit of 220,000 to 240,000 daltons. During storage of blood (a form of aging) the surface protein becomes denatured and can no longer be monomerized in 0.1% SDS. Monomerization requires SDS concentration ten times higher, yet since it can still be achieved with SDS it is obvious that the forces involved are not covalent and must instead be hydrophobic [109].

Another example of cellular death caused by alteration of the cell membrane is provided by the discovery of a nonspherocytic hemolytic anemia associated with an increase of phosphatidylcholine levels in the membrane probably as a result of defective membrane phosphatide catabolism [110]. The half life of the red cell was reduced to one-third of normal (approximately 10 days) and death results from a membrane defect. The red cell is incapable of protecting itself against ion and water influx and the sodium pump that is driven by ATP derived from glycolysis becomes exhausted.

Similarly, an alteration of the cell membrane is believed to cause hereditary spherocytosis probably as a result of a mutation in the DNA coding for tubulin protein [111, 112].

It is very likely that a large number of chemicals and possibly physical agents attack the plasma membranes. Until recently the methods for isolation and studies of the structure of the cell membrane were inadequate and no meaningful generalization on the macromolecular composition of the cell membrane was possible, except on the basis of morphology (see section on myelination, this chapter, and section on cancer metabolism, Chapter 16).

A classical example of a substance which appears to bind to the cell membrane and thereby modify its macromolecular structure is that of phalloidine. Phalloidine is a toxic cyclopeptide found in the toadstool *Amanita phalloides*. In some parts of the world, especially Europe, the collection of mushrooms is a sport. Mushrooms, when properly prepared, constitute a tasty dish whether they are poisonous or not.

Mushrooms are the reproductive organ or fruit of fungi. The fungus itself is mainly composed of filaments or hyphae that penetrate either the soil or other favorable media for growth. Plant fungi may be saprophytic and grow on dead wood, parasitic and grow on the roots of living plants, or symbiotic. In the last case both plant and fungus benefit, often in unknown ways, from the cohabitation.

Several species of mushrooms that are indistinguishable, except by an expert mycologist, produce toxins. The species of the genera *Clitocybe* and *Inocybe* produce muscarine that kills the victim in an hour or two. *Amanita muscaria* produces muscinol in addition to muscarine.

The species of the genus *Psilocybe* produce a hallucinogen and *Amanita phalloides* produces two groups of toxins: the phalloidines and the amanitines. We will discuss the effect of phalloidines here; amanitines is discussed in the section on liver injury. Both phalloidines and amanitines are cyclopeptides. The first is made of 7, the second of 8 amino acids. The details of the structural requirements for toxicity are still incomplete. It is not certain that the cyclopeptide constitutes the integral toxin. Some investigators believe that the original toxin is a much larger protein molecule called myriaphalloisin or myriamanin. Although the injection of phalloidine into experimental animals is fatal, ingestion may not be. It is not certain that phalloidines cause death in humans, yet their biochemical effect at the level of the cell membrane is interesting [160].

In experimental animals, phalloidine is deadly. In a matter of hours, it causes hemorrhagic necrosis of the liver. At autopsy, the striking finding is extreme swelling of the liver. Histologically, there is within 10 minutes marked vacuolization of the hepatocytes followed by necrosis. The mode of action of the toxin was investigated primarily in German laboratories. Tritium-labeled phalloidine was added to the perfusate of isolated livers and after differential centrifugation was found to bind to membrane fragments that sedimented with microsomes. When it became possible to obtain reasonably pure preparations of plasma membrane, it was shown that the labeled toxin preferentially binds to the plasma membrane. The toxin is believed to first bind to a glycoprotein receptor on the membrane surface [113]. The receptor has not been purified yet.

In vivo and *in vitro* electron microscopic studies of the plasma membrane after injection of phalloidine reveal the formation of numerous microfilamentous structures at the inner surface of the membrane [114]. It has been known, thanks to the studies of Palade and Farquhar [115], that the microfibrils seen at the inner aspects of the membrane are made of actin. Biochemical studies have established that those filaments are actin. If muscle actin is treated with phalloidine, it polymerizes to form F-actin filaments. Moreover, phalloidine binds to the actin and prevents its depolymerization [116].

It is not known how the polymerization of actin at the inner membranes causes the membrane distortion seen in phalloidine intoxication. Neither is it known how phalloidine penetrates the cell membrane to bind to the actin of the inner aspect of the membrane. In any event, the intoxication is followed *in vivo* by swelling and vacuolization of the hepatocyte. This vacuolization occurs *in vitro* by invagination, *in vivo* by protrusion of the membrane. The difference between the *in vivo* and *in vitro* results has been attributed to changes in the cell environment. *In vivo,* the pressure of the intercellular fluid would force the membrane to invaginate, while *in vitro,* it would be free to protrude. The membrane injury is further followed by elevated oxygen consumption of the damaged cells, loss of K^+ ions, and release of several enzymes.

Of course, as for most types of injuries, one must distinguish between a primary injury to the plasma membrane and its secondary effects. A report has appeared showing that the plasma membrane of rat livers given carbon tetrachloride or phenobarbital presented reduced 5′ nucleotidase activity and activation of the sodium potassium adenosine triphosphatase, two enzymes which are located in the plasma membrane. However, these events were detected only 24 hours after treatment and are likely to be several steps removed from the primary insult caused by carbon tetrachloride [117].

Role of Hydrolases in Cell Death

The sizes of nuclei, mitochondria, and fragments of the endoplasmic reticulum vary enough to permit these organelles to be separated by differential centrifugation. But a group of cellular organelles—the lysosomes and peroxisomes—have a density and size intermediate between that of mitochondria and microsomes. Before tissue fractionation methods were rigidly standardized, these organelles were sedimented with microsomes in some laboratories, and with mitochondria in others. Thus, some enzymes, like acid phosphatase and uricase, were considered by some to be located in small mitochondria; by others they were thought to be associated with large microsomes. By critically standardizing the fractionation techniques, de Duve and his collaborators [11–15] were able to separate a cell fraction containing approximately 10% of the total nitrogen and 40%—a high concentration—of the acid phosphatase activity. A special relationship between particle and enzyme was further demonstrated. The hydrolase activities were increased by decreasing osmotic pressure, by stirring the homogenate in the blender, or by adding Triton X-100 to the incubation mixture. Acid phosphatase was not the only enzyme associated with this cell fraction; several other hydrolases, all operating optimally at pH 5, were also present in the preparation.

On the basis of these findings, the Louvain group boldly assumed that they were dealing with a new type of cellular organelle delimited by a single membrane, responding to osmotic shock, and containing mainly acid hydrolases. The new granule that was born in the test tube of the biochemist was named lysosome, before the morphologist had a chance to look at it. Examining the pellet prepared by de Duve and his collaborators with the electron microscope, Novikoff discovered, among a large number of mitochondria, a few dense bodies that he suspected to be lysosomes surrounded by a single membrane. When it was later discovered that histochemically detectable acid phosphatase was present in these granules, it seemed clearly established that the small mitochondrial pellet prepared by de Duve's group also contained these dense bodies.

de Duve's group placed much importance on the fact that all hydrolases are released simultaneously by various means [15]. However, simultaneous release of all hydrolases occurs only under rather drastic conditions: in osmotic shock at 37°, in a blender, with strong detergents. When the release is more carefully controlled, such as osmotic shock at 0° or increasing concentration of detergents, some enzymes are released more rapidly than others. For example, as much as 50% of acid phosphatase remains sedimentable after osmotic shock in the cold. Therefore, it is not likely that the hydrolases are in solution in an osmotic bag; instead, the hydrolases probably are present in various degrees of attachment with the macromolecular framework of the organelle.

Repeated attempts using gradient centrifugation and preparations of serial pellets of liver homogenates to obtain a sample of lysosomes uncontaminated by mitochondria and microsomes increased the proportion of lysosomes associated with the pellet. Several laboratories attempted to separate granules rich in acid phosphatase from granules rich in cytochrome oxidase in tissues other than liver—such as brain, thyroid, spleen, thymus, and pancreas. In none of these tissues was a convincing separation achieved, although most morphologists could detect at least a few dense bodies in the electron micrograph prepared from these various sources. Using a combination of filtration and tissue fractionation, Straus [16] has separated an organelle rich in hydrolytic enzymes that also contains proteins resorbed by the kidney. However, the granules are heavily contaminated by cytochrome oxidase, suggesting contamination by mitochondria.

Leukocytes may well constitute the best source of lysosomes. These cells contain few mitochondria and are rich in granules that can be separated with minimal contamination by mitochondria, and which contain a large number of the hydrolytic enzymes that de Duve's group found associated with the liver lysosomes (see section on inflammation).

Role of Lysosomes in Cell Physiology and Cell Pathology

Biochemists and morphologists, each group with its own tools, attempted to grasp the physiological significance of the lysosomes. Since the granule was rich in hydrolytic enzymes, its function was naturally associated with digestion. Two main roles were proposed: (1) the lysosomes are pinocytic vacuoles formed by the movement of the cell membranes that engulf the normal or abnormal plasma components and introduce them to the cell, where these components may be later digested; (2) the lysosomes are "suicide bags" present in intact cells and are called into action in physiological or pathological autolysis.

Pinocytic Theory

The pinocytic theory rests on experiments in which easily traced proteins (ferritin) or other compounds like colloidal mercuric sulfide were used as markers. A classical experiment is that made by Palade on normal and nephrotic kidney. In nephrotic rats, ferritin penetrates the basal membrane and travels to the visceral layer of the epithelium where it accumulates in invaginations of the cell membrane. Later, the ferritin appears inside of small vacuoles, and it forms dense bodies. On the basis of these findings, it was assumed that the ferritin is trapped by invaginations of the membrane, which are later pinched off to form vacuoles that in turn coalesce to form dense bodies. Straus [17] found that horseradish peroxidase is trapped in cytoplasmic organelles called "phagosomes," which are devoid of acid phosphatase.

The findings made in experiments in which the kidney slides were stained simultaneously for acid phosphatase and peroxidase suggested that after peroxidase is engulfed, the phagosome (containing peroxidase) coalesces with the lysosome (containing the acid phosphatase) to yield a digestive vacuole (see below).

Daems [18] observed that after massive doses of dextran are injected, large cellular organelles containing the foreign material appear, some of which stain for acid phosphatase. The connection between the phagocytic granule and the lysosomes will be discussed further.

Examples of Physiological Roles of Lysosomes. Farquhar has studied the mechanism of feedback control of hormonal regulation in the hypophysis. She took advantage of the morphological heterogeneity of the cells of the anterior hypophysis in the rat that can be classified as: mammotrophs or lactogenes, somatotrophs, gonadotrophs, thyrotrophs, and adenocorticotrophs. Each cell type stores its reserves of a specific tropin in secretory granules.

The hormones are synthesized on the endoplasmic reticulum, packaged into vesicles in the Golgi and distributed in the cytoplasm where they accumulate at the periphery of the cell and are excreted in the pericapillary space in a manner similar to that of the secretion of zymogen granules in the pancreatic duct.

Milk secretion is suppressed in the lactating mother when the suckling young are removed. How is this achieved? The deprivation of the suckling stimulus signals the onset of secretion of releasing hormones in the hypothalamus, and secretory granules accumulate in the pituitary mammotrophs twenty-four hours after the suppression of lactation. Lysosomes appear in the cytoplasm of the mammotrophs and it is believed that the secretory granules fuse with primary lysosomes and are progressively digested. Similar observations were made when the secretion of other hypophyseal hormones was interrupted. The arguments in support of fusion of lysosomes (containing acid phosphatase, arylsulfatase, etc.) and secretory vacuoles are not compelling. They include occasional fusion image, which could result from sectioning overlapping granules and the presence of a single membrane surrounding the lysosome containing the vacuole. Other mechanisms of destruction such as segregation by membranes of the endoplasmic reticulum through a process of focal cytoplasmic degradation cannot be absolutely excluded.

In any event, the molecular mechanism triggering the digestion of the hormone remains to be discovered [118].

Thyroglobulin is believed to be phagocytized by follicular cells and digested by proteolytic enzymes to yield thyroxine; lysosomal enzymes have been implicated in the digestion. In the case of proinsulin, its conversion to insulin in the β cells seems to involve the Golgi and supernatant enzymes [119].

Hydrolases in Autolysis

Gross and histological examinations of necrotic tissue suggest that at least some forms of necrosis result in the lysis of cellular components, such as proteins and nucleic acid, and, as a result, hydrolases—especially nucleases and proteases—catalyze the process. In 1938, Bradley [19] reviewed what was known of the role of hydrolases in autolysis. The conclusions reached then are still relevant to modern understanding of the biochemistry of cellular death. Bradley proposed that the following sequence of events led to autolysis: (1) a decrease in oxidizing metabolism resulting from subnormal oxygen tension in the tissues; (2) an increase in the concentration of hydrogen ions resulting from the accumulation of acids including lactic acid, CO_2, and other metabolic products; (3) an increase in proteolytic activity.

Early students of autolysis were naturally intrigued by this seemingly paradoxical situation of a living cell storing large amounts of destructive enzymes. It seemed obvious that the hydrolases must exhibit no or little activity under normal conditions and must be activated during autolysis.

The mechanism of activation of proteases was not obvious, although it was already clear in 1932 through the work of Willstätter and Rohdewald [20] that all cathepsins in tissue do not exist in the free state, but that some remain permanently bound to insoluble proteins after attempts at extraction. The bound enzyme was called desmo-cathepsin, the free enzyme lyo-cathepsin. Liberation of the desmo form was achieved by either weak acid or moderate autolysis. A theory popular at the time proposed that in the absence of oxygen and in the presence of high concentrations of hydrogen ion, S-S groups would be reduced to SH groups, and thereby proteases would be activated. Reduced glutathione was assumed to be such an activator.

Berenbom and his associates [21, 22] examined the fate of a number of biochemicals in mouse livers that underwent autolysis in test tubes or after transplantation in the peritoneal cavity. The study included measuring the activities of peptidases, esterase, alkaline and acid phosphatases after various periods of autolysis. Whereas the activities of some electron transport enzymes, such as cytochrome oxidase and succinic dehydrogenase, had dropped to low values within a few hours after the onset of glycolysis, minimal changes in acid hydrolase activities took place.

The studies of the release of acid phosphatase and β-glucuronidase during autolysis *in vitro* have shed some light on the position of this release in the chain of events that starts when tissue is separated from the blood supply and ends with its autodigestion. The enzymes are released from their particulate support relatively late in the process of cellular death. Since when the lysosomes are ruptured, ATP is lost and oxidative phosphorylation is completely uncoupled, the release of the hydrolases is probably not the *primum movens* of cellular death [23, 24]. Such *in vitro* studies provide an exceptional opportunity for studying the effect of the enzymes on their substrates. Although the released acid phosphatase activity clearly hydrolyzed its substrate, DNase did not affect the DNA content of the nuclei even hours after the particulate enzyme had been released into the supernatant. Also, lysosomal enzymes were not released during pancreatic autolysis. All of these findings suggested that it is unlikely that autolysis is the reason for the lysosomes' existence.

The release of acid hydrolases observed in biochemical studies probably only reflects changes in the fragility of the lysosomes rather than their active participation in autodigestion. Electron microscopic studies of autolyzed tissues by Trump and his associates [25] demonstrate that the lysosomes remain intact for at least hours after the onset of autolysis, and cytoplasmic structures immediately surrounding these lysosomes are unaltered.

Latta and his associates [121] have studied the ultrastructural changes that take place in the proximal, distal, and collecting tubules of autolyzing rat kidneys. They observed the formation of myelin-like figures, fragmented mitochondria, and the development of light cytoplasmic bodies. However, none of these components could be related to lysosomes.

Hydrolases and Necrobiosis

Metamorphosis, organogenesis, and even adult development are associated with extensive histological reorganization, which is often accompanied by death of large groups of cells or even by resorption of entire organs. In some cases the role of hydrolases in digestion has been investigated.

An interesting form of necrobiosis is that which takes place when a larva undergoes metamorphosis in the adult form of the species. During the metamorphosis of tadpoles to froglets, the tail disappears. A number of fractions were prepared from tadpole tails by differential centrifugation. One fraction contained the myofibrils and the nuclei, another primarily mitochondria, another the microsome fractions, and a fourth the cytosol. Because the tadpole tail contains several different tissues—including muscle, connective tissue, and cartilage—it is difficult to homogenize. Consequently, only a small fraction of the lysosomal enzymes was found to be particulate bound. Nevertheless, the bound enzyme could be released by shearing, osmotic shock, or lowering of pH.

The demonstration of latent hydrolases in the tadpole tail raised the question of their participation in the resorption of the tail during metamorphosis. Interpretation of results *in vivo* is unfortunately complicated by the participation of lymphocytes and macrophages in resorption. Histochemical studies by Weber and his associates [26] clearly demonstrate that the major increase in enzyme activity resulted from macrophage invasion of the regressing tadpole tail. Resorption of tadpole tails can be brought about *in vitro* by adding thyroxine to the incubation mixture. Weber measured catheptic activities in control tails and in thyroxine-treated tails incubated *in vitro*.

In thyroxine-treated tails, cathepsin activity rises to values at least three times those measured in the control, but only after a 1- or 2-day lag period. Therefore, Weber concluded that thyroxine could not affect lysosomes, but rather the enzyme itself, indicating that the affinity of cathepsin for the substrate used in the experiment (casein-urea) increases during metamorphosis. Morphological examination of the cultured tail demonstrated that during metamorphosis no granules corresponding to lysosomes appeared. Thus, the possibility that the new cathepsin with greater affinity for its substrate results from proliferation of a new type of cell cannot be excluded. Macrophages are known to appear even in the cultured tail. They are derived through proliferation of preexisting macrophages or through transformation of other mesenchymal cells into macrophages.

Two embryonic structures of mesenchymal origin are involved in the development of the genitourinary tract of mammals: the primitive excretory tract (mesonephric or wolffian) and the paramesonephric or müllerian ducts. Both types of ducts are found in embryos of both sexes at early stages of development. In the female, the development of the excretory urinary tract develops from the mesonephric duct, and the müllerian duct grows and differentiates to yield the uterus, fallopian tubes, and the vagina. In contrast, in the male the müllerian ducts regress. The mesonephric ducts eventually connect with the testis, and both the genital and the urinary systems use a common pathway for excretion.

Brachet and his associates demonstrated an increase in lysosomal activity and a conversion of bound to free acid phosphatase during regression of the müllerian ducts. Scheib [27] measured the total and free acid phosphate, β-glucuronidase, cathepsin, and acid ribonuclease activity in homogenates of 8-, 9-, and 10-day-old chick embryos. The specific activity (per milligram of nitrogen) for all hydrolases is unchanged in the female, whereas it doubles in the male during that period.

Thus, although the müllerian canal grows and differentiates in the female, new hydrolases are synthesized, and the ratio of hydrolases to total proteins remains constant. In contrast, in the male hydrolases are not synthesized, but the ratio of hydrolases to other proteins increases as a result of protein degradation.

In the male, the ratios of free and bound hydrolases shift in the regressing müllerian duct. Scheib also tested the effect of steroid hormones on the release of hydrolases from their granule support in chick embryo homogenates and explants of müllerian ducts maintained in a standard medium for several days. Unfortunately, the hormonal effects were too small or too unspecific to permit definite conclusions as to their role in activating the lysosomal enzyme.

Necrobiosis occurs during development and in adult life as well as in the embryo. Breast tissue is resorbed in female mammals after lactation or during menopause. After painstaking efforts to develop adequate methods of homogenization, Slater and coworkers [28] established that rat breast contains particulate-bound hydrolases with structure-bound latency similar to that of lysosomes. During involutions of the mammary glands, the activity of succinic dehydrogenase, glucose-6-phosphate dehydrogenase, and glutamic aspartic transaminase decreases abruptly. In contrast, acid RNase activity increases slightly, β-glucuronidase activity remains unchanged, and cathepsin activity decreases after a short period of increase.

Interpretations of the results of the biochemical studies of acid hydrolases in necrobiosis are obscured by the near ubiquity of macrophages. Morphological data (as will be clear later) suggest that the invasion by macrophages is preceded by cellular autodigestion. Whatever the participation of the autodigestive vacuoles in necrobiosis may be, their appearance certainly results from cellular morbidity rather than being the determinant factor in cellular death.

Studies of necrobiosis in insect metamorphosis and chick embryo development have clearly established that cytonecrosis is programmed, and that the participation of acid hydrolase is a late event in the sequence of steps leading to cytolysis.

Some insects—*e.g.*, moths, butterflies, mosquitoes—develop in three stages. The larva is a caterpillar which, after molting several times, becomes a pupa. The amazing metamorphosis of a caterpillar into a butterfly takes place during this pupal stage. The various appendages (especially limbs and wings) originate from internal buds which, by a combination of cellular death and proliferation, are ultimately molded into the adult shape.

In Drosophila, the salivary gland of the larva undergoes histolysis 10 hours after the larva enters the pupal stage. The cytonecrosis that accompanies the histolysis is brought about by the hormones that induce metamorphosis. If the salivary gland of a larva that has not entered the pupal stage is transplanted to a metamorphosing larva, the graft will undergo histolysis. However, the stage of development of the larva from which the salivary gland is obtained is also important, because the salivary gland cells can respond to the hormone only after a certain stage of development (the second molt). If salivary glands obtained from a larva that has reached only the first molt are transplanted to a metamorphosing larva, they will not undergo histolysis.

Spinal ganglia of the early stages of the chick embryo seem to contain more neurons than are needed for adequate innervation of most of the adult body, except for those parts of the chick's body that include the wings and the limbs. Thus, although a large number of cells die in the ventral portions of the cervical and pelvic ganglia, few or no cells die in the brachial and lumbar ganglia. However, the cells of the lumbar and cervical ganglia die if the limbs are amputated.

The development of the chick embryo's wing bud is also associated with selective and rigidly scheduled cellular death. At a certain stage of the development of the chick embryo (sometimes before the 17th stage), a factor or factors introduce a change in some cells of the wing bud that makes these cells die at a scheduled time (the 24th stage). If these "condemned" cells are transplanted to another embryo that has reached a stage of development different from that of the donor embryo, the grafted cells die on schedule as if never transplanted.

The significance of these experiments has been summarized in a paper by Saunders and Fallon [29], and many of the metaphors used here are borrowed from that paper. These experiments clearly demonstrate that cells do not die by chance during necrobiosis, but that cell death is rather rigidly programmed in space and time. Some unknown intracellular or extracellular factors make certain cells, in due time, competent to die. From that moment, the competent cell follows a rigid course timed by a "death clock." Unfortunately, nothing is known of the molecular events that take place in the setting and unwinding of the "death clock." Yet the "death sentence" is executed with astounding punctuality. Morphological signs of cellular morbidity are not detectable until shortly before the cells are phagocytized by invading macrophages. At that time, typical focal cytoplasmic degradation develops in the dying cells. These observations indicate that the participation of acid hydrolases in cellular death is a late if not the last event in the sequence of steps that start with setting the clock and end with cytolysis.

Hydrolases in Experimental and Pathological Necrosis

The activity and intracellular distribution of lysosomal enzymes have been studied in experimental and pathological necrosis in animals and humans. Total free and bound activities of a number of acid hydrolases have been measured under various conditions of necrosis including ischemia, shock, nutritional imbalances, administration of toxins, and genetic dystrophies. Many of the reports have not included adequate morphological control studies and are hard to interpret. For example, it is often difficult to decide whether the reported changes in enzyme patterns result from a shift in the cellular populations of the organ under investigation. Such changes in liver, muscle, and other organs are the inevitable consequence of necrosis, exudation, and regeneration.

A moderate increase in the activity of three hydrolases was demonstrated in liver of animals exposed to shock and after ligation of the vascular pedicle of the left lobe of the liver. An increase in free hydrolases was also observed in livers of animals with deficient diets, after they were fed carbon tetrachloride, and after bile duct ligation.

Similar results were obtained in kidney after ligation of the renal pedicle. A small increase of the activity of free hydrolases was also observed in mouse spleen after the administration of total body doses of X-irradiation. In that case, the hydrolase was released after the block in DNA synthesis; therefore, release was most likely a consequence rather than a cause of cellular death. Lysosomal enzymes are released hours after the onset of necrosis in carbon tetrachloride- and thioacetamide-poisoned animals.

In conclusion, although the acid hydrolases probably participate in the autolytic process, they are unlikely to play a major role in the onset of cellular death. Furthermore, it cannot be excluded that nonlysosomal enzymes are, at least in the early stages of autolysis, as important as the acid hydrolases in the autolytic process.

As mentioned previously, acid hydrolases constitute only a small contingent of the large population of hydrolases in the cell. Nonlysosomal hydrolases are distributed among microsomes, supernatant, nucleus, mitochondria, Golgi, or plasma membrane. They catalyze a great variety of reactions, such as the hydrolytic splitting of ester, phosphoric diester, and sulfuric ester bonds; they may attack the peptide bonds of the N or carboxy terminal amino acid of the polypeptide chain or the endopeptide bonds of polypeptides or dipeptides. The substrate may be a vital but relatively small molecule like ATP or a large macromolecule such as DNA and proteins. The role that these enzymes play in the cellular economy is not always clear, let alone the role that they may play during cellular degradation. However, a primary injury that would interfere with bioenergetic or anabolic pathways would appear to make the substrates of the blocked pathway available for hydrolases. Since cell pH must be close to normal immediately after the primary injury, the enzyme with optimal pH for activity around neutrality might be expected to be fundamental in the early steps of cellular degradation. In fact, it is quite likely that the most specific of these hydrolases that act at a neutral pH might be critical in determining the irreversibility of necrosis, leaving the remains of their attack for the lysosomes. That enzymes other than the acid hydrolases can be involved in the early steps of cellular death is indicated by the role of trypsin in acute pancreatitis (see below).

Biochemical and Ultrastructural Correlation of the Lysosomal Concept

The lysosomal concept gained new impetus because of a discovery made in Porter's laboratory [30]. In the livers of animals perfused with glucagon, Porter discovered dense bodies delimited by single or sometimes double membranes containing intact mitochondria or endoplasmic reticulum. At about the same time, a group of investigators at the University of Chicago [31–33] examined livers and pancreata of rats and guinea pigs after the administration of several types of toxins, including amino acid analogs and compounds blocking cholesterol biosynthesis. They also investigated the changes in liver and pancreas induced by complete starvation and phenylalanine deprivation, and the effect of renal vein occlusion. They described various types of focal cytoplasmic degeneration, or areas—including vacuoles, Golgi vesicles, mitochondria, smooth and rough endoplasmic reticulum—that are sequestrated from the remaining intact cytoplasm by a membrane completely surrounding the degenerating cytoplasm (see Fig. 10-8).

In the early stages of the degeneration, the sequestered structures were highly recognizable, but later these structures reached various degrees of degeneration leading ultimately to the formation of dense bodies delimited by a single membrane. Histochemical tests for acid phosphatase demonstrated its presence in these areas of focal cytoplasmic degradation.* These are capital observations, both with respect to the mechanism of response to injury and the histogenesis of lysosomes. One of the most striking findings of this study is the uniformity of the response to various types of injury. The response to injury seems to be independent of the nature of the injurious agent and the organ. The lesion is identical after ischemia, starvation, or the administration of an amino acid analog. It is similar in pancreas, kidney, liver, intestine, adipose tissue, and other organs. Such a uniformity of the morphological response to injury suggests that this focal cytoplasmic degradation that ultimately leads to lysosome formation is several steps removed from the primary biochemical lesion. It is indeed unlikely that an amino acid analog and a cholesterol antagonist injure the cells in the same way.

Winborn and Bockman [34] studied the development of focal cytoplasmic degradation in the parietal

* These large vacuoles containing cytoplasmic debris at various stages of degradation were called lysosomes, cytolysosomes, areas of focal cytoplasmic degradation, cytosegresomes, autophagic vacuoles, glycogenosomes, autolysosomes, systeme macrovacuolaire heterogene geants. To distinguish this acid phosphatase-containing granule from the more traditional dense body (lysosome), investigators gave new qualifications to lysosomes, such as virgin, true, or primary lysosomes, or these lysosomes were called cytosomes.

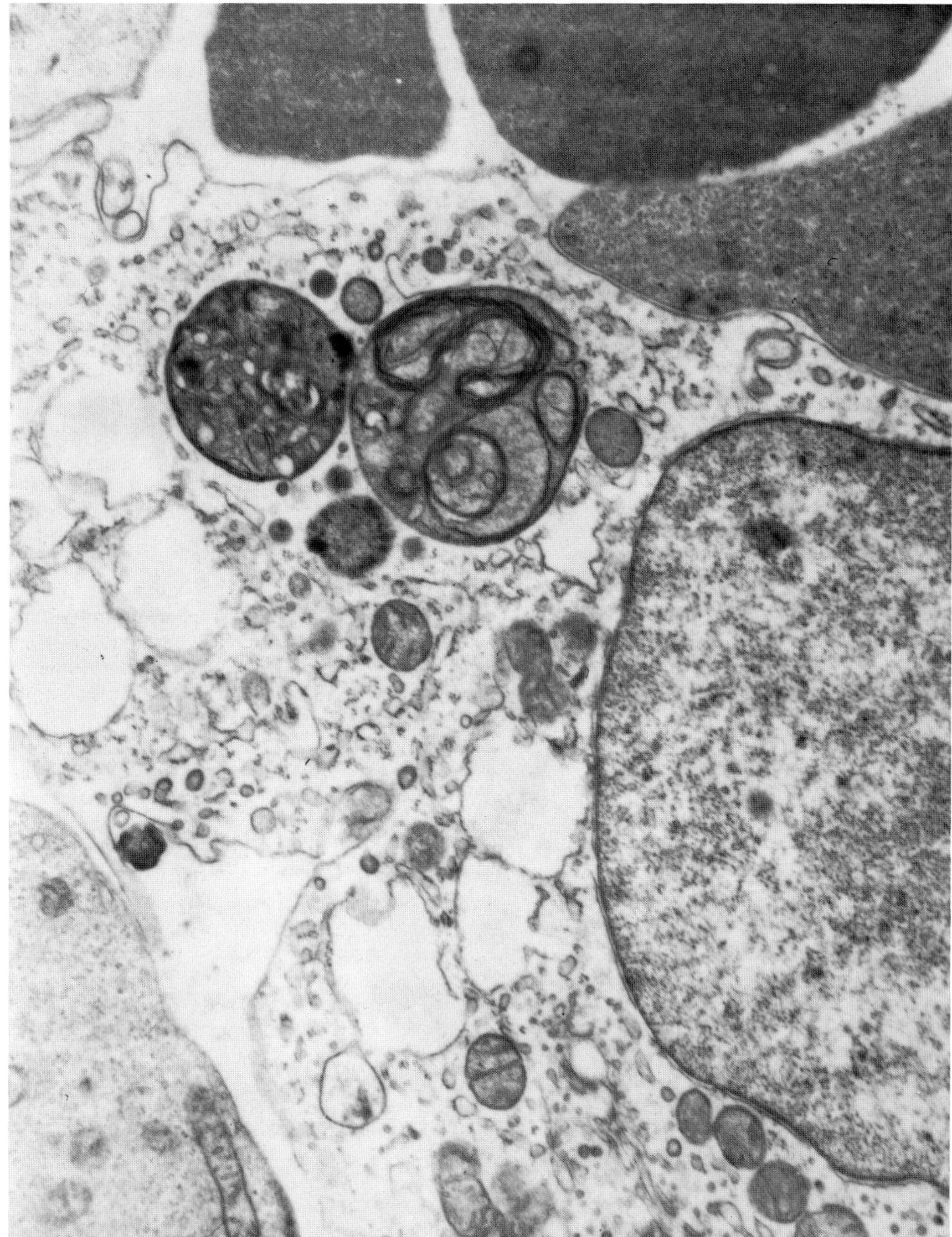

Fig. 10-8. Rat thymocyte showing focal cytoplasmic degradation after vinblastine administration

cells of hamster stomach, which seems to provide a simplified form of degradation because it involves only mitochondria. The authors described the surrounding of the mitochondria by a membrane and progressive disintegration of the organelle to yield myelin structures or granular dense bodies. However, the appearance of acid phosphatase could not be associated with transfer from Golgi or coalescence of primary lysosomes. These findings suggest that the dense granular bodies are similar to lysosomes and are also the product of mitochondrial degeneration. Thus, the morphological observations first made by the Chicago school and extensively confirmed by others support the impression acquired by the biochemical studies of autolyzed tissue—namely, that the appearance and rupture of the lysosome are consequences of necrosis rather than its primary motive.

The lysosomal concept proposes that the cell segregates pieces of cytoplasm for autodigestion by surrounding them with membranes. The cytoplasmic components are progressively digested within the membrane, and dense bodies are formed as a result. Thus, three stages in focal cytoplasmic degradation can be distinguished: formation of the autodigestive vacuole, conversion of the autodigestive vacuole into hetergeneous dense bodies (cytolysomes), and conversion of heterogeneous dense bodies into homogeneous dense bodies (residual bodies). The autodigestive vacuole is formed in three steps: formation of the segregating double membrane, the conversion of the double into a single membrane, and the progressive digestion of intravacuolar components.

What is the relationship between these areas of focal cytoplasmic degradation—a morphological concept—and the lysosome—a biochemical concept? One thing is certain, the areas of focal cytoplasmic degradation always exhibit positive acid phosphatase activity.

The formation of areas of focal cytoplasmic degradation thus raises a number of important questions: What critical factor determines that autolysis will take place in the restricted area? What signal tells the surrounding healthy cytoplasm that a portion of cytoplasm is to be digested? What is the origin of the membrane that surrounds the condemned portion of cytoplasm? What is the source of hydrolases that concentrate in the area of focal degradation? Only tentative answers to these questions can be given.

When the cell is exposed to graded injury, the cytoplasm could be selectively damaged from interference of the injurious agent with the supply of templates or substrates for biosynthetic or bioenergetic pathways in those areas of cytoplasm at the threshold of being deprived of these templates or substrates [35]. Such an interpretation proposes that the supply of templates and substrates is not continuous and uniform throughout the cell; on the contrary, these substances are delivered in packages to parts of the cytoplasm that have nearly or completely exhausted their stores of templates or substrates.

Membranes encircling the cytoplasm have many possible origins. The cell could elaborate a new membrane for each area of focal cytoplasmic degradation, or it could use a preexisting membrane to form the surrounding sac. A new membrane could be made at the site of injury or be elaborated in other cell structures and transported to the site of injury. Golgi vesicles or Golgi lamellae could constitute plausible precursors for such a newly formed membrane. The membrane could also be formed by distension of a preexisting membrane of the endoplasmic reticulum by the coalescence of smaller vacuoles (*e.g.* primary lysosomes—see below) or be supplied by engulfment of the condemned areas into a lysosome.

Determination of the membrane's origin is further complicated by the fact that areas of focal cytoplasmic degradation are surrounded by a double membrane at the beginning of the process and by a single membrane later.

Because the administration of actinomycin or puromycin does not interfere with the formation of the area of focal cytoplasmic degradation, it is believed that the membrane is not made *de novo*.

Arstila and Trump [36] have attempted to answer some of these questions by studying the formation of areas of focal cytoplasmic degradation (which they call autophagic vacuoles) in liver after glycogen administration. On the basis of a battery of histochemical tests, these investigators concluded that the membrane possesses the typical enzyme markers of the endoplasmic reticulum, but not those of the Golgi apparatus, the plasma membrane, or preexisting lysosomes. Measurements of the thickness of the membrane during the early stages of formation of areas of focal cytoplasmic degradation are compatible with this assumption.

Even if the endoplasmic reticulum is at the origin of the membranes surrounding the areas of focal cytoplasmic degradation, it is not clear how the double membrane is converted to a single one. Two different mechanisms have been proposed: cementation of inner and outer membranes and digestion of the inner membrane by hydrolases with concomitant thickening of the outer membrane.

Two principal approaches have been used to study the origin of the acid hydrolases found in the autodigestive vacuole: incorporation of labeled amino acid in enzyme purified from both microsomes and lysosomal fractions, and combined histochemical and electron microscopic studies.

In regenerating liver, the amount of acid phosphatase and that of β-glucuronidase associated with the microsomal fraction increase 184 hours after partial hepatectomy, when new proteins are synthesized.

Studies of β-glucuronidase binding demonstrated a different mode of attachment of the enzymes in lysosomal and microsomal fractions. These findings suggested that β-glucuronidase is a constituent protein of the endoplasmic reticulum, and that the increased microsomal β-glucuronidase activity after partial hepatectomy reflects *de novo* synthesis of that enzyme. Cytochemical demonstration of β-glucuronidase activity in the membranes of the endoplasmic reticulum supported this hypothesis. Because it was shown in several laboratories that β-glucuronidase may exist in multiple molecular forms, it was appropriate to consider whether different forms of these enzymes were present in microsomal and lysosomal fractions. Starch-gel electrophoresis of β-glucuronidase partially purified from mitochondria, microsome, cytosol, and regenerating rat liver yielded several protein bands associated with β-glucuronidase activity. However, only one band was obtained for enzymes purified from lysosomes and nuclei.

Mitochondrial, cytosol, and microsomal enzymes were purified until the preparation yielded single bands on polyacrylamide gel. The single band had a mobility similar to that of the purified lysosomal enzyme. β-Glucuronidase purified from mitochondrial, lysosomal, and microsomal pellets obtained from 24-hour regenerating livers were found to have similar catalytic and electrophoretic properties. The effects of substrate concentration, pH, thermal activation and inactivation are identical.

After labeled amino acids were injected, enzyme purified from the endoplasmic reticulum was rapidly labeled, but no label appeared in enzyme purified from lysosomal or other cell fractions. These findings suggested that in liver regeneration, the transfer of enzyme from endoplasmic reticulum to lysosomes was slow and, therefore, undetectable without special stimuli. However, label suddenly appeared in the lysosomal β-glucuronidase when animals were also subjected to prolonged periods of hypoxia (2 hours), an event known to be associated with focal cytoplasmic degradation.

Consequently, slow but not detectable transfer appears to take place from endoplasmic reticulum to lysosomes in the regenerating liver of nonhypoxic rats. Rapid incorporation of labeled amino acid in the endoplasmic reticulum β-glucuronidase without secretion or excretion of the newly made enzyme also suggests that a large amount of the new enzyme must remain associated with the endoplasmic reticulum.

Studies of Fishman and his associates [37] with mouse kidney clearly confirmed lysosomal and extralysosomal (mainly endoplasmic reticulum) localization of the enzyme. Histochemical studies of mouse kidneys injected with gonadotropins further revealed that the activity of β-glucuronidase expressed in function of the time of injection increased in the endoplasmic reticulum before it increased in the lysosomes. But because Fishman's group used a hormone to stimulate enzyme biosynthesis, their study has raised new questions about the origin and the intracellular sites of action of the hydrolases. The investigators measured the activity of β-glucuronidase and acid phosphatase in kidney and liver of male mice injected with gonadotropin and found that whereas the activity of β-glucuronidase increases, that of acid phosphatase remains unchanged. Furthermore, it was observed that β-glucuronidase activity uniformly increases (8 times) in all subcellular fractions, including lysosomes. Only lysosomal enzyme could, however, be released by freezing and thawing. Moreover, although the β-glucuronidase associated with endoplasmic reticulum could be released by hyaluronidase, acid phosphatase could not.

Polyacrylamide electrophoresis of lysosome enzymes suggests that these enzymes exist in two forms: acidic (A form) and basic (B form). Only the basic form is found in lysosomes; the acidic form is associated with microsomes. Partially purified ribosomal enzymes are believed to contain oligosaccharide components, and neuraminidase converts the acidic form into the basic form. In Tay-Sachs disease, apparently only the acid form of the enzyme is absent. The significance of these observations is still obscure.

The "Point of No Return"

Many types of injuries cause cellular death, which may ultimately result in bodily death or serious mutilation. To prevent injury is often impossible; therefore, the only hope for preventing the consequences of injury would be to reverse what seems to be an inevitable course. Although we know little of the chain of events in cellular death, it seems obvious from the preceding discussions that cell death is not instantaneous but is associated with the unwinding of a sequence of molecular and ultrastructural changes. The earliest changes probably are reversible; the latest are not. Before the changes can be reversed, we must determine which event separates the last reversible from the first irreversible step, and how soon that critical event occurs after the injury. The time at which this critical molecular change takes place is often called the "point of no return."* If diagnosis is prompt, the knowledge of what happens at that critical moment should permit physicians to reverse a sequence of cellular changes that would otherwise inevitably lead to cytonecrosis. *In vivo* necrosis is difficult to control, and autolysis of excised tissues is irreversible. Therefore, it is impossible to detect the point of no return in the succession of events leading to cellular death. One morphologically recognizable pathological condition is reversible: cloudy swelling. This is the earliest form of cellular degeneration recognizable with the light microscope. It is of little diagnostic value because it occurs during a delay between death and fixation of the tissue, but it can be a useful experimental tool. Fonnesu and his associates [38] have used it extensively to study early degenerative changes.

In cloudy swelling, the cell is enlarged, the membrane is often accentuated, the cytoplasm is pale and granular, and the tinctorial properties of the nucleus are considerably reduced. Under the electron microscope, the only recognizable abnormality is mitochondrial swelling. Such electron microscopic changes are not surprising. Indeed, they had been suspected from examinations of stained mitochondria on fixed preparations and from examinations of tissues showing cloudy swelling with the aid of the phase-contrast microscope.

Cloudy swelling can be produced in a variety of tissues by a wide range of toxins. Diphtheria toxin is often used to produce it experimentally. Fonnesu and coworkers investigated the biochemical changes associated with cloudy swelling. Among their findings is a reduction in the tissue's ability to convert inorganic phosphate into organic phosphate. Such findings reflect the inability of the injured organism to use inorganic phosphate for glucose phosphorylation, which, as may be anticipated, is associated with a reduction in the level of easily hydrolyzable organic phosphate derivatives, such as triphosphates. Among the triphosphates, ATP is particularly important as a source of chemical energy. In an injury caused by diphtheria toxin, direct measurement revealed a drop in tissue

* The "point of no return" refers to cellular and not bodily death. The body can tolerate extensive areas of cellular death. However, massive cellular death of vital organs (heart or brain) taxes the individual because integral restoration does not occur. Instead, the dead cells are replaced by scarring tissue.

ATP content. The reduced ATP level was shown to result from a partial blocking in oxidative phosphorylation, and it might not be pure chance that uncouplers like DNP produce cloudy swelling. (Studies of Trémolières and his associates [39] indicate that a similar mechanism operates in ischemia produced by the application of a tourniquet. The results of these experiments suggest that mitochondria must be important in many forms of cellular death. However, one should not conclude from these results that all forms of cellular death begin with mitochondrial damage.)

It has been proposed that the primary injury in cloudy swelling affects the mitochondria, which are swollen and unable to couple oxidative phosphorylation. How mitochondrial alterations lead to the overall swelling of the cell remains to be shown. Nevertheless, incubation of tissue slices under conditions in which cellular metabolism is blocked leads to similar changes, and then the swelling results from increased hydration. Furthermore, anaerobiosis, DNP, and cyanide cause reversible cellular swelling. These observations suggest that the cell membranes require energy to maintain their permeability.

On the basis of such observations, it seems logical to assume that cloudy swelling results from an increase in hydration. However, Fonnesu suggested that such a process plays a minimal role in cell enlargement. He proposes the alternative hypothesis that the increase in size results from accumulation of proteins in the cell. An increase in the amount of intracellular proteins could result from the introduction of plasma proteins into the cell or from *de novo* synthesis within the cell.

Fonnesu claims to have eliminated the possibility of inhibition by plasma protein on the basis of comparative electrophoretic studies of the protein present in normal and injured liver. In contrast, studies of the incorporation of [^{14}C]glycine and [^{14}C]leucine suggested that the increase in cell size is due to *de novo* protein synthesis.

Moreover, Fonnesu's finding in reversible cloudy swelling induced by small doses of toxin needs to be reconciled with more recent views on the mode of action of diphtheria toxin. Experiments in which doses of diphtheria toxin leading to necrosis were administered to mammalian cells *in vitro* revealed that the intact toxin binds to the cell membrane. No specific receptor site seems to be involved, and the attachment of the molecule involves only the B fragment (see Chapter 16). By mechanisms still unknown, the intact toxin molecule is split, and the A fragment penetrates the cell, where it catalyzes the breakdown of NAD to yield nicotinamide and adenosine diphosphate ribose. The latter compound binds effectively to and inhibits acetyl transferase II. Because that enzyme is essential to the GTP-dependent translocation step, its inhibition inescapably blocks protein synthesis at the level of translation. Whether or not the uncoupling of oxidative phosphorylation followed by the drop in ATP levels, mitochondrial swelling, and cytoplasmic hydration are consequences of an interference with protein synthesis or the result of a direct effect of the toxin on the coupling system remains to be established.

The accelerated protein synthesis during cloudy swelling is difficult to reconcile with the reduced activities of bioenergetic pathways. Fonnesu's observation that injected DNP stimulates protein synthesis contradicts the effect of DNP *in vitro*. The difference in amino acid incorporation observed in normal liver as compared with liver exhibiting cloudy swelling would seem to be related to differences in cellular permeability to the precursor. Indeed, the changes in permeability of the cellular membrane induced by cloudy swelling conceivably could lead to a more rapid resorption of the labeled amino acid by the liver cell, making more labeled precursor available for protein synthesis in the injured cell than in the normal cell, where the precursor may be produced endogenously. This question can be resolved only by studying amino acid penetration into normal and injured cells at various times after the labeled compound is injected.

Studies of Farber and his axsociates have revived the notion that protein synthesis might play a role in cellular death. The administration of cycloheximide was found to interfere with radiation necrosis of the intestine [122] or pancreatic necrosis induced with various toxins.

Similarly, Flaks and Nichols have shown that the administration of cycloheximide protects against the necrogenic action of 2 AAF, 3′-methyl-4-dimethylaminoazobenzene, and carbon tetrachloride, further suggesting that *de novo* protein synthesis may be involved in triggering the necrotic process [123]. In contrast, it was found that actinomycin D exacerbates radiation death [124] and we were unable in our laboratory to observe changes in the incidence of mitosis or nuclear damage in the intestine of rats irradiated and injected with cycloheximide.

Myocardial infarcts and strokes—two major causes of death in the western world—are associated with the development of ischemia. Because ischemia is such a frequent cause of death, the molecular changes that follow interruption of arterial circulation have intrigued many investigators. A convenient way to produce ischemia is to clamp an artery that is the only artery irrigating the organ under investigation. The renal artery is readily accessible and can easily be clamped or unclamped. Moreover, the biochemistry of the ischemic kidney can be compared with that of the contralateral kidney.

Van Lancker and Gottlieb [40] studied the ratios of bound and free acid phosphatase and β-glucuronidase in ischemic rat kidney and observed that no significant amounts of enzymes were released for as long as 1 hour of clamping of the renal artery. Such results clearly suggested that acid hydrolase release was not an early event in cell necrosis.

Studies of Vogt and Farber [41] amply support this view and also provide some clues as to the time and the events that are critical to recovery. Thus, in the absence of oxygen the ATP levels drop, and most of the ATP made must be derived from glycolysis. The morphological findings show that most cells can survive with these restricted sources of bioenergy for 20 minutes, but further oxygen starving causes a large number of the cells to die. What happens at 20 minutes to trigger the irreversible sequence is not known. The ATP levels are low but remain unchanged even after 2 hours of ischemia; but the lactic acid levels continue to increase, so it seems logical to implicate lactic acid accumulation as the factor that changes a reversible to an irreversible course of events.

However, administration of a glycolysis inhibitor reduced not only lactic acid levels but also ATP levels (2%–6% of normal) in the ischemic kidney, making the results of these experiments difficult to interpret. In any event, neither deoxyglucose nor iodoacetate administration made the ischemic kidney recover after 30 minutes of renal artery clamping.

Vogt and Farber further observed that the ability to generate ATP was 80% of normal after 20 minutes and 50% of normal after 30 minutes of clamping. Such a finding suggests that the ability to generate ATP determines whether the damage is reversible or not. Surprisingly, this ability to restore the ATP-generating system does not correlate with the ability of mitochondria to restore biochemical functions that are altered by ischemia. In fact, mitochondria could recover normal oxygen uptake and coupling of oxidation and phosphorylation even when they were obtained from kidney already doomed to necrosis (30 minutes ischemia plus 30 minutes recovery).

Two hours of ischemia induced a marked drop in DNP-stimulated ATPase activity in mitochondria. The study of ATPase activity is significant because it correlates well with the level of mitochondrial restoration. But again, the activity of DNP-stimulated ATPase returns to normal if the kidney is allowed to recover before the mitochondria are isolated.

Mitochondria obtained from ischemic kidney had not lost their ability to actively swell in the presence of calcium or to contract in the presence of ATP.

These results of Vogt and Farber suggest that the critical event separating the reversible from the irreversible sequence occurs 20–30 minutes after the onset of ischemia, and probably consists of an inability of the ischemic cells to restore their ATP stock to at least 80% of the preischemic levels. However, the inability of the cell to generate normal levels of ATP does not result from permanent mitochondrial damage since most of the mitochondrial damage is reversed even if the mitochondria are obtained from ischemic kidney already doomed to necrosis. Consequently, the event separating the irreversible from the reversible sequence appears to be the formation in the doomed cell of mitochondrial inhibitors or the activation of an ATP breakdown pathway.

The results of Vogt and Farber from studies with ischemic kidney compare favorably with previous findings made by Busch in ischemic liver, except that the liver seems to be able to sustain prolonged periods of ATP starvation without entering the irreversible path to necrosis. In liver, the ability to restore normal ATP levels is maintained even after 3 hours of ischemia. The ability to restore ATP levels drops to 40% of normal if the liver is kept ischemic for 4 hours, and all oxidative phosphorylation ceases after 5 hours of ischemia. Inosine infusion before restoring blood circulation makes the liver able to survive after 4 or even 5 hours of ischemia.

Thus, recovery of the ability to synthesize ATP appears to be essential for cell survival. Yet persistence of low ATP levels is unlikely to cause irreversible cellular death because hepatic cells are known to survive up to 48 hours in the presence of ATP levels even lower than those found in ischemic kidneys.

Obviously, too little is known of the molecular mechanisms of cellular death to permit the statement of a lasting working hypothesis on what constitutes the point of no return. Cells could be programmed to function with suitable levels of ATP (far above those actually needed for adequate performance), and as soon as the ability of the cell to maintain such levels has dropped to a certain threshold, the death clock could be set and the course to cytonecrosis would be inevitable. The setting of the death clock could be associated with protein synthesis.

The difference between kidney and liver cells' ability to survive at low levels of ATP would therefore not depend so much upon their respective ATP requirements as on their special programming for death. What determines programming in each cell type is not clear. The program could relate to the need of the body for the integrity of certain organs rather than others for survival. The fact that mammals have two kidneys and only one liver might be relevant to this assumption. The mechanism by which intracellular ATP levels could be brought to low threshold levels has been proposed by Judah and coworkers (see above) [42].

One of the best qualitative definitions of the point of no return was reached by K. Decker [120] in his studies on liver injuries induced by D-galactosamine. The biochemical mechanism of D-galactosamine liver necrosis will be described later. It appears that a level of deprivation of substrate (probably UTP) is critical. If deprivation is not maintained beyond a certain time, the lesion is reversible, but if it is maintained beyond that time, the lesion is irreversible. Such observations may be related to those of Vogt and Farber, since in the latter experiments it seemed that the cell was programmed for a level of aerobic ATP production.

Relationship between Spontaneous and Provoked Cellular Death

In describing cloudy swelling and autolysis, we have mentioned some of the reversible and irreversible changes that take place during cellular death in situations in which the passage from life to death takes a short time. Because the time is short, the individual steps of the sequence of events are difficult to dissociate. Our observations would be facilitated if the time required for passage from life to death were slowed down. We have seen that nature has provided numerous examples of deliberate cellular suicides for functional purposes. The skin cell slowly dies to become keratinized. The red cell, after having performed all the functions of a multipotential cell, deliberately destroys its genome and most of its bioenergetic pathways to become a hemoglobin-filled "bag," which has few functions other than those related to maintaining the integrity of hemoglobin. How many other cells partially mutiliate themselves to serve a function? Are polymorphonuclears and macrophages cells that have slowed down on the path to death to be able to kill foreign life or scavenge foreign material?

If the life of the adult human organism is associated with slow cellular death for functional purposes, embryogenesis involves sometimes widespread cellular death. Bending or twisting and branching of an organ is accompanied by focal necrosis. The areas to be destroyed are clearly marked in space and time. Disturbance in the position or schedule of the necrosis leads to congenital anomalies. Even in the growing child, the formation of adult bone configurations involves repeated destruction of the preexisting cartilaginous or bone structures. What mechanisms regulate this rigidly controlled destruction?

If we know little of what causes programmed death in the red cell, we know even less of what triggers it in the fetus where the programmed elimination of cells of various types is indispensable for development. Evidence from plants where programmed death is rigidly regulated could be helpful, but even then we know little about the mechanism that triggers death.

The vegetative growth of Xantium plants stops and the plants age dramatically after seeding. The removal of buds and flowers prevents senescence. It was believed that senescence was triggered by a feedback signal to cellular metabolism originating in the buds and the flower. This view has been challenged [125].

Studies of programmed death in plant cultures *in vitro* have suggested an involvement of cyclic AMP in the process. The exact role of cyclic AMP remains to be established [126].

The Role of Trypsin in Cell Death

Three groups of diseases are probably caused by disturbances of the mechanism activating proteolytic enzymes. The activation of trypsin plays a key role in the pathogenesis of acute pancreatitis, and the absence of an α-antitrypsin inhibitor may be responsible for some forms of chronic obstructive pulmonary diseases and liver cirrhosis.

Pancreatitis

The term pancreatitis is a misnomer because the ending *itis* suggests an infectious process, and in reality infections of the pancreas are rare. A mild local manifestation of a generalized infection (mumps, tuberculosis, congenital syphilis) may involve the pancreas. But pancreatitis usually is not infectious and simply results from autolysis of the organ. Three characteristics of pancreatitis are evident on gross examination of the involved abdomen are blood- and bile-stained fluid in the peritoneal cavity, foci of fat necrosis in the omentum (usually near the pancreas, but actually anywhere in the peritoneum), and a swollen, hemorrhagic pancreas with numerous foci of fat necrosis. Depending upon the severity of the disease and the time elapsed between onset of symptoms and intervention, the histological changes in the pancreas range from focal to massive necrosis and extensive hemorrhage.

Two symptoms of acute pancreatitis dominate the clinical picture: severe abdominal pain and shock. The pain starts suddenly, usually in the left upper quadrant; sometimes it extends to the back and is aggravated by breathing. Once established, pain persists, and pain that was localized at first spreads to the epigastrium and to the entire upper abdomen to become even more diffuse later. The pain is accompanied by rigidity of the abdominal wall, which is localized at first but soon spreads to a large segment of the abdomen.

In some forms of fulminating pancreatitis, circulatory collapse rather than pain dominates the picture. Physicians should consider acute pancreatitis as a possibility in all cases in which acute abdominal pain develops in association with severe shock.

Two steps can confirm the diagnosis: determination of blood serum amylase and lipase and an X-ray (see below).

If there is no pathognomic X-ray picture for acute pancreatitis, radiological examination will permit the exclusion of at least two acute conditions that could readily be confused with acute pancreatitis: rupture of pelvic ulcer (which is often associated with the appearance of air under the diaphragm), and acute intestinal obstruction (which should reveal fluid levels). In acute pancreatitis the pancreas may have a peculiar ground-glass appearance, with a dilated segment of the intestine.

The conditions most frequently associated with acute pancreatitis include gallstone, alcoholism, and hyperlipidemia (see Table 10-3). In none of these cases is the pathogenesis of pancreatitis known. In patients with gallstones, regurgitation of bile from the common channel in the pancreatic duct is believed to activate the conversion of trypsinogen to trypsin. The evidence for such mechanism is not convincing. In hyperlipidemia, the formation of a fat embolism has been proposed as the cause of pancreatitis with subsequent liberation of the free fatty acid as triglyceride contacts pancreatic lipase. However, it is difficult to conceive of a mechanism that would bring lipase and blood triglyceride in contact in the pancreatic cell. Whatever is the primary cause, the pathogenesis of acute pancreatitis is not settled.

Acute pancreatitis has long intrigued clinicians in pathology. Its onset is sudden and dramatic, and hospi-

Table 10-3. Factors associated with acute pancreatitis

Alcoholism
Mostly in municipal hospitals
Biliary tract disease
Mostly in private hospitals
Infections
Mumps
Coxsackie virus
Protein starvation
Kwashiorkor
Malabsorption syndrome
Sprue
Hereditary diseases
Cystic fibrosis
Hyperlipidemia
Hormonal diseases
Hyperparathyroidism (with calcification)
Administration of steroids (rare)
Trauma
Car accident
Crushing against spine
Whiplash of tail

talization and immediate intervention are required. The diagnosis is seldom simple, and pancreatitis may be confused with pneumonia and myocardial infarct as well as with other acute peritoneal crises. The central injury in acute pancreatitis is autodigestion of pancreatic macromolecules by digestive hydrolases elaborated and secreted by the pancreas. The consequences of acute pancreatitis are necrocytosis, necrosis, hemorrhage, inflammation, diffusion of enzymes in the peritoneal cavity, and distant necrosis by enzymes escaping in the bloodstream.

The enzymes involved in pancreatic tissue autolysis are those found in the zymogen granule: trypsinogen, chymotrypsinogen, carboxypeptides, lipase, and amylase. In the normal pancreas, these enzymes are kept inactive by three means: (1) they are surrounded by the protective membrane of the zymogen granule; (2) the active center of the proteolytic enzymes is trapped within a molecular structure that must be dismembered before the enzyme can become active; and (3) blood and tissue contain inhibitors of ribonucleases and trypsin. Once the peptidases are activated, they digest membranes and intracellular proteins, modify cellular permeability, and ultimately lead to cellular death simply by shifting the delicate balance between anabolic and catabolic pathways toward irreversible catabolism.

All cells exposed to the enzymes are autolyzed, but when the endothelial cells of capillaries and blood vessels are damaged, blood exudes into the tissue, leading to hemorrhage. Hemorrhage and necrosis are responsible for the inflammatory reaction observed in acute pancreatitis, which includes edema, vasodilatation, and leukocytic infiltration. (See section on inflammation.)

Lipase specifically attacks lipids and therefore primarily affects adipose cells, where it digests triglycerides to yield glycerol and fatty acids. At the basic pH of the cell, the fatty acids complex with bases such as calcium to form insoluble calcium soaps. Thus, spotty fatty necrosis develops wherever the lipase is made available, either because of leakage in the pancreatic tissue and the peritoneal cavity or because of transport of lipase through the bloodstream. The most common sites of fatty necrosis are in pancreas and the omentum, but sometimes fatty necrosis occurs at a distance, for example, in the bone marrow.

The release of amylase in tissues, peritoneum, and blood causes little injury, but as we shall see it is important for the diagnosis of the disease.

In some cases, pancreatitis is associated with massive ascites, the pathogenesis of which is unclear.

Most typical is the widespread fat necrosis. Although the fat necrosis appears in a broad zone of the omentum and the peritoneal wall, the lesions are usually relatively small, ranging in diameter from a few millimeters to several centimeters. The areas of fat necrosis appear as whitish-yellow-brown, poorly delimited placques resembling paraffin drippings or dried wax. They have a consistency intermediate between that of wax and ground chalk; in fact, they are a lipid-calcium complex.

Focal or generalized peritonitis with fluid in the peritoneal cavity, edema, and congestion of the omentum and the peritoneal wall may accompany severe pancreatitis. In typical cases, part or all of the pancreas shows marked anatomical changes. The tissue is softened and fragile, swollen, and filled with blood.

On section, the pancreas reveals brownish-gray zones of liquifying necrosis alternating with yellowish fat necrosis and hemorrhage. In severe cases, the entire pancreas may be transformed into a macerating mass of necrotic tissue; in the milder cases, hemorrhage and fat necrosis are not conspicuous, and the predominant change is pancreatic swelling. Cases of acute pancreatitis have been reported in which no visible anatomical changes could be recognized.

A wide variety of histologic changes appear including edema, diffuse leukocytic infiltration, hemorrhage, fat necrosis, cellular necrosis, digestion of the connective tissue of the blood vessel, and other alterations. Massive and sudden pancreatic necrosis leads to death. Untreated generalized but mild pancreatitis may result in total restoration with calcified nodules at the site of earlier fat necrosis. Intermediate forms may lead to a form of chronic pancreatitis with partial regeneration and fibrosis. Severe localized pancreatitis may lead to the development of large pancreatic hemorrhagic cysts due to the accumulation of blood and secretion within the necrotic area limited by a fibrous capsule.

Severe pancreatitis involving the entire organ is associated with a bandlike pain in the abdomen. The pain may be more localized if only a portion of the pancreas is affected. It will be in the left, middle, or right epigastrium when the head, body, or the tail of the pancreas is involved, respectively.

Leakage of the pancreatic enzymes in the peritoneum causes peritonitis, and absorption of the enzyme in the bloodstream leads to hyperenzymia and excessive urinary enzyme excretion. The amount of enzyme in the blood depends upon the amount of enzymes released in the pancreas, the rate of breakdown of enzyme in the blood, and the rate of urinary excretion of the enzyme. Although it is impossible to determine quantitatively how much each of these factors contributes to the levels of amylase, lipase, and trypsin in the blood, the patterns for amylase and lipase increase in pancreatitis are very different. Amylase* levels rise rapidly in the blood of patients with acute pancreatitis; the rise in the blood is followed by a rise in the urinary amylase levels, and the latter remain high long after blood levels have dropped. In contrast, lipase levels remain high in the blood, and little of the lipase appears in the urine. All forms of pancreatitis, however, are not associated with high amylase levels. The amylase level depends on the severity of the pancreatitis, although there is no rigid correlation between these two factors. The diagnostic value of serum amylase measurements is somewhat limited because high amylase levels are also found in a number of other abdominal diseases—such as perforated peptic, gastric, or duodenal ulcer, intestinal obstruction, and peritonitis. Moreover, increased serum amylase can also be detected in nonabdominal diseases—such as salivary gland infection (mumps) and renal disease—and often after the administration of drugs—such as morphine, codeine, and Demerol—that cause the sphincter of Oddi to contract. The normal levels of amylase activity expressed in Somogyi units per 24 hours is 5,000 in urine. In pancreatitis, these levels are increased. The increased urinary amylase levels appear sooner and persist longer than the increased levels of serum amylase. It is often said that the determination of serum lipase is of more significance for the diagnosis of acute pancreatitis than that of serum amylase because the levels of the serum lipase increase gradually and persist longer after the onset of the disease. Moreover, serum lipase levels are normal in salivary gland disease. The normal levels of serum lipase are between 0 and 1 unit; they increase 10–100 times in pancreatitis and pancreatic obstruction. Urinary lipase increases in hemorrhagic pancreatitis.

When the fat necrosis is extensive, so much calcium may be removed from the blood so fast that hypocalcemia may develop; this may be followed by tetany. Drops of calcium levels from 10 mg/100 ml to 7 mg/100 ml have been reported; this is equivalent to the formation of 4.25 g of fatty acid. Pancreatitis is almost always fatal when the blood calcium levels drop below 7 mg/100 ml.

Hormonal mechanisms have been invoked to explain the hypocalcemia. Glucagon is believed by some to cause the release of calcitonin. However, direct measurements of glucagon do not support this view. A deficiency of hypoparathyroid hormones has also been incriminated but without convincing evidence [148].

Trypsin is a very vigorous proteolytic enzyme that attacks preferentially the carboxyl groups of arginine and lysine residues involved in peptide formation. In the pancreas, trypsin exists in an inactive form called trypsinogen. Enterokinase activates trypsinogen to yield trypsin. Once trypsin has been formed, activation is autocatalytic.

Similarly, chymotrypsin exists in the form of chymotrypsinogen inside the zymogen granule and is activated to yield chymotrypsin under the catalytic action of trypsin. The specificity of chymotrypsin differs from that of trypsin in that chymotrypsin preferentially attacks carboxyl groups of tyrosine and phenylalanine residues involved in peptide bond formation.

Zymogen granules also contain a procarboxypeptidase, which under the influence of trypsin is converted to the carboxypeptidase, exopeptidase, which splits off the terminal amino acid possessing a free carboxyl group. In acute pancreatitis, trypsinogen is activated to trypsin, and as a result the chymotrypsinogen and the procarboxypeptidase are also activated. A direct method of measuring pancreatic functions consists of injecting the hormones that specifically stimulate pancreatic secretion: secretin, which stimulates the secretion of bicarbonate and pancreatic fluid, and pancreozymin, which mainly stimulates enzyme secretion. The injection of secretin with or without pancreozymin followed by measurement of the volume of duodenal secretion and enzyme activity in the pancreatic fluid may serve to distinguish between steatorrhea resulting from the loss of pancreatic function (cystic fibrosis) and steatorrhea of other origin (sprue). In acute pancreatitis, the combined injection of secretin and a drug that contracts the sphincter of Oddi (thus preventing the excretion of the pancreatic juice into the duodenum) will lead to an increase in serum amylase far in excess of what would be observed if the same procedure were used in a normal individual.

When symptoms of acute pancreatitis are present, the diagnosis may be difficult because the enzymes released in the acute necrotic process, especially trypsin, diffuse through the retroperitoneal space and in the peritoneal cavity down to the pouch of Douglas. The enzymes may irritate the nervous plexus (*e.g.*, celiac plexus) damaging such organs as the appendix. As a result, acute pancreatitis is often difficult to distinguish from perforated ulcer, appendicitis, generalized peritonitis, and other abdominal conditions.

Although the pathogenesis of acute pancreatitis is unknown [43, 44], the key event is obviously the activation of trypsinogen to trypsin. When there is massive trauma or necrosis, such as in severe accidents or infections or after the administration of certain drugs, the lysis of the cell and its intracellular organelles releases the trypsinogen, which can then be activated by peptidases in the autolyzing cell (cathepsin). But what triggers the conversion of trypsinogen to trypsin in other types of pancreatitis is much less clear. On the basis of the normal physiology of the pancreas, a number

* The normal amylase value for adults measured in Somogyi units in 100 ml of serum is 40. Values of about 500 are considered suggestive of pancreatitis.

of mechanisms can be proposed: (1) cellular necrosis; (2) lysis of the zymogen granules as a result of damage to the membrane (alcohol?); (3) inability to surround the enzyme with the protective membrane of the zymogen granule (in that case, the disease could be a disease of the Golgi apparatus); (4) elaboration of an abnormal trypsinogen molecule that is susceptible to activation; and (5) absence or elaboration of an abnormal trypsin inhibitor. Which mechanism obtains alone or in combination with others in each type of acute pancreatitis remains to be seen. For example, in alcoholic pancreatitis, it is not known whether alcohol causes cell necrosis first and pancreatitis second, or whether the cell necrosis is a consequence of the intracellular release of trypsin and trypsinogen by other mechanisms. Similarly, reflux of bile acid into the pancreatic duct as a result of increased intraduodenal pressure or because of obstruction of the common opening of a pancreatic bile duct at the sphincter of Oddi does not always lead to pancreatitis. When it does, how the activation of trypsinogen to trypsin takes place is unknown, although the injection of bile into the bile ducts clearly leads to trypsinogen activation. In some experiments, the common bile duct was anastomosed to the pancreatic duct, and although bile flowed abundantly in both pancreatic ducts under those conditions, acute pancreatitis never developed.

In conclusion, the only thing well established about the pathogenesis of acute pancreatitis was demonstrated first in 1908 by Polya [45], who injected diluted trypsin solution in the pancreatic duct of a dog and produced acute pancreatitis. This finding has been confirmed again and again, and there seems to be no doubt that trypsin activation explains most of the pathological and clinical changes in pancreatitis. The mechanism by which the activation takes place remains a mystery.

α_1-Antitrypsin Deficiency

The cellular mechanisms of protection against hydrolases were discussed above. Any defect in such a mechanism obviously might be catastrophic for the cell or the tissue involved. One form of protection devised by the cell against its own hydrolases is the elaboration of inhibitors. For example, species-specific protease inhibitors were found in serum, colostrum, urine, and pancreatic juice, in nasal and bronchial mucus, in saliva, and in a number of tissues.

Serum protease inhibitors are numerous and can be separated by electrophoresis into a number of fractions referred to as: postalbumin, α_1-globulin, inter α- and α_2-globulin fractions. The major antiprotease fraction is the α_1-antitrypsin fraction, a protein with a molecular weight of 60,000. The presence of the inhibitor is determined genetically (autosomal dominant) and is influenced by pregnancy and typhoid vaccine injection, both of which increase the levels of the inhibitor in the blood. Nothing is known of the metabolism of the α_1-antitrypsin protein and its site of synthesis and breakdown, although its half-life is believed to be 5–6 days. At least seven variants of the α_1-antitrypsin protein have been described in Scandinavians on the basis of studies with starch-gel electrophoresis. The presence of the variants is believed to be determined by the presence of codominant allelic genes [46, 47].

The inhibitor is a glycoprotein containing galactose, mannose, N-acetylglucosamine, and sialic acid. α_1-Antitrypsin has been found to inhibit several proteolytic enzymes including trypsin, plasmin, urokinase, the Hageman factor, cofactor elastase, collagenase, chymotrypsin, thrombin [127].

Binding of human α_1-antitrypsin and α and β bovine trypsin has been investigated. In each case inhibitor and enzyme form a stable complex which cannot be dissociated except by rather drastic methods. The binding is stoichiometric, one molecule of enzyme for one molecule of inhibitor. In the case of the binding of the inhibitor to the α-trypsin, it is believed that an acyl bond is formed between the carbonyl carbon of the inhibitor and the γ-oxygen of the Ser-183 of the enzyme [128].

Patients whose serum is low in α_1-antitrypsin protein have been described. The defect is hereditary. The serum levels are 10% of normal in the homozygote and 55% of normal in the heterozygote.

Although not all patients with homozygous α_1-antitrypsin deficiency are unhealthy, the incidence of so-called chronic obstructive lung disease (bronchitis, asthma, emphysema, bronchiectasis) appears to be significantly higher among such patients. The incidence of such lung disease is highest in deficient men, and the incidence seems to be modulated by exposure to irritants (including smoking) and by bronchopulmonary infections. It is not certain whether heterozygous levels of α_1-antitrypsin influence the health of the lung.

There have been a number of studies attempting to correlate levels of α_1-antitrypsin activity with pulmonary function. The results often conflict and are difficult to interpret. An extensive study done in Tucson seems, however, to establish that significant reduction in the α_1-antitrypsin activity (from 38 to 80%) does not affect the incidence of chronic obstructive disease [147].

Although it is established that heterozygotes do not develop overt lung disease, it can not be excluded that they might show mild functional pulmonary change. The lung appears to be the only organ susceptible to the α_1-antitrypsin defect; no convincing disease in other organs has been established.

Clearly, the elucidation of the pathogenetic mechanism of the disintegration of lung tissue in the absence of α_1-antitrypsin could tell much about the pathogenesis of chronic obstructive lung disease. Unfortunately, the pathogenesis remains a matter of speculation. In the absence of inhibitors, elastase, collagenase, or unspecific proteases of tissue, bacterial, leukocytic or macrophagic origin are thought to attack the elastocollagen skeleton of alveoli, bronchioles, and bronchi, thereby destroying their resilience.

Antitrypsin deficiency has also been described in young children with cirrhosis of the liver. The deficiency is transferred as a hereditary trait likely to be autosomal dominant. The disease affects only the homozygous. It is fatal, progressive, and culminates in liver cirrhosis with all its complications—esophageal varices, ascites, etc.

In those cases in which other causes of cirrhosis have been excluded, one finds: (1) large amounts of α_1-antitrypsin with the aid of immunofluorescent antibody; (2) accumulation in liver of amorphous material, visible on hematoxylin-eosin stains, but even more apparent on periodic acid-Schiff stains (yet the material is diastase resistant); (3) accumulation of large amounts of amorphous material in the endoplasmic reticulum but not in the Golgi or lysosomes.

Nothing of the pathogenesis of this disease is known. The defect in secretion has, at least in some cases, been linked to a deficiency in sialyltransferase [129]. It has been proposed that the α_1-antitrypsin accumulates in liver (the organ in which it is normally elaborated) because its normal pattern of excretion is interrupted. Thus, instead of being transferred from endoplasmic reticulum to Golgi and from Golgi to secretory granules, the α_1-antitrypsin glycoprotein accumulates in the endoplasmic reticulum. The mechanism of cirrhosis production is not known. It has been proposed that in the presence of extensive amounts of antitrypsin in the liver, fibrin and collagen that accumulate in cases of liver insult as a result of protease action are not eliminated normally. However, direct evidence supporting such an interpretation is lacking.

Conclusions and Comments on Cell Death

To understand cellular death, one must remember that the cell is an integrated functional and structural unit. Interaction between the various functional units is regulated by complex molecular events, but also by compartmentalization of the functions within the confines of semipermeable membranes. Direct damage to one or more components of the functioning units, whether there be transcription, translation, or production of energy, will necessarily be reflected in damage to other functional units and may even ultimately alter the structures of the individual membranes and lead to disruption of compartmentalization. In other cases, direct damage to either the plasma membrane or the membranes surrounding specific organelles may be the cause of the primary injury and result in distortion of other cellular functions. Therefore, in studying cellular death caused by a given agent one must distinguish between the primary insult which may occur at the level of a single molecule and the secondary consequences which may result in the distortion of one or more metabolic pathways, or in the disruption of compartmentalization.

It is conceivable that if noxious agents are withdrawn from the cell in time, the damage that they have caused may be reversible, while if they are left in the cell, they will inexorably lead to death. The distinction of the events that separate the reversible from the irreversible stage is, of course, critical to the management of patients exposed to injurious agents.

The mechanisms put in gear to kill a mammalian cell are likely to be very complex and obviously we know little of them. The sequence of events that lead to the conversion from the lysogenic to the lytic stage in *E. coli* infected with λ phage illustrates the complexity of the events involved in killing a bacteria and might be relevant to at least some aspects of mammalian cell death.

Phage λ, a temperate phage, either enters a replicative cycle or lysogenizes the cell after infection (see Chapter 16).

Lysogeny is maintained by the λ repressor which represses all viral genes except cI, the structural gene for the repressor and a so-called *rex* gene whose role is unknown, but is believed to determine the return from lysogen to lytic cycle. The *rex* gene effect is achieved by distortion of normal cellular controls of the host through proteins coded for by *rex* and by redirecting host function toward viral replication.

When a culture of *E. coli* which contains a mutant λ phage that produces a temperature sensitive repressor is heated to 40° C, three steps occur: reduction of prophage, replication of phage, and lysis of the host cells. The lysis is caused by an endolysin coded for by the phage that hydrolyzes cross-linkages in the cell wall. By itself the endolysin is unable to cause lysis because an integral cell membrane prevents the endolysin from reaching the cell interior. The λ phage produces, however, an S protein which in some way eliminates the block imposed by the cell membrane and thereby controls lysis. The events are rigidly timed. Replication goes on for 41 minutes. Endolysin is synthesized in the cytoplasm starting 20 minutes after infection and after that time 50% of the cells lyse. The S gene product is synthesized during the second half of the lytic cycle. Once a lytic cycle is started a rigidly timed sequence of molecular events takes place, as if a clock had been put in gear. Some of the time sequence can be distorted by metabolic inhibitors or mutations. Cyanide, dinitrophenol, and chloramphenicol accelerate the lysis; thus, in some way assisting the S gene product effects. Since the S protein is synthesized during the lytic process, the effect of chloramphenicol suggests that the S protein is not indispensable for lysis and that other regulators for lysing are needed, presumably the *rex* gene product.

Since cI, which produced the λ repressor, and *rex* are the only genes expressed in the lysogen, it would seem logical to conclude that the *rex* gene product is involved in the timing in the lysogenic effect.

Clearly there is much to be uncovered in the mechanism of lysogeny, but complex gene interactions are certainly involved and it cannot be excluded that the mammalian genome is also involved in the death sentence of cells [130].

Intracellular Macromolecular Deposits

We have reviewed forms of cellular death that may be associated with hyperdifferentiation and accumulation of large amounts of single macromolecules (keratin, hemoglobin, etc.), or with focal cytoplasmic degradation. But as the cell can sustain limited hydrolysis, it can also survive extensive intracellular accumulation of macromolecules, such as glycogen, mucopolysaccharides, cholesterol, cerebrosides, and triglycerides.

The intracellular accumulation of macromolecules often results from inborn errors of metabolism. Those have been discussed in another chapter. Other accumulations are the result of injury. The accumulation of triglyceride is prominent in that way.

Liver Steatosis

Steatosis, or intracellular fat accumulation in nonadipose cells, is a common form of cellular injury occurring in many organs: heart, liver, lung, kidney, and others. Its pathogenesis has been most extensively investigated in liver. Before the mechanism of production of the injury is described, the morphological changes that take place in fatty liver will be examined.

Light Microscopy and Ultrastructure

When a large amount of fat accumulates in the liver, the gross appearance of the liver changes. The organ is bigger than normal. The capsule is under tension and the cut surface bulges. The liver has a yellowish hue and is soft and greasy to the touch. Nevertheless, the presence of excessive amounts of fat in liver cannot always be recognized macroscopically.

The histological section prepared after embedding the tissue in paraffin or celloidin loses its lipid content (phosphatides and cerebrosides become insoluble in lipid solvent if they are treated with chromic salts), and the intracellular spaces, in which the fat droplets were lodged, appear as various-sized vacuoles. But if a tissue block is frozen and a thin section is made without submitting the tissue to the regular dehydration and embedding procedures, the intracellular lipids remain in place and can be stained specifically with liposoluble dyes such as shellac, Sudan III, Nile blue, chlorophyll, etc. When a liver cell has undergone a full-blown fatty infiltration, the hepatocyte may be difficult to distinguish from an adipose cell. The liver cell loses its cytoplasm, and its intracytoplasmic structures are relegated to the periphery of the cell, the central part of the cell being filled with a huge fat droplet; the nucleus is small, sometimes pyknotic, and is rejected from its central position to an extreme peripheral one. In the early stages of fatty infiltration, small fat droplets barely visible with the microscope appear in the cell cytoplasm and are believed to coalesce to form larger droplets (see Fig. 10-9).

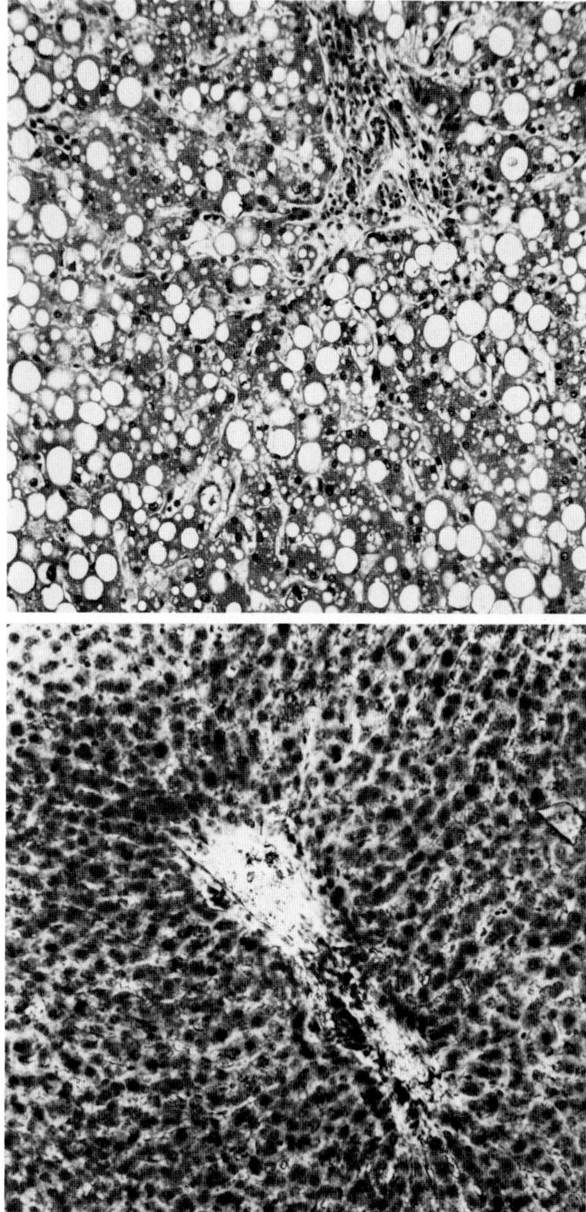

Fig. 10-9. Liver steatosis showing fat droplets in human hepatocytes in slide stained with H and E *(top)* and in rat liver stained with Sudan black *(bottom)*

Sometimes several cells loaded with lipids coalesce and form a larger lipid cyst, which itself may rupture into blood vessels and thereby may be responsible for lipid emboli formation.

All liver cells do not undergo fatty infiltration at the same time. In fact, the fat distribution may be restricted to certain parts of the hepatic lobule, depending upon the cause of the injury. A typical example is cardiac failure, which results in chronic passive congestion with anoxemia, likely to be most intensive at the periphery of the lobule. The cell layer surrounding the portal veins shows the first signs of fatty infiltration. In contrast, the fatty infiltration associated with the administration of toxins often affects the cell layer that surrounds the central artery.

Electron microscopists have described the sequence of ultrastructural changes that take place in liver steatosis. Fatty liver that develops after the administration of orotic acid, carbon tetrachloride, and ethionine, or as a result of choline deficiency has been studied with the electron microscope by a number of investigators (see Fig. 10-10).

In the early stages of fatty infiltration, tiny lipid droplets appear. They are close to the endoplasmic reticulum and are surrounded by a single membrane that is claimed to be in continuity with the membranes of the endoplasmic reticulum. These lipid granules are called liposomes. Small liposomes are thought to coalesce to yield giant liposomes. However, little direct evidence supports that assumption, and, to our knowledge, no available serial sections establish coalescence between the small granules and the large ones. Furthermore, the chemical similarity between small and large granules has not been shown. In fact, some electron microscopists believe that the small, clear vacuoles found in close relationship with the endoplasmic reticulum are proteins.

In addition to causing lipid droplet accumulation, the administration of orotic acid leads to further changes in the endoplasmic reticulum, which after the fourth day of an orotic acid diet vesiculates and later fragments. After 7 days of orotic acid administration, the vesicles contain a dark-staining, electron-opaque droplet. Yet the periphery of the vesicles continues to be studded with ribosomes. Occasionally, fat droplets have been described in the nucleus of liver undergoing fatty infiltration. Some believe that these droplets are present in the nuclear area only as a result of cytoplasmic hernia. Others think that they are native to the nucleus. For example, electron micrographs have been published showing fat droplets between the inner and outer membranes of the nucleus.

Not all forms of fatty infiltration result in the formation of large liposomes. Even as long as 2 years after orotic acid administration the lipid droplets remain separate as small, discrete liposomes. The steatosis associated with various types of intoxication (*e.g.*, tetracycline) or resulting from pregnancy causes multiple small droplets to form.

Handschumacher and his associates [48] isolated liposomes from the livers of rats fed orotic acid. The

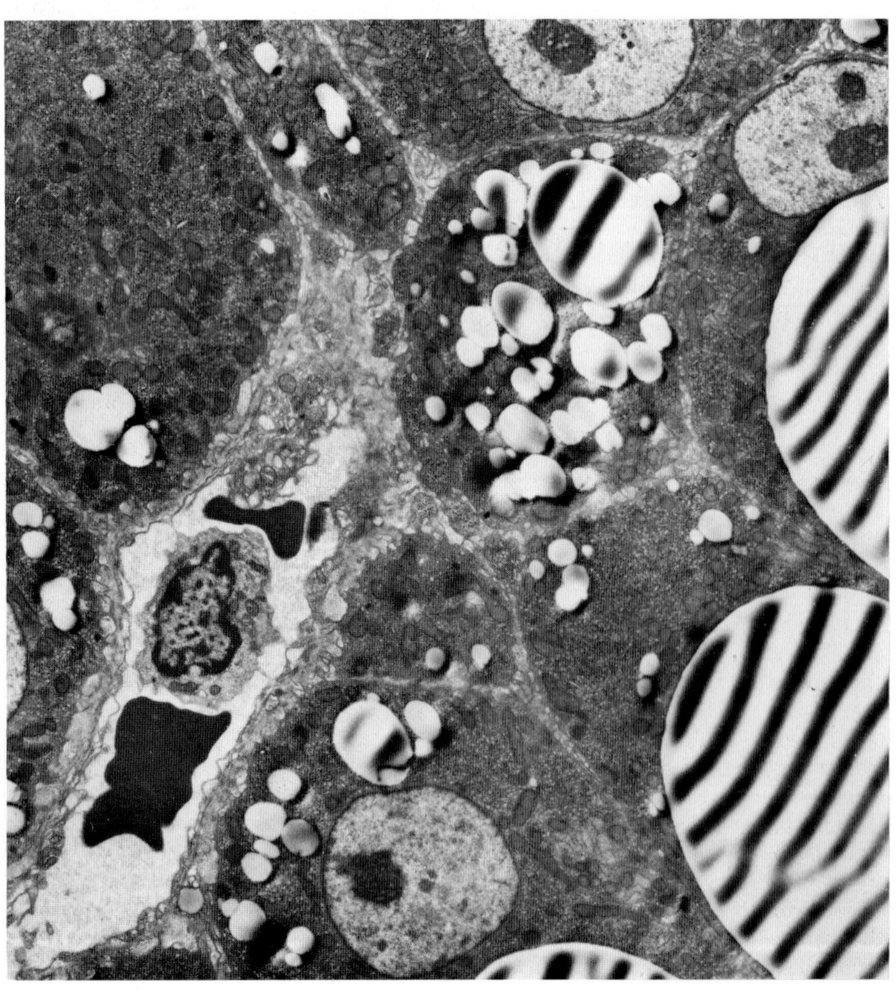

Fig. 10-10. Lipid degeneration of hepatic cell in a case of chronic alcoholism. The alternately dark and clear bands in the lipid droplets are sectioning artifacts (×4,000; from Zamboni)

macromolecular analysis of the granules suggests that in addition to lipoprotein, the granules contain the membranes of the smooth endoplasmic reticulum as well as ribonucleoprotein granules. The labeling patterns and the base ratio of the 28 ribosomal RNA's isolated from the liposomal fraction resemble that described for ribosomes associated with the membrane of the endoplasmic reticulum. Similar observations were made by Lombardi and his group [49, 50] in liposomes of animals injected with ethionine.

Origin of Lipids. Recent electron microscopic observations made by Japanese observers have again raised the question of lipophanerosis. Virchow, who was the first to recognize the presence of lipids in the hepatocytes, believed that steatosis could have a dual origin: (1) the degeneration of intracellular constituents rich in lipids yielding typical lipid droplets; and (2) introduction of lipids from extrahepatic sources. The first type of steatosis was referred to as lipophanerosis. Pathologists later excluded lipophanerosis as a possibility because it was observed that phosphorus intoxication mobilized lipids from adipose tissue and induced hyperlipemia. Experiments on dogs fed sheep fat seemed to establish conclusively that the liver lipids that accumulated after phosphorus intoxication were of extrahepatic origin.

When dogs are fed sheep fat, the fat of their adipose tissue acquires the physical and chemical properties of sheep fat. Furthermore, if toxic amounts of phosphorus are administered to dogs, their liver lipids have the properties of sheep lipids.

However, Japanese investigators recently have claimed that the lipids that accumulate in some cases of fatty liver are derived from degradation products of intracellular structures, *e.g.*, mitochondria and endoplasmic reticulum. This, of course, implies that in those cases there is no net gain in total lipids, in spite of progressive steatosis. Lombardi has wisely remarked that many cases of liver steatosis may result from a combination of early lipophanerosis later complicated by infiltration of exogenous fat.

Almost any type of liver injury results in steatosis, and, although in each case the pathogenesis may vary, the uniformity of the response to injury suggests that the liver contains highly sensitive targets somewhere along the pathway for lipid usage or synthesis.

Pathogenesis. The pathogenesis of liver steatosis can be understood only in the light of lipid metabolism. It is unnecessary to review all aspects of lipid metabolism here; only the mobilization of lipids from the fat deposits and lipid usage in the liver are relevant.

Adipose tissue triglycerides are hydrolyzed to free fatty acids and glycerol. In liver, the free fatty acids have a double fate—they are oxidized to form ketone bodies or reconverted to triglycerides. The ketone bodies are further oxidized by tissues other than liver.

Normally, triglycerides do not remain in the liver, but are transferred to the general circulation after having been complexed to a protein to form a lipoprotein. The protein moiety of the lipoprotein is probably synthesized by the endoplasmic reticulum of the liver cell.

Thus, at least two cell structures are involved in this rather restricted aspect of lipid metabolism: the mitochondria and the endoplasmic reticulum. In addition, the cell membrane probably is active in transporting nonesterified fatty acid into the liver cell and in transferring triglyceride from the hepatic cell into the circulation. Which of these three cellular elements is injured during the development of fatty liver? Because fatty livers resulting from carbon tetrachloride intoxication have been investigated most extensively, the pathogenesis of these kinds of fatty livers is discussed first.

Effects of Carbon Tetrachloride on Liver—Metabolic Alteration

Mitochondria were first thought to be the site of the primary hepatic injury after CCl_4 administration because swelling and mitochondrial distortion can be observed in fatty liver. However, the mitochondrial changes occur after the onset of lipid deposition.

Further experimentation brought various investigators to suspect the endoplasmic reticulum to be the site of the primary injury. At first, most of the evidence seemed only suggestive, but research in several laboratories provided direct support for this notion. Recknagel and associates [51, 52] injected both Triton X-100, a compound that produces lipemia by preventing the penetration of triglycerides into adipose tissue cells, and carbon tetrachloride, a compound known to lead to triglyceride accumulation in liver cells. When carbon tetrachloride is administered, the lipemia normally induced by Triton does not occur, but the triglycerides accumulate in the liver cell. This important observation led Recknagel to conclude that the primary injury induced by carbon tetrachloride involved triglyceride secretion.

Smuckler and his associates [53–56] reexamined the early changes in fatty liver with the aid of the electron microscope and observed that soon after CCl_4 is injected, the ribonucleoprotein particles are dissociated from the membranes of the endoplasmic reticulum of the liver cells. The cisternae of the endoplasmic membranes present various degrees of dilation and a loss of the parallel arrays. However, the most striking observation is a random dispersion of the ribonucleoprotein particles into the cytoplasmic matrix. Ribosomes may even be found within the space delimited by the endoplasmic reticulum membranes.

The Seattle group complemented their morphological studies by systematically studying the effect of CCl_4 on the cellular machinery for protein synthesis and found that the incorporation of injected labeled amino acids into liver proteins was reduced after CCl_4 administration.

Carbon tetrachloride depresses the incorporation of [^{14}C]glycine in albumin or fibrinogen. No effect of CCl_4 on the total amount or on the electrophoretic pattern of the albumins elaborated by the liver could be detected. The possibility that the difference in labeled amino acid incorporation into proteins results from a difference in the availability of the precursor (for example, due to a decreased blood flow or to changes in cellular permeability in liver of CCl_4-injected animals) was eliminated. Indeed, the specific activity of the acid-soluble fraction of the liver was found to be the same in normal and in CCl_4-injected animals.

The CCl_4-induced block in protein synthesis could result from interference with the biosynthesis of mRNA or from interference with the cytoplasmic template-enzyme complex responsible for protein synthesis. Carbon tetrachloride does not affect the incorporation of precursors into rapidly labeled nRNA, which is assumed to contain fractions that are homologous to the bacterial mRNA. The activities of the enzymes that activate amino acids are not impaired by CCl_4 administration; in contrast, the ability of the microsomes to incorporate labeled amino acid into protein is markedly inhibited after the CCl_4 administration *in vivo*.

Microsomal preparations obtained from noninjected animals, or animals injected with CCl_4, or both were incubated with liver supernatant, and all the coenzymes and precursors necessary for amino acid incorporation were added to the incubation mixture. The system obtained from CCl_4-injected animals differed from that of normal animals in its ability to incorporate amino acids into proteins. The rate of incorporation in the treated animals was lower than that in the normal animals, and the changes in the rate of incorporation were inversely related to the dose of CCl_4 administered.

The alteration in the rate of protein synthesis was attributable to the microsomes because when isolated microsomes obtained from treated animals were incubated with supernatant obtained from normal animals, the ability to incorporate the precursor was still reduced. The rate of incorporation was normal when microsomes prepared from normal animals were incubated with supernatant prepared from CCl_4-injected animals. Furthermore, when the entire polysomal population of the hepatic cell was extracted from CCl_4-injected animals and put on sucrose gradient, a decrease in the number of polysomes sedimenting at 200–80 S was observed, with a corresponding increase in the 50 S component. This suggested that CCl_4 disrupts the polysomal structure into smaller fragments and possibly breaks down the 80 S ribosomal unit into 50 S units.

The alteration of the endoplasmic reticulum is not restricted to the polyribosomal component. Meldolesi [57] has studied the incorporation of ^{32}P in the membranes of the endoplasmic reticulum after CCl_4 administration and has demonstrated an increased uptake of the isotope during the early hours after CCl_4 poisoning. Although the significance of this finding has not been explained, it is believed to reflect increased microsomal membrane synthesis.

In contrast to the early changes observed in the endoplasmic reticulum, alterations in mitochondrial enzyme activities occur late. However, remember that mitochondrial activity is not reflected only by the concentration of the enzymes present, but also by the close integration of the multiple-enzyme system involved in generating ATP and the integrity of the membrane transport system. Therefore, it cannot be excluded that a discrete primary effect of CCl_4 would be to alter the coupling of oxidative phosphorylation or modify ion transport. Smuckler and his collaborators have shown that the ATP levels drop to 65% of normal within 1 hour after CCl_4 administration and to 25% of normal 18 hours later. Yet, the ATP synthetic machinery appears to be intact for at least 3 hours after initiation of injury, and no changes in the mitochondrial structures can be detected. Therefore, the drop in ATP is more likely to result from accelerated breakdown or usage than from decreased synthesis.

The studies of Slater and Greenbaum [58] have shown that the lysosomes play no direct part in the onset of the injury. Indeed, no significant changes in lysosome stability or in the latency of the hydrolases are observed during the early stages of the intoxication, and the changes that take place even as long as 24 hours after intoxication are relatively insignificant.

Primary Molecular Injury of Carbon Tetrachloride

Although it seems now well established that CCl_4 affects the endoplasmic reticulum primarily and that this injury ultimately results in inhibition of protein synthesis, the primary molecular alteration caused by CCl_4 remains mysterious.

Two major hypotheses have been proposed to explain the molecular action of CCl_4. The first assumes that the alkene acts as a solvent. The solvent theory has been rejected on various grounds: (1) the effect of CCl_4 is organ specific; (2) its effects are manifested at doses so low that a solvent effect can hardly be implicated; and (3) the toxicity of lipid solvents does not correlate with lipid solubility in water.

The second theory proposes that the effect of CCl_4 on tissue results from the formation of toxic metabolites. Such a hypothesis can be substantiated only if it is clearly demonstrated that CCl_4 is metabolized in tissues, and that the products of that metabolism are toxic.

Eighteen hours after administration of ^{14}C-labeled CCl_4, 85% of the CCl_4 is converted to CO_2. A small fraction of the CCl_4 is dehalogenated to yield chloroform. When ^{14}C-labeled chloroform is administered, 70% remains unchanged; 4% is converted to CO_2.

Covalent binding of $^{14}CCl_4$ has been investigated in rats 15 minutes after injection of ^{14}C labeled carbon tetrachloride. The microsomal lipids are the first to be labeled and among the lipids both phospholipids and cholesterol are heavily labeled. Among the phospholipids the highest specific activity is in phosphatidyl serine and the lowest in phosphatidyl choline. Cholesterol esters have a specific activity ten times that of cholesterol itself [131].

When CCl_4 is administered, it is assumed that chloroform is an intermediate in the degradation to CO_2. It has been proposed that CCl_4 is dehalogenated to yield $CHCl_3$, which is further reduced to CH_2Cl_2. CH_2Cl_2 is converted to formaldehyde and formic acid by oxidation.

It has also been proposed that the rate-limiting step in CCl_4 degradation is the conversion of CCl_4 to $CHCl_3$. From then on, the conversion to methylene chloride and formic acid proceeds rapidly.

The degradation of CCl_4 and chloroform is inhibited by the classical metabolic inhibitors iodoacetate, fluoride, arsenate, and cyanide and is stimulated by citrate. Significant amounts of $^{14}CO_2$ are derived from chloromethanes only if pyridine nucleotides are added to the incubation mixture. All these findings suggest that chloromethane degradation involves a specific enzyme. It has been proposed that at least two enzymes are involved in chloromethane degradation, one of which is found in the microsome and the other in the supernatant.

The mechanism of CCl_4 dehalogenation is still not clear. It is not established whether this is an enzymic reaction. An nonenzymic reaction has been proposed by Butler [59], who assumes that CCl_4·dehalogenation results from the homolytic cleavage of the molecule to yield a dechlorinated free radical, which in turn reacts with the hydrogen of a sulfhydryl group. The replacement of the covalent bond between the carbon and halogen by a bond between carbon and hydrogen yields an electric dipole with electrostatic energy sufficient to assist heterolytic fission of the bond. Heterolytic fission of alkyl halides occurs when they are placed in water. In this type of molecular degradation, the halogen carries with it the two electrons involved in bond formation. (Two electrons from an outside source are needed to replace the chlorine with hydrogen.) In the homolytic breakdown of CCl_4, one of the bonding electrons is retained by each fragment of the fission product, and a neutral organic molecule and a neutral halogen atom with an outer electron appear.

The formation of free radicals from CCl_4 is easier to understand if free radical formation from water is considered. A water molecule can be dissociated to yield an anionic hydroxyl and a cationic hydrogen. The hydrogen carries the two electrons that were involved in combining the hydroxyl and the hydrogen to form water. However, water can also be split homolytically to form a hydrogen free radical and a hydroxyl free radical. The two electrons involved in bond formation are separated, one to accompany the hydrogen and the other, the hydroxyl group.

The fission of a molecule to yield free radicals usually requires energy. For example, in the splitting of water, energy can be provided by ionizing radiation. The free radicals are usually very short lived, and they have a tendency to recombine with each other to form covalent bonds.

Thus, in the homolytic splitting of CCl_4, a CCl_3 free radical and a chloride free radical are formed. The free radical could then cause cellular damage by attacking some vital molecule—proteins, lipids, or other macromolecules. The free radical derived from the homolytic fission of CCl_4 and chloroform could implement its toxic effect either by alkylating the sulfhydryl groups of enzymes, or by triggering lipid peroxidation. Cysteine and glutathione do not protect against CCl_4 toxicity; instead, compounds with typical antioxidant properties (α-tocopherol, methionine) prevent damage due to CCl_4. Therefore, the free radicals are believed to lead to lipoprotein peroxidation.

From what we know of the theories of rancidity, unsaturated fatty acids probably constitute a good target for the actions of free radicals formed by homolytic cleavage of CCl_4. Many fatty acids contain conjugated double bonds; polyunsaturated fatty acids contain more than one double bond. The polyunsaturated fatty acids are particularly important to human health because they cannot be synthesized by the body. Therefore, they are called essential fatty acids. The polyunsaturated fatty acids found in humans include linoleic, linolenic, and arachidonic acids. Linoleic is a straight-chain fatty acid with two double bonds, one between carbons 13 and 12, and another between carbons 9 and 10. Linolenic has three double bonds: one between carbons 16 and 15, one between carbons 13 and 12, and one between carbons 10 and 9. Arachidonic acid has 4 double bonds: between carbons 5 and 6, 8 and 9, 11 and 12, and 14 and 15. Also, the double bonds of the essential polyunsaturated fatty acids are not conjugated but are separated by methylene bridges.

In rancidification, the fatty acids are oxidized. This is assumed to result from an attack on the double bond by peroxide radicals, yielding unstable hydroperoxides, which, after decomposition, yield keto and hydroxyketo acids. These breakdown products are volatile and are responsible for the unpleasant odor of the degraded fatty acid.

Recknagel [60] has proposed a theory in which the trichloromethyl free radical attacks the methylene bridges of the unconjugated fatty acid bonds to yield an organic free radical and chloroform. Resonance within the organic free radical molecule leads to a large number of substitutes, many of which include -diene conjugation (maximum absorption at 233 mμ). Ultimately, organic peroxides would be formed.

To substantiate the theory, researchers have demonstrated that peroxides are found in livers of animals receiving CCl_4. This is difficult to achieve because of the short life of the free radicals. Recknagel has attempted to demonstrate lipid peroxidation in animals given CCl_4. When a free radical attacks the methylene bridge of an unsaturated fatty acid, an organic free radical is formed and resonance occurs. As a result, conjugated -dienes are formed. The conjugated -dienes (for example, [^{14}C]butadiene) have an absorption peak at 233 mμ. Therefore, the theory can be tested simply by measuring the absorption at 233 mμ of lipids extracted from the endoplasmic reticulum of liver of normal and CCl_4-injected rats. The results of such experiments established that conjugated -dienes were formed within 90 minutes after CCl_4 administration. The fatty acid composition of the microsome of CCl_4-injected animals demonstrated a decrease in arachidonic acid. The *in vivo* results obtained by Recknagel were further confirmed by the demonstration that CCl_4 acts as a peroxidant *in vitro*.

Yet, when an attempt was made to demonstrate an increase in the formation of malonyl dialdehyde (a degradation product of peroxidized fat), the results proved unsuccessful *in vivo*. Recknagel attributed this failure to the rapid breakdown of malonyl dialdehyde by mitochondria.

Dianzani [61] has studied the effect of what he claims to be physiological doses of CCl_4 on isolated mitochondria, microsomes, and lysosomes. Preincubation with CCl_4 practically abolishes microsomal glucose-6-phosphatase activity. Preincubation of mitochondria stimulates Mg^{++}-activated ATPase but inhibits NAD-activated ATP. Carbon tetrachloride releases lysosome enzymes from their structural support *in vitro*. The significance of these findings is difficult to evaluate. The *in vivo* findings are reminiscent of some of the *in vitro* findings. However, if CCl_4 acts *in vivo* after it has been metabolized, what is the fate of the toxin *in vitro*, and how can the *in vitro* results be compared with the *in vivo* results? Smuckler found no effect of CCl_4 added *in vitro* to a cell-free system capable of incorporating amino acid into proteins.

Stop flow spectrophotometry and pulse radiolysis measure reactions that occur in the millisecond range in the former and in the microsecond range in the latter (see chapter on radiation). Using these techniques to measure rapidly occurring reactions such as the formation of free radicals, Slater has been able to demonstrate that lipid peroxidation does occur *in vivo* through the formation of free radicals. In the case of carbon tetrachloride the CCl_3 radical is probably the primary species formed. Highly reactive radicals further initiate the lipid peroxidation and cause covalent binding of carbon tetrachloride with neighboring nucleotide thiols, etc. Damage to the endoplasmic reticulum decreases glucose-6-phosphatase activity and interferes with the activity of the mixed function oxidases [132].

Recknagel's theory is vulnerable to some of the objections used to reject the solvent theory—namely, the intracellular specificity of CCl_4. To obviate this objection, Recknagel further postulated that the homolytic breakdown of CCl_4 occurs in the liver only in an area close to the membrane of the endoplasmic reticulum.

Although Recknagel's studies include testing of liver of animals injured by means other than CCl_4, it should be kept in mind that Bernheim [62] demonstrated that although the amount of peroxidized fat in the liver of normal animals is low, these peroxides increase considerably in liver that has been injured. Peroxide formation in liver cells after injury depends on the presence of inorganic iron, which is liberated from protein or heme. Antioxidants such as vitamin E prevent the peroxidation.

Lipid peroxidation can be produced *in vitro* by incubating liver slices or cell fractions with various reducing agents, such as ferrous iron, mercurial compounds, hemoprotein, ascorbate, and cysteamine. The changes in the appearance of the vesicles of the endoplasmic reticulum (or so-called microsomes) are intriguing. First, the ribosomes detach from the surface of the vesicles. Later, the microsome vesicles lose their round shape and gradually become irregular. The membrane folds between the vesicles. Dense amorphous precipitates and membranous debris with myelinlike figures appear. At low magnification, the aggregates resemble lipofuscin observed in aging heart and brain [63].

Some Other Forms of Steatosis

There is credible evidence that steatosis associated with ethionine, puromycin, and phosphorus intoxication all result, at least in part, from interference with protein synthesis. Whether or not other factors, such as reduced levels of fatty acid oxidation, are also involved is not known.

Steatosis after orotic acid administration is unlikely to result from a block in protein synthesis with a subsequent block in lipoprotein excretion. After orotic acid administration, there is a marked depression in plasma lipids associated with the steatosis. Furthermore, the incorporation of labeled precursors in the low-density lipoproteins is markedly reduced.

Blocks in the coupling of protein to lipid or in the mechanism of transfer through the cell membrane have been postulated to explain lipid accumulation after orotic acid administration.

Intoxications are not the only cause of fatty livers. Hepatic steatosis occurs in association with diabetes, galactosemia, starvation, and cardiac insufficiency. Acute steatosis sometimes occurs in pregnancy (Sheehan's syndrome). The steatosis is then usually associated with severe jaundice and liver insufficiency. The prognosis is serious but not necessary fatal. The pathogenesis of such forms of steatosis is not known.

In conclusion, although the development of fatty livers after CCl_4 administration has been investigated intensively, many steps of the pathogenesis remain unknown. On the basis of available knowledge, it seems plausible that CCl_4 intake is followed by its spontaneous or enzymic homolytic split, leading to the formation of free radicals. The free radicals modify macromolecules, probably lipids, resulting in their peroxidation.

The damage to lipids of the endoplasmic reticulum is followed by a disruption of the normal relationship between endoplasmic reticulum membranes and ribosomes; this disruption interferes with protein synthesis. Although all protein synthesis is not inhibited, the synthesis of proteins that bind to triglycerides that are being secreted is; therefore, lipids are not secreted but accumulate in the hepatic cells.

Appealing as it may be, this interpretation of the mode of action of CCl_4 leaves important questions unanswered. An explanation of the selectivity in damage to lipoproteins of the endoplasmic reticulum and the selectivity in the block of protein synthesis is needed.

Synoptic View of Liver Steatosis. The liver receives lipids from and returns lipids to the blood. There are two sources of blood lipids that are transferred to the liver: those derived from lipolysis and those derived from dietary sources. Free fatty acids are derived from adipose tissue lipolysis, a process stimulated by growth hormone and epinephrine. (In contrast, insulin favors fatty acid deposition in adipose tissue. The fate of the dietary lipids is discussed in detail in the chapter on arteriosclerosis.)

In addition, the liver synthesizes fatty acid from acetyl-CoA, a process stimulated by insulin. The anabolic process competes with a catabolic breakdown of fatty acid (fatty acid oxidation), which takes place in mitochondria.

In the liver, the free fatty acids are esterified in the presence of glycerophosphate, which is mainly derived from glycolysis, but a small fraction may be derived from the direct phosphorylation of glycerol through the catalytic action of glycerokinase.

The newly synthesized triglycerides (there is no evidence that the triglycerides in chylomicrons are absorbed as such in liver) are coupled to proteins synthesized by ribosomes, and the freshly made lipoprotein is secreted back into the plasma through the channels of the endoplasmic reticulum.

In the plasma, the newly formed lipoproteins constitute the very low density plasma protein pool (see Chapter 11). When hepatic triglyceride production exceeds its rate of secretion in the plasma, fatty livers develop. This can result from: (1) excess delivery of triglyceride to the liver, which is unlikely because obesity is not associated with fatty liver; (2) retarded fatty acid oxidation (alcohol?); or (3) a block in lipoprotein synthesis as a result of a block in protein synthesis (CCl_4) or a block in the coupling of the lipid and protein moieties (orotic acid). Whether other mechanisms of liver steatosis exist is not certain.

Steatosis in Tissues Other Than Liver

As mentioned previously, steatosis does not occur in liver only, but appears in kidney, muscle, heart, and glial cells. When fat appears in organs other than liver, the disturbance is usually referred to as fatty degeneration, implying that the fat results from the breakdown of intracellular structures. This may be the case in the wallerian degeneration of nerves, but it is by no means certain that "degeneration" is the cause of fat deposition in kidney and heart.

When lipid is deposited in the kidney, it is usually found in the convoluted tubules. If the fat deposition is severe, the organ softens, swells, and becomes yellowish. Fatty degeneration of the heart is usually associated with a debilitating disease, especially anemia and generalized infection. The degeneration is of two types: in the first, the organ is patchy or streaky (tigroid), and yellow patches or streaks are found in the papillary muscle or in the myocardial fiber underlying the endothelium; in the second, the lipid distribution is diffuse and the heart is yellowish and flabby.

Fatty metamorphosis has also been observed in metabolically active immature glial cells of premature infants apparently as a result of hypoxia and acidosis.

Peroxidation of Lung Lipids. Lipid peroxidation may be of considerable importance to human health also when it occurs in lung lipids after exposure to nitrogen dioxide [64]. The exhaust products of private or public transport or industrial complexes contain a number of chemicals that interact with light to produce smog. Nitrogen dioxide is one of the many toxicants in smog. The toxic effect of nitrogen dioxide seems to be restricted to the lung where the gas induces typical ultrastructural changes in alveolar cells.

One part per million of NO_2 induces detectable signs of peroxidation in the lung of exposed rat. Peroxidation is measured by reading absorption spectra. The spectra are characteristic of -diene conjugation and typical for peroxidized polyenoic fatty acids. However, the peroxidative changes appear only 24–48 hours after exposure to the toxin. Peroxidation could then be the consequence of necrosis. Therefore, control studies with other lung toxicants are needed.

Liver Injuries in Humans

To illustrate the significance of steatosis in human disease and its relationship to cellular necrosis, various forms of liver injuries, such as alcoholism and acute hepatitis, as they occur in humans will be described.

Effects of Alcohol and Alcoholism

Only individuals with a perverted sense of taste would deliberately sacrifice the health of their hepatic cells to the regular consumption of CCl_4. For years one could hardly escape the occasional inhalation of chloroform or ether for the purpose of anesthesia, but even those hepatotoxins are now seldom used. Most westerners, however, daily assault their liver cells by adorning their diets with complex cocktail mixtures, varied wines with rich bouquets, tasteful thirst-quenching beers, and a myriad of liquors with flavors ranging from that the rose to turpentine. The concentration of alcohol varies considerably depending upon the type of beverage: it is around 100–180 proof in some spirits, and 40–60 proof in wines and beers. All these delicacies have one ingredient in common—ethyl alcohol. The ethyl alcohol contains in solution various proportions of other substances: acetaldehyde, ethyl formate, ethyl acetate, methanol, propanol, butanol, amyl alcohol. These additives are usually referred to as congeners. The proportion of congeners may vary from 0.265 mg/100 ml in vodka to 245.5 mg/100 ml in bourbon. In addition to these volatile components, the alcoholic beverage contains substances with high boiling temperatures, such as resins and caramels. The presence of congeners in alcoholic beverages may modulate the toxic effects of ethyl alcohol, but for the sake of clarity, the present discussion shall be restricted to the effect of ethyl alcohol.

Alcohol Metabolism

Alcohol is absorbed in the intestine and metabolized in the liver. Although in muscles pyruvate is reduced to lactic acid to conclude glycolysis, in other tissues pyruvate may be altered in various ways. For example, in yeast it is decarboxylated by the pyruvate decarboxylase to yield acetaldehyde and CO_2, and glycolysis is concluded by reduction of acetaldehyde to ethanol by alcohol dehydrogenase.

Alcohol dehydrogenase is a Zn-containing enzyme found in many forms of life, ranging from yeast to mammalian livers [65–67]. The enzyme has been purified and crystallized from liver.

Bäcklin [68] has shown that in the reversible reaction of alcohol dehydrogenase the equilibrium constant is:

$$\frac{[\text{NADH}]\ \text{acetaldehyde}\ (\text{H}^+)}{[\text{NAD}^+]\ \text{alcohol}} = 0.90 \times 10^{-11}.$$

Alcohol dehydrogenase has a broad substrate specificity and acts on a great variety of primary and secondary alcohols, aldehydes, and ketones. The exact role of the enzyme in liver metabolism remains unknown. The importance of this point will become clearer later.

Horse liver alcohol dehydrogenase was crystallized in 1948. The enzyme is composed of 374 amino acids. The amino acid sequences of the rat and yeast enzymes have been established [134], but the functional unit in the enzyme has not been conclusively identified.

The enzyme is a dimeric molecule, and the three-dimensional structures of the dimer and the monomer have been reconstructed from X-ray crystallographic studies. The monomer is itself composed of two parts: one forming the amino terminal third, composed of 120 amino acids and containing the coenzyme; the other forming the carboxy terminal segment and containing the Zn atoms. The monomeric polypeptide is folded in a complex fashion and as a result, one Zn molecule is brought close to the active site in proximity to the nicotinamide [135].

In presence of NAD acetaldehyde dehydrogenase, acetaldehyde is rapidly converted to acetate which can be utilized for fatty acid synthesis, broken down to CO_2 or enter the 2 carbon pool. In the sequence of the reaction involving alcohol dehydrogenase and acetaldehyde dehydrogenase, the conversion of ethanol to acetaldehyde is rate limiting. In fact, under normal conditions, the alcohol dehydrogenase functions as an acetaldehyde reductase converting acetaldehyde derived from pyruvate into ethanol, which is believed to be reoxidized to acetaldehyde by catalase. Thus the equilibrium of the alcohol dehydrogenase reaction lies far to the left and oxidation of ethanol proceeds only because acetaldehyde is continuously destroyed, as a result there is little alcohol excreted in the urine and the amount of acetaldehyde in the blood is very low unless acetaldehyde oxidation is blocked by disulfiram, also called Antabuse. Acetaldehyde is in part oxidized by the liver, but peripheral tissues play an important role in oxidation. Little is known of the organ distribution and the level of activities of acetaldehyde in the various tissues.

The levels of acetaldehyde have been measured in the blood of both alcoholic and nonalcoholic subjects. In either case the level increased with the amount of alcohol ingested until high levels of alcohol were administered. This suggests that with a high concentration of alcohol, the oxidation of acetaldehyde is accelerated either by existing extrahepatic mechanisms or by unknown metabolic pathways. The level of acetaldehyde was found to be higher in alcoholic than in nonalcoholic subjects, suggesting that the catabolism of acetaldehyde is impaired in alcoholics possibly as a result of mitochondrial damage [136].

At least three aldehyde dehydrogenases have been found in rat liver; two are unspecific and reduce acetaldehyde among other substrates. One is a specific betaine aldehyde dehydrogenase. The enzymes that reduce acetaldehyde are found one exclusively with the mitochondrial matrix, the other in the mitochondrial outer membrane, the endoplasmic reticulum and the cytosol. The betaine aldehyde dehydrogenase is a cytosol enzyme. The inner mitochondrial dehydrogenase has the greatest affinity for acetaldehyde suggesting that most of the acetaldehyde produced in the oxidation of alcohol is oxidized in mitochondria.

Although acetaldehyde dehydrogenase is found in both mitochondria (80%) and cytosol, the two enzymes are different; the K_m for acetaldehyde of the mitochondrial enzyme is much lower than that of the cytosol enzyme. Consequently, most of the acetaldehyde is oxidized in mitochondria utilizing intramitochondrial reducing equivalents and diminishing the need for transfer of NADH from cytosol to mitochondria for total oxidation of ethanol [137–138].

When ^{14}C-labeled alcohol is injected in rats maintained in a closed chamber, CO_2 is formed. The level of alcohol in blood and the expiration of $^{14}CO_2$ in the air pumped through the chamber at a constant speed can readily be measured. Blood alcohol levels drop as the $^{14}CO_2$ increases. Therefore, injected alcohol undoubtedly seems to be oxidized by alcohol dehydrogenase.

Nevertheless, a number of observations seem to suggest that in spite of the increased activity of alcohol dehydrogenase in alcoholics, there is no relationship between the activity of that enzyme and the rate of alcohol consumption. For example, the activity of alcohol dehydrogenase in various species does not account for the differences in tolerance to alcohol. The administration of [^{14}C]ethanol to alcoholic and nonalcoholic individuals reveals that the rate of $^{14}CO_2$ output is the same in both groups of individuals when amounts of alcohol leading to a plasma concentration of 50–60 mg/100 ml are administered. However, regular consumers undoubtedly can drink more and more alcohol without serious alteration of their behavior. Alcoholics that drink up to 900 ml of alcoholic beverages a day for several weeks can function well in perceptual motor tasks.

Since this tolerance cannot be related to increased alcohol metabolism, one would be inclined to accept the suggestion of Westerfield and Schulman that tolerance to alcohol is a function of central nervous system adaptation, rather than of a modification in ability to metabolize alcohol in liver.

Some strains of mice will voluntarily select ethanol rather than water. Although there seems to be no correlation between the genetic control of the levels of alcohol dehydrogenase and the resistance of these mice to alcohol, the strains that prefer alcohol seem to be those that are most resistant to alcohol injections in sleeping-time studies. But even if neurological adaptations are partially responsible for increased tolerance to alcohol, we shall see that other enzymic adaptations play a role as well.

Catalase and Alcohol Oxidation

Although most ingested alcohol is postulated to be oxidized through the alcohol dehydrogenase-acetaldehyde dehydrogenase pathway, catalase may also play a role.

Catalase is a large enzyme made of four identical subunits (mol wt 60,000), each containing one heme molecule. The entire molecule is assembled in three stages: formation of apoprotein, subunit and tetramer. The life spans of the two intermediates and the final product are very different. The respective estimated turnovers are 49, 17 and 3100 minutes. The enzyme is synthesized in the endoplasmic reticulum and most of it is channeled to peroxisomes (see Chapter 2).

Peroxisomes contain two types of enzymes: oxidases and catalases. The oxidases include L-α-hydroxyacid oxidase which attacks lactate and glycolate among other hydroxyacids, D-amino oxidase and uricase. In the presence of the appropriate substrate, the oxidase generates H_2O_2 which is converted to H_2O by catalase [139].

Catalase serves as a second pathway for alcohol oxidation. The H_2O_2 produced by the cell oxidases binds to catalase and causes a rearrangement of the molecular conformation around the heme. As a result, the H_2O_2 is reduced and the iron oxidized. To reduce H_2O_2 to H_2O an oxidant is needed, ethanol is the best known oxidant for H_2O_2 [140].

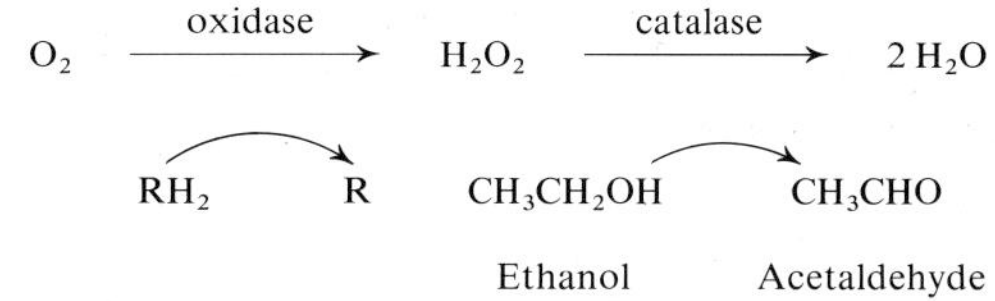

The microsomal mixed-function oxidases (see Chapter 16) were also suspected to oxidize ethanol. However, microsomal preparations devoid of catalase could not oxidize ethanol and therefore the participation of microsomes in ethanol oxidation probably results from their catalase content [141].

Alcohol and Diet

Alcohol can serve as a food, and indeed constitutes one of the major foodstuffs in the diet of many westerners. Hartroft [69, 70] and his associates estimate that alcohol provides 10% of the caloric intake in the average adult diet (teetotalers excluded). In contrast to the chronic alcoholic, the average adult drinker consumes no alcohol at breakfast. At lunch, he may drink two martinis, but no more, to conform to social convention. Two drinks are commonly taken during the cocktail hour, and wine or beer is usually drunk with dinner. During the evening, the average adult drinker usually has one or two more drinks.

The average drinker's life would be undisturbed if he didn't gain weight, but he does. When he consults his doctor about this matter, his physician may quote some of Hartroft's computations. To his surprise, the patient may then discover that the alcoholic beverages have provided 75% of his diet, or 1,800 calories. (One shot of whiskey provides 240 calories—10% of the average caloric intake.) If a drinker who weighs 70 kg wants to maintain his weight, he must restrict additional caloric intake to 600 calories, and if the diet is to be balanced (1 g of protein per kg of body weight), 280 calories must be provided by proteins. A normal caloric diet of 2,400 calories should consist of 12% protein, 40% fat, and 48% carbohydrate. Consequently, for a drinker to maintain his weight, he must reduce his caloric intake accordingly, and this usually leads to an unbalanced diet. Protein requirements can be satisfied by restricting the diet to a food in which 50% of the caloric value is provided by proteins. This is almost impossible, unless the diet consists of shellfish and skim milk only.

An obvious and important problem is whether the injuries observed in the liver of alcoholics are caused by dietary imbalances or by a direct effect of alcohol. Studies by Truitt and associates [71, 72] and Rubin, Lieber, and De Carli [73] suggest that in normal individuals alcohol toxicity is independent of the diet. When nonalcoholic volunteers received an isocaloric substitution of alcohol for carbohydrates with a high-protein diet, the high protein level did not prevent the development of fatty liver. The amount of alcohol used in these experiments replaced 5% of the caloric intake, and the level of alcohol in the blood of the volunteers was below the accepted legal limits for intoxication.

Acute Behavioral Effects

The acute effects of alcohol include behavioral alteration and fatty liver. The behavioral changes include impairment of intellectual activity and modification of emotional behavior with relaxation, euphoria, and finally alcoholic stupor and coma.

The behavioral changes are associated with the elimination of large amounts of urine and alterations in the serum electrolyte pattern that suggest a disturbance of water and electrolyte metabolism. Whether these events are related, and whether the finding that alcohol inhibits membrane transport and ATPase are relevant to these changes in electrolyte distribution are not certain [74–76].

Some of the pharmacological effects of alcohol are believed to result from its ability to release catecholamines from their storage sites. The injection of ethanol in human subjects is followed by a significant increase in urinary tryptamine. This increase is not explainable by increased biogenesis, nor can the increase be interrupted by inhibiting the monamine oxidase induced by alcohol. Whether catecholamine release affects behavior remains to be established.

Many of the deleterious effects of alcohol may not be due to ethanol *per se,* but to the metabolic product—acetaldehyde [72]. Acetaldehyde is seldom incriminated because only small amounts of the metabolite are formed at one time. However, considering that acetaldehyde exhibits a pharmacological effect similar to and 100 times greater on a weight basis than alcohol, the toxic potential of acetaldehyde becomes more obvious. Acetaldehyde is a potent hypnotic; it affects circulation, respiration, and the metabolism of many tissues, and can produce nausea, vomiting, and sweating. Metabolically, acetaldehyde interferes with the usage of pyruvate in the Krebs cycle and thereby reduces the level of mitochondrial oxidative phosphorylation. However, it seems unlikely that acetaldehyde duplicates the effects of alcohol. Indeed the inebriating effect appears immediately after alcohol ingestion, and then little acetaldehyde is formed. The effects of acetaldehyde are more likely to be manifested in chronic alcoholism or in the hangover effect that follows alcohol absorption.

Metabolic Alterations Caused by Ethanol

Alcohol is oxidized in the cytosol, acetaldehyde in the mitochondria. Both types of oxidation result in the formation of reducing equivalents. Thus, the ingestion of ethanol disturbs the regulation of the reducing power and the NADH/NAD ratios are increased in both compartments. The high levels of NADH in the cytosol and mitochondria are believed to be responsible for the metabolic effects of ethanol in liver: a shift in pyruvate lactate ratios, inhibition of the Krebs cycle, inhibition of gluconeogenesis, inhibition of fatty acid synthesis from carbohydrates, interference with the urea cycle.

The transfer of NADPH from mitochondria to cytosol is believed to contribute to the maintenance of a high reduction potential in the cytosol, the transfer takes place via an isocitrate transhydrogenase cycle.

The transhydrogenase catalyzes the reversible transfer of hydrogen between NAD and NADP (see Chapter 1).

$$\text{NADH} + \text{NADP} \rightleftharpoons \text{NAD} + \text{NADPH}$$

The transhydrogenase reaction is needed to maintain a concentration of NADPH sufficient to activate the isocitrate dehydrogenase. Isocitrate moves from mitochondria to cytosol where it is again oxidized generating more NADPH.

NADP linked isocitric dehydrogenases are found both in mitochondria and cytosol.

$$\text{Isocitrate} \underset{\text{NADP} \frown \text{NADPH}}{\overset{\text{Dehydrogenase}}{\rightleftharpoons}} \alpha\text{-oxoglutarate} + CO_2$$

Thus in presence of high levels of NADPH the NADP linked isocitric dehydrogenase will catalyze the reductive carboxylation of α-oxoglutarate to isocitrate.

In absence of an artificial electron transport acceptor for NADH, the excess cytosol NADH must enter mitochondria for oxidation through the electron transport chain. However, mitochondria are impermeable to NADH and therefore, several substrate shuttles are responsible for the transfer of the reducing equivalents from cytosol to mitochondria. They include: the α-glycerophosphate, the malate citrate, the malate aspartate and the fatty acid shuttles.

In the presence of α-glycerophosphate dehydrogenase the cytosol NADH can be oxidized.

$$\text{Dihydroxyacetone phosphate} \xrightarrow[\text{NADH} \frown \text{NAD}]{} \alpha\text{-glycerophosphate}$$

The glycerophosphate enters the mitochondria where it is oxidized in presence of FADH to yield dihydroxyacetone phosphate, which in the presence of FADH enters the respiratory chain.

	MITOCHONDRIA	CYTOSOL
Respiratory chain ←	dehydroxyacetone PO_4	dehydroxyacetone PO_4
FAD ← FADH	↑ FADH / FAD	↓ NADH / NAD
	α-glycerophosphate	← α-glycerophosphate

NADH generated in the cytosol by glycolysis or alcohol oxidation can also be transferred to mitochondria through the citrate-malate shuttle.

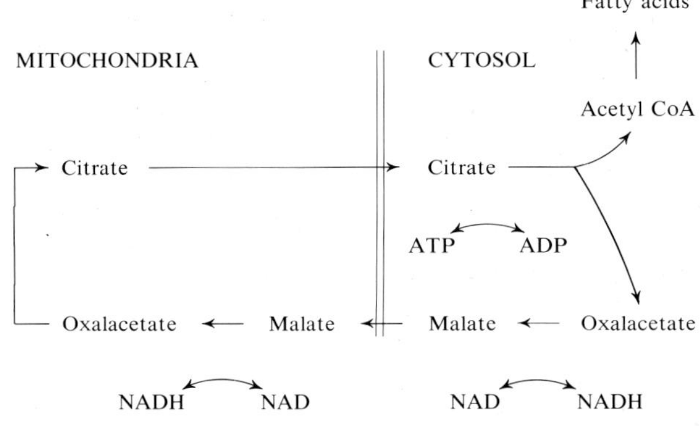

Citrate and malate can cross the mitochondrial barriers. Thus citrate generated in the Krebs cycle leaves the mitochondria for the cytosol where ATP citrate lyase cleaves citrate to acetyl CoA and oxalacetate. Malate dehydrogenase reduces oxalacetate to malate which is returned to the mitochondria where it is reconverted to oxalacetate.

Fatty acids may reduce the redox equivalent in the cytosol in the following fashion. The elongation of the fatty acid in the cytosol requires NADH and acetyl CoA. The extended fatty acid may be oxidized in mitochondria regenerating NADH and $FADH_2$ which may be further oxidized in the respiratory chain.

CYTOSOL | MITOCHONDRIA

Respiratory Chain

$R{-}\overset{O}{\overset{\|}{C}}{-}SCoA \longleftarrow R{-}\overset{O}{\overset{\|}{C}}{-}S{-}CoA$

ADH / AD

$CH_3\overset{O}{\overset{\|}{C}}{-}S{-}CoA \longleftarrow CH_3\overset{O}{\overset{\|}{C}}{-}SCoA$

NAD ← NADH

FAD ← FADH

$R{-}CH_2{-}CH_2{-}\overset{O}{\overset{\|}{C}}{-}S{-}CoA \quad RCH_2CH_2{-}\overset{O}{\overset{\|}{C}}{-}S{-}CoA$

Normally glucose is converted to pyruvate which enters the Krebs cycle where it will yield acetyl CoA. After ingestion of ethanol there is excess NADH and NADPH in the cytosol and as a result pyruvate instead of entering the Krebs cycle is reduced to lactate.

Similarly, ethanol probably inhibits gluconeogenesis by decreasing the substrate concentration for pyruvate carboxylase.

An extended concept of the citrate-malate is the malate-aspartate shuttle.

In the malate-aspartate shuttle, the cytosol NADH is oxidized in presence of oxalacetate, glutamate and malic dehydrogenase to yield malate which moves into the mitochondria where it is oxidized to oxalacetate. Oxalacetate can either enter the respiratory chain in presence of NADH or be converted to α-ketoglutarate in presence of glutamic oxalacetic transaminase. α-Ketoglutarate is transferred to the cytosol where it is deaminated to generate glutamate.

In mitochondria, glutamate is converted to aspartate in the following reaction:

$$\text{Glutamate} + 1\text{–}{}^{1}/_{2}\,O_2 \rightarrow \text{aspartate} + CO_2 + H_2O$$

The aspartate moves from mitochondria to cytosol where it is deaminated to regenerate oxalacetate.

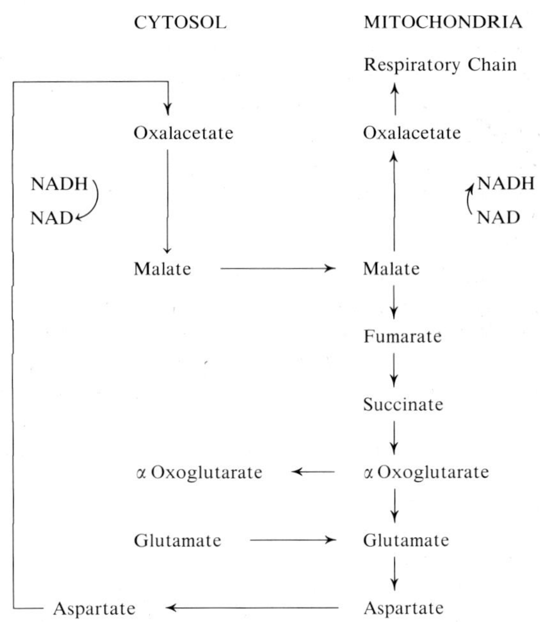

In rat, chronic alcohol intoxication results in increased rate of oxidation of alcohol, but decreased activity of aldehyde dehydrogenase. A possible mechanism for explaining the increased oxidation of ethanol after prolonged exposure is that the reducing equivalent in mitochondria is increased through one or several of the shuttle pathways, thus generating more NAD in the cytosol.

Rubin and Cederbaum [145] studied several mitochondrial properties in rats chronically intoxicated with alcohol, such as: the activity of succinic dehydrogenase and cytochrome oxidase, the permeability to NADH and to the various substrates of the shuttle pathways.

In chronic alcohol intoxication, there is a decrease in cytochrome oxidase, succinic dehydrogenase and α-glycerophosphate dehydrogenase with a decreased oxidation of NAD dependent substrates and inhibition of calcium uptake by mitochondria. Acetaldehyde was found to inhibit activity of the malate aspartate, the α-glycerophosphate and the fatty acid shuttle, oxidative phosphorylation and energy dependent calcium uptake in mitochondria. These observations suggest that if the increased oxidation of alcohol cannot be explained by activation of the shuttle, the accumulation of acetaldehyde might play a role in eliciting mitochondrial damage.

Chronic alcoholic intoxication inhibits the Krebs cycle in cell suspensions, liver slices and perfused livers. Both the mechanism and the target of the inhibition are under debate. It is generally assumed that the inhibition is caused by the increased reducing equivalents in both cytosol and mitochondria. Some believe that the target is citrate synthetase; others, α-ketoglutarate dehydrogenase [142–143].

When isolated liver is perfused and supplied with ammonia and ornithine, it produces urea. To provide the energy needed to synthesize carbamyl phosphate and argininosuccinate, ureagenesis requires oxygen. Inasmuch as alcohol increases the levels of NADH in mitochondria, one would expect alcohol intake to stimulate urea synthesis and vice versa. Urea synthesis should increase alcohol oxidation. In fact, these two pathways mutually inhibit each other Krebs *et al.* have investigated the effect of ethanol on the urea cycle. Alanine is one amino acid most readily metabolized by the liver, mainly through transamination with oxoglutarate. Later the carbon skeleton appears in glucose and lactate while the amino nitrogen appears in urea and ammonia.

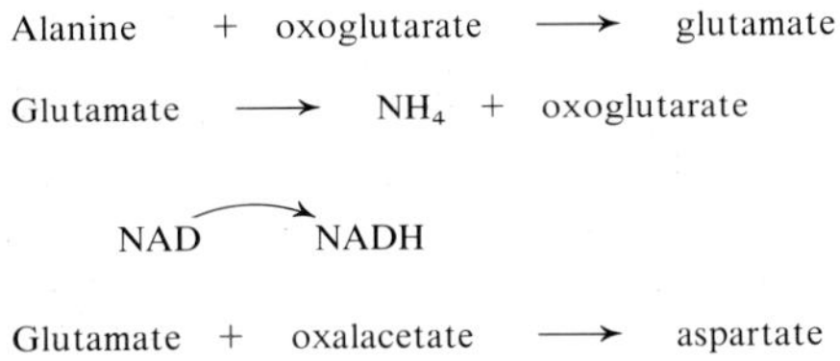

In absence of ornithine most of the nitrogen of alanine appears in the form of ammonia, but in presence of ornithine the nitrogen is used to form urea; thus, the availability of ornithine is one of the rate limiting steps of the urea cycle.

When ethanol is added to rat liver perfused with alanine, or with lactic acid and ammonia, glutamate and aspartate (two intermediates in the urea cycle) accumulate. Yet, except in severe liver disease, the activity of the enzymes of the urea cycle are capable of disposing of large excesses of ammonia.

Therefore, the rate limiting step in urea formation is not enzyme activity, but substrate availability.

It is not certain how alcohol distorts the regulation of the urea cycle. However, stoichiometric amounts of carbamyl phosphate and aspartate must be formed for the performance of the urea cycle. This balanced production of substrates is disturbed by alcohol, which is believed to divert some of the nitrogen normally used to make carbamyl phosphate to the synthesis of aspartate.

Since the substrate accumulation does not take place after the addition to the perfusate of pyrazole (a specific inhibitor of alcohol dehydrogenase), the interference of ethanol with the performance of the urea cycle has been linked with the oxidation of ethanol and the increase in reducing equivalents.

Acute Effects on Liver

Acute ethanol intoxication induces fatty liver. The exact mechanism of the steatosis is not clear. On the basis of studies on perfused liver several mechanisms have been proposed: enhanced lipolysis with esterification of the fatty acid in liver, reduced fatty acid oxidation, increased fatty acid synthesis in liver, interference with lipoprotein synthesis or secretions.

Studies on fatty acid synthesis in rat livers perfused with alcohol and ^{14}C uniformly labeled glucose and tritiated water indicate that the total rate of fatty acid synthesis is not affected by ethanol, yet most newly made fatty acids are derived from ethanol rather than glucose [149]. We have seen that alcohol inhibits fatty acid oxidation. The accumulation of fatty acids could explain that of triglycerides in liver.

Di Luzio [77] has accumulated evidence suggesting that a block in triglyceride oxidation might contribute to the steatosis in acute ethanol intoxication. On the basis of isotopic studies, Di Luzio's group has claimed that impaired oxidation can account for all the fat accumulated in liver. They found that the intoxicated liver presents a normal removal rate of fatty acid and normal uptake. The plasma triglyceride concentration is normal, and the liver responds normally to Triton injection. Di Luzio believes that the steatotic effects of acute ethanol intoxication can be prevented by the administration of antioxidants. He concludes that even though the metabolic alterations in liver metabolism are different after CCl_4 and ethanol intoxication, the primary injury in both is peroxidation.

To support of these views, Di Luzio's group demonstrated peroxide formation by spectrophotometric and iodometric analyses. However, Recknagel has challenged these findings.

Kiessling and Tobe [78] have established that rats consuming alcohol present biochemical alterations of their liver mitochondria. When a 15% alcohol solution is substituted for the drinking water for several months, the ability of liver mitochondria to oxidize glutamate and pyruvate is reduced in males and females. In contrast, the ability to oxidize succinate is reduced only in females.

Electron Microscopic Alterations in Alcoholism

Several groups of investigators have described the electron microscopic alterations found in experimental alcoholism. They include mitochondrial disfiguration, distortion of the endoplasmic reticulum, and the development of focal cytoplasmic degradation. However, changes observed in humans are often difficult to interpret because they are frequently blurred by dietary deficiencies, intake of other toxins, and superinfection, such as hepatitis [79, 80].

When rats are given a diet in which normal foods have been replaced calorie-for-calorie by alcohol, hepatic steatosis develops within hours. Within a week, the channels of the endoplasmic reticulum are distended and become vesicular, and the membrane-bound ribosomes decrease. Within 10 days, the mitochondria are considerably enlarged (15 μ in diameter), and the pattern of the cristae mitochondriales becomes severely distorted. Similar findings were made in human volunteers submitted to alcohol intake and liver biopsy.

Although there is no doubt that alcohol ultimately causes damage to mitochondria, the mechanism by which the mitochondrial alterations take place has not been clarified. Gordon has pointed out that under normal conditions 85% of the reducing equivalent for the respiratory chain is produced by oxidation of lipids. He further postulates that in the case of excessive ethanol intake, most of the reducing equivalents (NADH and NADPH) are produced by the reduction of alcohol to acetaldehyde and acetaldehyde to acetate in the two hydrogenase sequences already described. This switch in generation of reducing equivalent from lipids to ethanol increases the level of acyl CoA derivatives of fatty acids. Long chain acyl CoA derivatives of fatty acids inhibit the adenine nucleotide translocase and thereby prevent the penetration of ADP across the inner membrane of the mitochondria. Consequently there is a decreased flux of substrate of the tricarboxylic acid cycle, a shift in the oxidation reduction stage of the mitochondria to the more reduced level and a decreased rate of ADP synthesis. The chronic decrease in ATP synthesis could in turn be linked to other forms of damage in the hepatic cell. In view of the difficulties encountered in studying mitochondrial permeability and in establishing the role of ATP in cellular damage, appealing as it may be, the theory is very likely to be an oversimplification of the mechanism of mitochondrial and cellular injury in chronic alcoholism [150].

Ethanol, like many other liver toxins, seems to stimulate the development of the smooth endoplasmic reticulum. When rats are fed ethanol for 2 weeks along with regular or choline-deficient diets, lipids accumulate in the hepatic cells and the smooth endoplasmic reticulum proliferates. The increase in the smooth endoplasmic reticulum is associated with an increase in activities of hydroxylase, nitro reductase, and other drug-metabolizing enzymes [81].

Such observations are of practical importance because it is well known that alcoholics are frequently more resistant to drugs than other individuals. Alcohol appears to damage the endoplasmic reticulum in some way, stimulate the production of smooth endoplasmic reticulum, and activate some of the metabolizing enzymes, as well as increase the biosynthesis of cholesterol and neutral lipids.

Chronic Effects on Liver

Characteristic histologic alterations are frequently associated with alcoholism. The liver, muscle, and nerves are among the tissues most frequently affected. Steatosis of the liver cell is almost a constant finding in acute and chronic alcoholism. In chronic alcoholism, steatosis is associated with degeneration and necrosis of the hepatic cells, as well as regeneration of hepatocytes and fibrosis.

We have seen already that alcohol induces mitochondrial changes marked essentially by considerable enlargement. Pathologists have long known that livers of chronic alcoholics and of choline-deficient rats contain large eosinophilic hyalin masses called Mallory bodies (see Fig. 10-11). Correlated light and electron microscopic studies have suggested to some that the Mallory bodies are enlarged, distorted, and sometimes coalescent mitochondria. In reality, the origin of Mallory bodies is not known.

The morphological changes that take place in mitochondria of patients with chronic alcoholism are linked to functional alterations that include: interference with the biogenesis of the mitochondrial membrane, reduction in the concentration of certain components of the electron transport chain, decreased levels of mitochondrial protein synthesis, and decreased rates of respiration and fatty acid oxidation [82].

Although pathologists argue about the extensiveness of the necrotic process in liver of chronic alcoholics, there seems to be no question that some degree of necrosis takes place. Although the degree of hepatic regeneration in chronic alcoholics has not been quantitatively evaluated, the presence of mitosis, binucleate cells, and large nuclei indicates hepatocyte regeneration. Repeated insult to the liver cell, which induces steatosis, undoubtedly culminates in fibrosis. Although the names of many famous schools of pathology are associated with such observations, not all pathologists agree on the mode of development of fibrosis. Hartroft and his collaborators have proposed a form of pathogenesis in which the "fatty cyst" constitutes the pivot between fatty deposition and fibrosis. The fatty cyst is formed by the coalescence of lipid-laden hepatocytes. The cyst grows by adding more hepatocytes until it explodes. Then the lipids are released into the surrounding tissue and disappear, and the fibrous framework, which supported all the hepatocytes that formed the cysts, falls together in the process of condensation fibrosis.

According to Hartroft, this mechanism could explain most of the fibrosis that appears in the fatty liver except, of course, the formation of new collagen and reticulum fibers in regenerating nodules. However, other investigators demonstrated, with both light and electron microscopy, the apposition of fibrils around hepatocytes without cell loss. Vascular occlusion and endothelial proliferation have been found to participate in the genesis of fibrosis of chronic alcoholics.

The combination of necrosis, regeneration, and fibrosis distorts the liver's architecture and possibly its vascularization, and the new histological pattern is that of cirrhosis. The distribution and relative intensity of the elementary lesions, fibrosis, regeneration, and necrosis vary with the degree of alcoholism, the diet, and previous or simultaneous insults to the liver with toxins or viruses (hepatitis). Consequently, no

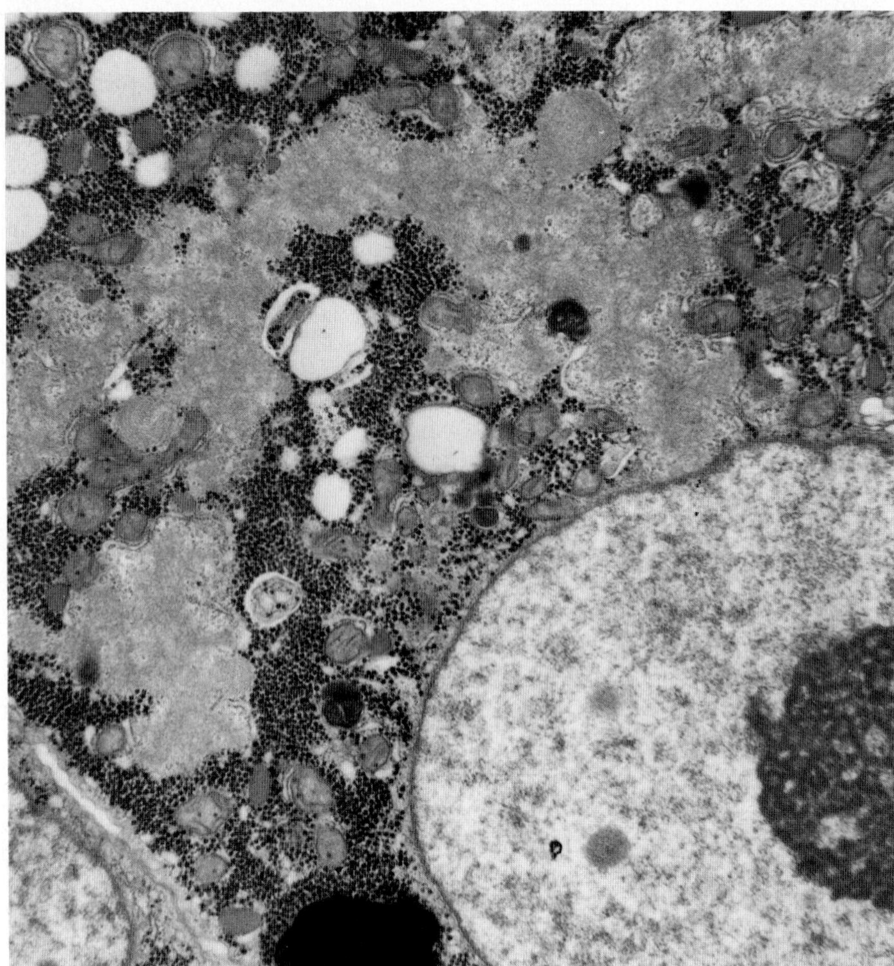

Fig. 10-11. A Mallory body in a hepatocyte in a case of primary biliary cirrhosis. The abnormal protein appears as a filamentous material of medium electron density occupying confluent areas of cytoplasm devoid of organelles (×9,700; from Zamboni)

histological picture is ubiquitous and consistent for alcoholic cirrhosis. Neither is a unique macroscopic pattern associated with alcoholic cirrhosis. Yet, typically, the liver appears grossly and microscopically in the form described as Laennec's, or portal, cirrhosis.

Gross Findings

The normal liver has a smooth surface covered by a thin capsule; the liver is cut easily, and the cut surface is smooth and regular. The surface of a cirrhotic liver is irregular and knobnailed with a thickened capsule; the liver is more difficult to cut, because of fibrous trabeculae. The cut surface is much harder than normal, and trabeculae of fibrous tissue of various thicknesses crisscross the surface of the liver in a lacework pattern; in the opening of the pattern, foci of hepatic cells, sometimes regenerating, are entrapped.

For a detailed description of the anatomopathological appearance of liver cirrhosis, consult such authorities as Gall, Baggentoss, and Popper. Suffice it to point out that alcoholism may be associated with two types of cirrhosis: portal and postnecrotic. In postnecrotic cirrhosis, the liver is most distorted; it is coarsely nodular, with a nodule appearing approximately every 30 mm. The diagnostic feature of postnecrotic cirrhosis is said to be the preservation of small areas of liver with normal anatomical relationships. Thus, normal portal tracts are found near normal hepatic vein radicals in the midst of the architectural distortion caused by cirrhosis.

Although the gross anatomical appearance may be less distorted in Laennec's cirrhosis (see Figs. 10-12 and 10-13), the overall histological architecture seems to be more profoundly disturbed. Granules are smaller and more regular (one 5 mm) than in postnecrotic cirrhosis. Microscopic examination reveals that the granules are made of regenerating hepatic cells, some fat laden, surrounded by fibrous tissue; central arteries or veins are completely lost or seldom seen.

In addition to liver disease, numerous other pathological conditions may be associated with alcoholism. There is a high incidence of pulmonary emphysema, pulmonary fibrosis, and bronchiectasis in alcoholism. Two hypotheses have been proposed to explain this high incidence of pulmonary disease. One assumes that it results from smoking, which is common among alcoholics; the other proposes that the pulmonary injury results from the direct effect of the alcohol that is

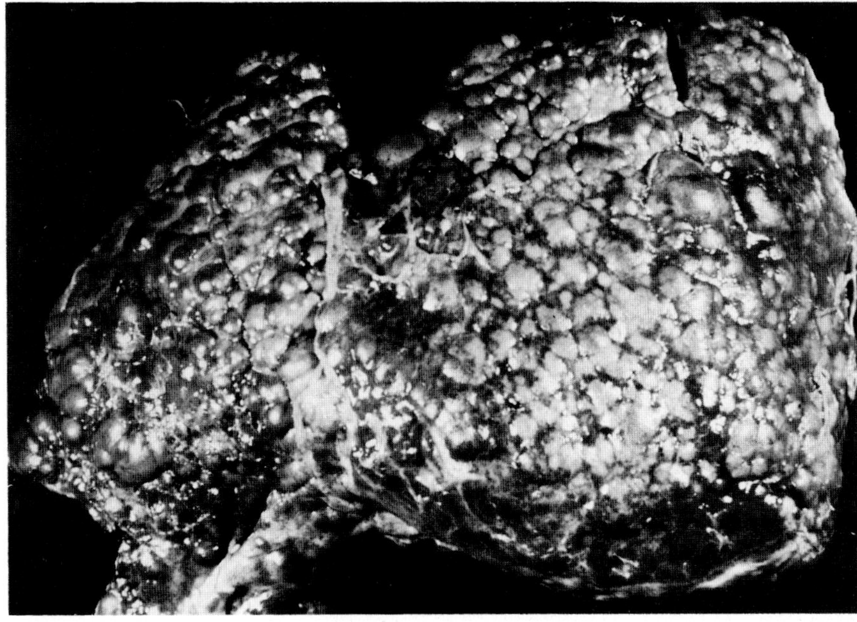

Fig. 10-12. Juvenile portal cirrhosis

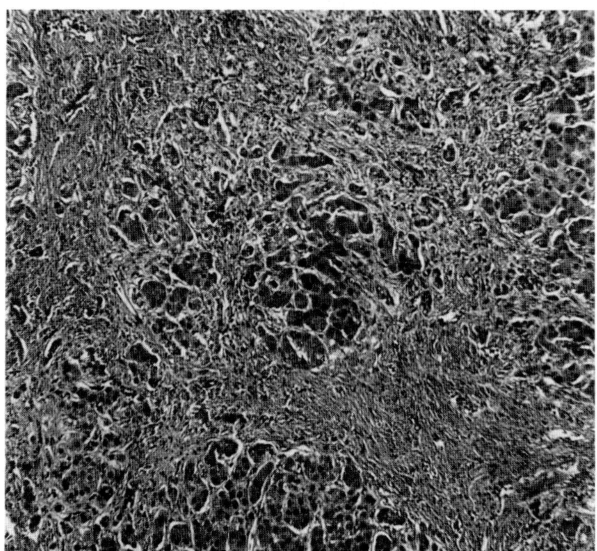

Fig. 10-13. Laennec's cirrhosis

eliminated from the lung passively during expectoration [83].

Myocardial disease has been described in alcoholics. Whether it results from the direct effect of alcohol or from the associated malnutrition and vitamin deficiencies is not clear. In any event, the disease, which in nonalcoholics is sometimes referred to as primary myocardial disease, evolves in the following manner. At first the patient has minimal symptoms and normal heart function, but he then develops concentric left ventricular hypertrophy with hypertension and all the symptoms of hypertensive heart disease. The disease evolves into left and frequently right ventricular hypertrophy and dilatation with congestive heart failure [84].

In addition to myocardial alterations, acute and chronic muscle injuries have also been described in alcoholics. Europeans have described an acute muscle syndrome in alcoholics consisting of hypoproteinemia associated with muscle edema, tenderness, and aching. Myoglobin appears in the urine, and glutamic transaminase increases in blood.

A more chronic type of alcoholic myopathy has been described in the United States. In this type of myopathy, the phosphorylase levels in muscle seem to be decreased, leading to a syndrome resembling hereditary McArdle's syndrome. The low phosphorylase is associated with glycogen deposition, poor lactic acid response, and cramps and tenderness with exercise. Myoglobin and other muscle proteins may appear in the urine. Creatine phosphokinase is increased in the serum. In contrast to the hereditary myopathy, alcoholic myopathy is reversible. The pathogenesis of acute and chronic alcoholic myopathy is not clear; both forms are associated with heavy drinking.

A great variety of central nervous system alterations have been described in association with chronic alcoholism, whether it is accompanied by liver cirrhosis or not. The most frequent alterations are thickening of the meninges with moderate cellular atrophy and demyelination in the frontal, central, and parietal cortices. Usually, these are simply forms of cellular degeneration (pigmentary degeneration without active astrocytic proliferation). However, some pathologists in the 1950's claimed that delirium tremens is associated with neuronal degeneration and astrocytic proliferation in the third layer of the frontal center.

Occasionally, alcoholism has been associated with degenerative processes in specific structures of the brain: cerebellum, corpus callosum, and cerebellopontile zone. It is never simple to decide whether the brain lesions associated with alcoholism result from damage of the brain by alcohol, or are secondary to malnutrition, arteriosclerosis, or cirrhosis of the liver. Also, nervous injuries, typical of vitamin B_1 and B_{12} deficiencies, have been found in the central nervous system of alcoholics.

Alcohol and Drugs

Physicians accustomed to treating alcoholics are often faced with paradoxical reactions of alcoholics to drugs, especially barbiturates. When he is sober, the alcoholic is resistant to the effect of drugs; inebriated, he is oversensitive. A group of New York investigators have provided at least a tentative explanation for this paradox. The chronic administration of alcohol, like that of phenobarbital, Dolantin, tolbutamide, and many other drugs, induces the proliferation of smooth endoplasmic reticulum with an increase in the microsomal fraction of the activity of drug-metabolizing enzymes. In the sober chronic alcoholic, the resistance to barbiturate therapy is explained by the increased activity in microsomal detoxifying enzyme.

In vitro, alcohol inhibits microsomal hydroxylase. This fact has been invoked to explain the higher sensitivity to barbiturates in the inebriated. The possibility that other factors, including inhibition of detoxifying enzyme by alcohol metabolites, may be responsible has not been excluded in these experiments. These drugs also stimulate *de novo* synthesis of a mitochondrial enzyme, α-aminolevulinic dehydrase, the enzyme that catalyzes the rate-limiting step in porphyrin biosynthesis. Whether this finding can be correlated with the acquired porphyria sometimes observed in cirrhosis remains to be seen.

A tragic consequence of chronic alcoholism is the outcome of pregnancy in chronic alcoholic women in whom the abuse of alcohol seems to interfere with fetal development and results either in high incidence of infantile mortality, or in abnormal physical features and mental retardation in the survival offspring [151].

Deterioration

During the regime of Mendès-France, a milk drinker, the French government campaigned against the increasing alcoholism that prevailed in that country. One of the tools of the propaganda was a poster (also used in the movie, *Le Grande Illusion*) that stated, "l'alcool tue lentement." A humor-loving Frenchman made counterposters that were placed next to the official posters stating "qui est pressé?". Although one hates to tarnish the flavor of a "bon mot", as a pathologist I cannot avoid remarking that the "humorist" was unaware of the miserable life led by chronic alcoholics.

In modern society, attitudes toward alcoholism vary according to individual philosophies. The moralists believe that it is a sin that deserves punishment. The educated and health-minded individual believes that it is a disease. F.A. Bourdeau, from the health ministry of Quebec, has given one of the most sensible definitions of alcoholism. "Alcoholism is a disease, because he who suffers from it does not know how to adapt his personality or his organism to a nonessential, habit forming chemical."

The diseased individual is one who does not successfully adapt to changes in his environment. The changes can be physical (trauma, radiation), chemical (intoxication, chemical allergies), biological (infections: virus, bacteria, parasites), or sociological. Sociological maladaptation may result from known chemical alteration in the organism (intoxication,* inborn errors of metabolism, etc.) or from unknown causes. In a disease such as alcoholism, it is difficult to determine whether the toxin is responsible for the mental attitude, or if mental inadaptation of an unknown cause is responsible for the alcoholism.

In any event, what distinguishes a normal from an excessive drinker is the fact that the excessive drinker is unable to control the intake. There is no obvious correlation between loss of control and drunkenness; one man can become drunk with one drink and be able to control further intake, and another man can be at the verge of drunkenness and not be able to control further intake, which although excessive, will not lead to shocking behavior. An important point about this aspect of alcoholism—loss of control—is that preventive therapy is ineffective unless the victim stops drinking altogether for life.

Of the people that drink alcohol, 12% are excessive drinkers and 4% are chronic alcoholics. Four stages can be distinguished in the development of alcoholism: prealcoholic, prodromic, alcoholism, and chronic alcoholism. The prealcoholic is a normal citizen who likes to go to parties to relieve the tension of daily life with the help of tasteful alcoholic drinks. During the prodromic stage, the victim likes alcohol for its effect rather than for the special taste of alcoholic drinks. At this stage, the victim drinks more than his friends, feels guilty about it the next day, and is not inclined to discuss the matter. During the frank alcoholic and the chronic alcoholic stages, the ability to control alcoholic intake further collapses and slowly develops into the abnormal pattern of behavior characteristic of chronic alcoholics.

Acute Viral Hepatitis

Epidemiology

The most typical form of acute hepatitis is usually caused by viruses, but the clinical manifestations of acute hepatitis may also be caused by toxic agents, and it is often difficult to distinguish between acute viral and toxic hepatitis.

* Intoxication is a temporary state resulting from alcohol in the blood.

Viruses are known to cause severe liver necrosis in humans. Two different types of viruses are believed to be involved: a so-called IH or A virus and an SH or B virus. The hepatitis caused by A virus is referred to as epidemic hepatitis; that caused by B is serum hepatitis. The two types of hepatitis are distinguished on the basis of differences in the epidemiology of the two types of disease rather than by differences in clinical symptoms.

Viruses causing hepatitis can survive relatively drastic environmental changes: for example, they are not killed by chlorine concentration up to 1% and resist temperatures as high as 60° C. The victims of epidemic hepatitis A usually acquire the disease through ingestion of food contaminated with the virus. The ingested virus is excreted in the feces. When foods are contaminated with human excretion and eaten raw (*e.g.*, clams, oysters), the live virus enters the host, and by the nature of its special tropism, the virus lodges itself and proliferates in the liver cells.

A typical epidemic developed in New Delhi in 1955 when sewage accidentally was allowed to flow into the water supply. Although heavy chlorination prevented the development of bacterial disease, it had no effect on the hepatitis virus, and 55,000 cases of acute hepatitis developed. This suggests a low incidence in relation to the general population of New Delhi, indicating that many were immunized as a result of previous contact with the virus.

Patients with epidemic hepatitis often have virus particles in their serum. Therefore, they can contaminate other humans with the agent of epidemic hepatitis A through a path similar to that by which serum hepatitis is transmitted. In epidemic hepatitis, virus is found in feces and blood during the incubation period and the acute phase, but rarely during convalescence. There is no evidence that viruses can be found in nasopharyngeal secretions. Neither has transfer through arthropods been shown. However, some evidence indicates that animal handlers in contact with recently imported monkeys are occasionally infected with the A virus.

Serum hepatitis (B) is transferred from the carrier to another victim through transfer of serum, sometimes in very minute amounts. Thus, the infection may follow blood transfusion, intravenous injections, tatooing, etc.

Both types of viruses (A and B) can be transferred in the serum. No clinical test distinguishes between IH and SH infection. In addition, the distinction is usually based on the duration of the incubation period, which is usually much longer with the SF infection (15–60 days in IH infection as opposed to 60–180 days in SH infection). Recently immunological tests for diagnosis of hepatitis B were developed.

Clinical Manifestation

Infectious hepatitis is by far the most common liver disease. It is benign and unique to men. In typical cases, the clinical manifestation can be divided into four successive periods. During the prodromal phase, the patient shows anorexia and malaise, nausea, vomiting, diarrhea, and often respiratory symptoms (which may predominate the symptomatology). The disease may or may not start with fever and chills. Physical examination at that time reveals a high temperature and a palpable, tender liver, but no jaundice. During the second stage, jaundice develops, increases progressively, and is associated with the emission of dark urine and light stool; pruritis may or may not exist at that stage. In the recovery period, jaundice fades away, the stool darkens, and the urine clears. This stage is followed by a period of convalescence.

In atypical cases, a form of hepatitis without icterus may develop. A fulminant type of hepatitis occasionally develops. In such cases the disease progresses rapidly and leads to death in a matter of days. The reasons for the differences in virulence and symptomatology are not known.

In acute hepatitis, the liver is usually enlarged and tender as a result of distension of the capsule of Glisson. Microscopically, changes can be observed in the hepatic and Kupffer cells. Two manifestations of injury are seen in the hepatic cells: necrosis and cytoplasmic degeneration. The cytoplasm is markedly enlarged with faint granularity. The nuclei reveal pyknosis or karyorrhexis. Similar lesions are seen in the Kupffer cells, which often contain finely granular, golden pigment (lipochrome). Cellular necrosis is associated with intense periportal histiocytic and lymphocytic infiltration. Necrosis may be followed by regeneration or fibrosis, which may ultimately culminate in a typical cirrhosis (see Fig. 10-14).

In 1968, hepatitis B (HB_sag Australia antigen) was isolated [153]. Dane [154] identified a viral particle about 410 A in diameter composed of an inner core of 270 A and an outer core which carries the hepatitis B antigen. The DNA, RNA viral core has been detected in hepatocytes of patients with viral hepatitis where it replicates. The core migrates from the nucleus where it is coated by viral proteins including the hepatitis B antigen. The coat proteins are produced in excess of core proteins; therefore the levels of B antigen are not an exact measure of the amount of effective virions. The coat forms particles with a diameter of approximately 200 A. The sera of patients with asymptomatic hepatitis contain only 200 A and none or few 410 A particles. In contrast, increased numbers of 410 A particles are found in symptomatic patients [155–156]. Recovery from type B hepatitis is usually associated with a decrease in the hepatitis B antigen. The core itself contains antigens (Hb_cAg). The antibody has been detected in two-thirds of patients with active hepatitis. The discovery of these antigens is certain to lead to much new research in the field and to a better understanding of the pathogenesis of the disease. The particles probably have an icosahedral configuration and contain a minimum of 162 protein subunits [157].

No antigenic marker is available for hepatitis A or infectious hepatitis. Antigens have been found in feces by immune electron microscopy and gel diffu-

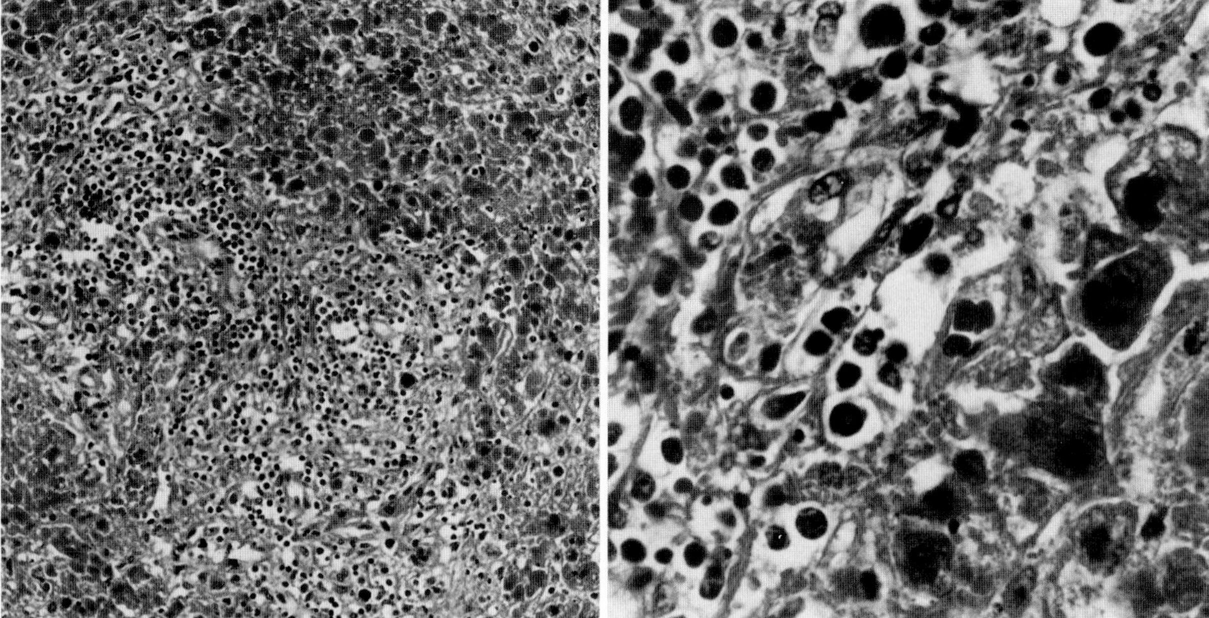

Fig. 10-14. Acute hepatitis; liver necrosis with leukopoietic infiltration

sion—the antigens are, however, not likely to be specific, because in acute and chronic liver disease titres against intestinal, bacterial, viral, and even dietary antigens are increased [158].

Drug Hepatitis

A number of drugs, such as iproniazid and trinitrotoluene, may cause symptoms and anatomical changes similar to those seen in acute viral hepatitis. The pathogenesis of drug-induced hepatitis is not known. The effect of drugs on hepatic cells should not be confused with drug-induced cholestasis, which results in biliary obstruction with jaundice. Chlorpromazine and para-aminosalicylic acid are prominent among cholestatic agents.

Chronic Hepatitis

Although chronic hepatitis is not restricted to young women and is observed even after menopause and in men, the typical patient with chronic hepatitis is a girl in her late teens or early twenties who experiences a collapse of her health. She loses her appetite, has spells of nausea, feels tired, and may become jaundiced. A physical examination reveals an enlarged and tender liver, and blood bilirubin and SGOT levels are elevated. After this stage the symptoms may disappear, worsen, or relapse after a period of relief. When the disease pursues its course, the patient develops either progressive hepatitis with little chance for recovery, or liver cirrhosis with its potential complications—jaundice, pruritus, spider angioma, and ascites.

In chronic hepatitis the hepatic cells undergo necrosis, fibrosis, and plasmo-lymphocytic infiltration. Dying hepatic cells are ballooned and may contain scattered eosinophilic bodies. In some cases, lupus erythematosus (LE) cells are seen in the patient's blood. Often the etiology of chronic hepatitis is not obvious. The various types are distinguished more on the basis of manifestations of the disease than on pathogenesis. Two pathogenetic mechanisms have been proposed, viral and autoimmune. Although each case may present symptoms that support either of these mechanisms, the true cause of the disease usually remains unknown.

Experimental Viral Hepatitis

Observations made on experimental infection of liver with viruses have helped investigators to understand the pathogenesis of viral hepatitis. The virus must first break down the natural barrier that separates the internal milieu from the environment. The path of the virus to its target (in this case the hepatocyte) is not exactly a promenade, but a constant and cunning struggle against the defense mechanisms which may act independently or synergetically. The defenses include phagocytosis by polymorphonuclears and macrophages, humoral and cellular immunity, the release of interferon, the production of fever and hypoxia. The virus must overcome each one of these defense mechanisms.

Viral infection succeeds only if the virus manages to proliferate in the phagocyte, to inhibit interferon production, secure immunosuppression or induce immunotolerance.

The number of viruses that are able to cause either mild or severe forms of hepatitis is quite large. We shall not attempt to list their properties, the reader is referred to the review article of Sabesin and Koff [159]. Hepatitis viruses include: the murine hepatitis virus (MHV), reoviruses which produce hepatitis in suckling mice; the infectious canine hepatitis virus (ICH); the rat virus hepatitis (RVH), this virus grows only in dividing cells and therefore causes hepatitis only in newborn rats or in adult liver after partial hepatectomy); the Rift Valley virus (an arbovirus which causes hepatitis in sheep, cattle and sometimes man); the ectromelia virus (a DNA virus which is a member of the poxvirus and causes hepatitis in man and animals); the yellow fever virus, which causes hepatitis in monkeys and humans; and the human type B viral hepatitis virus, which has been transferred to rhesus monkeys and chimpanzees; and the human type A virus, which has been transferred to marmosets.

The virus may circulate attached to cells, erythrocytes, lymphocytes or macrophages, or travel free. Whether it enters the blood or a body cavity, the virus is met by macrophages which patrol the body fluids and cavities for intruders. The virus may either escape phagocytosis or be phagocytized. When phagocytized, it may be destroyed or proliferate in the host. In the latter case, the macrophage which is free to circulate in blood, body cavities, or bone marrow may bring the criminal close to its choice victim. The virus also binds to innocent bystanders, the red cells and the lymphocytes, which are not always readily phagocytized by macrophage and thereby transport the virus to a more fertile terrain.

When the free virus reaches the liver, it first encounters the Kupffer cell, which may destroy the virus after phagocytosis or may become the primary site of viral infection and transfer the virus to the hepatocyte. In the latter case, the virus extrudes from the Kupffer cell into the hepatocytes. If the metabolism of the hepatocyte and the biochemical requirements of the virus are compatible (the molecular combination responsible for such compatibility is not known), the virus extruded from the Kupffer cell replicates in the hepatocyte.

In yellow fever there is an asymptomatic latent period after viral infection followed by fever, jaundice and the clinical symptoms of hepatitis. It is believed that the latent period coincides with the proliferation of virus in the Kupffer cells and in fact, the initial pathological change in experimental yellow fever is an acidophilic hyaline necrosis of those cells. Kupffer cells are unable to destroy the phagocytized Rift Valley fever virus or to support its replication, but they release the virus which then enters the hepatocyte where it causes massive cellular necrosis.

When MHV is injected intraperitoneally, the first visible histological change is enlargement of the Kupffer cells. This is followed by necrosis of the hepatic cell close to the reticuloendothelial cells. It is not certain whether the reticuloendothelial cell or the hepatocyte is the first target of the virus. Electron microscopic studies have been interpreted to indicate that MHV replication occurs in the hepatocyte which then releases the newly formed virions into the space of Disse, where they are then picked up by the Kupffer cells.

The role that the Kupffer cells play in the pathogenesis of human hepatitis is not clear; but there are a variety of alterations of the Kupffer cells. Light microscopic examination shows enlarged Kupffer cells, containing hemosiderin, lipofuscin, glycogen, and sometimes fragments of hepatocytes. The use of hepatitis B immunofluorescent antibodies has revealed the presence of virus B antigen in the Kupffer cells. Whether this is an indication that the Kupffer cell is the primary site of infection or whether it reveals an attempt of the reticuloendothelial cell to clear the dead hepatocytes is not known.

The immune system plays a central role during the regression of viral hepatitis. This has been established experimentally by transfer of lymphocytes sensitized to viral antigen, the administration of antithymocyte serum and neonatal thymectomy after infection with ectromelia virus. The administration of sensitized lymphocytes gradually rids the liver of the virus, and necrosis regresses. The administration of antithymocyte serum increases the mortality in mice infected with ectromelia virus. Similarly, neonatal thymectomy reduces the resistance of infected mice.

In human hepatitis, it would appear that cellular mediated immunity is necessary for both acute manifestation and regression of the disease. Although much of the role of cell mediated immunity in human hepatitis remains to be clarified, it is certain that the administration of corticosteroids produces chronic viremia with chronic hepatitis, and viral antigen (B type) appears in the blood.

The exact role of immunity in the pathogenesis of human hepatitis remains unknown. Antibodies to hepatitis B antigen have been found in serum of infected individuals, but it is not known whether the antibody is effective in controlling viral infection or whether it contributes to cell necrosis by the formation of immune complexes.

Although there is no evidence of hereditary or age dependent susceptibility to human hepatitis, such susceptibilities have been clearly demonstrated in certain strains of mice infected with MHV. Hereditary susceptibility to MHV infection is conditioned by the presence of a dominant gene which determines the susceptibility of the macrophages to infection.

As is often the case, immune reaction in viral hepatitis is a double-edged sword; it may either interfere with the development of the disease or may aggravate it. The immune reaction may result in the formation of circulatory antibodies or in the sensitization of thymocytes to viral antigens. When two different strains of mice, one resistant, the other sensitive to ectromelia infection, are inoculated with the virus neutralizing antibodies, cell-mediated immunity appears 24 hours earlier in the resistant mice. Similarly, the response of dogs infected with ICH depends upon the status of their immune defense. If it is highly effective, there is only mild symptomatology; if it is weak, the hepatitis is fulminant; if it is intermediate, the dog develops subacute and ultimately chronic hepatitis.

Moreover, the administration of serum containing high titers of antibodies against ICH in dogs with only minor signs of infection causes the disease to turn into a subacute or chronic hepatitis.

The mechanism by which viruses kill cells is not known. Several have been proposed: (1) depletion of substrates essential to the host's cell survival as a result of viral replication; (2) mechanical interference with normal metabolic flow by accumulating virions. (3) direct cytotoxic effect of the virus; (4) immunological reaction to the viral infected cells.

A number of experiments which include interference with viral replication or interference with protein synthesis have led to the conclusion that the elaboration of viral toxic proteins participates in killing the cell. The administration of p-fluorophenylalanine, an inhibitor of viral replication, does not prevent cellular injury caused by vaccinia virus or poliovirus in cultured cells. Inhibitors of protein synthesis, puromycin or cycloheximide, not only block virus replication, but also viral induced cell injury.

The role of lysosomes in viral infection is controversial. The possibilities fall in two major categories: the virus is entrapped in the lysosomes or it stimulates lysosomal development. The entrapped virus is stripped of its protein, facilitating the activation of the genome, or the lysosome loaded with the virus migrates toward the surface of the cell and releases the virus to the outside.

In contrast, the proposal was made that the cell killing by viruses results from stimulation of the development of lysosomal enzyme. Electron microscopic or biochemical evidence indicating that lysosomes play a central role in viral infection is controversial.

Mushroom Toxins

Some species of mushrooms are poisonous. In the United States, all poisonous mushrooms are of the Amanita family, and those that cause death most frequently are the *Amanita muscaria* (fly agaric) and the *Amanita phalloides* (destroying angel). The toxin in *A. muscaria* is the parasympathomimetic agent, muscarine. Intoxication results in symptoms similar to those observed in muscarine poisoning. *A. phalloides* contains a number of toxins: a hemolysin, phallin, and two groups of cytopathic toxins, the phalloidines and the amanitines. Phallin is destroyed by heat and gastric juices, therefore it is seldom a source of intoxication. The cytopathic agents are polypeptides. It is not certain whether phalloidine plays a role in mushroom intoxication in humans, although it does in some rodents (see section on damage to cell membranes).

In contrast, amanitines are known to be very toxic. The molecular mechanism of action of amanitine has recently been clarified, at least in part. After ingestion or intraperitoneal injection of α-amanitine, the liver is the primary target of the toxin, and the kidney is affected secondarily. An important manifestation of the effect of the toxin on the liver is a 50% reduction of the incorporation of orotic acid into RNA. This interference with RNA synthesis was demonstrated to result from inhibition of the activity of that type of RNA polymerase that is found in the nucleolus (see chapters on determination of specificity) [85, 86].

The interference with RNA synthesis is associated with condensation of chromatin in the hepatocyte nuclei, which suggests that chromatin is in the state characteristic of euchromatin only if it is transcribing DNA into RNA. The ultrastructural counterpart of these changes is fragmentation of the nucleoli into small, round or oval-shaped pieces. In the fragments, the granular and fibrillar components are segregated.

Amanitine is also reabsorbed in the proximal tubules of the kidney, where it concentrates in the tubular cell causing necrosis and functional disturbances.

Reye's Syndrome

The discovery of the Reye's syndrome by an Australian pathologist indicates that careful and patient observation of autopsy cases can still lead to the uncovering of new diseases.

Reye's syndrome is a rare children's disease of unknown etiology that evolves as follows. Usually after a prodromal period with symptoms resembling those observed in flu, there is repeated vomiting and rapidly progressive and severe deterioration of the central nervous system with hypoglycemia, high serum transaminase values, acidosis, stupor, and coma. Although the liver is enlarged, jaundice and signs of hepatic failure are characteristically missing; morphological features include intensive steatosis of the hepatocyte and of the renal tubule cell. The brain shows neuronal degeneration and edema.

Ultrastructural examination of liver biopsies or of liver fragments obtained at autopsy characteristically reveals the presence of dramatically swollen mitochondria, with loss of mitochondrial granules and expansion of the matrix space. At present, there is no experimental model for Reye's syndrome; viruses and toxins are suspected pathogenetic agents.

Viruses are suspected because the disease often follows a respiratory infection, and a number of viruses have been isolated from the victims' stools. In Japan, the disease is endemic in areas where aflatoxins contaminate the food. In Jamaica, a similar hypoglycemic syndrome develops after the ingestion of unripe akee fruit which contains a toxin called hypoglycin.

A link between ornithine-transcarbamylase deficiency and Reye's syndrome has been described.

Whether the deficiency plays an important pathogenic role in the disease remains to be established, but the administration of ornithine and arginine has been suggested as potential therapy for the disease [152].

Extracellular Accumulation of Degenerative Macromolecules

Organ degenerations are often associated with discrete or abundant accumulation of foreign material outside the cells. Sometimes the foreign material is suspected to be elaborated inside the cells (amyloid). Sometimes its origin is unknown (hyalin). Three different types of such accumulations are amyloidosis, hyalinization, and fibrinoid necrosis.

Amyloidosis

Amyloidosis is a pathological condition resulting from the accumulation of normal or pathological fibrous protein material called amyloid. Although the amyloid may be formed in cells, it is mainly found in extracellular locations.

Classification

Many attempts to classify amyloidosis have been made, but since types of amyloidosis cannot be classified on the basis of their pathogenesis, most schemes remain unsatisfactory. One of the first attempts at classification distinguished between primary and secondary amyloidosis, depending upon whether the amyloid deposition was an isolated event (primary), or whether it was secondary to a debilitating disease (*e.g.*, chronic suppurative infections). However, the term "secondary" implies a cause-effect relationship between the chronic infection and amyloidosis, and this is not always established. In 1929, Lubarsch [87] claimed that he could distinguish primary from secondary amyloidosis simply by using staining techniques. Yet when other investigators attempted to make this distinction, they failed and they found instead a great variability in the staining properties of amyloid in both groups. Moreover, a wide overlap in staining properties existed between amyloid accumulated in primary and secondary disease.

Attempts to distinguish between primary and secondary amyloidosis on the basis of the gross anatomical distribution of the disease, although sometimes useful, are not always consistent. Although parenchymal tissue (liver, spleen, and kidney) is the preferred site of deposition in secondary amyloidosis, and mesenchymal tissue (heart, lung) is preferentially affected in primary amyloidosis, it is impossible on the basis of anatomical examinations to distinguish primary from secondary amyloidosis in at least 25% of the cases.

Attempts to classify amyloidosis on a histological basis have not been much more convincing. Some investigators distinguish between amyloid deposits found near reticular fiber and those found near collagen fiber and claim that amyloidosis is related to infectious disease in one case and to vascular disease in the other. These assertions have not been confirmed.

All that is actually known about amyloidosis is that (1) amyloid exists; (2) all amyloid may not be the same; (3) in some cases amyloidosis is associated with debilitating disease (frequently purulent infection, but not always), in other cases, amyloidosis exists without any detectable preconditioning (acquired or hereditary familial form). In rare cases, amyloidosis is simply localized in one organ.

Whether all these situations are manifestations of a single disease or whether a small or even a large number of different types of amyloidosis exist is not known. Obviously, any attempt to present an integrated picture of the biochemical, substructural, anatomical, and clinical manifestations of amyloidosis would be artificial. Therefore, the morbid anatomy of amyloidosis as it appears in various organs will be described first, then the pathogenesis of the disease will be discussed, and, finally, an attempt will be made to integrate this information in a clinical picture.

Pathological Anatomy

All organs that contain connective tissue may be affected by amyloidosis. Some organs are affected with predilection (the spleen, liver, and kidney in secondary amyloidosis; the heart and lung in primary amyloidosis) but no organ system is immune. Amyloidosis has been described in the alimentary, respiratory, and urinary tracts; muscle; and the endocrine glands.

When an organ is affected by amyloidosis, it is as if molten wax had been poured on its connective tissue framework. Amyloid confers to the organ a whitish gray, translucent, glassy, homogeneous appearance. The deposits are firm but elastic in consistency. At first, small, fine streaks may be visible at close examination, but sometimes only special staining can confirm the diagnosis (see below). As more amyloid is deposited, it forms wide streaks that cross the organ in various directions and give it the appearance of sliced bacon or cooked ham (*e.g.*, spleen and heart), or amyloid may accumulate in small nodules (reminiscent of cooked sago) or diffuse plaques.

As the foreign material accumulates, it may compress the surrounding functional cells and lead to necrosis and loss of function in the organ (*e.g.*, renal and cardiac insufficiency). The normal histological architecture is distorted in the amyloid-containing organ by the appearance of streaks or plaques of material that stains pink with eosin, khaki or yellowish orange with van Gieson's stain, pale violet with PAS, metachromatic red with crystal violet, and pink with Congo red. The deposits are found in the connective tissues. In the early stages of amyloidosis, deposits

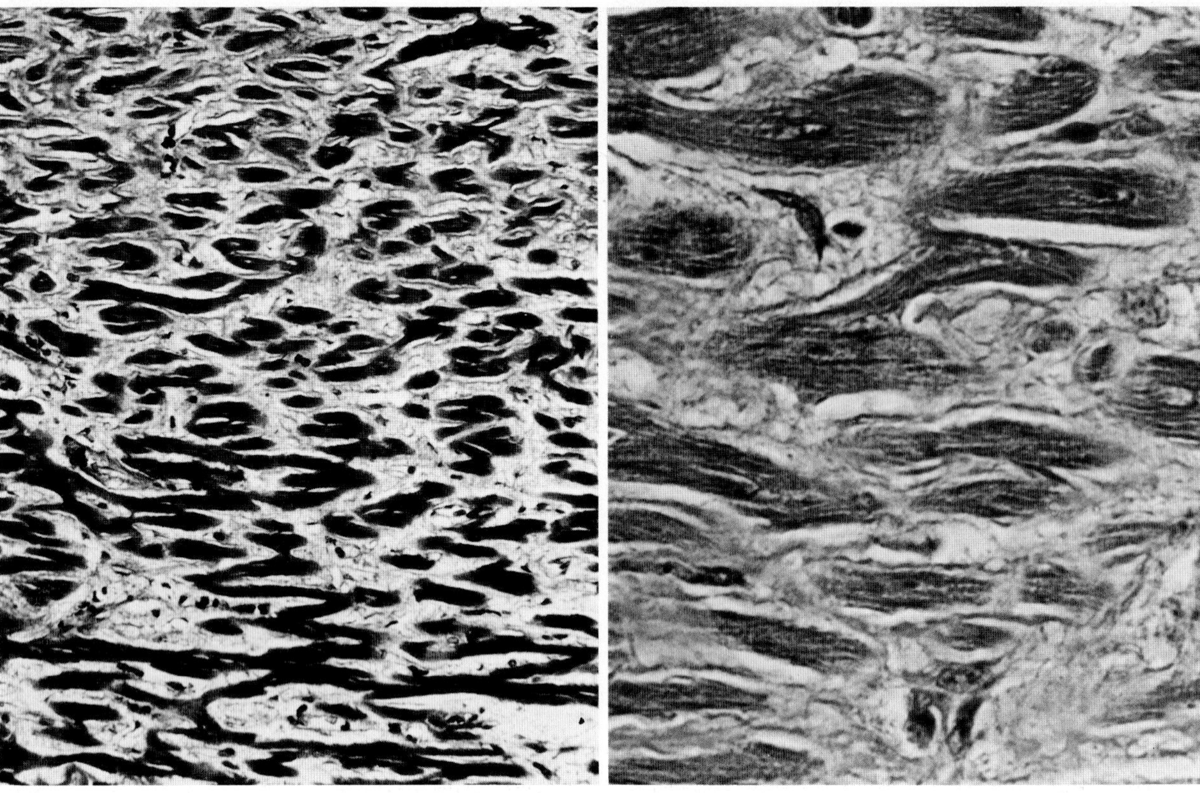

Fig. 10-15. Amyloidosis of heart; low *(left)* and high *(right)* power

form preferentially at the periphery of the small arteries.

At autopsy, the liver is regularly enlarged and firm; the cut surface is smooth, translucent, and shiny, as if it were covered with a thin layer of veneer. The spleen is similarly enlarged, firm, and translucent. Two distinct pathological types of spleen are found on section, depending upon whether the amyloid is distributed in diffuse streaks (*rate jambon* of the French) or in condensed small nodules (the sago spleen, or "sagomilz" of Virchow). Although the appearance of the amyloid liver and spleen is very typical, that of the kidney varies considerably depending upon the secondary reactions of necrosis, lipid degenerations, and other changes. Typically, the kidney is large and whitish. On section, the difference between cortex and medulla is accentuated; the cortex often appears waxy and translucent. The amyloid heart is enlarged and firm, almost rigid, as if it were fixed. It has a waxy, streaky appearance, which on section is reminiscent of sliced bacon. Massive involvement of the heart is usually associated with severe heart failure (see Fig. 10-15).

Amyloidosis in other organs may lead to diffuse infiltration, occasionally causing organ distortion—*e.g.*, macroglossia and pseudoscleroderma. Tumorlike formations caused by amyloid accumulations have been observed most frequently in the larynx, but also in the conjunctiva and the tongue. Hereditary amyloidosis is associated with small kidneys with irregular subcapsular deposits and extreme firmness.

Amyloid is deposited in three renal structures with varing degrees of frequency: the glomerulus, the basal membrane of the tubules, and the arteries (see Figs. 10-16 and 10-17). In the glomerulus, the amyloid accumulation begins in the basal membrane of the tufts; later the accumulations spread through the entire glomerulus, obliterating the capillary lumen and finally replacing the glomerulus by homogeneous, glassy, translucent amyloid plaques. Amyloid can also be detected in the basal membrane of the tubules. For reasons that are not immediately obvious, the parenchymal cells of the tubules swell, accumulate fat, and ultimately die. As a result, numerous nephrons are lost. Amyloidosis of glomeruli and tubules is frequently associated with amyloid deposition in the walls of the small renal arteries. Two types of casts are found in the tubules of patients with amyloidosis: an eosinophilic cast like that seen in any other renal condition, and weakly metachromatic, laminated casts that contain amyloid.

In the liver (see Fig. 10-18), amyloid is found at first in the hepatic chord, the connective tissue between the endothelium of the sinus and the hepatic cell. Usually as it accumulates at the periphery of the nodule, the amyloid compresses the liver cells and the sinusoids. As a result, the sinusoids narrow and the liver cells die.

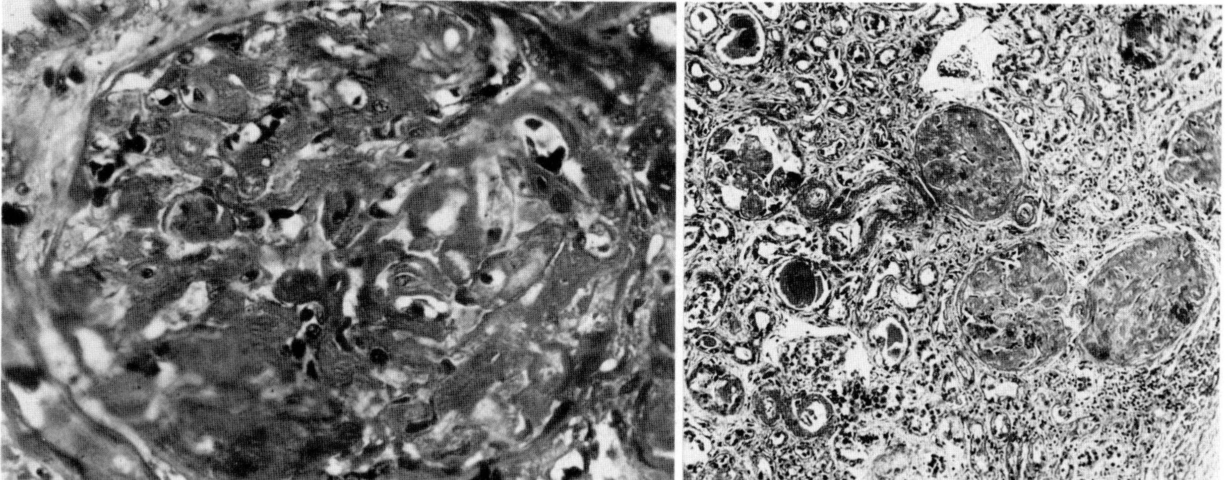

Fig. 10-16. Amyloidosis in human kidney; low *(right)* and high *(left)* power. Note glossy appearance of glomeruli and amyloid casts in tubules

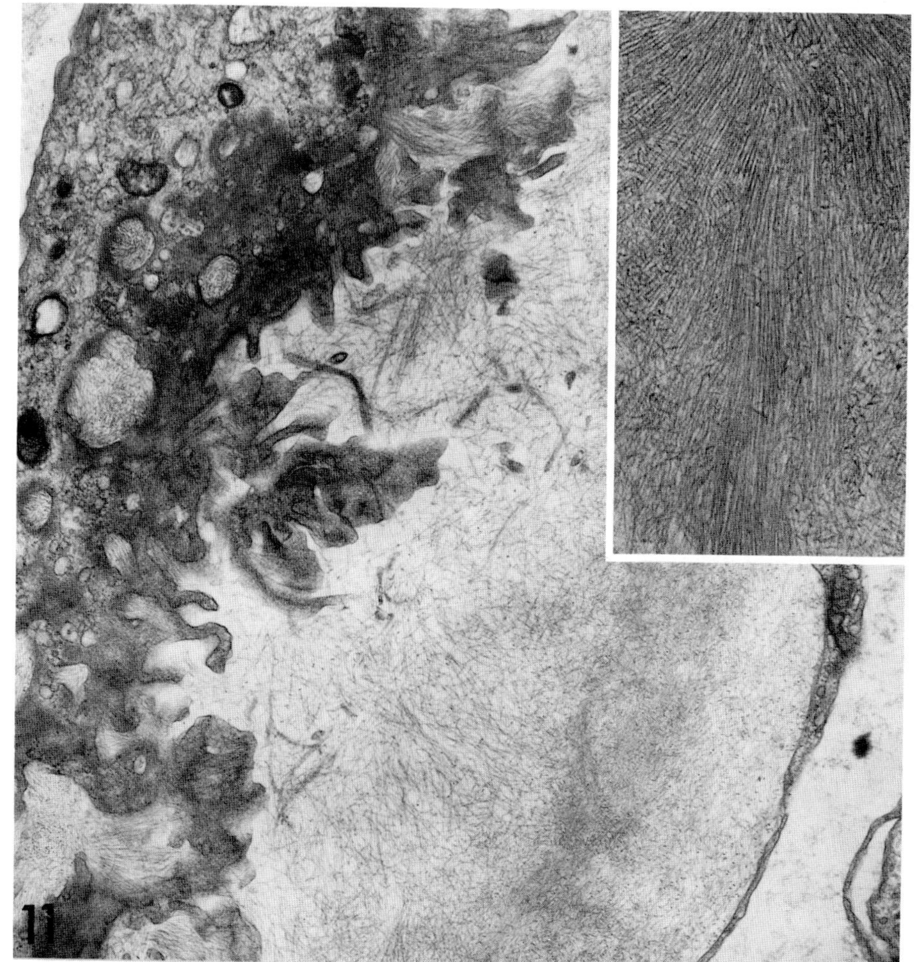

Fig. 10-17. Renal amyloidosis, segment of a glomerular capillary with increased thickness of the wall (×20,000). Inset shows the fibrillar structure of amyloid (×48,000; from Zamboni)

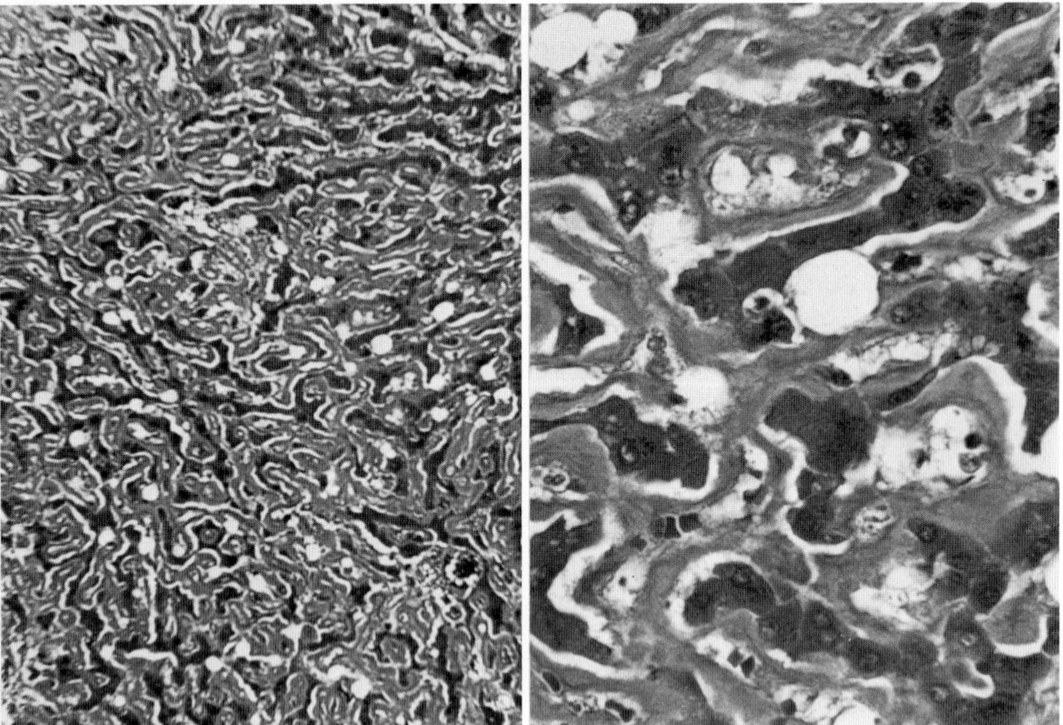

Fig. 10-18. Amyloidosis in liver; low *(right)* and high *(left)* power

In the spleen, amyloid is deposited first in the walls of the arteries of the malpighian body, and as it accumulates, amyloid spreads along the connective chords of the stroma of the red pulp or forms small nodules that replace the entire malpighian corpuscle. Diffuse, nodular amyloid distribution can be observed in a number of other organs containing connective tissues.

Pathogenesis

Three sources of information led to an elementary understanding of the pathogenesis of amyloidosis: (1) the incidence of amyloidosis; (2) electron microscopic studies of amyloidosis; (3) the chemical studies of isolated amyloid fibers [88–91].

In Rokitansky's day (1804–1878), lardaceous disease of the spleen, liver, and kidney must have been a common finding at autopsy since many died of chronic infection. Rokitansky described the gross changes by the term "lardaceious degeneration." Virchow changed the name because he observed that the material that accumulates in this disease would, like starch, take an intense coloration with iodide. Virchow coined the word amyloidosis, which has survived to our day, even though it is well established that amyloid is not a polysaccharide.

Amyloidosis has been observed in patients with chronic purulent infection. However, since the discovery of antibiotics, amyloidosis is much less common; consequently, most observed cases are either primary or secondary to other debilitating diseases, such as Hodgkin's disease, multiple myelomas, and rheumatoid arthritis.

Primary amyloidosis usually occurs after 50 years of age. The patient dies 3–7 years after the onset of the disease. Primary amyloidosis is twice as common in men as in women. The organs most frequently affected are the heart (10–15%), the brain (in senile plaques), pancreatic islets (6%), and the seminal vesicles (17–34%). Amyloidosis has been observed in dogs, cats, baboons, hamsters, and mice. It has been proposed that spontaneous amyloidosis reflects an accelerated autoimmune process more common in men than in women. Amyloidosis occurs more frequently than is ordinarily suspected in old age, when it can be discrete and well localized (*e.g.*, in the brain) or generalized.

In man, as in animals, amyloidosis (primary and secondary) is a progressive disease with usually a very poor prognosis. Renal biopsies often provide a convenient way of diagnosing amyloidosis.

Five parameters are known to influence the incidence of amyloidosis in humans: infection, heredity, cellular proliferation, hormones, and diet. In countries where tuberculosis is prevalent (India, Poland, USSR), it continues to be the major predisposing factor to amyloidosis. Leprosy the second predisposing disease, and a large number of lepers die from renal insufficiency resulting from amyloidosis.* In our country, chronic ulcerative colitis, chronic enteritis, pyelitis, cystitis, and especially rheumatoid arthritis constitute predisposing factors to amyloidosis.

Amyloidosis is associated with a number of hereditary diseases. Amyloidosis of the peripheral nerve is found in a Portuguese form of venereal polyneuritis. Severe cardiac amyloidosis is common in patients with a fimilial Mediterranean disease (periodic disease).

It has sometimes been claimed that all patients with primary amyloidosis necessarily have a form of plasma cell tumor. However, in contrast to multiple myeloma, the tumor is not associated with skeleton destruction. Moreover, only 1 in 30 patients with amyloidosis unquestionably presents a diffuse type of plasmocytosis. Myeloma and Hodgkin's disease tumors are most frequently associated with amyloidosis. Other cancers, except pelvic carcinomatosis, are seldom found with amyloidosis. It has been argued that in carcinomatosis, the amyloidosis results from urethral obstruction and subsequent pyeloureteritis.

There is no convincing evidence that hormones influence the incidence of amyloidosis. Amyloidosis of the endocrine organs understandably induces imbalances. Amyloidosis has been observed in the islet cells of the pancreas in association with diabetes, in the thyroid in association with myxedema, and in the hypophysis. Whether diabetes or myxedema in turn affects the development or the incidence of amyloidosis remains to be seen.

Experimental Production and Spontaneous Incidents

Amyloidosis may be produced experimentally in many animals in innumerable ways. To list all methods now available to induce amyloidosis would be cumbersome. Nevertheless, it is impossible to detect any common denominator that would explain the mode of action of all the agents. The agents causing amyloidosis can be divided into three major categories: bacteria and bacterial extracts, γ-globulin, and casein diets.

When administered repeatedly, various bacteria lead to amyloidosis. The bacillus pyocyanus, *Staphylococcus aureus,* the bacillus *E. coli, Neisseria gonorrhoeae,* hemolytic streptococci, and a host of other bacteria, as well as repeated injections of turpentine, have been used to produce amyloidosis in mice, rabbits, and dogs. In general, these procedures lead to a type of secondary amyloidosis with predominating involvement in the spleen and the kidney.

Associated with the development of amyloidosis and the bacterial infection is a rise in γ-globulin. Thus, it was assumed that amyloidosis results from overproduction of γ-globulin. Consequently, attempts were made to produce amyloidosis by direct injection of γ-globulin. In these experiments, amyloidosis was or was not produced depending upon the laboratory in which the experiments were done. Furthermore, there is no direct correlation between the incidence of amyloidosis and the levels of γ-globulin in the blood. In fact, the disease has been observed in patients with hypoglobulinemia. Thus, if there is a relationship between γ-globulin production and amyloidosis, it is not likely to be a simple one.

The prolonged administration of a casein diet seems to be one of the most efficient means of producing experimental amyloidosis. It is difficult to evaluate variations of casein diet because of the conflicting results. For example, some feel that a high-protein diet facilitates the development of amyloidosis; others think that it retards it. The mechanism of production of amyloidosis is not clear. Some have claimed that the fibrinogen levels have increased after casein injection, but there is no evidence that fibrinogen is converted to amyloid. Similarly, it has been claimed that casein induces hyperglobulinemia, especially in rabbits. However, amyloidosis was observed in rabbits with hypoglobulinemia, although at a much lower incidence.

One of the most significant contributions of the electron microscope to pathology may well have resulted from the observation of amyloid-containing tissue. This observation unquestionably established that amyloid has a fibrillar structure. The amyloid fibrils are composed of small beaded filaments with a diameter of 75 ($\pm$5) A and a 100-A longitudinal periodicity. The same fine structure is found in all tissue of animals with amyloidosis. Furthermore, similar fibrillar structures have been found in the reticuloendothelial cells of animals in which experimental amyloidosis has been produced. However, some investigators argued that the presence of intracellular fibrils is the result of phagocytosis rather than intracellular elaboration. Studies of cultures of spleen *in vitro* seem to exclude phagocytosis. Indeed, the filaments appear in the cell before they can be found in the extracellular medium. Studies with labeled amino acid, leucine, and tryptophan (pulsed and continuous labeling) reveal radiophotographically that the label appears in the cell before it is found in the extracellular medium.

The electron microscopic observations encouraged investigators to partially purify the amyloid substance. Virchow discovered that amyloid stained with iodine was like starch, and he believed that amyloid was a polysaccharide. He called it "amyloid," after amyline and starch. Virchow obstinately refused to acknowledge findings that suggested that amyloid was a protein because of the high nitrogen content in amyloid tissue. Virchow argued that the studies were made on whole amyloid tissue, and that the accumulating substances had to be purified before the properties of amyloid could be determined.

Because chondroitin sulfate was found in tissue affected by amyloidosis and histochemically was

* It has been claimed that amyloidosis among TB victims is less common in India than in the western countries. Similarly, lepers in Mexico have a lower incidence of amyloidosis than lepers in Louisiana. Whether these differences are the consequence of differences in the diet or the result of inadequate diagnostic procedures in developing countries remains to be seen.

detected in close association with amyloidosis, amyloid was believed to be a mucopolysaccharide. Since amyloidosis is frequently the result of chronic infectious processes, amyloid deposits were thought to be the product of an antigen-antibody reaction; therefore, it was assumed that these deposits would be rich in α-globulin.

The investigation of Cohen [88] clarified several of these points. Cohen first purified the amyloid fibroid from various sources by differential centrifugation of homogenates in saline. The fibers were then purified by sucrose gradient centrifugation. These studies clearly established that amyloid is a protein that doesn't contain chondroitin sulfate; is resistant to collagenase, sulfatase, and hyaluronidase; and is not an α-globulin. In addition, it was clearly established that amyloid contains hexosamine and uronic acid. The purified fiber may be a glycoprotein. Since the fiber cannot be readily solubilized, an exact analysis of amino acid composition is not available. However, partial solubilization was achieved [92]; the solubilized protein was found to have the electrophoretic mobility of an α-globulin. Yet, it was immunologically dissimilar to globulin, β_1-lipoprotein, fibrogen, thrombin, and many other blood proteins.

Ultracentrifugal studies have also been made on amyloid fibers treated with an alkaline phosphate buffer (pH 8). After the alkaline supernatant had been discarded, the residue was extracted with 0.01 M acetic acid and treated with 6 M urea. These fractions were then placed in the ultracentrifuge, and sedimentation values of 1, 6, 9, 16, and 23 were obtained. Again, immunological studies of the centrifugation product indicated that the prepared material did not react as the known blood protein. Electrophoresis on starch gel did not show any difference between the mobilities of the component of these extracts with secondary amyloidosis or those obtained from patients with primary amyloidosis.

Amyloid Fibrils

More recently, two kinds of amyloid fibrils have been described: protein A or AUO (amyloid of unknown origin), and protein B or AIO (amyloid of immunoglobulin origin). AIO is primarily found in patients with lymphoma and myeloma, whereas AUO is primarily found in patients with chronic inflammation, such as tuberculosis and rheumatoid arthritis. A number of different laboratories have reported partial amino acid sequences of AUO. The protein is believed to contain 76 amino acids with a stretch of 40 amino acids lacking proline, valine, threonine, and cystine. Since no immunoglobulin contains stretches of 40 amino acids free of these specific residues, AUO cannot be derived from immunoglobulin.

In contrast, AIO was found to have stretches of amino acid sequences similar to those found in light chains of γ-globulins or Bence Jones proteins (see chapter on immunopathology). A plausible interpretation of the formation of AIO fibrils is that they are formed by cells that make immunoglobulins. The soluble immunoglobulins are then phagocytized by macrophages, which yield an insoluble and undigestible fiber that may then be deposited in interstitial tissue, where the macrophages die.

An appreciation of the origin of the AIO fibers has considerable practical significance because if amyloidose could be detected before massive deposition, it might be possible to interrupt or completely stop amyloidosis by killing the cell of origin. In fact, such an approach is at the origin of immunosuppressive therapy in amyloidosis.

Amyloid was prepared from a patient with plasma cell dyscrasia without bone involvement; the amino acid composition and sequence of the fiber were found to be the same as those of Bence Jones protein. VL fragments of a light polypeptide chain (see Chapter 14) were isolated by immunological methods from the fibers obtained from a patient with primary amyloidosis and from fibers obtained from a patient with focal pulmonary amyloidosis. On the basis of such observations it has been concluded that in amyloidosis associated with occult or overt plasma dyscrasia, there is a monoclonal proliferation of plasma cells which elaborate a portion of the VL fragment of the light chain.

These observations which are still restricted to a few selected cases do not exclude the possibility that amyloidosis fibrils could also be derived from whole immunoglobulin molecules or portions of the heavy chain. In any event it is possible to reproduce *in vitro* fibers resembling amyloid fibers by treating Bence Jones protein light chains with proteases so as to separate their variable and constant regions. X-Ray crystallographic studies of the fibers revealed that the amyloid fiber protein existed in a β conformation.

In conclusion, immunoblasts may produce excess immunoglobulins which in some cases are captured by phagocytes where they undergo partial proteolysis. Some portion of the VL light chains have a tendency to form β pleated chains that resist further protease digestion, accumulate in the phagocyte and are excreted either through exocytosis or as a result of the death of the cell [161].

Hyalinization and Fibrinoid Necrosis

In addition to amyloid, a number of translucent substances with different staining properties accumulate under pathological conditions; they are referred to as hyalin depositions. The origin of the hyalin material is not known. Because hyalin material accumulates preferentially in the vascular wall when vascular permeability changes, hyalin is believed to be derived from blood proteins. Vascular hyalinization is found so frequently at autopsy that it is believed to be a manifestation of old age rather than a genuine disease process [93].

On a regular H + E-stained section, hyalin appears as a glassy, homogeneous, translucent, pinkish material not too different from amyloid. However, if the section is stained with PAS, hyalin can be distinguished from amyloid. Furthermore, the hyalin can be identified with special immunofluorescent methods. Hyalin accumulates in the vascular wall first of the small arteries, but later it invades the walls of the medium-sized arteries.

Although no artery is immune, preferred sites of hyalinization are the splenic, renal, pancreatic, and liver vasculature.

The special case of glomerular hyalinization observed in diabetes.

In a number of pathological situations—for example, hypertension and hypersensitivity—the vascular wall undergoes alterations distinct from those caused by amyloidosis or hyalinization. In such cases, there appears to be active necrosis of cells (endothelial cell, muscle fibers, or connective tissue cells) associated with accumulation of a fibrinoid material of unknown origin. In contrast to hyalinization, fibrinoid necrosis leads to distension rather than narrowing of the vascular lumen.

Elementary Lesions of the Nervous System

The Nerve Cell and Its Appendages

Nervous tissues are composed of at least two types of cellular elements: (1) the nerve cells and nerve fibers and (2) the neuroglia.

Nerve cells and their fibers are found in both the central and the autonomic nervous system. In the brain, nerve cells are found in the gray substance of the cortex and in the various nuclei. The spinal cord and the ganglia of the autonomic system also contain nerve cells. Only isolated nerve cells can be found in the sympathetic system.

Nerve cells vary considerably in size, ranging, for example, from 7 μ in the granular cells of the cerebellum to 80 μ in the Betz cells. Purkinje cells and those of the anterior horn and cerebral cortex are relatively large and contain abundant cytoplasm. The shape of these cells varies depending upon their location in the nervous system. They may be pyramidal (*e.g.*, efferent cells of the cerebral cortex and corpus striatum, and the motor nerve cells of the brain and spinal cord), spherical (cells of the dorsal and mesencephalic roots), bipolar (the cochlear, vestibular, olfactory, retinal, and ganglion cells), fusiform (cells of auditory cortex) or shaped like a flask (Purkinje cells). Before some of the properties of these cells are considered, it might be interesting to point out their almost unbelievable number—twenty million such cells are found in the brain.

The subcellular structure in the body of nerve cells resembles that in other cells. The nucleus is usually large, rich in nucleoplasm and chromatin, and often contains a well-developed nucleolus. The size of the nucleolus has been shown to correlate with the amount of Nissl substance (see below). In fact, when the Nissl substance is lost as a result of electrical stimulus, recovery of the Nissl substance in the cytoplasm is preceded by an increase in RNA synthesis in the nucleolus.

The nerve cell cytoplasm contains two kinds of subcellular structures. Some are identical to those found in all other cells (endoplasmic reticulum, mitochondria, Golgi, etc.), whereas others are specialized structures found only in nerve cells (Nissl substance, neurofibrils). The Nissl substance, also referred to in the past as tigroid substance, appears as flakes of basophilic material. Its overall staining properties vary with the physiological or pathological condition of the cell.

At first it was thought that the Nissl substance might be an artifact. But since the properties of Nissl substance varied with the cell's activity and size, it became clear that the Nissl substance must be important in cellular function.

The amount of Nissl material found in the brain varies with the size of the cell. The larger the cell, the larger the basophilic blocks of Nissl substance. Cajal also observed that the amount of Nissl substance increased with the number of cellular expansions. Finally, the size of the nucleolus seems to correlate with the amount of Nissl substance in the nerve cell.

Neurofibrillar structures are found in the body and the axoplasm of the neural cell. This neurofibrillar apparatus forms a sort of intracellular framework of thin fibers, which have been observed with the electron microscope and are 100–200 A thick. The fibers can be stained on histological slides by special methods, including the silver reduction technique developed by Cajal. The fibers appear in the dendrite as a bundle of parallel fibers. The bundle splits into numerous branches that are distributed in the ramifications of the dendrite. Sometimes only one fiber can be found in some of the branches of the most ramified dendrites. Toward the center of the cell, the fibers that constitute the dendritic bundle disassociate and form a tridimensional network at the periphery of the cytoplasm. The network of fibers is again recollimated to form a new bundle, which enters the cylindraxile of the cell.

Investigators argued about the function of the neurofibrillar apparatus. Whereas some believed that these neural fibers simply formed an intracellular skeleton to support the enormously extended cell, others believed that the fibers transmitted impulses. In the midst of the controversy were rebels who simply denied the existence of the fibers and claimed that they were fixation artifacts.

Although the neurofibrillar system has not been observed *in vivo* in vertebrates, in invertebrates fine threads in constant motion can be seen in the axoplasm *in vivo*. Furthermore, the appearance of the neurofibrillar system in the nerve cell coincides with its functional differentiation. Although the neurofibrillar apparatus is present at birth in the cells of the spinal cord and the brain stem, it appears postnatally in the cells of the cerebral cortex within 15 months.

Many investigators have been intrigued by the nerve cell. In the middle of the 19th century, Remak and Wagner recognized the polarity of nervous cells. A little later, Deiters distinguished two examples of cellular expansion—the cylindrax and dendrites. Yet, when Ehrlich invented the silver chromatic staining method, the intricacies of the interaction between the extensions of the nerve cell were unravelled.

One important aspect of the neuron's structure is its centralization. The cytoplasm of the neuron forms stretched-out and sometimes very long expansions that conduct afferent or efferent impulses.

In *in vivo* preparations, the axon is known to be made of substances with two different consistencies: a firm outer gel and a liquid core. The liquid is displaced under pressure. After fixation the axon is stainable. All axons are likely to be surrounded by a myelin sheet, and the so-called myelinate differ from demyelinated fibers (see below) primarily in the thickness of the myelin sheet. Although the axon contains mitochondria, it seems to be unable to synthesize protein. Therefore, it is assumed that most of the constituents of the axon must be brought to its extremity by a special liquid movement referred to as the axon flow. Some drugs interrupt this flow and thereby lead to swelling of the peripheral portions of the axon.

The axon terminates at the surface of another nerve cell near the dendrite extending from the neuron, or close to a nerve ending. The dendrites are short, ramified cytoplasmic expansions of the body of the nerve cell. They contain neurofibrils that extend throughout the dendrite, an endoplasmic reticulum, and a few mitochondria. Although Nissl substance may not be found within the dendrite, a mass of Nissl substance is often seen at its origin in the nerve cell.

In most organisms, impulse conduction involves a sequence of several neurons; therefore, the connection between neurons is especially important.

Researchers have tried to describe the pattern of these interneuron connections. To study the reproducibility of the pattern, they have also attempted to find out whether a pattern that disappears after neuronal injury reappears during regeneration. If mistakes are made during regeneration researchers wanted to find out how frequently they appear. Maybe the two most important features of the synaptic connection are lack of cytoplasmic continuity from the expansion of one nerve cell to another, and the presence of acetylcholine in the synaptic region of the afferent nerve. In fact, these findings are at the foundation of modern concepts of neurophysiology, which assumes that the transfer of the impulse from one neuron to the other involves the release of acetylcholine.

Types of Nerve Cell Injury

Neuronal damage caused by anoxemia, toxins, or other injurious mechanisms of unknown origin usually affects both nucleus and cytoplasm. The changes in the nucleus are similar to those described in other tissues. The chromatin tends to become more homogeneous, losing its normal granular appearance, and may condense and form pyknotic nuclei. The chromatin may also slowly disappear and lose its staining properties in the process of karyolysis. However, karyolysis is seldom observed in the central nervous system.

Mitoses are not observed in neurons. Nevertheless, binucleated and multinucleated cells have been described in the central nervous system, and a controversy has long existed as to whether the binucleated cells result from damage to the nervous system.

The changes in the nerve cell cytoplasm are of four types: (1) alteration of the Nissl substance; (2) alteration of the neurofibrils; (3) modification of the overall size of the cytoplasm; and (4) the formation of intracytoplasmic inclusions.

Cytoplasmic Nissl substance may change after injury through chromatolysis or densification. Chromatolysis is more common than densification and may be total or partial. Partial chromatolysis of the Nissl substance may be restricted to the perinuclear region, or it may develop in more peripheral areas of the cell. When chromatolysis is associated with cell injury, it usually parallels cytoplasmic swelling and vacuolization. During chromatolysis, the Nissl substance breaks down, and the debris is dispersed in a fine dust that may be absorbed by the neurofibrils, so that with proper staining methods, the fibers appear to be impregnated with the Nissl substance.

During densification, the debris, instead of dissolving, condenses into a voluminous mass that may occupy large portions of the cytoplasm.

These differences between chromatolysis and densification of the Nissl substance seem to result from different actions of hydrolytic enzymes. In densification, the hydrolases appear to be inactivated, or the Nissl substance may have become inaccessible to the enzymes. Generally, the neurofibrils are more resistant to injury than the Nissl substance of the brain, but again, they may undergo a dual fate. Neurofibrils may disintegrate or become more dense. Neurofibrillar disintegration is referred to as fibrolysis, and it is also more common than densification. Densification occurs in special pathological conditions, such as Alzheimer's disease. In this case, the fibers are thickened, curled, and form hornlike structures pasted together by a pathological substance that can be recognized with the aid of silver stains.

The overall size of the cytoplasm can be altered in two ways—the cell may swell or shrink. Acute swelling takes place, for example, in cases of acute infection or after heat strokes. Two stages of swelling are the reversible and irreversible stages. In the reversible stage, the neuroplasm of the cell body and sometimes that of the dendrites swells, and there is marked chromatolysis of the Nissl substance. When swelling passes into the irreversible stage, karyolysis, massive chromatolysis, and focal cytoplasmic degradation are seen in the cytoplasm. Shrinking takes place in a number of chronic and acute situations. It is associated with atrophy of the cell body and may or may not be followed by chromatolysis, cytoplasmic acidophilia, and nuclear pyknosis. A special variation of shrinkage observed in ischemia, hypoglycemia, hypoxia, and cardiac arrest consists of homogenization of the cytoplasm, which becomes pale, opalescent, and eosinophilic. The nucleus may undergo karyorrhexis with chromatin clumping around the nucleolus.

Different types of inclusion bodies may be found in the cytoplasm of the nerve cells: hematin, ferruginous material, bilirubin, hyalin, amyloid, and lipoid material.

Hematin inclusions are rodlike, black incrustations that resemble melanin deposits and should not be confused with ferruginous material. Hematin can readily be identified by the Prussian blue reaction, which is negative for hematin.

Ferrugination results from iron pigment accumulation, which may be intracellular, resulting from phagocytosis, or extracellular because the cell that phagocytized the iron pigment is dead. The iron pigment accumulation is stainable with Prussian blue, and more extensive histochemical examination may reveal that calcium is also present in areas of ferrugination.

Bilirubin impregnates the nerve cells in cases of severe jaundice in the infant. Some nuclei are stained preferentially and the condition is referred to as kernicterus (see section on bile pigment).

Round hyalin bodies (Lewy bodies) of unknown composition with a highly eosinophilic core and a pale peripheral crown are found in the nerve cell cytoplasm in a number of central nervous system diseases: status pigmentosum, idiopathic paralysis agitans.

Round, concentric amyloid bodies with staining properties similar to those of the corpora amylacea have been found in the cell body, the axon, and the dendrites of neurons. These bodies, called Lafora bodies, can be distinguished from Lewy bodies by their basophilia, which is manifested with all stains, and their ability to stain with PAS.

Lipoid material of varied composition (cerebrosides, sphingomyelin, and sphingosine) accumulates in a number of hereditary diseases (see Lipoidosis).

Nonconductive Elements

The nervous system contains a number of nonconductive elements of ectodermic or mesodermic origin. The ectoderm produces supportive cells, referred to as the neuroglia, and the special epithelia of the ependyma and the chorioplexus. In addition to blood vessels and connective tissue, the mesoderm produces phagocytic and supportive elements.

There are two types of neuroglial cells—astrocytes and oligodendrocytes. The two major forms of astrocytes are the fibrous, which resemble ordinary connective tissue, and the protoplasmic. Both types have a round or sometimes an ellipsoid-shaped body and emit protoplasmic processes. Fibrous and protoplasmic astrocytes differ in the type of processes extending from them.

The processes extending from fibrous astrocytes have primarily supportive properties. They are found in the outer cell layer of the cortex and around the penetrating arteriole.

Most of the astrocytes in the cerebral cortex are of the protoplasmic variety. They have shorter and wider processes that branch off into many fine fibrils. Astrocytes are found in the cortex, the various nuclei, the putamen and the granular layer of the cerebellum. Astrocytes emit protoplasmic processes that tend to adhere to adjacent surfaces. Those close to the surface of the cortex form processes that attach to the cells of the ependymal membrane. An important modification of the protoplasmic expansions of some astrocytes is referred to as the sucker feet—flattened protoplasmic expansions that surround capillary walls. The protoplasmic expansion of the astrocytes is believed to constitute the anatomical counterpart of the blood-brain barrier.

Histophysiologically, the astrocyte is to the nervous system what the fibroblast is to the rest of the body. However, there are important differences between the astrocytic system and the connective tissue. First, astrocytes are of ectodermic and connective tissue is of mesodermic origin. Second, the fibers of the astrocytes remain an integral part of the astrocytic cytoplasm, in contrast to collagen fibers, which, although they are emitted by the fibroblast, lose some of their intimate metabolic connection with the mother cell. There is no evidence that astrocytes possess phagocytic properties.

Two types of injury to the astrocytes are swelling and proliferation. Swelling may develop in an acute fashion or rather slowly. In acute swelling, the body of the astrocyte assumes an enlarged round shape, and the cytoplasmic expansion disappears. Examples of this acute swelling are found in the ameboid Alzheimer cells, and Cajal named the process clasmatodendrosis. In the more moderate form of swelling, the body and the dendrites enlarge simultaneously. Some of the dendrites may become lost and, in fact, seem to be phagocytized by the astrocyte itself; this situation is referred to as dendrophagia.

There are also two forms of proliferation—astrogliosis and astrocytosis. In astrogliosis, there is hyperplastic proliferation of the astrocyte cells similar to that observed in fibrosis during scar formation. But although astrogliosis often plays the role of fibrosis, collagenous scars can still appear in nerve tissue. In many nervous diseases—*e.g.*, multiple sclerosis—gliosis may be quite intense. In proliferating astrocytes, the nuclei may divide without comparable division of the cytoplasm. As a result, multinucleated giant cells form.

Oligodendrocytes outnumber all other cells of the nervous system. They have globular cytoplasm, with nuclei coarser than those of astrocytes, containing blocks of chromatin. Oligodendrocytes are smaller than astrocytes and have fewer cytoplasmic processes. Oligodendrocytes are found practically everywhere in the central nervous system and are concentrated in three primary sites: the perineural area in the gray matter (the collection of oligodendrocytes around the neuron is sometimes referred to as satellitosis), the interfascicular glia in the white matter (these oligodendrocytes are believed to elaborate the myelin found in the white matter), and around blood vessels.

The function of oligodendrocytes other than elaborating and maintaining myelin is not clear. They might be phagocytic with a special appetite for myelin under conditions of myelin breakdown.

Oligodendrocytes are the most sensitive cells of the central nervous system. Three types of oligodendrocytic injuries can be distinguished: (1) acute swelling with or without vacuolization; (2) accumulation of glycolipids and mucopolysaccharides; and (3) atrophy in which the oligodendrocyte appears as a small cell with emaciated cytoplasmic fibrils.

Oligodendrocytes must clearly be distinguished from the microglia, which are of mesodermic origin. Hortega first distinguished microglia, therefore these cells are often referred to as Hortega cells.

Microglia are to the central nervous system what the reticuloendothelial system is to the rest of the somatic tissue. During the resting phase microglia are small, but under pathological conditions they enlarge, emit cytoplasmic expansions, and incorporate within their cytoplasm a variety of substances by phagocytosis. Understandably, microglial cytoplasm contains lipid droplets and mucopolysaccharide clumps. When portions of neurons are engulfed by microglia, one speaks of neurophagia. Microglia are a type of first-line scavenger in the nervous system, monocytes being called into action only in the most severe cases of neurological infection or damage.

The response of the myelin sheath to injury can thus best be understood if the reader is familiar with the morphology, chemistry, and origin of the myelin sheath. The early anatomists and later histologists recognized two kinds of nerve fibers. The naked, amyelinic fibers, also called the fibers of Remak, are found in higher vertebrates in the autonomous system. In invertebrates and lower vertebrates, they may even be found in the olfactory nerve. It is not quite clear why such nerves function without a well-developed myelin sheath; traditional explanations are that (1) they constitute an inferior form of conductivity; (2) the path is so short that there is no need for strict isolation; and (3) the type of message that is conducted does not require isolation.

The fibers of Remak are long, thin, gray cylinders (102 μ) made of one or several axon fibrils surrounded by a thin sheath of Schwann cells. The distinction between unmyelinated and myelinated fibers was believed to be only a quantitative one, because when even the smallest nerve fibers are examined with the polarized microscope, they are found to be surrounded by birefringent material similar to myelin. Electron microscopic examination of amyelinated fibers confirmed these views.

Most of the peripheral nerves and the fibers of the white matter of the central nervous system are myelinated fibers. (Myelin is refractive, hence the white appearance of tissues made of myelin fibers.) When a freshly prepared small nerve is placed in a solute and examined under the microscope, thin, regular, cylindric fibers are dissociated. Each fiber is made of a central clear cylinder (the axon) surrounded by a birefringent girdle of myelin; the diameter of the fiber varies from 2–30 μ. The longest fibers are also the thickest. The birefringent layer that surrounds the axon is not continuous but intercepted by ringlike narrowings called the nodes of Ranvier. Even between two nodes, the glistening myelin sheath is not continuous. Discontinuities in the sheath, called the clefts of Schmidt-Lanterman, are oblique with respect to the long axis of the fiber.

A number of different staining methods permit the examination of the nerve fiber after fixation. The axon turns blue, brown, or black after fixation with silver stains. Osmic acid selectively blackens the myelin sheath. Examination of the fixed nerve after using one or more of such staining techniques reveals that the fiber is composed of four concentric cylinders: (1) the central axon; (2) a thin, clear layer of axolemma; (3) the membrane of Maűthner; (4) the myelin sheath; (5) the layer of Schwann cells.

The axons of the myelinated fibers are much larger than those of the unmyelinated fibers.

The Schwann cell is a rather large cell with an abundant but thin layer of cytoplasm that seems to adhere to the myelin sheath. The nucleus of the Schwann cell is well delineated and is usually located in a depression of the myelin sheath. Early histologists recognized within the Schwann cell a chondrioma and various granular inclusions including myelin droplets. They concluded that the Schwann cell "secreted" myelin. Myelin is a lipoprotein that blackens with osmic acid and surrounds the axon. The myelin sheath usually forms one-third of the diameter of the axon. A layer of clear cytoplasm separates the axon from the myelin sheath.

The axon is made of a bundle of neurofibrils that travel in a parallel fashion without forming anastomoses within the axoplasm (or neuroplasm), an extension of the nerve cell cytoplasm.

The fibers of the central nervous system have a structure similar to that of the peripheral fibers except that there are no recognizable Schwann cells at the periphery of the myelin sheath. As we shall see later, this does not imply that the mechanism of myelin formation in the central nervous system differs from that in the peripheral nerves.

Submicroscopic investigations of the myelin sheath were of considerable consequence in cell biology as well as in neurobiology because these studies have provided original or confirmed existing information on the structure of the plasma membrane. Again, the myelin sheath is birefringent when examined with polarized light. Klebs recognized this property of myelin in 1865. In the nerve fiber, birefringence requires a regular arrangement of anisodiametric structure with a refractile index different from that of the medium in which the fiber is immersed. If the repeated arrangement of the fundamental structure falls into the proper range (the size of a mole or atom), X-ray diffraction techniques can be used to analyze further the structural characteristic of the biological component under investigation. Then the results obtained on biological material can be compared with those obtained on purified chemicals.

On the basis of studies of the myelin sheath made with the aid of the polarizing microscope, Schmidt proposed that the myelin sheath was composed of concentric lipid and protein layers. In the lipid layers, the molecules were assumed to be arranged radially with respect to the long axis of the axon. Low-angle X-ray diffraction studies using fresh or dried amphibian or mammalian nerves revealed regular, radially oriented spacing. The distance between repeating units varied, however, with the source of the myelin. It was greater in fresh mammalian nerve (184 A) than in fresh amphibian (171 A). When the nerves were dried, values dropped to 159 A and 144 A, respectively.

Similar studies on lipids extracted from nervous tissues (total lipid) or sphingomyelin yielded spacing between repeating units of 63.7 A or 66.2 A, respectively. On the basis of such measurements, it was concluded that the spacing between repeating units in the dried myelin fiber (159 A) was filled by a double lipid layer (127 A), separated by a protein layer 20–30 A thick. The difference between fresh and dried myelin was assumed to result from hydration of the protein layer in the fresh myelin.

This molecular model of the myelin sheath was confirmed and extended when electron micrographs of the myelin sheath became available. Under the electron microscope, the myelin sheath appears to be formed of concentric layers; the structure varies depending on the mode of fixation. On osmium-fixed preparations, one can distinguish a 25-A thick main period and an interperiod. Each main period is separated by a clear space (100 A). Such pictures were interpreted with the following considerations in mind: (1) the concentration of lipid in the white matter of brain is high (64.4% of the dry weight); (2) lipid molecules tend to form double layers with facing hydrophobic sites; (3) such a double layer would be 50 A thick.

It is now believed that the area between two consecutive main periods is made of four layers of lipid molecules or of two sets of double layers, in each set of which the hydrophobic ends of the lipid molecules oppose each other and the hydrophilic ends face a water layer. The main period (25–30A) is made of stretch proteins; the inner period, of a thin layer of protein.

The discovery that the myelin sheath was an extension of the plasma membrane of the Schwann cell provided indirect information on the structure of the cell membrane. In 1954, Geren [94] observed that the myelin sheath is formed by the growth of one of the free edges of an invagination of the Schwann cell that surrounds the axon. This free edge is formed by two layers of the plasma membrane of the Schwann cell: the part of the membrane that forms the outer membrane of the Schwann cell and the part opposed to the axon. Both parts are, of course, in continuity at the free edge. The extension of the Schwann cell membrane grows in a spiral and forms concentric layers around the axon (see Figs. 10-19 and 10-20). It is debated whether the Schwann cell turns around the axon or stays in place while its membrane grows and spirals around the axon. The Schmidt-Lanterman clefts are believed to be areas

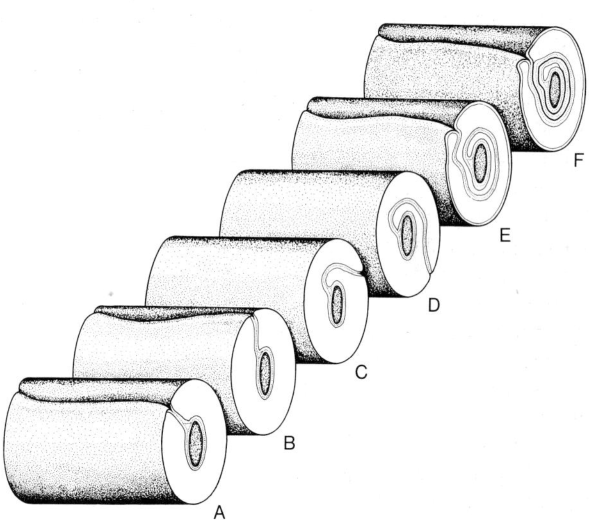

Fig. 10-19. Schematic illustration of the *growth* of the myelin spiral around the axon as observed at a cross section through the developing nerve. (From Sjöstrand [95].) Mechanisms of Demyelination (Pearson, C.M. and Rose, A.S., eds.) 1963, McGraw Hill, New York

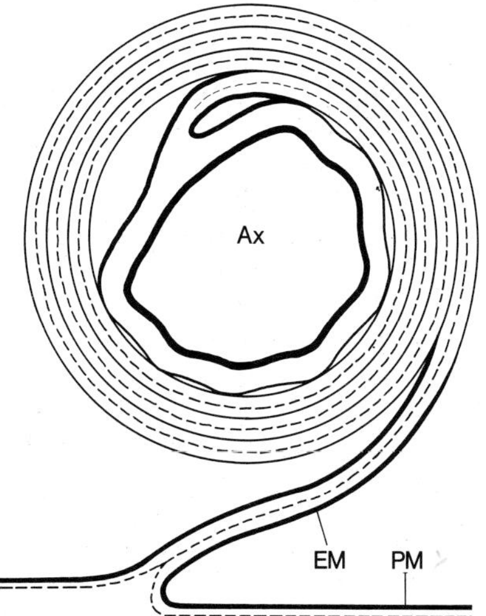

Fig. 10-20. Mechanism of demyelination. Schematic drawing showing the relationship between the Schwann cell plasma membrane (*PM*) and the myelin sheath. *EM* external mesaxon; *Ax* axon. (From Sjöstrand [95].) Mechanisms of Demyelination (Pearson, C.M. and Rose, A.S., eds.) 1963, McGraw Hill, New York

in which the two layers of plasma membrane are separated by cytoplasm derived from the Schwann cells. It is not known what role these clefts play, but it is believed that they favor diffusion of nutrients and waste products.

The kinetics and the detailed molecular mechanism of such extensive membrane growth are not known. Where are the enzymes involved in synthesizing lipids and proteins located? What is the source of energy? Where do the precursors come from? What directs the rigid structural arrangement of the macromolecules involved.

What are the ultrastructural characteristics of the nodes of the Ranvier, and how do they relate to the structure of myelin just described? The expansion of the membrane of the Schwann cell that forms the myelin sheath is not rolled around the axon in the same way as a carpet is rolled around a bamboo stick, but the spiral becomes wider as it becomes longer. As a result, less myelin layers are at the extremities of the long axis of the Schwann cells than are at the center. When the myelin sheath is stained, the nodes of Ranvier correspond to the extremities of the Schwann cells. Therefore, the formation of such nodes can be explained by assuming that the Schwann cells grow while they elaborate the myelin sheath, so that the turns of the spiral, which are expansions of the cell membrane, become wider and wider as the myelin sheath thickens. Such a process would explain the appearance of the node under the electron microscope: at the site of the nodes, a layer of myelin becomes thinner as the distance from the center of the Schwann cell increases.

The space separating the axon from the thin myelin sheaths is filled with infolds of the Schwann cell membrane, which is filled with Schwann cell cytoplasm. In fact, at the junction of two Schwann cells, the cytoplasmic processes of the adjacent cells often interdigitate. Thus, at the node of Ranvier, protection by the insulating myelin is reduced, but contact with Schwann cell cytoplasm is increased. Therefore, it has been proposed that the nodes of Ranvier might be important in conducting the impulse along the axon, and they may affect the axon's nutrition.

The central nervous system does not contain Schwann cells, yet it is rich in myelin fibers. What cell, then, elaborates the myelin? Is myelin production in the central nervous system comparable to its production in the periphery? Electron microscopic studies of myelin genesis in the central nervous system done in a number of laboratories have clearly established that the myelin of the central nervous system is formed by the expansion of membranes of the oligodendrocyte. However, there are two major differences between peripheral and central myelin formation. First, the membrane of the oligodendrocyte can, it is believed, form more than one lip and be at the source of myelin sheaths of several axons. Second, in contrast to the free plasma membrane of the Schwann cell, which is in contact with the extracellular space of the connective tissue, the oligodendrocyte's plasma membrane is more likely to be in contact with other glial cells.

Until about 1950, all analyses of the molecular composition of the brain were made on either whole white or all gray matter. But more recently information on the chemical composition of myelin has become available because myelin fibers can be isolated by density gradient fractionation of myelin-rich fractions. The myelin membrane contains much cholesterol and sphingolipid, and large saturated fatty acids.

When myelin is solubilized, it yields lipoproteins with an average molecular weight of 109,000, composed of 50% phospholipids and galactolipids, 30% proteins, and 20% cholesterol.

Lipid composition of human myelin

	μmoles/mg lipid
Cholesterol	0.775
Cerebroside	0.248
Lecithin	0.116
Cephalin	0.156
Plasmalogen[a]	0.236
Sphingomyelin	0.098
Triglyceride	—
Cholesterol ester	—

[a] Phosphatidyl ethanolamine (a plasmalogen) is a lipid characteristic of myelin; in contrast, choline is distributed equally between gray and white matter, and, although present in myelin, it is not characteristic of that structure.

The presence of the various types of lipids mentioned within myelin has been confirmed by histochemical studies. Histochemical methods used to stain lipids in brain include: (1) the perchloric acid naphthoquinone for cholesterol; (2) gold hydroxamate for cephalin and lecithin; (3) the plasma Feulgen reaction with mercuric chloride and the Schiff reagent; (4) the sodium hydroxide-osmium tetraoxide, D-naphthylamine method; (5) modification of the periodic acid-Schiff method that stains cerebrosides; (6) the cresyl violet acetic acid method that stains sulfatides metachromatically.

Myelin is composed of at least three major proteins: basic protein, proteolipid, and the Wolfgram protein. Two of these proteins form the major protein constituents, and the other exists in smaller amounts. The function of these proteins is unknown.

The basic protein, also called myelin membrane encephalitogenic, is extracted with weak acid and has a molecular weight of 18,000. The amino acid composition and sequence of the human proteins are given in Table 10-4. The sequence contains no cysteine but twelve prolines, and a stretch of four closely spaced proline residues are near the center of the linear sequence of the molecule. Therefore, these prolines are believed to generate a bend of the molecule to give it a hairpin shape. Amino acid substitutions reveal that the amino acid side chains are exposed

Table 10-4. Amino acid sequence of human myelin membrane encephalitogenic protein

Amino acid											
12	Ala	A	8	Gln	Q	8	Leu	L	19	Ser	S
19	Arg	R	1	Glu	E	12	Lys	K	8	Thr	T
1	Asn	N	26	Gly	G	2	Met	M	1	Trp	W
10	Asp	D	10	His	H	9	Phe	F	4	Tyr	Y
0	Cys	C	4	Ile	I	12	Pro	P	4	Val	V

					5					10					15
1	Ala	Ser	Gln	Lys	Arg	Pro	Ser	Gln	Arg	His	Gly	Ser	Lys	Tyr	Leu
16	Ala	Thr	Ala	Ser	Thr	Met	Asp	His	Ala	Arg	His	Gly	Phe	Leu	Pro
31	Arg	His	Arg	Asp	Thr	Gly	Ile	Leu	Asp	Ser	Ile	Gly	Arg	Phe	Phe
46	Gly	Gly	Asp	Arg	Gly	Ala	Pro	Lys	Arg	Gly	Ser	Gly	Lys	Asp	Ser
61	His	His	Pro	Ala	Arg	Thr	Ala	His	Tyr	Gly	Ser	Leu	Pro	Gln	Lys
76	Ser	His	Gly	Arg	Thr	Gln	Asp	Gln	Asp	Pro	Val	Val	His	Phe	Phe
91	Lys	Asn	Ile	Val	Thr	Pro	Arg	Thr	Pro	Pro	Pro	Ser	Gln	Gly	Lys
106	Gly	Arg	Gly	Leu	Ser	Leu	Ser	Arg	Phe	Ser	Trp	Gly	Ala	Glu	Gly
121	Gln	Arg	Pro	Gly	Phe	Gly	Tyr	Gly	Gly	Arg	Ala	Ser	Asp	Tyr	Lys
136	Ser	Ala	His	Lys	Gly	Phe	Lys	Gly	Val	Asp	Ala	Gln	Gly	Thr	Leu
151	Ser	Lys	Ile	Phe	Lys	Leu	Gly	Gly	Arg	Asp	Ser	Arg	Ser	Gly	Ser
166	Pro	Met	Ala	Arg	Arg										

to the solvent, suggesting that the protein may be shaped like a random coil.

Myelin membrane encephalitogenic protein represents 30% of the total myelin protein. It contains several antigenic sites and is the protein responsible for inducing experimental allergic encephalomyelitis (EAE). The active polypeptidic fragment that induces EAE in rabbits appears to be different from that which induces EAE in guinea pigs.

Proteolipid represents approximately 40% of the protein population of myelin. Proteolipid is a glycoprotein soluble in organic solvents (chloroform, ethanol 2–1) and contains 50% nonpolar amino acid—an amino acid composition found only in a few membrane proteins. Its molecular weight is 25,000 with glycine as an NH_2 terminal. Its location and function in the myelin membrane are unknown.

The third class of protein, Wolfgram protein, represents 20% of the total myelin protein. It has a molecular weight of approximately 50,000.

Proteolipids are abundant in white matter of the brain, where they constitute 2% of the fresh tissue weight. They seem to be associated with the myelin of the central nervous system and are absent in special nerves. Although fetal brain contains no proteolipid, the protein does appear when myelin develops. Solubilization methods have permitted investigators to separate three types of proteolipid cells and determine the basis of their lipid content. Cell types A, B, and C contain 15%–25%, 50%, and 75% of lipid, respectively.

Like many other functional proteins, myelin proteins can be phosphorylated. Apparently the phosphorylating enzyme is incorporated in the myelin membrane and catalyzes the transfer of the γ ^{32}P from ATP to the membrane protein. Phosphorylation has been achieved with purified myelin fractions *in vitro* and under *in vivo* conditions. ^{32}P seems to be transferred primarily to serine residues of the basic protein. Myelin obtained from adult rat is more readily phosphorylated than that prepared from 14 day old rats. The difference in phosphorylation between young and old rats seems to be due to the level of protein kinase activity because when rabbit muscle protein kinase was added to the native myelin preparation, the basic proteins of the young rats were as readily phosphorylated as the basic proteins of the old rats. Clearly phosphorylation of myelin seems to play an important role in myelin metabolism, but the exact significance of this role is not established [162].

In conclusion, myelin is composed of ordinary membrane substances such as phospholipids and cholesterol and specific myelin components such as the sphingolipids, glycoproteins and long chain unsaturated hydroxy fatty acids. The biosynthesis of myelin occurs in the oligodendrocytes in the central nervous system and in Schwann cells in the peripheral nerve. It involves two stages: the elaboration of the building blocks and the organization of the elementary component into the macromolecular complex referred to as myelin. Although a great deal is known of the biosynthesis of building blocks (see chapter on inborn errors of metabolism, arteriosclerosis, etc.) the details of the macromolecular assemblage are not known. Brady and Quarles [163] have, however, presented a hypothesis explaining the initiation of myelination. Both the axon and the surface of the oligodendrocyte are believed to be covered with special glycoproteins and gangliosides. During migration oligodendrocytes recognize the axolemmas of the neurons that need myelination. Once neurolemma and oligodendrocytes have come in contact, the neuronal cell produces an inducer, probably cyclic AMP, which triggers the biosynthesis of catabolic extracellular enzymes that convert complex gangliosides to more simple ones. This assumption is based on the fact that the glycoproteins in the immature myelin are made of numerous components while they are converted to a single component with a lower molecular weight in mature myelin. In the process the molecular weight of the glycoprotein changes from 125,000 daltons to 110 daltons. The conversion of the high molecular weight to a low molecular weight glycoprotein reduces the number of hydrophilic sites and thereby renders the glycoprotein more hydrophobic. This change assists the formation of lipid rich myelin lamellae. As myelin further matures more galactocerebrosides are incorporated, thus causing hardening and contributing to the stabilization of the myelin sheath.

Defective myelination could occur from interference with the biosynthesis of the building blocks. Interference with the elaboration of building blocks has been shown to occur in experimental animals under at least two different sets of circumstances. (1) In certain strains of rats with hereditary demyelination in which the following enzyme defects have been demonstrated: UDP-galactose sphingosine galactosyl transferase, UDP-galactose ceramide galactosyl transferase, sphingosine sulfotransferase, cerebroside sulfotransferase and 2′,3′-cyclic AMP 3′-phosphohydrolase [164]. (2) In experiments in which cerebroside antibodies were found to inhibit sulphatide synthesis [165]. In addition defective myelination could result from an inability to assemble the building blocks.

In at least one condition, referred to as dominant inherited hypertrophic neuropathy or Charcot-Marie-Tooth disease, defective myelinization seems to originate from an unknown inborn metabolic derangement in peripheral neurons. The exact nature of the metabolic disorder is not known, but it seems to involve either synthesis, packaging or transport of material needed for development and maintenance of the nerve cell. Because of this defect the axons atrophy with demyelination. Whether damage to the Schwann cells is also involved in the disease has not been determined [166].

Demyelinization

Demyelinization is a form of degeneration of the myelin fiber that may be focal or diffuse. It may be restricted to myelin or associated with death of nerve tissue cells. Demyelinization must be distinguished from absence of myelinization as it occurs in certain forms of inborn errors of metabolism or dysmyelination, that condition in which abnormal myelin is formed because of an enzyme defect (*e.g.*, leukodystrophy).

Numerous injurious agents can induce demyelinization: toxins, viruses, autoimmune diseases, hypoxia, ischemia, salicylate intoxication, encephalitis, anaphylaxis, and sonic trauma. Most diseases of the central nervous system are ultimately demyelinizing, but only relatively few diseases primarily affect the myelin. In diseases in which the damage is primarily in the myelin, referred to as demyelinating diseases, the myelin is injured first and the injury to myelin is preponderant.

The electron microscopic study of demyelination has been reviewed by Sjöstrand [95]. The first observable change is the focal dissociation of concentric myelin layers. Thus, on a transversal section of the myelin sheath, the neat, regular concentric arrangement of superposed myelin layers is interrupted in part, and several layers are separated from the underlying one by an empty space. Later, the layer of myelin that has been displaced from its concentric arrangement becomes irregular and wavy. As Sjöstrand pointed out, interpreted in molecular terms, these events suggest dissociation of the lipid bimolecular layers and distortion of the polar arrangement of the hydrophobic and hydrophilic groups. Such molecular distortions could result from partial hydrolysis of lipids or simply from modifications of the ionic environment.

Axon Degeneration

A simple model for observing demyelinization is axon demyelinization after sectioning of the dorsal root. When the dorsal root of a rat is cut, the axon degenerates within 48 hours after the injury. The myelin sheath splits and the Schwann cells hypertrophy between 48 and 96 hours after the injury. The Schwann cells appear stuffed with disorganized masses of fragmented myelin. However, the model has not permitted investigators to resolve the mechanism of demyelinization. For example, although it appears that degeneration of the axon may constitute a primary event in some forms of demyelinization, axon damage is not observed in all forms of demyelinization. In multiple sclerosis the axons remain remarkably unaffected, at least during the early stages of plaque formation. Even in cases in which axon injuries develop first, the existence of such injuries does not explain demyelinization. It is not known what events start the process.

Allergic Encephalitis

When rhesus monkeys are inoculated three times a week with rabbit or monkey brain, about 2–8 weeks after injection they show signs of paresis or paralysis of one or more extremities, ataxia, and diminution of vision or complete blindness. Although this symptomatology is consistent, the order of appearance of the symptoms is not always the same.

Gross examination of the monkey experimentally afflicted with allergic encephalitis usually reveals no conspicuous changes. Oval yellow, gray, or gray-pinkish plaques appear mainly in the white matter of the cerebrum, the pons, and the optic nerve, and seldom in the gray matter. The plaques are often studded with petechiae; rarely are they frankly hemorrhagic.

Three stages can be distinguished in the histological development of the lesion. In the first few days after onset of the experimental disease, the animals show signs of an acute inflammatory reaction: congestion, edema, polymorphonuclear margination, perivascular accumulation of polymorphonuclears and fibrin with a minimal degree of demyelinization. Thrombi are rarely seen, and perivascular hemorrhage occurs occasionally.

Demyelinization takes place in the perivascular area. At first the zones of demyelinization are discrete, but later they become confluent and large, well-delineated zones of demyelination develop.

Within a few days the acute signs retrocede and a more chronic type of inflammatory reaction is observed. The polymorphonuclears are replaced by lymphocytes and monocytes. Microglial proliferation also appears, but the demyelination persists.

Allergic encephalitis is a clinical model of autoimmune disease that resembles multiple sclerosis in its development. There are, however, major differences between allergic encephalitis and multiple sclerosis, the most striking difference being that the monkey disease has an acute course without relapsing events, whereas the human disease is chronic with relapsing episodes. In spite of these differences, it would appear that a plausible working hypothesis about the pathogenesis of at least some forms of multiple sclerosis is that an autoimmune mechanism causes the nerve tissue to be sensitized in such a way that myelin is destroyed.

Multiple Sclerosis

Multiple sclerosis is a chronic demyelinating disease of the cerebrum, the spinal cord, and the optical track. Clinically, it is characterized by the triad described by Charcot: nystagmus, intention tremor, and slurred speech. These symptoms occur in spurts that are often triggered by fatigue or stress. Because multiple sclerosis was not described by medieval physicians, it is sometimes said that it did not exist before the 19th century. Apparently, the first documented reference to multiple sclerosis is that of Gustave Dustay who suffered from the disease and described his own attacks during periods of remission. Whether the increase in incidence reported in the 19th and 20th centuries resulted from improvement in diagnostic methods or is the consequence of a genuine modification in the ways of life of modern man is not established. However, some believe that the increase in incidence is real and may result from alterations in dietary habits. Excluding psychogenic disorders, multiple sclerosis is the most common disease to affect the nervous system of younger women and men today.

Factors Influencing the Incidence of Multiple Sclerosis

Two factors seem to influence the incidence of multiple sclerosis significantly: heredity and geographic distribution. Multiple sclerosis occurs more frequently among the members of one family (*e.g.*, twins). Whether this reflects a genuine hereditary factor or the existence of well-entrenched familial habits has not been resolved. Curtius [96] believes that there is a genetic element in the etiology of the disease, and he has pointed out that although the incidence in the general population is 1.3–6/10,000, among the families of multiple sclerotics the incidence may be 62/10,000.

A study in New York indicated that the incidence of multiple sclerosis was the same in all racial groups except Negro. As was true for many other rare diseases, an awareness of the high incidence of multiple sclerosis was generated during the wars because of the systematic medical examination of all draftees. In the United States, for example, it soon became obvious that multiple sclerosis is much more common than was originally believed, and that the central northern states seem to be areas where the disease occurs with predilection. Michigan seems to have the highest incidence. Similar studies in Europe suggested that the northern part of a given country, even one as small as Switzerland, or in general the northern part of Europe, is where the disease is most common. In contrast, multiple sclerosis is rare in tropical areas and in Asia, including Japan. Thus, a climatic factor seems to be involved, and northern countries appear more favorable to the development of multiple sclerosis than the southern countries. It is not likely that these trends are due to racial characteristics rather than climatic factors.

Several explanations have been provided for the effect of geography on the incidence of multiple sclerosis. The presence of lead in the soil has sometimes been incriminated. But this explanation is of little value when one considers that some countries (like Spain) where the lead content of the soil is relatively high present a low incidence of multiple sclerosis. Another interpretation centers around the dietary habits in these countries. Fat consumption has often been incriminated, but such epidemiological studies are difficult to interpret.

The epidemiology of multiple sclerosis has also been correlated with the consumption of milk because dairy production and consumption are greater in colder climates than in the warmer climates. Whether or not human or bovine milk consumption can in any way help us understand the pathogenesis of multiple sclerosis remains to be seen [167].

Influenced by the similarities between the epidemiological distribution of multiple sclerosis and acute poliomyelitis, G. Dean has proposed that the former may be caused by a latent virus [97]. This suspicion was confirmed by the studies of the incidence of multiple sclerosis among migrants. Israel is one of the modern centers of immigration. The incidence of multiple sclerosis is low among those who immigrate there at an early age, even if these individuals came from areas where the incidence of multiple sclerosis is high. In contrast, if the person immigrates after the age of 15, the risk of developing multiple sclerosis remains the same as it was in his country of origin. These observations suggest that infection with the latent virus [98–99] must have occurred after the age of 15. The role of viruses in the pathogenesis of multiple sclerosis has not been completely clarified.

Antibody titers against three viruses were measured in patients with multiple sclerosis and normal individuals. No difference was found between the titers of antibodies to the M.S. 6/94 virus, a virus isolated from brain of patients with multiple sclerosis or the parainfluenza virus. Patients with multiple sclerosis did, however, present higher measles antibody titer. This finding differs from what is observed in subacute sclerosing panencephalitis, all three antibodies are pathognomonically increased. Thus, although the isolation of the M.S. 6/94 virus from brains of patients with multiple sclerosis is of interest, the relationship between the virus and the etiology of the disease remains to be clarified by other methods including sophisticated serological approaches [168].

Pathology of Multiple Sclerosis

Two conspicuous histological changes that take place in the brain and the spinal cord of patients with multiple sclerosis are: demyelinization and glial reaction.

Because most of the myelin is in the white matter of the brain, demyelinization primarily affects the white matter. Nevertheless, demyelinization in multiple sclerosis not infrequently involves some of the cortical fibers. In the brain, periventricular regions in the margin between the cortex and the white matter seem to be areas of predilection for demyelinization (see Fig. 10-21). As some pathologists pointed out, this is precisely the location for anatomical lesions such as blood-borne infection and metastatic cancers. The anatomical explanation for this location is simple. The pial arteries that have penetrated the cortex break into small branches, and impaction of small emboli is favored at the branching points.

In multiple sclerosis, demyelinization is usually complete. It starts in small foci, possibly around the venules, and ultimately develops into larger areas of demyelinization with sharp outlines. These larger, macroscopically visible areas (to be described later) are referred to as plaques. Sometimes demyelinization is incomplete and such areas of partially demyelinated tissues are referred to as shadow plaques.

Gliosis is dense in multiple sclerosis due to the accumulation of astrocytes and their fibrous expansions. Usually, oligodendrocytes have disappeared in the areas of a plaque. In contrast, the neurons that are trapped in a plaque or have demyelinated fibers passing through the plaque are remarkably intact, although conduction through the demyelinated axon is impaired.

The injuries that precede plaque formation are not known. The primary injury may involve the oligodendrocyte, which may be specifically damaged and thereby prevented from laying the myelin sheaths. But then why is damage to the oligodendrocytes so restrictive, as it is in multiple sclerosis, and why does it occur in bursts? Some have proposed that the proliferation of astrocytes precedes the myelin destruction. Although astrocyte proliferation is extremely intense, it is difficult to decide whether this is the cause or a result of multiple sclerosis.

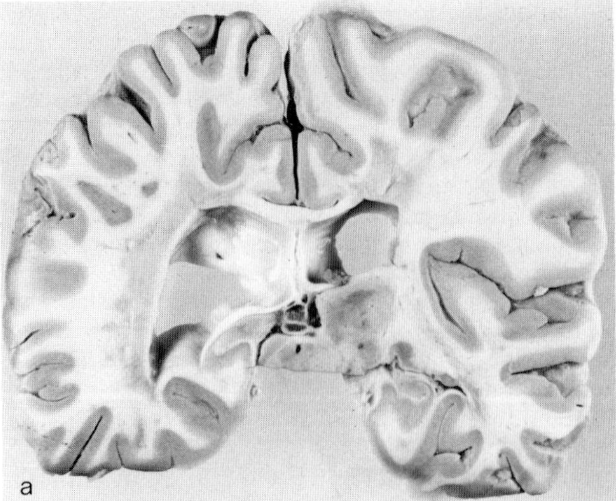

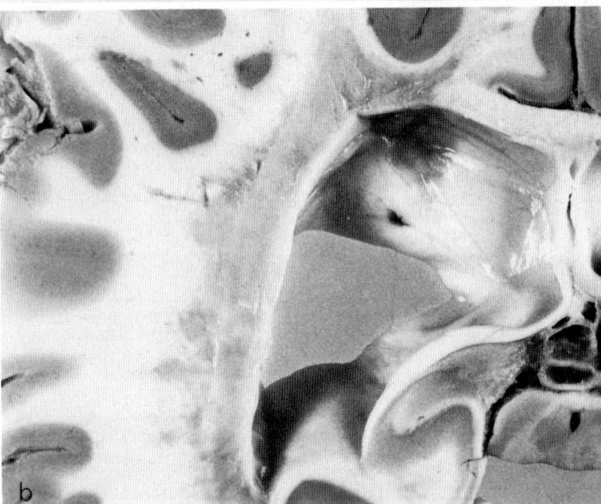

Fig. 10-21a and b. Multiple Sclerosis. (a) Sharply circumscribed zones of demyelination in the white matter adjacent to the ventricles. (b) A gray, irregular but sharply circumscribed zone of demyelination in the white matter adjacent to the ventricle. (From Cancilla)

In 1917, Dawson [100] provided an account of the histopathology of multiple sclerosis that has not been surpassed. Dawson observed that the loss of myelin precedes the infiltration of the area with microglial cells, which rapidly become laden with fat. Demyelinization and lipofibrocytosis are soon followed by proliferation of astrocytes. Dawson was particularly concerned with the vascular changes in multiple sclerosis and believed that dilatation and congestion of the blood vessels constituted the first observable injury in plaque formation. Careful studies brought him to conclude that the formation of small thrombi could be responsible for the development of the plaque. However, investigations on several continents by a number of competent pathologists, usually involving serial section of the spinal cord of patients with multiple sclerosis, have shown that thrombi are only a rare occurrence in multiple sclerosis. Moreover, those found in association with the disease are usually small, white platelet thrombi that do not change as the plaques age. Therefore, these thrombi are more likely to be a coincidental than a causal finding.

This description of the microscopic findings in multiple sclerosis should make it easier to understand the anatomical changes that take place in that disease. Punched-out plaques appear in the brain, the spinal cord, and other parts of the central nervous system. The histological examination of plaques of multiple sclerosis should include special stains for myelin (iron hematoxylin) and for glial fibrosis (crystal violet). Depending upon their age, the plaques may be soft, yellowish, and slightly pink, or hard, grayish, and translucent. The first type corresponds to the period of demyelinization; the second to that of gliosis. The plaques are found in the white matter in the brain. An area of predilection is around the lateral ventricles, especially close to the posterior horns. They can be found anywhere in the spinal cord, and the optical nerves, the optical track, and the chiasma are seldom spared.

To attempt to describe all the symptoms of multiple sclerosis would amount to writing a textbook of neurology because the elementary lesions just described—demyelinization and gliosis—may develop in most parts of the central nervous system. However, some symptoms occur more frequently and almost exclusively in multiple sclerosis, so that the disease can be recognized at some point in its development. Multiple sclerosis is a chronic neurological disease that affects adults and very rarely children or older people. The disease develops in a crisis, with periods of recovery and relapse. After each relapse the disease takes a more severe course, thus inevitably leading to complete degradation. Multiple sclerosis should be diagnosed before Charcot's triad of symptoms is observed. When the triad develops, it is almost a certain signature of multiple sclerosis. The disease affects the sensory and the motor nerves. Irritating paresthesia in the upper or lower limbs may be the first symptom, but alterations of the visual pathway are more typical. A transient blindness of one or both eyes is one highly characteristic symptom of multiple sclerosis. It results from bitemporal hemiatrophy of the optic disc. Characteristically, the patient describes the development of visual dimness that gradually increases in intensity. Within a week, the blindness disappears in a fashion which is the reverse of its development. In the advanced stages of multiple sclerosis, examination of the fundus reveals unilateral, bilateral, and temporal hemiatrophy of the optic disc.

Motor symptoms are always present in multiple sclerosis and may result from damage to the cerebellum. Nystagmus, intention tremor, and slurring of speech are manifestations of cerebellar injury. A common form of motor symptoms is the spastic paraplegia with weakness and stiffness in the lower limbs. The deep reflexes in the lower limbs may be increased and pathological reflexes may be elicited. Superficial reflexes such as Babinski's reflex may be present.

Normal superficial reflexes, particularly in the upper and lower abdomen, are diminished or absent. Usually the disease progresses slowly. Occasionally, it may develop very rapidly as in a rare acute form. The interval between crises varies. Sometimes a patient may live for 20 years without new symptoms. Sometimes the crises recur at short intervals, and the disease becomes fatal within a matter of months.

The fact that experimental allergic encephalitis can be produced by injection of extracts from the central nervous system has brought investigators to examine the possible autoimmune pathogenesis of multiple sclerosis.

Among the arguments invoked in favor of an autoimmune mechanism in the pathogenesis of multiple sclerosis are the observations: (1) that patients with multiple sclerosis contain complement fixing antibodies to the brain (there is, however, no correlation between antibody production and clinical manifestation of the disease); (2) that lymphoblastic transformation (a measure of cellular delayed hypersensitivity) has been demonstrated at least in a proportion of patients with multiple sclerosis; (3) that there exists a correlation between the production of migration inhibition factor (another measure of cellular hypersensitivity) to basic myelin protein and the clinical attacks in multiple sclerosis.

The basic encephalitogen of myelin extracted from either human or bovine brains transforms lymphocytes of patients with multiple sclerosis. The lymphocytes of the patients were exposed to the antigen *in vitro* and their proliferation was measured by the incorporation of tritium labeled thymidine. A positive stimulation was found in 20% of the patients. A correlation between the response to the antigen and the ineffectiveness of steroids in the treatment of the disease seems to have been established [169].

Lymphocytes from normal individuals and patients with multiple sclerosis were cultured in presence of basic myelin protein and the supernatants were assayed for the presence of migration inhibition factor on guinea pigs' peritoneal macrophages. Approximately a 20% drop in the migration inhibition test was observed in patients with multiple sclerosis. When patients with acute exacerbations were compared to convalescent patients, the drop was over 30% in the first group and 12% in the second suggesting a correlation between the cellular hypersensitivity and the development of the attacks [170].

Because multiple sclerosis could well be an autoimmune disease, attempts have been made to treat it by immunosuppression. The immunosuppressants used include intravenous antilymphocytic globulin, thoracic duct drainage, and administration of azathioprine and steroids. Claims have been made that among 20 patients treated with either one or a combination of these modes of therapy, 11 showed significant clinical improvement. A correlation between the level of lymphopenia achieved by the immunosuppressant and reduced symptomatology could be established [171].

Attempts have been made to relate the immunological and the viral component in multiple sclerosis. A virus with an unusually long latent period and replication phase, which preferentially attacks oligodendrocytes, is assumed to be the primary agent in multiple sclerosis. Free virions are undetectable because the viral particles are tightly bound to host cell compartments and no immune response to the virus is elicited in the host because of mechanisms that remain unexplained. The slow virus causes degeneration of the oligodendrocytes. The breakdown of the oligodendrocytes releases substances that are no longer recognized as self and a population of lymphocytes is sensitized. The cellular immune response accelerates the destruction of the infected cells and their myelin sheath eliciting an acute inflammatory response with plaque formation [172]. If the theory is correct, immunosuppression might accelerate oligodendrocyte destruction by the virus and immune stimulation might kill more cells containing the virus, but at the expense of extended damage to the central nervous system because of inflammatory reaction.

Amyotrophic Lateral Sclerosis

This chronic familial disease, described by Charcot, has a slow course that results from the progressive degeneration of the anterior horns of the cervical swelling of the spinal cord and, to a lesser degree, of the Betz cells of the cerebral cortex. In amyotrophic lateral sclerosis, the neurons shrink and decrease in number. There is active glial proliferation, and, as a consequence of neuronal destruction, the lateral and anterior corticopyramidal track atrophies, especially in the medulla oblongata. In fact, close examination of this track reveals demyelinization. The lower motor neurons on the cervical enlargement degenerate first. The small muscles of both hands atrophy with wasting of the thenar and hypothenar eminences. The thumb recedes dorsally as a result of flaccid paralysis and comes in line with the other fingers, giving the hand an ape-type appearance. As amyotrophic lateral sclerosis extends to the upper neurons of the cervical swelling, spastic paralysis of the upper limbs develops with further muscular atrophy. The course of the disease is slow, and as a rule it develops over a period of 10 years. It must be distinguished from muscular dystrophy, which usually involves muscles other than those of the upper limbs, the facial muscles, and the sternocleidomastoid. Amyotrophic lateral sclerosis is readily distinguished from anterior poliomyelitis, which is much more acute and affects primarily the lower limbs. Finally, a frequent source of confusion is syringomyelia, but that disease is frequently associated with sensory symptoms.

A number of degenerative diseases of the central nervous system result in degeneration of neurons at various levels of the central nervous system. The pathogenesis of these diseases is obscure; they may affect the sensory or the motor system. In the motor system, the pyramidal, extrapyramidal, or cerebellar tract can be affected. All these degenerative CNS diseases have the following common demonimator: unknown pathogenesis, system distribution, and effect on the neurons. To explain the occurrence of these degenerative processes in selective parts of the central nervous system, investigators have proposed that these neurons have inherent weaknesses or are unusually prone to develop them earlier.

Conclusion

In spite of much investigative effort, the pathogenesis of multiple sclerosis remains obscure. Two questions must be answered: what is the causative agent and how does demyelination develop? Clues to a plausible pathogenetic mechanism have been obtained from the similarities between the histogenesis of multiple sclerosis and experimental allergic encephalitis, and the discovery that viruses or viral antibodies are often associated with multiple sclerosis.

Both rabies and herpes viruses have been isolated from nerve tissues of patients with multiple sclerosis, but the role of these viruses as causative agents is in doubt.

Controversial reports have appeared on the possibility of transferring scrapie to sheep with brain extracts of deceased multiple sclerosis patients. Measle viruses seem to have emerged as the most popular causative agents. Patients with multiple sclerosis have been shown to have higher serum and cerebrospinal fluid antibody levels of measle virus than controls.

It has also been suggested that the lack of success in detecting the virus in multiple sclerosis is due to the presence of a defective virus that infects the victim at an early age and is activated later. It is, therefore, of interest that parainfluenza 1 virus could be isolated from brain cells of multiple sclerosis patients fused with monkey cells [19]. In these experiments, fusion with the proper cells is believed to have provided a favorable environment for the latent virus development.

Even if it is clearly established that multiple sclerosis is caused by a virus, the mechanisms of demyelination must still be explained. We have mentioned that an autoimmune mechanism has been proposed. How does such a pathogenetic cause relate to a viral infection? One theory suggests that the virus carries with it myelin antigens which, when introduced in the host, sensitize lymphocytes against myelin fibers. Although unproven, such a theory reconciles the evidence in favor of viral and autoimmune etiologies.

References

1. Tavassoli, M., Crosby, W.: Fate of the nucleus of the marrow erythroblast. Science **179**, 912–913 (1973)
2. Bessis, M.: Studies on cell agony and death: an attempt at classification. In: Cellular injury (de Reuck, A.V.S., and Knight, J., eds.). Ciba Foundation Symposium, p. 287–328. London: Churchill 1964
3. Bessis, M.: Cell death. Triangle **9**, 191–199 (1970)
4. Iyer, V.N., Szybalski, W.: Mitomycins and porfiromycin: Chemical mechanism of activation and cross-linking of DNA. Science **145**, 55–58 (1964)
5. Riva, S., Silvestri, L.G.: Rifamycins: A general view. In: Annual review of microbiology (Clifton, C.E., Raffel, S., and Starr, M.P., eds.), vol. 26, p. 199–224. Palo Alto, California: Annual Reviews Inc. 1972
6. Judah, J.D., Spector, W.G.: Reaction of enzymes to injury. Br. med. Bull. **10**, 42–46 (1954)
7. McLean, A.E.M., McLean, E., Judah, J.D.: Cellular necrosis in the liver induced and modified by drugs. Int. Rev. exp. Path. **4**, 127–157 (1965)
8. Trump, B.F., Bulger, R.E.: Studies of cellular injury in isolated flounder tubules. I. Correlation between morphology and function of control tubules and observations of autophagocytosis and mechanical cell damage. Lab. Invest. **16**, 453–482 (1967)
9. Trump, B.F., Bulger, R.E.: Studies of cellular injury in isolated flounder tubules. III. Light microscopic and functional changes due to cyanide. Lab. Invest. **18**, 721–730 (1968)
10. Trump, B.F., Bulger, R.E.: Studies of cellular injury in isolated flounder tubules. IV. Electron microscopic observations of changes during the phase of altered homeostasis in tubules treated with cyanide. Lab. Invest. **18**, 731–739 (1968)
11. de Duve, C.: A new group of cytoplasmic particles. In: Subcellular particles (Hayashi, T., ed.), p. 128–159. New York: Ronald Press 1959
12. de Duve, C.: General properties of lysosomes, the lysosome concept. In: Lysosomes (de Reuck, A.V.S., and Cameron, M.P., eds.). Ciba Foundation Symposium, p. 1–35. Boston: Little, Brown and Company 1963
13. de Duve, C.: From cytases to lysosomes. Fed. Proc. **23**, 1045–1049 (1964)
14. de Duve, C.: The separation and characterization of subcellular particles. Harvey Lecture Series **59**, 49–87 (1963–64)
15. de Duve, C., Gianetto, R., Appelmans, F., Wattiaux, R.: Enzymic content of the mitochondria fraction. Nature (Lond.) **172**, 1143–1144 (1953)
16. Straus, W.: Comparative observations on lysosomes and phagosomes in kidney and liver of rats after administration of horseradish peroxidase. In: Lysosomes (de Reuck, A.V.S., and Cameron, M.P., eds.). Ciba Foundation Symposium, p. 151–175. Boston: Little, Brown and Company 1963
17. Straus, W.: Methods for the study of small phagosomes and of their relationship to lysosomes with horseradish peroxidase as a "marker protein." J. Histochem. Cytochem. **15**, 375–393 (1967)
18. Daems, W.T.: Mouse liver lysosomes and storage. Thesis, Luctor et Emerge, Laden, Belgium 1962
19. Bradley, H.C.: Autolysis and atrophy. Physiol. Rev. **18**, 173–196 (1938)
20. Willstätter, R., Rohdewald, M.: Über desmopepsin (zu-kenntnis zellgebundener Enzyme der Gewebe und Drüsen) und desmo-kathepsin. Ztschr. J. Physiol. Chem. **308**, 258–272 (1932)
21. Berenbom, M., Chang, P.I., Stowell, R.E.: Changes in mouse liver undergoing necrosis *in vivo*. Lab. Invest. **4**, 315–323 (1955)
22. Berenbom, M., Chang, P.I., Betz, H.E., Stowell, R.E.: Chemical and enzymatic changes associated with mouse liver necrosis *in vitro*. Cancer Res. **15**, 1–5 (1955)
23. Van Lancker, J.L., Holtzer, R.L.: The release of acid phosphatase and beta-glucuronidase from cytoplasmic granules in the early course of autolysis. Amer. J. Path. **35**, 563–573 (1959)
24. Van Lancker, J.L., Holtzer, R.L.: The fate of nuclei, deoxyribonucleic acid, and deoxyribonuclease in the course of autolysis. Lab. Invest. **12**, 102–105 (1963)
25. Trump, B.F., Goldblatt, P.J., Stowell, R.E.: An electron microscopic study of early cytoplasmic alteration in hepatic parenchymal cells of mouse liver during necrosis *in vitro* (autolysis). Lab. Invest. **11**, 986–1015 (1962)
26. Weber, R.: Behaviour and properties of acid hydrolases in regressing tails of tadpoles during spontaneous and induced metamorphosis *in vitro*. In: Lysosomes (de Reuck, A.V.S., and Cameron, M.P., eds.). Ciba Foundation Symposium, p. 282–305. Boston: Little, Brown and Company 1963
27. Scheib, D.: Properties and role of acid hydrolases of the Müllerian ducts during sexual differentiation in the male chick embryo. In: Lysosomes (de Reuck, A.V.S., and Cameron, M.P., eds.). Ciba Foundation Symposium, p. 264–281. Boston: Little, Brown and Company 1963
28. Slater, T.F., Greenbaum, A.L., Wang, D.Y.: Lysosomes and pathological cell damage. Lysosomal changes during liver injury and mammary involution. In: Lysosomes (de Reuck, A.V.S., and Cameron, M.P., eds.). Ciba Foundation Symposium, p. 311–334. Boston: Little, Brown and Company 1963
29. Saunders, J.W., Jr., Fallon, J.P.: Cell death in morphogenesis. In: Major problems in developmental biology (Locke, M., ed.), p. 289. New York: Academic Press 1966
30. Ashford, T.P., Porter, K.R.: Cytoplasmic components in hepatic cell lysosomes. J. Cell Biol. **12**, 198–202 (1962)
31. Hruban, Z., Swift, H., Wissler, R.W.: Analog-induced inclusion in pancreatic acinar cells. J. Ultrastruct. Res. **7**, 273–285 (1962)
32. Hruban, Z., Swift, H., Wissler, R.W.: Effect of beta-3-thienylalanine on the formation of zymogen granules of exocrine pancreas. J. Ultrastruct. Res. **7**, 359–372 (1962)
33. Swift, H., Hruban, Z.: Focal degradation as a biological process. Fed. Proc. **23**, 1026–1037 (1964)
34. Winborn, W.B., Bockman, D.E.: Origin of lysosomes in parietal cells. Lab. Invest. **19**, 256–264 (1968)
35. Van Lancker, J.L.: Hydrolases and cellular death. In: Metabolic conjugation and metabolic hydrolysis (Fishman, W.H., ed.), vol. I, p. 356–418. New York: Academic Press 1970
36. Arstila, A.U., Trump, B.F.: Studies on cellular autophagocytosis. Amer. J. Path. **53**, 687–733 (1968)
37. Fishman, W.H., Goldman, S.S., DeLellis, R.: Dual localization of β-glucuronidase in endoplasmic reticulum and in lysosomes. Nature (Lond.) **213**, 457–460 (1967)
38. Fonnesu, A.: Changes in energy transformation as an early response to cell injury. In: The biochemical response to injury (Stoner, H.B., and Threlfall, C.J., eds.). Symp. Council Int. Org. Med. Sci., p. 85–104. Springfield, Ill.: Charles C. Thomas Publisher 1960
39. Trémolières, J., Derache, R.: Métabolisme des composés phosphorés et spécialement des nucléotides dans le tissu traumatisé. In: The biochemical response to injury (Stoner, H.B., and Threlfall, C.J., eds.). Symp. Council Int. Org. Med. Sci., p. 23–50. Springfield, Ill.: Charles C. Thomas Publisher 1960
40. Van Lancker, J.L., Gottlieb, L.I.: Unpublished results
41. Vogt, M.T., Farber, E.: On the molecular pathology of ischemic renal cell death: reversible and irreversible cellular and mitochondrial metabolic alterations. Amer. J. Path. **53**, 1–26 (1968)
42. Judah, J.D., Ahmed, K., McLean, A.E.M., Christie, G.S.: Ion transport in ethionine intoxication. Lab. Invest. **15**, 167–175 (1966)
43. Busch, H.: Chemistry of pancreatic diseases. Springfield, Ill.: Charles C. Thomas Publisher 1959
44. Wanke, M.: Experimental acute pancreatitis. Curr. Top. Path. **52**, 64–142 (1970)
45. Polya, E.: Die Wirkung des Trypsins auf das lebende Pankreas. Pflügers Arch. ges. Physiol. **121**, 483–507 (1908)
46. Guenter, C.A., Welch, M.H., Hammarsten, J.F.: Alpha_1 antitrypsin deficiency and pulmonary emphysema. Annu. Rev. Med. **22**, 283–292 (1971)
47. Sharp, H.L.: Alpha-1-antitrypsin deficiency. Hosp. Prac. **6**(5), 83–96 (1971)
48. Handschumacher, R.E., Creasey, W.A., Jaffe, J.J., Pasternak, C.A., Hankin, L.: Biochemical and nutritional studies on the induction of fatty livers by dietary orotic acid. Proc. nat. Acad. Sci. (Wash.) **46**, 178–186 (1960)
49. Lombardi, B.: Considerations on the pathogenesis of fatty liver. Lab. Invest. **15**, 1–20 (1966)
50. Lombardi, B.: Pathogenesis of fatty liver. Fed. Proc. **24**, 1200–1205 (1965)
51. Recknagel, R.O., Litteria, M.: Activation of acid phosphatase in carbon tetrachloride fatty liver. Fed. Proc. **18**, 125 (1959)
52. Recknagel, R.O., Lombardi, B.: Studies of biochemical changes in subcellular particles of rat liver and their relationship to a new hypothesis regarding the pathogenesis of carbon tetrachloride fat accumulation. J. biol. Chem. **236**, 564–569 (1961)
53. Smuckler, E.A., Iseri, O.A., Benditt, E.P.: Studies on carbon tetrachloride intoxication. II. Depressed amino acid incorporation into mitochondrial protein and cytochrome C. Lab. Invest. **13**, 531–538 (1964)
54. Smuckler, E.A., Iseri, O.A., Benditt, E.P.: An intracellular defect in protein synthesis induced by carbon tetrachloride. J. exp. Med. **116**, 55–72 (1962)
55. Smuckler, E.A., Iseri, O.A., Benditt, E.P.: Studies on carbon tetrachloride intoxication. I. The effect of carbon tetrachloride on incorporation of labeled amino acids into plasma proteins. Biochem. biophys. Res. Commun. **5**, 270–275 (1961)
56. Smuckler, E.A., Benditt, E.P.: Carbon tetrachloride poisoning in rats: alteration in ribosomes of the liver. Science **140**, 308–310 (1963)
57. Meldolesi, J., Vincenzi, L., Bassan, P., Morini, M.T.: Effect of carbon tetrachloride on the synthesis of liver endoplasmic reticulum membranes. Lab. Invest. **19**, 315–323 (1968)
58. Slater, T.F., Greenbaum, A.L.: Changes in lysosomal enzymes in acute experimental liver injury. Biochem. J. **96**, 484–491 (1965)
59. Butler, T.C.: Reduction of carbon tetrachloride *in vivo* and reduction of carbon tetrachloride and chloroform *in vitro* by tissues and tissue constituents. J. Pharmacol. exp. Ther. **134**, 311–319 (1961)
60. Recknagel, R.O.: Carbon tetrachloride hepatotoxicity. Pharmacol. Rev. **19**, 145–208 (1967)
61. Dianzani, M.U., Baccino, F.M., Comporti, M.: The direct effect of carbon tetrachloride on subcellular particles. Lab. Invest. **15**, 149–156 (1966)
62. Bernheim, M.L.: The effect of carbon tetrachloride, ethionine and chloretone on the ascorbic acid content of rat liver. Biochem. Pharmacol. **7**, 59–64 (1961)

63. Arstila, A.V., Smith, M.A., Trump, B.F.: Microsomal lipid peroxidation: morphological characterization. Science **175**, 530–532 (1972)
64. Thomas, H.V., Mueller, P.K., Lyman, R.L.: Lipoperoxidation of lung lipids in rats exposed to nitrogen dioxide. Science **159**, 532–534 (1968)
65. Theorell, H.: Function and structure of liver alcohol dehydrogenase. Harvey Lecture Series **61**, 17–41 (1965)
66. Forsander, O.A.: The role of metabolism in alcohol consumption. In: Biochemical factors in alcoholism (Maickel, R.P., ed.), p. 7–16. Oxford: Pergamon Press 1967
67. von Wartburg, J.P.: The metabolism of alcohol in normals and alcoholics: enzymes. In: The biology of alcoholism (Kissin, B., and Begleiter, H., eds.), vol. 1, Biochemistry, p. 63–102. New York: Plenum Publishing Corporation 1971
68. Bäcklin, K.I.: The equilibrium constant of the system ethanol, aldehyde, DPN^+, DPNH, and H^+. Acta chem. scand. **12**, 1279–1285 (1958)
69. Hartroft, W.S.: Alcohol, metabolism and liver disease. Nutrition Soc. Symp., Introductory Remarks. Fed. Proc. **26**, 1432–1435 (1967)
70. Porta, E.A., Hartroft, W.S., de la Iglesia, F.A.: Structural and ultrastructural hepatic lesions associated with acute and chronic alcoholism in man and experimental animals. In: Biochemical factors in alcoholism (Maickel, R.P., ed.), p. 201–238. Oxford: Pergamon Press 1967
71. Truitt, E.B., Jr., Duritz, G.: The role of acetaldehyde in the actions of ethanol. In: Biochemical factors in alcoholism (Maickel, R.P., ed.), p. 61–69. Oxford: Pergamon Press 1967
72. Truitt, E.B., Jr., Walsh, M.J.: The role of acetaldehyde in the actions of ethanol. In: The biology of alcoholism (Kissin, B., and Begleiter, H., eds.), vol. I, Biochemistry, p. 161–195. New York: Plenum Publishing Corporation 1971
73. Lieber, C.S., Rubin, E., DeCarli, L.M.: Effects of ethanol on lipid, uric acid, intermediary, and drug metabolism, including the pathogenesis of the alcoholic fatty liver. In: The biology of alcoholism (Kissin, B., and Begleiter, H., eds.), vol. I, Biochemistry, p. 263–305. New York: Plenum Publishing Corporation 1971
74. Kalant, H., Israel, Y.: Effects of ethanol on active transport of cations. In: Biochemical factors in alcoholism (Maickel, R.P., ed.), p. 25–37. Oxford: Pergamon Press 1967
75. Mendelson, J.H.: Biologic concomitants of alcoholism. I. First of two parts. New Engl. J. Med. **283**, 24–32 (1970)
76. Beard, J.D., Knott, B.H.: The effect of alcohol on fluid and electrolyte metabolism. In: The biology of alcoholism (Kissin, B., and Begleiter, H., eds.), vol. I, Biochemistry, p. 353–376. New York: Plenum Publishing Corporation 1971
77. Di Luzio, N.R., Poggi, M.: Pathogenesis of the acute ethanol-induced fatty liver. In: Biochemical factors in alcoholism (Maickel, R.P., ed.), p. 127–138. Oxford: Pergamon Press 1967
78. Kiessling, K.H., Tobé, U.: Degeneration of liver mitochondria in rats after prolonged alcohol consumption. Exp. Cell Res. **33**, 350–354 (1964)
79. Porta, E.A., Hartroft, W.S., Gomez-Dumm, C.L.A., Koch, O.R.: Dietary factors in the progression and regression of hepatic alterations associated with experimental chronic alcoholism. Fed. Proc. **26**, 1449–1457 (1967)
80. Rubin, E., Lieber, C.S.: Experimental alcoholic hepatic injury in man: ultrastructural changes. Fed. Proc. **26**, 1458–1467 (1967)
81. Rubin, E., Lieber, C.S.: Alcoholism, alcohol, and drugs. Science **172**, 1097–1102 (1971)
82. Rubin, E., Beattie, D.S., Toth, T., Lieber, C.S.: Structural and functional effects of ethanol on hepatic mitochondria. Fed. Proc. **31**, 131–140 (1972)
83. Kakihana, R., Brown, D.R., McClearn, G.E., Tabershaw, I.R.: Brain sensitivity to alcohol in inbred mouse strains. Science **154**, 1574–1575 (1966)
84. Burch, G.E., DePasquale, N.P.: Alcoholic lung disease—an hypothesis. Amer. Heart J. **73**, 147–148 (1967)
85. Kedinger, C., Gniazdowski, M., Mandel, J.L., Jr., Gissinger, F., Chambon, P.: α-Amanitin: a specific inhibitor of one of two DNA-dependent RNA polymerase activities from calf thymus. Biochem. biophys. Res. Commun. **38**, 165–171 (1970)
86. Mancino, G., Nardi, I., Covaja, N., Fruime, L., Marinozzi, V.: Effects of α-amanitin on Triturus lampbrush chromosomes. Exp. Cell Res. **64**, n37–239 (1971)
87. Lubarsch, O.: Zur Kenntnis unngewöhnlicher Amyloidablagerungen. Virchows Arch. path. Anat. **271**, 867–889 (1929)
88. Cohen, A.S.: Amyloidosis. New Engl. J. Med. **277**, 522–530 (1967)
89. Azar, H.A.: Amyloidosis and plasma cell disorders. Annu. Rev. Med. **17**, 49–62 (1966)
90. Cohen, A.S.: Preliminary chemical analysis of partially purified amyloid fibrils. Lab. Invest. **15**, 66–83 (1966)
91. Cohen, A.S.: The constitution and genesis of amyloid. Int. Rev. exp. Path. **4**, 159–243 (1965)
92. Ein, D., Kimura, S., Terry, W.D., Magnotta, J., Glenner, G.G.: Amino acid sequence of an amyloid fibril protein of unknown origin. J. biol. Chem. **247**, 5653–5655 (1972)
93. Dustin, P., Jr.: Arteriolar hyalinosis. Int. Rev. exp. Path. **1**, 73–138 (1962)
94. Geren, B.B.: The formation from the Schwann cell surface of myelin in the peripheral nerves of chick embryos. Exp. Cell Res. **7**, 558–562 (1954)
95. Sjöstrand, F.S.: The structure and formation of the myelin sheath. In: Mechanisms of demyelination (Rose, A.S., and Pearson, C.M., eds.), p. 1–43. New York: Blakiston Division, McGraw-Hill Book Company 1963
96. Curtius, F.: Multiple Sklerose und Erbanlage. Leipzig: Georg Thieme 1933
97. Dean, G.: The multiple sclerosis problem. Sci. Amer. **223**, 40–46 (1970)
98. Payne, F.E., Baublis, J.V., Itabashi, H.H.: Isolation of measles virus from cell cultures of brain from a patient with subacute sclerosing panencephalitis. New Engl. J. Med. **281**, 585–589 (1969)
99. Pette, E.: Measles virus: a causative agent in multiple sclerosis? Neurology (Minneap.) **18**, 168–169 (1968)
100. Dawson, J.W.: The histology of disseminated sclerosis. IV. Histological study, p. 47–166; V. Pathogenesis and etiology, p. 369–417. Rev. Neurol. Psychiat. **15** (1917)
101. Sobell, H.M.: The stereochemistry of actinomycin binding to DNA. Cancer Chemother. Rep. *58*, 101–116 (1974)
102. Tsai, M.-J., Saunders, G.F.: Action of rifamycin derivatives on RNA polymerase of human leukemic lymphocytes. Proc. nat. Acad. Sci. (Wash.) **70**, 2072–2076 (1973)
103. Decker, K., Keppler, D.: Galactosamine hepatitis: Key role of the nucleotide deficiency period in the pathogenesis of cell injury and cell death. Rev. Physiol. Biochem. Pharmacol. **71**, 77–106 (1974)
104. Reddy, J.K., Chiga, M., Harris, C.C., Svoboda, D.J.: Polyribosome disaggregation in rat liver following administration of tannic acid. Cancer Res. **30**, 58–65 (1970)
105. Bernelli-Zazzera, A.: Ribosomes in dying liver cells. IV. Workshop on experimental liver injury, "Pathogenesis and mechanisms of liver cell necrosis", Freiburg, November 9 and 10, 1974 (in print) (1974)
106. Seeman, P.: Ultrastructure of membrane lesions in immune lysis, osmotic lysis and drug-induced lysis. Fed. Proc. **33**, 2116–2124 (1974)
107. Whalen, D.A., Jr., Hamilton, D.G., Ganote, C.E., Jennings, R.B.: Effect of a transient period of ischemia on myocardial cells. Amer. J. Path. **74**, 381–398 (1974)
108. Kloner, R.A., Ganote, C.E., Whalen, D.A., Jr., Jennings, R.B.: Effects of a transient period of ischemia on myocardial cells. II. Fine structure during the first few minutes of reflow. Amer. J. Path. **74**, 399–422 (1974)
109. Conrad, M.J., Penniston, J.T.: Surface proteins of the erythrocyte membrane effect of aging. Vox Sang. (Basel) **26**, 1–13 (1974)
110. Shohet, S.B., Nathan, D.G., Livermore, B.M., Feig, S.A., Jaffé, E.R.: Hereditary hemolytic anemia associated with abnormal membrane lipid. II. Ion permeability and transport abnormalities. Blood **42**, 1–8 (1973)
111. Jaffé, E.R., Gottfried, E.L.: Hereditary nonspherocytic hemolytic disease associated with an altered phospholysed composition of the erythrocytes. J. clin. Invest. **47**, 1375–1388 (1968)
112. Jacob, H.S., Ruby, A., Overland, E.S., Mazia, D.: Abnormal membrane protein of red blood cells in hereditary spherocytosis. J. clin. Invest. **50**, 1800–1805 (1971)
113. Frimmer, M.: Phalloidin, a membrane specific toxin. IV. Workshop on experimental liver injury, "Pathogenesis and mechanisms of liver cell necrosis", Freiburg, November 9 and 10. 1974 (in print) (1974)
114. Govindan, V.M., Faulstich, H., Wieland, Th., Agostini, B., Hasselbach, W.: In-vitro effect of phalloidin on a plasma membrane preparation from rat liver. Naturwissenschaften **59**, 521–522 (1972)
115. Palade, G.E., Farquhar, M.G.: Cell junctions in amphibian skin. J. Cell Biol. **26**, 263–291 (1965)
116. Wieland, Th., Löw, I., Govindan, V.M., Faulstich, H.: Interaction of phalloidin with actin. IV. Workshop on experimental liver injury, "Pathogenesis and mechanisms of liver cell necrosis", Freiburg, November 9 and 10, 1974 (in print) (1974)
117. Kamath, S.A., Rubin, E.: Effects of carbon tetrachloride and phenobarbital on plasma membranes; enzymes and phospholipid transfer. Lab. Invest. **30**, 494–499 (1974)
118. Farquhar, M.G.: Lysosome function in regulating secretion: disposal of secretory granules in cells of the anterior pituitary gland. In: Lysosomes in biology and pathology (Dingle, J.T., and Fell, H.B., eds.), vol. 2, p. 462–482. Amsterdam: North-Holland Publishing Co. 1973
119. Steiner, D.F., Kemmler, W., Tager, H.S., Peterson, J.D.: Proteolytic processing in the biosynthesis of insulin and other proteins. Fed. Proc. **33**, 2105–2115 (1974)
120. Decker, K.: Quantitative aspects of biochemical mechanisms leading to cell death. IV. Workshop on experimental liver injury, "Pathogenesis and mechanisms of liver cell necrosis", Freiburg, November 9 and 10, 1974 (in print) (1974)
121. Latta, H., Osvaldo, L., Jackson, J.D., Cook, M.L.: Changes in renal cortical tubules during autolysis; electron microscopic observations. Lab. Invest. **14**, 635–657 (1965)
122. Lieberman, M.W., Verbin, R.S., Landay, M., Liang, H., Farber, E., Lee, T.-N., Starr, R.: A probable role for protein synthesis in intestinal epithelial cell damage induced *in vivo* by cytosine arabinoside, nitrogen mustard, or x-irradiation. Cancer Res. **30**, 942–951 (1970)
123. Flaks, B., Nicoll, J.W.: Modification of toxic liver injury in the rat; I. Effect of inhibition of protein synthesis on the action of 2-acetylaminofluorene, carbon tetrachloride, 3′-methyl-4-dimethylaminobenzene and diethylnitrosamine. Chem.-Biol. Interactions **8**, 135–150 (1974)
124. Smith, W.W., Carter, S.K., Wilson, S.M., Newman, J.W., Cornfield, J.: Joint lethal effects of actinomycin D and radiation in mice. Cancer Res. **30**, 51–57 (1970)

125. Krizek, D.T., McIlrath, W.J., Vergara, B.S.: Photoperiodic induction of senescence in Xanthium plants. Science **151**, 95–96 (1966)
126. Basile, D.V., Wood, H.N., Braun, A.C.: Programming of cells for death under defined experimental conditions: Relevance to the tumor problem. Proc. nat. Acad. Sci. (Wash.) **70**, 3055–3059 (1973)
127. Crawford, G.P.M., Ogston, D.: The influence of α-1-antitrypsin on plasmin, urokinase and Hageman factor cofactor. Biochim. biophys. Acta (Amst.) **354**, 107–113 (1974)
128. Moroi, M., Yamasaki, M.: Mechanism of interaction of bovine trypsin with human α_1-antitrypsin. Biochem. biophys. Acta (Amst.) **359**, 130–141 (1974)
129. Kuhlenschmidt, M.S., Yunis, E.J., Iammarino, R.M., Turco, S.J., Peters, S.P., Glew, R.H.: Demonstration of sialyltransferase deficiency in the serum of a patient with α-1-antitrypsin deficiency and hepatic cirrhosis. Lab. Invest. **31**, 413–419 (1974)
130. Rolfe, B.G., Campbell, J.H.: A relationship between tolerance to Colicin K and the mechanism of phage-induced host cell lysis. Molec. gen. Genet. **133**, 293–297 (1974)
131. Reynolds, E.S., Moslen, M.T.: *In vivo* covalent binding of $^{14}CCl_4$ metabolites in liver microsomal lipids. Biochem. biophys. Res. Commun. **57**, 747–750 (1974)
132. Slater, T.F.: The role of lipid peroxidation in liver injury. IV. Workshop on experimental liver injury, "Pathogenesis and mechanisms of liver cell necrosis", Freiburg, November 9 and 10, 1974 (in print) (1974)
133. Leech, R.W., Alvord, E.C., Jr.: Glial fatty metamorphosis. Amer. J. Path. **74**, 603–612 (1973)
134. Jörnvall, H.: Functional aspects of structural studies of alcohol dehydrogenases. In: Alcohol and aldehyde metabolizing systems (Thurman, R.G., Yonetani, T., Williamson, J.R., and Chance, B., eds.), p. 23–32. New York: Academic Press, Inc. 1974
135. Bränden, C.-I., Eklund, H., Zeppezauer, E., Nordström, B., Boiwe, T., Söderlund, G., Ohlsson, I.: Three-dimensional structure of the horse liver alcohol dehydrogenase molecule. In: Alcohol and aldehyde metabolizing systems (Thurman, R.G., Yonetani, T., Williamson, J.R., and Chance, B., eds.), p. 7–21. New York: Academic Press, Inc. 1974
136. Korsten, M.A., Matsuzaki, S., Feinman, L., Lieber, C.S.: High blood acetaldehyde levels after ethanol administration. New Engl. J. Med. **292**, 386–389 (1975)
137. von Wartburg, J.P., Berger, D., Bühlmann, Ch., Dubied, A., Ris, M.M.: Heterogeneity of pyridine nucleotide dependent alcohol and aldehyde metabolizing enzymes. In: Alcohol and aldehyde metabolizing systems (Thurman, R.G., Yonetani, T., Williamson, J.R., and Chance, B., eds.), p. 33–44. New York: Academic Press, Inc. 1974
138. Tottmar, S.O.C., Pettersson, H., Kiessling, K.-H.: Aldehyde dehydrogenases in rat liver. In: Alcohol and aldehyde metabolizing systems (Thurman, R.G., Yonetani, T., Williamson, J.R., and Chance, B., eds.), p. 147–160. New York: Academic Press, Inc. 1974
139. de Duve, C.: Intracellular localization, biosynthesis, and functions of rat liver catalase. In: Alcohol and aldehyde metabolizing systems (Thurman, R.G., Yonetani, T., Williamson, J.R., and Chance, B., eds.), p. 161–168. New York: Academic Press, Inc. 1974
140. Chance, B., Oshino, N., Sugano, T., Jamieson, D.: Role of catalase in ethanol metabolism. In: Alcohol and aldehyde metabolizing systems (Thurman, R.G., Yonetani, T., Williamson, J.R., and Chance, B., eds.), p. 169–182. New York: Academic Press, Inc. 1974
141. Oshino, N., Oshino, R., Chance, B.: The properties of catalase "peroxidatic" reaction and its relationship to microsomal methanol oxidation. In: Alcohol and aldehyde metabolizing systems (Thurman, R.G., Yonetani, T., Williamson, J.R., and Chance, B., eds.), p. 231–242. New York: Academic Press, Inc. 1974
142. Lundquist, F.: Influence of ethanol upon intermediary metabolism—Session eight. In: Alcohol and aldehyde metabolizing systems (Thurman, R.G., Yonetani, T., Williamson, J.R., and Chance, B., eds.), p. 564–565. New York: Academic Press, Inc. 1974
143. Williamson, J.R., Ohkawa, K., Meijer, A.J.: Regulation of ethanol oxidation in isolated rat liver cells. In: Alcohol and aldehyde metabolizing systems (Thurman, R.G., Yonetani, T., Williamson, J.R., and Chance, B., eds.), p. 365–381. New York: Academic Press, Inc. 1974
144. Krebs, H.A., Hems, R., Lund, P.: Some regulatory mechanisms in the synthesis of urea in the mammalian liver. In: Advances in enzyme regulation (Weber, G., ed.), vol. 11, p. 361–377. Oxford, England: Pergamon Press Ltd. 1973
145. Rubin, E., Cederbaum, A.I.: Effects of chronic ethanol feeding and acetaldehyde on mitochondrial functions and the transfer of reducing equivalents. In: Alcohol and aldehyde metabolizing systems (Thurman, R.G., Yonetani, T., Williamson, J.R., and Chance, B., eds.), p. 435–455. New York: Academic Press, Inc. 1974
146. Basile, D.V., Wood, H.N., Braun, A.C.: Programming of cells for death under defined experimental conditions: Relevance to the tumor problem. Proc. nat. Acad. Sci. (Wash.) **70**, 3055–3059 (1973)
147. Morse, J.O., Lebowitz, M.D., Knudson, R.J., Burrows, B.: A community study of the relation of alpha$_1$-antitrypsin levels to obstructive lung diseases. New Engl. J. Med. **292**, 278–281 (1975)
148. Acute pancreatitis, editorial. Lancet **1975I**, 205–206
149. Scholz, R., Kaltstein, A., Schwabe, U., Thurman, R.G.: Inhibition of fatty acid synthesis from carbohydrates in perfused rat liver by ethanol. In: Alcohol and aldehyde metabolizing systems (Thurman, R.G., Yonetani, T., Williamson, J.R., and Chance, B., eds.), p. 315–328. New York: Academic Press, Inc. 1974
150. Gordon, E.R.: Mitochondrial functions in an ethanol-induced fatty liver. J. biol. Chem. **248**, 8271–8280 (1973)
151. Jones, K.L., Smith, D.W., Streissguth, A.P., Myrianthopoulos, N.C.: Outcome in offspring of chronic alcoholic women. Lancet **1974I**, 1076–1078
152. Thaler, M.M., Hoogenraad, N.J., Boswell, M.: Reye's syndrome due to a novel protein-tolerant variant of ornithine-transcarbamylase deficiency. Lancet **1974II**, 438–440
153. Prince, A.M.: An antigen detected in the blood during the incubation period of serum hepatitis. Proc. nat. Acad. Sci. (Wash.) **60**, 814–821 (1968)
154. Dane, D.S., Cameron, C.H., Briggs, M.: Virus-like particles in serum of patients with Australia-antigen-associated hepatitis. Lancet **1970I**, 695–698
155. Nielsen, J.O., Nielsen, M.H., Elling, P.: Differential distribution of Australia-antigen-associated particles in patients with liver diseases and normal carriers. New Engl. J. Med. **288**, 484–487 (1973)
156. Hoofnagle, J.H., Gerety, R.J., Ni, L.Y., Barker, L.F.: Antibody to hepatitis B core antigen. New Engl. J. Med. **290**, 1336–1340 (1974)
157. Skikne, M.I., Talbot, J.H.: The identification and structural analysis of viral particles in serum hepatitis. Lab. Invest. **31**, 246–249 (1974)
158. Almeida, J.D., Gay, F.W., Wreghitt, T.G.: Pitfalls in the study of hepatitis A. Lancet **1974II**, 748–751
159. Sabesin, S.M., Koff, R.S.: Pathogenesis of experimental viral hepatitis. New Engl. J. Med. **290**, 996–1002 (1974)
160. Litten, W.: The most poisonous mushrooms. Sci. Amer. **232**, 91–101 (1975)
161. Glenner, G.G., Terry, W.D.: Characterization of amyloid. In: Annual review of medicine (Creger, W.P., Coggins, C.H., and Hancock, E.W., eds), vol. 25, p. 131–135. Palo Alto, Calif.: Annual Reviews Inc. 1974
162. Steck, A.J., Appel, S.H.: Phosphorylation of myelin basic protein. J. biol. Chem. **249**, 5416–5420 (1974)
163. Brady, R.O., Quarles, R.H.: The enzymology of myelination. Molec. Cellular Biochem. **2**, 23–29 (1973)
164. Mandel, P., Nussbaum, J.L., Neskovic, N.M., Sarlieve, L.L., Kurihara, T.: Regulation of myelinogenesis. In: Advances in enzyme regulation (Weber, G., ed.), vol. 10, p. 101–118. Oxford, England: Pergamon Press Ltd. 1972
165. Fry, J.M., Weissbarth, S., Lehrer, G.M., Bornstein, M.B.: Cerebroside antibody inhibits sulfatide synthesis and myelination and demyelinates in cord tissue cultures. Science **183**, 540–542 (1974)
166. Dyck, P.J., Lais, A.C., Offord, K.P.: The nature of myelinated nerve fiber degeneration in dominantly inherited hypertrophic neuropathy. Mayo Clin. Proc. **49**, 34–39 (1974)
167. Agranoff, B.W., Goldberg, D.: Diet and the geographical distribution of multiple sclerosis. Lancet **1974II**, 1061–1066
168. Nemo, G.J., Brody, J.A., Waters, D.J.: Serological responses of multiple-sclerosis patients and controls to a virus isolated from a multiple-sclerosis case. Lancet **1974II**, 1044–1046
169. Webb, C., Teitelbaum, D., Abramsky, O., Arnon, R., Sela, M.: Lymphocytes sensitised to basic encephalitogen in patients with multiple sclerosis unresponsive to steroid therapy. Lancet **1974II**, 66–68
170. Sheremata, W., Cosgrove, J.B.R., Eylar, E.H.: Cellular hypersensitivity to basic myelin (A_1) protein and clinical multiple sclerosis. New Engl. J. Med. **291**, 14–17 (1974)
171. Ring, J., Seifert, J., Lob, G., Coulin, K., Angstwurm, H., et al.: Intensive immunosuppression in the treatment of multiple sclerosis. Lancet **1974II**, 1093–1096
172. Adams, D.H., Dickinson, J.P.: Aetiology of multiple sclerosis. Lancet **1974I**, 1196–1199

Chapter 11

Blood Lipids in Arteriosclerosis and Hyperlipidemia

Atherosclerosis 679

Introduction 679

Morphology of the Arteries 679

Biochemistry 679

Arterial Regeneration 680

Elementary Lesions in Atherosclerosis 681

Edema 681
Endothelial Injuries 682
Smooth Muscle Proliferation 683
Lipid Accumulation 683
Fibrosis 683
Thrombosis 684

Fat Metabolism and Atherosclerosis 685

Fat Metabolism: Absorption of Fats 685
Blood Lipoproteins 687
Apoproteins
Blood Lipids 689
Origin of Blood Lipoproteins 690
Triglyceride Synthesis in Liver and Intestine

Cholesterol Metabolism 692

Exogenous Cholesterol 692
Endogenous Cholesterol 693
Mevalonic Acid Formation 693
Squalene Formation 694
Squalene Conversion
Regulation of Cholesterol Synthesis 696

Pathogenesis of Arteriosclerosis 697

Epidemiological Findings 697
Clinical Pathological Correlation and Experimentation 697
Effect of Hormones on Arteriosclerosis 698
Pancreatic Hormones
Adrenocorticoids
Experimental Arteriosclerosis 700
Blood Lipids and Arteriosclerosis 701
Hemodynamic Factors and Arteriosclerosis 702
Origin of Lipids

Consequences of Atherosclerosis 705

Coronary Occlusion and Myocardial Infarcts 705
Cerebral Consequences of Atherosclerosis 707

Embolism 707
Thrombus 707
Encephalomalacia 708
Brain Infarct 708
Cerebral Hemorrhage 708

Working Hypothesis on the Pathogenesis of Arteriosclerosis 709

Hyperlipidemia 710

Familial Hyperlipoproteinemia 710

Xanthoma
Foam Cells
Lipemic Retinitis
Pancreatitis

Tangier Disease and Abetalipoproteinemia 711

Conclusion 711

References 713

Atherosclerosis

Introduction

Atherosclerosis comes from the Greek words *αθηρη*, meaning "a porridge of meal," and *σκληρωσις*, meaning "hardening." It is characterized by progressive degeneration of the intima of the artery, in association with lipoid deposition and calcification. Although atherosclerosis was observed in the arteries of Egyptian mummies, only during the 17th, 18th, and 19th centuries was a correlation between the arterial injuries and angina pectoris or coronary diseases suspected. In the beginning of the 20th century, detailed morphological descriptions were made.

Atherosclerosis principally involves the aorta, the coronary arteries, and the cerebral arteries. The importance of atherosclerosis resides in its complications: occlusion of the coronary arteries (leading to myocardial infarcts) and the cerebral arteries (leading to stroke). Because modern concepts of atherosclerosis have led some to forget that the injury is primarily manifested in the arteries, it might be worthwhile to point out some characteristic features of the vascular organ system. The importance of the arterial system, some basic properties of the vascular system, and the morphological and chemical composition of the arteries will be reviewed.

Holman [1] pointed out that the total weight of the arteries in the body is equal to that of the liver and bone marrow combined. Impressive as such figures may be, the physiological significance of an organ is not measured by its weight, and only a small fraction of the entire arterial system is affected by atherosclerosis.

Morphology of the Arteries

Atherosclerosis affects the middle-sized or large arteries. Unlike the smaller arteries, middle-sized arteries have a distinct layer of smooth muscle in the media and a larger number of elastic fibers in the intima. In the large arteries the number of elastic fibers in the intima is even greater. These intimal fibers are disposed in concentric rings that are interconnected to form a dense network surrounding the tubular endothelium. The media of the large arteries also contains a thick layer of elastic fibers, among which smooth muscle fibers are found. In both middle-sized and large arteries the adventitia is formed essentially of loose connective tissue containing small, muscular-type arterioles called the vasa vasorum.

Electron microscopic studies have added new details to our information on arterial structure. Electron micrographs reveal a central layer of mononucleated endothelial cells with a distinct cell membrane, an endoplasmic reticulum, and mitochondria. An interesting characteristic of these cells is the presence of multiple vesicles and caveolae. Underneath the endothelium, Keech [2] describes a subendothelial layer that appears edematous. It is probably made of a collagenous granular substance, in addition to collagen fibrils and blunt processes extending from the lamina elastica. Keech suggests a double role for that subendothelial layer: it may serve as a lubricant that facilitates the sliding of the lamina elastica on the endothelium while longitudinal tension is applied on both structures,* or this subendothelial fluid accumulation may constitute a reservoir from which nutrients diffuse to the rest of the intimal structure or from which the metabolic product that needs to be eliminated can diffuse to the outside or be picked up by the endothelial cells by pinocytosis.

After the endothelium has been fixed and prepared, uniform gaps of 100 Å separate the plasma membranes of two neighboring cells. The gap may not be real because some substance or structure invisible to the electron microscopist may be present in the living endothelium. One of the most debated aspects of vascular endothelium morphology is the presence of "cement" between the individual endothelial cells. Zweifach [3, 4] and his associates claim that such a cement can be recognized between endothelial cells when the endothelium is stained with silver nitrate. The source or the molecular composition of the cement is not known. Some claim that it is the product of endothelial cell secretions. Others think that it is produced by the plasma cells. In fact, not all investigators [5] accept the existence of an intercellular cement.

The media is made of 7–11 elastic laminae, separated by an interlaminar space containing smooth muscle fiber. The fusiform muscle cells of the media are disposed obliquely to the elastic lamina of the aorta, to which they are attached by thickenings of the plasma membrane called desmosomes. Obviously, the obliquity of the smooth muscle cell may control the circumference of the arterial lumen. Therefore, it is significant that in lathyrism this obliquity is lost, thus leading to increased rigidity of the arterial circumference.

Biochemistry

Polysaccharide content and abnormal fat deposition are the only aspects of the biochemical composition of arteries that have been studied extensively. The mucopolysaccharides found in the arterial wall are elaborated by the fibroblast, which furnishes the enzymes and the building blocks necessary for their biosynthesis. The polysaccharides are found mainly in the ground substance of the connective tissue, where they constitute 5–10% of the total components. The presence of polysaccharides in the arterial wall

* The intermediate zone would thus reduce the stress on both structures. The sliding of one structure on another, however, is controlled by the elastic attachment between the endothelium and the lamina elastica.

is important in at least two respects. First, the amount of ground substance indirectly determines the rate of diffusion of metabolites from the vascular lumen to the fibroblast. Second, the chemical composition of ground substance influences the electrolyte composition of the arterial wall. At least two types of mucopolysaccharides, acid and neutral, have been found in the arterial wall. The groups responsible for the acidity are uronic acid and sulfates. Naturally, the acidic groups are prone to form complexes with anions, and bivalent anions like calcium combine more readily than monovalents. Therefore, calcium and acid polysaccharide levels are closely related, and the amount of polysaccharides in the arterial wall is definitely increased in atherosclerosis [6, 7].

The polysaccharide content of 30 human aortas has been investigated. Two polysaccharide acids were found: (1) a fast-moving fraction—with a mobility similar to that of chondroitin sulfate—containing 24% hexosamine (galactosamines), 25% uronic acid, and 24% sulfate; and (2) a slow-moving fraction that contains 22% hexosamine (56% of which is galactosamine and 44% glucosamine), in addition to 28% uronic acid and 16% sulfate.

Many laboratories have studied enzymes in the arterial wall. These investigations included analysis of the activities in the major energetic pathways and of hydrolytic enzymes. The arterial walls contain all the enzymes necessary for the glycolytic pathway, the hexose monophosphate shunt, the Krebs cycle, and the electron transport chain [8, 9].

The respiratory rate of the arterial wall is low. The respiratory quotient of 0.91 indicates that much of the energy is derived from carbohydrate oxidation. The rate of glycolysis is high in the aorta, and oxygen has only little effect in depressing glycolysis. This low Pasteur effect may be responsible for the accumulation of lactic acid in the arterial wall. This is of particular significance because it has been proposed that the acidification of the arterial wall is responsible for the calcium deposition. The enzymes of the glycolytic pathway are rather stable because the aorta can be preserved in the cold for many hours without appreciable loss of glycolytic activity. When the enzymes of the glycolytic pathway are assayed individually, and the enzymic activity is expressed in μM of substrate metabolized per gram of wet tissue per hour, it was found that the hexokinase activity is 0.013, aldolase: 0.056, enolase: 0.24, lactic dehydrogenase: 1.06, phosphoglucoisomerase: 0.85. Thus, hexokinase activity appears to be rate limiting in the arterial walls. In contrast, phosphoglucoisomerase, enolase, and lactic dehydrogenase have high activities, and the activities of these enzymes increase in arteries of older individuals.

Because human peripheral arteries contain a high concentration of glycogen, enzymes involved in glycogen anabolism and catabolism can be expected to be found in human aortas. Phosphoglucomutase and glycogen phosphorylase are present in appreciable amounts in aortic tissue. The activity of glycogen phosphorylase decreases with age, probably as a result of the atrophy of the smooth muscle tissue.

Glucose-6-phosphate dehydrogenase, 6-phosphogluconate dehydrogenase, and ribose-5-phosphate isomerase—three enzymes of the hexose monophosphate shunt—have been found in aortic tissue. The relative activity of glucose-6-phosphate dehydrogenase is 10 times greater than that of the 6-phosphogluconate dehydrogenase. The activity of the ribose phosphate isomerase increases with age. The significance of the existence of the hexose monophosphate shunt in aortic tissue resides in the fact that this pathway provides NADP, a coenzyme necessary for cholesterol and lipid biosynthesis.

Many enzymes of the tricarboxylic cycle are present in arterial tissue. Aconitase, isocitric, succinic, and malic dehydrogenase and fumarase have been assayed. The results suggest that the tricarboxylic acid cycle functions at a rather low rate in aortic tissue. The activity of these enzymes decreases in the atherosclerotic portion of human aortas. Diaphorase and cytochrome oxidase activities are low in the aortic tissue, and these activities decrease with age.

Hydrolases found in aortic tissue include lipase, phosphomonoesterase, aminoleucine peptidase, cathepsin, β-glucuronidase, phenol sulfatase, and ATPase. The activity of some hydrolases (β-glucuronidase, ATPase) increases with age; however, it is not known whether this results from focal degeneration. Others, like 5-nucleotidase and ATPase, decrease in activity with age and the decrease precedes atheroma formation. Many of the biochemical findings made on human aortas have been confirmed qualitatively by histochemical methods.

The metabolism of arterial lipids and phospholipids will be discussed in further paragraphs.

Arterial Regeneration

Until a certain age, vessels grow and can generate cellular energy and synthesize many products: proteins, lipids, polysaccharides, etc. Nevertheless, little is known of the adult artery's capacity to regenerate. Abundant physiological, pathological, and experimental information suggests that adult arteries are not inert organs. On the contrary, these elastic tubes are continuously influenced by a circular and longitudinal tension; they adapt to physiological and pathological changes.

Tension is due to the passage of the wave of circulating blood; the internal longitudinal tension results from friction of the liquid layers with an internal layer of the vascular canal. In many cases this friction causes the external wall of the vessel to slide against the surrounding tissues. Obviously, the longitudinal tension is marked at the convex aspect of the arterial curvature. In those areas the intima adapts itself to the pressure change by local thickening, and the elastica may even double. Such adaptations result in the formation of the salient spur often observed at arterial bifurcations. The uterine artery illustrates vascular adaptation to internal conditions. The uterine artery normally has many incurvations; therefore, it is under severe internal longitudinal tension so its intima is rather thick. In contrast, during pregnancy the artery becomes elongated and straight. Associated with this change in direction is a change in the thickness of the endothelium; during pregnancy, the intima is (by atrophy of the external elastica and thinning of the media) practically reduced to its endothelium, whereas the adventitia builds up new muscular, elastic, and conjunctive fibers. Pathologists are well acquainted with another example of arterial adaptation—namely, the medial changes in the branches of the pulmonary arteries during pulmonary hypertension.

When damaged, the artery can regenerate to a certain degree. Poole, Saunders, and Florey [10] studied the regenerative properties of the arterial wall. When patches of endothelial cells are removed from rabbit abdominal aorta, the denuded area is rapidly covered with small, round structures resembling platelets, accompanied by a few polymorphonuclear and mononuclear cells. Later, the endothelial cells at the periphery of the lesion spread, thus covering the denuded area with large cells containing sometimes 10 or more nuclei in their cytoplasm. These new cells lack orientation, contain silver-staining concretions in their cytoplasm, and have nuclei that vary in size, shape, and structure. Thus, endothelial cells undoubtedly can divide, but their regeneration is slow and restricted.

These changes are of interest because the atherosclerotic lesion is sometimes assumed to result from the deposition of thrombotic material, which is later covered by regenerating endothelium. In arterial walls of various origins, for example the aorta, the pulmonary and renal arteries, it was found that endothelial abnormalities possibly related to regeneration can be closely correlated with the age of the subject. Nevertheless, the incidence of atherosclerosis in these vessels does not correlate with that in abnormal endothelial patches.

Fibrous tissues grow readily within the media, as in the medial fibrosis that follows syphilitic aortitis. In contrast, little is known of the capacity of the arteries to regenerate their elastic fibers. If they regenerate the fibers at all, their capacity to do so must be limited because little of it is detectable. Carnes and his associates [11] found that young pigs maintained on copper-deficient diets for 2 or 3 months show signs of rupture of the elastic fibers, which are repaired upon administration of a normal diet.

Taylor and his associates [12] studied the regeneration of the aortas of young rabbits after freezing them for 1 hour with dry ice. After freezing, there were no visible alterations of the connective elastic structure; little inflammation developed, and all inflammation was restricted to the adventitia. Smooth muscle degenerated and was followed by calcium deposition, creating a mass of smooth muscle supported by a rigid, calcified shell. Next, fibroblasts proliferated in the intima, with collagenous and elastic fibers; then muscle cells appeared and a new aortic wall developed. Similar experiments in other rodents led to much less marked proliferation than that observed in rabbits, but the response to injury was qualitatively similar.

Rather similar findings were made in rabbit aortas repairing after a brief longitudinal injury. The manipulation obviously led to necrosis along the edges of the cut; this was followed first by polymorphonuclear migration and later by macrophages. The necrotic area became calcified rapidly and was surrounded by a fibrous capsule containing foreign body granulomas and capillary outgrowths. The site of injury was impregnated with lipids and also offered a favorable terrain for thrombi formation.

Although such experiments shed some light on the limitation of the arteries to repair their losses, their relevance to arteriosclerosis is uncertain because of the acuteness and the extensiveness of the injury [13].

Although our knowledge of the metabolism, ultrastructure, and even histophysiology of the great vessels is too incomplete and too scattered to permit an integrated presentation, it illustrates that blood vessels are living tubular structures rather than inert pipes. Many, if not all, of the macromolecules in arteries turn over. The arterial wall can generate the energy and synthesize the building blocks needed for its maintenance.

These properties make the blood vessel walls much more sensitive to injury than inert tubes might be, but they also confer on the vessel wall limited abilities to restore structure and function after damage.

Elementary Lesions in Atherosclerosis

Morphological observations of early lesions in the aortas of men and experimental animals have revealed a number of elementary lesions including edema, endothelial injuries, smooth muscle proliferation, lipid accumulation, fibrosis, and thrombosis.

Edema

Circumscribed gelatinous elevations are sometimes seen in the aorta. They are caused by intimal edema (serous or serofibrinous) which may remain superficial or extend deep in the intima. With the proper stain the lesions are metachromatic. The relationship of these lesions to the development of atherosclerosis is not clear, although it has been established that their incidence increases with hypertension. The pathogenesis of these lesions remains obscure. A plausible, but still unproven mechanism has been proposed [72].

The formation of sorbitol has been suspected to play a role in the pathogenesis of cataracts in diabetes and galactosemia in which the free entry of glucose and galactose would stimulate the formation of sorbitol [73].

Polyol NADP Oxidoreductase

Glucose ↔ Sorbitol

Galactose ↔ Dulcitol

NADPH ↶ NADP

L-iditol: NAD Oxidoreductase

Sorbitol + NAD ⇌ Fructose

NAD ↷ NADH

The accumulation of polyol derivatives, sorbitol and dulcitol, is associated with water uptake in the lens with loss of Na^+ and K^+, alteration of amino acid transport and decrease in the concentration of free myoinositol. On the basis of indirect evidence, polyol metabolism has been implicated in the early vascular changes in atherosclerosis.

Endothelial Injuries

Haust [74] remarks that two features are unique to the aortic wall: the mode of nutrition of the intima and the fact that the arterial system is never at rest until death. The intima is deprived of vascularization and therefore the nutrients must enter the intima from the blood. The diffusion gradient across the intimal wall will depend on the level of the blood pressure and the difference between systolic and diastolic pressure. The greater the systolic stretch and the diastolic recoil, the more effectively the nutrients are "pumped" through the arterial wall. In addition to intravascular pressure, the integrity of the subintimal acid mucopolysaccharide ground substance is important to the absorption and the clearing of nutrients because it acts as a sponge sucking in the diffused nutrients. In the healthy vessel, diffusion and clearing are balanced.

Because they operate under constant tension, arteries are often damaged and are not readily repaired integrally. There is little doubt that the intial atherosclerotic lesion is a subtle one which progresses slowly because neither cellular necrosis nor exudative reactions predominate in the early stages. Moreover, there is no damage beyond the intima. The primary insult could be either intraluminal or intramural. Hemodynamic factors could cause lesions of the endothelium, or the nutrients and possibly toxic substances could penetrate the intima without altering the endothelial cells, but directly causing damage to intimal components which in turn will cause endothelial damage.

Constantinides' [75] experiments illustrate the importance of endothelial injuries in atherogenesis. Injury to the endothelial wall results in rapid accumulation of lipids even with low lipemia, while little lipid accumulates when the endothelial cells are undamaged even in presence of high lipemia. Constantinides proposes that the normal arterial endothelium is impermeable to macromolecules and allows only the penetration of water, ions, glucose, fatty acids and maybe small proteins. Only when the endothelium is injured will large macromolecules accumulate in the intima. A large number of agents can interrupt the continuity of the endothelium either by crossing intercellular junctions or by directly damaging the cell, which then sluffs off leaving a gap behind.

A complete list of the agents capable of injuring the endothelium is probably not available, but it includes epinephrine, angiotensin, serotonin, tyramine, bile acids, calciferol, lysophosphatides, antigen antibody complexes, proteolytic enzymes, hyperlipemia, ketone bodies such as acetoacetic acid and β hydroxybutyric acid, EDTA and nicotine. The effect of these agents was studied by intra-arterial perfusion of the superficial femoral arteries of rats and rabbits. In most cases high doses of the substance under study were used. Although these agents are found in many conditions that influence the rate of development of atherosclerosis (hypertension, diabetes, cigarette smoking, etc.) it is not known how much they contribute to the pathogenesis of atherosclerosis in man.

Neither is it known what molecule or molecules in the endothelium constitute the target of the various injurious agents, but at least in the case of adrenalin and angiotensin immunofluorescence and scanning electron microscopy suggest that the contractile system of the cell is affected leading to the formation of blebs and the disruption of intercellular junctions [76].

Whatever their exact role may be in the pathogenesis of atherosclerosis, it seems unlikely that alterations of the endothelial cells are without effect on the development of the disease. Therefore, the kinetics and patterns of cell division in the arterial endothelium assume particular significance. Schwartz and Benditt [77] developed an elegant method for the purpose of investigating cell replication in the aortic endothelium. They found: (1) that the endothelial cells divide at a much faster rate in aortas of newborns than in three-month old animals; (2) that the endothelium is made of at least two groups of cells, some long lived ones with slow turnover, some short lived ones with high turnover. Investigations of the sites of cell division in the entire surface of large segments of the aorta revealed that the cell division is focal. Thus, after the administration of thymidine, heavily labeled foci alternate with large segments of the aorta in which the cell remains unlabeled.

The authors propose three explanations for the unequal distribution of cell division in the endothelium. The dividing cells have a more rapid turnover than the nondividing cell. The dividing cells are growing centers for the endothelium, similar to those found in the intestinal crypt, and the mature cell migrates from the point of growth to other areas in the aorta.

Finally, the foci of cell division occur in portions of the aorta which are still in a growing phase. In either case, the foci of endothelial proliferation could constitute weak spots in the endothelium, with permeability properties different from those of the mature endothelium and therefore, the observations of Schwartz and Benditt may go far in explaining the special localization of the early lesions in atherosclerosis.

Smooth Muscle Proliferation

Prior to the development of the atherosclerotic plaque there is a stage of proliferation of smooth muscle cells. Such proliferation has been shown to occur in humans, but it progresses rapidly in cholesterol-fed pigs (approximately six weeks). Geer and Haust [78] were the first to demonstrate that the proliferative lesions are largely composed of smooth muscle cells covered by intact endothelium. The smooth muscle cells have been identified by electron microscopy. The proliferation has been demonstrated by counting mitosis, measuring DNA increases, and following ^{3}H-thymidine incorporation by radioautography. As for most processes of cellular proliferation, the stimulus to proliferation is unknown. Whether cholesterol itself is responsible is not known. Moreover, when a piece of aorta obtained from a hypercholesteremic swine is transplanted to a normocholesteremic swine, smooth muscle proliferation persists for days after transplantation. Smooth muscle proliferation is associated with increased oxygen uptake. Whether or not this is coupled to increased ATP synthesis is not certain. Some investigators have claimed that oxidative phosphorylation is uncoupled in the wall of the arteries of hypercholesteremic animals, suggesting that either the chemical stimulus persists in the hypercholesteremic cell, or that the proliferative processes once stimulated are irreversible or take a long time to be reversed. No less intriguing is the fate of the smooth muscle cell. The smooth muscle cells are believed to differentiate into a fibroblast, which may either evolve into an even more primitive mesenchymal cell, or become lipid laden and ultimately die releasing the lipids into the surrounding tissues. The primitive cell may also redifferentiate into a smooth muscle cell [79].

Lipid Accumulation

A central, if not a primary, event in atherosclerosis is the accumulation of lipids in the intima. In 1856 Virchow discovered that lipids were present in the atherogenic plaque. The study of the lipid composition of the intima has only recently become possible [80, 81]. Lipids carefully extracted from the subintimal lesion are separated by thin layer chromatography. These investigations revealed two unexpected findings. Lipids accumulate in normal arteries and the lipid content varies with the type of injuries.

Undiseased intima accumulates lipids with age in an extra- and an intracellular form. The extracellular accumulation is found around collagen and elastic fibers; the intracellular in fat-loaded cells, probably multipotential smooth muscle cells. The fat filled cells contain sphingomyelin, lecithin, free cholesterol, and cholesteryl oleate. The composition of the extracellular lipid resembles plasma low density lipoprotein. Both extracellular and intracellular lipid accumulations contain cholesteryl esters, but while cholesterol linoleate is found in the extracellular, cholesteryl oleate is found in the intracellular accumulations. The reasons for these differences in the composition of the cholesterol esters are not understood. There is a positive correlation between the contents of cholesteryl esters and age. Thus, while the level of free cholesterol only doubles between the age of 20 and 80, that of esterified cholesterol increases 50 times during that period and the ratio of free to esterified cholesterol shifts from 4 to 0.5.

Among the early lesions of atherosclerosis are the fatty streaks. Grossly they appear as yellowish accumulations which can assume various shapes, but most often look like streaks underlying the intima. Histologically, the earliest event consists of the accumulation of fat-filled cells; this is followed by a fibrous reaction and later by the formation of pools of extracellular lipids. Analysis of the composition of the lipids in the fatty streak revealed it to be similar to that of the intracellular lipid found in undiseased aortas and thus the lesions are rich in cholesteryl oleate.

There is no major difference between the amorphous and the cellular pools of lipid except that the ratio of cholesterol to cholesteryl esters is higher in the extra- than in the intracellular pools [82].

Fibrosis

Some have described a reactive fibrosis around the lipid droplets, but others believe that no fibrosis occurs. In any case, the pearly gray elevation observed on close examination of a young aorta is mainly due to proliferation of spindle-shaped cells and young connective tissue immediately underneath the endothelium. Since the media of human aorta is thought to be devoid of fibroblasts and contain only multipotential smooth muscle cells, these smooth muscle cells must accumulate in the fibrous plaque. Geer and Haust and their collaborators [14, 15] have identified the spindle-shaped cells as smooth muscle cells. These proliferative plaques often undergo fibrolysis or hyalinization, and the elastic fibers of the intima are broken at their edges. Endothelial necrosis with ulceration covered by hemorrhage and thrombosis is followed by precipitation of calcium salts within the plaques, particularly in those areas containing lipids and hyalinized connective tissue [16] (see Fig. 11-1).

Again, observations made on copper-deficient pigs are significant. Copper deprivation in adult pigs leads

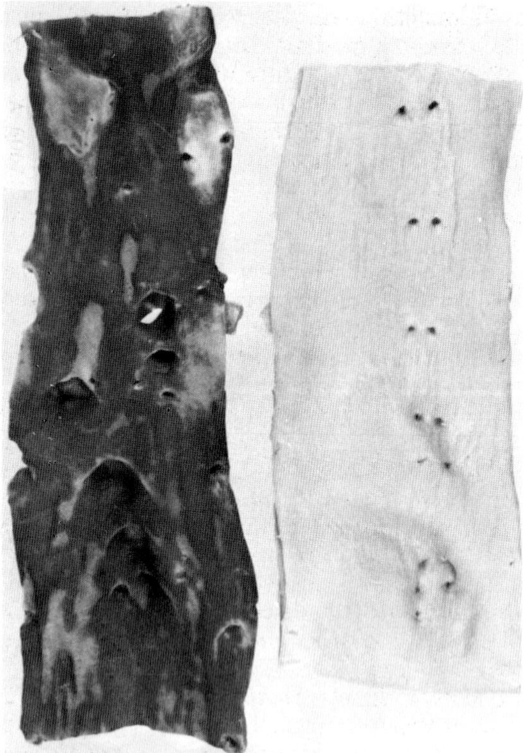

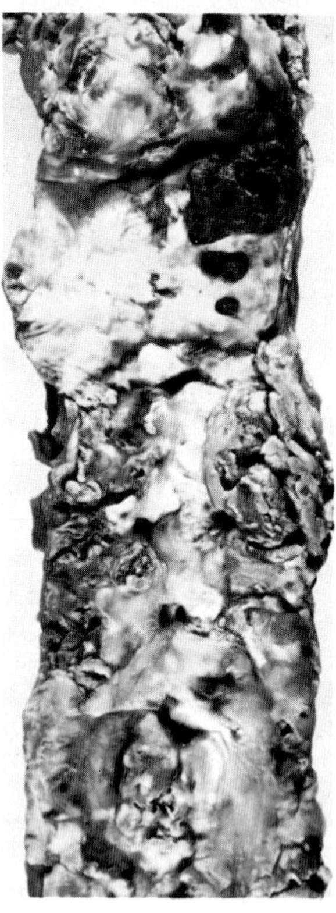

Fig. 11-1. Left and center: mild atherosclerosis in an elderly woman; aorta stained with oil red "O" (*left*) and unstained (*center*). Right: severe aortic atherosclerosis

to the rupture of elastic fibers and subendothelial migration and proliferation of muscle that resembles what Thomas [17] described as preatheromatous proliferative lesions. However, no lipids are found in association with the proliferative lesions described in copper deficiency.

In conclusion, the mechanism of development of fibrosis in atherosclerosis is not known. Again fibrosis could be among the primary lesions or a consequence of other insults. Among the factors suspected to cause fibrosis are the wear and tear caused by hypertension, the stimulation of fibrosis caused by platelet and fibrin encrustation and the sclerogenic effect of cholesterol and its esters. Adams believes the last contributes most to the fibrosis [84].

Thrombosis

Rokitansky was the first to propose that atherosclerotic lesions result from the deposition of fibrin at the surface of the intima.

A discussion on the role of thrombosis in the early stages of atherosclerosis should exclude the formation of large thrombi which are a consequence of vascular necrosis. At least two events associated with clot formation are related to the early stages of atherosclerosis: the intramural accumulation of fibrin and the endothelial aggregation of platelets. It is not known whether these changes constitute the primary injury in atherosclerosis or are a consequence of endothelial damage. While some believe that small mural fibrin platelet thrombi may form on the surface of healthy endothelium, others claim that such thrombi never occur unless the endothelium is damaged. The damage may or may not be detectable by modern electron microscopic methods. Using immunofluorescent techniques, Wissler was unable to detect fibrin in the early lesion.

The mechanism of formation of platelet aggregates on the surface of the arteries is similarly controversial. However, whatever their cause, fibrin and platelet aggregates contribute to the development of the atherosclerotic lesion. Both fibrin and platelet aggregates interfere with the nutrition of the endothelial cells. Moreover, the platelets release ADP which causes further aggregation and a number of factors modifying the permeability of the endothelial cells causing further accumulation of macromolecules in the intimal layer of the artery.

Some investigators believe that thrombosis can, at least in some cases, initiate the formation of the atherosclerotic plaque. This assumption is based on the observation that thrombi, occlusive or mural, are often incorporated into the vascular wall and covered by regenerating endothelial cells. Although unproven, such a view could at least explain some of the features of the atherosclerotic plaque. The appearance of the plaque would depend upon the composition of the thrombus. The presence of fibrin would stimulate fibrosis. The platelets would not only be a source of lipid, but their content would modify endothelial permeability and cause further lipid accumulation. Although small thrombi remain avascular, larger thrombi become vascularized, and damage to the vasculature causes hemorrhage and increases the accumulation of lipids. Thrombus organization would be associated with the proliferation of smooth muscle cells.

In conclusion, the engulfment of thrombi in the vascular wall may play a role in the pathogenesis of atherosclerosis, and in some cases they may even be the first event in plaque formation. However, experimental atherosclerosis suggests that such a mechanism is not likely to play a major role at the early stages of the disease [18, 85].

Although atherosclerosis is mainly a disease of the intima, when the plaque enlarges considerably it induces atrophy of or completely destroys the medial layer, leading to fibrosis, lipoid infiltration, and perivascular infiltration. When such lesions are present, atherosclerosis is sometimes difficult to distinguish from syphilis.

It is tempting to describe the sequence of events in the development of atherosclerosis on the basis of the morphological observations, but, as Holman [18] remarked, such a sequence must be established on solid experimental data. Those who attempt this after carefully observing a large number of autopsies do not always agree on sequence. Nevertheless, over the last two decades a consensus has been reached on the pathogenesis of atherosclerotic plaques. The modern concept of the pathogenesis of atherosclerosis will be easier to understand after we have reviewed lipid metabolism and its relation to arteriosclerosis.

Fat Metabolism and Atherosclerosis

Three groups of arguments support the concept that fat metabolism is altered in atherosclerosis: epidemiological studies, clinical investigations, and animal experimentation. The validity of these arguments can be reviewed only in the light of our understanding of fat metabolism in general.

Fat Metabolism: Absorption of Fats

About 40% of our total caloric intake is made of fat, mainly triglycerides. A large amount of the fat is hydrolyzed by the lipases of the gastrointestinal tract to glycerol and fatty acids (16–18 carbons) before absorption. At least two lipases, a gastric and a pancreatic, are found within the intestinal lumen. The known gastric lipase is of little importance in digesting ingested fats because its optimum activity is around neutrality and the gastric content is strongly acid. However, the fat that leaves the stomach is hydrolyzed to a certain extent (10–20%), but the enzyme responsible for that reaction is unknown.

When the alimentary bolus reaches the duodenum (pH around 7), the ingested fats are attacked by pancreatic lipase. Pancreatic lipase has been extensively purified (pH optimum 9). It is known to attack the ester linkage of the α-hydroxyl, but the β-hydroxyl is hydrolyzed as well. Therefore, if the enzyme specificity is restricted to the primary hydroxyl, then the fatty acid that is attached to the β-hydroxyl of glycerol must be shifted to the α position before the ester bonds can be split, and isomerization must precede hydrolysis.

The size of the fatty acid determines the affinity of the enzyme for the substrates. Esters of short fatty acids are more readily hydrolyzed than are those of long fatty acids.

The enzyme is not stereospecific and has no preference for one primary ester over the other (1 or 3). In spite of the lack of stereospecificity of the esterase, one should not conclude that the positions 1 and 3 in the substrate are equivalent.

Since triglycerides are water insoluble, solubilizing factors must exist in the intestine. Bile acid and the phospholipids probably play such a role. Borgström [19–21] studied the role of both these groups of compounds in intestinal absorption. He investigated the pH, the concentration of lipase, bile acids, and phospholipids in the intestinal content. The pH is constant in the small intestine. It is maintained between 6 and 6.5 in the small intestine 50 cm from its origin at the angle of Treitz to 1–1.5 meters from that point. The concentration of pancreatic lipase is high and constant (50 units per ml of intestinal content).

The bile acids of the intestine are conjugated to taurine or choline. Their metabolic origin was discussed in Chap. 9. They are present in high concentration in the duodenum (5 mg/ml). Distally to the duodenum, bile acid concentration decreases until it becomes constant in the more proximal portion of the small intestine. Borgström found that the concentration of bile was high in the intestinal content 30 minutes after a test meal and decreased progressively during the following hour. After extensive studies, Borgström could describe quantitatively the biochemical conditions in the proximal jejunum when lipids are hydrolyzed after a test meal. This permitted him to reconstruct an artificial system with the hope of clarifying our understanding of intestinal fat absorption.

Several questions remain unanswered. How can lipids be hydrolyzed in an intestinal content of pH 6 by an enzyme whose pH optimum is 9? Why is the hydrolysis incomplete? How are the unhydrolyzed triglycerides absorbed?

The physicochemical conditions in which ingested lipids are absorbed are now known. However, it has been suggested that triglyceride may be absorbed as such in the form of an emulsion in which the particle component is 5,000 A in diameter. Because the electron microscopist sees no holes or pores in the cell membrane of the intestinal epithelium, biochemists assumed that these particles are much too large to be absorbed as such. When so little is known of the physiology of the living cell and its membranes, it is difficult to evaluate the validity of such an objection. Nevertheless, Borgström has looked for alternative explanations by studying an artificially reconstituted system composed of pancreatic lipase, triglycerides, and bile acid. In such a system he found that the bile acids activate the lipase at the relatively low pH 6 (the lipase has a pH optimum of 9), and they solubilize the fatty acid to form mixed micelles of fatty acid and lower glycerides. It is not clear how much such a system may function *in vivo*, but the bile concentration needed in such an artificial system is much higher than that ever encountered within the intestinal lumen.

Although the exact mechanism by which the bile salts stimulate fat absorption is not known, the bile salt requirement is uniquely demonstrated in some classical pathological conditions in which bile salts are absent, because of an inborn error of metabolism or a mechanical shunt (fistula) in the normal excretory pathway. Under those conditions, steatorrhea occurs, and it can often be cured by the administration of bile salts.

Electron micrographs of intestinal mucosa suggest another process of fat absorption. Fat droplets are incorporated into the epithelial cells by pinocytosis and then transferred from the luminar to the peripheral surface of the cell through tubular channels of the endoplasmic reticulum. The droplets are then discharged in the intercellular space in the form of chylomicrons.

Experiments in Strauss' laboratory [22] seem to exclude the possibility of intestinal absorption by pinocytosis. Strauss incubated intestinal loops first at 0° with a suspension of monoglycerides, fatty acids, and bile salts, and then at 32°. He made electron micrographs of the epithelial cells and studied triglyceride biosynthesis. At 0°, absorption occurred without droplet formation, and intracellular fat droplets appeared only after incubation at 37°. Further studies of labeled fatty acid incorporation into triglycerides permitted Strauss to conclude that triglycerides were formed intracellularly. These observations finally reconciled the ultrastructural and biochemical findings.

Once fatty acids have reached the intestinal epithelial cells, all fatty acids with carbon chains longer than 10 carbons are reconverted into triglycerides through a chemical pathway similar to that which occurs in liver. The absorbed fats are transferred from the intestinal cell to the lymphatics or the veins of the intestines in the form of chylomicrons. Those chylomicrons that reach the lymphatics are first found in the thoracic duct, and from there they are poured into the left jugular and the subclavian veins. Chylomicrons that enter the portal vein reach the liver before they reach the general circulation.

Chylomicrons are huge fat globules (500 A) containing triglycerides, cholesterol, phospholipids, and small amounts of protein. Electron microscopic examinations of chylomicrons reveal a central structureless core surrounded by a thin electron-dense membrane. The peripheral coat can be separated from the core and is made of phospholipids (primarily phosphatidyl choline). Chylomicrons are responsible for the milkiness of the serum after a high-fat diet. They are water stable because they contain a specific lipoprotein secreted by the intestinal mucosa.

In the presence of ions, chylomicrons form a complex with a lipoprotein lipase. The enzyme attacks fats only when they are complexed with proteins in the presence of a fatty acid acceptor (albumin). Lipoprotein lipase yields a mixture of tri-, di-, and monoglycerides, lipoproteins, and lipoprotein lipase. Thus, in this reaction a water-soluble enzyme acts on a lipid-soluble protein. Ions are required in the formation of the enzyme-lipoprotein complex and during the hydrolysis. Although magnesium, calcium, barium, cesium, manganese, or ammonia is required for the latter, most ions are active in the former. This hydrolysis is responsible for plasma clearing, which occurs when 50% of the triglycerides have been hydrolyzed, because a mixture of tri-, di-, and monoglycerides and free fatty acids is much more soluble than the original triglycerides.

Lipoprotein lipase is not normally present in the blood, but appears only after ingestion of a meal rich in fat or during the intravenous administration of a fat emulsion. As a matter of fact, the blood concentration of protein lipase is so low that the enzyme that removes chylomicrons appears to be within or at the surface of some cellular structure. In rats, adipose tissue seems to be the main source of lipoprotein lipase, but it has also been prepared from liver, heart, lung, and skeletal muscle. The enzyme is easily precipitated at pH 5.5. It is inhibited by protamine, 0.5 M sodium chloride, detergents, and pyrophosphates.

Heparin administration is known to clear the blood after a fatty meal has been ingested. The exact mechanism of this clearing property of heparin is not clear. In addition to clearing the blood and producing a shift of the plasma protein from the low density to the higher density group, heparin injection also induces a rise in plasma free fatty acid that results from lipolysis of plasma lipids, and an increase in the electrophoretic mobilities of plasma albumin and α- and β-lipoproteins mediated by excess fatty acids.

Heparin activates *in vitro* an enzyme prepared from rat heart or adipose tissue. However, the enzyme prepared from chicken adipose tissue is not activated by heparin. Whatever the role of heparin may be in stimulating protein lipase, this property seems to be shared with a number of unrelated high molecular weight anions or heparinoids. Bernfeld and Kelly have proposed that the effect of polysaccharides on protein lipase depends on the relative number of N and O sulfate groups in the molecule. The polysaccharide composition of the aorta of older animals could be such as to interfere with protein lipase activity. Such an alteration in the arterial composition would be of considerable significance with respect to the development of atherosclerosis because several investigators have proposed that the incidence of atherosclerosis correlates with the blood levels of triglycerides more than with cholesterol levels.

Protamine inhibits all preparations of lipoprotein lipase, which indicates a requirement for anionic groups, but these need not necessarily be heparin. Lipase has been purified from mammalian adipose tissue, which contains no carbohydrate and is active without heparin.

Although triglycerides seem to require hydrolysis before they can enter adipose tissue cells, this might not be the general process of intracellular penetration. Electron micrographs demonstrate lipid particles identical to chylomicrons in liver cells, in macrophages, and in leukocytes after a fatty meal is ingested; this suggests that the fat globules may be absorbed by pinocytosis or phagocytosis without hydrolysis.

Such observations do not necessarily prove that the chylomicrons penetrate the cell unhydrolyzed because they could be reconstituted inside the liver cell. However, experiments with labeled triglycerides suggest that the triglycerides enter liver cells without appreciable hydrolysis.

All lipoproteins have a low density that is close to or even below that of water. Whereas most proteins have a density ranging between 1.26 and 1.38, the lipoproteins have a density of between 0.98 and 1.15 depending on their composition.

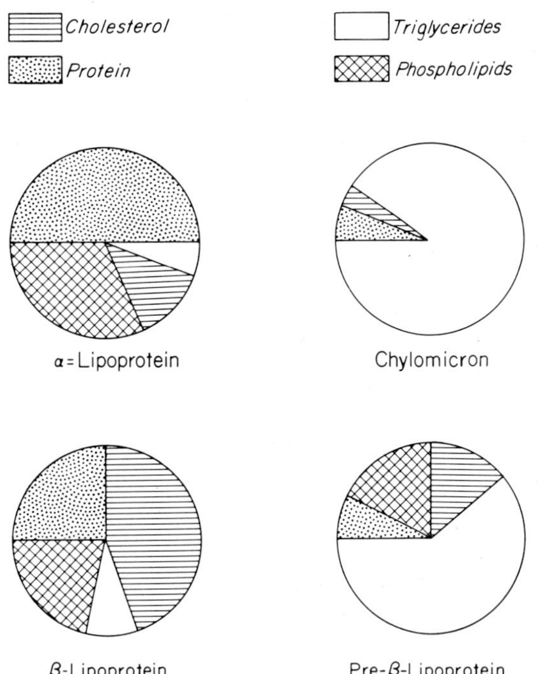

Fig. 11-2. Composition of blood lipoproteins

Blood Lipoproteins

The transport of lipids into a circulating fluid primarily made of water would seem to constitute an unusual challenge to traditional laws of physics and chemistry. Work of many laboratories has partially resolved this riddle in the recent decade [23–25]. The key to lipid transport is their complexion with protein to form lipoprotein. Moreover, most lipoproteins are not molecules in the traditional sense because the lipid can readily be separated from the protein moiety simply by extracting the lipid with solvents. Rarely are lipids and proteins covalently bound.

Lipoproteins have been divided according to their density, electrophoretic properties, ratios of proteins to lipids, and immunological properties (see Fig. 11-2).

The relationship between protein and lipid moiety in lipoproteins varies considerably depending upon the relative ratio of protein to lipid. When the protein constitutes less than one-third of the lipoprotein, the relationship appears to be mainly a phase distribution (chylomicrons). The lipoprotein forms a globule, the center of which is made of a core of hydrophobic lipids, while the periphery is coated with hydrophilic protein, thus permitting the lipid mass to circulate in the blood. In contrast, when the protein accounts for more than one-third of the lipoprotein molecule, the lipid moieties may lodge themselves within the groove of an unfolded protein.

Lipoproteins in which the ratio of protein to lipid is less than 1:3 are called micellar; those in which the ratio of protein to lipid is greater than 1:3 are called pseudomolecular because a genuine quaternary arrangement between protein and lipid is possible. Obviously, the density of the micellar lipoprotein is lower than that of the pseudomolecular type. Therefore, the micellar group includes the very low-density lipoproteins, whereas the low-density lipoproteins and the very high-density lipoproteins are pseudomolecular.

Lipoproteins occupy various levels of flotation when put in an adequate medium. The rate at which these levels of flotation are reached can be determined in the ultracentrifuge in a way similar to the determination of the rate of sedimentation of heavier particles. Therefore, a flotation constant can be calculated and expressed in Svedberg units. This has been done in various laboratories. Gofman determined the flotation constant of the lipoproteins in sodium chloride solution with a density of 1.063. Under those conditions, the Sf value (the sedimentation characteristic at a given concentration of the lipoprotein) is determined by the formula:

$$Sf = \frac{S^0f \cdot 0.00540\ (1.0360\text{-}D)d^2}{(1+kc)}$$

where: D = density of the lipoprotein; d = diameter of the lipoprotein molecule in A; k = a constant, characteristic for each lipoprotein (usually about 0.14), which can be determined only by measuring Sf of various lipoprotein concentrations; S^0f = the sedimentation constant extrapolated for a protein concentration tending to 0. $S^0f = Sf(1+kc)$.

Separation by flotation depends on the density of the lipoprotein under investigation (the lower the density, the higher the Sf value) and also on the size and shape of the particle containing the lipoproteins. In contrast, density-gradient centrifugation depends primarily and almost entirely upon the density of the lipoprotein. A gradient concentration of a given solute is established with special devices from bottom to top of a centrifuge tube. The lipoprotein is placed on top of the solution, and the tube is centrifuged at high speeds. The lipoprotein will band in that zone of the tube in which the density of the solution is in equilibrium with that of the lipoprotein. These methods have separated four major groups of lipoproteins in blood: high density, low density, and very low density lipoproteins, and chylomicrons.

Lipoproteins in blood resemble other plasma proteins in many respects. Lipoproteins have the mobility of globulins. Half of them move like the α-globulins and half move like β-globulins. The ratio af α- to β-lipoproteins is greatly influenced by sex or by androgen or estrogen injection. Paper and starch-block electrophoresis have become standard in separating various classes of lipoproteins, and in many cases changes in the electrophoretic patterns have provided invaluable diagnostic clues.

The solubility characteristics of blood lipoproteins are similar to those of other plasma proteins. The addition of alcohol decreases the solubility, whereas the addition of electrolytes increases it. Therefore, two main methods of separating α- and β-lipoproteins have been developed: one is based on the usage of various alcohol concentrations and the other consists of precipitating the various lipoproteins preferentially with zinc acetate or zinc glycinate reagents, or by adding high molecular weight dextran sulfates. These techniques do not yield highly purified proteins, but they allow concentration of the lipoprotein preparation so that it can be placed in the ultracentrifuge.

The lipoprotein-peptide moiety acts as a powerful antigen. The immunological reaction of lipoproteins can serve to identify classes of lipoproteins. Thus, anti-β-lipoprotein peptide serum (see below) precipitates both the low-density and the very low-density lipoproteins, whereas anti-α-lipoprotein peptide serum precipitates high-density lipoprotein.

There seem to be no rigid species specificities in the immunological reaction of lipoproteins. For example, an antihuman β-lipoprotein serum prepared from rabbits precipitates human β-lipoproteins and at least partially precipitates those of other animals, including primates and rodents.

With the aid of a battery of physicochemical and immunological techniques, at least four main classes of blood lipoproteins have been described. The α-lipoproteins (high-density lipoproteins or HDL), β-lipoproteins (low-density lipoproteins or LDL), pre-β-lipoproteins (very low-density lipoproteins or VLDL) and chylomicrons or VHDL (see Table 11-1). Each group is characterized by its protein and lipid contents, the structure of the apoprotein, its density, and its average molecular weight.

Table 11-1. Relative diameters of blood lipoproteins

Lipoprotein	Relative diameter	Flotation constant
Chylomicron	——————————	400 and above
Pre-β-Lipoprotein	———————	20–400
β-Lipoprotein	———	0–20
α-Lipoprotein	——	

The circulating lipids in plasma are cholesterol, phospholipids, triglycerides and free fatty acids. All are bound to globulins except for the free fatty acids which are bound to albumin. Half of the circulating cholesterol is found in association with LDL. Most of the remaining cholesterol is associated with HDL. HDL also contains more than half of the circulating phospholipids. Exogenous triglycerides are transported in chylomicrons while endogenous triglycerides are transported in very low density lipoproteins [83].

Apoproteins

Obviously in addition to the lipid composition, the type of apoprotein found in a class of lipoproteins will confer them special properties. A number of apoproteins have been described. Apoproteins have been purified, characterized with respect to their amino acid composition, carboxyl and amino terminals and immunological properties and in some cases even the amino acid sequence is known.

By tracing the amino acid terminal, by observing immunochemical reactions as well as by following the blood lipid pattern of patients missing apoproteins, investigators have determined which apoproteins are found in each class of lipoproteins. Although the lipoproteins of each density class contain one or two major apoproteins, they also contain a number of minor components. Moreover, an apoprotein found in one class of lipoproteins may also be found in another.

For example, apo HDL is composed of two major apoproteins, apoA-I and apoA-II. Both have a Gln-COOH terminal. ApoA-I composes 65 to 70% of the protein component of high-density lipoprotein by weight. It has a molecular weight of 25,000 to 28,000; its NH_2 terminal is aspartic acid. Its amino acid sequence is not known except for the first 39 amino acid residues. The amino acid sequence of apoA-II has been determined. In addition, HDL contains a number of smaller apoproteins referred to as C-I, C-II, C-III. The minor component represents about 10% of the total protein contingent of HDL. The amino acid sequences of C-I and C-III have been determined.

An apoB has been extracted from LDL. ApoB is believed to be a polymer made of several identical subunits. The N-terminal and C-terminal of the subunits are respectively glutamic acid and serine.

VLD lipoproteins also contain major and minor apoprotein components. LD apoprotein composes 40 to 50% of the protein contingent by weight. The remaining protein constituent is composed of a family of apoC proteins, which can be distinguished by their carboxy terminal amino acid, serine in apoC-I, glutamic in apoC-II, alanine in apoC-III and apoC-III_2. The difference between apoC-III and apoC-III_2 does not reside in their amino acid terminal or composition, but in their sialic acid content. C-III contains one and C-III_2 two sialic acid residues. The amino acid sequence of apoC-I has been determined. The protein contains 57 residues with an NH_2 terminal, threonine and COOH terminal serine [86, 87].

The identification of the various types of apoproteins is of significance. First because different apoproteins may play a different role in lipid transport and therefore affect the pathogenesis of some diseases. Second, because an understanding of the interaction between a specific protein and a specific lipid may lead to generalization with respect to protein lipid interaction. Except for the fact that the absence of some apoproteins leads to hyperlipidemia, little is known of their function.

Several attempts have been made to study lipid protein interaction of high density lipoproteins [88–90]. When the apoprotein is separated from its lipid component by organic solvents, it retains its capacity to bind to lipids, and the reconstituted particle has many of the physical properties of the original. Circular dichroism analysis has shown that the apoprotein loses some of its helical structure after delipidation and that the helical structure is restored after recombination. A study of the interaction of apolipoprotein serine (whose amino acid sequence is known) with phosphatidylcholine suggests that the phospholipid binding involves amphipathic helical regions of the protein molecule. Assmann and Brewer have proposed a model for the interaction of apoprotein and lipids which is analogous to that proposed by Singer for cell membranes [89] (see Chapter 16). It is now believed that the plasma lipoproteins are made by a core of triglycerides or cholesterol esters surrounded by a monolayer composed of phospholipids, apoproteins and cholesterol. The surface monolayer is 20–25 A thick or half the width of the cell membrane bilayer. Thus, in the plasma lipid as in the cell membrane, the proteins float into a sea of lipids.

Little is known about the chemical composition of the apoprotein found in chylomicrons, but overall amino acid composition and N- and C-terminal determinations have appeared. At least four major N-terminal residues seem to be in the apoprotein of chylomicrons: aspartic, glutamic, serine, and threonine. Such results suggest that there must be at least four apoproteins in chylomicrons. Although studies of amino acid composition (especially if the protein material is not homogenous at the start) cannot provide detailed information on the tertiary structure of the proteins, such investigation does tell something about the proteins binding capacity. Surprisingly, amino acid composition studies of the chylomicron protein suggest that there is no preponderance of hydrophobic residues. The amount of hydrophobic residues is 40%, which is similar to that found in nonlipid plasma proteins.

Blood Lipids

The lipid content of the blood can be determined by various analytical methods, including determinations of the total lipid, total esterified fatty acids, phospholipids, total cholesterol, cholesterol esters, neutral fats, and cerebrosides. The total lipid content is easy to determine. The lipid fraction of the blood is extracted with an organic solvent. The organic solvent is evaporated and the residue is weighed on a precise balance. The total lipid content of the blood in the postabsorptive plasma ranges from 50 mg/100 cc to about 800 mg/100 cc. The total cholesterol is determined after extracting the lipid with chloroform and reacting it with acetic anhydride in concentrated sulfuric acid. Cholesterol turns blue green depending on the cholesterol concentration and obeys the Beer-Lambert law. However, the color developed with cholesterol esters is not exactly the same as that with free cholesterol. Therefore, more accurate results may be obtained by precipitating the ester cholesterol with digitonin or by hydrolyzing all the esters into free cholesterol. The blood contains 135–260 mg of cholesterol per 100 cc. The amount of neutral fats is calculated by determining the difference between the total fatty acid and the sum of phospholipid and cholesterol ester. The lipid content of the plasma changes under physiological and pathological conditions. The composition of ingested foods is the most important physiological factor. After a fatty meal, the plasma level of neutral fats rises rapidly, reaching a peak between 6 and 8 hours after a meal and returning to normal 10 hours later. The rise in neutral fat is considerable: 30–130% of the normal value. This rapid rise in neutral fats is responsible for the milkiness of the serum after meals. The increase in phospholipid and cholesterol levels is relatively low: 20% in the former and 10% in the latter.

The glyceride composition of the lipoproteins varies with their mobility. α_2-Lipoproteins have a triglyceride composition similar to that of dietary triglyceride. In β-lipoprotein, the acid composition of the triglyceride is intermediate between that of body fat and dietary triglyceride.

The proportion of α- and β-triglycerides varies in hereditary or acquired lipemia depending upon the cause of the hyperlipemia. For example, in alcoholic, pancreatic, and fat-feeding hyperlipemia, α-type glycerides are found; in nephrosis or carbohydrate-induced lipemia, the β-type are found.

Because they represent only 5–10% of the total fatty acid, the importance of the nonesterified fatty acids in the plasma has long been underestimated. If all the organic acids of blood are treated with an acidified, aqueous solution and a hydrocarbon solvent, such as ester or petroleum ether, 90% of the long-chain fatty acids enter the nonpolar phase in a single distribution. These are not really free fatty acids; they are bound to albumin through an unknown association.* They move with albumin in the ultracentrifuge and have electrophoretic properties

* The antibacterial properties of the long-chain fatty acids are known; they would be relatively toxic if they were not bound to the albumin. In view of the role nonesterified fatty acids (NEFA) of the blood play in transporting fatty acids from adipose tissue to the utilizing cells, a mechanism for ketosis has been proposed, in which blood NEFA concentrations are utilized in diabetes.

similar to those of albumin. Apparently, 3 molecules of fatty acid are bound to 1 molecule of albumin. Oleic, palmitic, linoleic, and stearic acid represent 80% of the nonesterified fatty acid found in the blood. Isotopic studies have clearly demonstrated that nonesterified fatty acids are in the blood to be oxidized by the utilizing cells, not to be carried to the reserve or storage tissues. Indeed, when labeled palmitate is administered, it is rapidly converted into CO_2.

Various factors—including glucose, insulin, and epinephrine—influence the blood concentration of nonesterifying acids. Although glucose and insulin consistently decrease the amount of nonesterified fatty acids in the blood, epinephrine increases their concentration.

It has been assumed that in diabetes the mechanism controlling the release of nonesterified fatty acid from the storage tissues into the plasma is lost. Thus, excessive amounts of nonesterified fatty acid accumulate in the blood, leading to overloading of the liver and acetoacetic acid formation. This hypothesis is supported by the fact that in blood the nonesterified fatty acid concentration parallels the glucose concentration in hyperglycemia. Furthermore, in diabetic coma the increase in nonesterified fatty acid is considerable; it parallels the amount of ketone bodies found in the blood and also precedes the dangerous accumulation of keto acids. An alternative explanation for the accumulation of nonesterified fatty acid in the blood of diabetics may be that the storage tissues have lost their capacity to synthesize fatty acid in view of the lack of NADPH resulting from insulin deficiency.

Origin of Blood Lipoproteins

Blood lipids originate from food intake (exogenous), and synthesis in the liver (see Fig. 11-3).

In the intestine, ingested triglycerides are digested to fatty acids. The long-chain fatty acids are neutralized to form glycerides; short-chain fatty acids are transported as such.

Most of the dietary lipids—triglycerides, phospholipids, and cholesterol—are transported in the form of chylomicrons. Ethionine administration prevents chylomicron formation by interfering with protein synthesis. Indirect evidence suggests that ApoB and possibly ApoC are part of the chylomicron as it is elaborated in the intestine. ApoA is believed to be added later by exchange between HDL and chylomicrons in the blood.

Studies on hepatectomized and eviscerated dogs established that the β-lipoprotein (LDL) and the lipoprotein (VLDL) are made primarily in the liver, although some reports have appeared suggesting that small amounts of LDL and VLDL are made in the intestine.

Rat liver ribosomes were found to incorporate amino acids into a product with immunological properties of LDL, VLDL, and HDL, indicating that these three classes of lipoprotein are synthesized *de novo* in liver.

VHDL synthesis is stimulated by lipolytic factors (which liberate free fatty acids from the adipose tissue), alloxan diabetes, and feeding of carbohydrates. In contrast, VLDL and LDL production are inhibited by the administration of large doses of orotic acid

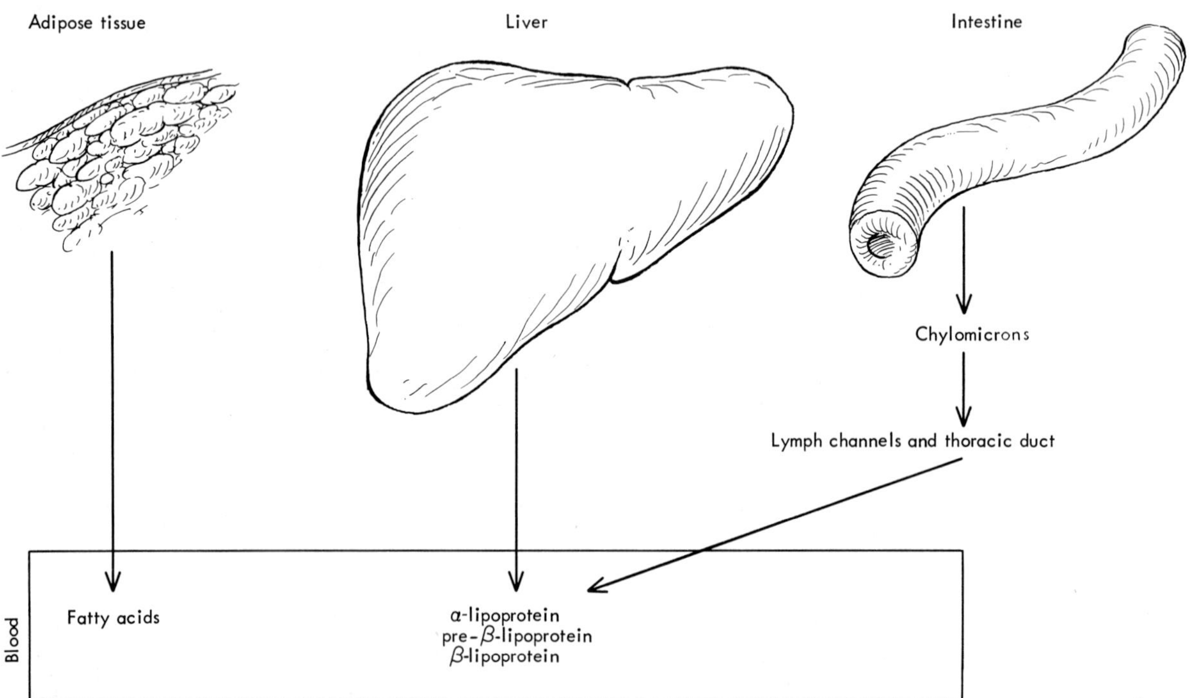

Fig. 11-3. Principal sources of blood lipoproteins

(see section on fatty livers). Part of the circulating LDL and HDL could be derived from the hydrolysis of chylomicrons and VLDL (endogenous particles) as the result of protein lipase action.

The protein moiety that is involved in forming pre-β_2-lipoprotein has not been identified with certainty. Some have proposed that a β-protein with unique properties forms the protein moiety of the pre-β_2-lipoproteins.

The β_2-lipoproteins have very low densities. The particles are lighter than plasma and have a density less than 1000 and *Sf* 20 to 400. The β_2-lipoprotein granules are sometimes called the endogenous granules to distinguish them from chylomicrons.

In addition to the VLDL, pre-β_2-lipoproteins derived from liver, the plasma appears to contain a VLDL in which the protein moiety is of the A type. These plasma lipoproteins are believed to originate in the intestine.

It has also been proposed that after VLDL is released into the circulation, the pre-β-lipoproteins, like the chylomicrons, pick up ApoA. The role of the bound ApoA is not clear. Some have proposed that it activates protein lipase and lecithin cholesterol acyl transferase.

The mechanism of lipoprotein transport differs depending upon the source of the triglyceride. Exogenous (dietary) triglycerides are packaged to form chylomicrons, which are transferred from the intestinal wall into the lymph, and from there into the blood. When the chylomicrons contact the endothelial walls of adipose tissue, heart, and other organs, they are attacked by protein lipase. The free fatty acids penetrate the cell membrane and are reused for triglyceride synthesis or oxidized.

Lipolysis or interference with glycerol esterification increases the levels of free fatty acids in the blood. Most of these free fatty acids enter the liver, where they are either metabolized or used for the biosynthesis of triglycerides, which are complexed with the pre-β_2-lipoprotein. The complex is excreted in the blood, where it contributes to the VLDL pool.

In addition, various amounts of triglycerides are transported in the blood as small complexes with two groups of proteins, the A and the B, which constitute the protein moiety of the α- and β-lipoproteins, respectively. A and B proteins are also believed to be present in chylomicrons. The α- and β-lipoprotein complexes and VLDL include cholesterol and phospholipids. Normally, these lipoprotein complexes account for 90% of the plasma cholesterol and the phospholipids.

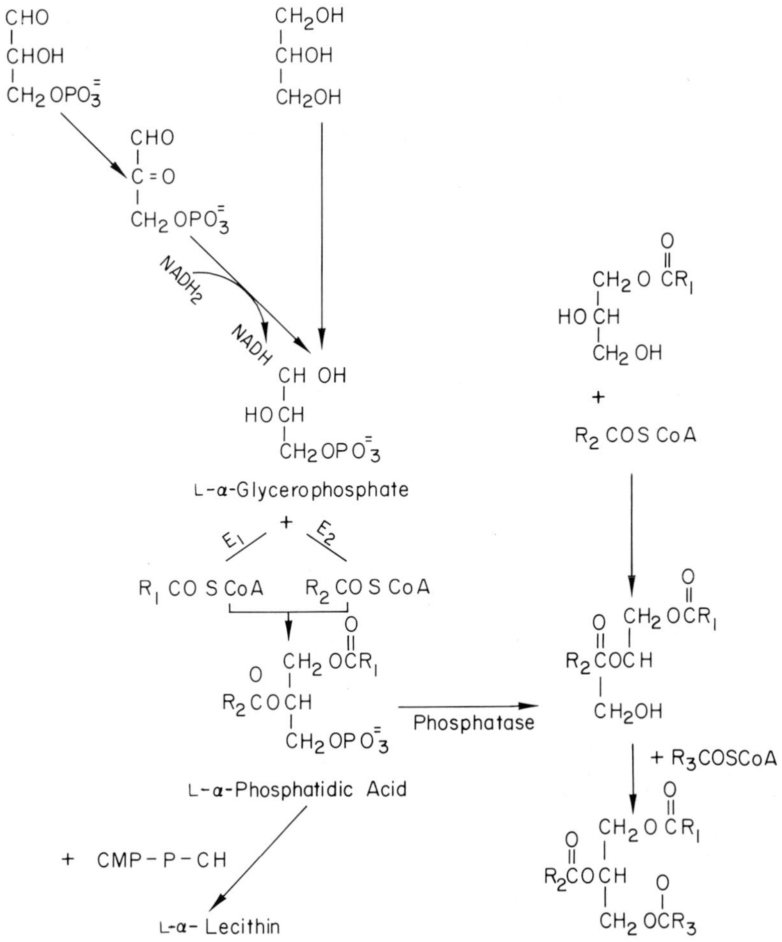

Fig. 11-4. Biosynthesis of triglycerides

Triglyceride Synthesis in Liver and Intestine

Although the hydrolysis of triglycerides to yield fatty acids and glycerol is accompanied by only a small loss of energy, the synthesis of triglycerides involves high-energy bonds [26]. In fact, triglyceride biosynthesis is reminiscent of that of phosphatides, which also involves high-energy bonds. The first step in the formation of triglycerides is α-glycerophosphate formation (see Fig. 11-4). L-α-Glycerophosphate can be generated in a reaction that involves glycerol and ATP and is catalyzed by a specific kinase, which selectively catalyzes the asymmetric phosphorylation of glycerol. Few of the glycerol moieties found in triglycerides are formed in that fashion, and most of the glycerol of the triglycerides is derived from D-phosphoglyceraldehyde, a product of the Embden-Meyerhof pathway. Phosphoglyceraldehyde is converted to glycerophosphate in the following way: In the cell, phosphoglyceraldehyde is in equilibrium with phosphodihydroxyacetone. In the presence of a specific dehydrogenase (operating in reverse), the dihydroxyacetone phosphate can be converted to the L-isomer. Two molecules of fatty acid are then added to the L-α-glycerophosphate to yield L-α-phosphatidic acid. In this reaction, the fatty acids are activated in the form of fatty acyl-CoA. Two enzymes are thought to be involved in converting L-α-glycerophosphate into L-α-phosphatidic acid: one with strict specificity which catalyzes the fixation of a fatty acid in position 2 of the L-α-glycerophosphate; a second with broad specificity which catalyzes the fixation of the fatty acid in position 1 of the L-α-glycerophosphate. In plants, the specificity of the first enzyme is restricted to unsaturated fatty acid; in mammals, that specificity is restricted by the chain length of the fatty acid. A phosphatase splits the phosphate moiety of the phosphatidic acid to yield the diglyceride. In the last step of triglyceride synthesis, the diglyceride reacts with an activated fatty acid to yield the triglyceride. In the intestine, in addition to the pathway just described, there is another pathway in which triglyceride biosynthesis starts with a monoglyceride. Thus, the monoglycerides react with the activated fatty acid to yield a diglyceride. This reaction is catalyzed by a microsomal enzyme, and it appears to be unique to the intestine.

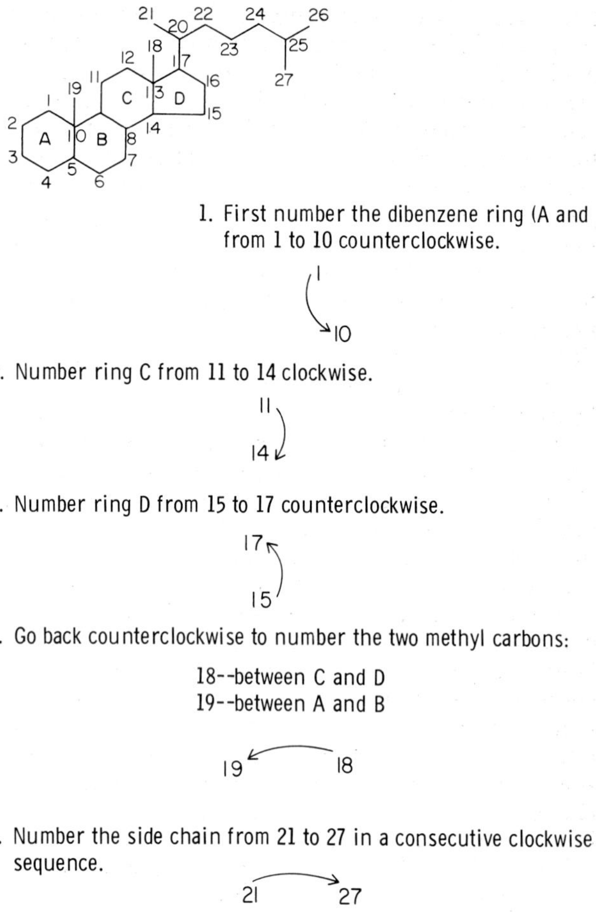

Cholesterol Metabolism

Exogenous Cholesterol

Among the blood lipids related to the development of atherosclerosis, cholesterol is of particular significance. The formula and numbering of the cholesterol molecule are given in Figure 11-5. The cholesterol found in the intestinal lumen comes from food and from cholesterol secreted with the bile. Even if esterification were essential for cholesterol absorption, this is not the case for all steroids: for example, cholesterone and the methyl ester of cholesterol are absorbed in the free form. Intestinal cholesterol is absorbed in the small intestine, probably in the jejunum. Cholesterol absorption in the intestine is facilitated by bile acid, esterifying enzymes, and the fat content of the intestine. Sitosterol, dehydrocholesterol, and such substances as ferric chloride, an extract of brain tissue, and mineral oil interfere with cholesterol absorption.

The exact role of bile in cholesterol absorption is not known. Two different hypotheses have been proposed.* One assumes that bile facilitates cholesterol absorption by emulsifying the lipids in the intestinal chyle, and the second postulates that bile activates the pancreatic esterase, which esterifies cholesterol before it is absorbed. The evidence in favor of the second hypothesis is based on the demonstration that cholesterol esters can be absorbed by the intestinal mucosa in the absence of bile. But it is not clear whether all cholesterol is absorbed in a free or esteri-

21 20 22 24 26
18 23 25
12 17
11 16 27
19 C 13 D
1 15
2 A 10 B 8 14
3 5 7
4 6
1. First number the dibenzene ring (A and B) from 1 to 10 counterclockwise.
1
10
2. Number ring C from 11 to 14 clockwise.
11
14
3. Number ring D from 15 to 17 counterclockwise.
17
15
4. Go back counterclockwise to number the two methyl carbons:
18--between C and D
19--between A and B
19 18
5. Number the side chain from 21 to 27 in a consecutive clockwise sequence.
21 27

Fig. 11-5. Numbering of the carbons of the cholesterol molecule

* Bile and cholesterol excretion in the feces can be altered by the administration of antibiotics. For example, neomycin has a hypocholesteremic effect. Excretion of bile acid and cholesterol is much higher in conventional than in germ-free rats [27].

fied form. Indeed, cholesteremia increases less after esterified cholesterol administration than after the administration of a cholesterol-free diet. Therefore, cholesterol probably is esterified within the intestinal cells, rather than in the lumen. If intraluminar cholesterol is esterified at all, the source of the esterifying enzyme remains to be established. Because an active pancreatic esterase exists, it is tempting to assume that the esterification is catalyzed by that enzyme after it is excreted in the pancreatic juice in the intestinal lumen. In conclusion, in experimental animals, neither the necessity for nor the site of the esterification of cholesterol has been solidly established.

Cholesterol absorption in humans has been studied by cannulating the thoracic duct. The results of these experiments suggest that cholesterol is absorbed in the jejunum and is esterified before absorption. The absorbed cholesterol may be transferred to the blood vessels (and from there reach the portal vein and the liver) or to the lymphatics and the thoracic duct.

Although the cholesterol in the thoracic duct is esterified at a rate of 50% of the total, the absorbed cholesterol in the blood is not esterified until several hours after absorption. The reasons for these differences are not clear. However, it has been assumed that whereas the lymph possesses a mechanism that esterifies cholesterol rapidly, the blood does not possess such a mechanism, and, therefore, the absorbed cholesterol in the blood is esterified only after it has been passed through the liver.

The cholesterol of the lymph is at first associated with chylomicrons, but it is rapidly transferred from chylomicrons to the β-lipoprotein fraction. The cholesterol that reaches the liver may be either converted into bile acid and excreted in the bile, or it may enter the biosynthetic pathways. That the choice between the anabolic and the catabolic pathways depends on the nature of the species and is hormonally influenced has been demonstrated by comparative experiments in dogs and rabbits. Although the dog normally oxidizes greater amounts of cholesterol than the rabbit, this pattern can be reversed by making the dog hyperthyroid.

Cholesterol is excreted in the feces in the form of cholesterol, coprostanol, and cholestanol. A small fraction (only a few milligrams) of cholesterol is also excreted in the urine, but the principal metabolic end products are bile acid conjugates.

Endogenous Cholesterol

Although exogenous cholesterol is readily absorbed, most animals synthesize cholesterol from very simple compounds: acetic acid, acetoacetic acid, propionic or isovaleric acid, etc. [28–32].

Mevalonic Acid Formation

Four successive steps can be distinguished in cholesterol biosynthesis: (1) formation of mevalonic acid; (2) squalene formation; (3) conversion of squalene to lanosterol; and (4) conversion of lanosterol to cholesterol (see Fig. 11-6).

The first reaction in cholesterol biosynthesis consists of a branching reaction that attaches a molecule of acetyl-CoA to the β-hydroxyl of the β-methylglutaryl-CoA. This is rapidly followed by the reduction of the product of the previous reaction to yield mevalonic acid. Then, the polymerization of several molecules of mevalonic acid leads to squalene formation. This polymerization is a complex reaction in which one reduction, six dehydrations, and six decarboxylations take place. Squalene is in turn cyclized in an oxidative process. Our knowledge of cholesterol biosynthesis is by no means complete. This biosynthetic process involves more than 20 steps, of which only a few have been identified.

The biosynthesis of cholesterol starts with acetyl-CoA, which is then converted to acetoacetyl-CoA. Acetoacetyl-CoA may be reduced to hydroxybutyric acid, which serves as a precursor for higher fatty acid synthesis or condenses with acetyl-CoA to yield β-hydroxymethylglutaryl-CoA.

Two enzymes are required for the formation of HMG-CoA from acetoacetyl CoA and acetyl CoA, a thiolase and a HMG-CoA synthetase. Both enzymes have been found in mitochondria and cytosol, but while the mitochondrial system serves to synthesize ketone bodies, the cytosol system is responsible for cholesterol synthesis.

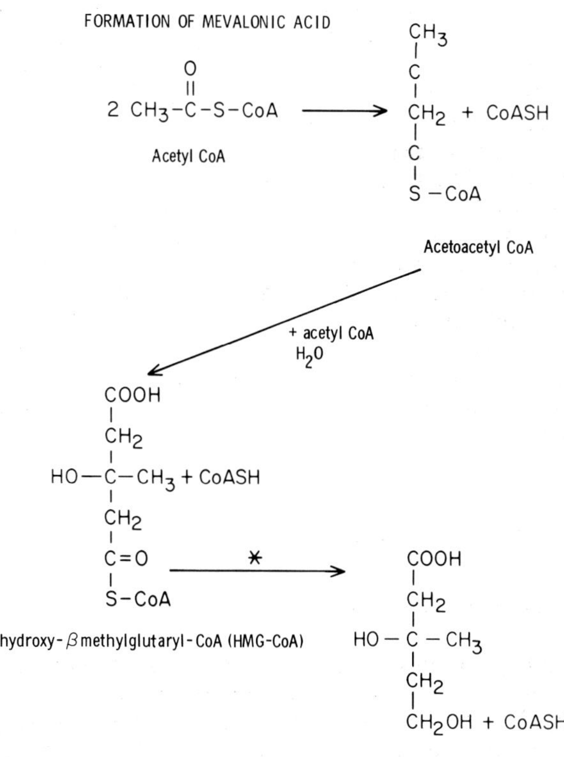

Fig. 11-6. Cholesterol biosynthesis. * Feedback inhibition by cholesterol

HMG-CoA reductase has been solubilized from microsomes. *In vivo* regulation of the activity of the enzyme is complex and still poorly understood. *In vivo* the enzyme activity fluctuates with the time of day, and it is affected by cholesterol concentration and the administration of hormones. The enzyme activity is lowest in the early morning and early evening and peaks around midnight. The molecular mechanisms involved in regulating the rhythm of activity are unknown. Cholesterol feeding depresses the enzyme activity. Insulin and thyroid hormones increase and glucagon and glucocorticoids decrease the enzyme activity [91].

The keto group of B-hydroxy-methylglutaryl-CoA is reduced to the aldehyde in the presence of a specific dehydrogenase and NADPH to yield mevaldic acid. That mevaldic acid is an intermediate in the biosynthesis of mevalonic acid has been demonstrated by isotopic dilution techniques, by direct isolation of the compound, and by its efficient incorporation into squalene. The aldehyde group of mevaldic acid is reduced to the alcohol group of mevalonic acid in the presence of a mevalonic dehydrogenase, the activity of which depends on the presence of $NADPH_2$.

Squalene Formation

Cholesterol synthesis from mevalonic acid occurs maximally if microsomes are combined with a high-speed supernatant. The system must, of course, be reinforced by adding NADH and small amounts of NADPH; ATP is not required. For maximum activity, both NADP and NADPH seem to be required. In the beginning, a boiled supernatant extract was also necessary for the reaction. Popják and his associates found later that a reducing substance, such as cysteine, glutathione, cysteamine or ascorbic acid, could substitute for the boiled extract. Inasmuch as glutathione and ascorbic acid both seem to be active reducing agents, it has been suggested that the oxygen-sensitive substances in the enzyme system were made of a reduced SH group. Further evidence for such a concept was provided by studies of the effect of mercuric chloride or parachloromercuribenzoic acid on the system. The mercurials block the reaction, and their inhibitory properties can be counteracted by adding reduced glutathione.

The structure of the precursor of squalene was not known until Tavormina and colleagues [33] demonstrated that mevalonic acid acted as an efficient precursor of squalene (see Fig. 11-7). Popják and his associates [34, 35] demonstrated by using degradation processes of the labeled squalene derived from mevalonic acid, labeled in its carbon 2, that mevalonic acid must lead to the formation of an isoprenoid unit, which undergoes polymerization to squalene without further degradation.

Paper and column chromatographic studies of the products of the incubation mixture of mevalonic acid and the liver enzyme have yielded a compound that separates from the original mevalonic acid. That compound is more polar than mevalonic acid and was shown to be a phosphorylated derivative of the latter. Indeed, the mevalonic acid derivative is formed in the presence of ATP. Furthermore, ADP and small amounts of AMP are formed in the reaction. Finally, a mevalonic kinase that has been prepared from yeast catalyzed the formation of 5-phosphomevalonic acid. The enzyme has been purified from yeast, mammalian muscle, and liver. The requirements of the enzyme purified from pork liver include cysteine or glutathione, ions (Mg, Mn, Ca, Co, Fe), and ATP or inosine triphosphate. Various biochemicals inhibit the enzyme, but its inhibition by farnesoate, a known inhibitor of cholesterol biosynthesis, is of particular interest.

The 5′-monophosphate is further phosphorylated in position 5 by an enzyme partially purified from pig liver (phosphomevalonic kinase). As for most kinases, magnesium is required for its activity.

The next step involves dehydration, decarboxylation, and isomerization of the mevalonic acid triphosphate. The first two of these transformations are probably performed by a single enzyme reaction; the enzyme purified from yeast requires a metal ion for activity (Mn, Mg, Fe, or Co). ATP is converted to ADP in that reaction, which yields isopentenyl pyrophosphate (5-diphosphomevalonic acid and hydrodecarboxylase). It is not clear why this occurs, but workers have postulated that mevalonic acid 5 pyrophosphate is phosphorylated in position 3 before dehydration and decarboxylation.

In the next reaction, isopententyl pyrophosphate undergoes an isomerization that shifts the double bond from the α- to the β-position to yield dimethylallyl pyrophosphate. There is indirect evidence that the isopentenyl pyrophosphate isomerase is an SH enzyme, but the exact mechanism of the isomerization is not clear.

Isomerization of the isopentenyl pyrophosphate to the dimethylallyl pyrophosphate provides the building blocks for the condensation of a 5-carbon unit into a 10-carbon unit. Thus, geranyl pyrophosphate is believed to be formed by the condensation of 1 molecule of dimethylallyl pyrophosphate with 1 molecule of isopentenyl pyrophosphate. PP_i is freed during the condensation. An additional condensation (in which another pyrophosphate is freed) of geranyl pyrophosphate and isopentenyl pyrophosphate yields farnesyl pyrophosphate.

Farnesyl pyrophosphate is a precursor of squalene. The conversion of farnesyl pyrophosphate to squalene has been demonstrated in yeast, liver, and several plants. It takes place without oxygen, and NADPH is required. The intermediates that appear during the conversion of farnesyl pyrophosphate into squalene are still unknown in spite of many attempts to identify them.

Popják [36] used 5-dideuteromevalonic acid as a precursor and carefully isolated the labeled squalene produced. The study established that: (1) 1 of the

4 hydrogen atoms on the C_1 carbon of one of the 2 farnesyl residues is lost during condensation; (2) the lost hydrogen is stereospecifically replaced by a hydride ion from NADPH; (3) the configuration is inverted, and the C_1 carbon of the farnesyl residue is not involved with hydrogen exchange.

A 30-carbon compound containing pyrophosphate ester of a tertiary alcohol and a cyclopropane ring was first believed to act as an intermediate between farnesyl pyrophosphate and squalene.

A hypothetical scheme for the formation of squalene from farnesyl pyrophosphate proposed that farnesyl pyrophosphate isomerizes to yield nerolidol pyrophosphate, and that squalene is formed by the reductive condensation of 1 molecule of farnesyl pyrophosphate with 1 molecule of nerolidol pyrophosphate.

Isolation and identification of the squalene precursor using nuclear magnetic resonance, mass spectrometry, and chemical degradation established that the squalene precursor is the cyclic pyrophosphoryl ester of squalene-10,11-glycol.

Edmond and Popják [92] have shown that the intermediates involved in the conversion of HMG-CoA to squalene may be diverted into another pathway culminating in the formation of trans-3-methylglutaconyl CoA which can then be converted to HMG-CoA. HMG-CoA may then be used for the formation of ketone bodies. The intermediate step of this shunt pathway will not be discussed, but the significance of the pathway is obvious, it provides another route for the utilization of cholesterol precursors and if the mechanisms which direct the precursors preferentially in one of the two pathways, squalene synthesis or the trans-methylglutaconate shunt, were known, a new mode of regulation of cholesterol and steroid synthesis could be uncovered.

Squalene Conversion

It is now well established that squalene is a precursor of cholesterol. Indeed, squalene fulfills all the conditions required for such a precursor. Acetate is incorporated in squalene, and sterols have been isolated from cells that synthesized squalene. Furthermore, the labeled acetate is distributed as it would be if squalene were an intermediate.

Squalene, a 30-carbon compound with a 22-carbon chain and an 8-methyl substitute, is converted to

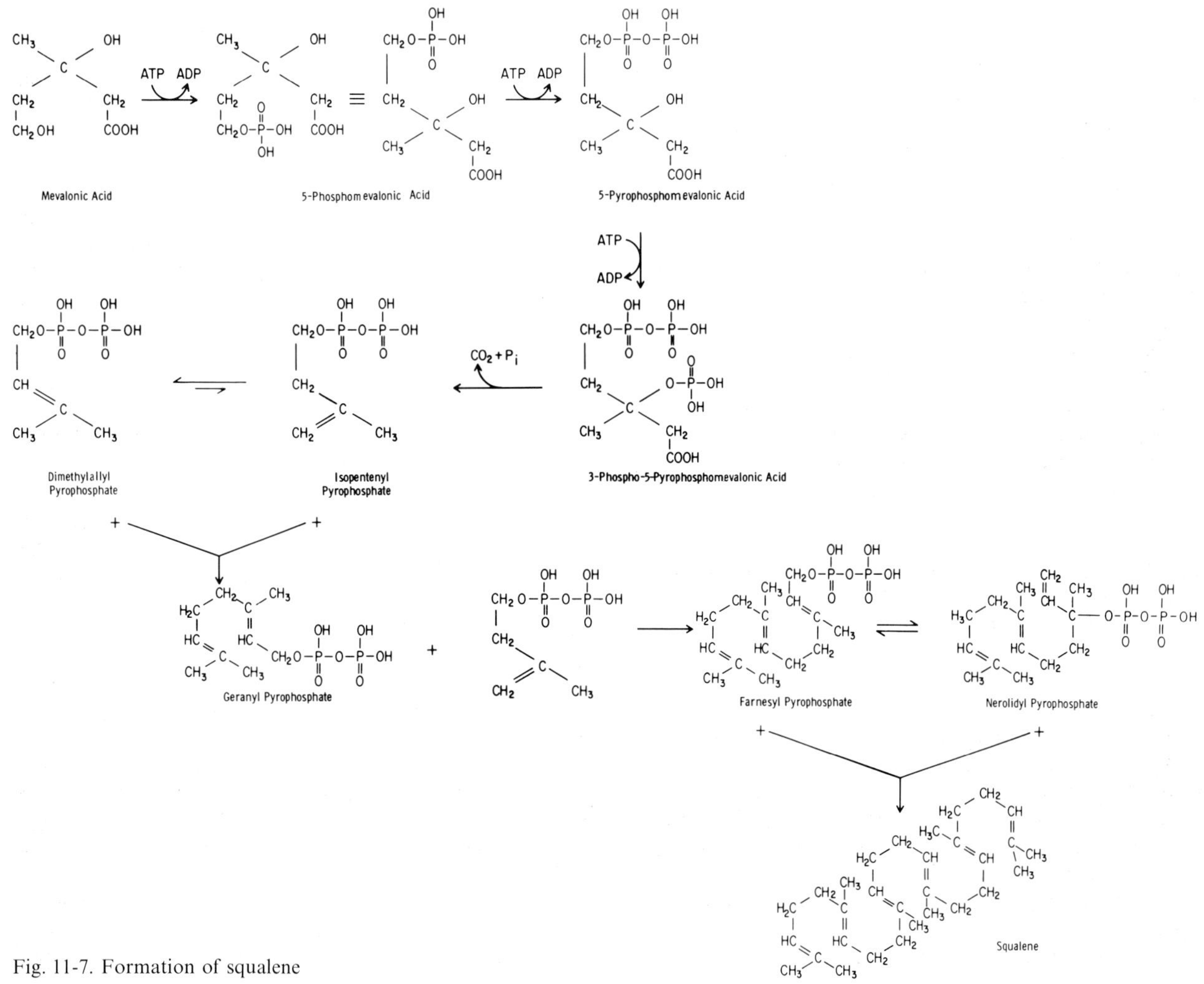

Fig. 11-7. Formation of squalene

lanosterol. The problem posed by the cyclization of squalene is that of converting a straight substituted chain into the cyclic cholesterol ring. This is one of the most puzzling reactions in biochemistry, and all the details of the intermediary steps are far from known. Only what seems to be the most plausible explanation of these molecular events is presented here.

Using ^{18}O, Bloch and Woodward demonstrated that the oxygen atom of carbon 3 of lanosterol was derived from oxygen and not from water. Moreover, when enzymic cyclization of lanosterol is allowed to take place in deuterated water, no deuterium is stably incorporated into lanosterol.

On the basis of these findings, Woodward and Bloch [37] have proposed that the enzymic reaction catalyzes a single molecular attack. The carbon in squalene that is destined to become the carbon 3 of lanosterol is attacked by the enzyme and molecular oxygen. This attack is then followed by electronic hydroyl and methyl shifts, and the molecule ultimately is stabilized by the release of the protein. The enzyme squalene oxidocyclase is believed to catalyze the reaction in two steps: conversion of squalene to its 2, 3-dioxide, and conversion of the oxide to lanosterol.

The conversion of lanosterol to cholesterol involves three groups of reactions: demethylations of the rings (one methyl in carbon 14 and two at carbon 4); isomerization of the Δ^8 to a Δ^7 bond; and reduction of the side chain. The side chain is believed to be reduced before any other change takes place. The demethylation of the 14-methyl group is likely to occur before demethylation of carbon 4. The removal of the methyl in carbon 14 is catalyzed by specific enzymes. The sequence of removal of the methyls in carbon 4 is specific, but it is not known which carbon is removed first.

Investigators have found Δ^8-Δ^7 isomerases in crude preparations of many tissues. The isomerase reaction occurs under anaerobic conditions and seems to be irreversible.

Because the intermediates of the reaction are relatively complex molecules with many common properties, identification and isolation are often difficult. Therefore, identification of the normal metabolite usually does not provide convincing evidence of its role as an intermediate. In most cases, it is necessary to synthesize the suspected intermediate and test its ability to act as a cholesterol precursor. The suspected intermediate must be proved to incorporate the simple precursor of cholesterol (acetate, mevalonic acid), to be the product of the conversion of the metabolite formed in the previous step, and to serve as a precursor for the next reaction in the scheme.

There are many potential intermediates between lanosterol and cholesterol, and the steps have not been mapped completely. The biochemist faces a monumental task that is quite relevant to our understanding of the pathogenesis of arteriosclerosis, and diabetes and myxedema as well.

Regulation of Cholesterol Synthesis

Knowledge of the regulation of cholesterol synthesis would seem to be essential to controlling the blood levels of cholesterol and possibly to lessening the incidence of myocardial infarct.

As we described the individual steps of cholesterol biosynthesis it became obvious that several points of the sequence that leads from acetate to cholesterol could constitute sites of regulation for cholesterol synthesis. One of the first regulating mechanisms discovered is the feedback inhibition of the conversion of hydroxymethyl glutarate to mevalonic acid [93].

Cholesterol intake decreases the levels of cholesterol biosynthesis in liver and in bone marrow, but not in other extrahepatic tissues.

The inhibition of the biosynthetic pathway of cholesterol in liver by the end product was the first example of negative feedback inhibition in mammals [38, 39]. The inhibited step is the reductive conversion of hydroxymethyl glutarate to mevalonic acid, an irreversible reaction in a point of the sequence at which the biosynthetic pathway for cholesterol branches off to become unique. Moreover, the conversion of hydroxymethyl glutarate to mevalonic acid is irreversible

The molecular structure of the inhibitor is not known. It is not believed to be cholesterol. Unidentified cholesterol metabolites, a cholesterol-protein complex, and bile acids have all been incriminated.

Because a large amount of cholesterol is derived from extrahepatic tissue, the relevance of hepatic cholesterol biosynthesis to blood cholesterol levels remains to be established.

If increased cholesterol intake decreases hepatic cholesterol biosynthesis, a low-cholesterol diet would cause increased cholesterol synthesis in liver. Moreover, a diet rich in lipids stimulates cholesterol biosynthesis. The mechanism by which the cholesterol metabolism is modified in these cases remains unknown.

Other regulatory mechanisms of cholesterol synthesis are likely to exist. HMG-CoA reductase activity is modulated by blood cholesterol levels and hormones. Cyclic AMP is believed to modulate the activity of one of the enzymes involved in mevalonate synthesis. A squalene sterol carrier protein has been discovered which is believed to play a critical role in the regulation of cholesterol and steroid biosynthesis. The protein is found in the cytosol of most cells investigated. It has been purified to homogeneity by electrophoresis on urea polyacrylamide gels. It binds water insoluble precursors before interacting with microsomal enzymes responsible for the synthesis of cholesterol and is therefore indispensable for conversion of water insoluble precursors to cholesterol. The mechanism regulating the availability of the protein is unknown, but the protein could clearly play a significant role in the regulation of cholesterol biosynthesis. For example, it has been shown that it is required for the conversion of farnesyl pyrophosphate to presqualene pyrophosphate and squalene [91, 93].

Pathogenesis of Arteriosclerosis

The hypothesis that metabolic factors are involved in the pathogenesis of arteriosclerosis rests on three groups of arguments: the epidemiological argument, clinical information, and experimentation in humans and in animals [40–42].

Epidemiological Findings

When caloric intake, the incidence of obesity, fat intake, cholesteremia, and the incidence of myocardial infarct are studied in specific racial, social, or national groups, a correlation is usually found between the high-fat diet and cholesteremia and the incidence of myocardial infarct. The incidence of arteriosclerosis is generally lower in economically underdeveloped countries than it is in the economically privileged.

Coronary disease is the only form of arteriosclerosis that correlates well with high dietary cholesterol levels. Therefore, some have suggested that dietary factors are not as important in inducing fat deposition as they are in modifying blood coagulability. However, as we shall later see, the effect of a high-fat diet on thrombogenesis and fibrinolysis remains controversial.

Within the economically underdeveloped countries, there are considerable group differences in the incidences of myocardial infarct that can be correlated with the standard of life. The incidence of arteriosclerosis is usually higher among those who enjoy a higher living standard. Epidemiological studies have been carried out on all continents and in many countries—Italy, the Scandinavian countries, the Lowlands, Japan, South Africa, the United States, and South America. Excellent reviews on the subject have been published.

Nevertheless, such data are sometimes difficult to interpret. Indeed, the correlation between arteriosclerosis and a high standard of living holds only for a few countries; for example, the correlation holds for Italy, the United States, and Japan, but not for Canada and Australia. Furthermore, Italy has a low per capita fat intake (animal or other) but has a greater incidence of myocardial infarct than the Scandinavian countries or the Lowland countries that have a high fat intake per capita. These discrepancies can be explained in various manners; *e.g.*, the Italians use mainly vegetable oils, which are usually consumed without waste, but Scandinavians and Lowlanders consume large amounts of animal fats that are often discarded in the kitchen. In that respect, it is interesting to point out that Trappist monks, who are strict vegetarians, have lower serum cholesterol than the Benedictines, who are omnivorous.

Thomas and his associates [43] reviewed the geographic aspects of arteriosclerosis. After a comprehensive survey of the literature, the authors reached the following conclusion:

"Our overall impression is that studies of geographical aspects of atherosclerosis are just emerging from their infancy. Very likely, important advances will be made in the future on the basis of geographical studies."

Clinical Pathological Correlation and Experimentation

Surveys of the hospital population in the United States and other parts of the world suggest that individuals with myocardial infarct or angina pectoris always have a higher blood cholesterol or β-lipoprotein level than other hospitalized groups. However, there are many individual variations, and a small percentage of patients with myocardial infarct have normal or low cholesterol levels, and *vice versa.* At least four groups of factors are known to affect blood cholesterol levels: heredity, diet, hormones, and disease. The effects of these various factors have been studied in humans and in animals.

Studies based on the pedigree of many patients with normal and elevated cholesterol levels and observations of monozygotic and dizygotic twins suggest that hypercholesterolemia is influenced by hereditary factors. The genes are transmitted as simple mendelian dominants; they are not sex linked. These observations are in agreement with the fact that both xanthomatosis and coronary diseases are apparently hereditary and are also transmitted as a simple mendelian dominants.

Absolute caloric intake, the relative proportion of fat in the diet, the nature of these fats, and the dietary intake of proteins or some amino acids all affect blood cholesterol levels. The reduction of fats in the diet will lead to reduced blood cholesterol levels. In addition, if unsaturated vegetable or marine oils are substituted for the saturated animal lipid content of the diet on an isocaloric basis, the blood cholesterol level drops sharply. This effect of unsaturated fat is observed when animal fats are completely substituted by vegetable fats, and also after partially substituting or supplementing an ordinary fat-rich diet with unsaturated oils. Some studies suggest that essential fatty acids may be important in correcting hypercholesterolemia The mechanism by which the unsaturated and the essential fatty acids act to modify blood cholesterol levels is not known. However, one experiment showed that if a normal *ad libidum* diet is replaced by a diet that includes 40% butter, plasma cholesterol rises immediately, reaching values around 300–500 mg/100 ml. This rise in plasma cholesterol is associated with a decrease in the fecal sterols. If corn oil is substituted for butter, there is no increase in blood cholesterol. Despite the high incidence of arteriosclerosis in this country, the American diet is not low in essential fatty acids. Consequently, if an essential fatty acid deficiency exists, it can only be relative to an exaggerated intake of other lipoprotein components.

Although the animal studies definitely confirm the arteriogenic properties of high-fat and high-cholesterol diets, they cast some doubt on the role of the various groups of fatty acids in the diet. Indeed, in animals, the administration of unsaturated vegetable oils associated with a cholesterol-rich diet seems to increase both cholesteremia and the incidence of atheromatous plaques instead of being hypocholesterolemic and reducing the rate of arteriogenesis. Furthermore, nonessential unsaturated fatty acids, such as oleic acid and others, stimulate hypercholesterolemia in rats. In rabbits, saturated, hydrogenated coconut oil has a similar effect. (Cholesterol feeding or alloxan diabetes accelerated the consequences of essential fatty acid deficiency in animals. Cysteine or taurine can replace choline in that respect.) However, when dietary saturated fatty acids are replaced by polyunsaturated fatty acid, the fatty acid moiety of cholesterol ester, phospholipids, and triglycerides becomes more unsaturated, and the total cholesterol levels fall. This is followed by increased excretion of bile acids and sterols in the stools.

In addition to the lipid composition of the diet, the plasma levels of β-lipoprotein and cholesterol are affected by the dietary intake of proteins, some amino acids, and some vitamins. Thus, a diet containing less than 25 g of protein per day seems to lower the β-lipoprotein content of blood even when large amounts of butter are added to the diet. When small amounts of choline or methionine are included in the diet, the plasma cholesterol drops to about one-third of its original value. Handler first observed the effect of choline and found that choline-deficient rats were hypercholesterolemic. It was later found that this is true in practically all species tested rigorously. A diet adequate in choline but low in methionine also causes hypercholesterolemia. Arteriosclerotic lesions have thus been produced by high cholesterol, high lipid, and reduced choline intake in both rats and monkeys.

In chicks, low-protein and low-methionine diets lead to severe hypercholesterolemia and arteriosclerosis. This effect of the low protein and methionine ratios is reversed by adding choline to the diet. Choline seems to be essential for the hepatic secretion of β-lipoproteins. In rats, lesions resembling those of human arteriosclerosis have been obtained by feeding diets low in choline or rich in fat and cholesterol with superimposed hyperthyroidism. In fact, myocardial infarcts were produced in rats by the concomitant administration of thiouracil, cholesterol, sodium cholate, and butter; 20% of the animals developed infarcts after about 14 weeks.

Several vitamins are thought to influence the incidence rf arteriosclerosis. Nicotinic acid lowers the blood cholesterol content 3–6 g/day. Nicotinamide has no effect. The effect of nicotinic acid is not clear; it may result from a stimulation of basal metabolism, but the drop in plasma cholesterol is too great to be explained by the relatively small rise in metabolism alone. Nicotinic acid probably affects the biosynthesis of endogenous cholesterol.

Ascorbic acid is assumed to reduce blood cholesterol. In monkeys, pyridoxine deficiency induces intimal fibrosis. Although pyridoxine deficiency alone does not lead to fat deposition in the arteriolar wall, the introduction of 5% cholesterol in the diet of rhesus monkeys leads to hypercholesterolemia, increased serum β-lipoprotein levels, xanthomatosis, and arteriosclerosis. After 4 years of such a diet, arteriosclerosis affects the aorta and its branches, the coronary arteries, and basal arteries of the brain. Thus, hypercholesterolemia and pyridoxine deficiency produce a form of arteriosclerosis in monkeys that closely resembles that in humans. Apparently, pyridoxine is required in the reaction that converts linoleate to arachidonic acid by the condensation of a molecule of acetate and a molecule of linoleate.

Diets deficient in vitamin E lead to calcification and fibrosis of the media in pigs and rabbits maintained on high levels of calcium, phosphorus, and vitamin D. Among the injuries observed are endothelial and smooth muscle fibroplasia, internal elastic lamellar fragmentation, and myocardial necrosis.

Effect of Hormones on Arteriosclerosis

Many hormones modify cholesteremia by an unknown mechanism and indirectly affect the incidence of arteriosclerosis [44]. Apparently, elevations in blood cholesterol levels alone are not sufficient to increase the incidence of arteriosclerosis, and typical arteriosclerotic plaques have never been produced by hormonal treatment alone in experimental animals or in humans.

The lower incidence [45, 46] of arteriosclerosis in women as compared to men is well known. Moreover, in patients treated with estrogen for prostatic carcinoma, the blood levels of cholesterol and the incidence of arteriosclerosis are considerably reduced. The administration of estrogen to cholesterol-fed cockerels has a prophylactic as well as a therapeutic effect on coronary arteriosclerosis in addition to decreasing the cholesterol-phospholipid ratio. Similar effects have been observed in rats; therefore, estrogen has been advocated as a prophylactic or therapeutic agent in arteriosclerosis.

Clinicians have known for a long time that blood cholesterol levels are elevated in hypothyroidism [47], and this has stimulated research in animals. Hypercholesterolemia was observed for the first time in 3 myxedematous patients in 1916. Hypercholesterolemia in these patients could be reversed by thyroxine administration. Twenty years later it was demonstrated that cholesterol-fed, thiouracil-treated dogs developed a form of arteriosclerosis that resembled the human disease histologically and anatomically. The administration of thyroid hormones reduces arteriosclerosis and cholesteremia in men and in cholesterol-fed rabbits and chicks. In animals, potassium, iodine, or dinitrophenol administration had no effect tn blood cholesterol levels, which suggests that the effect of tthyroid hormones in arteriosclerosis is not related to its effect on general metabolism. However, all forms of hypothyroidism do not have the same effect on blood cholesterol. Indeed, although hypothyroidism produced by labeled iodine administration or thyroidectomy reduces cholesterol synthesis in the liver, it has no effect on plasma cholesterol concentration. In contrast, thiouracil reduces hepatic cholesterol synthesis and has, at the same time, a hypercholesterolemic effect. The thiouracil-induced increase in blood cholesterol occurs even after thyroidectomy. Thus, thiouracil does not seem to act through the thyroid.

Whereas hypothyroidism increases blood cholesterol, hyperthyroidism or thyroxine administration reduces blood cholesterol. Triac is the only thyroxine metabolite that seems to affect blood cholesterol specifically. It reduces the amount of cholesterol circulating in the plasma and deposited in the arteries. Other metabolites, such as triiodothyronine or tectrac, when administered to rats, elevate the rate of hepatic cholesterol synthesis and increase oxygen consumption but have no effect on plasma cholesterol.

The mechanism by which thyroxine acts to reduce cholesteremia is not clear. Since no effect of dinitrophenol on the plasma cholesterol was observed, it was assumed that the hormone does not act on blood cholesterol through increasing metabolism. This conclusion is not entirely justified because the modes of action of dinitrophenol and thyroid hormones on general metabolism could result from completely different mechanisms. Also, the effect of the thyroid hormones is restricted to blood cholesterol. Although their administration may reverse hypercholesterolemia, they do not reverse established arteriosclerosis. In fact, at large doses thyroid hormones produce vascular injuries of the arteriosclerotic type.

Pancreatic Hormones

The relationship between diabetes and arteriosclerosis is discussed in more detail in the chapter devoted to diabetes. Only a few pertinent experimental and clinical observations are reviewed here.

Pancreatectomy in chicks leads to hypercholesterolemia. The pancreatectomized or alloxanized chick on a normal mash diet grows normally and does not develop hyperglycemia, glycosuria, hyperlipemia, ketosis, or acidosis. A diet containing 2% cholesterol and 5% cotton seed must be administered to induce hypercholesterolemia. With such a diet, the plasma cholesterol level doubles in the pancreatectomized animals as compared with controls, and this is associated with a high degree of aortic arteriosclerosis. Under these conditions, insulin has no effect. But if insulin is administered to chicks whose diet is changed from a cholesterogenic to a noncholesterogenic type, Katz and his associates found that the hormone interferes with the regression of arteriosclerosis. Furthermore, the same authors observed that insulin antagonizes the effect of estrogens on atherogenesis. However, these experiments are difficult to interpret because large doses of insulin were used, and they led to prolonged hypoglycemia. Similar effects of insulin on atherogenesis have been demonstrated in alloxan-diabetic rats. This condition induces a tremendous increase of atherogenesis of blood cholesterol with a normal cholesterol-phospholipid ratio, but no arteriosclerosis develops, except in one experiment Katz described in which insulin was administered to such animals. Katz has suggested that insulin might be the determining factor in the development of arteriosclerosis frequently observed in diabetic patients. This does not mean that therapeutic doses of insulin are atherogenic because, as mentioned previously, the doses of hormone used seem to be in excess of those needed for therapeutic purposes.

Adrenocorticoids

Severe disturbances of lipid metabolism accompany Cushing's syndrome and Addison's disease. Therefore, a role of the adrenal cortex in controlling lipid metabolism has been suspected for a long time. But no changes in serum cholesterol were observed in adrenalectomized animals in the early experiments, probably because these animals did not survive long enough. Now that deoxycorticosterone acetate is available and adrenalectomized animals can be kept alive, it has been possible to follow changes in the serum lipids under the influence of corticosteroids.

Bilateral adrenalectomy leads to a marked decrease (almost 50%) in plasma phospholipid and cholesterol concentrations. If cortisone or ACTH instead of deoxycorticosterone acetate is used to keep the animal alive, hypercholesterolemia and an increase in blood phospholipids occur, but no increase in the incidence of arteriosclerosis is observed. When cortisone administration is combined with alloxanization or pancreatectomy, it enhances the hyperlipemia that normally results from manipulating the endocrine pancreas; but the incidence of arteriosclerosis is not increased and the cholesterol-phospholipid ratio is maintained constant. These results with the adrenocorticoids or adrenal hormones were interpreted to indicate that the disturbance of the cholesterol-phospholipid ratio might be crucial in atherogenesis.

Although cortisone increases lipemia (cholesterol, phospholipids, and triglycerides) in rats and rabbits, this effect is of limited significance in dogs. Some investigators have also suggested that the hormones not only increase lipemia but also reduce the permeability of the arterial wall, thus preventing lipid deposition in the intima of the arteries. When hyaluronidase is administered to animals on a high-cholesterol diet, the permeability of the arterial wall to lipids increases, and this can be prevented by the concomitant administration of cortisone. However, the effect of hyaluronidase is restricted to the rabbit and has not been reproduced in chickens.

In conclusion, the mechanism of action of the adrenocortical hormones in regulating lipemia is not clear. Moreover, the effect of the hormones and plasma lipids varies from one animal to another, so it is impossible to extrapolate the experimental data to humans.

Stress has often been considered to be a major factor in the incidence of arteriosclerosis because the coronary patient is often active and ambitious [48].* As good a correlation can be obtained if job responsibility instead of dietary fat intake is plotted against the incidence of myocardial infarct. A study in Philadelphia indicates that the incidence of myocardial infarct is much lower among unskilled laborers than among executives. Rosenman and his associate [49, 50] followed proprietors for a period ranging from January through June. They measured blood cholesterol, weight, diet, and evaluated the degree of exercise and occupational and nonoccupational emotional tension. The subjects were divided into two groups: one was made of accountants exclusively, the other did not include accountants. Both groups were active. Both showed above average cholesterol levels during tax period, but only the accountant group showed blood cholesterol values above average during the inventory period in January.

Observations of Yudkin [51] indicate that the increase in television and automobile sales has paralleled the incidence of myocardial infarct much more closely than any other change in our environment, including diet. London bus drivers are more likely to develop coronary disease than are the conductors. This seems to indicate that the increased incidence of arteriosclerosis is related to the greater tension experienced by the driver. But closer examination indicates that factors other than stress may be responsible for the difference. Indeed, the bus drivers tend to be obese and short, whereas the conductor is more frequently tall and slender. An individual's education is thought to influence this tendency toward arteriosclerosis more than his occupation [52].

The mechanism by which stress may contribute to arteriosclerosis is not clear. Its effect may be mediated by epinephrine, which may act on the hemodynamics, or by liberating adrenocortical steroid. Obviously, the effects of stress are difficult to evaluate because stress cannot be measured accurately. However, the observations show that individual variations modify the incidence of arteriosclerosis; such factors should be considered in epidemiological studies on arteriosclerosis.

Several pathological conditions (diabetes, myxedema, and nephrosis) lead to hypercholesterolemia under some circumstances. The mechanisms by which these conditions lead to the development of arteriosclerosis are discussed in detail in other parts of this book.

A number of other epidemiological factors have been linked to the incidence of atherosclerosis. They include the use of soft water, the inhalation of carbon monoxide and cigarette smoking. Of these factors, only smoking seems to be related conclusively to ischemic heart disease. The mechanism by which cigarette smoking increases the risk of heart disease is not known, although carbon monoxide inhalation is suspected [94, 95].

Accelerated atherosclerosis develops in patients subjected to prolonged hemodialysis. The mechanism by which hemodialysis accelerates the disease is unknown [96].

Experimental Arteriosclerosis

The discussion above has already revealed that experimental arteriosclerosis has been produced in a variety of ways in many animals. The susceptibility of these animals varies considerably from species to species, and the animals respond differently to the mechanism of production of arteriosclerosis. However, a high-fat or cholesterogenic diet is indispensable to produce lesions that resemble those observed in arteriosclerosis. Therefore, these experimental procedures allow a certain degree of optimism with regard to comparison with the human disease.

Arteriosclerosis has been produced in animals of all kinds and of all types of dietary habits—omnivorous, carnivorous, and herbivorous. The rabbit and the chick seem to be susceptible species in which a diet supplemented with cholesterol alone can produce arteriosclerosis, whereas in less susceptible animals—like the dog, rat, and monkey—other factors are necessary, such as the administration of cholic acid or thiouracil. Although dissimilarities exist in different species, they are not in any way alarming. Indeed, the first stages of the injuries are similar in man and animals. Caulston and his associates have found in monkey aorta proliferative lesions similar to those found in the human. Furthermore, in some groups of animals, all stages in the development of the arteriosclerotic lesion are seen, and the final injury mimics that of human arteriosclerosis. This is the case in swine, dogs, monkeys, and rats; in rats, myocardial infarcts may be produced under adequate experimental conditions, despite the fact that only lipoic deposition occurs without true plaque formation. Popják has observed, very constantly, thrombosis in arteries of the stomach in hypercholesterolemic rabbits. And he suggests that if thromboses are

* Such an effect of stress does not correlate with the decrease in the incidence of arteriosclerosis during the war. This discrepancy has been explained in the following manner. Apparently, sociological changes experienced as a group do not cause stress; only individual sociological change leads to stress. The decreased incidence of arteriosclerosis during the war period probably cannot be linked to decreased fat consumption because the wartime reductions in the incidence of arteriosclerosis preceded restrictions on fat intake. In addition, arteriosclerosis was less common in the prewar period from 1935 to 1939, when the fat intake compared to previous years was normal. In Finland, fat intake was decreased from 1938 until 1947, but the incidence of arteriosclerosis does not follow the changes in fat intake. The incidence increased in 1938 to 1939, then decreased between 1939 and 1943, and increased again from 1943 to 1947. In Sweden, the incidence of arteriosclerosis changed between 1935 and 1940 without any concomitant change in fat intake.

not found in other animals, it is possibly because we do not examine all sites. A group of researchers of the Albany Medical School have accelerated the production of arteriosclerosis in swine by exposing the animals to irradiation. The mechanism of action of irradiation in this case is not understood.

In an attempt to test the hypothesis that immunologic injuries and a lipid rich diet can cause atherosclerosis, Murphy and his colleagues have fed high lipid diets to rabbits injected with foreign proteins and produced fatty proliferative fibromuscular intimal thickening resembling lesions in human atherosclerosis [97, 98]. Similarly, lesions resembling, but not identical to, atherosclerosis have been observed in arteries of transplanted organs. Such observations have led to an autoimmune theory of the pathogenesis of atherosclerosis [99]. In absence of more experimental evidence, the validity of such a pathogenic interpretation remains to be established.

Among the reasons for investigating the epidemiology of arteriosclerosis and for attempting to produce animal models are the hopes of preventing or reverting the course of the disease. It is not known whether atherosclerosis in humans can be reversed by changing dietary habits, but atherosclerotic lesions produced in Rhesus monkeys by feeding a diet supplemented with fat and cholesterol for 12 weeks regressed within 32 weeks after restoration of a basal diet [100].

Blood Lipids and Arteriosclerosis

The previous paragraphs have demonstrated that blood cholesterol levels are correlated with the incidence of arteriosclerosis. Attempts have been made to define which fraction of the blood lipoprotein is more specifically responsible for the disease. The serum concentration of β-lipoprotein, a protein that can easily be characterized electrophoretically, definitely correlates with the incidence of coronary disease.

In contrast, there seems to be no correlation between HDL, or α-lipoprotein, and the incidence of coronary disease. Gofman and his group [53, 54] have classified the plasma lipoproteins according to their flotation characteristics and found that all individuals have lipoproteins with a flotation constant of 3–8. Lighter components, with a flotation constant of 12–20, were absent in most individuals, but when present were more common in men than in women. They increased in diabetes and with age. Apparently, the increased serum concentration of the lighter lipoprotein group was related to the incidence of arteriosclerosis. In a further experiment, Gofman attempted to express the propensity toward arteriosclerosis in function of the lipoprotein fraction with a flotation constant of 12–400. The atherogenic index was calculated on a large number of normal individuals and those who had myocardial infarcts. This was based on the assumption that the severity of the infarct depends on the concentration of the serum β-lipoprotein.

The degree of arteriosclerosis observed at autopsy did not correlate with the atherogenic index during life. Furthermore, there is apparently no correlation between the development of arteriosclerosis and the development of myocardial infarct. A study of 500 necropsies in Jamaica shows that the incidence and degree of arteriosclerosis observed in that Negro population are the same as that observed previously in the Negro population of New Orleans. In contrast, the incidence of myocardial infarct is much lower in Jamaica than in New Orleans [55]. This would suggest that the development of coronary arteriosclerosis constitutes only a predisposing factor in the development of coronary artery disease.

These are not purely theoretical considerations. If arteriosclerosis and myocardial infarct are not related, research should be directed toward discovering the pathogenesis of myocardial infarct rather than arteriosclerosis. Also, myocardial infarcts may prove curable even if the cure leaves arteriosclerosis unaffected.

In conclusion, whenever the internal or external conditions lead to an increase in blood cholesterol levels, there is also an increase in the incidence of arteriosclerosis in humans, or some form of arteriosclerosis is experimentally produced in animals. Therefore, high blood cholesterol undoubtedly is correlated with the incidence of arteriosclerosis. Such a correlation does not imply a cause-effect relationship between high blood cholesterol and arteriosclerosis. Indeed, high blood cholesterol may constitute only a predisposing factor for arteriosclerosis. Some individuals with cholesteremia do not develop arteriosclerosis or myocardial infarct. Furthermore, cholesteremia in animals does not always lead to a form of arteriosclerosis comparable to that observed in humans. Finally, arteriosclerosis is sharply localized, so hemodynamics may affect this localization.

Immunohistochemical techniques in which antibodies were prepared against the apoproteins of the various plasma lipoproteins have helped to identify the lipids that accumulate in the arterial wall. Tissue sections treated with fluorescein-labeled anti-HDL antibody yield only slight staining of the intima. In contrast, marked fluorescein develops in atherosclerotic aortas that are treated with LDL antibody. LDL is not seen in children's aortas, and deposition is demonstrable only in the second decade of life. Accumulation proceeds with age, but there is evidence that the lipoproteins are degraded, leaving behind less metabolizable lipids such as cholesterol and its esters.

As the atherosclerotic lesion evolves, treatment of the arterial wall with antifibrinogen antibodies reveals the presence of fibrinogen even when no thrombus is visible. The significance of the fibrinogens or fibrin with respect to the evolution of the plaque is not lear.

The observation made by using the immunohistological technique of medial lipid accumulation has been at the origin of a new interpretation of the pathogenesis of arteriosclerosis. It is now believed that lipid droplets (whatever their origin) find their way into the media where they are phagocytized by the multipotential smooth muscle cells already described. The lipids are toxic for these cells, many of which die, but at the same time others proliferate invading the intima where they contribute to the thickening through (1) cell proliferation, (2) elaboration of collagen and elastin fiber, and (3) formation of mucopolysaccharide ground substance.

Since no vasa vasorum penetrate human coronary arteries and aorta, oxygenation of the arterial media and intima depends on oxygen diffusion from the lumen toward the periphery. Thickening of the intima evidently interferes with proper oxygenation, and this is conductive to necrosis of the arterial wall. Necrosis stimulates the cells at the periphery of the necrotic zone to proliferate, further contributing to intimal thickening.

Hemodynamic Factors and Arteriosclerosis

Arteriosclerosis affects those parts of the arterial system that receive the first shock of the cardiac impulse. In some arteries, like the pulmonary artery, arteriosclerosis never develops except when the right side of the heart is hypertensive. In coarctation of the aorta tension is elevated in the portion of the artery proximal to the constriction and reduced in the portion distal to the constriction; arteriosclerosis is minimal in the distal and maximal in the proximal portion. Even in veins—for example, the portal vein system—arteriosclerosis occurs when severe portal hypertension is induced, as in hepatic cirrhosis.

Portions of the saphenous veins are grafted between the aorta and coronary arteries to bypass obstructive lesions of coronary arteries. Atherosclerosis has been observed in implanted vein grafts older than six months [101].

The hemodynamic factors affecting the vascular wall include blood pressure, hydrostatic pressure, hydrostatic tension, cardiac thrust, vibration, and shearing forces.

Fry has developed semiquantitative methods to measure the reaction of the artery to mechanical stress and has shown that the development of structural or functional changes in the intima depends on the magnitude and the direction of the stress. Under moderate stress proteins and lipoproteins move in the subendothelial portions of the intima. Such influx occurs within minutes after the application of stress. If the stress is maintained for months or years, intimal fibrosis develops. More severe stress may lead to erosion of the endothelium [102].

The localization of arteriosclerosis in areas where the hemodynamic factors are preponderent suggests that lesions of the vascular wall contribute to arteriosclerosis [56, 57]. Any primary injury of arteriosclerosis could result from hemodynamic trauma. Indeed, the capillary proliferation and fibrosis might constitute attempts to repair traumatized walls. If, as some have stated, the small subendothelial thrombi are primary lesions of arteriosclerosis, the local trauma could injure the endothelium; this in turn leads to the formation of small thrombi, which are soon covered by the regenerating endothelial cells.

In view of the nature of the mechanical factors that operate in the arterial lumen, it seems that the internal elastica would be particularly vulnerable to hemodynamic injuries. In fact, splitting of the elastica has been observed in the aorta, the radial artery, and the cerebral artery of infants. However, the presence of such lesions in infants suggests that plaques develop extremely slowly and take an entire lifetime to become the classical lesions of arteriosclerosis, or that the elastical injury does not constitute the determining factor in disease development. In the latter case, the local injury would be only a predisposing factor, the determining factor of arteriosclerosis would appear only later in life and probably would be of a metabolic nature.

Trillo and Haust have studied the electron microscopic appearance of dog femoral arteries, of aortas of newborn and atherosclerotic pigs and of aortas of normal and hypertensive rats subjected to hemodynamic changes. They have discovered inside the smooth muscle and in the intimal and medial intercellular spaces, smooth round electron-dense granules surrounded by a membrane. These granules are more numerous in the atherosclerotic arteries and in hypertensive animals. The role of the granules is unknown, but it has been proposed that they are involved in the metabolism of elastic tissue by providing either elastin or enzymes involving cross linking of elastin (see Chapter 13) [103].

As a matter of fact, all types of wall injuries might occur as the early stage of arteriosclerosis and might each be the starting point of lipoic deposition. Such a concept might explain some of the individual differences observed in the development of coronary disease when large amounts of cholesterol are seen. Indeed, hereditary factors would undoubtedly play an important role in conditioning the resistance of the artery to hemodynamics by controlling the amount and structure of the cellular components of the wall. In conclusion, although it is improbable, as pointed out previously, that the injuries induced by the hemodynamic factor constitute the determining element in the outset of arteriosclerosis, they probably constitute an important predisposing factor.

Origin of Lipids

At the beginning of this chapter we reviewed some of the elementary lesions that compose the atherosclerotic plaque. Among these lesion two stand out: fibrosis and lipid accumulation. The pathogenesis of fibrosis was discussed; possible mechanisms include encrustation, reaction to trauma caused by hemodynamic stress, and the sclerogenic effect of cholesterol and its esters.

Here we will consider the origin of the lipids found in the arterial wall. Three groups of lipids are found in the atherosclerotic wall: triglycerides, phospholipids and cholesterol. Among those, cholesterol is by far the most abundant. The low levels of triglycerides in atherosclerotic lesions are believed to result from the high arterial lipase activity. The activity of the lipase decreases with age when calculated on a wet weight basis, but not when calculated on the basis of the surface area.

We have already mentioned that lipids penetrate the wall of healthy arteries. Since lipids do not accumulate in the normal artery, the influx must be balanced by the efflux. Therefore the accumulation of lipids in the diseased artery could result from increased influx from the lumen, decrease efflux, or active synthesis of the lipids in the artery leading to accumulation exceeding the ability of the wall to clear the lipids. We will consider the source of cholesterol and that of phospholipids.

The exact source of arterial cholesterol is not clear [58–61]. Because the blood lipoprotein concentration correlates with the incidence of arteriosclerosis, and because the arterial lipoproteins are similar to blood lipoproteins, it is often assumed that the blood lipoproteins are, with amendments, transferred to the arterial wall. This theory fails to account for two important morphological observations: (1) the restricted distribution of the injury to some areas of the vascular system; (2) the lack of correlation between cholesteremia and the development of arteriosclerosis in some individuals.

Furthermore, it has been suggested that the very identity of the relative concentration of the lipoprotein in the arterial wall and in the bloodstream constitutes an argument against the filtration theory. It is indeed highly improbable that a multilayer membrane such as the arterial wall would filter indiscriminately such diversified and large molecules as cholesterol and its esters. The blood lipids could be introduced in the intima by pinocytosis. Kinetic studies of the incorporation of cholesterol from blood into the aorta clearly indicate that cholesterol is transported from the aorta into the blood. Nevertheless, such studies have not permitted investigators to decide whether the penetration occurs by diffusion or pinocytosis. Whatever the significance for the pathogenesis of arteriosclerosis, reports have appeared suggesting increased aortic permeability in rabbits fed high-cholesterol diets [62].

An alternative hypothesis proposes that lipoproteins are synthesized within the arterial wall from simple molecules that diffuse easily, such as acetyl-CoA.

Calf aortas have been mounted on a special pump and their vasa vasorum perfused with defibrinated blood. Such conditions cause minimal trauma to the vessel when it is examined histologically or electron microscopically. These experiments showed that cholesterol was synthesized within the aortic wall from [^{14}C] acetate, that cholesterol accumulates within the arterial wall, and, finally, that the cholesterol accumulated within the arterial wall could be transferred from the aorta to the blood. Furthermore, when an intra-arterial pressure of 200 mm Hg was applied, the amount of cholesterol accumulating within the wall increased, whereas a pressure of 100 mm Hg has no such effect. The pressure effect was related to the initial concentration of cholesterol in the perfusing medium. There was also a correlation between glucose consumption and the accumulating cholesterol, which suggests that cholesterol accumulation is energy dependent. However, the energy could be used for the synthesis of cholesterol or for its transfer from the serum to the arterial wall. One could object that in such experiments part of the labeled cholesterol in the arterial wall may originate from cholesterol synthesized within the red cells. Indeed, those corpuscles are particularly active in synthesizing cholesterol. But this objection is invalid because the intra-arterial accumulation of labeled cholesterol is found even if the vessel is perfused with serum [63, 64].

Although such experiments indicate that the aorta is capable of cholesterol synthesis, they do not prove that aortic cholesterol accumulation is of endogenous origin. A plausible interpretation is that aortic cholesterol is of endogenous and exogenous origin.

The problem of arterial cholesterol accumulation could not be solved without the availability of labeled cholesterol. If all cholesterol in the arterial wall derives from plasma cholesterol, the specific activity of the arterial cholesterol should be identical to that of the plasma after injection of labeled cholesterol. This proved to be the case in early lesions of rabbits fed high cholesterol diets. Such findings do not exclude the possibility of *de novo* synthesis of cholesterol by the arteries, and as we have seen, there is a great deal of evidence that the arterial wall can synthesize cholesterol from acetate [104].

However, existing data strongly suggest that most of the cholesterol that accumulates in the diseased artery is derived from the plasma. Thus, [^{14}C]acetate is much more rapidly incorporated in the fatty acid than in the cholesteryl moiety of the cholesteryl esters that accumulate in the aorta.

If the accumulation of cholesterol is not caused by *de novo* synthesis, it must result from increased permeability of the arterial membrane to cholesterol, decreased efflux of cholesterol or decreased cholesterol catabolism in the arterial wall.

In spite of the efforts of many investigators, the mechanism of cholesterol accumulation in diseased arteries is uncertain. The finding that the specific activity of cholesterol in old atherosclerotic plaques remains low after the injection of cholesterol suggests that the exchange of cholesterol between the diseased artery and the plasma is lower than in the healthy artery. Such results could be explained by increased permeability to cholesterol, because of injury to the endothelial walls or by decreased metabolism of cholesterol to bile acid.

An accurate interpretation of cholesterol accumulation in the diseased artery must also take a number of related observations into account. Cholesterol penetrates the arterial wall more readily than esterified cholesterol. No energy is required for the penetration of cholesterol. The arterial wall is more permeable to free fatty acid which will serve to esterify cholesterol than to serum free cholesterol.

The cholesterol in normal or atherosclerotic aortas is esterified. Aortic enzymes are believed to contribute to the formation of cholesterol esters through the action of fatty acyl-CoA cholesterol acyl transferase. In pigeons, the rate of esterification of cholesterol is greater in atherosclerotic than in normal aortas [65].

Two enzymes capable of esterifying cholesterol are present in the wall, an acyltransferase and an acyl CoA dependent enzyme. Available evidence indicates that the CoA dependent enzyme is responsible for most of the esterification. The CoA dependent enzyme primarily catalyzes the esterification of cholesterol with oleate and thus, part of the esterified cholesterol is of the oleate type, but there is also a large amount of cholesterol linoleate.

We have seen that in early stages of infiltration of the artery, lipids accumulate in the form of extracellular droplets along collagen and elastic fibers. At that stage the linoleic esters predominate over the oleate 9 to 1. In the fatty streak, which contains fat-filled cells, it is the oleate ester that predominates. In the atheroma it is the primary linoleate ester that accumulates. The linoleate ester is the one found in plasma and therefore it is assumed that by some mechanism that is still unclear the plasma traverses the vascular membrane either by passing through gaps in the endothelial wall or by macrophage pinocytosis.

Among the two esters of cholesterol the oleate is the more fibrogenic, and its presence may therefore determine, at least in part, the degree of fibrosis associated with the lesion. In the fatty streak much of the cholesterol is intracellular. The mechanisms regulating the intracellular transport of cholesterol may have considerable bearing on the development of atherosclerosis.

Bailey [105] has studied cholesterol transport in tissue culture. Pinocytosis is believed to play only a minor part in the intracellular ingurgitation of cholesterol. During intracellular influx cholesterol binds to membrane receptors and enters the cytoplasm where it binds to a cytosol receptor. Efflux is believed to result from the reverse of this process. Influx and efflux seem to be regulated by external binding lipoprotein. The intracellular levels of cholesterol regulate cholesterol biosynthesis by feedback mechanisms [93].

There are thus three major mechanisms by which cholesterol may enter the arterial wall: extracellular uptake, intracellular uptake and *de novo* synthesis. The extracellular uptake probably occurs by penetration through gaps of the endothelium followed by binding of cholesterol to glycosaminoglycans (the major constituent of the intercellular matrix) or other acidic mucopolysaccarides. Glycosaminoglycans may retain blood proteins by either ionic bonding or molecular sieving. Dermatan sulfate is known to bind lipoproteins ionically. The glycosaminoglycans form a network of interconnected chains which may function as a molecular sieve for some of the larger molecules [106].

The possibility that the accumulation of cholesterol in the arteries does not result so much from abnormal uptake as from impaired efflux must be kept in mind. Two observations support this view; the accumulation of cholesterol in lysosomes and the low HDL levels in patients with hypercholesterolemia.

de Duve and his collaborators [107] have investigated some aspects of the biochemistry and the morphology associated with the transformation of the smooth muscle cell into a foam cell in aortas of rabbits fed a high cholesterol diet. Tissue fractionation studies revealed that in addition to accumulation of cholesterol esters, there was an increase in the activity of the lysosomal enzyme and catalase.

Electron microscopy showed that in normal smooth muscle cells acid phosphatase is associated with small vesicles located in the Golgi region. In the foam cell acid phosphatase is found in association with some, but not all, the lipid laden vacuoles.

The relevance of these findings to the primary insult in atherosclerosis may be that the changes in the activity of the lysosomal enzyme are secondary to the accumulation of cholesterol and constitute unsuccessful attempts to scavenge the remains of a dying cell. But it is also possible that the cholesterol esters are trapped in the tissue because the atherosclerotic artery is defective in cholesterol esterase.

The esterase is found in most animals investigated, even those that do not develop atherosclerosis. The results are conflicting; while some have claimed a decrease in activity in atherosclerotic rats and rabbits, this was not confirmed in monkeys. The intracellular distribution of the enzyme is also in question. While some have found the enzyme in the microsomes and the supernatant [108], others claim that it is found in lysosomes [109, 110].

HDL is believed to regulate cholesterol clearance from tissues. Cholesterol is synthesized in most tissues, but catabolized only in liver. Therefore, excess cholesterol must be transferred from the tissue to the liver. Only unesterified cholesterol exchanges readily between plasma lipoproteins and tissue [111].

Lecithin cholesterol acetyl transferase promotes the transfer of cholesterol from erythrocyte to plasma and the process is activated by the addition of HDL to the incubation mixture. Similarly, the efflux from ascites cell cholesterol is increased in presence of HDL apoproteins. The tissue pools of cholesterol increase in absence of HDL (Tangier disease).

These observations have led to the conclusion that the presence of HDL in the plasma is essential for cholesterol transport from tissue to liver and it has been further assumed that the accumulation of cholesterol in the arteries results, at least in part, from low HDL levels in the plasma. In fact, plasma HDL levels are low in high risk candidates for ischemic heart disease such as male versus female, obese and diabetic individuals and patients with hypercholesterolemia and hypertriglyceridemia.

In addition to cholesterol, phospholipids also accumulate in atherosclerotic arteries. In humans the sphingomyelin levels and in rabbits both sphingomyelin and lecithin levels are five times above normal. Isotopic studies have clearly established that in contrast to cholesterol, which is acquired primarily through influx from the plasma, the phospholipids that accumulate in the artery are synthesized *de novo*. Studies on isolated cells and radioautographic studies have shown that the phospholipids are synthesized in the aortic smooth muscle cells. The mechanisms triggering the increased rate of phospholipid synthesis are not known. The phospholipids may help to solubilize cholesterol [82, 104].

Japanese investigators have studied the incorporation of ^{32}P into rat aorta *in vitro*. When phospholipids of rat aorta are analyzed chromatographically on silica acid-impregnated paper, essentially eight spots can be identified. They include di- and triphosphoinositite, lysolecithin, phosphatidyl inositol, sphingomyelin, lecithin, phosphatidyl ethanolamine, and phosphatidic acid [66].

After incubation with ^{32}P, lecithin and phosphatidyl inositol and lysolecithin are highly labeled; in contrast, incorporation is low in sphingomyelin and phosphatidyl ethanolamine. So a phospholipid labeling pattern can be determined for the vessel under investigation. Labeling appears to vary with species, and within a species with the segment of the vessel. For example, phospholipid labeling is different in the aorta and the coronary artery.

The incorporation of phospholipid within a vascular segment also varies with the size of the vessel. Total phospholipids and the incorporation of ^{32}P into the total phospholipid of the arterial wall both increase with size, despite a reduction of ^{32}P incorporation in the acid-soluble phospholipids. Phospholipid accumulates in the arterial wall also as a result of atherogenic diets.

In conclusion, phospholipids appear to accumulate in arteriosclerotic arteries, and the increase in total phospholipids is associated with a modification of the pattern of incorporation of precursors into the various arterial phospholipids. The significance of these findings is not clear. For example, it is not known whether the phospholipids accumulate as a result of increased synthesis or because of interference with their breakdown.

Consequences of Atherosclerosis

Atherosclerosis would simply be part of the aging process if it did not interfere with blood flow by narrowing the artery and possibly leading to subsequent occlusion by thrombi. When ischemia is prolonged in such organs as the heart and brain, function is temporarily interrupted and life is threatened.

Coronary Occlusion and Myocardial Infarcts

The coronary arteries are muscular, medium-sized arteries that have two morphological characteristics: (1) they have no external elastica, so the only elastic layer is in subendothelial connective tissue and the media; (2) the intima is usually very thick, probably due to high blood pressure in those vessels. The right and left coronary arteries originate in the sinuses of Valsava and are richly anastomotic. The anastomoses increase in number and become wider after coronary artery occlusion; thus, anastomoses are important in the evolution of myocardial infarcts. Atherosclerosis may lead to coronary artery occlusion in various ways: first, by the development of the atherosclerotic plaque; second, by the formation of thrombi at the surface of the plaque (then the roughness of the endothelium and internal factors that modify the blood coagulability—such as slowing of the circulation, surgical trauma, infection, a high-fat diet—are responsible for the thrombi); third, by coronary artery rupture (the rupture occurs at the site of the plaque, leading to extrusion of the atheromatous material within the lumen); and, fourth, intramural hemorrhage of the vasa vasorum or the capillaries. Among these various mechanisms, thrombosis and intramural hemorrhage most often lead to coronary artery occlusion, whereas rupture of the atheromatous plaque is rarely responsible.

The left coronary arteries and their branches are occluded about twice as frequently as are the right coronary arteries. In both arteries, the first third of the artery after the origin is most often occluded.

The consequences of coronary artery occlusion are varied; they result mainly from the speed at which the occlusion occurs and the existence of an anastomosis at the time of the occlusion. If the occlusion is progressive, the two coronaries may anastomose and no severe consequences will ensue, except that eventually some repeated episodes of ischemia may develop when oxygen requirements are increased, leading to external pain called angina pectoris.

Occasionally, a narrowed artery may be occluded completely by a thrombus, embolus, hemorrhage, or rupture of an atheromatous plaque. The artery may be occluded so suddenly that the patient dies within 12 hours, before anatomical injuries are observed in the myocardium.

Coronary obstruction most often evolves into myocardial infarct; the site and extensiveness of the necrotic process will, of course, depend on the anatomical distribution of the artery that is occluded (see Figs. 11-8 and 11-9). When the descending branch of the left coronary artery is occluded it leads to infarcts of the anterior and lateral walls of the left ventricle. Right coronary occlusion leads to an infarct

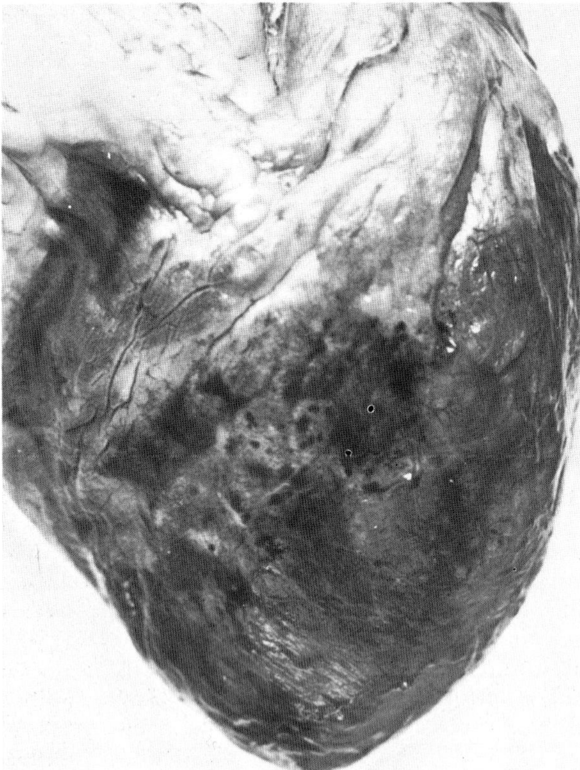

Fig. 11-8. Area of recent myocardial infarction

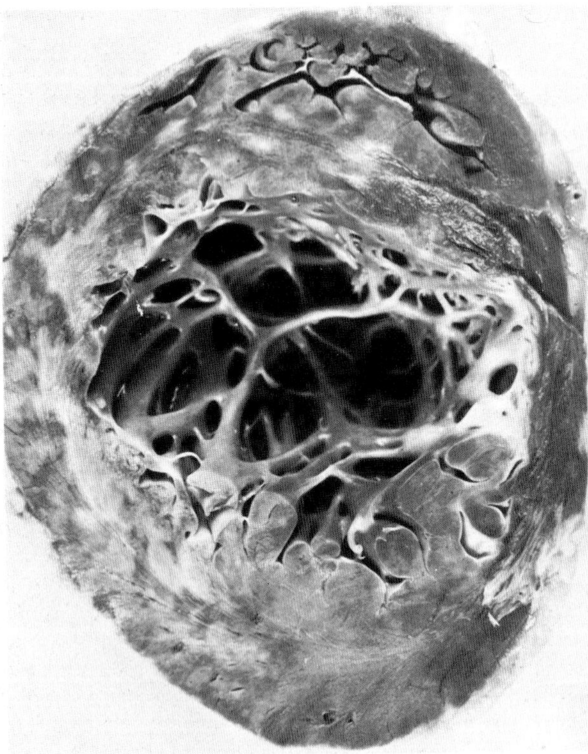

Fig. 11-9. Old myocardial infarct showing replacement of muscular fibers by fibrous tissue

of the posterior third of the septum and the posterior part of the left ventricle. Occlusion of the left or right circumflex results in infarcts of the lateral wall of the left ventricle. Depending upon the height at which the occlusion occurs in the arterial lumen, infarcts of the atrium or of the right ventricle may complicate left ventricular infarct.

The classical pathological appearance of the myocardial infarct can be seen in victims of coronary occlusion who died 2–15 days after the infarct. Although the disease is called myocardial infarct, it usually involves the three layers of the heart. At gross examination, a fraction of the heart is a tawny yellow-brown color, and it is more friable on sectioning than normal myocardium. The surface section is homogenous, and individual bundles of fibers can no longer be recognized. The pericardium is usually covered with a thin fibrinous layer, and the endothelium, with laminated thrombus. Histologically, three distinguishing features can be observed: (1) muscular degeneration characterized by hyalin degeneration of the fibers and pyknosis of the nuclei; (2) patches of hemorrhage throughout the infarcted area; and (3) polymorphonuclear invasion, especially at the edges of the infarcted area. The nucleus of the fiber may increase in size and become polyploid, or the fiber may become multinucleated. The necrotic area is usually populated with hemosiderin-loaded macrophages. Six to eight months after the myocardial infarct, the necrotic area is entirely replaced by fibrotic tissue.

The patient often dies from forward failure soon after the infarction, but sometime he survives, and then his life is threatened by the presence of mural thrombi (these do not organize; thus they are subject to autolysis, during which they constitute a permanent danger of emboli) or by rupture of the heart. The chances of the rupture depend on the extensiveness and on the stage of development of the infarct. The more softened the infarct, the greater the chance of rupture. The extensiveness of hemorrhage and polymorphonuclear infiltration are responsible for intramural softening of the heart. Naturally, hemodynamics are a determining factor in heart rupture. A person with a blood pressure over 140 mm Hg is three times more susceptible to heart rupture than a normotensive person.

If the infarct is not too extensive and the patient can be maintained under complete rest to avoid stress on the heart muscles, healing may occur. Healing does not consist of regeneration of the muscle fibers to restore the structural integrity of the heart, but it results in hypertrophy of the fibrous tissues associated with hypertrophy of some of the remnant fibers. In any case, these healed areas constitute weak points in the heart wall that bulge under the high blood pressure, leading to the formation of saclike areas called aneurysms of the heart. The aneurysms are favorite sites for mural thrombi formation. Of all cases of sudden death, 65% are due to cardiac failure, and 65% of the latter are due to coronary artery disease.

The clinical observations in acute myocardial infarct are revealing. An elderly individual, usually a man, experiences a sudden chest pain that cannot be relieved by the administration of vasodilating drugs. Severe dyspnea often develops. Ischemia impairs the heart's function, and blood pressure drops considerably, even in individuals with high blood pressure. The heart sounds are feeble, often with galloping rhythm and other arrhythmias. Furthermore, the condition for electrical conduction in the heart is modified, and the electrocardiographic pattern is altered.

The electrocardiographic findings are not always typical, but usually they develop within 2–12 hours after the onset of ischemia. The details of the electrocardiographic changes cannot be described here. Suffice to point out that they vary depending upon the location of the infarct in the heart walls. The extensive necrotic process causes some characteristic changes in the blood: polymorphonuclear accumulation, a drop in the sedimentation rate, and an increase in serum transaminase levels. (Coronary atherosclerosis and previous coronary occlusions were found in 90% of the hearts in a series of patients with angina pectoris who died of noncardiac causes.)

Associated with the increased levels of blood transaminase is an increase in catecholamines, particularly norepinephrine. But norepinephrine levels may be increased in cases of angina pectoris, whereas transaminase is not increased under such conditions.

Cerebral Consequences of Atherosclerosis

Stroke is the main consequence of cerebral arteriosclerosis, and it may be caused by hemorrhage or obstruction of an artery. Stroke by hemorrhage usually occurs in patients who have severe hypertension, and it may or may not be associated with arteriosclerotic lesions of the vessels. In any case, the primordial mechanism of injury in stroke by hemorrhage is hemodynamic stress on the artery rather than any local condition.

Embolism

Brain infarcts result from progressive or abrupt occlusion of the cerebral arteries. The pathogenesis of this injury is best understood if the vascularization of the brain is reviewed. The vessels of the brain stem from three main sources: the two carotid arteries and the vertebral arteries. The right and left carotid arteries divide at the level of the external angle of the optic chiasma to yield the anterior and median cerebral arteries. The vertebral arteries fuse to yield the basilar trunk, which divides to yield the two posterior cerebral arteries. The anterior, median, and posterior cerebral arteries are then welded in a continuous circle, called the polygon of Willis, by the anterior communicating artery connecting the two anterior cerebral arteries, and by the posterior communicating arteries connecting the posterior with the median cerebral arteries.

Obviously, the location of the brain infarct will depend upon the site of the occlusion.

Embolization is responsible for sudden occlusion, but thrombosis usually causes the slower forms of occlusion. Emboli may originate from various sources. Chronic pulmonary abscesses, pulmonary gangrene, and a fractured long bone may constitute a source of emboli that may enter the cerebral arteries. In the arteriosclerotic patient, the embolus usually originates from mural thrombi developing in arteriosclerotic plaques in the aorta or in the great vessels.

Due to their anatomical distribution, the vessels irrigating the left cerebral hemisphere are more susceptible to embolical occlusion than those of the right hemisphere. Whereas the left carotid artery emerges straight from the aortic arch, the right brachiocephalic trunk bends slightly before it yields the right carotid artery. This is also true of the anterior cerebral and the sylvian arteries. The anterior cerebral forms a right angle with the carotid stem, but the sylvian artery is on the direct course of the blood flow originating from the carotid, and therefore it is more likely to be occluded by emboli. If the emboli are large, they may occlude a large artery. If the emboli lodge in the median cerebral artery, severe clinical symptoms ensue: coma, complete hemiplegia, complete hemianesthesia, and total aphasia. But if the embolus is small, it enters smaller branches of the sylvian artery and localized damage results, such as motor aphasia, verbal deafness, verbal cecity, and monoplegia. In cases of massive embolism, the symptoms progress rapidly leading to the apoplectic ictus, which is characterized by coma associated with a slow pulse and a reduced temperature, at least in the beginning of the disease. Later the temperature increases and the patient is hyperthermic for several days. This increase in temperature usually coincides with autolysis of the brain tissue. Of course, if the embolus involves only a small artery, no ictus may occur and the functional symptoms may appear suddenly after a period of headache and dizziness.

Thrombus

The middle cerebral artery is one of the arteries most frequently affected by thrombosis. Thrombosis and emboli formation lead to the development of an infarct, the size of which depends on the location of the injury in the arterial tree and on the presence of an anastomosis. Autopsy findings show that the arteries of the circle of Willis are favorite sites for arteriosclerosis. The plaques may lead to progressive narrowing of the vessel, with localized anoxemia or thrombosis. In contrast to emboli, thrombi affect the right and left cerebral hemispheres equally. The occlusion produced by the thrombus is usually more progressive than that resulting from emboli, although it is not necessarily less extensive. However, sometimes the occlusion caused by thrombi may occur rather suddenly, and this usually results from associated spasms.

The superimposed spasm also explains how full or partial recovery is sometimes possible after thrombic occlusion. Thus, the focal symptoms are usually preceded by a period of diziness, headache, lack of concentration, and uncoordination. The symptomatology depends on the nature of the artery that is obliterated: if the anterior cerebral artery is affected, no significant symptomatology follows; if the posterior cerebral is affected, blindness develops; the median artery is affected, hemiplegia and hemianesthesia develop. If collateral branches are affected, various motor or functional systems are damaged.

An occlusion in a carotid artery or in one of its branches can be detected by temporal digital compression of the carotid at the site of the paralysis. If this procedure leads to syncope, the heterolateral carotid probably is occluded. Ophthalmotonometry, a more efficient and safer procedure for detecting carotid occlusion, consists of determining the pressure of the central retinal artery, a branch of the first important branch of the carotid—the ophthalmic artery. The therapy for thrombosis of the internal carotid involves combined thromboendarterectomy and anastomosis of the artery proximal and distal to the lesion with a dacron tube that bypasses the injury.

Encephalomalacia

When thrombi, emboli, or other forms of vascular occlusion involve small arteries, they cause encephalomalacia. This results from occlusion of smaller vessels irrigating the cerebral cortex, the striated nuclei, or the internal capsule. Occlusion of these terminal arteries leads to degeneration of the nerve cell, proliferation of glial cells, and fragmentation of the myelin sheath, the lipid components of which are phagocytized by macrophages. Under some circumstances, such reactions may lead to the development of a small glial scar or a cyst surrounded by a glial capsule. Particularly susceptible to encephalomalacia are the striatum, the hypocampus, the dentate nucleus, and the cerebral cortex. Obviously, the disease progresses slowly. For years no symptomatology is detected, but with time the patient loses memory, especially recent memories, his moods change, and he becomes tired rapidly and shows marked nervous depression. If the injuries are mainly in the corpus striatum, pseudobulbar paralysis may develop. The classical patient is an older person with an immobile face and a wide-open mouth (saliva drips from the corners of his lips), and he has difficulty swallowing food and articulating. He is excessively sensitive and cries or laughs easily. Lesions that cause exaggerated tendon reflexes and a positive Babinski reflex are often associated with these bulbar signs.

Brain Infarct

The site of a brain infarct will, of course, depend on the artery that is obstructed, and the extensiveness of the injury is a function of the density of the interarteriolar anastomoses and their degree of permeability. If the anastomoses are narrowed by arteriosclerotic processes or other types of injuries, the infarct will be extensive. Superficial infarcts are cone shaped with the base at the surface and the apex at the center; central infarcts are spherical.

Pathologists describe brain softening in three stages: white, red, and yellow. Such a subdivision is somewhat artificial because it is difficult to delineate one stage from another; however, such a classification has didactic advantages.

The period of white softening is short; during that time the brain bulges somewhat at the surface and an area of softening, although difficult to recognize on fresh material, becomes obvious after fixation.

Red softening results from a complex interaction of necrosis, hemorrhage, and lymphocytic infiltration. During red softening the neural cells degenerate, the myelin sheaths are fragmented, and their lipid components are phagocytized by invading macrophages and polymorphonuclear leukocytes. The entire brain substance autolyzes. This leads to hemorrhage and bulging of the involved area at the surface. The convolutions are flattened, and on sectioning the area appears brownish and friable.

In yellow softening, the entire mass of the brain is softened and replaced by a brownish-yellow material stained by the blood pigment. The infarcted area is not repaired, so at the end of the process when all tissues are autolyzed, all that is left is a shrunken cystic area surrounded by glial proliferation. The brain is smaller than normal, and the convolutions, particularly the frontal and parietal, are decreased in size; this is indicated by widening of the sulci.

Cerebral Hemorrhage

The exact mechanism of the development of cerebral hemorrhage is not so well established as to lead to unanimous agreement on its pathogenesis. At least three theories have been proposed. The first assumes that cerebral hemorrhages are of nervous origin. It postulates that temporary excitation leads to vasodilatation followed by vasoconstriction, during which an unknown mechanism causes red cells to travel from the vascular lumen into the extravascular spaces. The amount of red cell extravasation depends on the duration of the excitation. The second theory proposes that the mechanism triggering the cerebral hemorrhage resides in a vascular spasm, which leads to anoxemia followed by necrosis of the vascular walls and consequent hemorrhage. The third theory contends that the hemorrhage originates from the rupture of the vessel, either in areas weakened by arteriosclerosis or by the presence of congenital miliary aneurysm. Sudden ictus may well result from such a mechanism. Indeed, in ictus the hemorrhagic area does not truly infiltrate the nerve tissues and does not result from the confluence of smaller hemorrhages, as suggested by the previous hypotheses. The focus of hemorrhage in ictus is homogenous and pushes the normal nerve tissue toward the periphery.

Obviously, hemodynamic factors also determine the site and the time of the rupture. Consequently, cerebral hemorrhages occur more frequently among patients with hypertension, at times of excitement or episodes of coughing, sneezing, vomiting, or sometimes after a hearty meal or a cold bath.

Again, the branches of the median cerebral artery are most often the site of cerebral hemorrhage. The hemorrhage usually leads to apoplectic ictus, the patient falls, and severe coma follows. When he awakens, the patient is usually hemiplegic. His face is red, he is sweating, and he is breathing noisily or snoring. His pupils do not react to light and are dilated. Conjunctival and swallowing reflexes are missing. If he recovers, his reflexes reappear and his temperature increases, and when the coma has disappeared, the patients shows focal signs resulting from destruction of the basal ganglia and the internal capsule with total anesthesia and hemiplegia. It would be most useful to be able, on the basis of the evolution of the hypersensitive syndrome, to predict the chances of death from cerebrovascular accidents, because under those circumstances it might be possible to prevent the occurrence of the accidents. Unfortunately, this is impossible. In studies of large numbers of hypertensives who had cerebrovascular accidents, a pre-clinical history gave no clue as to the chances of developing stroke. The brain of a victim of cerebral hemorrhage is shown in Fig. 11-10.

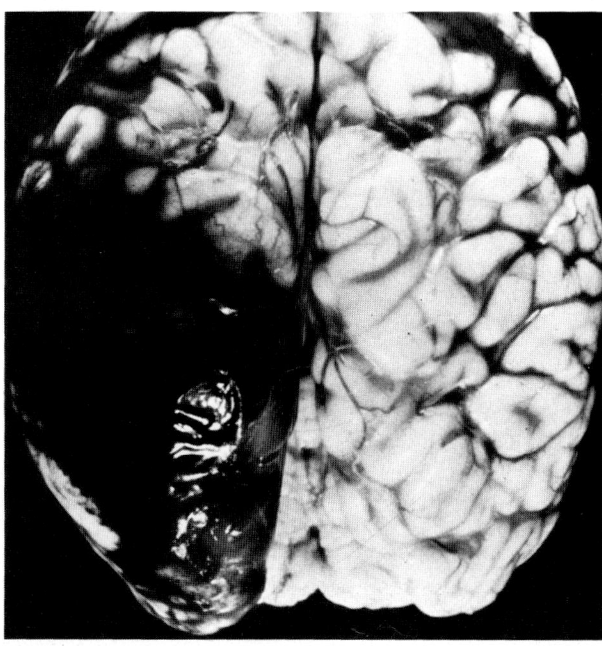

Fig. 11-10. Intracerebral hemorrhage

Working Hypothesis on the Pathogenesis of Arteriosclerosis

In spite of the difficulties encountered in identifying the epidemiological parameters of arteriosclerosis, the clinicopathological correlations between coronary heart disease detected by electrocardiography and blood cholesterol have established two important facts: (1) environment affects the incidence of arteriosclerosis in a number of different ways—diet and stress play key roles in influencing the risk of developing coronary heart disease; (2) although we do not know what level of blood cholesterol is safe, there is a close correlation between blood cholesterol levels and the incidence of arteriosclerosis.

Epidemiological studies have made it possible to describe the profile of high-risk individuals. Coronary heart disease is most likely to affect a man of average height who is slightly obese, middle-aged, and has high blood cholesterol and blood pressure. Such individuals usually eat too much rich foods, smoke, and are physically inactive. Because they are ambitious, they have many responsibilities, are anxious about them, and are constantly faced with new deadlines.

Using blood cholesterol as a measure of the risk, it is possible to manipulate the environment with the hope that such manipulations will reduce the incidence of arteriosclerosis. Consequently, any time a person is close to the arteriosclerotic profile described above, efforts should be made to modify his environment so that his profile differs from that of the typical arteriosclerotic. The candidate for heart disease should eat less, learn to relax, engage in controlled exercise, give up smoking, and plan ahead.

Because of the complexity of the pathogenesis of arteriosclerosis, it seems futile to attempt to weave all the factors involved in the pathogenesis of the disease into a coherent scheme. Yet such attempts are often helpful for planning further experimentation.

Robertson [67] and Whereat [68] are among those who have presented coherent pathogenic schemes. Such schemes aim primarily at providing an interpretation of the intimal lipid accumulation rather than at a comprehensive explanation of the pathogenesis of necrosis, etc. To enounce their working hypothesis, the workers take fundamental and unique properties of the arterial wall into account.

Atherosclerosis is a disease of the intima. The inner vascular wall is itself avascular and depends upon the vasculature of the media and diffusion for nutrients and elimination of by-products. One component that must diffuse through the media to reach the outer part of the intima is oxygen. Oxygen diffusion through the avascular wall will obviously be decreased as the the vascular wall thickens. Consequently, thickening of the arterial walls would appear to make the intima quite susceptible to anoxemia.

Another fundamental observation is that cholesterol accumulation in the arterial wall parallels cholesterol levels in the blood. We have seen that the intermediary metabolism of the arterial wall is somewhat unique. There is a high level of anaerobic oxidation of glucose with marked production of lactic acid. In contrast, aerobic generation of ATP is low in the arteries; moreover, oxygen has little of a depressing effect on anaerobic glycolysis in the arterial wall. In other words, regulation by the Pasteur effect is low in cells of the arterial wall. The activity of the pentose cycle enzymes is relatively high in arteries. Consequently, two pathways in intermediary metabolism produce reduced pyrimidine nucleotiddes, in the absence of the natural oxidative mechanism—the Krebs cycle—for oxidizing the pyrimidine nucleotides. Because reduced pyrimidine nucleotides are also valuable coenzymes for lipid biosynthesis, it is tempting to link lipid accumulation in the arterial wall with the accumulation of reduced pyrimidine nucleotides. Whereat has observed that anoxemia stimulates fatty acid synthesis in mitochondria. To explain the accumulation of cholesterol in the arterial wall, he postulates that cholesterol is driven in the intimal cell at higher than normal rates for the purpose of esterifying free fatty acids.

By studying the effects of anoxemia on tissue culture and organ cultures of aorta, Robertson found that low oxygen tension inhibited the biosynthesis of intracellular cholesterol from [^{14}C]acetate or mevalonic acid. But the squalene concentration increased and it was concluded that cyclization of squalene was impaired because of inadequate oxygen supply. Hypoxia was associated with an increased uptake of lipoproteins by the arterial cells. Thus, it would appear that any situation that would lead to focal anoxemia in the arterial wall—such as vasoconstriction, occlusion by thrombosis or emboli, or increased local pressure—could alter intermediary metabolism. The metabolic change may ultimately be responsible for the accumulation of cholesterol and other lipids as a result of secondary damage of the cell membrane, or because of a greater need for the substances inside the cell.

Hyperlipidemia

A number of hereditary diseases are characterized by excess lipids in the blood (familial hyperlipoproteinemia), others definitely result from deficiencies in either α- or β-lipoproteins (Tangier disease and familial β-lipoproteinemia) [25, 69–71].

Familial Hyperlipoproteinemia

The five types of familial hyperlipidemia are referred to as type I, II, III, IV, and V. The essential features of each type are as follows:

In type I hyperlipidemia, large amounts of chylomicrons appear in the blood after a fat diet, but the chylomicrons disappear if the patient is placed on a fat-free diet. The phenotype is expressed only in the homozygous for the defective autosomal gene. The inherited defect is believed to be an absence of protein lipase.

In type II hyperlipidemia, the patient has excessive amounts of β-lipoproteins. Glyceride remains within normal limits, but cholesterol and phospholipids are increased. The phenotype is expressed in the heterozygous, and the nature of the inherited defect is not known.

In type III, the patient has high levels of both β- and pre-β-lipoproteins while he is on a normal diet. The triglycerides in both of these lipoprotein fractions are of endogenous origin, so the hypertriglyceridemia may be carbohydrate induced. The symptoms of hypertriglyceridemia are clear-cut in the heterozygous. They are likely to appear at an early age in the homozygous. The biochemical defect is not known. Plasma cholesterol and phospholipid levels are elevated.

In type IV, cholesterol levels are normal and there are no changes in lipoprotein. However, there is an endogenous hyperlipemia that can be carbohydrate induced characterized by increased levels of pre-β-lipoproteins. The biochemical defect is not known.

In type V, both exogenous (chylomicrons) and endogenous (pre-β) lipoproteins are increased. Type V could result from a combination of the defect that prevails in types I and IV.

The clinical features of hyperlipidemia include formation of xanthomas, development of abdominal pain, pancreatitis, appearance of foam cells in tissues (hepatosplenomegaly), lipemic retinitis, and atheromatous disease in coronary and occasionally peripheral vessels. Frequent associated signs are hyperuricemia, gallstones, and abnormal glucose tolerance test.

Xanthoma

Xanthomas are subcutaneous or submucosal accumulations of lipid-laden cells. Naturally, the lipid droplets give the cytoplasm of these cells a foamy appearance. Sometimes the lipid-laden macrophages coalesce to yield giant cells, which are then called Touton cells. The most recent lesions are made primarily of xanthoma cells possibly infiltrated by a few neutrophils. In older lesions, fibrosis may be extensive. Xanthomatosis may be associated with hypercholesterolemia, hyperlipidemia, or normal blood chemistry.

Several clinical types of xanthomas have been described: eruptive, tuberous, tendon sheath, and xanthelasmas. In type I hyperlipidemia, xanthomas are eruptive and diffuse. They appear when hyperlipidemia prevails and disappear after a fat-free diet has been administered for some time.

The cutaneous xanthomas appear as yellowish nodules at the surface of the skin or mucosa; they have a yellow base delineated by dilated capillaries. They may appear anywhere—face, neck, buttocks, groin, etc. Xanthomatosis tuberosa, which usually occurs around joints, is characterized by yellow, tumorlike masses that usually are painless. Tendon sheath xanthomas appear as swollen, lipid-laden masses in tendons of the wrist or ankle. The achilles, patellar, and digital extensor tensor tendons are favorite sites for such lipid deposits. Xanthelasma is a specialized form of xanthomatosis in which the lipid-laden cells condense to form yellowish patches in the medial part of the eyelids (see diabetes).

Foam Cells

Histiocytes filled with lipid droplets appear in hyperlipidemias. These cells are often referred to as foam cells and are found in liver, spleen, lymph nodes, and bone marrow. They are not pathognomonic for hyperlipidemias, and they may be found in lipoidosis, Gaucher's disease, and Niemann-Pick disease, as well as in some diseases in which cholesterol accumulates in reticuloendothelial cells without associated hyperlipidemia, for example, eosinophilic granuloma or Hand-Schüller-Christian disease.

Lipemic Retinitis

A relatively simple way to examine the appearance of circulating blood is to look at the blood as it passes through the retinal vessels with the aid of an ophthalmoscope. When hyperlipidemia is severe, the retinal vessels may have a pale cast; ophthalmologists refer to this condition as lipemic retinitis.

Pancreatitis

The pathogenesis and pathology of acute pancreatitis are discussed in another section. The relationship between pancreatitis and hyperlipidemia is not clear. Most patients with pancreatitis do not have hypertriglyceridemia, and when it occurs, pancreatitis is thought to be associated with hyperlipidemia because of superimposed primary hyperlipidemia.

Tangier Disease and Abetalipoproteinemia

In addition to the five types of hyperlipidemia just described, there are two other types of hereditary disturbances of the blood lipids: Tangier disease, or HDL deficiency, and abetalipoproteinemia. Both are hereditary diseases transferred through autosomal genes. Both defects are associated with a pathognomonic profile of the serum lipoprotein and deposits of lipids in cells.

In Tangier disease, plasma HDL is almost completely absent, cholesterol and phospholipid levels are slightly reduced, and triglyceride levels are normal or slightly elevated. In abetalipoproteinemia, plasma LDL is absent. Tangier disease is usually a mild disease state compatible with normal life. Foam cells form and accumulate in tissue rich in reticuloendothelial cells in the liver, the spleen, and sometimes the lymph nodes. Foam cell agglomerates may also be found in the cornea and underneath mucosae. The pathognomonic sign of Tangier disease is tonsillar enlargement and discoloration. Characteristically, the normally red mucosa of the tonsils appears to be covered with an orange or white yellow film. A similar light orange discoloration is also seen in the rectal mucosa, again as a result of submucosal accumulation of foam cells. Examination of the eye with a slit lamp might reveal foam cell infiltration of the corneal stroma. It is not known what biochemical defect causes Tangier disease, but defective synthesis of the HDL apoprotein has been proposed to be responsible for the symptomatology.

Abetalipoproteinemia is more serious than Tangier disease. It is associated with steatorrhea, neuromuscular disease, and abnormal erythrocytes. Steatorrhea appears in early childhood and is associated with the pathognomonic engorgement of intestinal epithelial cells with triglycerides, resulting in the foamy appearance of almost every cell of the villi. Lipid is found also within the intercellular space and in the connective tissue stroma. The cerebellum and the posterolateral columns are progressively demyelinized, nuclei in the Betz cells of the cerebral cortex are lost, and the peripheral nerve undergoes focal demyelinization. A prominent symptom associated with the neurological defect is a progressive ataxia beginning in childhood. Defects in the structure of the lipoprotein membranes of the erythrocytes are responsible for the peculiar crenation observed in this disease. The primary biochemical defect remains unknown.

The manifestations of the various types of hyperlipidemias are summarized in Table 11-2.

Conclusion

Despite extensive morphological, metabolic, and epidemiological studies on atherosclerosis, a definite pathogenetic mechanism is not yet known. However, present knowledge provides us with a sensible working hypothesis. Exogenous and endogenous lipids enter the intima probably at a very early age, leading to the formation of fatty streaks; this may or may not be reversible. In the early stages of arteriosclerosis, light lipoprotein fractions accumulate in the wall of the arteries, later the proportions of phospholipids and cholesterol are increased. This is probably due in part to the breakdown of the light lipoproteins and possibly to the endogenous elaboration of cholesterol and cholesterol esters. Contrary to previous belief, lipids are not restricted to the intima; small amounts may be found in the media. Lipid accumulation seems to lead to proliferation of the multipotential smooth muscle cells—apparently the only type

Table 11-2. Hyperlipidemias

Type	Blood lipoprotein	Remarks	Genetic	Pathogenesis	Symptoms
I	Normal diet Excessive amounts of chylomicrons in serum Low α- and β-lipoproteins	Fat = free feeding Excess chylomicrons disappear after a few days Appearance of prelipoproteins	Autosomal recessive	Defects in lipoprotein lipase and in regulation of 3-hydroxy-3-methylglutaril CoA reductase	Eruptive xanthoma Abdominal pain Hepatic and splenic enlargement usually in a child less than 10 years old
II	Familial hypercholesterolemia Increased concentration of β-lipoproteins ↗ cholesterol [a] Normal phospholipids		Dominant	Unknown [b] Increased cholesterol synthesis? Increased levels of apoprotein? (seems to have been excluded by immunological studies)	Lipemic retinitis Xanthoma Arteriosclerosis occasionally fatal involvement of coronaries in early years of life in 50% of cases
III	↗ β-lipoprotein ↗ Pre β-lipoprotein ↗ cholesterol phospholipid in plasma The increase is directly related to carbohydrate intake	Hypercholesterolemia as in type II Associated with endogenous hypertrigluceridemia, which is carbohydrate induced	Dominant	1. Increased conversion of glucose → lipids? 2. Excessive input of FFA from adipose tissue 3. Inability to remove β-lipoprotein from plasma	Xanthoma Atheromatosis Ischemic heart disease Abnormal glucose tolerance Hepatosplenomegaly Hyperuricemia Gallstones
IV	↗ pre β-lipoprotein Normal phospholipids Normal cholesterol	Endogenous hyperlipidemia, which is carbohydrate induced		Same as III	Usually detected in childhood Abnormal glucose tolerance Xanthoma Ischemic heart disease
V	Normal diet Hyperchylomicronemia Hyperprelipoproteinemia Normal or low lipoprotein	Combined exogenous and endogenous hyperlipidemia		Inability to clear chylomicrons	Diabetes Abdominal pain Xanthoma No striking history of ischemic heart disease
Tangier disease	Complete absence of high density lipoprotein Slightly increased cholesterol and phospholipid Normal or slightly decreased triglycerides			Defect HDL apoprotein	Foam cells {liver, spleen, lymph nodes} Submucosal deposition ↓ Orange discoloration of {tonsils, rectum}
Abetalipoproteinemia	Complete absence of low density lipoprotein			Unknown	Steatorrhea Intestinal loading of cells Degeneration of cerebellum and posterolateral columns Crenation of erythrocytes

[a] Sometime evident before the age of 10.

[b] A defect in the regulation of 3-hydroxy-3-methyl-glutarate CoA reductase has been suggested as a cause of familial hypercholesterolemia. HMG CoA reductase is feedback inhibited by LDL or VLDL. The enzyme activity was found to be increased in cultured fibroblasts of patients with familial hypercholesterolemia as a result of the inability of the enzyme to respond to feedback inhibition. There were no alterations in the molecular properties, suggesting that the enzyme feedback inhibition may interfere with enzyme synthesis. However, the interference cannot occur at the level of the structural gene, but must involve regulatory genes that have not been identified [112].

of cell in the media. The stimulus of the proliferative process is not known. Some think it is associated with destruction of some of the smooth muscle cells, either through a direct toxic effect of the lipids that reach the media, or as a result of some hemodynamic factors (high blood pressure, etc.) that are involved in localizing the lesions of arteriosclerosis. The combination of lipid accumulation and smooth muscle proliferation in the intima—which because of the absence of vasa vasorum is dependent upon diffusion for oxygenation—leads to anoxemia, cellular death, and erosion of the surface of the endothelium and proliferation of smooth muscle cells at the periphery of a zone of fat necrosis. Calcium accumulation and mural thrombi formation appear to be consequences of the degenerative process.

References

1. Holman, R.L., McGill, H.C., Jr., Strong, J.P., Geer, J.C., Guidry, M.A.: The arterial wall as an organ. In: Hormones and atherosclerosis (Pincus, G., ed.), p. 123–129. New York: Academic Press 1959
2. Keech, M.K.: Electron microscope study of the normal rat aorta. J. biophys. biochem. Cytol. **7**, 533–538 (1960)
3. Zweifach, B.W.: Structural makeup of capillary wall. Ann. N.Y. Acad. Sci. **61**, 670–677 (1955)
4. Zweifach, B.W.: Structure and behavior of vascular endothelium. In: The arterial wall (Lansing, A.I., ed.), p. 15–45. Baltimore: The Williams & Wilkins Company 1959
5. French, J.E.: Atherosclerosis in relation to the structure and function of the arterial intima, with special reference to the endothelium. Int. Rev. exp. Path. **5**, 253–353 (1966)
6. Kirk, J.E., Wang, I., Dyrbye, M.: Mucopolysaccharides of human arterial tissue. IV. Analysis of electrophoretically separated fractions. J. Geront. **13**, 362–365 (1958)
7. Bertelsen, S.: The role of ground substance, collagen, and elastic fibers in the genesis of atherosclerosis. In: Atherosclerosis and its origin (Sandler, M., Bourne, G.H., eds.), p. 119–165. New York: Academic Press 1963
8. Kirk, J.E.: Intermediary metabolism of human arterial tissue and its changes with age and atherosclerosis. In: Atherosclerosis and its origin (Sandler, M., Bourne, G.H., eds.), p. 67–117. New York: Academic Press 1963
9. Zemplenyi, T., Lojda, Z., Mrhova, O.: Enzymes of the vascular wall in experimental atherosclerosis in the rabbit. In: Atherosclerosis and its origin (Sandler, M., Bourne, G.H., eds.), p. 459–513. New York: Academic Press 1963
10. Poole, J.C.F., Saunders, A.G., Florey, H.W.: Further observations on the regeneration of aortic endothelium in the rabbit. J. Path. Bact. **77**, 637 (1959)
11. Coulson, W.F., Carnes, W.H.: Cardiovascular studies on copper-deficient swine. IX. Repair of vascular defects in deficient swine treated with copper. Amer. J. Path. **50**, 861–868 (1967)
12. Taylor, C.B., Baldwin, D., Hass, G.M.: Localized arteriosclerotic lesions induced in the aorta of the juvenile rabbit by freezing. Arch. Path. **49**, 623–640 (1950)
13. Björkerud, S., Bondjers, G.: Arterial repair and atherosclerosis after mechanical injury. Part 2. Tissue response after induction of a total local necrosis (deep longitudinal injury). Atherosclerosis **14**, 259–276 (1971)
14. Geer, J.C., McGill, H.C., Strong, J.P.: The fine structure of human atherosclerotic lesions. Amer. J. Path. **38**, 263–287 (1961)
15. Haust, M.D., Balis, J.U., More, R.H.: Electron microscopic study of intimal lipid accumulations in human aorta and their pathogenesis. Circulation **26**, 656 (1962), Abstract, Council on Arteriosclerosis
16. Scott, R.F., Morrison, E.S., Jarmolych, J., Nam, S.C., Kroms, M., Coulston, F.: Experimental atherosclerosis in rhesus monkeys. I. Gross and light microscopy features and lipid values in serum and aorta. Exp. molec. Path. **7**, 11–33 (1967)
17. Thomas, W.A., Jones, R., Scott, R.F., Morris, E., Goodale, F., Imai, H.: Production of early atherosclerotic lesions in rats characterized by proliferation of "modified smooth muscle cells". Exp. molec. Path. **2**, Suppl. 1, 40–61 (1963)
18. Holman, R.L., Brown, B.W., Gore, I., McMillan, G.C., Paterson, J.C., Pollak, O.J., Roberts, J.C., Wissler, R.W.: An index for the evaluation of arteriosclerotic lesions in the abdominal aorta. A report by the Committee on Lesions of the American Society for the Study of Arteriosclerosis. Circulation **22**, 1137–1143 (1960)
19. Borgström, B.: Absorption of triglycerides. In: Lipid transport (Meng, H.C., ed.), p. 15–21, Proc. Int. Symp. Springfield, Ill.: Charles C. Thomas Publisher 1964
20. Borgström, B.: Studies on intestinal cholesterol absorption in the human. J. clin. Invest. **39**, 809–815 (1960)
21. Hofmann, A.F., Borgström, B.: Physico-chemical state of lipids in intestinal content during their digestion and absorption. Fed. Proc. **21**, 43–50 (1962)
22. Strauss, E.W.: Morphological aspects of triglyceride absorption. In: Handbook of physiology (Code, C.F., ed.), vol. 3, Intestinal absorption, sect. 6, Alimentary canal, p. 1377–1406. Washington, D.C.: American Physiology Society 1968
23. Levy, R.I., Fredrickson, D.S.: Heterogeneity of plasma high density lipoproteins. J. clin. Invest. **44**, 426–441 (1965)
24. Schumaker, V.N., Adams, G.H.: Circulating lipoproteins. Ann. Rev. Biochem. **38**, 113–136 (1969)
25. Fredrickson, D.S., Levy, R.I., Lees, R.S.: Fat transport in lipoproteins. An integrated approach to mechanism and disorders. A review. New Engl. J. Med. **276**, 34–42, 94–103, 148–156, 215–225, 273–281 (1967)
26. Greenberger, N.J., Skillman, T.G.: Medium-chain triglycerides. Physiologic considerations and clinical implications. New Engl. J. Med. **280**, 1045–1058 (1969)
27. Eyssen H., Vanderhaeghe, H., De Somer, P.: Effect of polybasic antibiotics and sulfaguanidine on absorption and excretion of cholesterol and bile salts. Fed. Proc. **30**, 1803–1807 (1971)
28. Bloch, K.: The biological synthesis of cholesterol. Science **150**, 19–28 (1965)
29. Bloch, K.: Biosynthesis of cholesterol. In: Hormones and atherosclerosis (Pincus, G., ed.), p. 1–6. New York: Academic Press 1959
30. Clayton, R.B.: Biosynthesis of sterols, steroids, and terpenoids. I. Biogenesis of cholesterol and the fundamental steps in the terpenoid biosynthesis. Quart. Rev. **19**, 168–200 (1965)
31. Frantz, I.D., Jr., Shroepfer, G.J., Jr.: Sterol biosynthesis. Ann. Rev. Biochem. **36**, 691–726 (1967)
32. Rothblat, G.H., Kritchevsky, D.: The metabolism of free and esterified cholesterol in tissue culture cells. A review. Exp. molec. Path. **8**, 314–329 (1968)
33. Tavormina, P.A., Gibbs, M.H., Huff, J.W.: The utilization of β-hydroxy-β-methyl-δ-valerolactone in cholesterol biosynthesis. J. Amer. chem. Soc. **78**, 4498–4499 (1956)
34. Popják, G., Goodman, D.S., Cornforth, J.W., Cornforth, R.H., Ryhage, R.: Studies on the biosynthesis of cholesterol. XV. Mechanism of squalene biosynthesis from farnesyl pyrophosphate and from mevalonate. J. biol. Chem. **236**, 1934–1947 (1961)
35. Popják, G., Goodman, D.S., Cornforth, J.W., Cornforth, R.H., Ryhage, R.: Studies on the biosynthesis of cholesterol. XVI. Chemical synthesis of 1-$H_2{}^3$-2-C^{14}- and 1-D_2-2-C^{14}-trans-trans-farnesyl pyrophosphate and their utilization in squalene biosynthesis. J. biol. Chem. **237**, 56–61 (1962)
36. Popják, G., Edmond, J., Clifford, K., Williams, V.: Biosynthesis and structure of a new intermediate between farnesyl pyrophosphate and squalene. J. biol. Chem. **244**, 1897–1918 (1969)
37. Woodward, R.B., Bloch, K.S.: The cyclization of squalene in cholesterol synthesis. J. Amer. chem. Soc. **75**, 2023–2024 (1953)
38. Siperstein, M.D., Fagan, V.M.: Studies on the feedback regulation of cholesterol synthesis. Advanc. Enzyme Regul. **2**, 249–264 (1964)
39. Dietschy, J.M., Wilson, J.D.: Regulation of cholesterol metabolism. In. New Engl. J. Med. **282**, 1128–1138 (1970)
40. Katz, L.N., Stamler, J., Pick, R.: Nutrition and arteriosclerosis. Philadelphia: Lea & Febiger 1958
41. Dock, W.: Cardiovascular disease (atherosclerosis), Ann. Rev. Med. **10**, 77–87 (1959)
42. Olson, R.E.: Nutrition, Ann. Rev. Biochem. **28**, 467–498 (1959)
43. Thomas, W.A., Lee, K.T., Daoud, A.S.: Geographic aspects of atherosclerosis. Ann. Rev. Med. **15**, 255–272 (1964)
44. Pincus, G. (ed.): Hormones and atherosclerosis. New York: Academic Press 1959
45. Pick, R., Stamler, J., Katz, L.N.: Influence of estrogens on lipids and atherosclerosis in experimental animals. In: Hormones and atherosclerosis (Pincus, G., ed.), p. 229–245. New York: Academic Press 1959
46. Katz, L.N., Stamler, J.: Experimental atherosclerosis. Springfield, Ill.: Charles C. Thomas Publisher 1953
47. Oliver, M.F., Boyd, G.S.: Thyroid and estrogen treatment of hypercholesterolemia in man. In: Hormones and atherosclerosis (Pincus, G., ed.), p. 403–422. New York: Academic Press 1959
48. Friedman, M., Uhley, H.: Experimental stress, blood lipids, and atherosclerosis. In: Hormones and atherosclerosis (Pincus, G., ed.), p. 205–211. New York: Academic Press 1959
49. Rosenman, R.H., Friedman, M.: Change in the serum cholesterol and blood clotting time in men subject to cyclic variation of emotional stress. Circulation **17**, 931 (1957)
50. Rosenman, R.H., Friedman, M.: The possible relationship of the emotions to clinical coronary heart disease. In: Hormones and atherosclerosis (Pincus, G., ed.), p. 283–300. New York: Academic Press 1959
51. Yudkin, J.: Diet and coronary thrombosis. Hypothesis and fact. Lancet **1957I**, 155–162
52. Hinkle, L.E., Jr., Whitney, L.H., Lehman, E.W., Dunn, J., Benjamin, B., King, R., Plakun, A., Flehinger, B.: Occupation, education and coronary heart disease. Science **161**, 238–246 (1968)
53. Gofman, J.W.: The nature of the relationship of disturbance in blood lipid transport with the evolution of clinical coronary heart disease. Trans. Amer. Coll. Cardiol. **4**, 198–220 (1954)
54. Tamplin, A.R., Strisower, B., DeLalla, O.F., Gofman, J.W., Glazier, F.W.: Lipoproteins, aging and coronary artery disease. J. Gerontol. **9**, 404–411 (1954)
55. Robertson, W.B.: Atherosclerosis and ischaemic heart disease. Lancet **1959I**, 444–446
56. Blumenthal, H.T.: Response potentials of vascular tissues and the genesis of arteriosclerosis. II. (C). Hemodynamic factors. Geriatrics **11**, 554–568 (1956)

57. Texon, M.: The role of vascular dynamics in the development of atherosclerosis. In: Atherosclerosis and its origin (Sandler, M., Bourne, G.H., eds.), p. 167–195. New York: Academic Press 1963
58. Swell, L., Treadwell, C.R.: Interrelationships of lipids in blood and tissues. In: Atherosclerosis and its origin (Sandler, M., Bourne, G.H., eds.), p. 301–347. New York: Academic Press 1963
59. Newman, H.A., McCandlees, E.L., Zilversmit, D.B.: The synthesis of C^{14}-lipids in rabbit atheromatous lesions. J. biol. Chem. **236**, 1264–1268 (1961)
60. Kahn, S.G., Slocum, A.: Enzyme activities in aortas of rats fed atherogenic diets. Amer. J. Physiol. **213**, 367, 373–379 (1967)
61. Gofman, J.W., Young, W.: The filtration concept of atherosclerosis and serum lipids in the diagnosis of atherosclerosis. In: Atherosclerosis and its origin (Sandler, M., Bourne, G.H., eds.), p. 197–229. New York: Academic Press 1963
62. Stefanovich, V., Gore, I.: Cholesterol diet and permeability of rabbit aorta. Exp. molec. Path. **14**, 20–29 (1971)
63. Jensen, J.: A further study of the kinetics of cholesterol uptake at the endothelial cell surface of the rabbit aorta *in vivo*. Biochem. biophys. Acta (Amst.) **173**, 71–77 (1969)
64. Jensen, J.: An *in vitro* method for the study of cholesterol uptake at the endothelial cell surface of the rabbit aorta. Biochim. biophys. Acta (Amst.) **135**, 532–543 (1967)
65. Hashimoto, S., Dayton, S., Alfin-Slater, R.B.: Esterification of cholesterol by homogenates of atherosclerotic and normal aortas. Life Sci. **12**, 1–12 (1973)
66. Nakatani, M., Sasaki, T., Miyazaki, T., Nakamura, M.: Synthesis of phospholipids in arterial walls. I. Incorporation of ^{32}P into phospholipids of aortas and coronary arteries of various animals. II. Effects of age and the addition of adrenalin and acetylcholine on the incorporation of ^{32}P into phospholipids of rat aortas. Atherosclerosis **7**, 747–757, 759–766 (1967)
67. Robertson, A.L.: Metabolism and ultrastructure of the arterial wall in atherosclerosis. Cleveland Clin. Quart. **32**, 99–117 (1965)
68. Whereat, A.F.: Recent advances in experimental and molecular pathology. Atherosclerosis and metabolic disorder in the arterial wall. Exp. molec. Path. **7**, 223–247 (1967)
69. Brown, W.V., Levy, R.I., Fredrickson, D.S.: Studies on the proteins of very low density lipoproteins. Fed. Proc. **28**, 666 (1969)
70. Gotto, A.M.: β-apoprotein sufficiency and function. New Engl. J. Med. **280**, 1297–1298 (1969)
71. Levy, R.I., Fredrickson, D.S.: Diagnoses and management of hyperlipoproteinemia. Amer. J. Cardiol. **22**, 576–583 (1968)
72. Jones, R.J. (ed.): Atherosclerosis. Proc. Second Int'l Symp. Berlin-Heidelberg-New York: Springer 1970
73. Kinoshita, J.H.: Cataracts in galactosemia. Invest. Ophthal. **4**, 786–799 (1965)
74. Haust, M.D.: Injury and repair in the pathogenesis of atherosclerotic lesions. In: Atherosclerosis (Jones, R.J., ed.), Proc. Second Int'l Symp., p. 12–20. Berlin-Heidelberg-New York: Springer 1970
75. Constantinides, P.: The important role of endothelial changes in atherogenesis. In: Atherogenesis (Shimamoto, T., Numano, F., Addison, G.M., eds.), vol. II, p. 51–65, Second Int'l Symp. on Atherogenesis, Thrombogenesis and Pyridinolcarbamate Treatment. Amsterdam: Excerpta Medica 1973
76. Shimamoto, T., Sunaga, T.: The contraction and blebbing of endothelial cells accompanied by acute infiltration of plasma substances into the vessel wall and their prevention. In: Atherogenesis (Shimamoto, T., Numano, F., Addison, G.M., eds.), vol. II, p. 3–31. Amsterdam: Excerpta Medica 1973
77. Schwartz, S.M., Benditt, E.P.: Cell replication in the aortic endothelium: A new method for study of the problem. Lab. Invest. **28**, 699–707 (1973)
78. Geer, J.C., Haust, M.D.: Smooth muscle cells in atherosclerosis. In: Monographs on atherosclerosis (Pollak, O.J., Simms, H.S., Kirk, J.E., eds.), vol. 2. Basel, Switzerland: S. Karger AG 1972
79. Scott, R.F., Jarmolych, J., Fritz, K.E., Imai, H., *et al.*: Reactions of endothelial and smooth muscle cells in the atherosclerotic lesion. In: Atherosclerosis (Jones, R.J., ed.), Proc. Second Int'l Symp., p. 50–58. Berlin-Heidelberg-New York: Springer 1970
80. Adams, C.W.M.: Tissue changes and lipid entry in developing atheroma. In: Atherogenesis: Initiating factors (Ciba Foundation Symp. 12, new series, p. 5–37. Amsterdam: Associated Scientific Publishers 1973
81. Bowyer, D.E., Gresham, G.A.: Arterial lipid accumulation. In: Atherosclerosis (Jones, R.J., ed.), Proc. Second Int'l Symp., p. 3–5. Berlin-Heidelberg-New York: Springer 1970
82. Stein, Y., Stein, O.: Lipid synthesis and degradation and lipoprotein transport in mammalian aorta. In: Atherogenesis: Initiating Factors (Ciba Foundation Symp. 12, new series), p. 165–183. Amsterdam: Associated Scientific Publishers 1973
83. Smith, E.B., Slater, R.S.: The lipoproteins of the lesions. In: Atherosclerosis (Jones, R.J., ed.), Proc. Second Int'l Symp., p. 42–49. Berlin-Heidelberg-New York: Springer 1970
84. Adams, C.W.M.: Local factors in atherogenesis: An introduction. In: Atherosclerosis (Jones, R.J., ed.), Proc. Second Int'l Symp., p. 28–34, Berlin-Heidelberg-New York: Springer 1970
85. Chandler, A.B.: Thrombosis and the development of atherosclerotic lesions. In: Atherosclerosis (Jones, R.J., ed.), Proc. Second Int'l Symp., p. 88–93. Berlin-Heidelberg-New York: Springer 1970
86. Scanu, A.M.: The structure of human serum low- and high-density lipoproteins. In: Atherogenesis: Initiating Factors (Ciba Foundation Symp. 12, new series) p. 223–249. Amsterdam: Associated Scientific Publishers 1973
87. Jackson, R.L., Sparrow, J.T., Baker, H.N., *et al.*: The primary structure of apoliprotein-serine. Biol. Chem. **249**, 5308–5313 (1974)
88. Assmann, G., Brewer, H.B., Jr.: A molecular model of high density lipoproteins. Proc. nat. Acad. Sci. (Wash.) **71**, 1534–1538 (1974)
89. Assmann, G., Brewer, H.B., Jr.: Lipid-protein interactions in high density lipoproteins. Proc. nat. Acad. Sci. (Wash.) **71**, 989–993 (1974)
90. Jackson, R.L., Morrisett, J.D., Sparrow, J.T., Segrest, J.P., *et al.*: The interaction of apolipoprotein-serine with phosphatidylcholine. J. biol. Chem. **249**, 5314–5320 (1974)
91. Dempsey, M.E.: Regulation of steroid biosynthesis, in Annual Review of Biochemistry (Snell, E.E., Boyer, P.D., Meister, A., Richardson, C.C., eds.), vol. 43, p. 967–990. Palo Alto, California: Annual Reviews Inc. 1974
92. Edmond, J., Popják, G.: Transfer of carbon atoms from mevalonate to n-fatty acids. J. biol. Chem. **249**, 66–71 (1974)
93. Brown, M.S., Goldstein, J.L., Siperstein, M.D.: Regulation of cholesterol synthesis in normal and malignant tissue. Fed. Proc. **32**, 2168–2173 (1973)
94. Peacock, P.B.: Atherosclerotic heart disease and the environment. Trans. N.Y. Acad. Sci. **35**, 631–635 (1973)
95. Editorial.: Can I avoid a heart-attack? Lancet **1974I**, 605–607
96. Lindner, A., Charra, B., Sherrard, D.J., Scribner, B.H.: Accelerated atherosclerosis in prolonged maintenance hemodialysis. New Engl. J. Med. **290**, 697–701 (1974)
97. Minick, C.R., Murphy, G.E.: Experimental induction of atheroarteriosclerosis by the synergy of allergic injury to arteries and lipid-rich diet. II. Effect of repeatedly injected foreign protein in rabbits fed a lipid-rich, cholesterol-poor diet. Amer. J. Path. **73**, 265–300 (1973)
98. Hardin, N.J., Minick, C.R., Murphy, G.E.: Experimental induction of atheroarteriosclerosis by the synergy of allergic injury to arteries and lipid-rich diet. III. The role of earlier acquired fibromuscular intimal thickening in the pathogenesis of later developing atherosclerosis. Amer. J. Path. **73**, 301–327 (1973)
99. Mathews, J.D., Whittingham, S., Mackay, I.R.: Autoimmune mechanisms in human vascular disease. Lancet **1974II**, 1423–1427
100. Eggen, D.A., Strong, J.P., Newman, W.P., III, Catsulis, C., *et al.*: Regression of diet-induced fatty streaks in Rhesus monkeys. Lab. Invest. **31**, 294–301 (1974)
101. Barboriak, J.J., Pintar, K., Korns, M.E.: Atherosclerosis in aortocoronary vein grafts. Lancet **1974II**, 621–624
102. Fry, D.L.: Responses of the arterial wall to certain physical factors. In: Atherogenesis: Initiating factors (Ciba Foundation Symp. 12, new series), p.93–125. Amsterdam: Associated Scientific Publishers 1973
103. Trillo, A., Haust, M.D.: The granulovesicular bodies of the arterial wall. Lab. Invest. **32**, 105–110 (1975)
104. Zilversmit, D.B.: Metabolism of arterial lipids. In: Atherosclerosis (Jones, R.J., ed.), Proc. Second Int'l Symp., p. 35–41. Berlin-Heidelberg-New York: Springer 1970
105. Bailey, J.M.: Regulation of cell cholesterol content. In: Atherogenesis: Initiating factors (Ciba Foundation Symp. 12, new series), p. 63–92. Amsterdam: Associated Scientific Publishers 1973
106. Iverius, P.-H.: Possible role of the glycosaminoglycans in the genesis of atherosclerosis. In: Atherogenesis: Initiating factors (Ciba Foundation Symp. 12, new series), p. 197–222. Amsterdam: Associated Scientific Publishers 1973
107. Shio, H., Farquhar, M.G., de Duve, C.: Lysosomes of the arterial wall. IV. Cytochemical localization of acid phosphatase and catalase in smooth muscle cells and foam cells from rabbit atheromatous aorta. Amer. J. Path. **76**, 1–10 (1974)
108. Brecher, P., Kessler, M., Clifford, C., Chobanian, A.V.: Cholesterol ester hydrolysis in aortic tissue. Biochim. biophys. Acta (Amst.) **316**, 386–394 (1973)
109. Takano, T., Black, W.J., Peters, T.J., de Duve, C.: Assay, kinetics, and lysosomal localization of an acid cholesteryl esterase in rabbit aortic smooth muscle cells. J. biol. Chem. **249**, 6732–6737 (1974)
110. Peters, T.J., Takano, T., de Duve, C.: Subcellular fractionation studies on the cells isolated from normal and atherosclerotic aorta. In: Atherogenesis: Initiating factor (Ciba Foundation Symp. 12, new series), p. 197–222. Amsterdam: Associated Scientific Publishers 1973
111. Miller, G.J., Miller, N.E.: Plasma-high-density-lipoprotein concentration and development of ischaemic heart-disease. Lancet **1975I**, 16–19
112. Goldstein, J.L., Brown, M.S.: Familial hypercholesterolemia: Identification of a defect in the regulation of 3-hydroxy-3-methylglutaryl coenzyme A reductase activity associated with overproduction of cholesterol. Proc. nat. Acad. Sci. (Wash.) **70**, 2804–2808 (1973)

Chapter 12
Radiation

Physical Phases of Biological Effects of UV and X-Irradiation 717

Photoelectric Effect 718
Compton Effect 718
Excitation and Ionization 720
Radiolysis of Water and the Hydrated Electron 722
Fate of the Radiation-Produced Holes 723
G Value
Photochemistry of Nucleic Acid Bases 723

Biological Effects of UV Irradiation 724

Base Alteration 724
Effects of UV Irradiation on Hydrogen Bond 725
Effects of UV Irradiation on Skin 726
Molecular Repair of UV Damage to DNA 727
Extent and Limitations of Excision Repair in Mammalian Tissues 729
Postreplication Repair 730
Dimers and Function 731
DNA Repair and Disease 731
DNA Repair and Aging 732

Biological Effects of Ionizing Radiation 733

Types of Exposures 733
Effects on Skin 733
Effect on Mammary Glands 735
Effect on Gonads 735
Effect on Ovaries 735
Effect on Hematopoietic Organs 735
Effects on the Gastrointestinal Tract 736
Miscellaneous Radiation Lesions 737
Causes of Death after Administration of Whole Body Doses of X-Irradiation 737
Criteria for Prognosis after Radiation Injury 738

Radiation Carcinogenesis 740

Sunlight and Cancer 740
Professional and Accidental Cancer Produced by Radiation 742
X-Ray Carcinogenesis 742
Experimental Radiation Carcinogenesis
Radiation and Leukemia 743

Biochemical Effects of Ionizing Irradiation 746

Nuclear Versus Cytoplasmic Radiosensitivity 746
Site of Lesions (Ionizing Radiation) 746
Effect of Irradiation on Enzymes *in Vitro* 746
Effect of X-Irradiation on DNA Synthesis 749
Effect of X-Irradiation on Mitosis 751
Effect on Chromosomes 753

Irradiation of DNA *in Vitro* 753
Effects of Ionizing Irradiation on DNA *in Vivo* 755
Repair of X-Ray Damage in Mammalian Cells 756

Conclusion 757

References 758

Physical Phases of Biological Effects of UV and X-Irradiation

We have seen previously that atoms are made of a central nuclear charge that is positive and that the positive charge of the nucleus is exactly counterbalanced by identical numbers of negative charges in peripheral electrons. These electrons are characterized by four quantic numbers that define: (1) the level of their orbital around the nucleus, (2) the shape of the orbital, (3) the direction taken by the electron within the orbital, and (4) the direction of the spin of the electron. The electrons have a characteristic charge, mass, and radius: the charge is 4.77×10^{-7}, u escgs; the mass is 9.04×10^{-20}; and the radius is 10^{-30} cm [1–5].

The production of the electromagnetic waves concerns the electron shelves; thus, although the motion of one electron around the nucleus within its normal orbit does not generate energy, the displacement of an electron from one orbital to another produces electromagnetic waves. Electromagnetic waves can be produced by a number of means, and the energy and the wavelength of the resulting electromagnetic waves depend on the nature of the original impact. The gamut of electromagnetic waves encompasses all wavelengths from radio waves to gamma rays. The velocity of all electromagnetic waves is constant; it equals C, the speed of light (300,000 km/sec).

To produce that special type of electromagnetic wave called X-irradiation, the atoms of a metal with a high melting point are bombarded with an electron beam. Thus, the X-ray tube is made of a glass shell in which a vacuum has been induced. One end of the tube contains the anode, and the other contains the cathode. The cathode is a tungsten filament the extremities of which are connected to a source of low voltage. The anode is usually made of a piece of metal with a high melting point—for example, tungsten—and is connected to a source of positive potential with respect to the cathode. The electrons that have been accelerated at the anode move toward the cathode because of the vacuum in the tubes, and when the electrons hit the electron shells of the atoms that compose the anode, they eject energized particles called photons.

The mechanism of X-irradiation production explains the relationships between the differences in electrical potential, the kinetic energy of the electrons emitted at the cathode, and the energy of the photon emitted at the anode. This relationship is expressed in the equation of Einstein-Planck, $E=(mV^2/2)=hv=eW$. 64.0.1234 A. Since $V=1/\lambda$, the relationship between wavelength and kilovoltage becomes obvious, as is expressed in the equation $\lambda=12.34/hv$. The equation tells us that the wavelength shortens as the kilovoltage applied to the X-ray tube increases.

Thus, theoretically, if one were to operate an X-ray machine at a kilovoltage of 100, the wavelength should be 0.1234 A. Practically, however, since the vacuum is never perfect within the tubes, many of the incident electrons are retarded in their displacement from the anode to the cathode by molecules in the tube. Consequently, different electrons reach the anode with different incidental kinetic energies, so the wavelengths of the photons produced are of different magnitudes. Therefore, the X-irradiation produced is never monochromatic but polychromatic. The spectrum of the wavelengths of the X-irradiation (as studied with diffraction crystals) is a continuum until a limit value of λ_0 is reached. This limit value is precisely the one that is defined by the Duane equation: $\lambda_0=1{,}2{,}3{,}4\ hv$.

Since most of the electrons have been retarded in their process to the anode and very few reach this limit value, the intensity of the beam with that characteristic wavelength λ_0 is very low. For practical purposes, it is more important to know the wavelength of the beam with the maximum intensity, or the λ maximum. There is, fortunately, a very simple relationship between λ maximum and λ_0: $\lambda_{max}=\omega\lambda_0$. Omega is a constant, roughly equal to 1.5.

Electromagnetic waves propagate as particles associated with waves; therefore, the laws of propagation of a photon are those that govern waves in motion and propagation of particles.

One very important law with respect to the propagation of X-irradiation is that of the square of the distances. The dispersion of the radiation is similar to that of light. If we consider the original source of light to be punctiform, the beam that emerges becomes broader and broader as the distance between the source and the target increases. Thus, while only small areas are illuminated close to the source, larger areas are illuminated as the distance between source and target increases. The intensity decreases with the distance according to a mathematical rule, which is expressed as follows: the intensity of X-rays decreases as a function of the square of the distance that separates target from source, $I_2=I_1 \times d_1{}^2/d_2{}^2$. The greater the distance, the smaller the intensity. This law is, of course, of the greatest practical importance in radiotherapy, radiodiagnosis, and in calculating doses received.

The absorption of X-irradiation by matter will depend on the wavelength of the incident source, on the incident rate, and on the thickness and the atomic number of the irradiated material. It is expressed by the equation: $I_x=I_0e^{-\mu x}$.

The laws of absorption are of particular importance to radiotherapy. If we imagine an internal tumor located 10 cm from the skin, and if we assume that the X-ray source is placed 20 cm from the tumor, the dose at the skin will be twice as high as the dose at the tumor. Obviously, the ratio of skin dose to tumor dose can be considerably reduced by increasing the distance between source and target.

Because the X-irradiation used in therapy is not monochromatic, the shorter wavelengths must be filtered; otherwise, the softer rays would be absorbed by the superficial tissues and burn the skin instead of killing the tumor cells. Aluminium and copper filters are placed between the source of X-irradiation and the target to eliminate the low wavelength radiation.

This is not the place to discuss the historical evolution of the theories on light. The student remembers that after Newton had proposed a "particulate" nature of light, Fresnell suggested the wave theory of light, which seemed to explain many of the phenomena associated with the propagation of light interference, polarization, diffraction, and other factors. Later, deBroglie reconciled the corpuscular and the wave theory of light. deBroglie assumed that light was made of small units called photons. The resting photon has no mass and thus can achieve maximal velocities (300,000 km/sec).

With X-irradiation, the particle and the wave find their way among the atoms and permeate electron orbitals. This travel is full of adventures including diffusion, the photoelectric effect, the Compton effect, and pair formation. To understand these effects, assume that the surface of a large sphere of plastic material is perforated by many holes. In the center of the sphere is a large compact mass of positive charge. At the periphery of the sphere are a number of concentric orbitals to which small masses of negative charge gravitate. If through one of the openings of the sphere a marble is thrown toward the center with a certain strength, that marble will progress in a specific direction with kinetic energy defined by its mass and equal to $mv^2/2$. The marble may skid on one of the electronic orbitals and be deviated from its original course without losing its initial energy (this is diffusion), or the Thomson effect, or it may transfer part of its energy to the electron that it hits, and the latter then acquires an electrical energy equal to the difference between the energy of the incident photon (the marble) and the residual photon (the marble after it has been slowed down). This is the Compton effect. The photoelectric effect is a particular form of the Compton effect, in which the difference between the energy of the incidental photon and the residual photon is 0, and all incident electromagnetic energy is transferred to the electron in the form of kinetic energy. The Compton and the photoelectric effects are mainly responsible for the biological effects of X-irradiation.

In the Thomson effect, the photons hit the atoms and bounce back without loss of energy. The capacity of matter to generate Thomson effects is proportional to the number of electrons, the charge of these electrons, the mass of the resting electrons, and the volume. The diffusion effect is important in radiotherapy because it makes it impossible to delineate exactly the irradiated field, and the real field irradiated is greater than the one originally delineated. Furthermore, because of this simple process of diffusion, called the Thomson effect, the dose at the target will always be higher than the dose calculated on the basis of absorption.

Photoelectric Effect

When matter is bombarded with electromagnetic waves, the energy of the wave may be, under special circumstances, transferred to peripheral electrons that are ejected from their orbitals. When certain metals or gases are exposed to visible or UV light, they emit electrons. The incident quantum thus disappears, and in its place a photoelectron and an excited atom appear.

The number of electrons that are emitted under the influence of a monochromatic source of light is proportional to the intensity of the incident light. The number also increases as the wavelength decreases and drops to zero below a certain threshold level. When visible light is used as a source, special metals, such as sodium and potassium, must be irradiated *in vacuo* for light to be converted into electricity. In contrast, X-rays generate photoelectrons with all metals.

The photoelectric effect can be seen as a reversal of the Einstein-Planck equation or it can be considered as a special form of the Compton effect.

If electrons endowed with an energy equal to ev can generate photons with an energy hv, it is quite conceivable that a light beam with energy hv can generate a photoelectron with energy ev. The kinetic energy of the photoelectron equals $mv^2/2$; thus in the emission of photons, $ev = {}^1/_2\, mv^2 = hv = h(e/\lambda)$. The photoelectric effect can also be looked upon as a special form of the Compton effect in which the wavelength of the diffused photon is so great that the energy of the photon tends to equal 0 (see below).

The applications of the photoelectrical effect in radiophysics and radiobiology are of considerable importance. The photoelectrical effect explains why an X-ray can charge or discharge an electrometer, an instrument that has been used to measure X-rays. The photoelectric effect is responsible for ionization of gases, which led to the use of ionization chambers to measure X-rays. Finally, most of the biological effects of X-irradiation result from the photoelectric effect.

Compton Effect

In the Compton effect, the interaction between the incident photon (hv) and the electron involves a partial transfer of energy from the photon to the electron with the emission of a residual photon with reduced energy. Obviously, the wavelength of the residual electromagnetic wave will be greater than that of the incident beam. Compton discovered this phenomenon in 1923, and the discovery confirmed the concept of Einstein, who had proposed that light was composed of small quanta called photons, or hv.

Thus, Compton discovered that the interaction between a monochromatic incident beam and the electron generates a new type of radiation, a secondary radiation with a wavelength greater than that of the primary radiation. The observable effect is different from the photoelectric effect, in which the quantum of energy that hits the electron disappears and is entirely converted into kinetic energy.

Compton assumed that the observed effect resulted from the elastic collision between photon and electron.

In such a collision, the total energy and the total momentum are conserved. Thus, not only does the diffused photon have a reduced energy level, but its direction is also changed, and the path of the diffused photon forms an angle with that of the incident photon.

The law of conservation of energy requires that in the collision, the energy of the incident photon ($h\nu$) equals the energy of the diffused photon ($h\nu^1$) and the kinetic energy of the ejected electron (W): $h\nu = h\nu^1 + W$. The theory of relativity tells us that

$$W = m_0 c^2 \left(\frac{1}{\sqrt{1-\beta^2}} - 1 \right)$$

when m_0 = mass of the electron and

$$\beta = \frac{v}{c} = \frac{\text{velocity of the electron after collision}}{\text{speed of light}}.$$

Thus,

$$h\nu = h\nu^1 = m_0 c^2 \left(\frac{1}{\sqrt{1-\beta^2}} - 1 \right).$$

The law of conservation of momentum requires that the momentum of the incident photons equals that of the diffused photon and that acquired by the ejected electron.

The equation of Einstein states e/c^2 = mass.

The energy of a quantum of light $= h\nu$; consequently, the mass of the quantum $= m = h\nu/c^2$, and the momentum $= m/c = h\nu/c$. The momentum of the electron

$$= \frac{m_0 v}{\sqrt{1-\beta^2}}.$$

Thus, in the direction of the propagation of the incident photon,

$$\frac{h\nu}{c} = h\nu^1 \cos\theta + \frac{m_0 v}{\sqrt{1-\beta^2}} \cos\theta_1,$$

and in a direction orthogonal with respect to the incident photon (a plane which includes the direction of both the scattered photon and the electron),

$$0 = \frac{h\nu^1}{c} \sin\theta + \frac{m_0 v}{\sqrt{1-\beta^2}} \sin\theta_1.$$

By eliminating θ_1 and v in the three equations, one can write

$$\frac{\nu^1}{\nu} = \frac{1}{1 + \frac{h\nu}{m_0 c^2}} (1 - \cos\theta).$$

Since $\nu = c/\lambda$

$$\lambda^1 - \lambda = \frac{h}{m_0 c} (1 - \cos\theta)$$

or, expressed in A,

$$\Delta\lambda = \lambda' - \lambda = 0.0243\,(1 - \cos\theta).$$

This important equation expresses the increase in wavelength that occurs when an incident beam with a wavelength λ is scattered at an angle θ. The wavelength λ' of the scattered beam exceeds that of the incident beam by a quantity of $0.0243\,(1-\cos\theta)$. $\Delta\lambda$ is thus independent of the composition of the irradiated material and of the incident wavelength. It varies only with the direction of the scattered beam. Thus, $\Delta\lambda$ is the same for all types of radiation used, be it X-rays or γ-irradiation.

The kinetic energy of the recoil electrons E can be calculated in a similar fashion:

$$E = h\nu \frac{\left(\frac{h}{m_0 c \lambda} \right) (1 - \cos\theta)}{1 + \left(\frac{h}{m_0 c \lambda} \right) (1 - \cos\theta)}.$$

In conclusion, the Compton effect manifests itself by: (1) a decrease in the energy of the incident beam (expressed by increased wavelength); and (2) the expression from matter of an electron with a kinetic energy proportional to the difference between the energy of the incident photon and that which holds the electron within its orbital.

Elastic Shock Between Photon and Electron

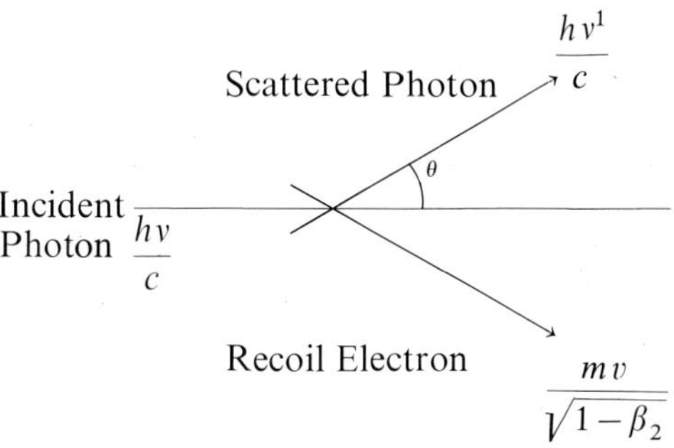

The Compton effect is readily demonstrable by projecting an X-ray beam into a Wilson chamber. The path of the electron can be photographed and the wavelength of the X-ray beam can be measured before and after it passes through the chamber.

Such an observation shows that because of the Compton effect, there is little advantage in using X-ray sources capable of operating beyond 400 kv for radiotherapy unless the generator operates at kilovoltages exceeding one million. Indeed, between 400 and 1,000,000 kv, the loss of energy of the incident photon is so great that increasing the potential is of little value. With potentials of 1,000,000 or above, the energy of the residual photon is often great enough to be effective in therapy; furthermore, the energy acquired by the target electrons is great enough to generate new X-rays.

In fact, if the potential of the generator is large enough (3 mv or more), the courses of the incident photon, the electron, and the residual photon will remain in a straight tract, and, as a result, the deleterious effects of diffusion are eliminated and the depth dose may be higher than the skin dose.

Excitation and Ionization

By either the photoelectric or the Compton effect, photons penetrate matter and remove electrons. These negative charges in motion generate electromagnetic fields and ionize the obstacles that they meet on their path. Atoms are neutral; the number of protons (+charges) equals the number of electrons (−charges). In contrast, ions are charged particles. In an ionized atom, one or more positive or negative charges have been eliminated. Since the proton is much heavier than the electron, much more energy is necessary to free a proton than to free an electron. Thus, ionization is mainly the result of an electron loss or gain.

An atom is excited when an electron shifts from a central to a more peripheral orbital as a result of a new increment of energy. The excitation state is unstable, and the electron soon returns to the orbital from which it came. In returning from the excited to the stable state, the electron releases an amount of energy equal to that absorbed.

Owing to their greater energy content, excited atoms are usually more reactive than nonexcited atoms. However, their life span is very short (10^{-7} to 10^{-8} seconds), and, as a result, few excited molecules interact [6–8].

The increment in energy that may produce excitation is thermal, visible, or UV light and ionizing radiation. Photochemical reactions differ from ordinary thermal reactions in a very important way. Whereas the free energy of the reacting system always decreases in ordinary thermal reactions, it increases in some photochemical reactions.

A most important biological example of photochemistry is the process of photosynthesis. In photosynthesis, electromagnetic energy light (hv=quantum) is converted into chemical potential; consequently, CO_2 reacts with water to yield carbohydrates and molecular oxygen.

$$CO_2+H_2O \rightarrow (CH_2O)n+O_2.$$

Before we consider radiochemical events, it would be wise to refresh our knowledge of elementary principles of photochemistry, not only because there are many analogies, but also because there are important differences between these two forms of chemistry [9, 10].

For example, when light hits a molecular compound in solution, all the electromagnetic energy is not converted into chemical energy, but part of the incident light may be converted to heat and part may be reemitted as light with a different frequency (fluorescence). Only the light that is absorbed by the reacting system is converted into chemical potential.

When molecules are hit by the incident light, they are usually at their lowest vibrational state. The light excites the peripheral electron for a period of 10^{-8} seconds. If, during this time, the excited molecule does not collide with another molecule, it releases part, but not all, of the absorbed energy. Since after fluorescence the molecule remains in a vibrational state greater than normal, the fluorescing light usually has a greater wavelength and a smaller frequency than the incident light. However, when atoms are hit by light, since they have no vibrational state, the return from the excited to the ground state is associated with emission of fluorescing light of the same wavelengths as the incident light:

	Ground State	
2537 A	S_0	2537 A
	Excited State	
	3p	

Thus, if mercury vapor is irradiated with UV (2537 A) light and the pressure is maintained low enough to prevent collision (conversion to kinetic energy), the vapor will fluorescence UV light of the same wavelength as the incident beams.

The addition of hydrogen to the mercury vapor quenches the fluorescence. If molecular hydrogen is added to the mercury vapors and the mixture is irradiated with 2537 A UV light, the molecular hydrogen decomposes. Therefore, the energy is transferred from the atom of mercury to the molecule of hydrogen in a collision of the second kind (inelastic collision). Such reactions are referred to as photosensitized reactions.

In photochemistry, the intensity of the chemical reaction is related to the quantity of light absorbed. For every quantum absorbed, one molecule is involved in the chemical reaction (provided, of course, that there are no side reactions). If hv is a quantum of energy, the energy absorbed is $E=Nhv$; $E=Nhv=Nhc/\lambda$ ergs$=2.859\times10^5/\lambda$ kilocalories per mole.* The formula indicates: (1) that the value of E (energy absorbed) varies with the wavelength of the incident light (E increasing as λ is shorter), and E is constant for a given wavelength; and (2) that whenever the law of physical equivalents is rigidly obeyed, the ratio of the number of molecules decomposed to the number of quanta absorbed should equal:

$$\phi=\frac{\text{number of molecules decomposed}}{\text{number of quanta}}=1.$$

* N=Avogadro's number$=6.023\times10^{23}$; $h=6.624\times10^{27}$; $c=2.9977\times10^{10}$; and 1 kilocalorie$=4.184\times10^{10}$ ergs.

As pointed out, this happens only when the reaction is instantaneous, and no secondary reaction takes place.

The interaction between radiation and matter is very different when ionizing radiation is used. These interactions are coulombic and involve the movement of charged particles. Consider an electron or β-particle moving rapidly along track *ab* (see Fig. 12-1). Let's assume that there is a water molecule in *d*. A β-particle with an energy of 0.5 mev will traverse distance *ab* (40 A) within 10^{-17} seconds. The electrons attached to the water molecule in *d* will be repelled along *ad* and *bd*. The components of the repelling forces that are parallel to the track of the fast electrons will cancel out, and only those perpendicular or oblique to the original track will actively repel. As a result, the electron located in *d* at the periphery of a water molecule will receive an impact perpendicular to that of the track of the primary electron. If the energy of the impact is great, the electron is ejected and the molecule is ionized. Weaker impacts only bring the electron to higher energy levels and excite the molecule. Still weaker impacts have no effect. Thus, the track of the β-particle is surrounded by three zones: a zone of ionization, one of excitation, and an unaffected zone.

The consequences of such a distribution of events are twofold. First, the original particle loses energy as it goes through matter and, as a result, is decelerated and finally stops. Interaction between fast electrons and molecular electrons is finite in space and time, and such interactions occur only in the immediate vicinity of the primary track. Second, since the force that acts on the molecular electron is purely coulombic, the action of ionizing radiations on molecules cannot be selective. It follows that this effect will not be merely a function of the concentration of a given molecule, but the number of ionizations and excitations will also be proportional to the electronic density in the path of the fast electron. The effect on a given molecular component depends upon the fraction of the electron population that is contributed by that component.

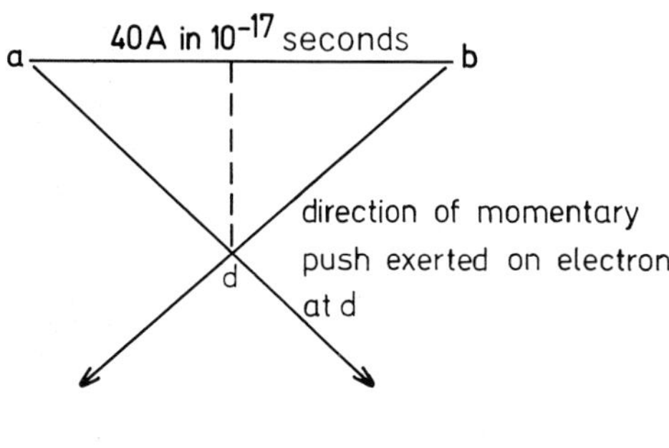

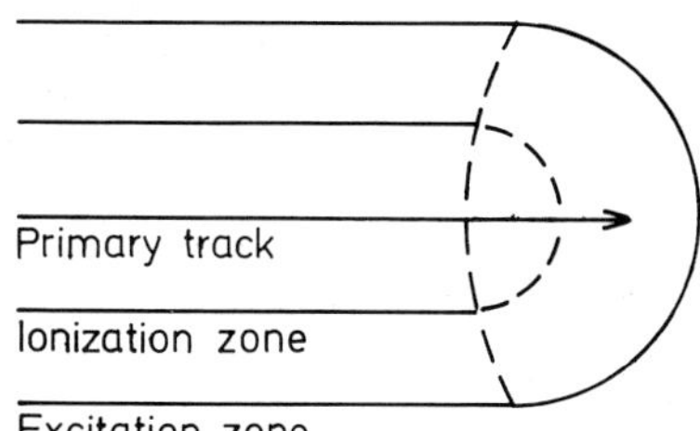

Fig. 12-1. Interaction between beta-particles and matter

Although the primary impacts are different in radiation and photochemistry, both types of processes yield the same primary chemical species; for example, OH and e_{aq}.

In conclusion, although the chemical reactions that are triggered by the administration of X- or gamma rays are analogous in principle, they differ in their manifestations in three ways.

First, the absorbed photons are quanta of considerably greater energy than the quanta of light. The photons of light have energy approximating a few electron volts, whereas those of ionizing radiation are of the order of thousands or millions of electron volts.

Second, photochemical effects are essentially molecular events and depend upon the energy of the incident photon and properties of the absorbent molecule. The absorption is of the resonant type and obeys the Beer-Lambert law. A photon generated by a source of ionizing radiation enters matter, and the impact between the electron and the incidental photon is great enough to ionize any molecules. Consequently, the absorption of ionizing radiation depends upon the electron density of the absorbent rather than on its number of molecules.

Third, although photochemical reactions are relatively simple and are explainable in terms of atoms and free radicals produced by decomposition of the excited molecules, the chemical reactions resulting from the absorption of ionizing radiation are much more complex, because in addition to primary excitation and free-radical formation, secondary electrons and ions are produced which move with various kinetic energies. It is usually estimated that half the energy absorbed is spent in producing ions while the other half is spent in producing excited molecules.

The interaction between high-energy radiation and matter occurs in three stages. In the first stage, a number of excited atoms or molecules, positive ions, and moving electrons are produced. The free electrons increase in number at first, and then decrease as the time between the absorption of the original quantum and the electronic release increases. The energy of these electrons is not known with certainty, but is estimated at around 1805 electron volts. Thus, the first stage of the interaction between incident radiation and matter involves activity in the electronic shells, and little of the absorbed energy is converted into heat.

In the second stage, however, the kinetic energy of the electron is degraded to thermal energy. The energy of the electron is no longer great enough to interact with the electronic system of the atom, and now these electrons with lower energies interfere with atomic movement; consequently, their energy is converted to heat. This is followed by a third stage in which chemical reactions take place as a result of collision between reactive atoms, free radicals, or molecules.

From this description, it appears that electronic events that follow ionizing radiation can be divided into fast and slow reactions. The fast electrons may interact with matter in either inelastic or elastic collision. Only the inelastic collision results in energy transfer. However, the elastic collision influences the path of the electron. With slow electrons, inelastic collision with electronic oscillation is excluded because of the principle of conservation of energy. The slow electrons do not have enough energy to dislodge electrons from their atomic orbital. Thus, the interaction of slow electrons involves atomic oscillations. Slow-moving electrons may also influence the dipolar structure of the medium.

Radiolysis of Water and the Hydrated Electron

Most of the biological molecules that are irradiated *in vivo* or *in vitro* are either in solution or suspended in water. The effect of ionizing radiation on water is therefore of considerable importance in radiation biology.

For years it was assumed that the chemical radiolysis of water resulted in a split of the original molecule into H and OH, the H and OH then recombining to yield H_2 and H_2O_2 [11–13]:

$$\begin{aligned} H_2O &\xrightarrow{h\nu} H + OH \\ OH + OH &\longrightarrow H_2O_2 \\ H + H &\longrightarrow H_2 \\ OH + H_2 &\longrightarrow H_2O + H \end{aligned}$$

On theoretical grounds, Platzman has excluded the possibility of a direct interaction between secondary electrons and water molecules and proposed that the thermalized electron imposed radial polarization on surrounding water molecules [11, 12]. The polarization of the water molecules around the electron generates an electrical potential, which has been referred to as the potential well. Electrons trapped in such wells may have one or more quantitized energy levels. The passage from one level to another, or transfer of the energy to the surrounding water molecule, should be detectable by absorption spectrography, and this was indeed achieved almost 10 years after Platzman's original prediction. In the meantime, radiation chemists established that a reducing agent other than H appeared in irradiated water.

However, when radiochemists attempted to investigate the kinetics of such reactions generated by the irradiation of water they found that there was a discrepancy between the rate constant of the H atom formed in $OH+H_2 \rightarrow H+H_2O$ and in the rate of the reaction of the reducing species with H_2O_2 in $H+H_2O_2 \rightarrow H_2O+OH$. The second reaction occurred much too fast to make it possible for the reducing agent to be supplied by the first. However, a reaction involving a hydrated electron e_{aq} as a reducing agent had a rate 500 times greater than the one involving H.

$$e_{aq} + H_2O_2 \rightarrow OH^- + OH$$

Although the formation of the hydrate electron was predicted on theoretical grounds and was suspected on a kinetic basis, direct evidence for this became available only in the early 1960s.

The lifetime of the hydrated electron is of the order of microseconds only; therefore, special equipment was necessary to detect them. Such special equipment includes: (1) a machine that can accelerate electrons and deliver them in short pulses; and (2) spectrographic instruments capable of recording the "flash absorption" resulting from the formation of transient species.

The short pulses are delivered by Van de Graaff accelerators. For example, some of these accelerators produce electron pulses of 3, 10, 30, and 100 nsec with an intensity of 1.5 amp. Hunt and Homes have redesigned the more traditional accelerators, and their new machine can produce pulses of 5 amp in 1 nsec.

Two types of pulse radiolysis detection systems have been used—flash spectroscopy and kinetic spectroscopy. In light-flash absorption spectrophotometry, the delivery of short electron pulses is synchronized with the production of a light flash produced by a continuous light source. The electrode tips of such a source are usually made of uranium. The transient species formed during the irradiation with the electron will absorb light at specific wavelengths, and if a sensitive photographic plate is placed on the path of the light, absorption bands appear and the intensity of the bands can be measured with a densitometer. Then a quartz cell (60 mm long) containing the sample is placed between the light source and the photographic plate and is irradiated with the electron source.

In kinetic spectroscopy, a continuous light source is used. The light is led through a monochromator, and from there to a photomultiplier, which is connected to an ossilograph. The advantage of the kinetic over the flash method is that the kinetic method yields better time resolution and is more sensitive, because the absorption of even small amounts of light is sufficiently amplified to be readable on the ossilograph.

The absorption spectrum of the hydrated electron [13] was observed for the first time by Hart and Boag [14] in 1962. A deaerated aqueous solution of sodium bicarbonate (0.05 M) was pipetted in a special quartz cuvette with a special syringe. The solution was activated with an electron beam of 1.8 MeV in a pulse of 2 μsec. At the same time, a spark of uranium light (5 μsec in duration) was generated from uranium electrodes. The absorption spectrum was recorded on a photographic plate. The spectrum of the pulse of the irradiated solution presents an intense, but transient absorption with a peak at 7000 A. The absorption band does not show in a photograph of flashes taken 30 μsec after the pulse irradiation. Three lines of evidence indicate that the absorption spectrum which appears during pulse radiolysis results from the formation of hydrated electrons: (1) enhanced electrical conductivity; (2) similarity between the absorption spectrum of water radiolysis and that of ammonia of alkali metal radiolysis, in which the solvated electron is stable; and (3) interference with the development of the spectrum by the addition of scavengers of hydrated electrons (H^+, O_2, CO_2, H_2O_2, etc.). These new methods have permitted the identification of the primary species in radiolysis, and they have helped investigators obtain more information on the reaction of the hydrated electron.

The transient hydrated electron is a highly reactive species. Since its charge is negative, it reacts preferentially with excessive positive charges. Under acidic conditions during water radiolysis, the hydrated electron is captured by H^+ and forms H; but at the pH of the living cell the hydrated electrons react with H_2O to split it into H and OH.

$$
\begin{aligned}
2\,H_2O &\rightarrow H_2O^+ + e_{aq} \\
e_{aq} + e_{aq} &\rightarrow H_2 + 2\,OH^- \\
OH + OH &\rightarrow H_2O_2 \\
e_{aq} + OH &\rightarrow OH_{aq} \\
e_{aq} + H_3O^+ &\rightarrow H + H_2O \\
e_{aq} + H &\rightarrow H_2 + OH_{aq} \\
H + H &\rightarrow H_2
\end{aligned}
$$

Although there seems to be no doubt that e_{aq} is the principal reducing agent in radiolyzed water, arguments have been presented against the hydrated electron being the sole precursor of H_2. Indeed, since reaction $e_{aq}+e_{aq}\rightarrow H_2+2\,OH^-$ should compete with reaction $e_{aq}+H_3O\rightarrow H+H_2O$, pH changes should consequently affect the production of H_2 and H; but this is not the case. Thus it cannot as yet be excluded that the second reducing species H is produced directly by the reaction $H_2O\rightarrow H+OH$ or indirectly by the formation of an excited molecule of H_2O. The exact mechanism of formation of the hydrated electron is not known.

Fate of the Radiation-Produced Holes

If ionizing or other forms of radiation eject electrons from water molecules to yield hydrated electrons, what is the fate of the positive ion $(H_2O)^+$ that is left? The lifetime of the $(H_2O)^+$ hole is believed to be much shorter than that of the electron, and the positive ion is thought to react with neutral water molecules to yield OH radicals and H_3O^+: $(H_2O)^+ + H_2O \rightarrow OH + H_3O^+$. The existence of the positive ions has been demonstrated in experiments in which ice was irradiated with γ-rays. For further detail, refer to the paper by Weiss* on ionization and excitation [8].

* Weiss has, however, proposed that under some circumstances, these positive ions are not so insoluble and may interact with such molecules as benzene to hydroxylate them.

For a recent review on the radiation chemistry of aqueous solutions see the paper by Schwarz [152].

G Value

It appears from the preceding information that the irradiation of water produces a number of new substances, hydrated electrons, free radicals, and peroxides (H_2O_2). Water radiolysis induces changes in the molecules in solution; irradiation of the dried solute also modifies it chemically. Radiochemists have defined a unit that expresses the yield of the new substance formed, to be called the G value. The G value expresses the number of specific events per 100 eV of energy absorbed. The molecular event under consideration can be a number of things: activation of an enzyme, radiolysis of water or other compounds, hydration of a purine, formation of a thymine dimer, formation of hydrogen peroxide, etc. Examples of some of the G values for a number of radiochemical events are presented below:

Event	G Value
Production of H	3.7
Production of OH	2.7
Production of H_2O_2	0.7
Inactivation of trypsin	0.12–0.44
Sugar-phosphate rupture	0.45
Single-strand breaks	10
Double-strand breaks	0.12–0.15
Base alteration	2
Cross-linking	0.08

Photochemistry of Nucleic Acid Bases

The nucleic acids are made of five principal heterocyclic conjugated structures: thymine, uracil, adenine, cytosine, and guanine. Thus, one of the most fundamental biological substances is made of resonating molecules with delocalized electrons. This electron delocalization gives the molecule an increment of stability referred to as "resonance energy" (see below).

Resonance Energy in Kilocalories per Mole

Porphyrins	200
Purines	50–80
Pyrimidines	30–40

Adenine has the highest resonance energy, and thymidine the lowest. Pullman and his associates [15] have established that a close relationship exists between the resonance stabilization energy and the resistance to X-ray and UV damage. It is, therefore, of considerable interest that nucleic acids irradiated with UV-, X- or α-radiation elicit electron spin resonance signals corresponding to the development of a free radical of thymine.

On this basis, one would expect that thymine would be the most radiosensitive of the bases in DNA, a fact that is indeed corroborated by the finding that thymidine dimers formed after UV irradiation of DNA involve precisely the formation of covalent bonding between C5 and C6. Furthermore, although thymine dimers are not formed when frozen thymine solution is X-irradiated *in vitro*, the thymine molecule is disrupted and urea is formed.

Hydrogen bonding may also lead to resonance stabilization. This stabilization is 1 Cal greater for the guanine-cytosine pair than for the adenine-thymine pair. This fact explains the relative resistance to UV light of DNA rich in guanine-cytosine pairs. As mentioned previously, this resonance stabilization explains the greater resistance of the guanine-cytosine pair to heat denaturation.

Extensive photochemical studies of the effect of UV and X-irradiation on bases, nucleosides, and nucleotides have confirmed the conclusion that the purine ring is not as readily altered with electromagnetic radiation as is the pyrimidine ring. The following mean G values have been reported for the splitting of the various bases: adenine—0.12; guanine—0.19; cytosine—0.28; and thymine—0.44.*

Electron spin resonance studies have indicated that no unpaired electrons appear in irradiated purine, although signals develop in irradiated pyrimidines. Nevertheless, relatively weak signals are detected when the purine nucleosides or nucleotides are irradiated.

Thus, pyrimidine bases are twice or four times as sensitive to the effects of UV radiation as the purine bases, and it is generally accepted that the most significant biological alterations of nucleic acid result from changes in the pyrimidine molecules. The reasons for these differences between the responses of purine and pyrimidine molecules will become apparent later.

Biological Effects of UV Irradiation

Many biological molecules absorb UV light, but the nucleic acids are particularly efficient. (The UV absorption spectrum of nucleic acids ranges from 200 to 300 mμ with a peak between 250 and 280.) They derive this property from the presence of purine and pyrimidine bases in the macromolecules. There is a good correlation between capacity to absorb UV light and inactivation of viruses or bacteria. In man, UV damage includes sunburn and eye injuries. The skin damage reaches catastrophic proportions in a hereditary disease called xeroderma pigmentosum.

Between 1950 and 1960, an unexpected uniformity in the molecular injury caused by UV light and response to that injury was discovered in the simplest to the more complex forms of life. In this section, we will describe the molecular injury and its repair in bacteria and viruses and establish the relevance of these findings to human skin.

Base Alteration

UV light inactivates the transforming factor of DNA and RNA viruses. But all wavelengths of UV light are not equally effective in inactivating the nucleic acid, and one can plot the effectiveness of inactivation of the transforming factor, or virus, versus the wavelength. Such a curve expresses the "action spectrum" of the UV light. The plot obtained for such an "action spectrum" can be superimposed almost exactly over the curve obtained for the UV absorption by nucleic acid. Such findings clearly suggest that the inactivation of the biological material results from absorption of UV light by the nucleic acid. As we have seen already, the purine and pyrimidine bases are responsible for the UV absorption properties of the nucleic acid. There is a clear correlation between UV absorption by biological material and biological inactivation.

Three major molecular alterations have been described in UV-irradiated pyrimidine: deamination, hydration, and dimerization. The discovery of the formation of thymine dimers after UV irradiation of a frozen solution of thymine by Beukers and Berends [18, 19] may well constitute one of the most important contributions to photobiology.

Beukers and Berends found that the irradiation of [^{14}C]thymine in aqueous solution yielded a photoproduct separable by chromatography. However, the yields (1–2%) were too low to permit isolation and characterization of the new photoproduct.

High yields of the photoproduct were obtained when frozen aqueous solutions of thymine were irradiated. The new compound has a molecular weight between 240 and 250, with only a low absorption at 260 mμ. The photoproduct is stable in 12N PCA even at 100° for 1 hour or at 37° for 16 hours. Since the UV irradiation product is practically insoluble in absolute alcohol, it can readily be separated from thymine by repeated washing with absolute alcohol. The photoproduct crystallizes in the rhombic system, and elementary analysis revealed that each unit cell contains 16 molecules of thymine. Inasmuch as the rhombic system usually results from the crystallization of 8 molecules, Beukers and Berends suggested that the new compound was a dimer of thymine (see Fig. 12-2). Further physiochemical studies led these investigators to propose the following structure for the photoproduct.

Beukers has suggested a simple explanation for the fact that dimers form in frozen but not liquid water.

* Emmerson and others [16] have published different G values: thymine—0.33; adenine—0.25; cytosine—0.23; and guanine—0.18. In these studies, the sensitivity of thymine was found to be only 1.5 times greater than that of adenine, which was almost the same as that of cytosine.

Smith and Hanawalt [17] have remarked that the differences obtained in G values in different laboratories are not surprising. The effect of X-irradiation on molecules depends on a number of variables including ionic strength, presence of oxygen, pH, concentration of impurities, and other factors. Unless all variables are rigidly controlled, variance is to be expected.

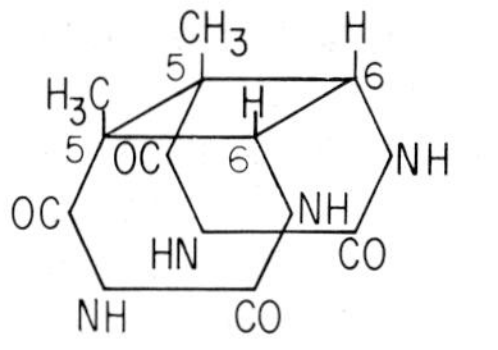

Fig. 12-2. Formula of thymine dimers

Thymine has no strong polar group; hence, when in solution it does not orient the water molecules, and charges are not transferred from one thymine molecule to another. In contrast, in frozen solution the thymine molecules are surrounded with structured water molecules, and charges are transferred. As a result, the molecule with the lowest potential energy forms; namely, the dimer.

The impact of this simple photochemical observation on radiobiology has been considerable. Indeed, thymine residues are often in close proximity in the DNA sequence; consequently, a thymine dimer can be expected to form after UV irradiation of DNA.

Beukers and his associates were able to demonstrate the formation of dimers in UV-irradiated apurinic acid, poly T, and DNA. Several investigators were also able to establish a correlation between the formation of dimers and the survival of UV-irradiated bacteria or phages. Irradiation of primer DNA with UV interferes with the enzymic replication of the DNA, possibly as a result of dimerization.

In the DNA molecule, however, two different types of dimerization must be considered: dimerization of two consecutive thymine molecules in a single strand and interstrand dimer formation. Although interstrand dimerization seems to be impossible in double-stranded DNA, it is possible when the two strands are separated during replication.

UV irradiation of aqueous solutions of thymidylyl (3′,5′)-deoxyadenosine results in a decrease of UV absorption due to the formation of thymine dimers. Another type of thymine dimer has been observed in poly dA-T or after irradiation of dry DNA. In this type of dimer, an oxygen atom bridges two molecules between each carbon 4 atom of thymine. Reversal of dimerization by UV irradiation is not possible, but dimerization is reversed by heat. Testing of the reversal of dimerization by UV and heat clearly distinguishes thymine dimers involving the formation of oxygen bridges from those resulting from carbon-to-carbon bonding, because the latter are not sensitive to heat but are reversed by UV [19].

Dimers are formed from uracil, orotic acid, and cytosine. Thus, at least four pyrimidine dimers have been described in addition to the traditional thymine-thymine dimers: cytosine-cytosine, uracil-cytosine, uracil-thymine, and cytosine-thymine. Detection and identification of some of these dimers are not simple. For example, the formation of a uracil dimer is complicated by hydration, and cytosine dimers are regularly converted to uracil dimers by deamination of cytosine. (Cytosine deaminates readily when the 5–6 bond is hydrolyzed.)

When uracil, cytosine, or cytidylic acid is exposed to UV light its absorbency decreases. Heat or acid treatment restores the absorbence spectrum to normal. It was established that the reversible drop in UV absorption of uracil results from the hydration of the 5–6 double bond, leading to 6-hydroxy-5-hydro derivatives. It is expected, although not directly established, that 6-hydroxy-5-hydro derivatives of cytosine are formed also. The formation of hydration products of cytosine has been demonstrated in irradiated DNA and polycytidylic acid.

The exposure of cytosine or uracil to UV irradiation (260 mμ) leads to the addition of a molecule of water at the 5–6 double bond. When irradiated in ^{3}H-labeled water, the cytidine incorporates amounts of tritium compatible with hydration. When compared to UV absorption in the original base, that of the new photoproduct is reduced. Absorption can be partially restored by heating or acidifying the solution. UV irradiation of uracil in the presence of tritiated water also induces the formation of hydrated uracil. In contrast, thymine, adenine, and guanine are not hydrated when exposed to doses of UV irradiation that hydrate cytosine or uracil [20].

When poly U is irradiated with UV 2500 A, the phenylalanine incorporation in the acid-insoluble fraction is decreased, but serine incorporation is increased. Normal coding by poly U was partially restored by heating; thus, it was concluded that UV irradiation of poly U leads to dimerization and hydration of uracil residues. Both forms of base alteration interfere with phenylalanine incorporation into ribosomal protein, and hydration alters coding for phenylalanine to serine [21].

UV irradiation of poly C leads to a changing of coding from guanylic to adenylic acid. The increase of AMP incorporation is heat reversible, and, again, hydration products probably are formed. However, hydrates are not found in double-stranded DNA, so they probably play a lesser role when resting DNA is irradiated. But during DNA synthesis, double strands are converted to single strands; therefore, interstrand dimerization and hydration of cytosine could be important in increasing the sensitivity of DNA to UV light during mitosis.

Effects of UV Irradiation on Hydrogen Bond

UV irradiation ruptures hydrogen bonds through altering the base structure or simply by uncoiling the two strands. In practice, it is impossible to evaluate whether the hydrogen bonds are broken as a result of alterations of basic structure or by direct interference with the bond.* However, the overall loss in

* Hydrogen bonds cannot be broken irreversibly without damaging the bases because broken hydrogen bonds reform as soon as the perturbance is removed. Thus, UV does not, in reality, break hydrogen bonds, but it initiates hydrogen bond breakage.

helical structure can be estimated by: (1) measuring the melting point of the DNA or other polynucleotides before and after radiation, and (2) following the increase in the relative absorbence of the DNA molecule at low pH.

When DNA passes from the helical structure of the double strand to a looser structure as the pH is lowered, UV absorption increases at 2537 A. Much less acid is needed to bring about the uncoiling of the double helix after UV irradiation. Another means of measuring uncoiling of the double strand is to measure directly the number of free amino or free keto groups that are made available after radiation. Formaldehyde reacts with the exposed amino group, whereas acridine reacts with the keto group. Both techniques have revealed increased hydrogen bond rupture after UV irradiation.

When dry DNA is irradiated, dimerization between the pyrimidine of adjacent molecules brought together by the removal of water is possible, and, as a result, the DNA acts as a gel when put in solution. The dimerization may involve pyrimidine residues of different strands. Interstrand cross-linking probably results from the formation of a type of dimer, and the incidence of cross-linking increases with the adenine-thymine content of the DNA. As pointed out previously, interstrand cross-linking does not occur unless the double strands separate. Consequently, the incidence of interstrand cross-links increases as the temperature of the DNA is raised to approach the temperature of half-maximal strand separation (TM).

We have seen that dimerization of pyrimidine nucleotides may lead to the formation of intermolecular and interstrand cross-links. The biological significance of these alterations is difficult to evaluate, but studies on bacteriophage and even mammalian DNA suggest that interstrand cross-links are at least in part responsible for the biological effects of UV irradiation.

Nevertheless, interstrand cross-linking is not believed to contribute appreciably to the lethal effects of UV light on DNA or in altering the biological activity of bacterial or mammalian DNA. Possibly of more consequence to the biological response to X-irradiation is the damage caused by cross-linking between the DNA and the protein. In the intact cell, the DNA and protein are in close contact. It is, therefore, interesting that when cysteine and uracil are irradiated together, a cysteine-uracil dimer is formed. Moreover, 5-formyluracil has been isolated after irradiation of thymine in solution. The 5-formyluracil formed readily combines with the amino groups of protein, leading to covalent links between the DNA and protein [22].

Effects of UV Irradiation on Skin

UV irradiation produces three types of skin lesions: sunburn, hyperkeratinization, and cancer. The link between these three types of injuries is not known, although, as mentioned previously, repeated exposure of unprotected skin to sunlight results in keratosis and wrinkling, and skin cancer usually develops at the site of senile keratosis.

Sunburn is one form of injury that most Caucasians and even Blacks have experienced one or more times in their lives. Three elementary lesions develop partly in sequence after excessive exposure to UV light: erythema, edema, and desquamation. The erythema followed by edema results from vasodilation and changes in capillary permeability. Experts still debate whether the erythema results from injuries to the corium or the epithelium or both.

Although it seems excluded that the primary injury of UV radiation of the skin results in the damage of protein or an enzyme, two schools of thought remain. One believes that on the basis of what is known of UV injuries in bacteria and mammalian cell cultures, the erythema results from damage to DNA. The other suspects, on rather shaky experimental evidence, that the primary injury involves the phospholipid of membranes and incriminates "lysosomal" rupture as the cause of erythema and edema.

At present, the most plausible interpretation of the pathogenesis of erythema and edema in sunburn is that UV irradiation damages DNA, and this interferes with transcription. The consequence is a reduction in the rate of mitosis in some cells and death in others. The release of hydrolases is likely to be a consequence, rather than a cause, of cell death.

Experimental production of erythema with UV light reveals that human skin is affected by UV radiation ranging between 2500 and 3150 A in wavelength. Investigators report varying peaks of effectiveness of the UV radiation. Two different types of curves have been reported: the standard curve and the erythema action curve. Studies by Hausser and Vahle in 1927 [23, 24] suggested that UV radiation with a wavelength of 2800 A was the most effective in producing erythema. In fact, according to these studies, the effective wavelength belongs to a narrow band between 2700 and 2970 A. More recent data assembled in Blum's and other laboratories are in conflict with the results of Hausser and Vahle and indicate that wavelengths between 2500 and 2600 A are the most effective in producing erythema. Effectiveness drops sharply between wavelengths of 2600 and 2900 A. The effectiveness of UV radiation with wavelengths ranging between 2900 and 3000 A is 75% of the maximum (between 2500 and 2600 A).

The oxygen in the atmosphere absorbs UV radiation and forms ozone, which itself absorbs all UV light with wavelengths smaller than 2900 A. Consequently, radiation with wavelengths ranging between 2900 and 3000 A is erythemogenic during exposure to sunlight.

A number of factors modify the effects of sunlight; some of these originate in the atmosphere: the composition of the atmosphere, the distance traveled through the atmosphere, or the reflection of light by the ground surface. Other factors are generated in the exposed individual; these include genetic differences and adaptation. In addition, empirical and scientific methods of protection against sunburn have been developed.

No UV light with a wavelength below 290 mμ reaches the earth because the ozone in the upper layer of the atmosphere absorbs all such UV radiation. (Absorption by ozone ranges between 210 and 300 mμ; the ammonia of the atmosphere absorbs wavelengths of 220 mμ.) On the other end of the spectrum, the wavelength of the infrared rays that reach the earth does not exceed 6 mμ. Thus, the electromagnetic radiation that emanates from the sun and reaches the earth ranges in wavelength from 290 to 6 mμ.

The energy of the radiation is not constant throughout this range. The maximum is at 530 mμ for light coming from the sun and at 430 mμ for the light originating from the blue sky. At 350 mμ, the energy has dropped to 10% of the maximum, and it continues to drop for radiations with smaller wavelengths. Yet, these small components are responsible for some of the skin alterations seen after prolonged exposure to sunlight.

At sea level at noon, the sun is at the zenith, the highest point above the horizon. More prosaically, the air mass is arbitrarily referred to as an air mass of 1. (The air mass equals 2 at 4 PM and 3 at 5 PM.) At noon, the distance radiation travels through the atmosphere is shortest, the intensity of sunlight is greatest, and the sun rays contain the highest proportion of short waves. Early in the morning and late in the afternoon, the distance radiation travels through the atmosphere is much greater. As a result, only radiation with the longest wavelengths (yellow, orange, and red) reaches the ground, and the erythemogenic effect of sunlight is markedly reduced before 9 AM and after 4 PM.

The presence of water vapor in the atmosphere and atmospheric pollution with dust, carbon, and other substances modify the composition of the sunlight that reaches the exposed individual. A ground covered with sand or snow reflects radiation more effectively than vegetation or water. As a result, the erythemogenic effect of sunlight is intensified in the desert and on ski slopes.

The effectiveness of sunlight in producing sunburn is illustrated by the following: at 30° latitude north at noon (air mass of 1) at 50 feet above sea level in mid-June, erythema develops in the average Caucasian within 5 to 10 minutes after exposure to the sun. Because of the high content of melanin in their skin, black and pigmented people are less sensitive than whites to sunburn. We shall see that a genetic deficiency in repair enzymes is responsible for unusual sensitivity to UV radiation.

Human skin adapts to exposure to sunlight in at least two ways: pigmentation and keratinization of the skin. Darkening of the skin occurs in two steps—a rapid one, which results in the oxidation of preexisting bleached pigment, and a slower one (4 to 5 days) resulting from the activation of tyrosinase, possibly by the destruction of a tyrosinase inhibitor.

Keratinization of the skin leads to thickened skin, which prevents UV penetration in the deeper layers of the skin. Whether or not resistance to sunburn can be developed by activation or *de novo* synthesis of repair enzymes remains to be seen.

Protection of skin against sunburn is achieved either by wearing clothes or by applying antisunburn lotions. Such lotions contain compounds that either absorb sunlight of all wavelengths (opaque preparations of zinc or titanium oxides) or absorb selectively (para-aminobenzoic acid, which absorbs wavelengths between 2900 and 3150 A).

Molecular Repair of UV Damage to DNA

At the beginning of life, it might have been an advantage to have a copying mechanism for DNA that included mistakes, because such mistakes brought about mutations which sometimes provided strains of viruses or bacteria with better chances of survival. Stabilization of the biosphere required, however, that the copying mechanism of the genetic material become strictly faithful. Some experiments were performed using bacterial culture maintained in a steady state of growth. This permitted the investigators to extrapolate the incidence of spontaneous alteration of the base sequence as expressed by mutation. Even after 100,000,000 replications, the chances that one gene be altered are still only 50%.

Although the DNA molecule has unusual conformational properties (a double helix held together by a hydrogen bonds and stacking forces), the force which confers stability to DNA cannot prevent DNA alterations resulting from chemical interaction and from UV or ionizing radiation. Consequently, even if the enzymic mechanisms involved in DNA replication were perfect, the base composition would change as a result of the effect of chemical or physical mutagenic agents.

Nature has reduced chances for such mistakes by providing the cell with repair mechanisms. The molecular aspects of repair have been investigated in detail in bacteria after the administration of UV radiation, but we shall see that similar mechanisms exist in mammalian cells.

UV-irradiated DNA may be repaired by four mechanisms: simple photoreactivation, enzymic photoreactivation, enzymic dark repair, and repair replication [25–31, 153].

The formation of covalent bonds between two thymidine molecules is reversible, and irradiation with UV light at 275 mμ of a DNA previously irradiated with UV reversibly splits some of the covalent bonds and converts the thymine dimers to the free thymidine. Thus, UV-irradiated transforming factor can be partially photoreactivated by new exposure to UV light. However, direct photoreactivation does not occur in the intact bacteria.

When bacteria are irradiated with UV light, they may lose their infectivity or viability. Infectivity and survival can be restored by exposing the bacteria to a source of visible light. Thanks to the work of Claud S. Rupert [32], it is known that photoreactivation *in situ* involves DNA binding enzymes, the catalytic properties of which depend upon visible light for energy. The exact mechanism of action of the enzyme is not known. As Kendrick pointed out, it is puzzling that 3 eV photons are used to repair damage promoted by 5 eV photons (UV). Whether the enzyme excises the thymidine dimer or simply monomerizes the dimer is not known. The enzyme, which has been extensively purified from yeast or *E. coli*, combines only with UV-irradiated DNA or synthetic polynucleotide. Competition studies between irradiated synthetic nucleotides, such as poly dA-dT and poly dG-dC, have indicated that the enzyme attacks all pyrimidine dimers but that its affinity is greatest for thymine dimer. The photoreactivating enzyme is widely spread in nature, and has been found in mammalian tissues. The significance of the enzymic reaction in mammalian cells is not known.

Some strains of *E. coli* are much more sensitive to UV light than others [33]. Later Ruth Hill [34] found a radio-resistant strain. Two important observations were then made by Setlow, who discovered that the effect of UV light on DNA synthesis was greatest in the sensitive strain and that thymidine dimers were released when resistant bacteria were incubated after UV irradiation. The dimers were not released from UV-sensitive bacteria. Genetic studies showed that resistant bacteria contain 3 genes which, when transferred to radio-sensitive bacteria (by bacterial mating), made them radio resistant. The biochemical and genetic observations led to the cut-and-patch hypothesis for repair, which proposes that: (1) an incision enzyme recognizes the thymine dimers and cuts off a nucleotide chain (including the dimers) from the remaining strand; (2) an excision enzyme eliminates the nucleotide sequence including the dimer; and (3) the denuded portion of the complimentary strain serves as a template for reconstruction of the interrupted chain.

We have seen how Meselson and Stahl [35] demonstrated that DNA replicates semiconservatively. Pettijohn and Hanawalt [36] used similar techniques to establish non-semiconservative replication of DNA after UV irradiation. They studied the incorporation of bromouridine (BUDR) into the DNA of UV-irradiated bacteria, and, after extraction of the DNA and strand separation on cesium chloride gradients, they found that the pattern of BUDR distribution in the DNA strands was not compatible with semiconservative replication. Details of the experiment can be found in Smith and Hanawalt's book [17]. When the bacteria are resistant to radiation, dimers are formed but the dimer is not replaced; however, some degree of semiconservative DNA synthesis can take place. Howard-Flanders and associates [37] have shown that when DNA containing a UV-induced pyrimidine dimer replicates, the new strands have a lower molecular weight. Thus, it would appear that when the two strands separate for replication, small polynucleotide chains are used as templates, and each chain is as long as the distance that separates the two gaps.

The enzyme involved in the first steps of the repair of DNA irradiated with UV light was investigated in Japan by Takagi and his associates [38] and in the United States by Grossman and his collaborators [39]. In 1962 Strauss had shown that crude extracts of *Micrococcus lysodeikticus* selectively inactivated the transforming DNA preexposed to UV radiation. Later, Strauss and his coworkers [40] showed by zone sedimentation analysis that the extract induced endonucleolytic breaks in UV-irradiated DNA. Nakayama and his associates [41] established in 1967 that the degradation of UV-irradiated DNA required two fractions: fraction A, which exhibits only endonuclease activity without releasing acid-soluble material (endonuclease?), and fraction B, which has exonuclease activity.

Takagi and his associates purified (360-fold), from crude extracts of *M. lysodeikticus*, an endonuclease specific for UV-irradiated DNA. The enzyme acts on double-stranded and single-stranded DNA. According to Takagi, magnesium is not necessary for the reaction.

The endonuclease was further purified by Grossman, who also devised an assay based on the fact that the enzyme causes single-strand breaks by hydrolyzing phosphodiester bonds in UV-irradiated double-stranded [^{32}P]DNA. In addition, Grossman purified (approximately 100 times) an exonuclease, which also attacks only the UV-irradiated DNA. Thus, the combination of the UV endonuclease incision enzyme and the UV exonuclease excision enzyme appears to release

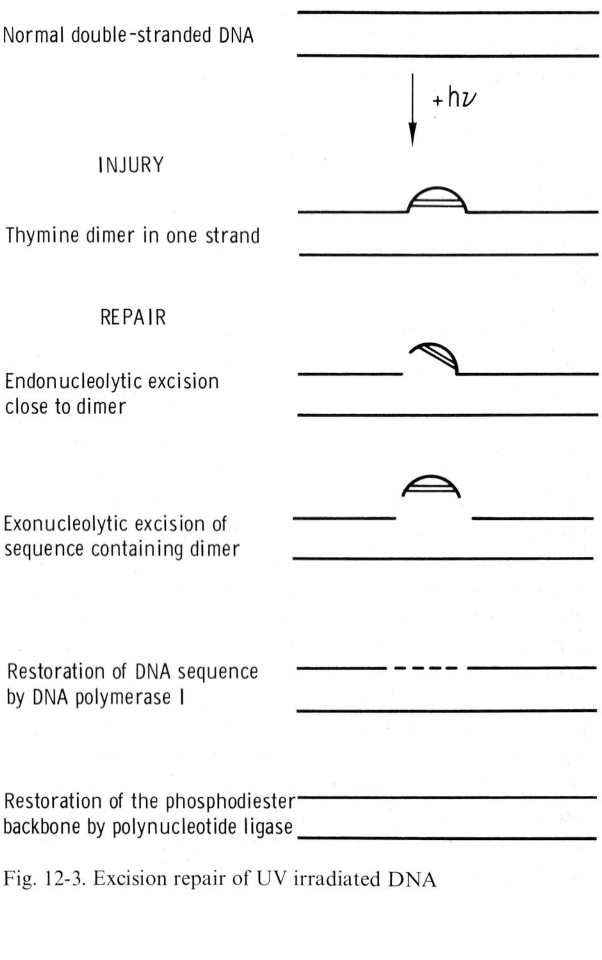

Normal double-stranded DNA

$+h\nu$

INJURY

Thymine dimer in one strand

REPAIR

Endonucleolytic excision close to dimer

Exonucleolytic excision of sequence containing dimer

Restoration of DNA sequence by DNA polymerase I

Restoration of the phosphodiester backbone by polynucleotide ligase

Fig. 12-3. Excision repair of UV irradiated DNA

the portion of the polynucleotide chain that contains the dimer. An important feature of the endonuclease is that its specificity is not dictated by the molecular configuration of the dimer, but rather by distortions of the DNA molecule. Therefore, the endonuclease might well be the enzyme responsible for the repair mechanism observed in DNA extracted from bacterial or animal sources treated with nitrogen mustards, X-irradiation, etc. However, direct evidence for such an activity of the bacterial endonuclease is lacking, except in the ease of X-irradiated DNA.

This cut-and-patch model further proposes that after excision of the nucleotide sequence which contains the dimers, DNA polymerase is responsible for repairing the nucleotide sequence, and polynucleotide ligase ultimately seals the repaired sequence within the strand (see Fig. 12-3). Kornberg and his collaborators [42] have suggested that because of its 5′,3′-exonuclease activity, DNA polymerase can catalyze both the excision and the repair of irradiated DNA. Consequently, Kornberg proposed a simplified model which would require only UV-specific endonuclease, DNA polymerase, and polynucleotide ligase. Van Lancker and Tomura have purified to electrophoretic homogeneity a repair endonuclease from rat liver [43]. For further details on the enzymology of excision repair in bacterial and in mammalian cells see [154]. The steps involved in excision repair of DNA are schematically shown in Fig. 12-3.

Extent and Limitations of Excision Repair in Mammalian Tissues

Three different methods have been used to determine excision repair in mammals: (1) direct measurement of the removal of thymine dimers; (2) incorporation of ^{3}HTDR into DNA in absence of semi-conservative DNA synthesis and (3) photolysis of incorporated BUDR. The last procedure is based on the following principle.

Cells are incubated with ^{3}HTDR and then UV irradiated. The irradiated cells are then incubated again with the thymidine analog, bromouridine (BUDR), which during unscheduled DNA synthesis is incorporated into the DNA sequence in positions normally occupied by thymidine. The cells are then exposed to 333 mμ UV radiation which renders the BUDR regions sensitive to single strand breaks when the DNA is exposed to alkali. This procedure is not only extremely sensitive (it permits the detection of one repair event for 10^8 daltons of DNA), but it also allows one to estimate the size of the oligonucleotide chain excised.

Using the BUDR procedure, Regan and Setlow [155] distinguished between two types of DNA repair: that involving short sequences and that involving long sequences. The short sequence repair occurs after γ radiation and probably involves single strand breaks. The breaks are followed by the exonucleolytic excision of a few nucleotides followed by DNA polymerase restoration of the sequence and sealing of the gap by polynucleotide ligase.

The long sequence repair is associated with excision repair. The prototype is the excision of thymine dimers in UV irradiated DNA. The agent which injures the DNA does not cause strand breaks, but results in the endonucleolytic incision of the chain, followed by exonucleolytic removal of a long polynucleotide chain, DNA polymerase restoration and polynucleotide ligase sealing of the patch. A number of chemical agents, such as acetylaminofluorene, ethylmethane sulfonate, and 4-nitroquinolineoxide bind to DNA bases. The damage to the bases can be repaired, at least in part. The process involves long patch DNA repair and the number of bases excised differs with the injury. For example, 100 and 140 nucleotides are excised per average repair region after UV irradiation and N-acetoxy-AAF, respectively. For further information on DNA repair and carcinogenesis see Chapter 16.

Unscheduled DNA synthesis in UV irradiated cells is incomplete, nonrandom and at least in lymphocytes occurs at different rates.

Meltz and Painter [156] have studied the distribution of repair of thymine dimers using the Cot technique of Britten and Khone. The results indicate that the repair is random throughout the DNA molecules. Such findings suggest that there are no preferential zones for DNA repair. Thus according to Meltz and Painter the damage caused by UV light and the repair of such damage are randomly distributed in spite of the variability in the DNA sequence and in spite of the variable interaction between DNA and proteins. Yet, these findings do not exclude the possibility that small portions of the DNA are inaccessible to repair. Persistent damage is not likely to be detected by the Cot method. Moreover, these findings are in conflict with those of other studies.

Brunk studied the effects of low doses of UV radiation on the formation of thymine dimers in bacterial DNA and found that most dimers were formed in long pyrimidine tracts and consequently the distribution of the dimers in the UV irradiated DNA was nonrandom [157].

Only 40 to 50% of the thymine dimers produced in the DNA after low fluence of UV irradiation are excised. Wilkins and Hart [158] irradiated human fibroblasts *in vitro* and subjected them to the *Micrococcus luteus* UV endonuclease to evaluate the repair ability. They found that chromatin treated with 2 M sodium chloride is much more susceptible to the endonuclease than untreated chromatin. The authors concluded that the presence of proteins interferes with the DNA repair.

Using radioautography, Harris et al. [159] measured excision repair in DNA directly in nuclei of fibroblasts exposed to UV irradiation and carcinogens and found that excision repair is nonrandom and occurs in clusters. Repair was more intensive in the inner core of the nucleus, believed to be composed primarily of euchromatin, than in the outer core, which is believed to be composed of heterochromatin.

In UV irradiated human lymphocytes unscheduled DNA synthesis occurs in two stages: a fast and a slow stage. The first is complete within an hour, the latter takes at least five hours for completion.

Berliner et al. [160] have studied by radioautography the incorporation of ^{3}HTDR into nuclei isolated from human lymphocytes after UV irradiation. They examined three different kinds of lymphocytes referred to as homogeneous, inhomogeneous, which contained masses of condensed DNA at the periphery of the nuclei, and inhomogeneous containing masses of heterochromatin, both at the periphery and the center of the nucleus. They counted the grains in three concentric regions in the nucleus. The distribution of grains was similar for all three types of cells and most of the grains were found at the periphery of the nucleus, whether the heterochromatin is condensed at the periphery or dispersed in the interior of the nucleus. Their findings suggest that the restriction to unscheduled DNA synthesis is not related to the structural organization of the DNA (euchromatin versus heterochromatin), but rather to the spatial distribution of the DNA in the nucleus. The peripheral DNA is more accessible to the repair enzymes.

Some cultured cells lose their ability to repair DNA. For example, primary cultures of golden hamster cells have a greater ability to perform excision repair than continuous cultures. When such cells are infected with DNA or RNA viruses, the host repair system repairs the UV irradiated virus and as a result viral survival rates increase.

Studies on UV irradiated mitochondria of *Saccharomyces cerevisiae* suggest that although pyrimidine dimers can be repaired by photoreactivation, excision repair does not occur. Similar observations were made in mammalian mitochondrial DNA [161]. Mammalian mitochondrial DNA is made of close circular DNA and although its base composition differs somewhat from that of nuclear DNA, one might expect that mitochondrial DNA would be susceptible to the same damage by UV light and by carcinogens as nuclear DNA. Clayton et al. [162] have, however, given evidence that pyrimidine dimers are not removed in mammalian mitochondria.

Postreplication Repair

The replication of the eukaryotic chromosome is undoubtedly a complicated phenomenon. It involves replication of DNA, histones and nonhistone proteins with quaternary interaction of the macromolecule permitting the genotype to be expressed into the phenotype of a specifically differentiated cell. Even if the DNA forms a continuous chain in the chromatid, its synthesis does not start at one end and terminate at the other. There are, in the mammalian chromosome, various points of replication leading to polynucleotides of various lengths. These segments of newly synthesized DNA are called replicons. They have a specific site called the origin at which DNA replication begins and both parental strands are duplicated. The elegant experiments that led to the description and the evaluation of the number of replicons per chromosome or per cell will not be described. The reader is referred to the review by Painter [163]. It is estimated that 100 replicons exist per chromosome and 1.5 to 2×10^5 replicating units exist per cell with an average size of 30 μm. Little is known of the initiation of DNA synthesis in the replicon. It is, however, established that the elongation of the chain is discontinuous and that 4 S fragments (200 nucleotides long) are formed

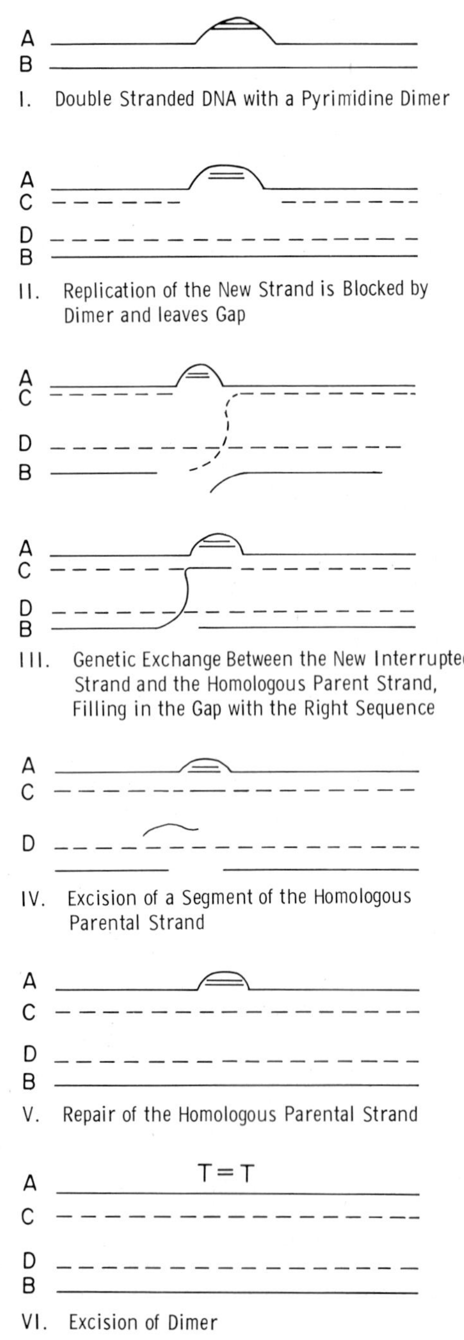
A
B
I. Double Stranded DNA with a Pyrimidine Dimer
A
C
D
B
II. Replication of the New Strand is Blocked by Dimer and leaves Gap
A
C
D
B
A
C
D
B
III. Genetic Exchange Between the New Interrupted Strand and the Homologous Parent Strand, Filling in the Gap with the Right Sequence
A
C
D
IV. Excision of a Segment of the Homologous Parental Strand
A
C
D
B
V. Repair of the Homologous Parental Strand
T=T
A
C
D
B
VI. Excision of Dimer

Fig. 12-4. Recombination repair of DNA containing pyrimidine dimers (after Howard-Flanders)

and later united (the Okazaki fragments in *E. coli* are 1000 nucleotides long) [164]. Essentially nothing is known of the termination of DNA synthesis in the replicon.

The molecular weight of DNA synthesized in UV irradiated *E. coli* is smaller than that of DNA synthesized in nonirradiated bacteria. The cells are believed to make small DNA fragments because the continuation of the elaboration of the DNA is at least temporarily blocked by the pyrimidine dimers leaving a gap in the new strands facing the dimers. Later the strands are filled in by new bases. According to Howard-Flanders the pyrimidines are not excised. The postreplication gap is filled by genetic exchange with an intact portion of the intact homologous parental strand. A portion of the parental strand not involved in filling the gap is excised, now leaving a gap in the homologous parental strand (B). The gap in (B) is repaired with DNA polymerase and polynucleotide ligase. The thymine dimers present in the new duplex are excised by the regular excision process [153] (see Fig. 12-4).

Dimers and Function

A number of experiments suggests that the presence of thymine dimers can interfere with cell function; only a few examples will be presented here.

Tan et al. [165] observed that DNA irradiated with UV light is a potent immunogen in rabbits. The authors developed a method by which rabbit antiserum to UV irradiated DNA could be used to detect UV damage to DNA in tissues by immunofluorescence. This technique allowed them to demonstrate changes in the DNA of human skin immediately after exposure to UV light.

Seaman et al. [166] developed a radioimmunoassay for the detection of thymine dimers that can be performed directly on the DNA extracted from the cells. This method enabled them to correlate the loss of transforming activity with the number of dimers present.

When vaccinia virus, a double-stranded DNA virus, is UV irradiated and plated on fibroblast derived from xeroderma pigmentosum cells, the virus grows poorly. Plating on normal fibroblast yields normal rates of growth. This finding suggests that the host cells repair the damage to viral DNA. In contrast, the growth of the RNA encephalomyelitis virus is the same as that of xeroderma pigmentosum or normal fibroblast [167].

Repair of DNA can restore interrupted cell functions. UV irradiation of monkey kidney cells *in vitro* interferes with interferon synthesis. Synthesis resumes after repair of the DNA either because of excision or replication repair [168]. Some chemicals are carcinogenic (*e.g.*, acetylaminofluorene). An endonuclease which triggers the excision of the DNA bound carcinogen has been purified to electrophoretic homogeneity [43]. The repair endonuclease activity was measured at various times after partial hepatectomy. It increases after operation, reaches a peak six hours after hepatectomy and drops to values 50% of those of controls forty-eight hours after the operation. The decrease in DNA repair may be related to the increased ability to produce cancer in regenerating liver.

DNA Repair and Disease

A number of diseases are associated with defects in DNA repair.

Radioautographic studies and DNA centrifugation in cesium chloride have led Cleaver to conclude that fibroblasts obtained from patients affected with xeroderma pigmentosum lack the ability to repair base damage to DNA, but are able to restore strand breaks. The finding suggests that xeroderma pigmentosum is an inborn error of metabolism in which the UV endonuclease is missing. The lack of such an endonuclease remains to be demonstrated by direct methods. Whether the low activity or absence of repair enzyme is the sole cause of sensitivity to sunlight and high incidence of skin cancer remains to be seen.

It is intriguing that the fusing of different fibroblast strains of patients with xeroderma pigmentosum yields a binuclear heterokaryon with a greater capacity for unscheduled DNA synthesis than the unfused cell. The complexity of the genetic events involved in this phenomenon cannot be discussed. The molecular basis for such complementation is unknown, but the event illustrates the difficulties involved in explaining a single inherited syndrome in simple molecular terms [169].

Like many hereditary diseases, the syndrome associated with xeroderma pigmentosum is not restricted to one single type of enzyme defect; geneticists distinguish four classes of genetically distinct forms of xeroderma pigmentosum and numerous variants have been described.

Three variants have normal levels of DNA excision repair, but present a slowing down of semiconservative DNA. This is expressed by a delay in the conversion of low into high molecular weight DNA. Furthermore the conversion is actively inhibited by caffeine which has no such effect on normal cells.

To explain the difference in sensitivity to caffeine some have proposed that while caffeine binds strongly to the gap region opposite the pyrimidine dimers in the xeroderma pigmentosum patients, in normal UV irradiated fibroblasts the binding of the inhibitor is prevented by the strong attachments of the enzyme to the gap region [170].

Clearly polynucleotide ligase must be involved in the last step of postreplication repair as it is in semiconservative and excision repair. Inasmuch as rejoining of single strand breaks, after radiation and excision repair, is normal in the xeroderma pigmentosum variant, a defect in polynucleotide ligase is unlikely.

Until recently enzymic photoreactivation of UV induced cyclobutyl pyrimidine dimers in DNA was not believed to occur in mammalian cells. Activity of the photoreactivating enzyme was found in human leukocytes by Sutherland et al. [171]. Low activity of the enzyme was found in fibroblasts of patients with xeroderma pigmentosum. The combination of both defects could result from a mutation of a gene controlling both the excision and the photoreactivating enzyme or from two independent mutations.

Bloom syndrome, Fanconi syndrome and progeria are other hereditary diseases in which the chromosome sensitivity is associated with a predisposition to cancer.

Bloom syndrome is transmitted as an autosomal recessive trait. In addition to sunlight sensitive telangiectasia, it is characterized by retarded growth in utero and after birth and defective immune response. The karyotype of cultured lymphocytes and fibroblasts obtained from homozygous individuals is unstable. The interchange of chromatids between homologous chromosomes is typical of the disease, resulting in a metaphase quadriradical distribution of the chromosome. Similar chromosomal alterations can be produced with mitomycin C or other chemicals that damage chromosomes. A study of the formation of new DNA chains in the replication units showed that replication is slower in the chromosome of Bloom syndrome than in normal chromosomes. The molecular mechanism responsible for the chromosomal anomalies is not understood [172].

Fibroblasts and lymphocytes of patients with Fanconi's syndrome show increased chromosome breakage and susceptibility to transformation *in vitro* by SV 40, and therefore a defect in DNA repair was suspected. Alkaline sucrose gradient studies of UV irradiated DNA or 4-nitroquinoline-N-oxide suggested that the defect in repair did not involve the repair endonuclease since the application of the injury was followed by the formation of single strand breaks.

When the number of thymine dimers was measured immediately after UV irradiation in fibroblasts of normal individuals and those of Fanconi's patients, the number of thymine dimers was the same. At later periods of exposure, the incidence of thymine dimers is decreased in normal fibroblasts, but not in patients with Fanconi's syndrome. The results suggest that the repair defect involves a specific exonuclease involved in the excision of thymine dimers. Similar studies, using larger doses of UV radiation, did, however, suggest that fibroblasts of patients with Fanconi's syndrome were able to excise thymine dimers. The reasons for the discrepancies are not clear. The dose of UV radiation used might be responsible. The fact is that in contrast to patients with xeroderma pigmentosum, patients with Fanconi's syndrome are not usually sensitive to UV radiation or to the development of cancer of the skin [173].

The evidence that DNA damage causes cancer is circumstantial (see Chapter 16). Setlow and Hart [174] have attempted to demonstrate that pyrimidine dimers are the cause of cancer. They cultured fish liver cells, irradiated them *in vitro* with UV light and reinjected the cells in fish derived from the same clone. The injected cells are claimed to produce cancer. If, however, UV irradiated cells are exposed to light, the photoreactivating enzyme, which is abundant in fish, monomerizes the dimers specifically, but does not modify other DNA damage produced by UV irradiation. When UV irradiated and photoreactivated cells are injected into fish, no tumors develop. These findings suggest that the presence of pyrimidine dimers in DNA is responsible for the carcinogenic process.

The results are, however, puzzling because they are complicated by the development of tuberculous granulomas and moreover, injected UV irradiated liver cells yield thyroid carcinomas, a surprising switch in the original phenotype!

DNA Repair and Aging

One possible definition of aging is that it is a universal progressive departure from ideal organismal performance which in most cases places the individual at a physical disadvantage over the healthy adult.

A number of theories have been proposed to explain such alterations. They include somatic mutation, immunological deterioration, widespread free radical damage, genetic programmed death, error catastrophy and cessation of growth. These various pathogenetic mechanisms could work separately or cooperatively, but none at this point can be excluded.

If somatic mutations are part of the cause of aging, DNA damage must play a key role in the genesis of aging. Even in an optimal environment, damage to DNA of skin and possibly blood cells can be caused by UV radiation and all cells are susceptible to damage by X, gamma and cosmic rays. Moreover, exposure to chemicals that bind to DNA is almost inescapable even if one were to survive on a vegetarian organic diet.

In absence of repair, damage to DNA will markedly modify the course of cellular life by interfering with DNA synthesis and transcription causing mutation, cellular death and possibly enhanced DNA antigenicity. However, some, but not all, DNA damage can be repaired. The restrictions imposed upon repair are not known.

However, one may expect a correlation between aging and the ability to repair DNA. DNA damage caused by UV radiation, ionizing radiation and chemicals includes strand breaks, intrastrand and interstrand cross-links and base alterations.

Hart and Setlow [175] measured excision repair in mammals with broadly different life spans (man, elephant, cow, hamster, rat, mouse and shrew) and found that unscheduled DNA synthesis was approximately proportional to the life span. As pointed out by these investigators, although the correlation is of considerable interest, it does not explain all aspects of the aging process. Patients with xeroderma do not age faster than normal, while progeria patients have no defect in excision repair.

Clarkson and Painter studied strand rejoining and repair of replication in cultured diploid cells which are known to be maintainable in culture only through a limited number of generations. They found no difference in the repair mechanism and cell aging [176]. Similarly, there seems to be no correlation between repair replication and aging *in vitro*.

Repair of strand breaks has been studied in chick lymphocytes and erythrocytes, in rat muscle, and in dog neurons. Young chicken red cells have less breaks after X-radiation than old red cells, but the red cells are apparently unable to repair the breaks. Old rat muscles are less effective in repairing strand breaks than young ones. Retinal and neuronal cells do not divide, but in the dog they were found to repair strand breaks produced by ionizing radiation as effectively as fibroblasts [177].

Progeria, or the Hutchinson-Gilford syndrome [178], is a disease characterized by greatly accelerated aging. The afflicted child may grow normally during the first year; later growth is impaired, but intelligence is normal. He develops a large and sometimes bold head, the face is small with flat eyebrows, beaked nose and receding chin. The remainder of the body is also distorted with a protruding abdomen and a narrow chest. The patient often presents atherosclerosis with heart and brain disease in his early teens. The average life span is 16 years. Epstein et al. showed that the fibroblasts of such patients were unable to repair single-strand breaks after exposure to γ radiation [179, 180]. Progeria cells have, however, normal repair replication after UV irradiation.

Biological Effects of Ionizing Radiation

Since its discovery, X-irradiation has been surrounded with an aura of mystery, possibly because it reveals, in seemingly harmless ways, many of the secrets of the living body. One can hardly imagine the thrills of Roentgen when he saw the picture of the bones of his hands on the fluorescent screen that he was irradiating with his then primitive X-ray generator. Within less than 10 years after Roentgen's discovery, it became clear that those who were indiscriminately exposed to the new rays developed incurable burns and died of mysterious anemias. In 1945, what had been a tool for diagnosing disease and curing cancer became the greatest threat humanity has ever known, and the mystery of yesterday became the nightmare of tomorrow. To protect humanity from a cataclysmic exposure to lethal doses of radiation is not only the task of the scientist, but it is the responsibility of all human beings. The immediate concern of the modern student of the effect of radiation is to discover the nature of the primary injury and then to attempt to use his knowledge to prevent and cure radiation damage, or to improve the effect of radiation in curing cancer.

Types of Exposures

Mankind is constantly exposed to X-irradiation in subtle and involuntary ways (cosmic rays, space travel), in deliberate and controlled ways (radiodiagnosis, radiotherapy), or in unwanted catastrophies (industrial accidents* and atomic warfare). Thus, exposure can be acute or chronic, and doses can be continuous or fractionated [44].

The effect of radiation on the victim varies with the mode of administration. Specialists have recently recommended the consideration of two major classes of radiation exposure—the short- and long-term exposures. The short term may be repeated, as it is in diagnosis and therapy, but it has been arbitrarily decided that less than 50 rads is a low exposure.

When all or part of the body is exposed to continuous or repeated radiation for long periods of time, this mode of exposure is referred to as long-term exposure. In such cases, it is more convenient to express the amount of radiation received in rads per week than in the total amount of radiation received. The integral dose is then the total radiation energy that is absorbed within a biological specimen after a prolonged period of time.

Relatively large or frequently repeated doses in restricted parts of the body lead to local radiation damage followed by a reaction of the surrounding tissue. Single and relatively low doses of whole-body irradiation cause radiation sickness and death. Small whole-body doses, single or repeated, may have long-range effects, such as causing cancer or aging.

The arsenal of the modern radiotherapist and the radiobiologist includes sources of electromagnetic waves (γ- and X-rays) and sources of corpuscular radiation (α- and β-particles, protons, and electrons). Both the corpuscular and electromagnetic radiation ionize matter as they are absorbed, and we have seen how the energy levels of the positive ions and the electrons are thermalized and converted into chemical energy, which causes the chemical changes in the biological substrate. Many investigations have been performed on relatively simple biological units, such as proteins, nucleic acid, viruses, bacteria, and cell cultures. The relevance of these studies to the pathology of radiation is not always immediately obvious, and it will be understood better if one is familiar with the cellular and histological changes that take place in the irradiated organism.

Effects on Skin

In 1896 Stevens [45] described changes in the skin of radiologists, and in the same year Daniel [46] described the loss of hair in a child whose skull was explored fluoroscopically for a long time. Compared with the radiosensitivity of such organs as the bone marrow and the spleen, that of the skin—despite constant replacement of the superficial layer—is relatively

* There are three major sources of industrial accidents with radiation. One is the unexpected activation of an active source, as happens primarily with atomic piles. A second is caused by unawareness of an active source, as in the case of a Wisconsin student who carried a source of cobalt until he received large total body doses of irradiation. A third industrial accident with radiation is fallout, as in the case of the atomic explosion, which released a cloud of calcium oxide formed from the incineration of the calcium carbonate of an atoll in the Pacific. Overexposure as a result of therapy (iatrogenic) is usually restricted to limited areas of the body.

low. The skin will be restored, except for its hair follicles, after the administration of up to 1600 to 2000 R in a single dose, or 3000 to 6000 R in fractionated doses [47–50].

After such doses are administered, a complex pattern of injury and reaction to injury develops slowly. The pattern includes inflammation, necrosis, repair, and pigmentation. Erythema develops in two stages: first, the exposed areas become mildly erythematous a few hours after irradiation; then erythema subsides during the day of the exposure, and a second, more severe erythema develops within approximately a week after exposure. At that time the skin is warm and swollen, yet there is little if any pain. Histologically, there is vasodilatation, moderate edema of the connective tissue, and mild lymphocytic migration. In the middle of the second week, enough edema fluid has accumulated so that the superficial layers of the skin become detached from the basal layer, thus yielding blisters similar to those observed in second-degree burns. These blisters become enlarged, the distended skin cracks, the fluid escapes, and the hemorrhagic naked dermis appears at the surface. This stage of ulceration is almost immediately followed by repair through epithelialization as it occurs in wound healing. The irradiated skin heals slowly, and a month may pass before the corium is covered again with the thin new epithelium. Fig. 12-5 illustrates a case of secondary radiodermatitis in a patient treated for cancer of the breast.

The hair starts to fall out a week after exposure to 1600 to 2000 R. Such doses sterilize the hair follicles and the new skin remains hairless. In contrast, pigmentation is stimulated by such a dose of X-irradiation. But the pigmentation produced by X-irradiation is not always permanent, and often it does not last for much longer periods than after UV irradiation.

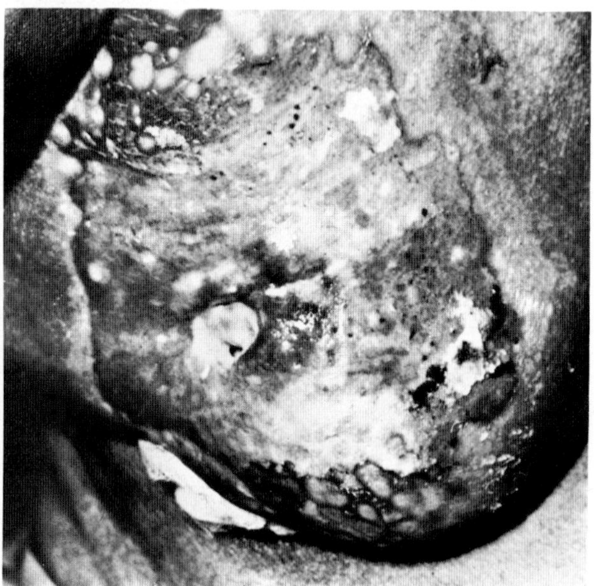

Fig. 12-5. Secondary radiodermatitis of the skin of the breast which developed as a result of radiotherapy. Notice the superficial ulceration and the congestion of the skin. These lesions, if properly treated, will fully disappear without severe scarring, within approximately six weeks

Thus, the administration of more than 2000 R in a single dose is not compatible with the integral repair of the irradiated skin. With doses slightly higher than 2000 R, the skin may still be epithelialized, but the epithelium is thin and fragile. The pattern of the underlying vascular connective tissue is distorted, scar tissue sometimes accumulates, and telangiectasis develops. When the single dose administered to the skin exceeds 2500 R, permanent damage usually results. Such doses kill most of the cells of the basal layers, and they also lead to necrosis of the connective tissue and sometimes of cartilage and bone. As a result, deep wounds are produced containing large masses of necrotic tissue. Necrotic tissue is not easily eliminated because many of the vascular channels are closed by thrombi. Moreover, since few polymorphonuclears reach the necrotic zone even when the radionecrosis is superinfected, little suppuration takes place.

Poor vascularization, distorted patterns of the connective tissue, and extensive necrosis of the basal layer of the epithelium are not conducive to integral restoration. Sometimes the skin will not repair at all; but if it does, the epithelium is thin, fragile, and readily subject to new ulcerations. The fibrosis and disorganized distribution of the connective fibers lead to disfiguration, scars, and keloids and are believed to constitute favorable ground for the development of cancer, either of the skin or of connective tissue. Although radionecrosis usually appears within a few days after high doses are administered, it may also appear belatedly several weeks or months after the administration of lower doses.

Repeated irradiation of the skin—for example, that of the fingers and hands of the early radiologists and radiochemists—leads to various degrees of radiodermatitis. Depending on the total dose administered, radiodermatitis may range from hyperacanthosis and telangiectasis to severe ulceration. The irradiated skin may even become cancerous; usually squamous cell or, more rarely, basal cell carcinoma develops. In rare cases, sarcomas have developed after severe skin irradiation.

These descriptions of the effect of the area doses of irradiation on the skin illustrate several of the concepts that have emerged in radiobiology: radiolesions, repair, and radiosensitivity.

The microscopic events that we have described after irradiation of the skin are obviously several steps removed from the primary molecular injury; therefore, it is not surprising that the histological manifestations are necrosis and inflammation. These reactions to injury are, after irradiation, essentially the same as in other types of injury except for special modalities—for example, the low level of suppuration or the intense fibrosis. Similarly, repair after an irradiation injury results primarily from cell proliferation, as it would in wound healing, but repair is slower if damage to the small vessels of the irradiated area of fibrosis is great, so scarring is common. This form of repair by cell proliferation and elaboration of connective tissue should not be confused with the molecular form of the repair that takes place in irradiated DNA, which will be discussed later.

Various responses of the cellular components to identical doses of X-irradiation are illustrated by the response of the sebaceous and sweat glands to X-irradiation. Temporary epilation results after administration of 400 to 500 R, and hair grows again after 4 to 5 weeks. Permanent epilation occurs after a dose of 1500 to 2000 R. This dose also leads to exfoliative radiodermatitis of the epithelium, but it is usually compatible with integral repair. The sebaceous glands are permanently destroyed within 3 to 4 weeks after the administration of a dose of 1500 to 2000 R, but it takes 2500 R to destroy the sweat glands permanently.

Effect on Mammary Glands

The mammary gland is a gland of epidermal origin, and its growth is controlled by estrogens. A spontaneous burst of estrogen secretion takes place at puberty. The cellular proliferation that follows can be prevented by irradiating the mammary gland before puberty, but relatively large doses are required to block growth completely. A dose of 700 to 1500 R will only slow mammary gland growth; it takes about 4500 R to block proliferation completely. However, the radiosensitivity of the mammary gland can be increased considerably simply by stimulating cellular proliferation by administering estrogens to the impubic rabbit. Then 2800 R is required to block the development of the mammary gland at puberty. This suggests that proliferating tissues are more radiosensitive than nonproliferating tissues. This basic concept will emerge again when we study the effect of irradiation on other tissues.

Effect on Gonads

We shall consider only the effect of irradiation on the germinal cell. In the testicles, the germinal cells proliferate from puberty to old age and sometimes until bodily death. The sperm cell is the spermatogonium. After division, it matures through various morphological steps and ultimately becomes a spermatocyte. The genital cells are the most sensitive cells in the testicle. As little as 50 R temporarily interferes with cell division but does not kill the cells. At least some of the cells die after exposure to 250 to 300 R, but it takes up to 800 R to deplete the male gonad of all its germinal cells. In fact, male sterilization requires relatively large doses. In monkeys, whole body doses that kill half of the irradiated population do not sterilize the survivors. In mice, temporary sterility is overcome 5 to 6 months after a local dose of up to 4000 R.

Effect on Ovaries

The effect of irradiation on ovaries is different from its effect on testicles. The ovaries contain a finite stock of ovocytes, which divide only after fertilization in the uterus. It must be quite a disappointment for the heroic spermatozoon, who among 500,000 competitors alone finds its way to an irradiated ovocyte, only to discover that its mate will no longer divide.

Ovocytes are not isolated. They are part of the histocellular complex of the follicle. The follicles go through various degrees of maturation, ranging from the small primordial follicle to the large mature graafian follicle, the roundness of which bulges at the surface of the functional ovary.

After a dose of 1200 R, all types of follicles are damaged—the large one more consistently than the primordial follicles. The first visible damage usually develops in the ovocyte, where the nucleus presents pyknosis and later chromatolysis, and the cytoplasm shows granular alteration or clumping. The damage extends to the follicular cell, which also degenerates, and ultimately the follicular structure disappears. As a result, a few months after X-irradiation, the gross appearance of the ovary is modified. The organ is small and white with a smooth surface; histologically mature follicles have disappeared; and only a few primordial follicles with seemingly intact ovocytes remain. When these follicles start to mature several months later, many degenerate soon after the first burst of cellular proliferation, but others develop into normal graafian follicles, and at that time sexual function (which will have been inoperative for 3 to 5 months) is usually reestablished. Permanent radiological castration requires doses ranging between 2000 to 2500 R.

Effect on Hematopoietic Organs

The blood contains a number of corpuscular structures that circulate in the vascular system in suspension in plasma. Some of these elements (polymorphonuclears and lymphocytes) have all the attributes of the cell: a membrane, a nucleus, an endoplasmic reticulum, etc. Many of these cells are capable of dividing (lymphocytes) while in the bloodstream. In contrast, other cells, like the red cells, have reduced their structural components to the strict minimum needed for function and have retained only a membrane and a rudimentary stroma. The circulating white and red blood cells are made in specialized hematopoietic organs: spleen, bone marrow, thymus, lymph nodes, bursa of Fabricius, and liver in the embryo. Polymorphonuclears, lymphocytes, and monocytes made in the lymphopoietic tissue may migrate in the interstitial tissue, especially under pathological conditions, such as inflammation, hypersensitivity, or an autoimmune reaction. If the source of the circulating and migrating cell is destroyed, then the blood count will drop and the cell will not react to injury.

The hematopoietic organs are among the most radiosensitive organs. Doses as low as 5 R are believed to lead to the blocking of mitosis in spleen and thymus. The stem cells of lymphocytes, platelets, and erythrocytes are all radiosensitive. The sequence of events is the same in all cases: mitotic arrest, cellular death, cellular elimination, and regeneration. For example, in the spleen 30 minutes after the administration of 300 to 600 R, irradiated cells show signs of nuclear pyknosis and karyorrhexis, which may be followed by cellular death. Usually, the damage at first is prominent in the center of the malpighian corpuscle, but later it spreads to its periphery. Within a day or two the entire organ is depleted of its lymphopoietic cells, leaving only the stroma with wandering histiocytes stuffed with necrotic white or red cells and a few intact immature cells. The spleen is markedly reduced in size; after irradiation in rats and mice, the formerly plump organ resembles a thin, elongated, stringy, reddish-blue ribbon. The medulla and the cortex of the thymus and the germinal centers of the lymph nodes or the Peyer patches also shrink. These organs are emptied of their cellular contingent soon after irradiation, and they are reduced to a vasculoconnective stroma.

Regeneration is more or less rapid, depending upon the dose administered. If the animal is of low sensitivity to a whole-body dose, or if a single dose has left enough immature cells untouched so that they can recolonize the organ, regeneration takes place and the organ recovers its normal histological appearance and its weight. Thus, the irradiated organ, which a few weeks earlier was a desert of vasculoconnective tissue, is quickly repopulated by normal cellular contingents properly arranged to reconstruct normal histology. In fact, in the spleens of those animals which normally have no erythropoietic activity, foci of vicarious erythropoiesis may appear in the form of conglomerations of 20–50 cells. A few of the cells are immature precursors of the red cells. Most are nucleated erythropoietic cells at various stages of maturation. Similarly, foci of granulopoietic activity may also be found.

Nothing is more impressive than the effect of irradiation on the bone marrow. Within a few days after exposure, the bone marrow, rich in cells with various functions, is reduced to a fine network of reticular fibers with a few interdispersed fibroblasts and scattered immature cells. The precursors of erythrocytes, granulocytes, lymphocytes, and platelets are all sensitive to irradiation. However, there seem to be identifiable differences in their individual radiosensitivity. Although there is not a uniform agreement as to which cell is most radiosensitive, the precursors of granulocytes seem to be more sensitive than those of erythrocytes. Precursors of lymphocytes are next in radiosensitivity, and those of megakaryocytes are the least radiosensitive. If the animal survives the exposure, within 2 or 3 weeks the few immature cells remaining in the bone marrow actively proliferate into small colonies and slowly repopulate the entire organ, which may even be hyperplastic for a short period of time.

It has been established using chromosome markers that stem cells migrate from the shielded area to the irradiated marrow [181].

From this description of the changes in spleen and bone marrow after X-irradiation, the alteration of the blood cell count can be predicted, provided that one keeps in mind that: (1) the life span of circulating cells varies; (2) white cells migrate from the vascular system into the intercellular tissue; and (3) some of the mature circulating cells are also radiosensitive.

Since the lymphocytes have a short life span, emigrate from the vascular tree, and, as we shall see, are directly sensitive to irradiation, the lymphocyte count drops rapidly after irradiation with hypolymphemia and increased levels of polymorphonuclears in the blood.

This early drop in the level of circulating lymphocytes may be followed, after the administration of whole-body doses of X-irradiation, by a secondary and mild hyperleukocytosis. This is only a transient event, and, after the secondary rise, the white blood cell counts drop consistently to values of one-half, one-third, or even one-tenth of the normal value. For each species there is a critical level below which the drop in the white blood cell count is no longer compatible with survival.

The red cells have a relatively long life span. They do not leave the bloodstream unless the vasculature is ruptured. They are relatively radioresistant; consequently, they may continue to circulate long after exposure to irradiation. Nevertheless, red cells that have reached the end of their normal life span and are eliminated by the normal process of red cell phagocytosis in the spleen are not immediately replaced after a dose of irradiation because of severe depression of the erythropoietic activity in the bone marrow.

Effects on the Gastrointestinal Tract

Because the epithelial cells of the gastrointestinal tract are constantly replaced, the lining of the gastrointestinal tract can be expected to be especially sensitive to radiation. Damage to the epithelium of the large intestines is of special clinical importance. The epithelial wall separates an internal, essentially aseptic, milieu from the lumen of the intestine, which communicates with the exterior milieu and harbors varied and large bacterial populations. The collapse of this epithelial barrier between exterior and interior environment may lead to bacterial invasion of blood and other tissues resulting in septicemia. The effect of X-irradiation on the intestinal mucosa is the same as that on the hematopoietic tissue, except, of course, for the functional consequences.

The cells of the crypts of Lieberkühn are the germinal cells from which the surface cells are derived. The crypt cells divide very rapidly, providing enough new cellular elements to replace all surface cells, which are shed in the lumen every other day. A dose as low as 50 R temporarily blocks mitosis in those cells. If the doses are small, the temporary arrest of mitosis in the crypt cell seems to be linked with prolonged life span in the surface cell, as if a feedback information loop existed between surface and crypt cell (see necrosis). At higher doses (between 300 and 600 R in rodents, possibly even less in primates and humans), mitotic inhibition is followed by necrosis of the crypt cell. Consequently, when the surface cells have reached the end of even a somewhat prolonged life span, they are shed in the lumen without being replaced by fresh mature layers of epithelial cells.

The combination of destruction of the germinal cells and shedding of the superficial layers leads to epithelial denudation. Denudation is to the intestine what depopulation is to the hematopoietic system. In fact, when the surface epithelium is lost in the intestinal wall, the Peyer patches simultaneously are reduced to masses of connective and reticular tissue containing few lymphocytes. Intestinal damage does not always lead to death. If the dose is not excessive, bodily survival may be secured with proper treatment of an experimental animal or therapy for a human. The restoration of the epithelium starts with DNA synthesis and mitosis in the crypt, followed by reepithelialization of the wall. Sometimes restoration is somewhat distorted in the squamous epithelium, and transitional metaplasia may take place.

The duodenum and jejunum appear to be the most radiosensitive segments of the small intestine. Irradiation of the mucosa of the colon and rectum results in histological changes similar to those already described in the small intestine, except that these segments of the intestines are more radioresistant than the small intestine. Consequently, epithelial denudation is rare unless a single large dose is delivered. The rectum is exposed to repeated therapeutic doses more frequently than any other segment of the intestine (*e.g.*, in treatment of cancer of the cervix), and severe post-therapeutic radiorectitis with fibrosis of the wall and narrowing of the lumen has been observed.

The effect of X-irradiation on the histology and the function of the stomach is of particular interest because of the possible implication of radiation damage to the stomachal mucosa in the development of radiation sickness. In general, both glandular and chief cells of the stomach are radioresistant. The epithelium is altered only if doses above 1 000 R are administered. Between 1920 and 1925, investigators studied the effect of irradiation on the secretion of the gastric juices in dogs prepared with either a gastric fistula or a Pavlov pouch. HCl secretion is blocked and pepsin secretion is markedly reduced within 1 or 2 weeks after repeated irradiation of the stomach with small doses.

Miscellaneous Radiation Lesions

Some organs which were believed to be radioresistant show severe and sometimes irreparable damage when they are included in the radiation field outlined for radiotherapy. For example, the parotid glands are often included in the radiation field for treatment of cancer of the neck, and patients may develop acute sialadenitis and xerostomia of variable duration. Yet, the gland has a low mitotic rate and therefore would be expected to be radioresistant. Therefore it was generally assumed that the adenitis was secondary to microvascular damage. Studies by Sholley et al. established that radiation causes direct damage to the acinar cells [182].

In 1962, Groover et al. [183] described radiation pneumonitis in patients irradiated for cancer of the breast, lung or for other intrathoracic tumors. The pneumonitis does not develop immediately, but it usually occurs 3 to 6 months after therapy is completed; it may either subside or it may progress to irreversible fibrosis. The lesion usually starts after 10 to 60 days with exudation and ends 200 days to a year after therapy with fibrosis. It is not clear whether or not the injury is caused by direct damage to the lung cells or results from indirect damage to the vasculature. The exudation state is followed by infiltration with lymphocytes, polymorphonuclears, etc. The elimination of the cellular infiltrate is associated with a temporary recovery. Late progressive fibrosis develops. The fibrosis may be focal or diffuse and may or may not be associated with calcification [183–185].

Similarly in 1962, Luxton [186] described a radiation nephritis and showed that the kidney was a radiosensitive organ whose enclosure in the field of therapy could compromise the therapy of abdominal tumors. Again the lesion is delayed, the histological changes will develop at four months after the administration of therapy and will progress over the years. The lesions affect the proximal and the convoluted tubules primarily, but will also lead to necrosis of the glomeruli and hyalinization of the arterioles. Depending upon the severity of the histological changes, radiation nephritis may be associated with proteinuria, uremia, renal deficiency and hypertension. If only one kidney has been irradiated, the hypertension can be corrected by unilateral nephrectomy [187]. Arneil et al. [188] have studied the effects of the combined administration of 1 500 and 2 000 rads and actinomycin to the single kidney of children nephrectomized for neuroblastomas. Radiation nephritis ensued suggesting that the combination of these two modes of therapy may accelerate nephritis. This finding conflicts with experimental data which suggest that actinomycin D protects against radiation damage.

Delayed radiation damage also occurs in bone, cartilage, skin, etc. Laryngeal or nasal cartilages and maxillar bones undergo necrosis several years after exposure to radiation.

The molecular pathogenesis of these events is not known. A primary lesion must be imprinted in many or a few cells of one or more types. The damage may involve vascular cells. The consequences of the primary lesions are not expressed for a long time either because the injured cells have a long life span or because the cells may undergo several divisions before cell death. Necrosis results in an inflammatory reaction which may be aseptic at first, but will often be superinfected. Restoration of the lost cells does usually not occur and reparation can only occur through fibrosis.

Causes of Death after Administration of Whole-Body Doses of X-Irradiation

The causes of death after the administration of acute dose of radiation vary, depending upon the dose. After receiving doses of X-irradiation greater than 10,000 R, animals die within an hour or two as a result of severe damage to the central nervous system.

After the whole-body administration of 2000 to 5000 R, animals will die within 3 to 5 days, primarily because of septicemia resulting from gastrointestinal damage. Doses from 300 to 1000 R lead to death within the second or third week after the exposure because of severe depression of the hematopoietic system, principally the bone marrow.

When the dose is below 1000 R, dose mortality curves can be plotted. The dose at which 50% of the animals die is referred to as the LD 50. Since most experimental animals that will die in an experiment die within 30 days after exposure, one usually observes the animals for 30 days and refers to the LD 50 as 30 days or LD 30 abbreviated. The LD 30 varies, depending upon the animal used for the experiments. It is approximately 250 R for dogs and 600 R for monkeys. Two values have been reported for humans; the most plausible LD 30 is believed to be around 360, but several investigators have proposed that the LD 30 in humans may range around 700 R. Observations on human victims of accidents suggest, however, that death occurs at much lower doses. For example, in the accident in which inhabitants of the Marshall Islands were exposed to nuclear fallout, it was estimated that the victims received only 175 R. Yet their hematopoietic systems were severely depressed, and cases of purpura were beginning to be reported. Such clinical observations suggested that an increment of 50 R could have brought the victims within the lethal range. Similarly, 1 of the 5 Yugoslavs who had been exposed to radiation after an atomic pile explosion died after receiving a dose of 350 R.

Criteria for Prognosis after Radiation Injury

Although diagnosis of radiation injury after exposure is seldom a problem, prognosis is of considerable importance, especially in a large population catastrophe. Therefore, attempts have been made to develop criteria for classifying the victims according to their chance of survival. The criteria used are based essentially on the intensity of some of the gastrointestinal symptoms experienced by the exposed individuals. These criteria have been reviewed by Cronkite [44]. Usually after a large exposure, it is proposed to divide the population into three groups: survival improbable, survival possible, and survival probable. The improbable group includes those who present intractable nausea and diarrhea very soon after exposure; the probable develop the same symptoms with lesser severity and at a later time, that is to say, 1 or 2 days after exposure. This symptomatology is likely to be followed by a period of well-being. However, relatively soon after exposure, the hematopoietic systems of these individuals become depressed. The probable survivors are individuals who have no initial symptoms, may present a transitory drop in their white blood cell and possibly red cell count, but otherwise show no symptoms.

The individuals categorized as possible survivors require further attention. The development of radiation disease can be followed two ways: measuring the bone marrow mitotic index and taking the blood count. When the bone marrow is taken at 10 AM, the bone marrow mitotic index is of the order of 0.9%. It will drop to a relatively low value if the victim is exposed to even as low as 50 to 200 R; with doses above that, the bone marrow mitotic index may drop to zero. Blood counts, especially counts of polymorphonuclears and monocytes, may help considerably in following the course of radiation sickness. The significance of the lymphocyte count is more difficult to evaluate because relatively small doses (300 R) bring the lymphocyte count to almost zero.

In general, treatment of radiation sickness resembles that for pancytopenia; however, there is a potential for restoration in the former, which does not always exist in cases of pancytopenia of another origin. One of the physician's functions in treating patients exposed to whole-body doses of irradiation is to attempt to carry the patient through the critical period. The therapeutic arsenal includes antibiotics, blood transfusion, platelet transfusion, and, in some cases, marrow transfusion. Some of the pathological manifestations of radiation are illustrated in Figs. 12-5, 12-6, 12-7, 12-8, and 12-9.

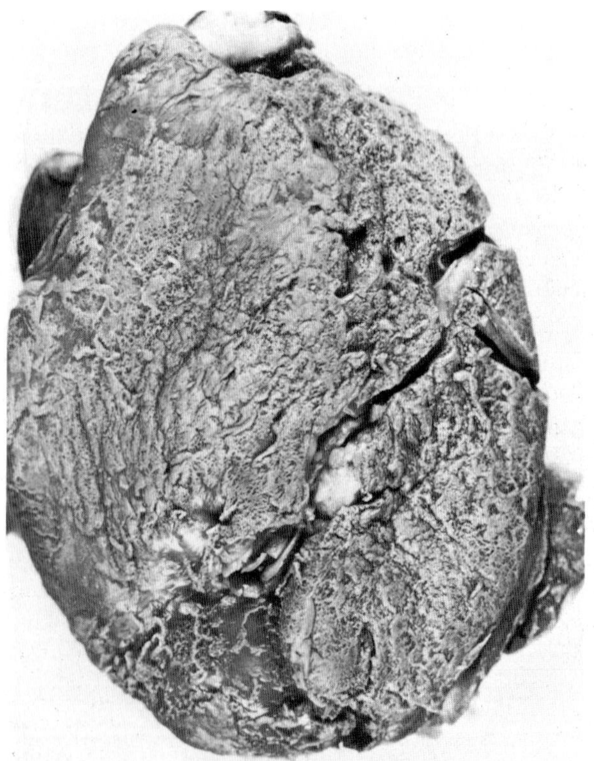

Fig. 12-6. Fibrous pericarditis caused by radiation after therapy for chest cancer

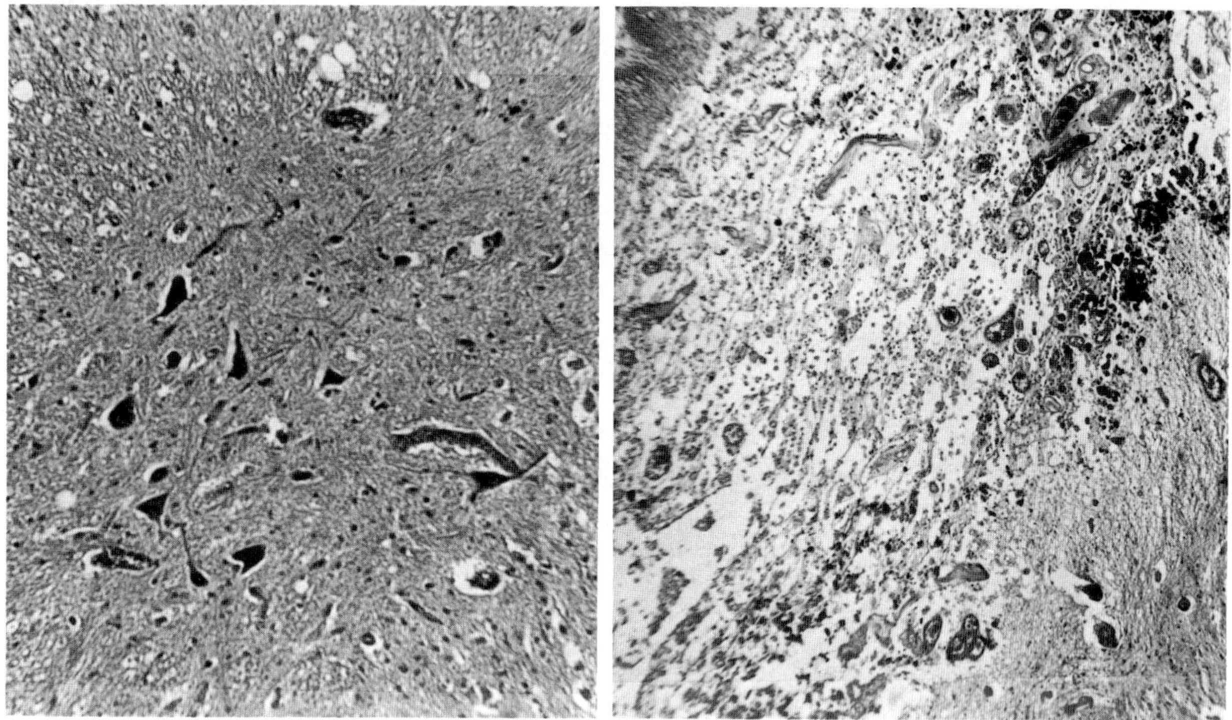

Fig. 12-7. Normal spinal chord (*left*) and spinal chord showing necrosis (*right*) after the administration of 6200 rads, given in 44 divided doses as therapy for cancer of the larynx. The spinal chord was shielded, and the maximum chord dose was estimated to be 2200 rads. Myelopathy developed 1 year after irradiation, and the patient died 2 years later

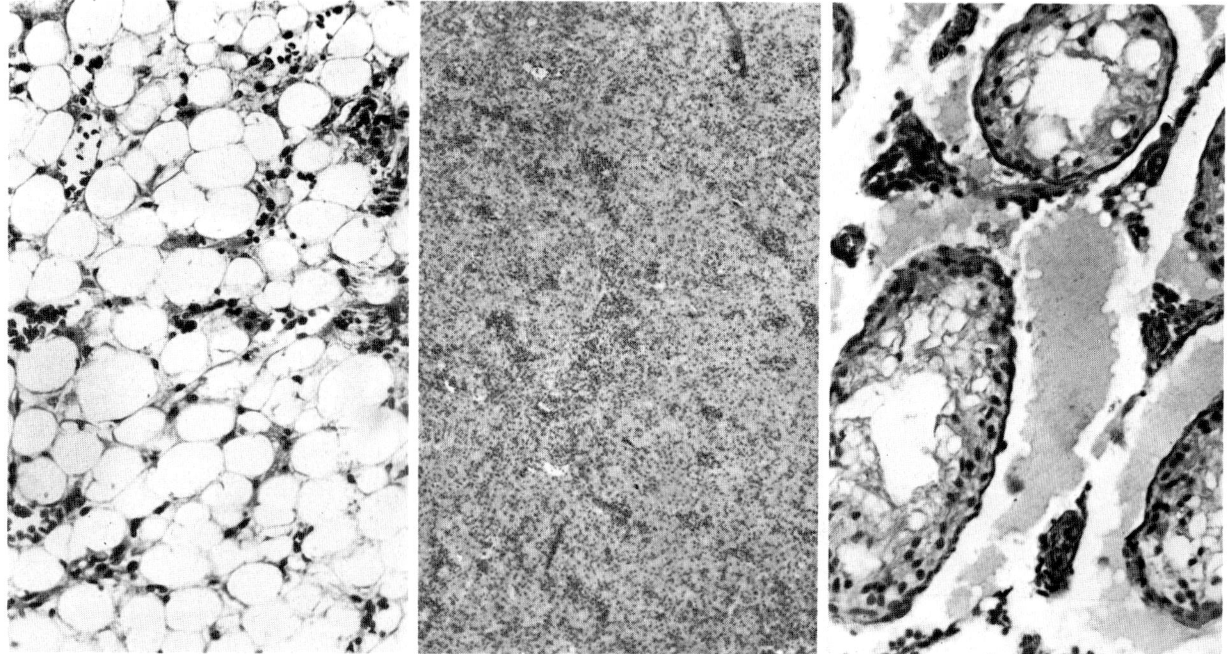

Fig. 12-8. Bone marrow (*left*), spleen (*center*), and testicles (*right*) of a rat given 700 rads; note the disappearance of hematopoietic, lymphopoietic, and germinal cells

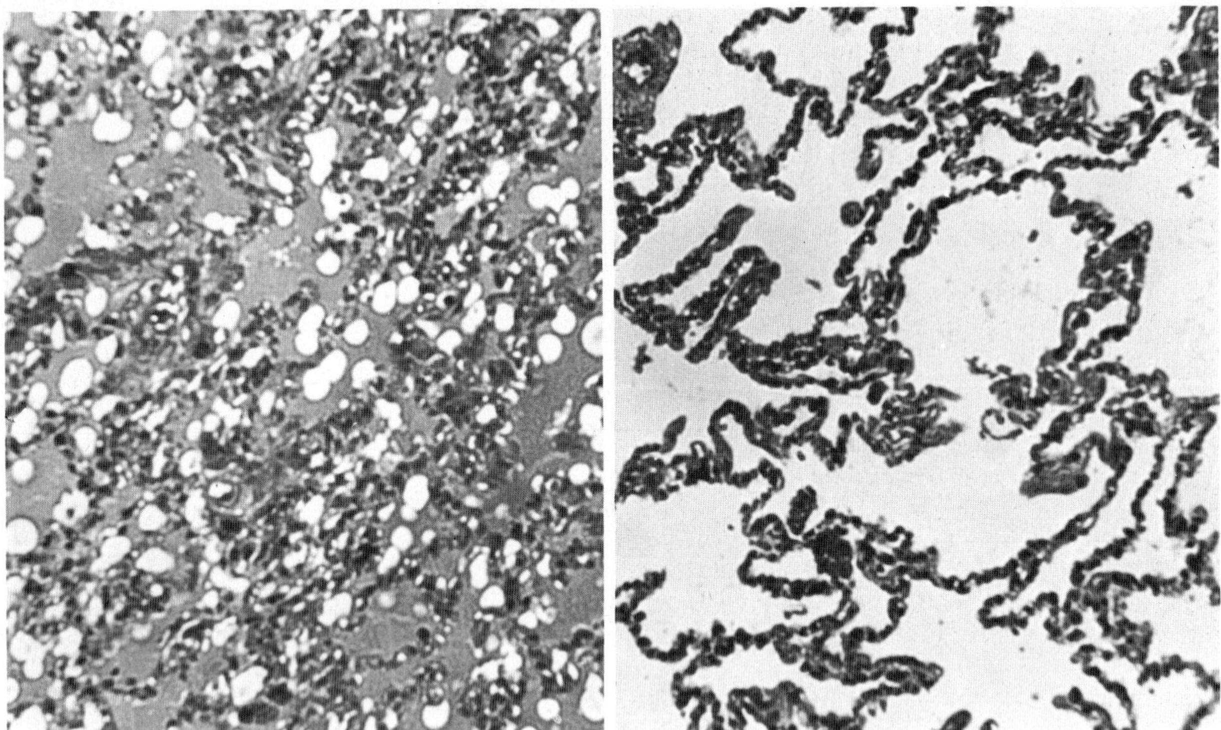

Fig. 12-9. Radiation pneumonitis was found in an area adjacent to a portion of lung that had been irradiated with 6000 rad for bronchial carcinoma. *Right*, normal alveoli; *left*, alveoli filled with edema fluid

Radiation Carcinogenesis

Sunlight and Cancer

Among electromagnetic radiations, infrared, ultraviolet, and ionizing radiations have all long been suspected of being carcinogenic. Although the carcinogenic effects of infrared rays may be doubted, those of UV and X-irradiation are unquestionable.

The physicians of ancient Egypt knew that deep scars caused by burns were a field favorable for the development of skin cancer (see Fig. 12-10). The observations of antiquity have been repeatedly confirmed in modern times, and the incidence of squamous cell carcinoma of the skin appears to be greater in scarred areas than in normal skin. Thus, on scarred skin, cancer develops in areas where cancers ordinarily are not observed. Kangri (India) and kairo (Iran) cancers have now become classical examples of the relationship between burns and skin cancer. In many parts of Asia where the climate is cold, the shepherds and farmers wear a basket or an earthpot filled with hot coals underneath their garments to keep them warm. This procedure frequently burns the skin of the abdomen, and scars may form. An unusually high incidence of skin cancer has been observed among these people. Whether the cancer is caused by the infrared rays *per se* or is the consequence of scarring is debatable. Similarly, cancer of the mouth has been observed among some people in India who habitually smoke cigars with the lit end in their mouths.

Adequate or convincing experimental data on the carcinogenic potential of infrared rays are lacking. Few experiments have been done, and most have been poorly controlled. There is no conclusive evidence that simple exposure to infrared rays causes cancer in the absence of scarring.

The situation is very different with respect to skin cancer caused by sunlight. Special features of farmers' skin and the frequency of "seaman's carcinoma" have been known for more than a century. The combination of aging and exposure to sunlight causes the skin to become pigmented, thickened, and wrinkled. Brown or gray warty, irregular lesions develop ranging in size from 1 mm to 2 cm. Histologically, the lesions reveal epithelial hyperkeratosis and moderate lymphocytic infiltration of the chorion. These senile hyperkeratoses are favorite sites for the development of skin cancer in the exposed areas. Blacks are practically immune to such lesions, and blond and red-haired Caucasians are most susceptible. Mediterraneans and Orientals are of the middle range of susceptibility. Skin cancer seldom develops in unexposed areas.

Two kinds of cancer occur: basal cell and squamous cell carcinoma. The histological difference between these two types is important, primarily because of the biology of the cancer. Basal cell carcinoma invades but seldom metastasizes, whereas squamous cell carcinoma readily metastasizes to regional nodes. Basal cell carcinoma occurs more frequently on the lateral aspects of the nose, the temporal regions, the jaws, the chin, and the eyelids. Squamous cell carcinoma

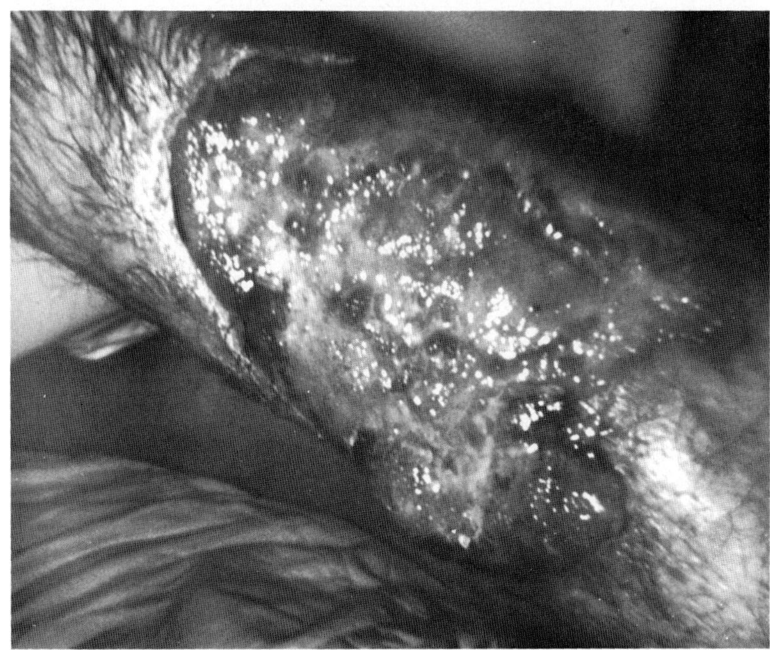

Fig. 12-10. Squamous cell carcinoma developing in an area of chronic inflammation, resulting from a skin burn. (From Guillard)

affects the lobule of the ear, the lower lip, and the forehead.

Unless the skin has been exposed to chemical carcinogens, most skin cancer results from exposure to natural sources of electromagnetic radiation. Which of these sources of radiation causes skin cancer?

Living beings must either succumb or adapt to two major sources of electromagnetic radiation: light* and cosmic rays. Under more unusual conditions, they might also be exposed to X- and γ-rays and be bombarded with α- and β-particles or neutrons. We shall consider here only the effects of light on the human skin. During the day, the sun and the skies are the major source of light. Light emitted at night by the moon and the stars, although of great importance for some biological systems, is of no relevance to skin cancer. The sun gives off three major types of radiation: visible, ultraviolet, and infrared.

Many investigators attempted to produce skin cancer in mice, rats, and rabbits with the aid of artificially produced UV light. But a systematic study of the carcinogenic effect of UV light was not available until Rusch and Baumann [51] clearly defined UV carcinogenesis in quantitative terms. These investigators established that the carcinogenic wavelength ranges between 290 and 334 mμ. Moreover, they established that below a critical energy level (30×10^7 ergs/cm^2), no cancer appears.

Increasing the dose level not only increases the incidence of cancer, but also reduces the latent period between exposure and appearance of cancer. When the wavelength used ranges between 290 and 334 mμ, 160×10^7 ergs/cm^2 are needed to produce skin cancer in 50% of the mice.

Blum and coworkers [52, 53, 54] studied the effects of dose fractionation on the incidence of cancer produced with UV light. No greater number of cancers is obtained when the skin is irradiated five times weekly with doses of 0.7×10^7 ergs/cm^2. However, the latent period is markedly reduced if higher energy levels are used.

These results are puzzling when considered in the light of modern knowledge. If we assume that UV carcinogenesis results from alteration of the DNA molecule, then the formation of thymine dimers and their repair might be related to the process. The presence of dimers could lead to somatic mutation: (1) directly by miscoding for all abnormal or ineffective messengers, or (2) indirectly after mispairing when the polynucleotide chain is reconstructed during repair. Again, the result would be nonsense coding or miscoding. If a structural gene is to be affected, a point mutation would lead to the formation of an abnormal protein, or the gene would not be translated at all and a protein would be deleted. The altered or missing protein could be an enzyme, a structural protein, or a regulatory protein. In any event, this form of injury would be one or several somatic mutations, which would resemble one or several inborn errors more than cancer.

In contrast, if one or more regulatory genes, and possibly structural genes, are all affected at the same time, anything can happen in the cell. Some cells may die, some may hyperdifferentiate, some may be modified in such a way that one or more properties of cancer are assembled (disdifferentiation, invasion, etc.) in a cell still able to reproduce.

The high incidence of cancer in cases of xeroderma pigmentosum suggests that damage to DNA may in

* At least two environmental factors have been claimed to contribute to an increase in the incidence of cancer of the skin by UV light: reduction of the ozone levels of the stratosphere and the exhaust products of supersonic aircraft and the fluorocarbon of spray cans.

some way be involved in skin carcinogenis. Xeroderma pigmentosum is a rare hereditary skin disease first described by Kaposi in 1870. The disease is transmitted as an autosomal characteristic, both sexes are equally affected, and the first symptoms develop, in most cases, during the first or second years of life.

After a moderate exposure to sunlight, the baby with xeroderma pigmentosum develops an unusually severe sunburn. In addition, the skin becomes edematous and bullae form, especially on the exposed parts of the body: the hands, arms, legs, and face. Within 3 or 4 years, the skin of the affected child is aged and resembles that of an old farmer. The skin of the face and hands has a spotty appearance (*peau bariolée*), and some pigmented spots of telangiectasia alternate with whitish-pink areas of atrophic skin. Histologically, the lesions resemble senile atrophy of the skin.

Patients with xeroderma pigmentosum are unusually susceptible to skin cancer. Basal cell and squamous cell carcinomas with metastases have been observed at an early age. Some young patients have several types of skin cancer at the same time.

Professional and Accidental Cancer Produced by Radiation

Roentgen discovered X-rays in 1825. Within 7 years, the first radiation cancer was described by Frieben [55], a manufacturer of X-ray tubes. He tested his product by placing his hand between the source and the fluoroscope. Consequently, Frieben developed first a severe radiodermatitis and later an epidermoid carcinoma with metastasis to the lymph node. In 1910, Marie Clunet and Roulot Lapointe produced sarcomas in the rat with the aid of X-irradiation [56].

After this early observation, case reports of radiation cancer followed in the literature. Large-series studies were reported by Porter in 1909 and by Hesse in 1911. Two groups of people were victims of radiation cancer: repeatedly exposed personnel and treated patients. Hesse's report covered 54 cases of so-called *roentgen karcinom*, 4 of which occurred in patients, 26 in physicians, and 24 in radiation technicans.

Few therapeutic agents have been as abused as X-rays. In the first part of this century, X-rays were used to treat a wide spectrum of ailments: psoriasis, lupus, parasitic infection of hair, angiomas, eczema, and even for epilation of excessive hair in young girls. In most cases, the therapy was applied skillfully, and no or few complications were observed. Nevertheless, in a few cases radiodermatitis was produced, and epitheliomas or sarcomas developed. Presumably, radiation therapy may be responsible for the development of new cancers. But convincing statistical studies on the subject are not available, primarily because of the long latent period that elapses between the application of therapy and the development of cancer. It has been proposed that radiation therapy for fibromyoma of the uterus or cancer of the cervix may sometimes be responsible for the development of fibrosarcoma. Cancer of the larynx has been reported in women after irradiation of the thyroid. Beck observed osteosarcomas in 1922 in patients with bone tuberculosis treated with ionizing radiation.

Now that radiotherapy is used only to treat otherwise fatal diseases, the decision to apply radiotherapy is seldom agonizing for at least two reasons: the incidence of cancer that will develop after radiotherapy is low, and the latent period often exceeds the patient's life expectancy. Yet, when radiotherapy is used in young patients with curable cancer, the carcinogenic potential of the agent must be kept in mind, and a careful follow-up must be planned.

The classical example of cancer produced by radiation therapy is cancer of the thyroid following irradiation of the neck. Duffy and Fitzgerald [54] were the first to report that of 28 children with cancer of the thyroid, 10 had received radiation therapy for thymic hypertrophy.

X-Ray Carcinogenesis

From 1949 to 1960, 17,000 children who were immigrants to Israel were irradiated for the fungal scalp infection tinea capitis. Eleven thousand of these children were followed up retrospectively. They showed a significant increase in the incidence of benign and malignant tumors of the head and neck, especially in the brain, the parotid gland and the thyroid [189].

These findings were confirmed on larger groups in the United States, Great Britain, and France. According to Delawater and Winship [58] the incidence of cancer of the thyroid is increased only in patients under 19 years old when irradiated. However, Zeldis and coworkers [59] reported that the incidence of cancer of the thyroid is increased among atom bomb casualties. The incidence is 3 times greater than normal among those within a 1400-m radius of the hypocenter at the time of the explosion.

Today's physician need not be concerned so much with the carcinogenic effect of therapeutic doses of radiation as with that resulting from exposure to ionizing radiation because of accidental or premeditated contamination of the environment with radioisotopes and use of X-rays or isotopes for diagnostic purposes.

The role that diagnostic radiation may play in human carcinogenesis is debatable. Repeated breast fluoroscopy and radiography have been claimed to increase the chances of breast cancer developing in women, but not in men. Some question the data assembled on the victims of the atom bomb, which are interpreted to indicate that the incidence of breast cancer is increased among those who received even relatively small doses of irradiation. Neither is it certain what the relationship between repeated radiation exposures, radiation diagnosis, and the incidence of leukemia is. It is not known whether ^{131}I, which is used for diagnosing thyroid diseases, is carcinogenic for the thyroid.

Radioactive substances are sometimes ingested, inhaled, or injected. Accidents produced by radioactive substances introduced into the body are classified as industrial or iatrogenic accidents.

The classical industrial accident occurred in Newark, New Jersey, in 1924, in a factory of luminous clock and watch dials. Theodore Blum [60], a New York dentist, observed a young girl working in that factory who had an unusual case of osteitis. He described the disease as the "radium jaw." Later, 12 similar cases were reported, and the mechanism of the production of disease was established. The paint used to mark the numbers on these luminous dials contained a mixture of gum, zinc, sulfur, radium, mesothorium, and radiothorium. To increase the efficiency of the paintbrushes they used, the girls who painted the dials used to sharpen the brush by wetting it with their lips. By so doing, they absorbed 3 to 4 μg of radioactive material a day. Most of the radioactive material remained in contact with the mucosa of the gums and caused severe pyorrhea and osteitis. Some of the radioactive material was stored in viscera, especially the liver, the spleen, and in bone. Therefore, it is not surprising that the girls working in the factory developed, in spite of the light work, severe palor due to anemia and osteitis. In a few cases, osteosarcomas were also observed. Osteosarcomas of the bone have been produced in rodents and dogs fed a diet containing ^{90}Sr or after injection of plutonium.

For a long time, it was known that the miners of Erzgebirge, a mountain range located between Bohemia and Saxony, died young due to respiratory disease. One side on the mountain is called a Schneeberg and is in Germany; the other side, Joachimstahl, is in Czechoslovakia. A number of minerals are extracted on both sides, but since the discovery of radioactivity by Madame Curie, the miners of Joachimstahl have concentrated on extracting uranium. In 1879 Härting showed that the pulmonary disease of these patients was lung cancer. Since then, it has been debated whether the cancer was caused by radioactivity or by inhalation of other mineral dusts.

In the beginning of the 20th century, several mineral resorts added radioactive radon to their mineral water because low levels of radioactivity had been found in some of the water of the traditional spas of Europe. By 1935, at least one victim of the use of such radioactive water had been reported, a man who had habitually drunk radioactive mineral water and who had in 5 years ingested 2.8 mg of radioactive material. He developed maxillary necrosis and died.

Thorium oxide (Thorotrast) was introduced in radiology to mark tissues—such as the liver, the spleen, and the bone marrow—for radiodiagnostic purposes. It soon was observed that the Thorotrast was trapped in the liver and caused liver cirrhosis and blood dyscrasia. In 1934, Roussy and Oberling [61] showed that the substance was carcinogenic for animals. Soon many cases of cancer of the liver were reported in patients who had received Thorotrast for radiodiagnosis of the gall bladder.

Experimental Radiation Carcinogenesis

It would serve no purpose to describe the innumerable animal experiments that established the carcinogenic properties of ionizing radiation. Since the first experiment of Marie Clunet and Roulot Lapointe, radiation cancers have been produced in many species, including monkeys, at almost every body site and by a great variety of methods. In fact, ionizing radiation may well be the most reliable and most versatile carcinogen known.

In 1923 Bruno Block [62, 63] produced squamous cell carcinomas of the rabbit ear after exposure to 32,000 R. Radiation sarcomas and carcinomas have been produced in guinea pigs and mice. Large doses of radiation have been used to produce chondrosarcomas and osteosarcomas in rabbits and chickens.

In 1918 Lazarus Barlow produced skin cancer in mice injected with radium trapped in pulverized mica. The introduction of radioactive substances into various parts of the animals' bodies has produced osteosarcomas (injection of radium mixed with vaseline in the medullary cavity of the femur, administration of diets containing ^{90}St), liver sarcomas in rats and mice (injection of mesothorium), and skin sarcomas and carcinomas in mice (subcutaneous implantation of radon tubes). Squamous cell carcinomas of the skin with lymph node metastases have been produced by local irradiation in monkeys.

Perhaps a case reported by Ross in 1932 best illustrates the carcinogenic efficacy of radiation. A form of treatment of breast cancer was, and still is in some places, the implantation of radium needles within and around the cancerous mass. Each needle is tied to the skin by a silk thread to keep it from being lost in the soft tissue. In the case Ross reported, one needle became loose, traveled to the heart, and became lodged in the interventricular septum. The patient died from heart failure. The patient's liver, the area that had been most exposed to radiation, contained a malignant hemoendothelioma. One could argue that the presence of the tumor was, in this case, a coincidence. Ross, however, was able to produce osteosarcomas, squamous cell carcinomas, and fibrosarcomas in rabbits in which 0.1 mg of radium was implanted in various parts of the body.

Maldague [64] has shown that total body doses of X-irradiation markedly increase the incidence of cancer in rats, and he believes that the development of the cancer results from local absorption of the dose. Total body doses of irradiation increase the incidence of cancer of the prostate, the seminal vesicles, the mammary glands, the ovaries, the adrenal glands, the stomach, the small bowel, the colon, the salivary glands, and the kidneys.

Radiation and Leukemia

Leukemia can be produced by low doses of radiation, and a clarification of radiation leukemogenesis may

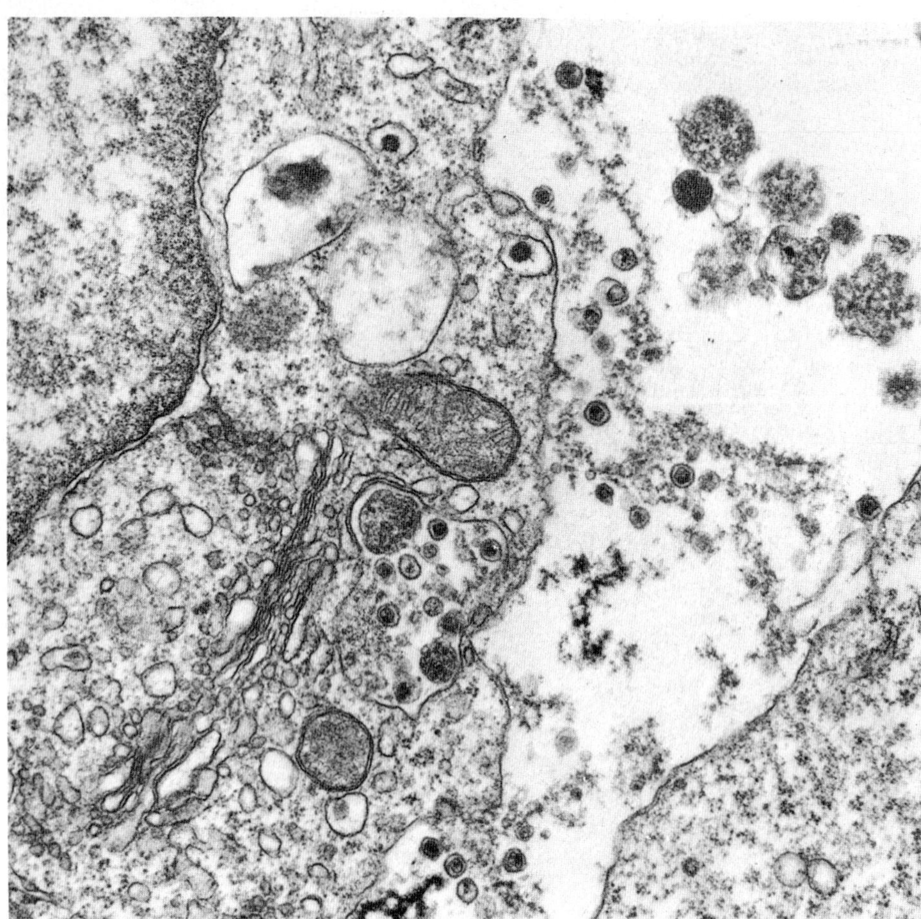

Fig. 12-11. Type-C extracellular and type-A intracisternal viruses in cell culture ($_1$M, clone 7) of a Rad LV-induced lymphoma of a C57 BL mouse. Osmium fixation; uranyl acetate and lead hydroxide stain; magnification 30,000. (From M.L. Hart)

contribute considerably to an understanding of carcinogenesis as a whole [65–68].

German physicians reported two cases of lymphoid leukemia among radiologists. Larger numbers of cases were soon reported by Aubertin [69] and Lacassagne [70]. In 1944 Henshaw and Hawkins [76] found that leukemia is a more frequent cause of death among physicians (1.7 times) than among the general population; it was further established that radiologists are more prone to develop leukemia than is the rest of the physician population [67]. However, reports of the United Nations Scientific Committee suggest that this trend was reversed after 1960.

A clear relationship between the dose of radiation received and the incidence of leukemia was observed among the victims of the atom bombs in Hiroshima and Nagasaki. Acute rather than chronic leukemia predominates among atom bomb casualties. The peak incidence developed 6 years after the explosion.

The dose-response relationship is believed to be linear. However, the reliability of the estimation of the dose received in each case is questionable, especially at lowest dose levels. Therefore, it cannot be determined whether a threshold dose exists, below which the incidence of leukemia is not increased. In general, doses below 100 R are believed to have no influence on the incidence of leukemia.

Radiation therapy at low, but frequently repeated, doses was and still is in some centers advocated as therapy for ankylosing spondylitis. Large segments of the bone marrow of such patients are irradiated.

Court-Brown [72, 73] investigated the incidence of leukemia among such patients and again established a linear relationship between the incidence of leukemia and the dose absorbed. No leukemogenic effect was observed at doses below 54 R. The older the irradiated patient, the greater are his chances of developing leukemia.

The human studies reported above clearly establish that relatively large whole-body or even local doses of X-irradiation are leukemogenic for men, and that there is a coarse linear relationship between dose received and incidence of leukemia. Nevertheless, the data do not allow us to determine whether there is a threshold dose level below which no leukemogenic effect is observed. If the dose relationship observed could be extrapolated to zero, such a relationship would: (1) support the theory that a somatic mutation is a mechanism of pathogenesis, and (2) allow physicians to estimate a patient's risk of developing leukemia after exposure to diagnostic doses of radiation.

Investigators do not know whether exposure to a dose of less than 100 R is leukemogenic, except maybe in young children or the fetus irradiated *in utero*. Leuk-

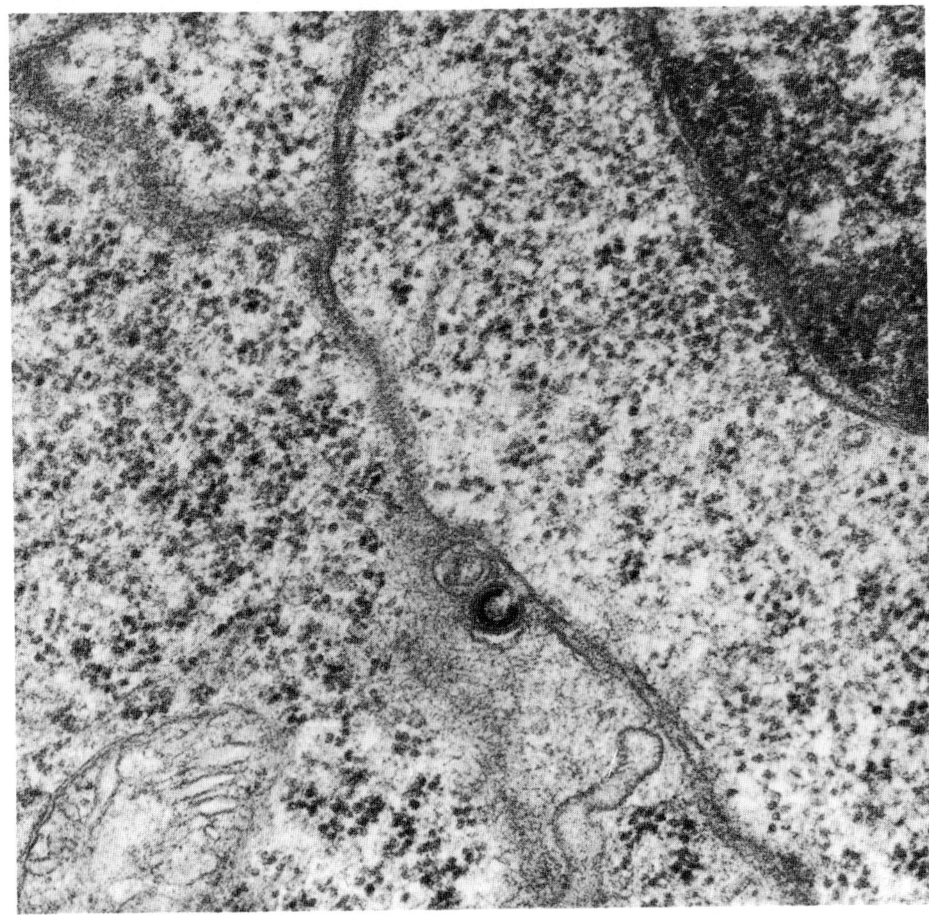

Fig. 12-12. Plasma membrane budding type-C virus in primary thymic lymphoma of C57 BL mouse induced by irradiation (400 R) plus Rad LV inoculation. Osmium fixation; uranyl acetate and lead citrate strain; magnification 60,000. (From M.L. Hart)

emia has been reported among patients who received therapeutic doses of ^{131}I.

In the early 1930s, Krebs and associates [74] observed that the incidence of lymphosarcoma was 5 times greater in irradiated (150–300 R) than in nonirradiated mice. After confirming Krebs' findings, Furth and Butterworth [75] established (using strains with various degrees of susceptibility to the development of spontaneous leukemia) that X-irradiation not only increased the incidence of leukemia but also accelerated the appearance of the disease. By manipulating strain and X-ray doses, these workers increased the incidence of experimental leukemia in mice. Kirschbaum, using CBA mice with 3% of spontaneous leukemia, raised the incidence to 50% by giving repeated fractionated doses of 80 R up to a total dose of 400 R.

In the 1940s it became obvious that the thymus was essential to the pathogenesis of leukemia in at least some strains of mice; indeed, work from Furth's [77], Kaplan's, and other laboratories [76, 78, 79, 80, 81] established that thymectomy reduced the incidence of leukemia produced by X-irradiation and methylcholanthrene [82]. The incidence of lymphoid tumors could, however, be restored to normal in thymectomized mice by implantation of an autologous or homologous thymus [83].

Yet, paradoxically, when C57 BL mice (a strain with low spontaneous incidence of leukemia but high susceptibility to lymphoid tumors after whole-body irradiation) are irradiated directly on the thymus, the incidence of leukemia drops to almost 0 [84].

All these observations indicate that the thymus plays a central role in the pathogenesis of mouse leukemia. Kaplan and Brown demonstrated that the tumors arise in the thymus—whether the thymus is *in situ* or grafted—and disseminate to other tissues (lymph node, spleen, and liver).

Tumors develop in thymectomized irradiated animals, even if the thymus implant is obtained from a nonirradiated mouse. The conclusion seems inescapable: the thymus is essential because that is where the tumor starts. Yet nonthymic factors are involved in transforming the normal thymus into a cancerous organ. Further evidence for the existence of extrathymic factors in the pathogenesis of leukemia in AKR or C57 BL mice was provided when it was established that shielding of a thigh or injection of bone marrow interferes with leukemogenesis.

The administration of estrogen, urethane, or turpentine after irradiation increases the incidence of leukemia, and the susceptibility to leukemia varies markedly with the animal's age at the time of irradiation—younger mice are much more susceptible than older ones.

A new parameter in mouse radiation leukemogenesis was added when it was shown in several laboratories [85] that radiation-induced leukemia could be transmitted by filtrates prepared from organs of leukemic mice. Again, thymectomy before or after administration of the filtrate interfered with leukemogenesis. Group C-type RNA viruses have been seen even before birth in AKR or C58 mice, inbred strains with a high incidence of leukemia (see 12-11 and 12-12).

Irradiation is now believed to initiate a multistage process of leukemogenesis. The first step is the "unleashing" of a virus, which may then transform susceptible cells—*e.g.*, the thymus cell in AKR or C57 BL mice (see cancer virus).

According to Huebner [86], events in the mouse leukemia are typical for all cancers.

An infectious virus is normally transmitted horizontally. It infects neighboring cells and other animals of the species. Huebner proposes that the oncogenic virus is special in that it is not infective in the ordinary sense of the word, because it is transmitted *vertically* instead of horizontally. Thus, the virus is transmitted from mother to daughter cell, from parents to progeny. The mode of transfer of the oncogenic virus resembles that of a gene more than that of an infectious agent.

To explain this special mode of transfer of the oncogenic virus, Huebner proposes that the virus exists in all cells of possibly all vertebrates in a "repressed" form. Whether the repressed virus is expressed is determined by a number of factors—the host's genetic makeup, exposure to radiation or other carcinogens, and aging.

Huebner believes that the oncogenic virus is a C-type RNA virus. Of course, nothing is known of the chemistry of the repressor, the mechanism of derepression, or the mode of transfer from mother to daughter cell.

Biochemical Effects of Ionizing Irradiation

Nuclear Versus Cytoplasmic Radiosensitivity

The task of identifying the site of radiation would be considerably simplified if we were able to decide at which level of the cell X-irradiation causes maximum damage. Morphological observation, focal irradiation of nucleus versus cytoplasm, and nuclear transplantation experiments all suggest that the nucleus is more radiosensitive than the cytoplasm [87–90]. The first morphological alteration produced by radiation occurs within the nucleus. Of course, it can be argued that such nuclear changes are the consequences of the elaboration of toxic substances formed in the cytoplasm. However, this possibility seems to have been excluded in experiments in which narrow beams of protons were used to irradiate the cell. Although only a few protons administered to the chromosome produce considerable damage, such as chromosomal rupture, more than 1000 protons are without effect on the cytoplasm.

Elegant nuclear transplantation experiments demonstrated that nucleated and irradiated ameobas survive normally if a nonirradiated nucleus is transplanted inside of the irradiated cytoplasm. In contrast, a nonirradiated cell died rapidly when an irradiated nucleus was implanted. These experiments clearly established that a dose which kills the cell when administered to the nucleus is not lethal when administered to the cytoplasm [91, 92].

These findings suggest that the biochemical effect of X-irradiation is somewhat specific. The nucleus and cytoplasm have many of the same biochemical constituents: proteins (albumin, globulins, lipoproteins, enzymes), ribonucleic acid, and coenzymes. The constituent unique to the nucleus (except for small amounts in mitochondria and possibly in the endoplasmic reticulum) is DNA. Consequently, it seems logical to propose that DNA is the biochemical constituent most sensitive to the effect of irradiation.

Site of Lesions (Ionizing Radiation)

Tobleman and Cole compared the biological effects of electron beams that penetrate only one-tenth or one-half of the cell thickness to fully penetrating beams. The weaker beams were three to ten times more effective in killing the cells and causing DNA strand breaks than the stronger beams. This led the authors to suggest that radiosensitive sites are located close to the nuclear membrane [190].

Effect of Irradiation on Enzymes *in Vitro*

Before we provide evidence for the notion that DNA is the radiosensitive molecule, we must first reconcile this fact with *in vivo* and *in vitro* observations indicating that the metabolism of numerous biochemical constituents is altered by X-irradiation. The effects of radiation on some single-enzyme and multiple-enzyme systems will be briefly reviewed.

The literature contains many studies of inhibitions of enzymes irradiated *in vitro* [84, 93]. For example, variable doses were used to inhibit hyaluronidase. The amount of X-irradiation needed to inhibit an enzyme depended in part on the purity of the preparation. Catalase is inhibited by high doses of X-rays, and the sensitivity of the enzyme to X-rays depends on the pH (the enzyme is more sensitive in acid than in alkaline solutions), and on the solution's physical state (catalase is less sensitive in the frozen than in the liquid state).

Dale was among the first to investigate *in vitro* enzyme inhibition by X-irradiation [94, 95]. He irradiated crystalline or partially purified enzymes, such as carboxypeptidase, polyphenol oxidase, and amino acid oxidase, and established inhibition of the catalytic properties by X-irradiation. The doses Dale used were large and did not correspond to biological realities because the enzymes investigated were unusually radioresistant or because the partially purified enzyme preparation contained components that protected the enzyme from the effect of radiation.

If the biological significance of studies on enzymes irradiated *in vitro* is not always immediately obvious, the studies have yielded important information on the mode of action of enzymes. Of particular interest is the influence of absorption on enzyme sensitivity to radiation. A number of investigators have studied modifications in enzyme radiosensitivity, depending upon whether or not the enzyme is absorbed.

The effect of absorption varies according to: (1) the type of interphase that has been generated and (2) the enzyme—some are more sensitive, others less sensitive after absorption. Of course, the determining factor is the degree of dissipation of the excitation energy in the absorbent medium. Consider, for example, the effect of X-irradiation on DNase. Deoxyribonuclease has been irradiated in a solution of water, as a dry powder, in suspension after absorption on a resin, and as a dried enzyme-resin complex. The dehydrated DNase-resin complex is 10 times more sensitive than DNase in solution. In contrast, when the DNase-resin suspension is irradiated, the DNase is much more sensitive to radiation.

In 1949 Barron and Dickman [96, 97] established that a few hundred roentgens inhibited succinoxidase activity *in vitro*. Assuming that the effect was due to oxidation of SH groups, the authors protected the enzyme from radiation simply by adding glutathione to the incubation mixture. Although the *in vitro* results were of limited significance, they served as a working hypothesis for others who later succeeded in devising chemicals efficient in preventing radiation damage.

These inhibitory effects of the activities of "SH enzyme" were later largely confirmed by irradiating solutions of hexokinase, ATPase, phosphoglyceraldehyde dehydrogenase, urease, trypsin, and other enzymes. In all cases (except for phosphoglyceraldehyde dehydrogenase and urease) inhibition could be reversed by adding glutathione to the incubation mixture. Moreover, when parachloromercuric benzoate was in the incubation mixture during irradiation, activity could be restored later by adding glutathione. These findings led Barron to propose that the active SH groups were protected by the parachloromercuric benzoate.

In conclusion, many enzymes are inhibited by ionizing radiation, and the mechanism of inhibition is likely to vary depending upon the enzyme and the conditions of incubation.

Although in most cases it is not possible to describe in detail the molecular alterations in the irradiated enzyme, it is easy to imagine the various mechanisms that could be responsible for enzyme degradation after exposure to ionizing radiation. Through promoting the formation of free radicals, X-irradiation could oxidize a group essential to the catalytic performance of the enzyme—such as SH groups, hydroxyl radicals, or amino groups; free radicals could rupture hydrogen bonds or convert an SH to a tight SS bond. An interesting example is that of the effects of X-irradiation on the activity of aspartic transcarbamylase. The administration of kilo doses of X-irradiation to aspartic transcarbamylase interferes with the binding of both the substrate and the allosteric inhibitor. The catalytic site is three times more radiosensitive than the allosteric site. The loss of catalytic activity is due to breakdown of the enzyme molecules into smaller subunits.

The mode of action of X-rays on the enzymes *in vitro* will, of course, not be understood until the active center of the enzyme and the role of other molecular fractions indispensable to the catalytic effect are known.

Protein denaturation and enzymic inactivation by X-ray or γ radiation probably result in part from disturbances of the secondary and tertiary structures. The use of infrared spectroscopy and the determination of deuterium-exchange processes have shown that after γ-radiation the secondary structures of lysozyme, α-chymotrypsinogen and ribonuclease are altered. Ribonuclease irradiated in solution shows a progressive destruction of the α helical structure and loss of intramolecular hydrogen bonds. Studies by Marciani and Tolbert [192] suggested that in lysozyme there is, in addition to disruption of the α and β helical regions, a destruction of the hydrophobic regions which maintain the tertiary structure of the protein.

On the basis of these *in vitro* results, it is tempting to conclude that the biological action of X-rays is due to inhibition of enzyme activity, but this conclusion could be reached only if inhibition of enzyme activity could be demonstrated *in vivo*. The activities of a large number of enzymes have been studied in many animal tissues irradiated *in vivo*. The results can be summarized as follows: either the enzyme activity is not modified, or it is modified too late and must be considered an effect secondary to the initial irradiation injury.

The effect of ionizing irradiation on enzymes has been described in several reviews [98–100, 191]. Therefore, we shall only emphasize here several points relative to our discussion on the molecular pathology of irradiation. Only constitutive and not induced enzymes will be considered.

In contrast to what happens *in vitro*, irradiation *in vivo* has no effect on such enzymes as hexokinase or succinic dehydrogenase. Inhibition of lactic dehydrogenase but not of triose phosphate dehydrogenase has been described.

The activity of certain hydrolases—such as DNase, RNase, acid phosphatase, and β-glucuronidase—is increased after irradiation. This increase is not observed in all tissues, and the increase usually develops late after exposure. The mechanism of the enzyme increase is not clear. In some cases, release from particulate support (see below) is likely to take place; in others, the activation must be of a different origin.

The radiosensitivity of an enzyme varies from one species to the other and with the animals' stage of development. The administration of whole-body doses of X-irradiation to rodents interferes with the activity of liver catalase in mice, but not in rats. Hickman and Ashwell [101] have shown that the administration of 1000 R interferes with the activity of lactic dehydrogenase of mouse spleen in both the adult and the embryo, but the lactic dehydrogenase activity seems to be more sensitive in embryonic than in adult tissues. Whether this effect on the dehydrogenase is a direct one on the enzyme or secondary to other molecular alterations is not known.

Although revealing, the study of the effect of X-irradiation on enzymes is far from complete. First, the activities of a relatively small number of enzymes have been measured after irradiation. Secondly, the significance of the changes in activity that have been observed is difficult to evaluate in the absence of detailed knowledge of the different factors that regulate enzyme activity *in vivo*.

One means of gaining broader information on the effect of X-irradiation on enzymes is to study the effect of X-irradiation on the yields of the final product of multiple-enzyme pathways, for example, lactic acid, ATP, and glycogen.

Controversial results were obtained in studies of the effect of X-irradiation on glycogen production in liver. Whereas some investigators found an increase in glycogen levels, others found them to be decreased. It is not known whether irradiation affects glycogen synthesis or glycogen breakdown. Moreover, it is not clear whether changes in glycogen metabolism observed after irradiation are direct consequences of the irradiation or are secondary to other disturbances caused by the exposure. The administration of 500 to 2000 R to rats immediately reduces the glycogen level of liver, but is without effect on the glycogen level in testicle. Within 3 hours after irradiation liver glycogen levels increase, and this effect persists even if the liver or the hypophysis is shielded during exposure. Similarly, glycogen levels increase 24 hours after exposure in liver of guinea pigs irradiated with 1000 to 500 R, yet the liver glycogen decreases 6 to 8 days after exposure. No interference with glycogen synthesis and no correlation between glucose level in blood and glycogen levels in liver has been demonstrated.

The effects of X-rays on oxygen consumption and CO_2 elimination are insignificant with respect to the nature of the primary injury if one keeps in mind that relatively large doses are needed to affect these processes, and that the changes occur late after irradiation. The results can be summarized as follows: respiration of liver, kidney, heart, and brain obtained from animals irradiated with 10,000 to 20,000 R is somewhat decreased, but no effect is observed at lower doses. However, irradiation with as little as 400 R reduces respiration of thymus slices within an hour. A temporary decrease in respiration is also observed in irradiated unicellular structures. Dry barley seeds were irradiated and respiration measured during the first week of germination. No effect was observed with doses below 2500 R.

Massive doses of radiation are necessary to reduce respiration* in irradiated but otherwise intact animals. Oxygen consumption is, however, increased within 24 hours after exposure to irradiation. Oxygen consumption then returns to normal, but it increases again between 6 and 14 days after exposure. Because this increase in metabolism is too far removed from the moment of irradiation to be considered a primary effect, some have implicated the thyroid or TSH to explain these metabolic effects on oxygen consumption.

Using the sequential blocking technique described by Potter in 1951 [103], DuBois, Cochran, and Doull [104] and later Ord and Stocken [105] demonstrated that irradiation decreases the amount of citric acid that accumulates in thymus, bone marrow, intestinal, and pancreatic homogenates after a fluoroacetate block. These findings suggest that acetic acid biosynthesis is inhibited at a rate proportional to the dose of X-rays administered.

Such results are in agreement with the observations of Hevesy and Forssberg [106] who observed a reduction in CO_2 formation at the expense of radioactive glucose. But others have reported increased production of $^{14}CO_2$ in the bone marrow of irradiated animals. DuBois further observed that although citric acid synthesis was inhibited in a number of other tissues, it was increased in the liver of irradiated animals. In contrast to the female, the male rat does not accumulate citrate after treatment with fluoroacetate but citrate accumulates in the castrated male.

In conclusion, these experiments on citric acid accumulation suggest that irradiation affects citric acid accumulation indirectly and through hormones.

In 1952 Potter and Bethell [107] discovered that within 1 hour after 800 R of whole-body irradiation is administered, spleen mitochondria lose their ability to couple oxidation and phosphorylation. Van Bekkum [108] reported similar findings, although differences between the mitochondria of normal rats and the mitochondria of irradiated rats were small.

The effect of different dose levels at various times after exposure was further investigated by Scaife and Hill [109], who reported results similar to those of previous investigators. The interference with oxidative phosphorylation could not be prevented by prior administration of aminoethylisothiouronium (AET). A direct effect of irradiation on oxidative phosphorylation *in vitro* could not be demonstrated. John F. Thompson [110] studied the oxidative phosphorylation capacity of mitochondria prepared from livers of rats exposed for 4 hours to total whole-body doses of 1000 R. Thompson could detect no effect on oxidative phosphorylation using various substrates and different mitochondrial preparations. Alteration of oxi-

---

* Fructose-1,6-diphosphate accumulates in thymocytes irradiated with kilo doses of X-irradiation. This is believed to result from enhancement of the activity of phosphoglucokinase. There seems to be a correlation between the accumulation of fructose-1,6-diphosphate and the decrease in ATP, which is small below 4000 R but rises rapidly between 4000 and 32,000 R [102].

dative phosphorylation by X-irradiation is unquestionably an interesting finding. If the pathogenesis of the molecular injury were elucidated, our understanding of the relationship between ATP synthesis and subcellular death would be improved. Whether more information on the coupling mechanism would also emerge from such studies remains to be seen. In any event, it is difficult to define the position of uncoupling of oxidative phosphorylation in the sequence of biochemical lesions triggered by whole-body irradiation. Investigators do not know whether the alterations result from a direct or an indirect effect, or whether they occur early enough in the sequence of changes to cause cellular death or are simply a step toward it.

We have seen previously that Allfrey and Mirsky demonstrated the occurrence of oxidative phosphorylation in thymus nuclei. Creasy and Stocken [111] found that within 3 to 5 minutes, and surely within 1 hour after exposure to 100 R, nuclear oxidative phosphorylation in the thymus and the spleen was reduced 50%–80%. These findings seemed, however, to be restricted to the thymus, and Klouwen's studies [112] have indicated that nuclear oxidative phosphorylation in lymphosarcoma cells changes only after the administration of 1000 R, and then within 2 hours after exposure. There is no correlation between interference with ATP synthesis in the nucleus, DNA synthesis, and mitotic index. Nuclear ATP synthesis has never been observed in nuclei of tumors or of regenerating liver or other proliferating tissues. Klouwen and Betel [113] studied ATP synthesis *in vivo* using ^{32}P. The changes in specific activity of ^{32}P, ATP, and inorganic phosphate, isolated from nuclei and total thymus, indicated that at least part of the nuclear ATP is supplied by the cytoplasm.

It also remains to be established whether the effect of radiation on ATP synthesis in the nucleus is a direct one, or whether it results, for example, from DNase release. Moreover, as mentioned previously, DNA synthesis does not seem to be correlated with inhibition of nuclear ATP synthesis. In any event, delayed effects of X-irradiation would be difficult to explain in terms of reduction of nuclear ATP synthesis.

A increase in RNase activity was found 24 and 48 hours after the administration of 400–1000 R in a number of rat organs, but not in liver and kidney. The total increase of the enzymic activity was assumed to result from either removal of inhibitors or rupture of mitochondria. Although X-irradiation modifies the chemical properties and the permeability of the red cell membrane, the doses required far exceed doses that are lethal *in vivo*. Similar results were obtained with populations of lymphocytes [193].

Effect of X-Irradiation on DNA Synthesis

Once it was established that ^{32}P is readily incorporated in the nucleic acids of growing cells and that the rate of incorporation is related to the rate of cell proliferation, a number of investigators studied ^{32}P-incorporation into the nucleic acid of growing bacteria and mammalian cells after irradiating the cells *in vivo* or *in vitro*. Laboratories scattered on several continents all agreed that X-irradiation interferes with ^{32}P-incorporation into DNA of proliferating cells in plants, bacteria, and mammals [114–119].

Once pyrimidine precursors of nucleic acid became available, the findings made with ^{32}P were largely confirmed on a variety of tissues. When methods for separating DNA and RNA were developed, the effect of X-irradiation on the incorporation of precursor in each of the nucleic acids was studied separately.

Although results assembled in various laboratories on the incorporation of precursors into RNA were somewhat controversial, the results obtained on the incorporation of precursors into DNA were clear-cut. X-Irradiation interferes with the incorporation of precursors into DNA. We shall see later how the availability of methods for separating various types of RNA finally resolved the inconsistencies with respect to incorporation of precursors into RNA.

The effect of X-irradiation has been investigated in a great variety of proliferating cells, but all these experiments [117–119] cannot be described here. Interference with DNA synthesis is one, if not the most, important biological effect of radiation; therefore, the molecular alteration responsible for blocking DNA synthesis should be determined. We shall concentrate on the interference with DNA synthesis in mammalian tissues.

The most systematic studies on the molecular mechanism responsible for blocking DNA synthesis in mammalian cells has been pursued in regenerating liver and cells in culture. The radiosensitive cells of the body (the cells of the spleen, bone marrow, intestine, mucosa and skin) seem to be the most appropriate material for studying the effect of X-irradiation on DNA synthesis. Unfortunately, these organs contain a heterogeneous population of cells, many of which are at different stages of cell division.

Moreover, these tissues are often difficult to manipulate (*e.g.*, homogenization), so little is known of their biochemistry. As is pointed out in Chapter 15, although the liver contains a great variety of cells, after partial hepatectomy only the hepatic cells divide, and the metabolic steps that lead to DNA synthesis and cell division occur in synchrony in many cells. Consequently, regenerating liver provides a unique material to study the effects of X-irradiation on each of the steps of the sequence that culminates in DNA synthesis and cell division. Studies made in Kelly's and Holmes' [121] laboratories established that X-irradiation interferes with the incorporation of ^{32}P in DNA.

In the early 1950s we studied the effect of X-irradiation on DNA synthesis on 24-hour regenerating liver after orotic acid incorporation into DNA. The animals were partially hepatectomized; irradiated 6, 12, 18, and 24 hours after partial hepatectomy; injected with orotic acid 29 hours after operation; and killed 1 hour later. The effect on DNA synthesis was the same whenever the animals were irradiated. In fact, interference with DNA synthesis took place even if the livers were irradiated before partial hepatectomy. These findings led to the inescapable conclusion that the radiosensitive molecules were present in the cell at all times, even during interphase. There was some indication that the cell lost its sensitivity to radiation with respect to DNA synthesis 16 hours after irradiation, but these experiments were difficult to interpret because the time lapse between irradiation and sacrifice was not constant in controlled and irradiated animals.

It remained to be established which was the radiosensitive substance. Considering the mode of action of X-irradiation (formation of free radicals, excitation, ionization), one might expect that many, if not all, macromolecules would be damaged by X-irradiation. Nevertheless, Butler calculated that only one out of 10,000 protein molecules is likely to be damaged by X-irradiation at minimum lethal doses [122]. Moreover, the free radicals are short-lived, and many are likely to be trapped before they hit sensitive molecules. Finally, damage to all molecules probably is not functionally equivalent because most catalytic molecules, except those that are rate limiting, are available in excess of the cellular needs.

Clues as to the nature of the radiosensitive component in regenerating liver were obtained unexpectedly. X-Irradiation was found to interfere with the biosynthesis of enzymes and other proteins involved in the last steps of DNA synthesis. In addition, the incorporation of precursors is markedly reduced in the polydispersed portion of the nRNA, and orotic acid incorporation is reduced in 16-S cytoplasmic RNA—a population of cytoplasmic RNA that some researchers believe contains mRNA. Therefore, the sequence of DNA transcription and mRNA translation appears to be interrupted. Of course, direct demonstration of transcription of the DNA segment into a messenger for a specific protein and translation of that messenger into a specific polypeptide chain was not possible in liver. However, stimulation of amino acid incorporation into ribosomes with nRNA can be measured. Amino acid incorporation, when stimulated by regenerating liver RNA, was the same in ribosomes of irradiated and nonirradiated animals. Moreover, nRNA, whether it was obtained from irradiated or nonirradiated animals, on a weight basis, illicited the same stimulation of amino acid incorporation into ribosomes.

One other experiment was of considerable significance for the interpretation of the results. Again, irradiation of normal liver interferes with DNA synthesis in the regenerating liver if the animal is partially hepatectomized after irradiation. It is not likely that all the messengers for thymidylic kinase and cytidylic reductase are present in normal livers since these enzymes are never made in extensive amounts, especially not cytidylic reductase. Consequently, a direct effect of X-irradiation on the messenger seemed to be excluded. Among the macromolecules involved in the coding and transcription of proteins involved in the last steps of DNA synthesis in regenerating liver, only DNA appears to be present in liver before hepatectomy. Thus, the inescapable conclusion is that X-irradiation damages the DNA molecules and thereby interferes with their transcribing properties and possibly with their priming abilities for new DNA synthesis. Studies by Markov et al. confirmed that X-radiation interferes with the biosynthesis of messenger RNA in regenerating liver and led the authors to conclude that ionizing radiation does not suppress transcription per se, but interferes with gene expression [194].

Direct damage to the DNA molecule was demonstrated and will be discussed in another section.

Even if DNA molecules are the primary site of radiation injury, it remains to be explained how damage, which is likely to involve all DNA molecules, is ultimately expressed selectively—mainly through interference with transcription of the mRNA of proteins involved in the last steps of DNA synthesis. The solution to this problem can best be understood if one first questions the difference between the DNA which codes for the proteins involved in the last steps of DNA synthesis and all other DNA molecules in liver. DNA is repressed in normal liver (not transcribed) and becomes derepressed (transcribed) in regenerating liver. Consequently, the repressed DNA must be more sensitive to X-irradiation than derepressed DNA. Some experiments from our laboratory [119] and many previous observations made in others support this conclusion.

Repressed DNA could be more radiosensitive than derepressed DNA for many reasons. For example, the presence of the repressor could radiosensitize the DNA by facilitating cross-link formation. It is also possible that all DNA is damaged but that derepressed DNA is rapidly repaired while the presence of the repressor or other proteins prevents repair (see Fig. 12-13).

The studies of Pederson and Robbins [195] may be relevant to the mechanism of restriction of DNA repair. These investigators have measured the binding of [^{3}H]actinomycin to the chromatin of synchronized HeLa cells and found against all expectations that the binding capacity decreases progressively during the S and G2 phases and mitosis. There are stages when one would expect the chromatin to be expanded and DNA to be more accessible to actinomycin than during interphase when one expects the chromatin to be condensed.

The finding that chlorambucil treatment results in the progressive removal of histones from chromatin, as a result of inhibition of histone synthesis, may explain the results of Pederson and Robbins. Thus, the effects of both X-irradiation and actinomycin suggest that the DNA of the interphase cell is more susceptible to damage. Whether this is the case because of interference with DNA repair remains to be shown. The histones are later replaced by nonhistone proteins.

It is not known at what stage of the process of DNA synthesis X-irradiation exerts its blocking effect

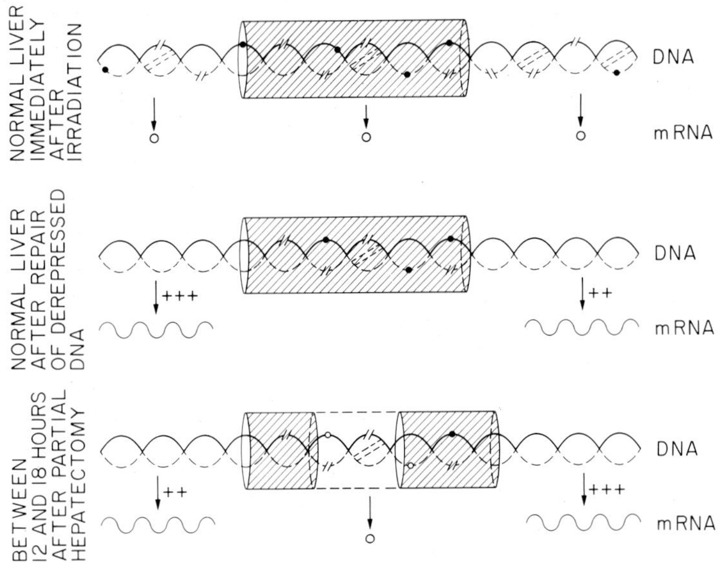

Fig. 12-13. Events after irradiation. The DNA is damaged immediately after irradiation. The damage includes strand breaks (⫽) base distortions (●), and possibly cross-links (⩵). Shortly after irradiation is terminated, derepressed DNA is repaired but repressed DNA is not. Consequently when the DNA coding for protein indispensable for DNA synthesis is called upon to become derepressed, it either remains repressed or as indicated in the graph is derepressed but not transcribed

on DNA synthesis. If one accepts modern views that chromosomes are made of multiple replicating units (replicons, see below) and that there are at least three steps in DNA synthesis (initiation, chain growth and termination), radioautographic studies suggest that the step sensitive to ionizing radiation is the initiation step rather than chain growth [196].

Results similar to those obtained in liver stimulated to proliferate after partial hepatectomy were obtained when the effect of X-irradiation was studied on organs with normally low or no proliferative activity that were stimulated to proliferate. Such systems include kidneys stimulated to grow after unilateral nephrectomy [123], the uterus stimulated to proliferate after the administration of estrogens [124], and lymphocytes stimulated by phytohemagglutinin [125]. In all cases, irradiation during G0 interferes with DNA synthesis after application of the proliferative stimulus. These findings suggest that in nonproliferative organs of intact mammals, DNA coding for the biosynthesis of proteins involved in DNA synthesis is repressed during interphase. The early observations on the effects of X-irradiation on antibody formation might well be explainable in a similar fashion [126]. Formation of antibodies is blocked if irradiation precedes the administration of antigen, and antibody formation continues if irradiation follows the administration of antigen.

Studies by Pollard and Davis [127] in which radiation was applied before and after induction of β-galactosidase in special strains of bacteria confirmed the findings made in the mammalian system, except for the fact that much larger doses of irradiation are needed to affect transcription in bacteria than in the mammalian system. Thus, radiation applied before induction interferes with galactosidase synthesis, whereas after induction it has no or little effect on the appearance of the enzyme. Setlow and coworkers made similar observations in UV-irradiated bacteria.

Studies by Stryckmans and associates [128] have shown that the lymphocytes of leukemic patients submitted to extracorporeal radiation were more radioresistant than normal lymphocytes. The radioresistance has been linked to increased turnover of the lymphocyte. These results illustrate the relevance of our hypothesis to radiotherapy. The survival of lymphocytes could depend on constant replacement of one or more species of RNA. That RNA could be coded for on a DNA which is alternately repressed and derepressed. If the periods of derepression are short compared to those of repression, the lymphocytes would obviously be highly radiosensitive. If the mechanism controlling repression were lost causing the period of repression to be shortened or inhibiting production of repressors, the lymphocytes would be more radioresistant. Interestingly, increased resistance of lymphocytes obtained from patients with chronic lymphocytic leukemia has been observed, and the turnover of the messenger is increased in the leukemic cells. The increased turnover could result from acceleration of transcription, which could be caused by modification in the regulation of repression and derepression in the leukemic lymphocyte [128].

Effect of X-Irradiation on Mitosis

Because of the special radiosensitivity of rapidly growing tissue, the effects of radiation on cell division were investigated from the beginning of radiation biology and led in 1906 to the enunciation of the law of Bergonié and Tribondeau.

The law states that the effect of radiation on cells increases in intensity with the proliferative capacity of the cells and with their potential to divide during their life span; furthermore, the effect of radiation is inversely related to the cells' degree of differentiation.

Clearly, ionizing radiation interferes with cell reproduction because many of the irradiated cells are killed, but a direct effect on the mitotic process also has been observed. Mitosis can be blocked with sublethal doses of X-irradiation.

If cells present different degrees of sensitivity to radiation depending upon their stage in the DNA-synthesizing and mitotic cycles,* then cell population kinetics is important in determining the responses of normal and malignant tissues to irradiation.

Cell population kinetics refers to the sequence of changes in the composition or size of the cell population as a result of growth, differentiation, aging, or recovery from an insult. Thus, the life span of a cell can be divided into various cycles, and all the cells that are in a given cycle belong to the same so-called compartment. The compartment concept is a functional and not an anatomical one. For example, the bone marrow dividing and undividing cells are mixed anatomically, but these cells can be separated into a dividing and an undividing compartment on a functional basis.

The key molecular event in cell division is DNA synthesis, usually referred to as S. It is preceded by a G1, or presynthetic, period and a G2, or postsynthetic, period. G2 is followed by mitosis. Between the mitotic time and the G1 of the next cycle, a period referred as G0 may exist. The length of G0 varies depending upon the tissue—it is minimal in rapidly dividing cells, of intermediate length in such apparently static tissues as normal liver, kidneys, etc. (see Fig. 12-14), and lasts for the life of the individual in brain cells.

To understand the importance of cell population kinetics in radiation biology, consider a simple situation in which all stages—G0, G1, G2, and M—are sensitive to radiation except the S-phase. Obviously, the number of cells that will be damaged by radiation will depend on the number of cells that have entered S. In the absence of any special stimulus, the number of cells that will be in the S state at a given time

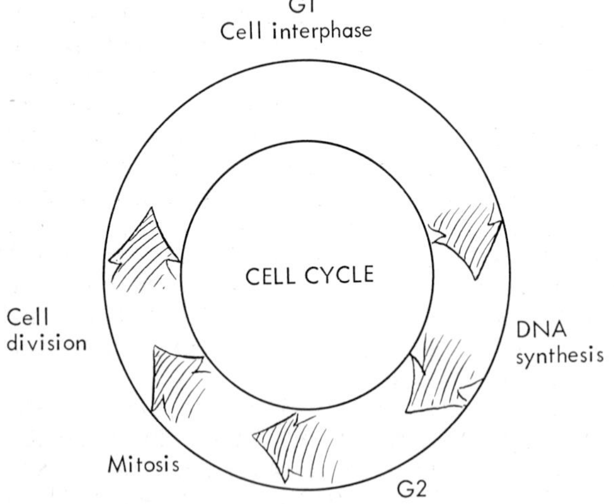

Fig. 12-14. The cell cycle

* A critical technical step in the development of cellular radiation biology was the development by Puck, Marcus, and Cieciura in 1956 of a plating technique, which permitted accurate determination of the proliferative capacity of mammalian cells.

will depend on the length of G0+G1—G2+M and be directly proportional to the duration of S. For each type of cell cultured, this method made it possible: (1) to measure the dose response in terms of cellular proliferation, and (2) to plot on a logarithmic scale the capacity for clone formation versus the dose on the linear scale.

Several laboratories have studied the relative cellular radiosensitivities as a function of the various stages of the cell cycle. Sinclair [129] evaluated some of these investigations and stated that several radiation responses are modified depending upon the position of the cell in the generation cycle.

Sinclair investigated three of these responses: survival, division delay, and modification of DNA synthesis in mammalian cell lines synchronized *in vitro*. In Chinese hamsters with long G1, the survival varies with the position of the cell in the generation cycle in the following fashion. G1 can be divided into two stages—an early one, which is radioresistant, and a later one, which is radiosensitive. The S period is the least sensitive, while the G2 period is the most sensitive.

X-Irradiation also induces mitotic delay in culture cells. The pattern of division delay depends upon the position of the cell in its generation cycle during irradiation. The delay is maximal when the cells are irradiated during the S period, and shortest when the cells are irradiated in G1. The delay is still considerable for cells irradiated during mitosis and declines when the cells are irradiated in G2. No definitive molecular explanation is available for these complex events; however, any attempt to explain radiation damage on a molecular basis must explain selective radiosensitivity during the different stages of the cell cycle.

Irradiation of culture cells during periods G1 and G2 of the generation cycle does not affect DNA synthesis markedly. But when the irradiation occurs during the S period, it reduces the rate of DNA synthesis without, however, modifying the total amount of DNA synthesized. Such findings are in agreement with those made in regenerating liver, and they suggest that the DNA coding for the proteins involved in the biosynthesis of DNA is derepressed during the entire cycle except during G0. The slowing down of DNA synthesis when irradiation is administered during the S period is likely to result from an alteration of replication or transcription of the irradiated DNA.

The molecular mechanism responsible for the changes in radiosensitivity during the cell cycle is not known. Dewey and his associates [197, 198] have measured the radiosensitivity of Chinese hamster Don cells in preparations synchronized during various stages of the cell cycle by removing cells in metaphase. Radiosensitivity was measured by determining the incidence of chromosomal aberrations. The study established that the cells in S phase are 2.6 times less sensitive than the cells in mitosis. They further established that the decrease in radiosensitivity correlates with the dispersion of chromatin which was determined by electron microscopy. Although the findings agree with those of Pederson and Robbins, they do, however, not discriminate between two possible interpretations. Either the tightness of the chromatin facilitates clusters of injuries to DNA and cross-links between the DNA and proteins, or the dispersion of chromatin facilitates DNA repair.

Effect on Chromosomes

X-Irradiation may cause chromosome breaks or abnormal distribution of chromosomes to daughter cells after telophase. Chromosome breaks may be repaired integrally, or they may result in a number of chromosomal anomalies of the various types discussed in Chapter 1.

The consequence of these anomalies is either cellular death or mutation, and the ultimate effect will, of course, vary depending upon whether the mutation affects a somatic or a germ cell (see Chapter 3).

Irradiation of DNA *in Vitro*

Because it is suspected that most, if not all, of the histological effects of ionizing radiation result from damage inflicted to DNA, the results of *in vitro* irradiation of dry DNA or DNA in aqueous solution have been extensively investigated [130–135, 199].*

When the quantum hits DNA in solution, it generates free radicals in the DNA and in the medium. The free radicals in the medium may in turn react with the DNA.

The free radicals are short lived, but their appearance leads to the development of more stable chemical alterations. Studies on the effect of ionizing radiation on DNA *in vitro* have been concerned with both the free radicals formed in nucleic acid and the stable chemical changes.

Much progress has been made in the study of free radicals, thanks to the development of ESR and pulse radiolysis. As a result, $H^{\bullet}$ and $OH^{\bullet}$ attacks on bases, pentose sugars, and nucleic acid are reasonably well understood [136]. Thus, in nucleic acid, radicals formed by $H^{\bullet}$ attacks result from the addition of $H^{\bullet}$ to the bases and from the abstraction of hydrogen from the pentose sugar; similarly, $OH^{\bullet}$ adds to the bases and abstracts hydrogen from pentoses to give organic free radicals.

The radicals formed by direct absorption of radiation by the nucleic acid are, however, not as well known, in part because the free radical spectrum that emerges after irradiation of DNA is not the same as that which is obtained by irradiating the constituents. Electron-spin resonance spectra have revealed that free radicals are formed in the irradiated DNA, but for most radicals it is not known what type is formed [133–135].

Several investigators have sought to identify the intermediate species that are formed before the preradical [135]. In the beginning of this chapter, we saw that electromagnetic waves (light, UV, or X-ray) may be transmitted, refracted, scattered, or absorbed.

Chemical changes are produced by absorbed quanta. When any molecule absorbs a quantum of light, it can lose that excess energy in a number of processes, some of which are considered to be physical (quenching, fluorescence, phosphorescence, internal conversion) and others chemical (radical and nonradical) reactions. When one of the DNA bases absorbs a quantum of energy, hν, a π or regular electron is promoted to an unfilled π orbital without changing the direction of its spin. Under those circumstances, only paired electrons are present, all spins cancel, and an excited singlet state develops.

If the excited state is quenched by other molecules, the energy of excitation is dissipated in a radiationless process. In fluorescence, the transition from the excited to the base state is accompanied by emission of radiation. Some excited single states decay to a metastable triplet state.* In this case, the electron in the excited orbital flips its spin.

The passage from one electronic species (singlet) to another (triplet) is referred to as intersystem crossing. The triplet state has two paired electrons in the excited orbital.

The interaction of the free radicals produced by radiolysis in presence of oxygen leads to the formation of stable radiation products in the purine and pyrimidine bases. Most of the studies have been directed at the identification of the radiation products of thymine. Téoule and Cadet [200] separated 21 different thymine products by paper chromatography. All products have not been identified, but they include hydroxyperoxide, pyruvyl urea, hydroxybarbutiric acid and thymine glycols. Among thymine radiation products the hydroxyperoxides have received most of the investigators' attention. The hydroxyperoxides are formed by the saturation of the pyrimidine 5–6 double bond. Scholes et al. [201] have proposed a mechanism for their formation *in vitro*. In their scheme $OH^{\bullet}$ radicals are added to C_5 and C_6 of the pyrimidine ring, molecular oxygen reacts rapidly with the thymine $OH^{\bullet}$ radical to ultimately yield the hydroxyhydroperoxide (Fig. 12-15). Hariharan and Cerutti [202] have demonstrated that hydroperoxides of thymine are formed in DNA irradiated *in vivo*.

A sensitive assay was developed to measure 6-hydroxy-5-hydroxy-5-6 dihydrothymine by reduction with sodium bromide to yield urea and 2 methyl glycerol. Thus, if thymine labeled in the methyl group

* The effects of ionizing radiation of DNA irradiated *in vitro* vary considerably depending upon the conditions of irradiation. One modulating factor is the concentration of the irradiated DNA. As pointed out, the alteration of DNA molecules may result from the formation of free radicals in water or from direct hits of the molecules. Obviously, the incidence of direct hits increases with the concentration of DNA.

* The multiplicity of an electronic species is given by the formula $2S+1$, in which S is the total electron spin. In the singlet state, $S=0$; in the triplet state, the excited level includes two electrons with a parallel spin of $^1/_2$. Thus, $S=^1/_2+^1/_2=1$, and the multiplicity of the state $=2\times1+1=3$.

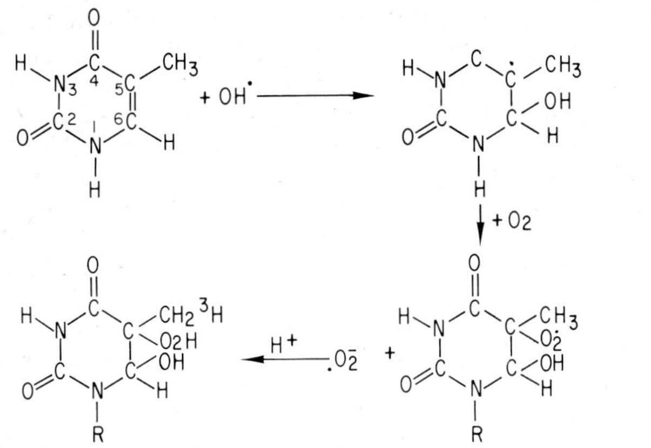

Fig. 12-15. Hydroxyhydroperoxide formed from thymine in presence of oxygen

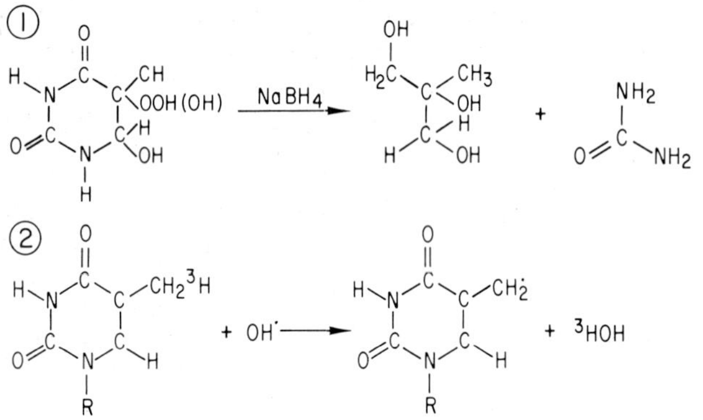

Fig. 12-16. *1* Reduction of thymine radiolysis product with sodium borohydride. *2* Exchange of ^3H of thymidine methyl group with H_2O (after Hariharan and Cerutti)

is used, the product of the reduction is 2 methyl glycerine, also labeled in the methyl group.

The loss of hydrogen from the methyl group can also be measured by using thymine labeled with tritium in the methyl group. The methyl hydrogen reacts with the OH$^\bullet$ radical yielding tritiated water, and ultimately 5-hydroxymethyluracyl and 5-hydroperoxymethyluracyl are formed from the thymine radical (see Fig. 12-16). The concentration of the base damage is modulated by the macromolecular association of DNA. Double-stranded DNA is less sensitive than single-stranded. This is because the bases are sterically protected from the free radical attack inside the double helix.

Thus, Swinehart and his associates [203] have studied the production of γ ray induced thymine damage, 6 hydroxy or hydroperoxy-5,8-dihydrothymine and thymine demethylation, in mononucleotide mixtures and single and double stranded DNA, and Ward and Urist [204] have studied the destruction of adenine in polyriboadenylic acid. Both groups found that the sensitivity of the bases to γ radiation was greater in single than in double stranded DNA, indicating that the structure of the double helix protects the DNA.

Roti Roti et al. [205] have studied the effects of γ radiation on four different preparations of chromatin: native chromatin, reconstituted chromatin, reconstituted DNA histone complexes and reconstituted nonchromosomal protein DNA complexes. They measured induced formation of tritiated water from methyl [^{3}H]thymine to evaluate the effect of irradiation of the thymine methyl group and the formation of 5-hydroxy-6-hydroxy peroxide hydrothymine. The results indicated that (1) chromosomal proteins shield DNA bases from free radical attack triggered by γ radiation; (2) the amount of base damage is the same whether chromatin is native or reconstituted; (3) partially reconstituted DNA, whether it be with histones or nonhistone protein, is much more sensitive to base damage than native or totally reconstituted chromatin; (4) the methyl group of thymine is more sensitive to γ radiation than the thymine ring.

These important observations confirm a long lasting suspicion that chromatin shields DNA. They do, however, not explain why low doses of γ radiation can cause such severe damage to intact cells, while much higher doses are needed to cause damage in purified DNA. The fact that the thymine methyl group is more sensitive to irradiation than the thymine ring is not surprising. In the DNA double helix the thymine ring is intercalated toward the helical center and therefore more effectively protected by the nucleoprotein. In contrast, the methyl group sticks out at the periphery of the helix and therefore is believed not to be shielded as effectively by nucleoproteins.

Although it is likely that other base products are formed in irradiated DNA, little has been done to identify them. Cytosine forms stable peroxide at low pH through the attack of the C_5, C_6 double bond by OH$^\bullet$ radicals. Adenine OH$^\bullet$ adducts are also believed to be formed, but they are believed to revert to adenine. Only a small number of the OH$^\bullet$ radicals are believed to react with the sugar moiety.

Summers and Szybalski [137] devised a method for scoring single-strand breaks in polydispersed DNA samples. DNA in which the two complementary strands have been cross-linked with mitomycin or with nitrous acid becomes resistant to heat denaturation. Thus, when the cross-linked DNA is heated, a hyperchromic effect is observed. But upon cooling, the DNA renatures and bands in cesium chloride exactly as it did before being heated. If such polydispersed cross-linked DNA includes single-strand breaks, strand fragments will fall out as the DNA is temperature denatured, and these fragments can be separated by sedimentation from the remaining part of the molecules.

In conclusion, if it can be proven that the primary injury of X-irradiation affects DNA molecules, the following sequence of events can be assumed to occur. The quantum of energy, $h\nu$, may excite the DNA directly or excite it indirectly through the formation of preradicals generated through water radiolysis. The excited state in the DNA molecule may yield a stable photoproduct, or it may give birth to a short-lived free radical, which in turn yields a stable photoproduct. The stable photoproduct is responsible for the biological effects of irradiation.

Effects of Ionizing Irradiation on DNA *in Vivo*

Identified damage to DNA molecules *in vitro* includes base alterations and strand breaks. Both types of lesions have now been shown to occur *in vivo*. We have already mentioned that the formation of thymine adducts was demonstrated in DNA of irradiated cells.

Dalrymple et al. have shown that the ability of X-irradiated DNA to compete in DNA:DNA hybridization is reduced, indicating that the X-irradiated DNA is incapable of recognizing complementary regions on the nonirradiated DNA. This may result from alteration of bases or destruction of the sugar backbone [206]. Similar findings were made by Tomura et al. [207]. However, large doses of irradiation were needed and no alteration in DNA:DNA reassociation was observed when the DNA was extracted from liver of irradiated animals. The findings suggest that either the base alteration *in vivo* is to sparce to be detected by DNA:DNA reassociation or is rapidly repaired.

We have already seen that Hariharan and Cerutti provided direct evidence for the formation of thymine hydroxyperoxides in DNA of irradiated cells in culture.

The irradiation of DNA *in vitro* leads to a decrease in viscosity which was believed to be associated with a reduction of molecular weight. Several different techniques including enzymic treatment of the DNA and sedimentation on alkaline sucrose have revealed that single-strand breaks occur in DNA irradiated *in vitro*.

Studier [138] developed the alkaline sucrose methods for studying strand breaks. In neutral media, single-strand breaks are not readily detectable because they do not alter the molecular weight of the DNA significantly. Nevertheless, they can be detected if the DNA is sedimented on a mild alkaline sucrose gradient. The alkaline milieu separates the two strands and permits detection of the components with lower molecular weights. Single- and double-strand breaks can be differentiated by comparing results of centrifugation in alkaline sucrose with results obtained in neutral sucrose.

During preparation from bacteria, the DNA fiber is subjected to shear, which could cause more breaks than are produced by X-irradiation. To avoid shear, bacterial cells are gently layered on top of either alkaline or neutral sucrose, and the DNA is allowed to sediment in the ultracentrifuge.

Freifelder [139] studied the relationship between strand breaks and viral survival after X-irradiation. After studying the incidence of single- and double-strand breaks in several phages, Freifelder concluded that inactivation results almost entirely from the production of strand breaks. For T4, T5, T7 double-strand breaks accounted for about half of the killing.

Williams and McGrath [140] gave fixed doses of X-rays to *E. coli* and showed that X-irradiation causes single-strand breaks, which are repaired during the 40 minutes of postirradiation incubation. Kaplan [141] further established that double-strand breaks are not repaired and are probably responsible for cellular death. Strand breaks will be considered further in the discussion of DNA repair after X-irradiation.

The biological significance of the formation of single-strand breaks is debatable. By irradiating cells in presence of various concentrations of oxygen, Johansen et al. [208] found that oxygen renders the DNA 16-fold more sensitive to strand breaks without a corresponding increase in lethality.

DNA extracted from the liver of irradiated rats does not contain single-strand breaks, suggesting that either single-strand breaks do not occur in organs of irradiated animals, or that they are repaired within a few minutes. After irradiation a low molecular weight double-stranded DNA appears suggesting that X-irradiation leads to double-strand breaks. The incidence of double-strand breaks is dose dependent and it is not altered even a week after irradiation, suggesting that at least in the interphase cell the double-strand breaks are not repaired. A mechanism for the formation of such strand breaks has been proposed [209].

The molecular alterations associated with the formation of single-strand breaks in DNA exposed to ionizing radiation are not known. A direct break at the 3′ hydroxyl 5′ phosphoryl bond has been excluded by some. There is evidence that some of the deoxyribose moieties are destroyed at least with large doses of irradiation and that base alterations occur after irradiation with ionizing radiation *in vitro*. These lesions are excised as short nucleotide strands. The lesion to the deoxyribose moiety leads to the formation of a monoaldehyde-like material. Payes labeled the aldehyde with NaB^3H_4 and traced the release of the altered deoxyribose by a partially purified nuclease. The enzyme requires calcium and is inhibited by Ca^{++} and PCMB [210].

It has been objected that the formation of the monoaldehyde is not associated with strand breaks, but occurs at sites where damaged bases have been released. Kapp and Smith [211, 212] have shown that all strand breaks have a 3′-PO_4 terminus; other experiments have yielded 90% of breaks with 5′ PO_4 termini. It is also debated whether the strand breaks are directly produced by irradiation. There is evidence that ionizing radiation produces alkali labile bonds. Irradiation in presence of oxygen rather than nitrogen increases the incidence of alkali-sensitive bonds.

In any event the incidence of strand breaks varies with the level of oxygenation. It is generally assumed that it is due to differences in the amounts of free radical formed. The possibility that the difference in radiosensitivity between oxygenated and anoxemic cells results from differences in ability to repair damage has been eliminated by rapid irradiation of *E. coli* (100 milliseconds 4 MeV electrons) in presence and absence of oxygen [213].

Time-lapse cinematography of HeLa cells irradiated with 500 R have established that all cells can complete a second round of mitosis and the generation time is the same as for unirradiated cells. However, increasing fractions of the irradiated cell population fail to divide in the next generation. The first round of mitosis after irradiation is, however, abnormal in that the amount of DNA synthesized during the S phase is 30 to 40% below normal. Hopwood [214] has also proposed that the interference with DNA synthesis results from damage to the DNA itself. Potential radiation damage includes single and double-strand breaks, base damage, hydroperoxide formation and cross-linking. Among these, single and double-strand breaks and the formation of hydroperoxides have been demonstrated to occur *in vivo*. Single-strand breaks are very rapidly repaired (within a few minutes after irradiation), but double-strand breaks persist for at least a week [209] and therefore may form the basis for the interference with DNA synthesis. Indeed, if double-strand breaks occur, they would disrupt the replicating unit and initiation of DNA synthesis might be blocked.

Repair of X-Ray Damage in Mammalian Cells

In 1966 Kimball [142] showed that the incidence of mutation (lethal or slow growth) in paramecium differed depending upon the mode of irradiation. The highest incidence was obtained when single large doses were administered. The incidence was lowest when the same dose was fractionated and the time elapsing between each fraction was greatest. The results were interpreted to mean that between the administration of the dose fractions, sensitive molecules had an opportunity to be repaired. Consequently, the mutations caused by irradiation were eliminated. This potential for repair was demonstrated for X-irradiation, γ-radiation, UV radiation, and the administration of α-particles and alkylating agents. Dose rate effects on mice spermatogonia and oocytes also led to the conclusion that repair mechanisms must exist in mammalian systems.

The most convincing indication that repair occurs in mammalian tissue came from the remarkable studies of Elkind and Sutton [143], who compared the effects of single and fractionated doses of irradiation on cells in tissue culture. In Elkind and Sutton's experiments, Chinese hamster cells were irradiated in two exposures separated by various intervals. The survival increased with the time interval between the two doses; survival was maximal when that interval was 1 hour. There are at least two possible explanations for these results. One is that all cells are equally sensitive; some are repaired, and others are not. Then a molecular mechanism of repair must be postulated. The other explanation is that at the time of exposure the cells presented different degrees of sensitivity to radiation. The difference in sensitivity could depend on the stage reached in the DNA-synthesizing cycle. Inasmuch as the cell population used in these experiments was not synchronized, restoration probably was the consequence of a combination of molecular repair and differences in sensitivity.

The studies of Elkind and Sutton did not determine whether the changes in survival resulted from repair or from selective radiosensitivity of the cell due to its stage in maturation (G1, S, G2). Using the two dose fractionation technique, Sinclair and Morton [144] were able to distinguish recovery after the administration of X-irradiation to HeLa cell from changing response resulting from varying cell age. Recovery (with respect to survival) was quite definite for cells in S, but whether it occurs when irradiation is administered during other stages of the cell cycle was not determined.

Similarly, Dewey and Humphrey [145] studied chromosomal restitution of radiation damage in fibroblasts and demonstrated that restitution occurred over a period of 2 to 3 hours when the cells were irradiated in both S and G1 phases, although no clear-cut recovery could be demonstrated for cells irradiated in the G2 phase.

Pettijohn and Hanawalt's [36] demonstration that UV irradiation of bacteria was followed by non-semiconservative replication of segments of the DNA strand greatly enhanced our understanding of repair of UV damage in bacteria. Painter and Cleaver [146] were the first to use a modification of that technique to demonstrate non-semiconservative DNA synthesis in HeLa cells. The dose needed to demonstrate repair replication, however, far exceeds lethal doses. More recently Painter and Cleaver were able to correlate this form of unscheduled DNA synthesis with the incidence of repair from UV or X-irradiation. A notable exception to this repair is namely that of the skin of patients with xeroderma pigmentosum, in which there is no repair and no unscheduled DNA synthesis.

The factors modifying repair have been investigated in several laboratories. Phillips and Tolmach [147] have irradiated synchronous populations of HeLa S3 cells with 300 and 600 rads. Such doses do not cause cell death but are potentially lethal in that further administration of fluorodeoxyuridine, hydroxyurea, or deoxyadenosine and postirradiation incubation of these cells at 29° C decrease the fraction of surviving cells. When administered alone, none of the postirradiation treatments affects the viability of the cell. The postirradiation treatments are administered during G1, and no time during G1 is more sensitive than any other. However, when the various treatments described above are administered 5 hours after irradiation, the irradiated cells lose their sensitivity to the treatment. A somewhat unexpected observation is that cycloheximide increases cell survival when administered postirradiation. To explain the effects of the DNA inhibitors, it was postulated that repair involves DNA synthesis and that inhibition by DNA inhibitors resulted from interferences with the repair mechanism.

The effect of cycloheximide has been interpreted to result from protection of the repair mechanism as a consequence of selective inhibition of protein synthesis. Thus, cycloheximide might interfere with the biosynthesis of some proteins but not with that of others. Conflicting results have been obtained by

Djordjevic and Kim [148], who studied the effects of hydroxyurea and puromycin on the modification of the radiation response of synchronized populations of HeLa cells.

Cleaver [149] further established that compounds which prevent the formation of DNA precursors inhibit semiconservative replication but do not interfere with repair replication. In contrast, compounds that bind to the DNA inhibit both semiconservative and repair replication. Repair seems to depend further upon metabolic activity since iodoacetate, a glycolysis inhibitor, and cycloheximide, an inhibitor of protein synthesis, inhibit both semiconservative and repair replication. Thus, the recovery period after irradiation damage cannot be explained by interference with the repair mechanism.

These results are of considerable significance because they shed some light on the molecular mechanism of repair in mammalian tissue. The findings suggest that the nucleotide pool is not rate-limiting, that the enzyme is present and active even when semiconservative DNA synthesis does not take place, and that binding between enzyme and DNA—and possibly uncoiling of DNA—is needed for repair in mammalian tissue. Moreover, the fact that cycloheximide inhibits both semiconservative and non-semiconservative DNA synthesis suggests that new protein synthesis (not likely to be the repair enzyme) is needed for molecular repair. Whether the needed protein is the same in semiconservative and repair DNA synthesis cannot be predicted.

Hariharan and Cerutti have attempted to investigate the molecular mechanism of DNA repair in DNA of irradiated *E. coli*. They were concerned with the 5,6-dihydroxy-dihydrothymine products which constitute major products of γ induced lesions *in vivo* and *in vitro*.

They used poly A-T as a substrate to avoid mismatching of the bases or looped-out regions during renaturation and to reduce the incidence of lesions involving other bases. The substrate was incubated with a crude enzyme preparation of *E. coli*. The result suggested that the altered bases were excised. However, the details of the mechanism of excision will remain unknown until the enzymes responsible for the excision are purified [215].

Tomura and Van Lancker have demonstrated that X-irradiated DNA is a susceptible substrate for a purified mammalian repair endonuclease and that treatment with the endonuclease restores the priming ability of the DNA for DNA polymerase. These findings suggest that damaged bases are excised [216].

Dalrymple and his associates [150] studied the effect of 2,4-dinitrophenol on the repair of irradiated L cells. The radiosensitivity of L cells cultivated in the presence of DNA was lower than that of cells grown in normal culture media. Investigation of the repair component indicated that it was not modified by DNP, even though almost all ATP and macromolecular synthesis had ceased. Such findings led Dalrymple to conclude that repair processes occur in spite of a marked block in macromolecular synthesis or interference with the bioenergetic pathway. Thus, these investigators suggested that before exposure to irradiation, a repair mechanism exists as a "cork spring" which is autocatalytically released after the injury.

Polynucleotide ligases close breaks with 3′ OH and 5′-PO_4 termini. Dalrymple and his associates have suggested that X-irradiation (1000 R) produces DNA breaks in mouse liver and L cells. The breaks are of the 5′-PO_4 termini type and are repairable *in vitro* by polynucleotide ligase [150]. These findings, however, conflict with previous studies made by K. Smith in bacteria. Moreover, as we mentioned before it seems unlikely that X-irradiation would produce only breaks yielding 5′-PO_4 termini, and it cannot be excluded that the breaks detected by Dalrymple are not the direct result of radiation, but are a step in the repair process.

Since polynucleotide ligase requires ATP for activity, it is not surprising that complete repair of single-strand breaks or excision repair requires ATP. Masker and Hanawalt [217] and Hadden et al. [218] using either *E. coli* poly A mutants made permeable to deoxynucleotide triphosphates with toluene or frozen and thawed *B. subtilis* have established that DNA repair is ATP dependent [219].

Burrell et al. [220] have investigated the repair of double-strand breaks in DNA of X-irradiated *Micrococcus radiodurans*, a radioresistant bacteria. These bacteria were found to be able to repair a great number of double-strand breaks and the process involves attachment of DNA to the cell membrane.

Wolff and Scott [151] have studied repair of chromosome breaks in *Vicia faba*, in hamster cells, and in patients with xeroderma pigmentosum. Chromosomal repair took place in the absence of unscheduled DNA synthesis, which led the authors to conclude that chromosomal repair after X-irradiation does not involve the dark repair mechanism.

Studies in adult animals have shown that small fractions of the initial injury caused by irradiation are not repaired. Furthermore, irreparable damage after exposure of the fetus is considerably greater than that observed in a similarly exposed mature animal. The potentialities of many of the fetal cells often remain unexpressed in the phenotype until days or weeks after birth. Although many different mechanisms may work separately or synergically to bring about differentiation, derepression of repressed DNA is likely to be one of them. If the repressed DNA irradiated *in utero* is not repaired, harmonious differentiation of all cells is impossible, and dysfunction of cells, organs, and entire organisms may take place. It is not surprising, therefore, that the incidence of irreparable injuries would be greater after irradiation *in utero* [152].

Conclusion

Although much is known of the mechanism of absorption of ionizing radiation in biological matter and of the conversion of radiant energy into chemical energy, little is known of the actual chemical alterations that are responsible for the biological effect of radiation.

Therefore, any attempt to organize existing knowledge into a pathogenic scheme is likely to be ephemerous; still, such efforts help to organize our thoughts about the mechanism of action of ionizing radiation.

Clearly, free radicals must be generated in all parts of the cell and many molecules must be altered, but damage to DNA molecules appears to be one change that is responsible for the various manifestations of cellular injury observed after the administration of ionizing radiation.

The changes in the DNA molecule include single- and double-strand breaks, base alterations, and possibly cross-links. These molecular injuries may or may not be repaired. If not repaired, transcription of DNA into RNA is altered. Depending upon the mode of alteration of transcription, the following consequence may obtain: cellular death, block in DNA synthesis, delay in mitosis, or distortion of gene expression. For reasons that are not completely clear, the coding for those proteins indispensable for DNA synthesis and mitosis is particularly sensitive to ionizing radiation, and the blocks of DNA synthesis and mitosis are linked with cellular death. As a result, populations of rapidly dividing cells are depleted after exposure to X-irradiation.

References

1. Castelfranchi, G.: La Physique Moderne, II, Paris: Dunod 1949
2. Bergman, P.G.: Basic Theories of Physics, Heat, and Quanta. New York: Dover Publications 1962
3. Jones, H.E.: The Phsics of Radiation Therapy. Springfield, Ill.: Ch.C. Thomas 1953
4. Lapp, R.E., Andrews, H.L.: Nuclear Radiation Physics, Prentice-Hall, New York: Englewood Cliffs 1948
5. Richtmyer, F.K., Kennard, E.H., Lauritsen, T.: Introduction to Modern Physics. New York: McGraw-Hill Book Co. 1955
6. Pollard, E.C.: Physical considerations influencing radiation response. In: The Biological Basis of Radiation Therapy (Schwartz, E.E., ed.), p. 1–30. Philadelphia: J.B. Lippincott Co. 1966
7. Stein, G.: Excitation and ionization: some correlation between the photon and radiation chemistry of liquids. In: The Chemistry of Ionization and Excitation (Johnson, G.R.A., and Scholes, G., eds.), p. 25–34. London: Taylor Francis, Ltd. 1967
8. Weiss, J.J.: Electron transfer processes in radiation-induced reaction. In: The Chemistry of Ionization and Excitation (Johnson, G.R.A., and Scholes, G., eds.), p. 17–23. London: Taylor Francis, Ltd. 1967
9. Smith, K.C., Hanawalt, P.D.: Molecular Photobiology. New York: Academic Press 1969
10. Vles, G.: Introduction a la Photochimie Biologique, Paris: Nigot Freres 1942
11. Platzman, R.L.: Initial energy transfer from incident radiation to matter, In: Basic Mechanisms in Radiobiology. II. Physical and Chemical Aspects (Magee, J.L., Kamen, M.D., and Platzman, R.L., eds.), p. 1–21. Washington: National Research Council 1953
12. Platzman, R.L.: Energy transfer from secondary electrons to matter. In Basic Mechanisms in Radiobiology. II. Physical and Chemical Aspects (Magee, J.L., Kamen, M.D., and Platzman, R.L., eds.), p. 22–50. Washington: National Research Council 1953
13. Hart, E.J.: The hydrated electron. Science **146** (3640), 19–25 (1964)
14. Hart, E.J., Boag, J.W.: Absorption spectrum of the hydrated electron in water and in aqueous solutions. J. Amer. chem. Soc. **84**, 4090–4095 (1962)
15. Pullman, B., Pullman, A.: Quantum Biochemistry. New York: Interscience Publ. 1963
16. Emmerson, P., Scholes, G., Thomson, D.H., Ward, J.F., Weiss, J.: Chemical effects of ionizing radiations on nucleic acids and nucleoproteins. Nature (Lond.) **187**, 319–320 (1960)
17. Smith, K.C., Hanawalt, P.C.: Molecular Photobiology Inactivation and Recovery, Mol. Biol. Int. Ser. Monogr. and Textbooks. New York: Academic Press 1969
18. Beukers, R., Berends, W.: Isolation and identification of the irradiation product of thymine. Biochim. biophys. Acta (Amst.) **41**, 550–551 (1960)
19. Beukers, R., Berends, W.: The effects of UV-irradiation on nucleic acids and their components. Biochim. biophys. Acta (Amst.) **49**, 181–189 (1961)
20. Johns, H.E., Pearson, M.L., Helleiner, C.W., Logan, D.M.: The effects of ultraviolet light on thymine, uracil, and their derivatives, in Cellular Radiation Biology, Proc. Symp. Fundamental Cancer Res., p. 29–51. Baltimore: Williams & Wilkins Co. 1965
21. Doudney, C.O.: Ultraviolet light effects on deoxyribonucleic acid replication, in Cellular Radiation Biology, Proc. Symp. Fundamental Cancer Res., p. 120–141. Baltimore: Williams & Wilkins Co. 1965
22. Shooter, K.V.: The effects of radiations on DNA biosynthesis and related processes, Progr. Biophys. **17**, 289–323 (1967)
23. Hausser, K.W., Vahle, W.: Sonnenbrand und Sonnenbräunung, Wiss. Veröff. Siemens Konzern. **6**, 111–113 (1927)
24. Hausser, I.: Sonnenbrand und Sonnenbräunung. Naturwissenschaften **26**, 137–139 (1938)
25. Setlow, R.B.: Physical changes and mutagenesis. J. Cell. Comp. Physiol. **64** (1), 51–68 (1964)
26. Setlow, R.B.: Repair of DNA. In: Regulation of Nucleic Acid and Protein Biosynthesis (Koningsberger, V.V., and Bosch, L., eds.), p. 51–62. Amsterdam: Elsevier Publishing Company 1967
27. Setlow, R.B.: The photochemistry, photobiology, and repair of polynucleotides. Progr. Nucleic Acid Res. Mol. Biol. **8**, 257–295 (1968)
28. Ginoza, W.: The effects of ionizing radiation on nucleic acids of bacteriophages and bacterial cells. Ann. Rev. Microbiol. **21**, 325–368 (1967)
29. Hanawalt, P.C.: Cellular recovery from photochemical damage. In: Photophysiology: Current Topics (Giese, A.C., ed.) Vol. 4, p. 203–251. New York: Academic Press 1968
30. Stauss, B.S.: DNA repair mechanisms and their relation to mutation and recombination. Curr. Top. Microbiol. Immunol. **44**, 1–85 (1968)
31. Howard-Flanders, P.: DNA repair. Ann. Rev. Biochem. **37**, 175–200 (1968)
32. Rupert, C.S.: Photoreactivation of ultraviolet damage. In: Photophysiology: Current Topics (Giese, A.C., ed.), vol. 2, p. 283–327. New York: Academic Press 1964
33. Kelner, A., Bellamy, W.D., Stapelton, G.E., Zelle, M.R.: Symposium on radiation effect on cells and bacteria. Bact. Rev. **19**, 22–44 (1955)
34. Hill, R.F.: A radiation-sensitive mutant of Escherichia coli. Biophys. biochem. Acta (Amst.) **30**, (3), 636–637 (1958)
35. Meselson, M., Stahl, F.W.: The replication of DNA in Escherichia coli. Proc. nat. Acad. Sci. (Wash.) **44**, 671–682 (1958)
36. Pettijohn, D., Hanawalt, P.: Evidence for repair-replication of ultraviolet damaged DNA in bacteria. J. molec. Biol. **9**, 395–410 (1964)
37. Howard-Flanders, P., Rupp, W.D., Wilkins, B.M., Cole, R.S.: DNA replication and recombination after UV irradiation. Cold Spr. Harb. Symp. quant. Biol. **33**, 195–207 (1968)
38. Takagi, Y., Sekiguchi, M., Okubo, S., Nakayama, H., Shimada, K., Yashuda, S., Nishimoto, T., Yoshihara, H.: Nucleases specific for ultraviolet light-irradiated DNA and their possible role in dark repair. Cold Spr. Harb. Symp. quant. Biol. **33**, 219–227 (1968)
39. Grossman, L., Kaplan, J.C., Kushner, S.R., Mahler, I.: Enzymes involved in the early stages of repair of ultraviolet-irradiated DNA. Cold Spr. Harb. Symp. quant. Biol. **33**, 229–234 (1968)
40. Strauss, B., Searashi, T., Robbins, M.: Repair of DNA studied with a nuclease specific for UV-induced lesions. Proc. nat. Acad. Sci. (Wash.) **56**, 932–939 (1966)
41. Nakayama, H., Okubo, S., Sekiguchi, M., Takagi, Y.: A deoxyribonuclease activity specific for ultraviolet-irradiated DNA: a chromatographic analysis. Biochem. biophys. Res. Commun. **27**, 217–223 (1967)
42. Kelly, R.B., Atkinson, M.R., Huberman, J.A., Kornberg, A.: Excision of thymine dimers and other mismatched sequences by DNA polymerase of Escherichia coli. Nature (Lond.) **224**, 495–501 (1969)
43. van Lancker, J.L., Tomura, T.: Purification and some properties of a mammalian repair endonuclease. Biochim. biophys. Acta (Amst.) **353**, 99–114 (1974)
44. Cronkite, E.P.: Radiation injury in man. In: The Biological Basis of Radiation Therapy (Schwartz, E., ed.), p. 163–207. Philadelphia: J.B. Lippincott Co. 1966
45. Rowland, S.: Report on the application of the new photography to medicine and surgery. Injurious effects on the skin. Brit. med. J. **1**, 997–998 (1896)
46. Daniel, J.: Depilatory action of the x-rays. Med. Rec. (N.Y.) **49**, 595–596 (1896)
47. Lacassagne, A., Gricouroff, G.: Action des Radiations Ionisantes sur L'Organisme, 2nd ed. Paris: Masson et Cie 1956
48. Krayevskii, N.A.: Studies in the Pathology of Radiation Disease, English Translation. London: Pergamon Press 1965
49. Bloom, W.: Histopathology of Irradiation from External and Internal Sources, 1st ed. New York: McGraw-Hill Book Co. 1948
50. Upton, A.C.: Pathologic effects. In: The Biological Basis of Radiation Therapy (Schwartz, E., ed.), p. 126–162. Philadelphia: J.B. Lippincott Co. 1966

51. Rusch, H.P., Baumann, C.A.: Tumor production in mice with ultraviolet irradiation. Amer. J. Cancer **35**, 55–62 (1939)
52. Blum, H.F., Grady, H.G., Kirby-Smith, J.S.: Limits of accuracy in experimental carcinogenesis as exemplified by tumor induction with ultraviolet radiation. J. nat. Cancer Inst. **3**, 83–89 (1942)
53. Blum, H.F.: Accuracy and reproducibility in induction of tumors with ultraviolet radiation. J. nat. Cancer Inst. **4**, 75–79 (1943)
54. Blum, H.F.: Some fundamental aspects of tumor development illustrated by studies with ultraviolet radiation. J. nat. Cancer Inst. **3**, 569–581 (1943)
55. Frieben: "Vereine und Kongresse. Ausstellung Arztliche". Eine umschaltevorichtung fur einfache und stereoskopische rontgendurchleuchtungen mit gleichzeitig wirkender vorichtung zur unterdruckung der schliessungsinduktionsstromme. Fortschr. Röntgenstr. **6**, 99–114 (1902)
56. Marie, P., Clune, J., Raulot-Lapointe, G.: Contribution a l'etude du developpement des tumeurs malignes sur les ulceres de roentgen, Bull. Ass. franç. Cancer **III**, 404–426 (1910)
57. Duffy, B.J., Jr., Fitzgerald, P.J.: Thyroid cancer in childhood and adolescence; report on 28 cases. Cancer **3**, 1018–1032 (1950)
58. Delawater, D.S., Winship, T.: Follow-up study of adults treated with roentgen rays for thyroid disease. Cancer **16**, 1028–1031 (1963)
59. Zeldis, L.J., Jablon, S., Ishida, M.: Current status of ABCC-NIH studies of carcinogenesis in Hiroshima and Nagasaki. Ann. N.Y. Acad. Sci. **114**, 225–240 (1964)
60. Blum, T.: Osteomyelitis of the mandible and maxilla. J. Amer. dent. Assoc. **11**, 802–805 (1924)
61. Roussy, G., Oberling, C., Guerin, M.: Action cancérigène du dioxyde de thorium chez le rat blanc. Bull. Acad. nat. Méd. (Paris) **112**, 809–816 (1934)
62. Bloch, B.: Experimental roentgen-ray cancer. Schweiz. med. Wschr. **54**, 857–865 (1924)
63. Bloch, B.: De l'importance de la pigmentation pour l'etude des naevocarconomes, Congres des Dermatologistes et Syphiligraphes de Langue Français, p. 121. Strasbourg 1923
64. Maldague, P.: Radiocancérisation expérimentale du rein par les rayons x chez le rat. I. Les radiocancers du rein. Pathol. Eur. **1**, 321–409 (1966)
65. Upton, A.C.: Biological effects of ionizing radiations. Int. Rev. exp. Path. **2**, 199–240 (1963)
66. Stein, J.J.: The carcinogenic hazards of ionizing radiation in diagnostic and therapeutic radiology. Progr. clin. Cancer **4**, 231–241 (1970)
67. Miller, R.W.: Delayed radiation effects in atomic-bomb survivors; major observations by the Atomic Bomb Casualty Commission are evaluated. Science **166**, 569–574 (1969)
68. Brown, P.: American Martyrs to Science Through the Roentgen Rays. Springfield, Ill.: Ch.C. Thomas Publisher 1936
69. Aubertin, C., Ambard, L.: Blood eosinophilia and medullary transformation of the spleen without intestinal eosinophilia, produced by repeated injections of secretin. C.R. Soc. Biol. (Paris) **62**, 263–265 (1912)
70. Lacassagne, A.: Les Cancers Produits par des Rayonnements Electromagnétiques, Hermann et Cie, Paris 1945
71. Henshaw, P.S., Hawkins, J.W.: Incidence of leukemia in physicians. J. nat. Cancer Inst. **4**, 339–346 (1945)
72. Court-Brown, W.M.: Nuclear and allied radiations and the incidence of leukemia in man. Brit. med. Bull. **14** (2), 168–173 (1958)
73. Court-Brown, W.M., Doll, R.: A prospective study of the leukemia mortality of children exposed to ante-natal diagnostic radiography. A preliminary report. Proc. roy. Soc. Med. **53**, 761–762 (1960)
74. Krebs, K., Rask-Nielsen, H.C., Wagner, A.: Origin of lymphosarcomatosis and its relation to other forms of leucosis in white mice. Acta Radiol. (Suppl.) **10**, 1–53 (1930)
75. Furth, J., Butterworth, J.S.: Neoplastic diseases occuring among mice subjected to general irradiation with x-rays; ovarian tumors and associated lesions. Amer. J. Cancer **28**, 66–95 (1936)
76. Kaplan, H.S.: Preliminary studies of effectiveness of local irradiation in induction of lymphoid tumors in mice. J. nat. Cancer Inst. **10**, 267–270 (1949)
77. Furth, J., Furth, O.B.: Neoplastic diseases produced in mice by general irradiation with x-rays; incidence and types of neoplasms. Amer. J. Cancer **28**, 54–65 (1936)
78. Kaplan, H.S.: On etiology and pathogenesis of leukemias: a review. Cancer Res. **14**, 535–548 (1954)
79. Kaplan, H.S.: Radiation-induced leukemia in mice: a progress resport. In: Radiation Biology and Cancer, Ann. Symp. Fund. Cancer Res., p. 289–302. Austin: University of Texas Press 1959
80. Kaplan, H.S.: The nature of the neoplastic transformation in lymphoid tumor induction, in Carcinogenesis, Mechanisms of Action, p. 233–248. London: Ciba Foundation Symposium 1959
81. Kaplan, H.S.: Some possible mechanisms of carcinogenesis. In: Cellular Control Mechanisms and Cancer (Emmelot, P., and Mühlbock, O., eds.), p. 373–382. Amsterdam: Elsevier Publishing Company 1964
82. Arnesen, K.: Preleukemic and early leukemic changes in the thymus of mice. A study of the AKR/O strain. Acta path. microbiol. scand. **43**, 350–364 (1958)
83. Kaplan, H.S., Brown, M.B., Paull, J.: Influence of postirradiation thymectomy and of thymic implants on lymphoid tumor incidence in C57BL mice. Cancer Res. **13**, 677–680 (1953)
84. Kaplan, H.S., Brown, M.B., Paull, J.: Influence of bone-marrow injections on involution and neoplasia of mouse thymus after systemic irradiation. J. nat. Cancer Inst. **14**, 303–316 (1953)
85. Berenblum, K.: The possible role of a transmissible factor in leukemia induction by radiation plus urethan. In: Viruses, Nucleic Acids, and Cancer, p. 529–543. Ann. Symp. Fundamental Cancer Res. Baltimore: Williams & Wilkins Co. 1963
86. Huebner, R.J., Todaro, G.J.: Oncogenes of RNA tumor viruses as determinants of cancer. Proc. nat. Acad. Sci. (Wash.) **64**, 1087–1094 (1969)
87. Brachet, J.: Cytoplasmic and nuclear structure in relation to metabolic activities. In: Ionizing Radiations and Cell Metabolism, p. 3–24. London: Proc. Ciba Symp., Churchill 1956
88. Errera, M.: The probable role of the cytoplasm in radiobiology. Adv. biol. med. Phys. **12**, 333–339 (1968)
89. Scaife, J.F.: Early biochemical changes in lymphatic cells following ionizing radiations, in The Cell Nucleus—Metabolism and Radiosensitivity, p. 309–323. London: Taylor Francis, Ltd. 1966
90. Errera, M.: Biochimie et radiobiologie du noyau cellulaire. In: The Initial Effects of Ionizing Radiations on Cells (Harris, R.J.C., ed.), p. 165–172. New York: Academic Press 1961
91. Daniels, E.W.: Cell Division on the giant amoeba, *Pelomyxa carolinensis,* following x-irradiation. II. Analysis of therapeutic effects after fusion with nonirradiated cell portions. J. exp. Zool. **127**, 427–461 (1954)
92. Zirkle, R.E., Bloom, W.: Irradiation of parts of individual cells. Science **117**, 487–493 (1953)
93. Augenstine, L.G.: The effects of ionizing radiation on enzymes. Advanc. Enzymol. **24**, 359–413 (1962)
94. Dale, W.M.: Effect of x-rays on aqueous solutions of biologically active compounds. Brit. J. Radiol. **16**, 171–172 (1943)
95. Dale, W.M.: The effects of ionizing radiations on enzymes *in vitro*. In: Ionizing Radiations and Cell Metabolism, p. 25–37. London: Churchill 1956
96. Barron, E.S.G., Dickman, S., Muntz, J.A., Singer, T.P.: Studies on the mechanism of action of ionizing radiations. I. Inhibition of enzymes by x-rays. J. gen. Physiol. **32**, 537–552 (1949)
97. Barron, E.S.G., Dickman, S.: Studies on the mechanism of action of ionizing radiations. II. Inhibition of sulfhydryl enzymes by alpha-, beta-, and gamma-rays. J. gen. Physiol. **32**, 595–605 (1949)
98. Errera, M., Herve, A.: Mécanismes de l'action biologique des radiations. Paris: Masson et Cie 1951
99. DuBois, K.P., Petersen, D.F.: Biochemical effects of radiation. Ann. Rev. Nucl. Sci. **4**, 351–376 (1954)
100. Shapiro, B.: Biochemical mechanisms in the action of radiation. In: The Biological Basis of Radiation Therapy (Schwartz, E.E., ed.), p. 31–59. Philadelphia: J.B. Lippincott Co. 1966
101. Hickman, J., Ashwell, G.: Effect of irradiation by x-ray upon anaerobic glycolysis in spleen homogenates. J. biol. Chem. **205**, 651–659 (1953)
102. Yamada, T., Ohyama, H.: Accumulation of fructose-1,6-diphosphate in x-irradiated rat thymocytes. Int. J. Radiat. Biol. **14**, 169–174 (1968)
103. Potter, V.: Sequential blocking of metabolic pathways *in vivo*. Proc. Soc. exp. Biol. Med. **76**, 41–46 (1951)
104. DuBois, K.P., Cochran, K.W., Doull, J.: Inhibition of citric acid synthesis *in vivo* by x-irradiation. Proc. Soc. exp. Biol. Med. **76**, 422–427 (1951)
105. Ord, M.G., Stocken, L.A.: The biochemical lesion *in vivo* and *in vitro*. In: Mechanisms in Radiobiology (Errera, M., and Forssberg, A., eds.), vol. I, p. 259–331. New York: Academic Press 1961
106. Hevesy, G., Forssberg, A.: Effect of irradiation by x-rays on the exhalation of carbon dioxide by the mouse. Nature (Lond.) **168**, 692 (1951)
107. Potter, R.L., Bethell, F.H.: Oxidative phosphorylation in spleen mitochondria. Fed. Proc. **11**, 270 (1952)
108. van Bekkum, D.W.: The disturbance of oxidative phosphorylation and the breakdown of ATP in spleen tissue after irradiation. Biochim. biophys. Acta (Amst.) **16**, 437–438 (1955)
109. Scaife, J.F., Hill, B.: The uncoupling of oxidative phosphorylation by ionizing radiation. Canad. J. Biochem. **40**, 1025–1042 (1962)
110. Thompson, J.F.: Effects of total-body x-irradiation on phosphate esterification and hydrolysis in mitochondrial preparations of rat spleen. Radiat. Res. **21**, 46–60 (1964)
111. Creasy, W.A., Stocken, L.A.: Biochemical differentiation between radiosensitive and nonsensitive tissues in the rat. Biochem. J. **69**, 17 (1958)
112. Klouwen, H.M.: Radiosensitivity of nuclear ATP synthesis and its relation to inhibition of mitosis. In: Cellular Radiation Biology, Proc. Symp. Fundamental Cancer Res., p. 142–166. Baltimore: Williams & Wilkins Co. 1965
113. Klouwen, H.M., Betel, I.: Radiosensitivity of nuclear ATP-synthesis. Int. J. Radiat. Biol. **6**, 441–461 (1963)
114. Nygaard, O.F.: Effects of radiation on nucleic acid metabolism: a review of current concepts. In: The Effects of Ionizing Radiations on Immune Processes (Leone, C.A., ed.), p. 47–73. New York: Gordon and Breach, Science Publishers, 1961
115. Quastler, H.: Physiological importance of radiation effects on DNA synthesis. In: Actions Chimiques et Biologiques des Radiations (Haissinsky, M., ed.), p. 184–185. Paris: Masson et Cie 1963
116. Kanazir, D.T.: Radiation-induced alterations in the structure of deoxyribonucleic acid and their biological consequences, Prog. Nucleic Acid Res. Mol. Biol. **9**, 117–222 (1969)
117. van Lancker, J.L.: Cytochemical injury of x-radiation. Fed. Proc. **21**, 1118–1123 (1962)

118. van Lancer, J.L.: Control of macromolecular synthesis in regenerating liver and its alteration by x-radiation. In: Biochemistry of Cell Division (Baserga, R., ed.), p. 155–177. Springfield, Ill.: Ch.C. Thomas Publisher, 1968
119. van Lancer, J.L.: Recherche sur la nature moleculaire de la radiosensibilité cellulaire, Report of the Symp. on Radiosensitivity, Basic Research Clinical Applications, **34** (1), 63–68. Laval Medical Inc., Quebec 1963
120. Kelly, L.S., Hirsch, J.D., Beach, G., Palmer, W.: The time function of P^{32} incorporation into DNA of regenerating liver; the effect of irradiation. Cancer Res. **17** (1), 117–121 (1957)
121. Holmes, B.E.: Influence of radiation on metabolism of regenerating rat liver. In: Ionizing Radiation and Cell Metabolism, p. 225–238. London: Churchill 1956
122. Butler, J.A.V.: The action of ionizing radiations on biological materials, facts and theories. Radiat. Res. **4**, 20–32 (1956)
123. Threlfall, G., Cairnie, A.B., Taylor, D.M., Buck, A.T.: Effect of whole-body x-irradiation on renal compensatory hypertrophy. Radiat. Res. **27**, 559–565 (1966)
124. Perrotta, C.A.: Effect of x-irradiation on DNA synthesis in the uterine epithelium. Radiat. Res. **28**, 232–242 (1966)
125. Schrek, R., Stefani, S.: Radioresistance of phytohemagglutinin-treated normal and leukemic lymphocytes. J. nat. Cancer Inst. **32**, 507–521 (1964)
126. Benjamin, E., Sluka, E.: Antikörperbildung nach Röntgenstrahlen. Wien. klin. Wschr. **21** (10), 311–313 (1908)
127. Pollard, E.C., Davis, S.A.: The action of ionizing radiation on transcription (and translation) in several strains of Escherichia coli. Radiat. Res. **41**, 375–399 (1970)
128. Stryckmans, P.A., Chanana, A.D., Cronkite, E.P., Greenberg, M.L., Schiffer, L.M.: Studies on lymphocytes. X. Influence of extracorporeal irradiation of the blood on lymphocytes in chronic lymphocytic leukemia: apparent correlation with RNA turnover. Radiat. Res. **37**, 118–130 (1969)
129. Sinclair, W.K.: Cyclic x-ray responses in mammalian cells *in vitro*. Radiat. Res. **33**, 620–643 (1968)
130. Szybalski, W.: Molecular events resulting in radiation injury, repair and sensitization of DNA. Radiat. Res. (suppl.) **7**, 147–159 (1967)
131. Hutchinson, F.: The inactivation of DNA and other biological molecules by ionizing radiations. In: Cellular Radiation Biology, Proc. Symp. Fundamental Cancer Res., p. 86–99. Baltimore: Williams & Wilkins Co. 1965
132. Freifelder, D.: Lethal changes in bacteriophage DNA produced by x-rays. Radiat. Res. (Suppl.) **7**, 80–96 (1966)
133. Wacker, A.: Molecular mechanisms of radiation effects. Progr. Nucleic Acid Res. **1**, 369–399 (1963)
134. Muller, A.: The formation of radicals in nucleic acids, nucleoproteins, and their constituents by ionizing radiations. Progr. Biophys. Mol. **17**, 99–147 (1967)
135. Eisinger, J., Gueron, M., Shulman, R.G.: The excited states of DNA. Advanc. biol. med. Phys. **12**, 219–238 (1968)
136. Myers, L.S., Jr.: Free radical damage of nucleic acids and their components by ionizing radiation. Fed. Proc. **32** (8), 1882–1894 (1973)
137. Summers, W.., Szybalski, W.: γ Irradiation of deoxyribonucleic acid in dilute solutions. I. A sensitive method for detection of single-strand breaks in polydispersed DNA samples. J. molec. Biol. **26**, 107–123 (1967)
138. Studier, F.W.: Sedimentation studies of the size and shape of DNA. J. molec. Biol. **11**, 373–390 (1965)
139. Freifelder, D.: Physicochemical studies on x-ray inactivation of bacteriophage. Virology **36**, 613–619 (1968)
140. McGrath, R.A., Williams, R.W.: Radiobiology: reconstruction *in vivo* of irradiated Escherichia coli deoxyribonucleic acid: the rejoining of broken pieces. Nature (Lond.) **212**, 534–535 (1966)
141. Kaplan, H.S.: DNA-strand scission and loss of viability after x-irradiation of normal and sensitized bacterial cells. Proc. nat. Acad. Sci. (Wash.) **55**, 1442–1446 (1966)
142. Kimball, R.F.: Repair of premutational damage. Advanc. Radiat. Biol. **2**, 135–166 (1966)
143. Elkind, M.M., Sutton, H.: X-ray damage and recovery in mammalian cells in culture. Nature (Lond.) **184**, 1293–1295 (1959)
144. Sinclair, W.K., Morton, R.A.: Survival and recovery in x-irradiated synchronized Chinese hamster cells. In: Cellular Radiation Biology, Proc. Symp. Fundamental Cancer Res., p. 418–422. Baltimore: Williams & Wilkins Co. 1965
145. Dewey, W.C., Humphrey, R.M.: Radiosensitivity and recovery of radiation damage in relation to the cell cycle. In: Cellular Radiation Biology, Proc. Symp. Fundamental Cancer Res., p. 340–375. Baltimore: Williams & Wilkins Co. 1965
146. Painter, R.B., Cleaver, J.E.: Repair replication in HeLa cells after large doses of x-irradiation. Nature (Lond.) **216**, 369–370 (1967)
147. Phillips, R.A., Tolmach, J.L.: Repair of potentially lethal damage in x-irradiated HeLa cells. Radiat. Res. **29**, 413–432 (1966)
148. Djordjevic, B., Kim, J.H.: Modification of radiation response in synchronized HeLa cells by metabolic inhibitors: effects of inhibitors of DNA and protein synthesis. Radiat. Res. **37**, 435–450 (1969)
149. Cleaver, J.E.: Repair replication of mammalian cell DNA: effects of compounds that inhibit DNA synthesis or dark repair. Radiat. Res. **37**, 334–348 (1969)
150. Dalrymple, G.V., Sander, J.L., Baker, M.L., Wilkinson, K.P.: The effect of 2,4-dinitrophenol on the repair of radiation injury by L cells. Radiat. Res. 90–102 (1969)
151. Wolff, S., Scott, D.: Repair of radiation-induced damage to chromosomes. Independence of known DNA dark repair mechanism. Exp. Cell Res. **55**, 9–16 (1969)
152. Schwarz, H.A.: Recent research on the radiation chemistry of aqueous solution. In: Advances in Radiation Biology (Augenstein, L.G., Mason, R., and Quastler, H., eds.), vol. 1, p. 1–32. New York and London: Academic Press 1964
153. Howard-Flanders, P.: DNA repair and recombination. Brit. med. Bull. **29**, 226–235 (1973)
154. van Lancker, J.L., Tomura, T.: Purification and some properties of a mammalian repair endonuclease. Biochim. biophys. Acta (Amst.) **353**, 99–114 (1974)
155. Regan, J.D., Setlow, R.B.: Two forms of repairs in the DNA of human cells damaged by chemical carcinogens and mutagens. Cancer Res. **34**, 3318–3325 (1974)
156. Meltz, M.L., Painter, R.B.: Distribution of repair replication in the HeLa cell genome. Int. J. Radiat. Biol. **23**, 637–640 (1973)
157. Brunk, C.F.: Distribution of dimers in ultraviolet-irradiated DNA. Nature [New Biol.] **241**, 74–76 (1973)
158. Wilkins, R.J., Hart, R.W.: Preferential DNA repair in human cells. Nature (Lond.) **247**, 35–36 (1974)
159. Harris, C., Connor, R.J., Jackson, F.E., Lieverman, M.W.: Intranuclear distribution of DNA repair synthesis induced by chemical carcinogens or ultraviolet light in human diploid fibroblasts. Cancer Res. **34**, 3461–3468 (1974)
160. Berliner, J., Himes, W., Aoki, T., Norman, A.: The sites of unscheduled DNA synthesis within irradiated human lymphocytes. Radiat. Res. (in press)
161. Waters, R., Moustacchi, E.: The fate of ultraviolet-induced pyrimidine dimers in the mitochondrial DNA of *Saccharomyces cerevisiae* following various post-irradiation cell treatments. Biochim. biophys. Acta (Amst.) **366**, 241–250 (1974)
162. Clayton, D.A., Doda, J.N., Friedberg, E.C.: The absence of a pyrimidine dimer repair mechanism in mammalian mitochondria (pyrimidine dimer endonuclease). DNA repair/DNA replication/density gradient centrifugation. Proc. nat. Acad. Sci. (Wash.) **71**, 2777–2781 (1974)
163. Painter, B.: Eukaryotic replicons. In: Handbook of Genetics, vol. 5. New York: Plenum Press (in press)
164. Okazaki, R.: Short-chain intermediates in DNA replication. In: DNA Replication (Wickner, R.B., ed.), vol. 7, p. 1–32. New York: Marcel Dekker, Inc. 1974
165. Tan, E.M., Stoughton, R.B.: Ultraviolet light induced damage to desoxyribonucleic acid in human skin. J. invest. Derm. **52**, 537–542 (1969)
166. Seaman, E., van Vunakis, H., Levine, L.: Serologic estimation of thymine dimers in the deoxyribonucleic acid of bacterial and mammalian cells following irradiation with ultraviolet light and postirradiation repair. J. biol. Chem. **247**, 5709–5715 (1972)
167. Závadová, Z.: Host-cell repair of vaccinia virus and double stranded RNA of encephalomyocarditis virus. Nature [New Biol.] **233**, 123 (1971)
168. Coppey, J.: Repair of interferon synthetic capacity in ultraviolet-irradiated normal and hybrid mammalian cells. Nature [New Biol.] **234**, 14–15 (1971)
169. Kraemer, K.H., Coon, H.G., Petinga, R.A., Barrett, S.F., Rahe, A.E., Robbins, J.H.: Genetic heterogeneity in xeroderma pigmentosum: Complementation groups and their relationship to DNA repair rates. Proc. nat. Acad. Sci. (Wash.) **72**, 59–63 (1975)
170. Lehmann, A.R., Kirk-Bell, S., Arlett, C.F., Paterson, M.C., Lohman, P.H.M., deWeerd-Kastelein, E.A., Bootsma, D.: Xeroderma pigmentosum cells with normal levels of excision repair have a defect in DNA synthesis after UV-irradiation. Proc. nat. Acad. Sci. (Wash.) **72**, 219–223 (1975)
171. Sutherland, B.M., Rice, M., Wagner, E.K.: Xeroderma pigmentosum cells contain low levels of photoreactivating enzyme (DNA repair/ultraviolet light damage/pyrimidine dimers). Proc. nat. Acad. Sci. (Wash.) **72**, 103–107 (1975)
172. Hand, R., German, J.: A retarded rate of DNA chain growth in Bloom's syndrome (DNA replication/chromosomes/Fanconi's anemia/DNA fiber autoradiography). Proc. nat. Acad. Sci. (Wash.) **72**, 758–762 (1975)
173. Poon, P.K., O'Brien, R.L., Parker, J.W.: Defective DNA repair in Fanconi's anaemia. Nature **250**, 223–225 (1974)
174. Setlow, R.B., Hart, R.W.: Direct evidence that damaged DNA results in neoplastic transformation—a fish story, from the Proceedings of the 5th International Congress of Radiation Research, at Oak Ridge National Laboratory, Oak Ridge, Tennessee. New York: Academic Press, Inc. (in press)
175. Hart, R.W., Setlow, R.B.: Correlation between deoxyribonucleic acid excision-repair and life-span in a number of mammalian species (aging/UV irradiation/unscheduled DNA synthesis). Proc. nat. Acad. Sci. (Wash.) **71**, 2169–2173 (1974)
176. Painter, R.B., Clarkson, J.M., Young, R.: Ultraviolet induced repair replication in aging diploid human cells (WI-38). Radiat. Res. **56**, 560–564 (1973)
177. Wheeler, K.T., Lett, J.T.: Formation and rejoining of DNA strand breaks in irradiated neurons: *in vivo*. Radiat. Res. **52**, 59–67 (1972)

178. Gilford, H.: Progeria; a form of senilism. Practitioner, London **73**, 188–217 (1904)
179. Epstein, J., Williams, J.R., Little, J.B.: Deficient DNA repair in human progeroid cells (Hutchinson-Gilford progeria syndrome/X-irradiation/DNA strand breaks/senescence). Proc. nat. Acad. Sci. (Wash.) **70**, 977–981 (1973)
180. Epstein, J., Williams, J.R., Little, J.B.: Rate of DNA repair in progeric and normal human fibroblasts. Biochem. biophys. Res. Commun. **59**, 850–857 (1974)
181. Feher, I., Antal, S., Gidali, J.: Correlation between circulating stem cell count and stem cell regeneration in locally irradiated bone marrow. Radiat. Res. **58**, 516–523 (1974)
182. Sholley, M.M., Sodicoff, M., Pratt, N.E.: Early radiation injury in the rat parotid gland. Reaction of acinar cells and vascular endothelium. Lab. Invest. **31**, 340–354 (1974)
183. Groover, T.A., Christie, A.C., Merritt, E.A.: Observations on the use of the copper filter in the roentgen treatment of deep seated malignancies. South med. J. **15**, 440–444 (1922)
184. Holsti, L.B., Vuorinen, P.: Radiation reaction in the lung after continuous and split-course megavoltage radiotherapy of bronchial carcinoma. Brit. J. Radiol. **40**, 280–284 (1967)
185. Wara, W.M., Phillips, T.L., Margolis, L.W., Smith, V.: Radiation pneumonitis: A new approach to the derivation of time-dose factors. Cancer **32**, 547–552 (1973)
186. Luxton, R.W.: Radiation nephritis. A long term study of 54 patients. Lancet **1961 II**, 1221–1224
187. Phillips, T.L., Ross, G.: A quantitative technique for measuring renal damage after irradiation. Radiology **109**, 457–562 (1973)
188. Arneil, G.C., Harris, F., Emmanuel, I.G., Young, D.G., Flatman, G.E., Zachary, R.B.: Nephritis in two children after irradiation and chemotherapy for nephroblastoma. Lancet **1974 I**, 960–963
189. Modan, B., Baidatz, D., Mart, H., Steinitz, R., Levin, S.G.: Radiation-induced head and neck tumours. Lancet **1974 I**, 277–279
190. Tobleman, W.T., Cole, A.: Repair of sublethal and oxygen enhancement ratio for low-voltage electron beam irradiation. Radiat. Res. **60**, 355–360 (1974)
191. Augenstein, L.G., Brustad, T., Mason, R.: The relative roles of ionization and excitation processes in the radiation inactivation of enzymes. In: Advances in Radiation Biology (Augenstein, L.G., Mason, R., and Quastler, H., eds.), vol. 1, p. 227–266. New York and London: Academic Press 1964
192. Marciani, D.J., Tolbert, B.M.: Structural damage in γ-irradiated lysozyme. Biochim. biophys. Acta (Amst.) **351**, 387–395 (1974)
193. Nikesch, W.: Studies of radiation induced membrane damage in lymphocytes using fluorescent probes (Ph.D. thesis, in press)
194. Markov, G.G., Dessev, G.N., Russev, G.C., Tsanev, R.G.: Effects of γ-irradiation on biosynthesis of different types of ribonucleic acids in normal and regenerating rat liver. Biochem. J. **146**, 41–51 (1975)
195. Pederson, T., Robbins, E.: Chromatin structure and the cell division cycle. J. Cell Biol. **55**, 322–327 (1972)
196. Watanabe, I.: Radiation effects on DNA chain growth in mammalian cells. Radiat. Res. **58**, 541–556 (1974)
197. Dewey, W.C., Noel, J.S., Dettor, C.M.: Changes in radiosensitivity and dispersion of chromatin during the cell cycle of synchronous Chinese hamster cells. Radiat. Res. **52**, 373–394 (1972)
198. Dettor, C.M., Dewey, W.C., Winans, L.F., Noel, J.S.: Enhancement of X-ray damage in synchronous Chinese hamster cells by hypertonic treatments. Radiat. Res. **52**, 352–372 (1972)
199. Ward, J.F.: Molecular mechanisms of radiation-induced damage to nucleic acids. In: Advances in Radiation Biology (Lett, J.T., and Adler, H., eds.), vol. 5, p. 181–239. New York: Academic Press 1975
200. Téoule, R., Cadet, J.: Peroxides produced from thymine by γ-irradiation in aerated solution. Biochim. biophys. Acta (Amst.) **238**, 8–26 (1971)
201. Scholes, G., Ward, J.F., Weiss, J.J.: Mechanism of the radiation induced degradation of nucleic acids. J. molec. Biol. **2**, 379–391 (1960)
202. Hariharan, P.V., Cerutti, P.A.: Formation and repair of γ-ray induced thymine damage in Micrococcus radiodurans. J. molec. Biol. **66**, 65–81 (1972)
203. Swinehart, J.L., Lin, W.S., Cerutti, P.A.: Gamma-ray induced damage in thymine in mononucleotide mixtures, and in single- and double-stranded DNA. Radiat. Res. **58**, 166–175 (1974)
204. Ward, J.F., Urist, M.M.: γ-irradiation of aqueous solutions of polynucleotides. Int. J. Rad. Biol. **12**, 209–218 (1967)
205. Roti Roti, J.L., Stein, G.S., Cerutti, P.A.: Reactivity of thymine to γ-rays in HeLa chromatin and nucleoprotein preparation. Biochemistry (Wash.) **13**, 1900–1904 (1974)
206. Dalrymple, G.V., Sanders, J.L., Moss, A.J., Jr., Baker, M.L., Nash, J.C., Wilkinson, K.P.: Radiation alters the ability of mammalian cell DNA to compete in a DNA:DNA hybridization system. Biochem. biophys. Res. Commun. **47**, 938–943 (1972)
207. van Lancker, J.L., Tomura, T.: Alterations of liver DNA after X-irradiation. Reassociation and hybridization with nuclear RNA. Int. J. Rad. Biol. (in press)
208. Johansen, I., Gulbrandsen, R., Pettersen, R.: Effectiveness of oxygen in promoting X-ray-induced single-strand breaks in circular phage λ DNA and killing of radiation-sensitive mutants of *Escherichia coli*. Radiat. Res. **58**, 384–397 (1974)
209. van Lancker, J.L., Tomura, T.: Alterations of liver DNA after X-irradiation. Cancer Res. **34**, 699–704 (1974)
210. Payes, B.: Enzymatic repair of X-ray-damaged DNA. I. Labeling of the precursor of a malonaldehyde-like material in X-irradiated DNA and the enzymatic excision of labeled lesions. Biochim. biophys. Acta (Amst.) **366**, 251–260 (1974)
211. Kapp, D.S., Smith, K.C.: Lack of *in vitro* repair of X-ray-induced chain breaks in DNA polynucleotide-joining enzyme. Int. J. Rad. Biol. **14**, 567–571 (1968)
212. Kapp, D.S., Smith, K.C.: Chemical nature of chain breaks produced in DNA by X-irradiation *in vitro*. Radiat. Res. **42**, 34–49 (1970)
213. Johansen, I., Brustad, T., Rupp, W.D.: DNA strand breaks measured within 100 milliseconds of irradiation of *Escherichia coli* by 4 MeV electrons. Proc. nat. Acad. Sci. (Wash.) **72**, 167–171 (1975)
214. Hopwood, L.E.: Cause of deficient DNA synthesis in generation 1 of X-irradiated HeLa cells. Radiat. Res. **58**, 349–360 (1974)
215. Hariharan, P.V., Cerutti, P.A.: Excision of damaged thiamine residues from gamma-irradiated poly(dA-dT) by crude extracts of *Escherichia coli*. Proc. nat. Acad. Sci. (Wash.) **71**, 3532–3536 (1974)
216. Tomura, T., van Lancker, J.L.: the effect of a mammalian repair endonuclease on X-irradiated DNA. Biochim. biophys. Acta (Amst.) (in press)
217. Masker, W.E., Hanawalt, P.C.: Ultraviolet stimulated DNA synthesis in toluenized *Escherichia coli* deficient in DNA polymerase I. Proc. nat. Acad. Sci. (Wash.) **70**, 129–133 (1973)
218. Hadden, C.T., Billen, D., Corrigan, K.: Stimulation of non-conservative DNA synthesis by ultraviolet light in freeze-treated *Bacillus subtilis*. Biochim. biophys. Acta (Amst.) **324**, 461–471 (1973)
219. Waldstein, E.A., Sharon, R., Ben-Ishaei, R.: Role of ATP in excision repair of ultraviolet radiation damage in *Escherichia coli*. Proc. nat. Acad. Sci. (Wash.) **71**, 2651–2654 (1974)
220. Burrell, A.D., Feldschreiber, P., Dean, C.J.: DNA-membrane association and the repair of double breaks in X-irradiated *Micrococcus radiodurans*. Biochim. biophys. Acta (Amst.) **247**, 38–53 (1971)

Chapter 13

Inflammation

History 765

Inflammatory Process as a Whole 765

Phase I: Hemorrhage Necrosis 765
Phase II: Vasodilation, PMN Migration, and Pus Formation 765
Phase III: Repair 765

Vascular Reaction to Inflammation 766

Axon Reflex 766
Capillary Dilation 766
Increased Permeability: Morphological Alteration of the Wall 767
Chemical Mediators 768

Histamine
5-Hydroxytryptamine in Inflammation
Proteins, Peptides, and Capillary Permeability

Kinins—Structure and Metabolism 771

Kinins in Disease 774

Epinephrine 774

Prostaglandins 775

Metabolism 775
Miscellaneous Functions 777
Role in Inflammation 777
Role in Essential Hypertension 778
Conclusion 778

Cellular Changes in Inflammation 778

Leukocytic Migration 778

Diapedesis
Chemotaxis

Phagocytosis 782
Polymorphonuclears and Phagocytosis 784
Bacteriostatic Agents 788
Eosinophils 788
Plasmocytic and Lymphocytic Migration 789
Macrophages 789
Defective Leukocytic Response in Inflammation 791

Gross and Histological Appearance of Inflammation 792

Acute Inflammation 792
Chronic Inflammation 795

References 799

History

The ancients did not fail to recognize the pertinent symptoms of inflammation. Descriptions of inflammatory processes can be found in Egyptian papyrus, and it was Hippocrates who coined the word "erysipele." Later, Celsus enounced his famous description of the inflammatory process in the concise Latin way: "Signae vero inflammationis sunt quatuor rubor et tumor cum colore et dolore."

Despite the addition of a few more symptoms by Galen, little progress was made in the study of inflammation until Virchow examined inflamed tissues and concluded erroneouusly that inflammation is a local cellular reaction. The widespread significance of the inflammatory process, however, was revealed by Cohnheim's famous experiment on frog mesentery, which clearly demonstrated the participation of the vascular system and blood cells in the reaction.

Some of the greatest names of science have since been associated with the study of inflammation. By his discovery of bacteria and viruses, Pasteur described an important class of agents responsible for inflammation. Metchnikoff discovered phagocytosis, and although he undoubtedly exaggerated the importance of that process in the overall inflammatory reaction, it is because of this discovery that he remains one of the prominent figures in pathology.

Inflammatory Process as a Whole

The description of the evolution of a small wound is probably the most convenient way to review the inflammatory process in its entirety. The causes of inflammation are varied; they may be physical, chemical, or biological. The reaction that follows the trauma of the skin may be divided into three phases: (1) the degenerative stage; (2) the vascular reaction; and (3) the repair or proliferative stage.

Phase I: Hemorrhage and Necrosis

If one examines a fresh wound within an hour after injury, the most striking event is the cellular destruction that occurs in the traumatized area. In a sterile cut, a wedge opening stretches from the surface of the epithelium to various depths in the derma, depending upon the extent of the trauma. In the course of the injury, various vessels are destroyed and hemorrhage ensues. In fact, hemorrhage is beneficial because it blocks any further bleeding by exerting pressure on the surrounding tissues. Compression in the hemorrhage area leads to cellular necrosis; the epithelial cells and some of the fibroblasts swell, their cytoplasm becomes vacuolized, and their nuclei undergo pyknosis and karyorrhexis.

Phase II: Vasodilation, PMN Migration, and Pus Formation

Thus, in the first moments after trauma, the main results are hemorrhage and necrosis. These passive phenomena are then followed by active tissular and cellular reactions, namely, vascular dilatation and polymorphonuclear migration; active congestion develops at the edges of the wound. This alteration is responsible for the heat and redness observed in inflamed areas by the ancient physicians. A section of the injured area demonstrates vastly dilated capillaries in addition to an increase in capillary number. Capillaries that normally are invisible can easily be recognized because they are engorged with blood. Extravasation of serous fluid from the lumen of the dilated vessels in the extravascular spaces soon accompanies the vasodilatation, giving rise to local edema.

The second reaction to inflammation is the migration of polymorphonuclears into the injured area. First, the polymorphonuclears increase in number within the lumen of the vessel. This is referred to as leukocytic margination. Later, the white cells migrate from the lumen of the vessel into the surrounding tissues by a process called diapedesis. The polymorphonuclears now form a thick cuff that surrounds the necrotic tissue in the congested area.

The vasodilatation and PMN migration are followed by an interaction between the invading polymorphonuclears and the necrotic tissue, resulting in active lysis. The injured tissues liquify and the fluids originating from the necrotic process mix with the serous material that extruded from the vessels, yielding a characteristic material called pus.

The destructive process results from the release of proteolytic enzymes and from the engulfing of the debris into the polymorphonuclears or monocytes by phagocytosis.

Phase III: Repair

The proliferative stage is the last phase of the inflammatory reaction. It includes the proliferation of capillaries, young fibroblasts, and epithelium. Young capillaries proliferate actively in the bottom of the wound and bulge at the surface; they are accompanied by young fibroblasts, which soon elaborate collagen fibers. These meaty buds that become visible at the bottom of the wound and bleed easily make up the granulation tissue. While the granulation tissue develops to fill the wedge of the wound, the epithelium regenerates at the surface.

Thus, the classical process of inflammation is the sum of several elementary reactions; namely, necrosis, vasodilation, edema, diapedesis and polymorphonuclear mobilization, phagocytosis, proliferation of macrophages, repair, and regeneration. Necrosis and regeneration are discussed in other chapters. The pathogenesis of the other elementary reactions in inflammation will be reviewed.

Vascular Reaction to Inflammation

Vascular congestion is the first event in inflammation. It is an active type of congestion and is restricted, at least in the beginning, to the injured area. In some inflammations—for example, erysipelas and some viral lobular pneumonias—the congestion is so important that it becomes of diagnostic value. In the beginning congestion is active, but in the later stages active congestion may be aggravated by superimposition of a passive form of congestion due to local thrombosis. The pathogenesis of the vasodilatation associated with inflammation is not completely understood, but the problem can be clarified somewhat if a distinction is made between vasodilatation of the arterioles and that of the capillaries.

Axon Reflex

The arterioles are innervated by vasomotor nerves that follow the parasympathetic branches of the posterior spinal roots and by vasoconstrictor nerves, which are sympathetic fibers arising in the lumbar chain. These nerves act by relaxing or contracting the circular smooth muscle fibers surrounding the arterioles. Vasodilatation may be a result of stimulation of the sympathetic nerves through an axon reflex. Chemical substances, usually called (H) substances because of their relationship with histamine, are liberated at the site of the inflammatory reaction and are responsible for the nervous stimulation.

The effects resulting from stroking the skin with a blunt instrument, which Lewis [1] has studied in detail, have provided an unusually simple model of the vascular reaction in inflammation. If the stroke is light, a white line appears in the area of the contact between instrument and skin. Moreover, morphological studies have established that nerves are not involved in the process because the effect will be seen even in denervated areas.

The response to a more forceful stroke to the skin is somewhat different. Lewis has distinguished three stages: the red line, the flare, and the wheal. The red line at the site of the stroke results from capillary dilation, possibly induced by chemostimulators (histamine or a histaminelike substance). The flare results from increased blood flow in an area several times the size of the original point of contact. The flare is caused by arterial dilation; it is mediated through nervous stimuli referred to as the axon reflex (see below). The area of the flare is red and the temperature of the area is higher than that of the surrounding skin. The wheal forms along the initial line of the stroke and is due to changes in capillary permeability.

Although everyone will develop these wheals after a stroke with a blunt instrument, some people are particularly sensitive to such a reaction. This phenomenon is called dermographism. In patients afflicted with dermographism, rubbing the skin of the back or the chest vigorously with a blunt instrument results first in the development of a zone of constriction, followed by the appearance of a red line which broadens until it is 1 or 2 cm wide. Within 1 or 2 minutes after the stroke is applied, an edematous band develops in the middle of the red line, and it may reach 3 or 5 cm in height. Unlike urticaria, this dermographism can be produced any time without any stimulus other than trauma. There is no agreement as to how these effects are mediated. Although serotonin and bacterial endotoxin elicit the nerve-mediated vasomotor response, the exact role of these compounds in the development of the axon reflex in inflammation is not clear.

Numerous scientists of great repute and of varied disciplines have studied the vasodilatation occurring in inflammation. Stricker in 1876 found that stimulation of the posterior roots that contribute nervous fibers to the sciatic nerves induces vasodilatation of the hind foot. Bayliss [2] demonstrated that the neurons from which these fibers originate are located in the dorsal root ganglia. Thus, if the fibers are sectioned between the ganglion and the spinal cord, the peripheral nerve fibers will not degenerate; but if they are sectioned peripheral to the ganglion, wallerian degeneration will take place. Furthermore, exclusion of the sympathetic fibers distributed to the leg or destruction of the lumbosacral ventral roots does not affect the vasodilatation of the hind legs.

Bruce [3] investigated this phenomenon more extensively by studying the effect of applying croton oil to the conjunctival epithelium. The sensitory nerves of that epithelium originate from the fifth nerve. Sectioning the fifth nerve between the spinal cord and its ganglion does not interfere (even a long time after sectioning) with the development of vasodilatation after the irritant is applied. In contrast, if the nerve is sectioned peripheral to the ganglion and enough time is allowed for complete degeneration of the peripheral nerves, then the vasodilatation reaction is abolished. These experiments demonstrate that the reflex could not be of central origin. Instead, the irritant stimulates the ending of the sensory branch, and afferent fibers conduct this impulse centrally. At a point of bifurcation of the central fiber, the impulse is conducted antidromically from one branch to another (the latter being the vasodilatation branch). This mechanism of nerve impulse transfer is called the axon reflex.

Capillary Dilation

The molecular mechanism responsible for physiological or pathological vasodilatation is not completely understood. The available evidence can best be presented in the light of a brief review of the physiology and the anatomy of the capillaries.

During inflammation the capillaries participate in the vasodilatation process. The capillaries of the inflamed area are more numerous and are engorged with blood. This vascular reaction is not surprising because it occurs frequently under physiological conditions.

The surface of the capillary bed in man is 6,300 m^2. Thus, the total number of capillaries is extremely large, and if all capillaries were filled with blood at the same time, the normal blood volume would have to be increased considerably (300 ml). In muscles, the capillaries could occupy 5% of the total mass if they were all open at once; however, normally only 1% of the muscle's capillary bed is functional. In active muscles, the capillary bed's surface increases, but it is not known to what extent.

The pressure in the capillaries is 20–25 mm Hg, and this pressure is maintained for some time after the heart has stopped beating. It is not known why the blood flows at one time into one set of capillaries and at another time into a different capillary bed; for example, frog glomeruli seem to alternate in forming the glomerular filtrate.

The opening and closing of capillaries is controlled indirectly by two muscular systems: (1) the muscular cuff that surrounds the metarteries or arteriovenous capillaries; and (2) the arterial muscles just at the origin of the capillaries. The contraction or dilatation of these capillary branches that directly connect the vein to the artery controls the resistance to flow not only in the lumen of these branches but also in the lumen of the subsidiary branches or true capillaries. Although true capillaries are not provided with smooth muscles and receive none or only a few nerve fibers, these are vessels of a diameter so small that minor changes in tension alter it.

It also appears that the endothelial wall of the capillary can contract passively, and that the loss of normal endothelial tone might itself be responsible for vasodilatation. Although we have described the sites (the muscular cuffs and the endothelial cell) that, within the capillary walls, may be affected by the factors controlling capillary diameter, the nature of that control mechanism remains unexplained.

During inflammation, vasodilatation is associated with an increase in capillary permeability. Various factors may induce these changes: (1) passive dilatation resulting from the increased blood flow in the arteriole; (2) a direct dilating effect of the injurious agent on the capillary wall; and (3) the release of toxic substances with vasodilating properties in the inflamed area.

Before an attempt is made to discuss the physiological chemistry of the changes in capillary permeability, it will be useful to examine briefly the morphological alterations that accompany the changes in capillary permeability.

Increased Permeability: Morphological Alteration of the Wall

Capillaries are made of endothelial cells completely surrounded by a cellular membrane and containing all the classical constituents of all cells: a nucleus, mitochondria, and the endoplasmic reticulum. The endothelial cells are hooked together by an intercellular cement the origin of which is not established but is probably cellular. The endothelial layer is supported by a basal membrane. The changes in capillary permeability observed in inflammation result from alterations either of the cells (cytoplasm or membrane) or of the cement. At the present time, it is impossible to determine which of these structures is involved. It is often argued in favor of the extracellular origin of the changes in capillary permeability that any cell losing as much protein as is lost during inflammation would have to be at the verge of death. Even if it is assumed that the changes in permeability result from endothelial cell injury, the mechanism by which this occurs remains to be demonstrated. Is it the result of increased pinocytosis, increased permeability of the cell membrane, or dilatation of channels that extend from peripheral membrane to the intraluminar membrane of the cell?* The distinction between "cellular" and "cement"** injury is likely to be academic because the intercellular cement is probably elaborated by the cell. Thus, the changes observed in the intercellular cement when capillary permeability is increased (softening, stickiness, and fluffing of cement) probably reflect some primary injury at the cellular level. Some investigators object that the changes in capillary permeability are too sudden to be explainable by primary cellular injury. Such argumentation is of little value because neither the susceptibility of the endothelial cell to injury nor the turnover of the cement is known.

In any event, in inflammation electron microscopic changes occur in the endothelial cell; they first appear in the thin wall of the vessels that are devoid of a muscular coat, and the changes are mainly of two types: (1) the development of intraluminal cytoplasmic processes, probably related to leukocytic infiltration; and (2) the development of large intracytoplasmic vesicles. Like the vesicles normally observed in the endothelial cells, the intracytoplasmic vesicles originate from infolds of the plasma membrane. However, the vesicles developing in inflammation are much larger than those appearing under normal conditions (1 μ). It seems reasonable to assume that the appearance of intracellular vesicles results from increased permeability of the capillaries to proteins and other chemical structures.

On the basis of morphological and physiological observations, various models have been proposed to explain the changes in capillary permeability to proteins. It is assumed that 0.2% of the surface of the endothelial walls is pierced by channels filled with water, with openings measuring from 12 A–40 A in

* Morphological investigations, carried out primarily with the aid of the electron microscope, indicate that some of the above mechanisms are probably operating in some tissues. We shall see later that one of the first morphological changes in endothelial cells of capillaries during inflammation is the appearance of large vacuoles.

** Some investigators have seriously questioned the existence of "cement," believing that it may be an artifact of staining methods.

diameter. Since 40 A is larger than the maximum dimension of even the largest plasma proteins, such a model could explain the extrusion of even the largest plasma proteins under pathological conditions. The model is not without faults. Such large openings could not prevent the extrusion of protein under physiological conditions, and no account is made of any control of these apertures.

In any case, the model implies that under pathological conditions increased permeability results from: (1) alteration of the pore itself; (2) alteration of the protein in solution within the pores; or (3) an increase in the total number of pores [4–7].

Chemical Mediators

Even if the physical mechanism of increased capillary permeability were explained, it would still be necessary to demonstrate the molecular mechanism triggering those changes. The trigger appears to be a chemical one, and many different substances ranging from complex polypeptides to simple amino acids have been implicated.

Histamine

Among those substances capable of increasing capillary permeability, histamine seems to be essential. Therefore, an understanding of histamine metabolism will be useful to the elucidation of the production and therapy of inflammation.

Histamine Metabolism. Histamine is the β-4-imidazolylethylamine; it is found in most tissues and in the blood, but it reaches highest concentrations in the large mast cell, where under normal conditions histamine is present in granules that contain also 5-hydroxytryptamine and heparin. When mast cells are grown in tissue culture, histamine and serotonin can be extracted from the granules. The presence of these compounds, however, is not strictly related to the development of such granules because some of the cells growing in tissue culture may produce granules that resemble the histamine granules morphologically but are devoid of histamine or serotonin.

Histamine is produced in animals by the decarboxylation of histidine. Histidine decarboxylase has been prepared in a soluble form from rabbit platelets. It was purified from mast cells of peritoneal fluid and mouse mastocytomas [8–11].

The activity of the enzyme purified from mastocytomas was unaffected by 24-hour dialysis. However, after 60-hour dialysis, the enzyme activity was lost, and pyridoxal phosphate had to be added to restore activity. These findings suggest that the coenzyme is tightly bound to the enzyme, and that prolonged dialysis is required to release all the bound coenzyme.

The exact role of pyridoxal phosphate in the decarboxylase reaction is not known, but the addition of the coenzyme reverses the inhibition of enzyme activity that occurs when hydroxylamine is present. Therefore, the carboxyl group of the coenzyme is assumed to be involved. Histidine decarboxylase activity can be induced by substrate administration, and an "unbound" form of histamine is then produced. The activation of the decarboxylase appears to be correlated with the histamine effects in the animal. It is not known where the induced decarboxylase is synthesized, but the available evidence suggests that mature mast cells are not involved in that process. Researchers have proposed that the "induced" histamine is formed in the endothelial cells of the small capillaries [12].

The administration of glucocorticoids affects histamine production in the lung, liver, and skin of the rat. Whereas the effect on lung and liver apparently results from a reduction in histamine decarboxylase activity, the effect on skin does not seem to involve histamine decarboxylase. It is not known which of the steps in the conversion of histidine to histamine in skin is inhibited by the glucocorticoids.

Histamine has multiple fates in mammalian organisms [13–15], including decarboxylation, methylation, or acetylation of the base. Histamine may be oxidized to yield β-imidazole acetaldehyde, ammonia, and hydrogen peroxide in the presence of water, oxygen, and an amino oxidase. This enzyme has a broad specificity and attacks substrates other than histamine; namely, putrescine, cadaverine, and even monoamines.

The properties of the enzyme that decarboxylates histamine have been debated for a long time. Kapeller-Adler [13] claims to have purified a specific histaminase that acts on histamine 1-methyl-4-(β-aminoethyl)-imidazole and 1-methyl-5-(β-aminoethyl)-imidazole; but not on putrescine, cadaverine, or hexamethylene diamine. Kapeller-Adler claims that her histaminase is a flavoprotein which requires pyridoxal phosphate for activity. Zeller [16] maintains that histaminase and diamine oxidase are identical enzymes. He interprets the failure of decarboxylating putrescine and cadaverine with histaminase as the result of impurities, including histidine residues, which slow down the oxidation of putrescine and cadaverine by the enzyme. Zeller thinks that the catalytic properties of the diamine oxidase depend upon the presence of copper in the protein molecule, and he has proposed that the copper forms a chelation complex with one ring of nitrogen and with the primary amino group. The new orbital situation that develops in the copper atom after the metal is chelated facilitates hydrogen transfer between indigocarmine and hydrogen peroxide (see methods for histaminase assay).

When histaminase and diamino oxidase preparations were subjected to repeated fractionation procedures, the ratio of diamino oxidase to histaminase activity remained constant, suggesting that the two enzymes were identical. Whether or not histaminase and diamino oxidase are a single molecule is more than of academic interest. If a specific enzyme exists the sole purpose of which is to catabolize histamine, then it seems proper to postulate that at least one of the histamine catabolic pathways involves decarboxylation.

The role of an unspecified decarboxylase in physiological or pathological histamine catabolism is less evident. To illustrate this point, Zeller cites the example of the brain. In brain, diamino oxidase is scarce or absent; therefore, catabolic pathways other than decarboxylating ones are likely to exist in brain.

The broad specificity of the decarboxylase may play a significant role in the onset of inflammation. When local conditions are such that a large amount of other substrates, in addition to histamine, are present in the medium, these substrates may interfere with the attack of the amino oxidase on histamine, and thus intensify the inflammatory reaction.

The enzyme is widely distributed. It is found in bacteria, plants, reptiles, birds, and mammalians alike.* The product of the amino oxidase reaction, β-imidazole acetaldehyde, is further oxidized by either aldehyde oxidase or xanthine oxidase to imidazole acetic acid, which may be excreted as such or in the form of its ribosides.

The methylation is catalyzed by an enzyme called N-methyltransferase, which has been partially purified from mouse liver and guinea pig brain. This enzyme does not methylate histidine. Thus, the methylhistidine found in urine derives from other sources, including azaserine. S-Adenosylmethionine might serve as a methyl donor in this reaction. Methylation of histamine seems to be the preponderant detoxifying pathway in humans.

The conversion of histamine to methylhistamine was investigated in mice after the injection of [^{14}C]histamine. The injected histamine rapidly disappears from blood and tissues, and methylhistamine is formed. The administration of serotonin, bufotenin, and chlorpromazine interferes with methylhistamine formation, possibly by blocking the methylation step. The administration of aminoguanidine, an inhibitor of diamino oxidase, enhances methylhistamine formation.

An enzyme that catalyzes the formation of imidazoleacetic acid ribotide from imidazoleacetic acid, ATP, and phosphoribosyl pyrophosphate has been purified from liver.

The exact contribution of histamine catabolism to the *in vivo* pools of imidazoleacetic acid ribotide is difficult to measure because imidazoleacetic acid is also produced in transamination from histidine. The reaction yields imidazolepyruvic acid, which by decarboxylation yields imidazoleacetic acid.

NADases catalyze the displacement of the nicotinamide moiety of the pyridine coenzyme by histamine, yielding histamine AD. There is no conclusive evidence that the conversion of histamine to histamine AD occurs in the intact animal. Yet, intriguing speculations have been made about the role of HAD. The first proposes that HAD is a storage form of histamine, the second that HAD is a precursor of the histamine ribose nucleoside found in tissues. If HAD were a storage form, one would expect the HAD to be split to histamine *in vitro* or *in vivo*. But the histamine-ribose bond is very stable, and no enzymes that catalyze the breakdown of histamine riboside have been found. Therefore, if HAD is formed at all *in vivo*, it seems likely to be a precursor of the histamine ribosides that have been found in the urine of rats, guinea pigs, and mice. No enzyme was found to catalyze the condensation of histamine and PRPP (Fig. 13-1).

Histamine Release. At first it was assumed that histamine is released only after cytolysis until some substances were observed to release histamine without greatly altering cellular structure. Such an observation is of interest to physiologists and pathologists because it demonstrates the release of the content of intracellular organelles without cellular death, a situation analogous to that observed in the secretion of the zymogen granules [17–23].

A large number of organic or inorganic substances release histamine (*e.g.*, detergents, large proteins and polysaccharides, proteolytic enzymes, trypsin or snake venom, basic peptides or their derivatives, peptides or amino acids, and organic bases). A compound that is frequently used to release histamine is an organic base referred to as 48/80. Five minutes after such a compound is added to the mast cells, the granules start moving in the cell toward the cell membrane. Then the granules appear to pass through the membrane and cluster at the exterior surface of the cell membrane. This degranulation process leaves an empty and shrunken cell.

The degranulation effect is a function of the concentration of releasers of pH, ionic strength, and temperature. The process is inhibited by anoxia, dinitrophenol, cyanide, thyroxine, and azides. Such findings suggest that at least the triggering of the degranulation process is energy dependent.

The mechanism by which histamine is released from cells is only partly clear. It may involve changes in ionic charge, the rupture of polar linkages, changes in permeability of the membrane to histamine, or, finally, release of histamine under the influence of some enzyme that has been specifically activated. Inasmuch as trypsin and other proteolytic enzymes induce histamine release, activation by a proteolytic enzyme has been suspected, but this has never been adequately substantiated. Benditt and his associates [24] have found proteolytic enzymes in association with the mast cell granule. At least two such enzymes were found. One hydrolyzes casein, albumin, and insulin and operates at an alkaline pH. Its specificity for esters is similar to that of chymotrypsin. The other proteolytic enzyme found in the mast cell granule is homospecific with trypsin. Chymotrypsin induces mast cell degranulation, and no energy is required for the process.

Uvnäs claims that phospholipase A is the enzyme responsible for histamine release, and that the

* Apparently, low concentrations of benzene activate histidine decarboxylase in rat kidney. This observation has not been extensively exploited. It might, however, lead to interesting clues with respect to the mechanism of histamine production.

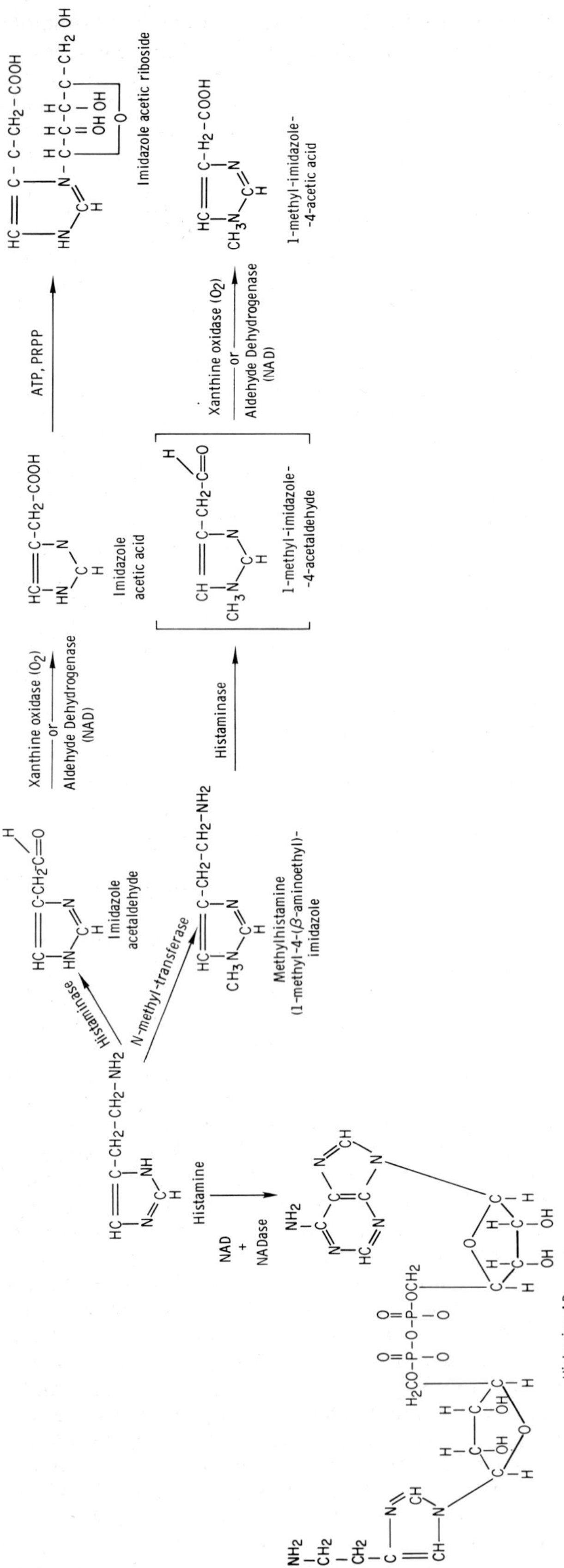

Fig. 13-1. Histamine metabolism

degranulation effect of phospholipase A requires oxygen and glucose. Phospholipase A is a hydrolytic enzyme that splits saturated fatty acid moieties from such phospholipid molecules as lecithin. In histamine degranulation, the effect of phospholipase A is specific. Other phospholipases (B, C, D) are without effect. When the morphological response of a mast cell is observed on a television screen, vigorous intracellular movements push the granules in a package toward the cell surface; from here the granules are ultimately expelled in a single package or as a chain of beads. Once out of the cell, the granules remain together in a single mass close to the cell surface. After degranulation, the cell appears wrinkled and deflated. The morphological changes are not unique to phospholipase A—they also occur with other degranulation agents 48/80. The active phospholipase A contains free NH_2 groups, which are masked in the inactive enzyme.

A unified hypothesis of mast cell degranulation has been proposed. The hypothesis postulates that chymotrypsin acts by earmarking the NH_2 groups in the phospholipase A. The lipase modifies the permeability of the cell membrane, and at the same time vigorous intracellular movements are generated.

Esterase is another enzyme that has often been suspected to be activated during histamine release, and some investigators have claimed that organic bases release histamine by interfering with an inhibitor that normally maintains esterase inactivation. Recently, cyclic 3′,5′-AMP has been implicated in histamine release, primarily because methyl xanthine and catecholamines, compounds that increase the intracellular levels of cyclic AMP, also inhibit histamine release induced with antigens [21].

Although histamine undoubtedly is released by the substances listed above and the release of the base triggers phenomena reminiscent of inflammation, there is no unequivocal evidence that histamine is responsible for the changes in capillary permeability observed in inflammation.

The study of the release of histamine and other granular contents is further complicated by the finding that in presence of releasing agents, part of the histamine or other granular content is lost from the granule into the cytosol [85].

Electron microscopic studies suggest that the histamine loaded granules are located in cavities in direct contact with the exterior. The addition of 48/80 to the mast cell results in the formation of pores at the surface of the membrane. The pores themselves communicate with the channels that contain the histamine granule [86]. These observations have led to a simple theory for the release of histamine. Degranulation is based on an ion exchange mechanism between histamine in the granule and cations (especially sodium) in the extracellular fluid.

Available evidence suggests that cyclic AMP modulates histamine release in patients with ragweed hay fever. The initial stimulus for the release of histamine from basophils is the binding of the antigen to an IgE antibody. Compounds such as epinephrine or theophylline, which modulate the synthesis of cyclic AMP, prevent the histamine release from leukocytes of patients with ragweed hay fever. Substances that stimulate adenylate cyclase (prostaglandin E, β-adrenergic catecholamines) inhibit the release of histamine. In contrast, substances that inhibit cyclic AMP synthesis, such as propranolol and burimamide, do not interfere with histamine release.

In allergic humans the sublingual administration of isoproterenol inhibited the wheal and flare response observed on the skin of patients injected with the appropriate antigen, but the response to an injection of histamine could not be inhibited, indicating that the hormone acts primarily by interfering with histamine release.

5-Hydroxytryptamine in Inflammation

The importance of 5-hydroxytryptamine in medicine does not stem from its possible role in inflammation. In contrast to histamine, 5-hydroxytryptamine is a potent vasoconstrictor, and therefore it is suspected of playing an important role in the pathogenesis of hypertension. Whereas a vasoconstrictor effect is observed when 100 μg of 5-hydroxytryptamine is injected under the skin of rats, capillary permeability is increased and edema develops if the compound is injected at lower doses. Therefore, it has been suggested that the inflammatory reaction results from a chain of events triggered by the release of 5-hydroxytryptamine, which in turn releases histamine. Such conclusions cannot be generalized because mice and rats respond to hydroxytryptamine injection with increased vascular permeability, but guinea pigs and rabbits do not. Therefore, it seems that if 5-hydroxytryptamine acts as an intermediate or a mediator in rats, in other animals other permeability factors must exist [24].

Proteins, Peptides, and Capillary Permeability

In 1890 Massart and Bordet [25] demonstrated the role of peptides and proteins in the inflammatory process. In the last decades, a number of polypeptides have been isolated that are able to increase capillary permeability, as demonstrated by the extrusion of intravenously injected dye at the administration site of the permeability factor. The mechanism by which these polypeptides affect capillary permeability is not clear. Under normal conditions they are poor histamine liberators; thus, if they play any role in the development of inflammation, it is likely to be by a mechanism different from that of histamine release. This class of polypeptides includes leukotaxine, exudime, bradykinin, kaleidin, plasmin, and GF [26–30].

Leukotaxine is a compound discovered by Menkin [30, 31] obtained from alkaline inflammatory exudates. It increases capillary permeability, but also exerts a chemotactic effect on leukocytes and facilitates the migration of polymorphonuclear and mononuclear phagocytes to the injured area. The chemotactic effect is greater for neutrophils than for monocytes. These effects of leukotaxine are demonstrable in a medium with neutral or alkaline pH. They can be inhibited by the administration of cortisone, but not by that of ACTH. After a rather crude tissue fractionation study of macrophages obtained by injecting turpentine in the pleural cavity of dogs, Menkin concluded that leukotaxine is a particulate compound located in the "mitochondrial-microsomal" fraction of the cell.

Exudine, another substance described by Menkin, is recovered from exudates obtained at later stages of the inflammation process when the pH of the medium is acidic. It differs from leukotaxine in at least two ways: (1) Its effects are repressed by ACTH but not by cortisone, and (2) it does not induce chemotactic effects on leukocytes. According to Menkin, exudine is localized in the nuclear and supernatant fractions of his leukocytic preparation. The presence of leukotaxine in sterile exudates produced by turpentine injection has been challenged in some laboratories. Although leukotaxine has been occasionally but not consistently crystallized, its chemical nature is unknown. The compound has precipitated virulent controversies, and the reader is referred to Menkin's monograph for a detailed discussion of the subject.

It is not established whether leukotaxine and exudine are specific polypeptides with a highly specialized role in inflammation or a class of unspecific polypeptides produced during the inflammatory reaction but not participating in its establishment.

Kinins—Structure and Metabolism

Bradykinin is a physiological vasodilator first obtained by treating the α_2-pseudoglobulins from blood plasma with trypsin and snake venom. Since bradykinin is derived from the α_2-globulin fraction, it is found in all tissues. Rocha e Silva has classified bradykinin among kinin hormones, a class of polypeptides characterized by marked physiological or pharmacological activities, not secreted by any specialized gland, but formed from inactive precursors present in the plasma or other tissues.

The exact physiological function of bradykinin is not clear. The vasodilatation of the skin observed after exposure to heat and the triggering of sweat secretion, salivation, and possibly exocrine pancreatic secretion by vasodilatation of the gland's capillaries are assumed to result from bradykinin release. Bradykinin may also play a role in increasing capillary permeability and vasodilatation, in the migration of leukocytes, and in the production of pain in inflammation. The release of kinins, among them bradykinin, could contribute to the bronchial constriction observed in asthma. Bradykinin antagonists (phenazone and aminopyrine) have been used in Germany as antiasthmatic drugs. Indeed, bradykinin produces bronchiolar constriction in the guinea pig and is known to be released during anaphylactic shock.

Bradykinin was first purified in Rocha e Silva's laboratories [32] using ion exchange chromatography on amberlite IRC 50. The purification procedure yielded a homogeneous peak with respect to ninhydrin color after hydrolysis and biological activities (5000 units per mg).

In 1959 [33] the amino acid composition of bradykinin was established and later bradykinin was believed to be an octapeptide with the following amino acid sequence: H-Arg-Pro-Pro-Gly-Phe-Ser-Phe-Arg-OH. A group of investigators in Boissonnas' [34] laboratory hurried in synthesizing the octapeptide, but their product proved to be physiologically inactive. The Swiss group first synthesized the octapeptide with an amino sequence similar to that proposed. The affinity of chymotrypsin for the synthetic compound was different from its affinity for natural bradykinin, a finding suggesting differences in the amino acid sequences of the natural and synthetic compounds. Since the sequence of the two first and two last amino acids had been solidly established, only that of the four central amino acids could be different. This still left 24 possible combinations; fortunately, 21 of them could be eliminated either on logical grounds or because the synthetic compound was found to be inactive. Among the three remaining sequences, only one of the synthetic octapeptides had physiological activity, yet it was only 2% of that of natural bradykinin. Full activity could be demonstrated only when one proline was added to the octapeptide. Thus, by combining clever deduction with skillful techniques, the same group finally succeeded in synthesizing a nonapeptide that contained one more proline than the peptide originally proposed by Elliott and had all the biological properties of bradykinin. In the meantime, Elliott [35] had shown that the physiological bradykinin contained one more proline residue than he suspected. Attempts were made to modify bradykinin's structure to either increase its activity or dissociate the bronchoconstrictor activity from the hypotensive activity. A large number of derivatives were prepared by Nicolaides and his associates, and among them a few derivatives are of some importance: the 8-para-fluorophenylalanine bradykinin, which exhibits a bronchoconstrictive and hypertensive activity about 150% of that of physiological bradykinin, and the 9-citrulline and 9-histidine bradykinins, which are strongly hypertensive but only weakly bronchoconstrictive. Further studies done in Bodansky's laboratory demonstrated that the strong cationic character of the terminal arginine, although indispensable for full activity, was not an absolute requirement for bradykininlike activity. The length of the chain is also an important feature of bradykinin's structure, and only the nonapeptide presents full activity.

The nonapeptide bradykinin and the octapeptide angiotensin both contract smooth muscle after a lag period of 25–50 seconds. A comparative study of the effects of these two polypeptides on smooth muscle contraction could therefore give some clues as to their mechanism of action. Whereas bradykinin acts directly on smooth muscle in isolated rat uterus and intestine, angiotensin acts through the intermediate of acetylcholine, which is released by stimulation of the Auerbach plexus. It is not known how the differences in the mode of action of the two polypeptides relate to differences in tertiary structure. Although angiotensin probably has a helical structure held together by hydrogen bonds, a helical structure is incompatible with the amino acid sequence of bradykinin. The hypothetical tertiary structures of angiotensin and bradykinin are presented in Fig. 13-2.

Although angiotensin activity is inhibited by incubation in 15% urea or arginine at room temperature for 10 minutes, such a treatment does not affect the biological activity of bradykinin. On the basis of such

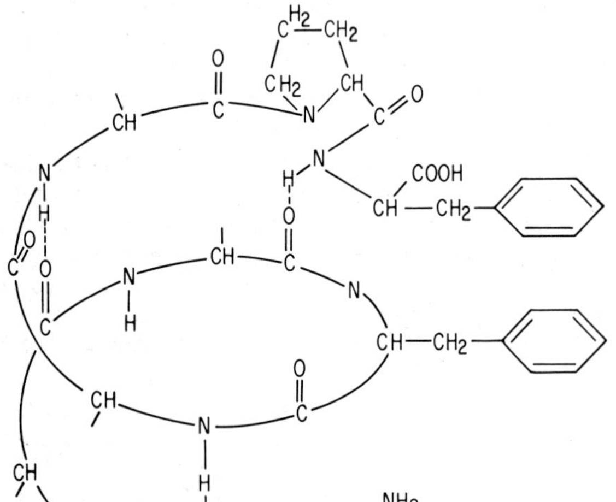

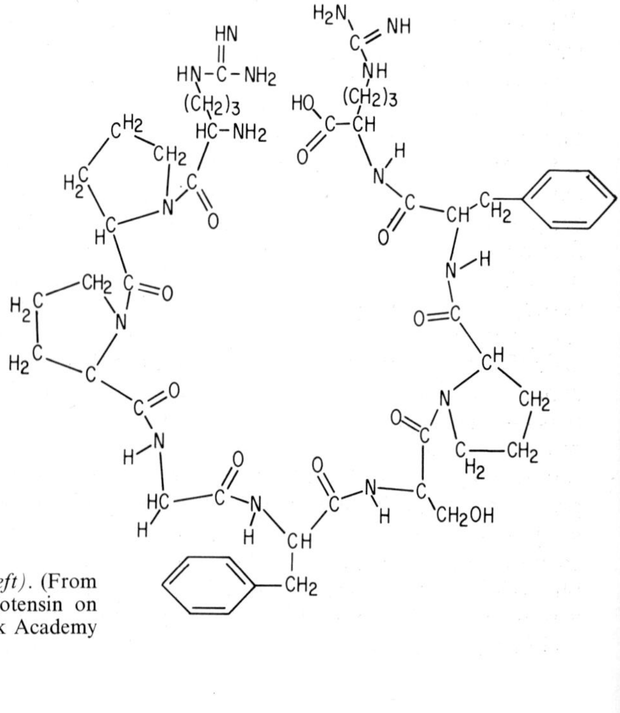

Fig. 13-2. Tertiary structures of bradykinin *(right)* and angiotensin *(left)*. (From Khairallah, P.A., and Page, I.H., Effects of Bradykinin and Angiotensin on Smooth Muscle, pp. 212–221, Figs. 4 and 5, Annals of the New York Academy of Sciences, Vol. 104, Art. 1, 1963.)

findings, it has been proposed that angiotensin has a helical structure held together by three hydrogen bonds, while helical structure is not necessary for bradykinin activity. In fact, helical structure is incompatible with the amino acid sequence of bradykinin (3-proline in sequence).

Angiotensin and bradykinin are compounds with such vigorous physiological activities that large tissue and blood concentrations would lead to dramatic consequences; therefore, it is not surprising that instead of the active form, a precursor of the active compound, referred to as angiotensinogen or bradykininogen, is present in tissues and fluid. Once released, the active compound is rapidly hydrolyzed by a catabolic enzyme.

Before the postulated mechanism for bradykinin activation can be discussed, it is necessary to review briefly the properties of a few other compounds, namely, kallikreins, kallidins, kininases, and the permeability factor/dilute.

Kallikreins are proteolytic enzymes originally found in the pancreas. They act on unknown substrates, kallidinogens (which are present in the α_2-globulin fraction of the plasma), to yield hypotensive substances, kallidins. The kallikreins have been purified from submaxillary glands, pancreas, urine, and sera of hogs, humans, and horses. The purified enzymes manifest two types of catalytic properties—proteolytic and esterolytic. They will thus act on casein, hemoglobin, benzylarginine, and α-tosylarginine. Kallikreins are assumed to have such high specificity that only the kallidinogens present the optimal amino acid sequence of a susceptible substrate [36].

Diniz and Carvalho [31] devised a micro method for bradykininogen determination, which permitted them to demonstrate the presence of kininogen in blood plasma of all species tested. In plasma, the kininogen is associated with the α_2-globulin fraction. Plasma kininogen levels are reduced in some pathological conditions, such as liver disease (cirrhosis, hepatitis, liver metastasis), induced experimentally in animals by carbon tetrachloride administration, or induced or occurring spontaneously in humans. Studies with carbon tetrachloride suggest that a correlation exists between the reappearance of bradykininogen in the plasma and the restoration of the liver injury. This finding suggests that bradykininogen is synthesized in the liver. Although the mechanism involved in converting bradykininogen to bradykinin is not conclusively elucidated, it has been suggested that bradykinin is liberated from the plasma by enzymes with tryptase properties. These enzymes, normally inactive in the plasma, can be activated under various physiological or pathological conditions, including heat, cold, injection of trypsin, and the effects of snake venom. This process is of interest with respect to shock, which has long been associated with the release of proteolytic enzymes. Such shock is produced by hemorrhage, anaphylaxis, or the administration of trypsin, snake venom or antitoxins, kallikrein, or peptone. Interestingly enough, in hemorrhagic shock, after an initial rise in bradykininogen levels, there is a rapid drop to values lower than those normally found under preshock conditions, suggesting that the kininogen has been excreted in the circulation, perhaps by spleen contraction or liver secretion, and then rapidly degraded to the bradykinin under the influence of proteolytic enzymes. Similar observations were made after the injection of antigen, producing anaphylactic shock.

At least two active peptides are formed if acid-treated plasma is subjected to the action of human urinary kallikreins. The acid treatment not only destroys the inhibitor of kallikrein and inactivates the kininase activities of the plasma, but it also activates kallikrein itself. This treatment of α_2-globulins yields two different kallidins, kallidin 10 and kallidin 9. Kallidin 9 is a nonapeptide with an amino acid sequence identical to that of bradykinin. Kallidin 10 is a decapeptide identical to kallidin 9 except for the addition of a lysine residue.

The sera of most animals, including humans, contain inhibitors of kallikreins that act optimally at pH 7.5. These inhibitors are assumed to be enzymes that destroy the kallikrein.

Two enzymes are known to hydrolyze the C-terminal arginine of bradykinin or kallidin. One, carboxypeptidase-N, is found in plasma. The other, carboxypeptidase B, is found in pancreas. Both enzymes have similar catalytic properties but are known to be structurally different. Both "kininases" are inhibited by chelating agents and are reactivated by the addition of zinc or cobalt.

In addition to the kallidin-kallikrein-kininase system, two other plasma permeability factors need to be considered: the Hageman factor and the permeability factor dilute. The role of the Hageman factor in the intrinsic clotting mechanism is described elsewhere. The Hageman factor is also believed to play an important role in the activation of the PF/dil, which is a vasoactive protein found in plasma. It can be clearly separated from kallikrein by chromatography, and is believed to activate kallikrein.

The sequence that has been proposed for the formation of kinins is outlined in Fig. 13-3.

Although all the molecular events responsible for the formation of plasma kinins are far from known, plausible models have been proposed. In the first step the Hageman factor (factor XII) is in presence of col-

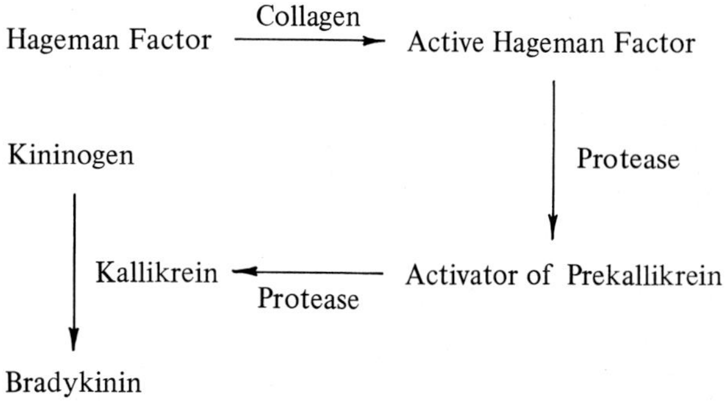

Fig. 13-3. Sequence in the formation of kinins

lagen activated to yield the active Hageman factor or factor XIIa. The molecular interactions between the Hageman factor and collagen are unclear, but it appears that both the intactness of the triple helical structure and the presence of glutamic and aspartic free carboxyl groups of the collagen molecules are prerequisites for activation.

$$\underset{\text{Hageman factor}}{\text{Factor XII}} \xrightarrow[\text{Collagen}]{} \underset{\text{Active Hageman factor}}{\text{Factor XIIa}}$$

In the second step factor XIIa is partially split and yields a polypeptide which is a potent activator of prekallikrein.

$$\text{Factor XIIa} \xrightarrow[\text{Protease}]{} \text{Activator of prekallikrein}$$

In the third step, prekallikrein, a protein synthesized in liver, is converted to kallikrein.

$$\text{Prekallikrein} \xrightarrow[\text{Protease}]{} \text{Kallikrein}$$

In the fourth step, kininogens are activated to bradykinin and in the last step a kinase activates the bradykinin.

$$\text{Kininogen} \xrightarrow[\text{Kallikrein}]{} \text{Bradykinin} \xrightarrow[\text{Kinase}]{} \underset{\text{Bradykinin}}{\text{Active}}$$

Plasma contains several protein inhibitors of kallikrein; one is identical to the protein that inactivates the plasma precursor of the first component of complement. The inhibitor is lacking in angioneurotic edema, the other inhibitors are antiprothrombin III and α_2 macroglobulin which is active in presence of heparin. Plasma contains polymeric forms of several different kininogens; two monomeric kininogens (I and II) are known, both contain the bradykinin sequence, in I at the carboxyl end, and in II near the carboxyl end of the molecule [87].

In conclusion, tissues appear to contain a large number of biochemical compounds that differ in their molecular composition and can trigger changes in vascular tonicity and permeability. Which of these substances are effective under normal physiological conditions or in inflammation and the exact sequence of events that follow the application of the inflammatory agent remain to be established. The cell protects itself against the unwanted effect of vasoactive polypeptides by making sure that the effect results from a cascade of reactions including several inhibitory feedback loops. The biochemical mechanism just described for the kinin-kininogen system resembles the sequence of the reaction that makes blood clot.

Kinins in Disease

Although kinins undoubtedly exist and are produced in the body through a complex sequence of reactions, their role in producing disease, especially human disease, remains obscure. Kinins have been suspected to play a pathogenic role in a number of conditions involving vascular disturbances, inflammation, and hypersensitivity [31, 39].

Although kinin levels and symptoms are not rigidly correlated, kinin release is believed to be at the origin of the flushing observed in association with the development of carcinoid tumors or of other neoplasms that cause flushing. Carcinoid tumors develop at the expense of the argentaffin cells: 70% of them in the appendix, 20% in the small intestine (ileum), and 10% in the stomach and rectum. Carcinoids produce a number of vasodilating substances (5-hydroxytryptamine, histamine, and bradykinin). Although the 5-hydroxytryptamine is believed to be responsible for the diarrhea and malabsorption observed in patients with such tumors, kinin release is thought to cause the flushing. Yet, although in some cases kinin levels are increased in the blood, no strict correlation between flushing and kinin release has been observed.

Occasionally, neoplasms other than carcinoids are accompanied by flushing (*e.g.*, carcinoma of lung, carcinoma of thyroid, retroperitoneal neuroblastoma). Whether kinin release causes the flushing in these cases remains to be seen.

The development of kininlike activity in anaphylactic shock has been demonstrated, but whether it is related to the pathogenesis of the disturbance is uncertain. The transfusion of plasma rich in fibrinogen or antihemophilic factors in humans is often associated with the development of shock. The cause of hypotension has been attributed to the kallikrein and esterases in the plasma preparation.

The plasma of patients with hereditary angioneurotic edema contains a permeability factor (derived from kallikrein) the appearance of which is inhibited by soya bean trypsin inhibitor, a potent inhibitor of esterases.

We have already seen that the precise role played by the kinins in the inflammatory reaction remains obscure. Although plausible, the proposed role of kinins in acute pancreatitis and the inflammatory reaction associated with gout and arthritis remains to be conclusively established.

Deficiencies in factor XII (Hageman factor, which activates intrinsic blood coagulation pathway), the complement system, the kininogen pathway, the plasminogen system, and prekallikrein have been described. None of these conditions leads to detectable clinical symptoms.

Epinephrine

Epinephrine biosynthesis has already been discussed. Because of its vasoconstrictive properties, epinephrine is believed to be released during inflammation to normalize vascular permeability. Unfortunately, the inflammatory process is also associated with the release of enzymes capable of breaking down epinephrine and thereby antagonizing its anti-inflammatory effect (see Fig. 13-4).

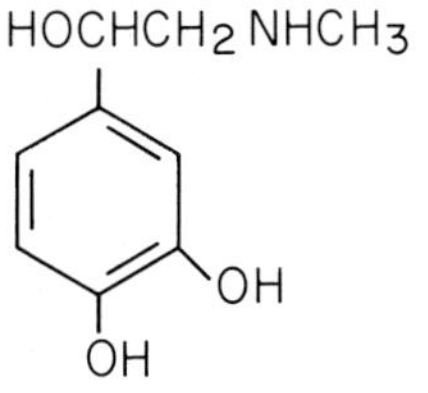

$HOCHCH_2NHCH_3$ (benzene ring with OH, OH)

Fig. 13-4. Formula of epinephrine

There are two major steps in the breakdown of epinephrine: oxidation by monoamine oxidase and methylation by catechol 0-methyltransferase. The belief that epinephrine acts as an anti-inflammatory hormone was further strengthened when it was discovered that monoamine oxidase inhibitors also have anti-inflammatory effects. Yet, monoamine oxidase interferes with inflammation, even in adrenalectomized animals; consequently, medullar epinephrine cannot be the source of the anti-inflammatory hormones.

Dopa and dopamine were later discovered to have anti-inflammatory properties, and it has therefore been proposed that monoamine oxidase, dopa decarboxylase, and dopamine β-oxidase mediate the inflammatory response by inactivating the anti-inflammatory amine.

The activity of these enzymes is believed to be increased after injury. The significance of all these observations with respect to the pathogenesis of inflammation is still not clear.

Prostaglandins

The biochemistry and the physiological function of prostaglandins will be discussed here because of their special role in inflammation. However, it should be kept in mind that prostaglandins affect many physiological functions, and a complete catalog of their functions probably is far from available [40–48].

Prostaglandins are relatively small and simple molecules soluble in lipid solvents at a high pH. They are derived from essential fatty acids, and they have an extraordinary range of physiological functions. In contrast to other hormones (e.g., biogenic amines) they are not stored, but must be made available when needed. During the first 3 decades of this century, a number of investigators associated prostaglandin function with a variety of tissue extracts. Thus, Falk discovered that an extract of intestinal walls induced smooth muscle contraction. The compound was uncommittedly called "darmstof." Extracts of the retina (retin) were found to have similar effects. However, an observation by two New York gynecologists led to the discovery of prostaglandins. In 1930 Kurzrok and Lieb reported that fresh human seminal fluid contained a substance capable of relaxing or contracting nonpregnant human uteri. Goldblatt and Von Euler discovered almost simultaneously that the active substance was an acid lipid. Using a standard smooth muscle contractility bioassay, Bergstrom later succeeded in isolating what is now referred to as prostaglandin E_1, a 20-carbon hydroxy fatty acid with an unusual cyclopentane ring. Fourteen prostaglandins have been described (thirteen in humans); they differ in the structure of their 5-membered ring.

Metabolism

Although the exact tissue concentration of prostaglandins is often difficult to measure, it is accepted that in most tissues the level of prostaglandins is very low; therefore, it must be assumed that prostaglandins are rapidly synthesized under some stimulus that elicits their effects and then is quickly destroyed. The molecular details of prostaglandin synthesis are not known. However, unsaturated fatty acids are known to be the precursors: homo-γ-linolenic acid (8,11,14-eicosatrienoic acid) and arachidonic acid (5,8,11,14-eicosatetraenoic acid) for prostaglandin E_2, and 5,8,11,14,17-eicosapentaenoic acid for prostaglandin E_3. (The most abundant among the essential fatty acids is arachidonic acid.) It is believed that the fatty acids exist in a bound state and are released by a phospholipase A close to a prostaglandin synthetase system found in microsomes. The phospholipase A exists in an inactive form and is activated under the stimulus that would ultimately release the prostaglandin.

When converted to prostaglandins, the 20-carbon long-chain fatty acids containing 3, 4, and 5 double bonds, respectively, become cyclized and take up molecular oxygen.

The prostaglandin synthetase system was found first in sheep and bull seminal vesicles, but it seems to be a ubiquitous enzyme. Prostaglandin synthetase has been described in the renal medulla, human skin, rat skin, rat stomach, and other organs. Although the enzyme system has not been extensively purified, available evidence suggests that its mechanism of action is similar in all tissues investigated. It is an insoluble microsomal enzyme system that catalyzes a number of reactions. The enzymic steps are not completely known, but the precursor fatty acid is converted to primary prostaglandin (prostaglandins E_1, E_2, E_3, $F_{1\alpha}$, $F_{2\alpha}$, and $F_{3\alpha}$) by hydroxylation of carbons 11 and 17 and double-bond isomerization. The PGA's are then produced by the loss of the elements of water from the 5-member ring of the PGE's. The PGE's are derived from PGA's by isomerization of the ring double bond.

The prostaglandins are attacked by a number of enzymes, which convert them to other metabolic types. An almost ubiquitous prostaglandins-specific dehydrogenase oxidizes the allylic alcohol group of carbon 15. A prostaglandins reductase, which requires a carbonyl L group at carbon 15 for activity, catalyzes the reduction of the $\Delta 13$ double bond. In addition to oxidation of the carbamyl fat chain, the ω-oxidation of the alkyl side chain and hydroxylation of carbons 19 and 20 have been observed. The relationships between the various types of prostaglandins and their

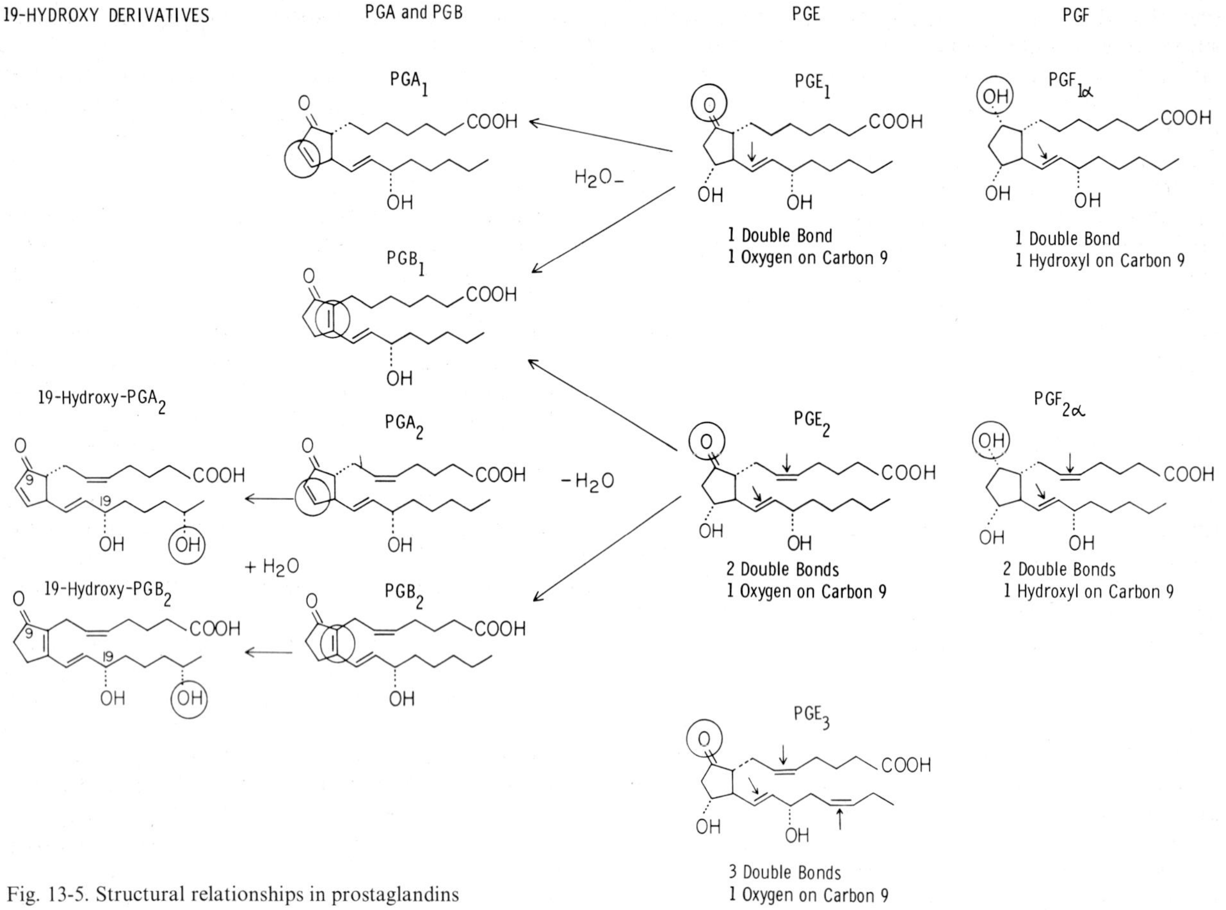

19-HYDROXY DERIVATIVES PGA and PGB PGE PGF

PGA1 PGE1 PGF1α COOH OH H2O−

PGB1 1 Double Bond 1 Oxygen on Carbon 9 1 Double Bond 1 Hydroxyl on Carbon 9

19-Hydroxy-PGA2 PGA2 PGE2 PGF2α −H2O + H2O

19-Hydroxy-PGB2 PGB2 2 Double Bonds 1 Oxygen on Carbon 9 2 Double Bonds 1 Hydroxyl on Carbon 9

PGE3 3 Double Bonds 1 Oxygen on Carbon 9

Fig. 13-5. Structural relationships in prostaglandins

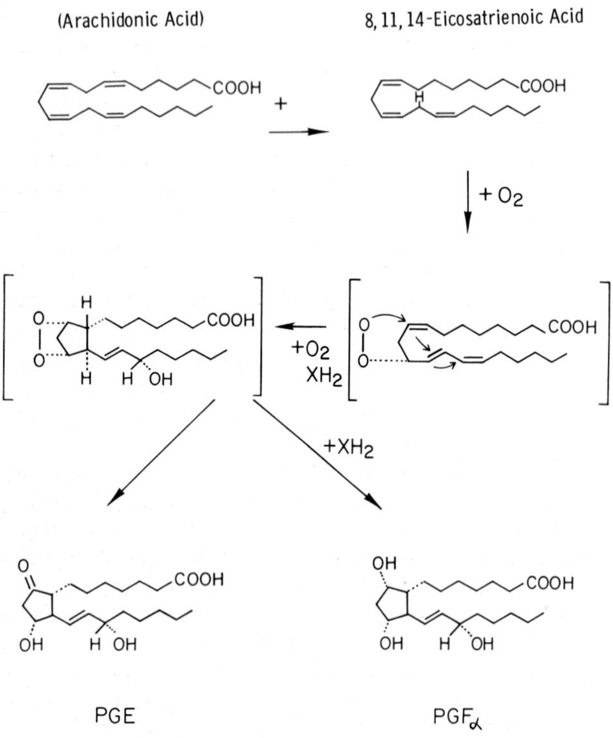

(Arachidonic Acid) 8, 11, 14-Eicosatrienoic Acid COOH + $+O_2$ XH_2 $+XH_2$

PGE PGFα

Fig. 13-6. Biosynthesis of PGE and PGF from arachidonic acid

biosynthesis are illustrated in Figures 13-5 and 13-6, respectively.

Although it can be suspected that the biosynthesis of such highly active compounds must be tightly regulated, little is known about such regulatory mechanisms. A number of factors have, however, been found to modulate the formation of prostaglandins.

Glutathione increases the production of prostaglandin E; cupric ions and dithiol compounds raise the levels of prostaglandin F at the expense of prostaglandin E. Also, the spectrum of prostaglandins produced varies from tissue to tissue. For example, whereas the largest amount of prostaglandin E is produced in seminal vesicles, prostaglandin F is produced predominantly in the uterus.

The lung is not usually thought of as an organ involved in anabolism or catabolism of metabolites other than those needed for the function and maintenance of the type 1 (squamous cell), the type 2 cell (the cell involved in the elaboration of surfactant and restoration of alveolar lining) or the endothelial cells. Yet in recent years it has become obvious that because of its geographical location between the splenic and general circulation, the lung is often the receptacle of hormones that have been rejected by the target organ. As a result the lung is, with the liver, a primary site of hormonal activation or degradation. We have seen that the activation of angiotensin I to angiotensin II occurs primarily in the lung. The lungs also contain the machinery needed to generate and destroy kinins. Similarly, the lungs are the major site for synthesis, degradation and release of prostaglandins. Degradation of prostaglandins in the lungs occurs only if they do not directly enter the portal circulation (through the gut or the spleen) in which case they are inactivated by the liver. The degradation of prostaglandins in the lungs varies with the type of prostaglandins, while the lungs seem to have little effect on prostaglandin A they rapidly degrade prostaglandins E and F [88].

Miscellaneous Functions

The number and the variety of physiological actions that are believed to be stimulated by prostaglandins are simply baffling. Moreover, the effects are often antagonistic; therefore, at this point it is difficult to present a logical and coherent description of the mode of action of prostaglandins. Among the effects ascribed to prostaglandins one must include: (1) an action as mediator of functional hyperemia, that is to say, in eliciting an increased blood flow in active muscles, (2) a role in the transport of water and electrolytes. Although it has been repeatedly claimed that prostaglandins play a role in the transport of ions and water across the cell membranes, the direction of such action varies with the tissue under investigation. In the toad bladder, prostaglandins stimulate sodium transport and inhibit water flow induced by vasopressin and theophylline, but they do not affect the water flow induced by cyclic AMP. Some of the roles of prostaglandins in controlling electrolyte transport are more directly related to clinical situations. It has already been mentioned that a natriuretic hormone, other than aldosterone, that simulates sodium reabsorption and is released in response to blood volume expansion acts either directly on the renal tubular sodium transport or indirectly by stimulating vasodilatation of the renal vascular bed. Prostaglandin A has been proposed for that role.

A number of neural or hormonal stimulations, trauma and shock are often associated with prostaglandin elaboration. Several natural compounds inhibit prostaglandin secretion, for example arachidonic and decanoic acids. Aspirin and several other nonsteroidal anti-inflammatory agents have also been found to inhibit prostaglandins.

The oral administration of prostaglandin E produces diarrhea; this is believed to result from inhibition of water transport across the mucous membrane. Prostaglandins are believed to be involved in the diarrhea elicited by cholera and enterotoxin. The toxin is thought to stimulate the synthesis of prostaglandin E_1 and prostaglandin E_2, which in turn activate adenyl cyclase, which then stimulates the secretion of chloride through the intestinal epithelium. If such a pathogenic mechanism obtains, drug inactivation of prostaglandin should stop the dehydration, which is the cause of death in cholera.

Medullary carcinoma of the thyroid and neural crest tumors contain large amounts of prostaglandins E_2 and $F_{2\alpha}$. These prostaglandins are thought to be involved in eliciting the diarrhea associated with the development of these tumors.

Prostaglandins seem to act as second messengers in eliciting hormonal action and thus in some ways mimic many of the effects of cyclic AMP. Whether this effect is direct or is mediated through the release of cyclic AMP is not entirely known. Moreover, the effect of prostaglandins on cyclic AMP concentrations varies depending upon the tissue involved. Although prostaglandin reduces the level of cyclic AMP in adipose tissue and toad bladder, it seems to stimulate cyclic AMP in most other tissues. Confusing as the data may be, there is evidence that: (1) prostaglandins stimulate the mode of action of cyclic AMP in many cases, and (2) they modulate hormonal reaction, and this modulation involves the cell membrane and calcium.

In addition to those hormones that regulate the reabsorption of water and sodium, the hormones that affect reproductive functions are among those most frequently suspected to be influenced by prostaglandin secretion. Here again, changes in prostaglandin concentration have been found to have some clinical significance. A correlation between the prostaglandin level in human semen and fertility as well as sperm migration has been observed.

We have already mentioned that the seminal plasma of men contains large amounts of prostaglandin. Prostaglandin can induce the luteolytic effect (regression of corpora lutea) normally prevented by hysterectomies in a pseudopregnant rat by reducing the length of the pseudopregnancy from 14 to 7 days. Prostaglandins E_2 and $E_{2\alpha}$ are believed to be involved in the rhythmic expelling of menstrual fluid from human uterus through inducing rhythmic contractions. Prostaglandins $F_{2\alpha}$ isolated from pregnant human myometria have been used clinically to induce parturition, and evidence suggests that the prostaglandins are elaborated from the decidual cells for that purpose.

Prostaglandins have also been suspected to function as mediators of synaptic transmission.

Role in Inflammation

Willis and his colleagues have studied the role of prostaglandin in inflammation produced by the carrageenin-induced paw swelling in rats and have established that: (1) prostaglandins induce most of the signs of inflammation, erythemia, pain, and edema; (2) the inflammatory process is associated with the release of prostaglandins at concentrations that indicate a potential role in the inflammatory reaction; and (3) the inhibitors of the synthetase aspirin and indomethacin interfere with the inflammatory process. Thus, PGE_1 and PGE_2 induce vascular permeability. It is, however, not known whether this action is due to a direct effect on the microvasculature or to histamine release. While in some strains of rats it seems to be a direct action, in others histamine release is likely to take place.

PGE has been shown to be chemotactic for polymorphonuclears in rats. Aspirin and indomethacin are potent inhibitors of the prostaglandin synthetase in guinea pig homogenates, and it has therefore been proposed that their antipyretic and analgesic effects result from interference with prostaglandin synthesis.

Similarly, PGE causes prolonged erythemia in normal human cutaneous vessels, and several prostaglandins induce wheal and flare responses in human skin.

Role in Essential Hypertension

Prostaglandins E and A lower arterial blood pressure of all mammalian species. Prostaglandins F increase blood pressure by causing peripheral vasoconstriction. In patients with essential hypertension, prostaglandins A_1 and A_2 reduce blood pressure. This may result from either general vasodilation or increased renal excretion of sodium, potassium, and water.

Prostaglandin A_1 is believed to reduce hypertension either by stimulating intrarenal vasodilation or by reversing renal vasoconstriction. The fall in renal vascular resistance that follows is responsible for the reduced arterial blood pressure.

Increased levels of prostaglandin E have been detected in the renal venous blood of humans with hypertension and in dogs following renal ischemia. The severity of the hypertensive state is not correlated with the levels of prostaglandin A in blood or kidney tissue.

Conclusion

We are clearly dealing here with a relatively simple group of chemicals present in all tissues, elaborated by a biochemical mechanism very similar in all these tissues, and manifesting extraordinarily potent and variable physiological functions. A common demoninator for the mode of action of prostaglandins has not yet been established, except for the fact that their action is likely to involve the cell membrane and that they often mimic the action of cyclic AMP. Whether prostaglandins act as first messengers, like hormones or intermediates between the action of the hormone and cyclic AMP, or are second messengers, like cyclic AMP, remains to be seen.

It goes without saying that the regulation of production and breakdown of compounds of such an intense physiological activity must involve numerous enzymic steps, which are allosterically controlled by activators and inhibitors. Here again, very little is known of the regulatory mechanism, but there can be no doubt that the elucidation of the mode of action, biosynthesis, catabolism, and regulation of prostaglandins will open many new avenues in diagnostic and therapeutic medicine. For further information, read Lee's work [89].

Cellular Changes in Inflammation

In the first part of the discussion of inflammation, the alterations in vascular tone and permeability associated with the inflammatory process were considered. This section deals with the cellular events: leukocytic migration and phagocytosis. Necrosis and tissular elimination were discussed in the section on necrosis.

Leukocytic Migration

Three stages can be distinguished in leukocytic migration: (1) the adhesion of leukocytes to the endothelial wall; (2) the penetration of leukocytes through the endothelial wall; and (3) the migration of leukocytes in the extravascular tissues. Soon after an injury has been inflicted, leukocytes move from the center of the bloodstream to the periphery. This shift in the intravascular distribution of leukocytes is responsible for the phenomenon histologists describe as leukocytic margination. Obviously, adhesion must result from interference with the normal relationship between leukocytes and endothelial cells. Whether these alterations result from modification of the endothelial cell, the leukocyte, or the mechanism that separates leukocytes from endothelial cells, or from a combination of the above factors is not known. What is certain is that any mechanism invoked to explain the adhesion of leukocytes to the endothelial wall must explain why adhesion occurs only after injury and is restricted to leukocytes.

A volume could be written on leukocyte stickiness. Such an endeavor could well constitute an invaluable contribution to pathology because it could unify concepts on the relationships between the membrane structures of different cells. Here we must restrict ourselves to a panoramic review of the concept [49].

Experiments on leukocytic adhesion in inflammation have generated two groups of theories. The first involves the elaboration of a chemical substance at the surface of the endothelial cells capable of trapping blood cells. Convincing evidence for elaboration of such a specific glue is not available. The second theory proposes that injury alters the endothelial or the leukocyte membrane, or both, in such a manner that the distribution of the surface charges, the site of hydrogen bonding, or the sources of the van der Waal's forces are altered.

Perhaps the most appealing among these theories is the one proposing that electrostatic charges bind the leukocyte to the endothelial cells by the intermediate of calcium bridges. Changes in the surface distribution of the charges—for example, by the formation of pseudopods on both leukocytes and endothelial cells—could reduce the energy of repulsion of the two types of cells by reducing the radius of curvation and cause the calcium bridges to form.

Obviously, adhesion of leukocytes is another of these instances in which much more needs to be known about the structure of the cell membranes before an acceptable molecular explanation will become available.

Most inflammatory agents induce leukocytic infiltration of the extravascular spaces, implying that the cells pass through the capillary membrane. Several different mechanisms have been invoked to explain the passage of the leukocyte through the capillary wall. Intercapillary spaces called stomas have been described in the normal capillary membrane. Leukocytes may enter the extravascular spaces by passing through these openings. The swelling of the endothelial cell observed in inflamed tissue would accelerate cellular exudation by dilating the normal channels. The fact that changes in permeability are often induced by those chemicals that stimulate cellular exudation would be in agreement with such assumptions. However, simultaneous effects on cellular exudation and capillary permeability are not a general rule, and the two effects are sometimes dissociated. For example, exudine is claimed to stimulate the extravasation of fluid without influencing leukocytic migration or diapedesis. An aqueous extract has been prepared from uteri of mice receiving estrogens which strongly stimulates leukocytic migration without affecting capillary permeability.

Diapedesis

In inflammation, long, thin infolds that are irregular in size and sometimes curled, measuring 8×1 μ develop and protrude in the capillary lumen. They are made of membranes with cytoplasmic cores, containing a few small vesicles but no specific organelles. Within the capillary lumen, these protrusions form a sort of spider web in which circulating leukocytes are caught. Once caught, the cells are soon surrounded by the endothelial cytoplasm. After the leukocyte has been enclosed within the cytoplasm, a new basal membrane develops from the edges. It pushes the cytoplasmic processes outward and surrounds the leukocytes. The rupture of the basal membrane at the peripheral aspect of the endothelial cell finally releases the entrapped leukocyte into the intercellular space.

These electron microscopic observations are in agreement with light microscopic observations demonstrating: (1) leukocytes adhering to the capillary wall; (2) roughness of the surface and irregularity of capillary endothelial cells; and (3) leukocytic margination within the capillary lumen. If these electron microscopic observations were a constant phenomenon, they would satisfactorily depict the ultrastructural changes accompanying leukocytic margination. Unfortunately, these observations cannot be generalized. Although they are obvious in the inflammatory reaction of the dog pancreas, cytoplasmic processes do not develop in acute inflammation of rat skins. Neither do they appear constantly in experimental inflammation produced in other tissues of the dog. Mechanisms involving the formation of intracellular gaps have also been invoked to explain diapedesis.

Electron microscopic studies of the earliest fine structural changes of the blood tissue barrier after the application of heat or turpentine indicate that the inflammatory response involves the formation of gaps between endothelial cells. If carbon particles are injected (in addition to the application of the inflammatory agent), they accumulate in the gap. Furthermore, polymorphonuclears, monocytes, and red cells were observed to fill the gap, suggesting that leukocytes migrate through the gap of the capillary endothelium.

In conclusion, there are two main concepts with respect to the passage of leukocytes through the endothelial membrane. The first proposes that the cells are thrust through the substance of the endothelial cells. The second suggests that leukocytes enter between the endothelial cells, either because the space separating endothelial cells is enlarged, or because the leukocyte can repel endothelial cells on the path that leads to the extravascular space.

Chemotaxis

Leukocytes, like protozoa, have chemotactic properties. Once leukocytes have reached the extravascular spaces, they are distributed at random if no specific substance directs their movement. However, in inflamed tissues the leukocytes concentrate in specific areas. This selectivity in leukocyte movements is explained by the existence of chemoreceptor centers responding to specific chemical substances, which induce the leukocytes to move toward or away from the highest concentration. Chemotaxis, which has been studied *in vivo* and *in vitro,* is assumed to result from the effect of chemicals normally present in bacteria or formed in the sterile inflammatory exudate [50–53].

Any pathology student who has looked at histological slides of inflamed areas is well aware of the accumulation of leukocytes occurring as a result of injury. In most acute inflammations, polymorphonuclears accumulate. Yet in some cases (typhoid fever, tuberculosis), monocytes are brought to the site of injury. Parasites selectively call upon one type of polymorphonuclear, and eosinophils predominate in the inflammatory exudate.

The leukocyte could be brought to the injured area passively or actively. For example, the polymorphonuclears circulating in the bloodstream could be drained through the gaps of the endothelium in the inflamed interstitial tissues, or they could be brought there by responding to specific "chemical" signals emanating from the injured area. Conceivably, the injured area could send signals to repel the leukocytes or to mobilize them against a concentration gradient. Therefore, positive and negative chemotaxis should be distinguished, although, practically, only positive chemotaxis has been observed.

Bacteria exhibit three types of chemotactic effects: They may stimulate, they may inhibit it, or may have no effect at all. Various pathogenic bacteria induce a positive chemotactism, among them some of the most effective are *Streptococcus pyogenes, Micrococcus pyogenes, Diplococcus pneumococci, Bacillus anthracis, Salmonella typhosa, Escherichia coli,* and *Corynebacterium diphtheriae.* Other bacteria, in particular those secreting toxins *(Clostridium tetani)*, inhibit leukocytic migration. However, this antagonistic effect can be eliminated by washing the toxin out of the culture medium.

For a long time, examination of histological sections constituted the only possible means of investigating chemotaxis *in vivo*. On the basis of such experiments, Menkin [21] claimed to have prepared from the exudate of inflamed tissue a biological compound leukotaxine, probably polypeptic in nature, that attracted leukocytes in the inflamed area. But when Harris was later able to photograph the leukocytic migration continuously and to follow the movements of the leukocyte in the extravascular space step by step, he concluded that although some substances extracted from bacteria are definitely chemotactic, no products prepared from inflammatory exudate presented such properties. Harris' results [52] suggest that polymorphonuclear migration results from the random distribution of polymorphonuclears that extrude through the intravascular wall into the extravascular space by the process of diapedesis. (Although the presence of leukotaxine in the sterile turpentine inflammatory exudates has not been confirmed, the leukotaxinelike substance has been found in necrotic muscles.) Harris' experiments explain the formation of polymorphonuclear layers around some bacterial lesions, but they shed no light on polymorphonuclear migration in areas of aseptic necrosis (*e.g.*, accumulation of eosinophils in bronchial asthma).

Movements of leukocytes can be observed on a cover slip dipped in heparinized blood for 30 minutes. The white cells move at random at a speed of 29–34 μ per minute. Their mobility can be modified by altering the condition of the medium. At least three components of the blood are known to stimulate the movement of PMN, namely, calcium, complement, and a γ-globulin fraction the nature of which is still unknown. (The γ-globulin fraction is missing in calcified citrated plasma.) In contrast, the mobility of the white cells is inhibited by a β-lipoprotein fraction in the plasma, by anesthetics, and by metabolic inhibitors.

Two aspects of the chemistry of chemotactism need to be considered: (1) the nature of those substances that attract the leukocytes in the inflamed area; and (2) the metabolic changes that are associated with the leukocytes' mobility. The chemical nature of those substances responsible for chemotactism has seldom been investigated thoroughly, in only a few cases is the gross nature of these substances known.

In pneumococci, the chemotactic properties result from the presence in the capsule of a polysaccharide, which has been purified. No chemotactic properties could be demonstrated for liposaccharide fractions and the phosphatides extracted from the bacillus of Koch. In contrast, proteins and polysaccharides prepared from the same source exhibited positive chemotactic properties.

The *Staphylococcus aureus* exerts its chemotactic effects on polymorphonuclear leukocytes in the absence of serum. Thus, although it is not known which molecular component in the bacteria is responsible for the chemotactic effect, serum factors such as complement seem to be unnecessary.

Studies done in Ward's laboratory have contributed much to our understanding of the mechanism by which bacteria exert their chemotactic effect. Bacteria release during replication either small chemotactic peptides with a molecular weight of 1,000, or enzymes that cleave C3 or C5 into chemotactic fragments [90].

Viruses also exert their chemotactic effect for polymorphonuclears in similar ways. Either they elaborate fully formed chemotactic factors which are not associated with virus particles, or they elaborate substances which release lysosomal enzymes that cleave C3 and/or C5 [91, 92].

Polymorphonuclears are well known to be attracted in areas of tissue necrosis. The chemotactic factors involved fall into two categories: breakdown products of collagen and fibrin and the release of cleaving enzymes that form C3 and/or C5.

Harris had claimed that only compounds of bacterial origin could elicit chemotactism toward polymorphonuclears. Yet, already in 1939 McCutcheon had shown that colloidin particles were chemotactic for polymorphonuclears. This intriguing observation was not adequately understood until Boyen developed more adequate techniques to compare the chemotactic properties of various substances. He devised a small plastic chamber, divided into two compartments by a porous membrane. The pores were small enough to keep resting leukocytes from crossing the membrane. But once the leukocytes are stimulated to "migrate," they can go through the pores. The chemotactic substance is placed on one side of the membrane, the cells on the other; and the cells that pass from one compartment to the other are counted after the membrane is fixed and stained. With this technique, it was established that colloidin particles are strongly chemotactic for rabbit polymorphonuclears. Moreover, if cellulose particles were incubated at 37° with serum and then separated by centrifugation, the supernatant serum proved to be strongly chemotactic. Further experiments established that a heat-labile substance present in normal rabbit serum combines with the cellulose particle. The complex cellulose heat-labile factor then activates other heat-labile components of serum. The complex heat-labile substance or the heat-labile substance activated in the serum is not chemotactic *per se,* but it releases a heat-stable chemotactic principle from tissues.

Various groups of investigators have provided evidence for the existence of precursors of chemotactic agents in plasma. The precursor is believed to be affected by cellular activators. Many tissues seem to contain such activators (liver, cardiac muscle), but granulocytes seem to be especially effective. Because the active substance is nondialyzable and digestible by trypsin, it is believed to be a protein. Granulocytic substances capable of eliciting leukocytic movements have been described. Such substances could be responsible for the late mobilization of leukocytes in the inflammatory process. The serum factors have chemotactic properties toward PMN that far exceed those of bradykinin, cationic proteins of PMN, or kallidin, indicating that chemotactism and changes in vascular permeability are mediated through different mechanisms. Kallikrein has been shown to be chemotactic for neutrophils and monocytes.

In studies of the pathogenesis of immunological vasculitis and acute glomerulonephritis, researchers showed that serum complement is required for the lesions to develop, and that serum complement binds with the deposits of antigen and antibody within the vascular wall to yield a potent agent chemotactic toward polymorphonuclears. It now appears that the chemotactic factor found in complement is a trimolecular complex consisting of C′5, C′6, and C′7 (see section on immunopathology).

The exact mechanism by which the molecular complex is activated *in vivo* is not known. *In vitro,* treatment with EAC′1a, 4, 2a, 3 or C4, 2a, 3 will yield the active complex in a readily reversible reaction. Similarly, the mechanism by which the molecular complex exerts its chemotactic effects on leukocytes is not known. It has been suggested that it activates a membrane protease, which might be involved in directing the movement of the polymorphonuclears. Treatment of a C3 fragment with streptokinase, trypsin, C′4, 2a factor, or C3 inactivator complex has yielded a compound with chemotactic properties.

Two inhibitors of chemotactism have been found in serum. One migrates on electrophoresis as a β-globulin and has a sedimentation constant of 7 S and seems to be directed against the C3 fragment. The other has the mobility of an α-globulin, a 4 S sedimentation constant, and it inhibits the C5 fragment. Available evidence suggests that the inhibitors act as protease. The levels of the serum inhibitors of chemotactism are increased in Hodgkin's disease and decreased in α_1-antitrypsin deficiency.

However, after the fifth component of guinea pig complement (7.85 S) was split into two fragments (7.4 S and 1.5 S), the smaller component (15,000 mol wt) exhibited chemotactic properties [54].

The relationship between this 15,000 mol wt chemotactic agent and the C′5, C′6, and C′7 complex or a low chemotactic factor that appears in guinea pig serum after endotoxin injection is not known.

In conclusion, polymorphonuclears can be attracted to the site of inflammation by three different sources of chemotactic agents: bacteria and viruses, serum compounds and tissue factors. In some cases the chemotactic effect is exerted without the complement, in others breakdown of C3 and/or C5 is required [93].

Polymorphonuclears are not the only cells to migrate to the inflamed area. Monocytes accumulate also either in the early stages of the inflammatory reaction (as in typhoid fever or tuberculosis) or after the polymorphonuclear accumulation has disappeared. Available evidence suggests that the monocytes (lymphocytes, macrophages, histiocytes, and epithelioid, giant, and plasma cells) are of hematogenous rather than tissular origin.

Yet the specific factors responsible for selective mononuclear accumulation are not now known. Various mechanisms have been proposed, but none is supported by substantial factual information. The theories include selective effects of pH and selective chemotactic agents. For example, it has been proposed that the mononuclears are attracted by a substance released by the polymorphonuclears. Such a hypothesis would not explain the monocyte accumulation that takes place at the outset of the inflammation, as in typhoid fever and tuberculosis. Some investigators have claimed, however, that in tuberculosis and brucellosis, polymorphonuclear accumulation precedes the mononuclear accumulation.

Harris [52] has proposed that the polymorphonuclears and the monocytes leave the bloodstream at the same time as a result of the vascular damage, but that the monocytes survive longer than the polymorphonuclears. Spector claims that the selectivity results from immobilization at the site of infection. When polymorphonuclears predominate, the monocytes pursue their course undamaged. When monocytes predominate, the polymorphonuclears leave the scene unaffected.

Monocytes respond chemotactically to a number of factors including bacterial chemotactic factors, kallikrein, fragments of C3 and C5, basic peptides derived from lysosomal granules and a lymphokine substance produced by antigenically stimulated lymphoid cells.

Chemotaxis does not affect only mammalian cells. Bacteria can also be attracted or repelled by chemical substances such as minerals, organic nutrients, and oxygen. Bacteria seem to be able to move toward the environment that provides them with the most appropriate supply of nutrients necessary to maintain the activities of the bioenergetic and biosynthetic pathways. Adler [55] has studied the phenomenon by planting mobile *E. coli* into a capillary tube containing an energy source, such as galactose and oxygen nitrate. For example, when excess galactose was used, Adler observed that two bands were formed—the first band using part of the sugar and all of the oxygen, and the second consuming the sugar anaerobically. These studies may prove useful in understanding chemotaxis in mammalian cells.

Chemotactic agents are also believed to be involved in the formation of mycobacterial aggregates during fruiting body formation.

The nature of the mechanism that directs the movement of the leukocyte against a concentration gradient of a chemotactic substance is completely obscure. The important aspect of chemotactism can probably best be understood by the close cooperation of the physicochemist and the biologist. What chemical features do all chemotactic agents have in common? The suggestion is often made that chemotactism is the result of differences in charges between the active chemotactic agent and the surface of polymorphonuclears; but this leaves unexplained the specificity of the chemotactic relationship. There seems to be no obvious common denominator in all agents capable of eliciting chemotactism. Boyden's suggestion that chemotactism is an expression of "self, nonself" discrimination seems quite plausible. The recognition of nonself is made not by the polymorphonuclear alone, but by the concerted action of polymorphonuclears and humoral factors.

After chemotactic agents have been released and when the cell has put in gear its source of energy needed for movement, what mechanical events are responsible for such displacement? Little is known of the machinery which brings the cell to respond to the call of the chemotactic agent, but one can list a number of components likely to be involved; for example, the actin filaments of the hyaline ectoplasm and the microtubules of the endoplasm. During polymorphonuclear or macrophage movement the hyaline ectoplasm protrudes in the direction of the movement. The ectoplasmic protrusions contain filaments 6 nm in diameter and glycogen particles. Similar filaments are found underneath the membrane of mast cells, they are made of actin and are believed to be involved in cell movement.

The arguments suggesting that microtubules may also be needed in the movement of polymorphonuclears include the observations that microtubules attach to the actin filaments, that microtubules increase in number during chemotactic movement and colchicine inhibits polymorphonuclear migration.

Since neither cyanide (0.011 M) nor sodium azide (0.005 M) interferes with cellular movement in the presence of a chemotactic substance, an aerobic source of energy is not required for these movements; and if energy (chemical) is needed at all, it can be provided by glycolysis. It has been further shown that *S. albus* attracts leukocytes in the absence of glucose, raising the question of need for metabolites. Moreover, chemotactism persists even in the presence of chelating agents, a finding that eliminates a role for calcium or magnesium in the process.

Two arguments associated with the development of movement of the phagocytes might be of significance. Complement derived chemotactic agents stimulate calcium influx and modulate the ratio of cyclic GMP to cyclic AMP. Although the sequence of events leading to the mobilization of polymorphonuclears remains unknown, one could imagine the following. After the cell has received the signal from the chemotactic agent it first builds the microtubular skeleton needed to perform the movement possibly under the influence of a shift in the relative concentration of cyclic AMP versus cyclic GMP.

The influx of calcium is responsible for biochemical events similar to those observed in contraction of skeletal muscle: actin reacts with myosin and ATP. ATP is hydrolyzed leading to the contraction of the myosin-actin filaments. A myosin with structural and enzymatic (ATPase activity) properties similar to that of muscle myosin has been purified from polymorphonuclears and macrophages.

Before we leave the subject of chemotactism, it is important to consider its relation to the general process of inflammation. What types of cells are attracted, and are phagocytosis and chemotactism closely related? Clearly, chemotaxis is most frequently manifested toward polymorphonuclears, but under some circumstances it may also involve mononuclears. This has been demonstrated in *Micrococcus pyogenes,* in *S. pyogenes,* and in *Mycobacterium tuberculosis.* Furthermore, chemicals like starch and glucose have been claimed to have a positive chemotactic effect on mononuclears. (There are no well-established examples of negative chemotactism despite previous reports to the contrary.)

Although generally chemotactism brings the bacterium and phagocytes in contact and may therefore facilitate phagocytosis, phagocytosis does not necessarily follow.

Phagocytosis

When Metchnikoff [56–59] sensed for the first time the importance of phagocytosis in biology, the phenomenon had already been known for many years. Hoeckel, Recklinghausen, Hiam, Schultz, and Grawitz all had described phagocytosis at some time between 1860 and 1880 [60]. The significance of Metchnikoff's contribution resides in the demonstration of the universality of phagocytosis.* Whereas in protozoa and primitive metazoa phagocytosis provides the sole mechanism for food ingestion, in higher animals with specialized intestinal tracts, the role of phagocytosis is restricted to mechanisms of clearing or defense.

A most fascinating observation of Metchnikoff, one which constituted the basis of his theory on phagocytosis, is that made on daphnia, or water lice. This transparent insect carries a disease produced by a small fungus called monospora biscupidata. The fungus has sharp spores that penetrate the digestive tract of the daphnia. Metchnikoff observed that these spores are

* The universality of the phenomenon was demonstrated by Metchnikoff and his student Cancatuzene, a Rumanian bacteriologist who gracefully combined vacation on the French seashore with productive research. Cancatuzene followed the ingestion of numerous types of bacteria in various invertebrates. Phagocytosis was further demonstrated in unicellular elements such as amoeba, which ingest foreign materials for nutrition; and although the nutritional role of phagocytosis is still preponderant in simple metazoa, such as sponges and earthworms, specialized cells seem to be involved in the process. In sponges, the cells lining the epithelial cavity (chromocytes) engulf the bacteria floating in the water that flows continuously into the central cavity. However, the bacteria are digested in a different type of cell called an amoebocyte. Even the simplest cells are capable of selectivity in the choice of the foreign material that they ingest. Amoeba are known to ingest some flagellates in preference to others.

engulfed and digested by phagocytes as soon as the spores enter the digestive tract. He further demonstrated that the severity of the disease was closely correlated with the survival of the spores. If all the spores were engulfed into phagocytes, the animals would not die; but if some escaped phagocytosis, death would soon ensue. Metchnikoff demonstrated phagocytosis in worms, arthropods, mollusks, tuna, crustaceans, insects, and vertebrates. He then proposed a general theory of inflammation; the inflammatory reaction is considered to be a defense mechanism in which phagocytosis of the deleterious agent plays the principal role.

Metchnikoff's theory of inflammation differs from that of Cohnheim, who proposed that inflammation results from the vascular reaction, and from that of Virchow who considered inflammation to be a deleterious mechanism endangering the victim's life.

The relationship between phagocytosis and infection was further confirmed in 1890 by Wagner, who demonstrated that if phagocytosis is inhibited artificially (by general anesthesia or by lowering the body temperature), susceptibility to the bacterial attack is increased. Furthermore, if the polymorphonuclear lineage is wiped out by a relative increase of lymphocytes—as in lymphocytic leukemia or after X-irradiation—or if the polymorphonuclears are immature—as in myeloid leukemia—the resistance to infection is considerably reduced [60–66].

Soon after phagocytosis was observed in mammalian tissues, various types of cells were shown to manifest such properties. However, cells' phagocytic capacities differ depending upon their nature. There are three main groups of phagocytic cells: (1) polymorphonuclears, (2) monocytes, and (3) the cells of the reticuloendothelial system. (More details on the various types of cellular elements will be given in other chapters.) We will consider here the anatomical and physiological features of phagocytosis and the fate of the engulfed particles.

Phagocytosis consists of four main steps: (1) contact between the phagocytes and pathogenic agents; (2) adhesion of the phagocyte and the pathogenic agent; (3) engulfment of the pathogenic agent within the phagocyte; and (4) digestion of the foreign material.

The contact between the phagocyte and its victim depends upon the density of the bacterial population and the phagocytic ability of the leukocytes. Adhesion apparently depends on the deposition of specific or unspecific proteins on the surface of the bacteria. The exact mechanism by which this occurs is not clear, but if bacteria are put in the serum of animals vaccinated against that bacteria, several alterations of the bacterial membrane occur—including stickiness of the membrane, an increase in the electric potential differences, and a decrease in the membrane's wettability by oil.

The facilitation of the phagocytic process by modification of the bacterial surface has been called opsonification and is due to opsonins (from the Greek *οψον* "appetizer"). Sir Homer Edward Wright observed that bacteria placed in serum of immunized individuals were more susceptible to phagocytosis. This susceptibility was enhanced if complement was added to the system.

In 1902 Mouton [67] demonstrated that amoeba secrete substances that trap microorganisms and make them adhere to the surface of the amoeba. The term opsonin, however, was used for the first time by Wright and Douglas [68, 69], who showed that components of normal serum sensitize bacteria to phagocytosis. Early in the study of phagocytosis, it was established through research with absorption techniques that most opsonins were specific for a given bacteria. For example, if tuberculosis bacilli are incubated with serum of humans and then centrifuged, the serum is left without the ability to opsonify for tuberculosis bacilli while it can still opsonify for staphylococci. Heat lability of opsonin was observed, but complement is responsible for that. Already in 1907 Cowie and Chapin established that opsonins require complement for activity.

Macrophages and reticuloendothelial cells phagocytize not only bacteria, but they are also capable of engulfing inert material, such as colloid particles, and dead cells, such as red cells. At first it was believed that phagocytosis by macrophages and reticuloendothelial cells did not require opsonification; even now this remains unsettled. Although Jenkin and Karthigasu's work suggests that "auto-opsonins" are needed for the phagocytosis of aging red cells, the studies of Vaughan and Boyden show that recognition of aged red cells by macrophages does not require opsonification.

Removal of carbon particles by reticuloendothelial cells has also been claimed to require opsonification. Some believe that particles are caught in these cells because a thin film of fibrin forms at their surface, making the particles stick to the cell walls. If, for some reason, the fibrin film is not formed, phagocytosis does not occur. This may explain the deleterious effect of heparin when it is administered before the injection of particles. In accordance, heparin has no effect when it is injected after the particles are administered because then the reticuloendothelial cells have already been coated.

There seems to be little doubt that opsonins are involved in the phagocytosis of bacteria. Whether the opsonification simply results in the release of chemotactic agents is not known, but the phagocyte holds its victim in a deadly, firm embrace before engulfing and digesting it. In conclusion, the mammalian polymorphonuclear cannot recognize "notself" without serum, but opsonification for macrophage phagocytosis is unsettled, except in the case of phagocytosis of microorganisms.

The phagocytosis of bacteria by polymorphonuclears is facilitated by a specific opsonin, a specific antibody for a given bacteria, and an unspecific opsonin, namely, complement (heat labile 56°). The simultaneous presence of the two types of opsonins secures optimum conditions for phagocytosis.

In addition to opsonins, other factors are known to facilitate phagocytosis. Histamine activates the removal of India ink by the reticuloendothelial system and stimulates phagocytosis by blood leukocytes *in vitro*. It is therefore not surprising that antihistamines depress the activity of the reticuloendothelial system and facilitate the development of bacteremia in local injection.

In addition to an effect similar to that of histamine on the reticuloendothelial system, choline also appears to facilitate the proliferation of that system. Mucin and levan reduce the sensitivity of microorganisms to phagocytosis. For example, the injection of levan increases the susceptibility of mice to intraperitoneal injection of microorganisms. This effect probably results from their effect on properdin. Indeed, mucin, levan, and some dextrans combine with the properdin of the blood (see chapter on immunopathology).

The sensitivity of the phagocyte to factors other than opsonin may also explain the relative sensitivity of some tissues to infection. A case in point is kidney infections. The kidney's sensitivity to infection could result from the high osmolarity in the medullary portion of the kidney. Man's renal medulla is particularly vulnerable to bacterial infection. High concentrations of salt and glucose, comparable to ranges encountered in man, have been shown to interfere with the phagocytic efficiency of the leukocytes [69].

Once the victim and the phagocyte have established contact, a series of maneuvers of the phagocyte brings the foreign material within the confines of the cell membrane, and, provided that the foreign material is susceptible to attack by the intracellular enzymes, it is ultimately digested. Because the phagocytic abilities of polymorphonuclears are different from those of macrophages, the events that take place during phagocytosis by macrophages and polymorphonuclears must be distinguished.

Bacterial adhesion to the plasma cell membrane of the polymorphonuclear cell is followed by alteration of the physicochemical properties of the membrane, resulting in the emission of pseudopods. The pseudopods, which first spread out in a winglike fashion on all sides of the victim, soon converge and completely envelop the bacteria. Invagination of the extruding membrane, which now contains the bacteria, brings the victim inside the cell. Amazingly little is known of the biochemistry of engulfment. Two aspects of metabolism need to be considered in relation to that important event: (1) the biochemical alterations of the membrane, and (2) the metabolic source of the energy required for the deployment of the pseudopods and the ultimate engulfment of the bacteria.

Whether it be a monocyte or the polymorphonuclear, the cell is selective about its prey. It will not attack an intact erythrocyte, but will readily eat dying red cells. It will avoid encapsulated bacteria, but will relish bacteria which have been exposed to fresh serum in the process of opsonization. Again, we know very little of the molecular events that alter the cell surfaces of the prey and the predator in such a fashion that engulfment of the prey becomes possible. The first question that comes to mind is what causes opsonization? Serum contains at least two components capable of facilitating the engulfment of the particle. One is heat labile and is derived from complement, the other one is heat stable and is derived from immunoglobulin. Obviously the serum of an animal which has not previously been exposed to the invading agent will contain little of the specific immunoglobulins and therefore will primarily contain the heat labile opsonins. A small quantity of antibody capable of opsonization activates C1, C4, and C2 to yield C1, C4, C2 complex, which in turn activates the properdin system. Either the C1, C4, C2 complex or the properdin system activates C3, the active fragment of which is then deposited on the surface of the particle to which it binds through firm hydrophobic bonds. The molecular weight of the active fragment is 70,000. Among the various types of immunohemoglobins found in the serum only those of the IgA type (more specifically IgA 1 and IgA 3) are capable of opsonization. Both the Fc and Fab fragments of the immunoglobulin must be intact to opsonize and it is apparently the Fab fragment that attaches to the particle. It is believed that the immunoglobulin and the C3 fragments attach each to specific receptors and like hormones trigger the machinery involved in the engulfment of the victim.

When ingestion is completed the foreign body finds itself entrapped inside of the body of the leukocyte surrounded by remnants of leukocyte membrane. This complex of foreign bodies and membranes forms the phagosome. The phagosome may or may not be digestible. In any event, there will in most cases be an attempt on the part of the predator to digest the prey. Both polymorphonuclears and monocytes contain large numbers of granules loaded with acid hydrolases. These granules are believed to fuse with the phagozome and thereby introduce the digestive enzyme in direct contact with the prey. Often the content of the granules will be found at the outside, either because of destruction of the predator, or because of release through an intact membrane.

The factors directing the movement of the granules toward the phagosomes are not known, but cyclic nucleotide and microtubules have been suspected to play a role. Indeed, extracellular degranulation is impaired by agents that increase intracellular cyclic AMP concentrations and by substances that interact with microtubules.

Polymorphonuclears and Phagocytosis

Polymorphonuclears are highly specialized cells that apparently derepress a large proportion of their genome to maintain only essential functions. Polymorphonuclear nuclei are multilobular. They are formed by two, three, or more sausage-shaped masses of chromatin, linked by thin chromatin threads. The molecular interactions responsible for this most special structure are not known. Neither is the purpose of such a special shape understood. Metchnikoff gave an imaginative but unconvincing interpretation: he believed that the appearance of multilobulated nuclei was a feat of evolution that took place when animals with circulatory systems developed. The oddly shaped nucleus of the polymorphonuclear is more readily bent than are the spherical nuclei of other cells, and, as a result, capillary migration of polymorphonuclears is made easier.

DNA is not synthesized in polymorphonuclears, and rather puzzling reports have suggested that [^{14}C]formate is not incorporated into polymorphonuclear RNA, although ^{32}P is. If such observations can be confirmed, they suggest that in polymorphonuclears, *de novo* synthesis is impossible. Thus, ^{32}P must be incorporated through the lengthening or turnover of existing RNA chains, or through synthesis via the salvage pathway. The high concentrations of free amino acids found in polymorphonuclears remain unexplained.

During phagocytosis, the metabolism of polymorphonuclear leukocytes is altered. The leukocytes normally have a high aerobic glycolytic rate and contain large amounts of glycogen. When *S. albae* and polymorphonuclears are put in a medium that contains 10% fresh rabbit serum and 0.1% glucose with air as the gas phase, the staphylococci are rapidly killed. Ninety per cent of the bacteria are killed within 3 hours after exposure to the polymorphonuclears. The bacterial destruction results from rapid phagocytosis and intraleukocytic digestion. The rate at which the bacteria are phagocytized can be modified by changing the medium or by adding metabolic inhibitors. The presence of rabbit serum is essential to phagocytosis. Without serum, the rate of phagocytosis is low and is not influenced by glucose. In contrast, when serum is present, the addition of glucose to the serum stimulates phagocytosis. When all the glucose has been used, phagocytosis persists; endogenous glycogen may be the source of energy.

The experiments described above suggest that glucose provides the energy needed for phagocytosis. Glucose could be used through glycolysis and the hexose monophosphate shunt, or the products of glycolysis can be further utilized through the Krebs cycle. All these biochemical pathways could yield ATP, which could then be a source of energy for phagocytosis. Studies with metabolic inhibitors suggest that glycolysis is essential to phagocytosis. Thus, the addition of iodoacetate or sodium fluoride to the medium prevents phagocytosis, whereas cyanide, antimycin A, and dinitrophenol have no such effect. Since glycolysis is essential for phagocytosis, it is not surprising that insulin given together with glucose stimulates phagocytosis.

Although glycolysis is essential for phagocytosis, when phagocytosis occurs, other pathways are also stimulated. The rate of respiration and the oxidation of the carbon 1 of glucose through the hexose monophosphate shunt are also stimulated. Results obtained in Evans' laboratory indicate that during the first 5 minutes after the onset of phagocytosis, glucose usage is markedly accelerated. This is followed during the next 20 minutes by acceleration of the oxidation of the carbon 1 of glucose which goes on for 45 minutes after the onset of phagocytosis.

The respiration rate seems to be stimulated from the onset of phagocytosis until 90 minutes later. The marked stimulation of the rate of activity of the hexose monophosphate shunt that occurs during phagocytosis has been interpreted to result in the production of NADPH, which is needed for phospholipid biosynthesis. The new phospholipids presumably are important in controlling the movements of the membranes involved with engulfing the agent within the phagocyte.

Phagocytosis is associated with changes in the biosynthetic pathway. In discussing these changes, we must distinguish between those that occur during and after ingestion. During ingestion, the only pathway that seems to be stimulated is the biosynthesis of phospholipids. The turnover of the neutral lipids and of the phosphatides is accelerated, a finding which might be relevant to the membrane movements associated with phagocytosis. The incorporation of [^{14}C]leucine into proteins or of [^{14}C]glucose into glycogen or RNA is not stimulated during ingestion, but 30 minutes after the onset of phagocytosis, glycogen synthesis is accelerated. Yet the phagocytic properties of polymorphonuclears toward pneumococci are not reduced in alloxan-diabetic rats, but bactericidal power of the blood is considerably reduced.

More detailed studies on the changes in phospholipid metabolism performed in Karnovsky and Hokin's laboratories have shown that the enhancement of incorporation of glucose and acetate in phospholipids includes the phosphatidic acid, phosphatidyl inositol, phosphatidyl serine, and phosphatidyl ethanolamine fractions, but not the phosphatidyl choline.

Since the increased incorporation of ^{32}P into phosphatidic acid and phosphatidyl inositol brought about by phagocytosis was not associated with elevated specific activity of ATP, Hokin suggested that the increased synthesis of phosphatidic acid occurred at the expense of α-glycerophosphate, possibly through the action of diglyceride kinase and lysophosphatidic acid cylase [70–75].

A small Golgi, a few mitochondria, and a sparce endoplasmic reticulum form the meager cytoplasmic contingent of the polymorphonuclear. But it is a special granule found in its cytoplasm that makes the polymorphonuclear unique. Under the light microscope the granules appear large; they pick up neutral, eosinophilic, or basophilic stains. Under the electron microscope the neutrophils appear as round, dense masses that are finely granular but otherwise structureless and are bound by single membranes. Inasmuch as little is known of basophil and eosinophil function, the properties of neutrophils will be discussed primarily. Neutrophils have been isolated by differential centrifugation. They contain few nucleic acids and proteins but are rich in acid hydrolases, which exhibit structural latency. In spite of some conspicuous differ-

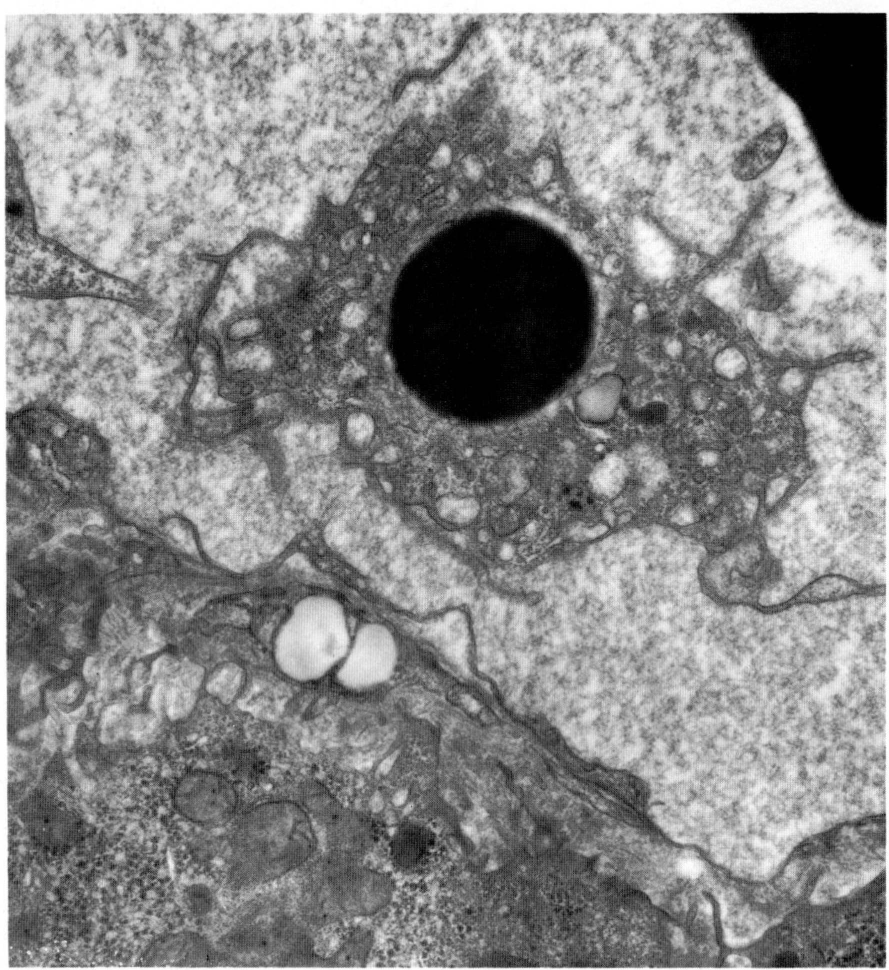

Fig. 13-7. Phagocytosis of an erythrocyte by a Kupffer cell lining the sinusoidal wall of a human liver. The ingested spheroidal erythrocte is contained within a phagocytic vacuole in the Kupffer cell cytoplasm (×11,500; from Zamboni)

ences between polymorphonuclear and hydrolase-rich granules found in other cells, the analogy between polymorphonuclear granules and liver lysosomes is striking [76–78].

Important differences between preparations of polymorphonuclear granules and liver lysosomes exist, although the most puzzling discrepancies have been clarified by further investigation. Polymorphonuclear granules were found to contain phagocytin, a bactericidal basic protein that kills both gram-positive and gram-negative microorganisms, and a number of enzymes not usually found in the lysosomal pellets obtained from other tissues, including lysozyme, peroxidase, alkaline phosphatase, lipase, and NADH oxidase. Classic liver lysosomes were assumed to contain only acid hydrolases, and therefore the finding of alkaline phosphatase in the lysosomal pellet was puzzling. Bainton and Farquhar [79, 80] examined polymorphonuclear granules histochemically and after combining histochemical and electron microscopic findings, concluded that the polymorphonuclear contains at least two types of granules: the lysosomelike granule, which has acid phosphatase and other acid hydrolases, and a special granule, which contains alkaline phosphatase and lysozyme. It is somewhat disturbing that peroxidase is found in lysosomelike granules, and that small levels of acid phosphatase activity are associated with the special granules. Using zonal centrifugation, Zeya and Spitznagel [81] separated from the lysosomelike and the special granule another type of granule that is low in enzyme and contains six cationic proteins not found in macrophages or in liver cells. Hirsch and his collaborators [82], in a combined morphological and biochemical study, essentially confirmed the above findings.

The presence of NADH oxidase in polymorphonuclear granules prepared from guinea pig lymphocytes has been demonstrated, and the enzyme has been implicated in phagocytosis. Although rabbit leukocytes do not seem to contains NADH dehydrogenase, Tappel and his collaborators claim to have purified liver lysosomal preparations containing an NADH dehydrogenase different from the enzyme found in mitochondria, but which shares some of the properties of the microsomal enzyme. Although the presence of the lipase in polymorphonuclear granules is not surprising, all attempts to demonstrate the presence of lipase in liver lysosomes have failed.

The mechanism by which the phagocytized agent is digested is still debated. Among the enzymes stored within granulocytes, lysozyme is the only one that has definitely been demonstrated to act on bacteria. (Lyso-

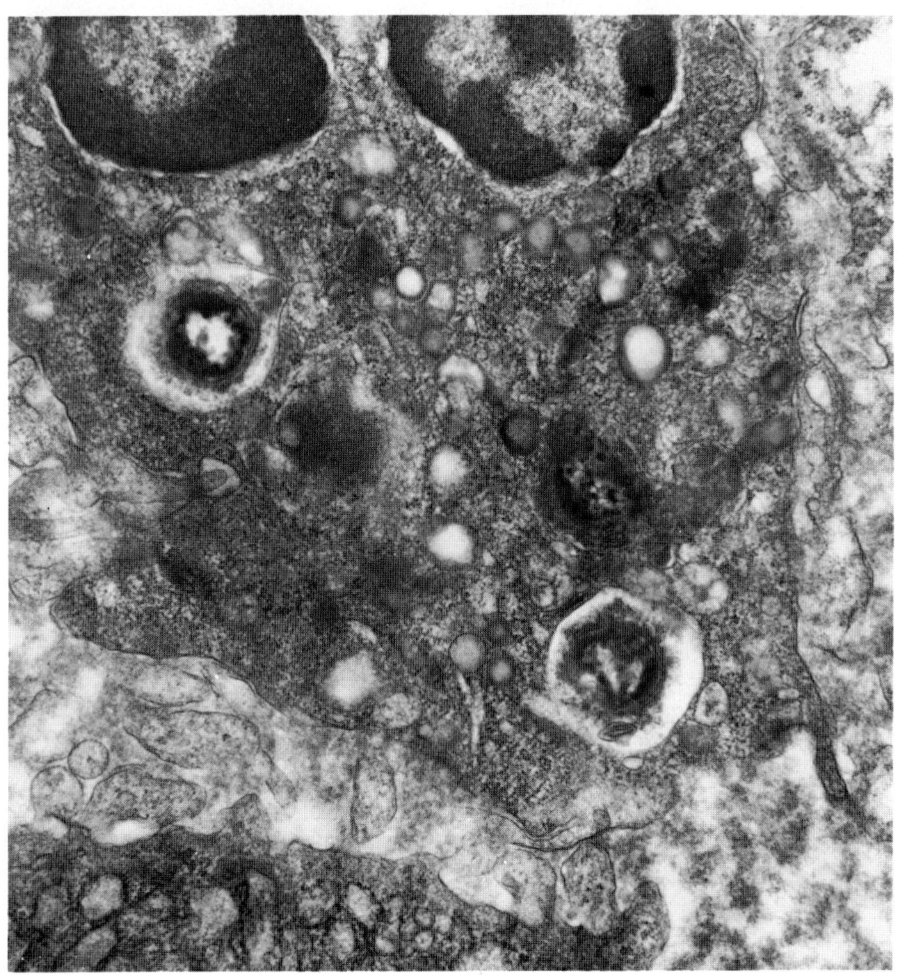

Fig. 13-8. Neutrophilic leukocyte in the nasal mucosa of a patient with rhinoscleroma. Two of the microorganisms (von Fritz's bacilli) responsible for the disease have been phagocytized and are easily identifiable within vacuoles in the neutrophil's cytoplasm (×24,000; from Zamboni)

zyme is an enzyme acting mainly on acetylamino polysaccharide. It is found in many tissues, but its concentration is particularly high in granulocytes and in inflammatory exudates. Lysozyme is inhibited by the presence of some acid polysaccharides, but it is activated by ketone.)

One observation made by Metchnikoff might be relevant to a role of the acid hydrolases in the digestion of bacteria. Metchnikoff observed that after phagocytosis, the color of the granule that picks up the litmus indicator changes from neutral to acid. It is not known whether this change in pH is the cause or the consequence of death of the polymorphonuclear, which inevitably follows phagocytosis.

The mechanism by which the enzyme-containing granule and the vacuole originally derived from the plasma membrane make contact is not certain (see above). But if the enzymes are to act on the engulfed bacteria, they must in some way be released. There are two possible mechanisms: (1) rupture of the granule and release of the enzymes into the cytoplasm (either indiscriminately or close to the phagocytic vacuole), an event likely to kill the cell; or (2) fusion of the membrane of the phagocytic vacuole with that of the polymorphonuclear granule. Cinematographic studies after bacterial engulfment indicate that the enzymes contained in the polymorphonuclear granule are released into the phagocytic granule after the two membranes fuse.

Hirsch and his collaboraters have contributed remarkable cinematographic studies on the fate of polymorphonuclear granules after attack by streptolysin A. Almost immediately after streptolysin A attacks, the polymorphonuclear granules explode and probably release their enzyme content into the surrounding cytoplasm. A few minutes later, morphological signs of cellular death are seen (formation of filamentous processes in the membrane, liquefaction of the cytoplasm, and clumping of the nucleus). The effect of streptolysin S is similar to that of streptolysin A, except that degranulation occurs late (15 to 30 minutes) after streptolysin S application.

The studies of Hirsch strongly suggest that streptolysin kills the polymorphonuclear and that polymorphonuclear death is in some way associated with degranulation, although Hirsch's observations do not exclude a primary effect on the cell membrane.

Evidence that the structure of the cell membrane is of consequence in phagocytosis is provided by experiments in which the effect of surfactants on phagocytosis was studied, and by studies of the uptake of macromolecules by Ehrlich ascites cells.

We have mentioned already that the phagocytic process, although most conspicuous in polymorphonuclears and macrophages, also takes place in other cells. Cancer cells are sometimes very active phagocytes. Cells of the Ehrlich ascites carcinoma take up extracellular proteins from the surrounding media and use them for nutrition. The kinetics of uptake and utilization follows Michaelis-Menten relationships, suggesting that the proteins enter the cell by an active process rather than by simple diffusion. Treatment of the membrane with neuramidase or pronase abolishes the phagocytic properties, which suggests that integrity of glycoproteins in the membrane is required for successful phagocytosis. Two examples of phagocytosis are illustrated in Figs. 13-7 and 13-8.

Bacteriostatic Agents

The polymorphonuclear contains three groups of antimicrobial agents: (1) metabolic products: lactic acid and H_2O_2; (2) cationic proteins, principally phagocytin and leukin and possibly others such as lactoferrin; and (3) enzymes, lysozymes, and myeloperoxidase. In general, the deterrent capacity of the leukocyte generously excedes its needs under ordinary conditions of infection. The mode of execution of the bacteria varies with the type involved. For example, H_2O_2 accumulation is most important in killing staphylococci, whereas a deficiency in H_2O_2 generation is compatible with the killing of pneumococci.

Leukocyte deficiencies in lactic acid production, lysozyme, and cationic proteins have not been described. In contrast, defects in myeloperoxidase and H_2O_2 production have been observed.

A number of patients have been described in whom the peroxidase was absent from polymorphonuclears and monocytes as a result of a mutation in an autosomal gene. To date, only one of the patients with MPO deficiency has been reported to have defective bactericidal and fungicidal mechanisms. In other patients, the bactericidal effect was the reverse of that in normal patients insensitive to azide. That azide blocks the bactericidal properties of normal leukocytes is understandable since azide is a potent inhibitor of myeloperoxidase. But then by what mechanisms are bacteria killed in MPO-deficient cells? An azide-insensitive mechanism appears to have been developed in those cells. One such mechanism is believed to function as follows: in the absence of myeloperoxidase, H_2O_2 is not used and a bactericidal effect results from H_2O_2 accumulation.

During the first year of life, some children develop a puzzling sensitivity to infections. The susceptibility is restricted to *S. aureus* and a number of gram-negative agents; these children resist infections by streptococci, lactobacilli, and pneumococci. The disease is hereditary and is linked to a mutation of the X chromosome. Without adequate prevention and therapy, the susceptibility to infection increases and the child dies at an early age. At autopsy, the critical findings are widespread abscesses, granuloma formation, and lipid-laden histiocytes.

Evaluation of leukocyte function of patients with this disease reveals a decrease in (1) bactericidal activity for *S. aureus* and gram-negative agents, (2) virucidal and fungicidal activity, and (3) O_2 consumption and H_2O_2 production. Although the pathogenesis of the disease is not known in all cases and phagocytin deficiency and abnormal vacuolization have been incriminated as pathogenic agents, it now appears that the decrease in H_2O_2 formation is responsible for the loss of bactericidal effect. However, it is not known which segment of the H_2O_2 generating system is altered in these patients with chronic granulomatous degeneration. Deficiencies in NADH oxidase and GSH peroxidase have been described in some patients, as has an increased lability of glucose-6-phosphate dehydrogenase.

Eosinophils

Not much is known about the role that eosinophils play in inflammation. Modern notions of their role rest on circumstantial evidence, which includes the special concentration of eosinophils in the healthy, the effect of hormones on the body distribution of eosinophils, and the tissue distribution of eosinophils in disease [82].

In the healthy organism, eosinophils are found in highest concentration in the mucosa that separates the internal from the external environment: the lungs, the intestines, and the skin. In fact, because of the high concentration of eosinophils in the intestines, it has often been proposed that these cells participate in digestion. The functional relationship that links eosinophils to cortisone is not known; what is certain is that cortisone administration reduces eosinophil levels in blood without affecting their number in bone marrow.

The role that eosinophilic granules play in inflammation is not clear. Yet it seems that the special features of the granules must be linked to unique functional properties. Inflammatory reactions resulting from parasitic infection or from allergy often contain cellular exudates rich in eosinophils. The eosinophilic granules vary in size: they are large (1 μ) in the horse, small in the rat (0.2 μ). In humans, the size of the eosinophilic granule is intermediate between rat and horse. To prepare pellets of clean eosinophilic granules, it is necessary to separate the eosinophilic from the neutrophilic polymorphonuclears. Hirsch has successfully separated the two types of cells and has prepared eosinophilic granules by differential centrifugation. Like neutrophilic granules, eosinophilic granules contain latent hydrolases. The two types of granules differ, however, in at least three ways. After most of the content of the eosinophilic granule is solubilized, the acid phosphatase and peroxidase remain tightly bound to the structural remains. As already mentioned, the eosinophil is rich in peroxidase and

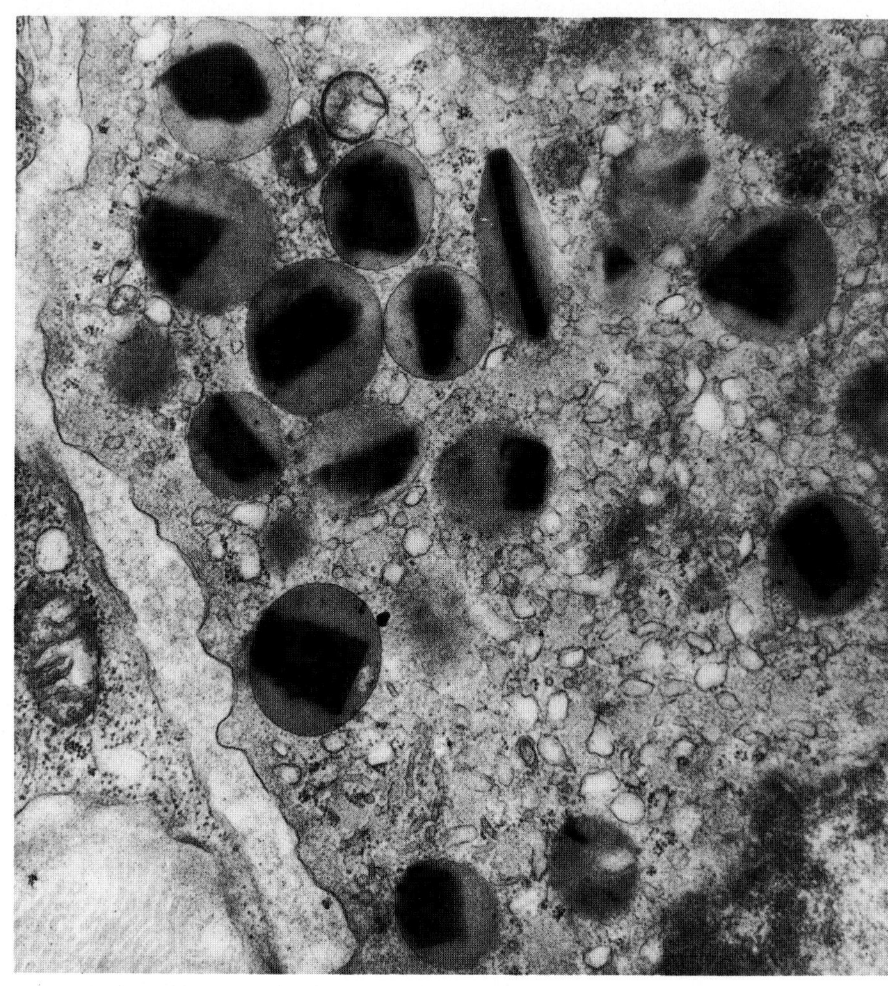

Fig. 13-9. The granules of the eosinophilic leukocyte contain a crystalloid with highly electron-dense material of uncertain chemical composition (×27,800; from Zamboni)

contains a crystalline structure, the composition and role of which remain unknown. Under the electron microscope, this crystal occupies the center either as a rectangle or as a band spanning the entire width of the polymorphonuclear, an otherwise structureless granule (see Fig. 13-9).

Thus, eosinophils contain a number of special substances—such as peroxidase, plasminogen, and digestive enzymes. Roles of eosinophils in inflammation have therefore been postulated that are in keeping with their biochemical composition, namely, carrier of peroxidase, source of plasminogen, etc. One hypothesis that has gained increasing support suggests that eosinophils carry antigen from the site of phagocytosis to the site of elaboration. (This view will be examined in more detail in the section on immunopathology.)

As we shall see later, some types of inflammatory reactions, especially those associated with anaphylaxis or parasitic invasion, are characterized by the presence of many eosinophils. It would seem that such a selective accumulation of inflammatory cells must result from special chemotactic properties. Although eosinophils will respond chemotactically to C3 and C5 fragments as well as to bacterial chemotactic agents, chemotactic factors specific for eosinophils have been discovered. One, called eosinophilic chemotactic factor of anaphylaxis (ECF-A) is a small peptide stored in granules of basophils or mast cells which is released when the antigen is introduced in a sensitized individual. The other, much more complex, develops in antigen stimulated cells but becomes active only after incubation of the lymphokinine with the immune complex. The existence of a chemotactic factor for eosinophils originating in the lymphocytes may explain the frequent association of lymphoid cells and eosinophils in inflammatory reactions.

Plasmocytic and Lymphocytic Migration

Inflammation is further characterized by the infiltration of the inflamed tissue by lymphocytes and plasmocytes. The role of lymphocytes and plasmocytes in inflammation is discussed in the Chapter on immunity.

Macrophages

The macrophages constitute a wide population of different cells distributed throughout the body, but all derived from a single marrow precursor, the promonocyte. A major characteristic of these cells is their marked ability for phagocytosis. The population of cells involved in macrophagia is sometimes referred to as the mononuclear phagocytic system.

Although earlier work suggested that macrophages may be derived from lymphocytes, there is no doubt left that all forms of macrophages are derived from a bone marrow precursor cell, the promonocyte. These bone marrow precursors migrate at different sites of the body to form the different types of macrophages: the monocytes of the blood and the serous cavities, the Kupffer cells of the liver, the litoral cells of the spleen, the histiocytes in the connective tissue, the epithelioid cells and the giant cells of the inflammatory granuloma.

If an animal receives a bone marrow transplant with appropriate chromosome markers at a specified time after partial hepatectomy, the new Kupffer cells of the liver will contain the marker, indicating that the Kupffer cells were derived from bone marrow cells.

Macrophages are involved in both acute and chronic inflammation. They are attracted to the inflammatory site by specific chemotactic mechanisms. In acute inflammation the mononuclear infiltration is short-lived (approximately a week). In chronic inflammation the monocytes may accumulate for long periods. The origin of the monocyte population in chronic inflammation has been investigated in detail. All kinetic experiments cannot be described here. Suffice to point out that the monocyte population behaves in three ways: the granuloma cells may die or migrate and be replaced by circulating monocytes, they may proliferate *in situ* through active cell division, or they may form a pool of immobile, long-lived nondividing cells [94].

The macrophage's appetite makes it much less discriminatory than the polymorphonuclear toward foreign material. In addition to bacteria, macrophages phagocytize dead cells and so-called inert materials, such as colloid particles, India ink, and fat globules. Several morphological features of the macrophage suggest that these cells metabolically are much more active than the polymorphonuclears. Macrophages are larger than polymorphonuclears and have a bean-shaped nucleus and chromatin that appears as a fine granular structure. Nucleoli are often prominent; the cytoplasm is abundant and contains a well-developed Golgi apparatus, endoplasmic reticulum, and numerous mitochondria. Ribosomes stud the membranes of the endoplasmic reticulum.

Like the polymorphonuclear, the macrophage contains special granules. Little is known of the synthetic ability of macrophage; however, the cell probably is capable of extensive biochemical synthesis since macrophages are known to divide and sometimes they proliferate actively, even *in vitro*.

Because blood monocytes have not been successfully separated, most studies on the bioenergetic activities of macrophages have been performed using peritoneal, rather than the peripheral, macrophages. The peritoneal macrophage survives adequately under anaerobic conditions. Even in the presence of oxygen, macrophages continue to have a high rate of glycolysis, and most of their energy is derived from the conversion of glucose to lactic acid. In contrast, alveolar macrophages take up three times as much oxygen as the peritoneal macrophages. However, in anoxemia, peritoneal macrophages also can respond quickly by increasing lactic acid production. The role of macrophages in immunity is discussed in Chapter 14.

Although phagocytosis is a property manifested by both polymorphonuclears and macrophages, the metabolic changes observed during phagocytosis differ with cell type. The metabolic reactions have been compared in polymorphonuclears, peritoneal macrophages, and alveolar macrophages. All three types of cells respond by an increase in respiratory activity, but whereas the increase is considerable in polymorphonuclears and peritoneal macrophages, it is small in alveolar macrophages. Interference with electron transport blocks phagocytosis in alveolar macrophages, but is without effect on polymorphonuclears and peritoneal macrophages, which depend mainly on glycolysis for activity. Changes in the metabolism of complex phosphatides could not be detected in alveolar macrophages. Whether the metabolic changes are specific to phagocytosis or are simply manifestations of membrane alteration is not certain. However, surface-active agents may induce metabolic changes similar to those observed during phagocytosis without recognizable vesiculation.

Special granules rich in acid hydrolases have been prepared from macrophages, and the acid hydrolases contained in these granules are believed to participate in digesting the engulfed material. Again, little is known of this mechanism of digestion. If one cannot exclude that the bacteria engulfed in the polymorphonuclear are digested as a result of rupture of the polymorphonuclear granules, and that the bacteria die because of the polymorphonuclear suicide, such an interpretation is untenable for macrophages. Macrophages have been known to phagocytize bacteria repeatedly; therefore, it is unlikely that the enzymic content of their granules is extruded in the cytoplasm. Consequently, it would appear that in macrophages, the phagocytic vacuole must fuse with the acid hydrolase granules. Whether the macrophage can, like the amoeba, use a breakdown product for sustenance remains to be seen.

Wiseman and Corn have studied the uptake of latex beads of various sizes by macrophages in tissue culture. Phagocytosis was prevented by inhibitors of oxidative phosphorylation, such as azide and dinitrophenol. In contrast, the glycolysis inhibitors fluoride and iodoacetate had little effect on phagocytosis. As the authors pointed out, such findings prove that phagocytosis is possible in the presence of aerobic sources of energy; but they do not imply that oxidative phosphorylation is indispensable for phagocytosis because it cannot be excluded that severe macrophage morbidity follows the administration of oxidative phosphorylation inhibitors. The kinetics of the phagocytic process are dictated by the size of the bead. Apparently, the phagocyte prefers to engulf beads of a given volume. Particles of a size smaller than that of the critical volume are aggregated in sufficient numbers on the surface of the membrane. The contact between the membrane and the beads is so intimate that all material in solution, including water, is excluded. On the basis of such observations, it has been proposed that the formation of the phagocytic vesicle is determined by special structural features of the plasma membrane.

Defective Leukocytic Response in Inflammation

Once the role of leukocytes in the inflammatory reaction became known, disorders resulting from defects in the inflammatory response, especially phagocytosis, could be identified. Such disorders fall into several major categories: defective cell production, interference with cell movement, interference with digestions of the prey and interference with the ability to kill the bacteria [95–96].

Defects in inflammatory cells can be divided into three major groups: decrease in total number, defects in function, quantitative defects which may result either from an absolute decrease in all types of granulocytes or from a relative takeover of the bone marrow space by other types of blood cells or by immature cells.

Absolute decreases are caused by agents that preferentially destroy rapidly growing cells such as X- or γ-radiation, most antimetabolites or specific antibodies. The term granulocytopenia is used when the granulocyte count in the blood drops to 3,000 per cu mm. When the count reaches 1,000 per cu mm the patient is vulnerable to bacterial infections. In some cases the granulocytopenia results from excessive breakdown. This is believed to be the case in the granulocytopenias that accompany pernicious anemia or the Chediak-Higashi's syndrome.

Conditions which result in unbalanced proliferation within the hematopoietic tissue of cells other than mature granulocytes will lead to neutropenia. Such conditions include polycythemia vera, chronic and acute leukemia, erythroleukemia, thrombocytopenia.

Decreased resistance to infection may occur with a granulocyte population normal in numbers, but with reduced function. The defect may involved motility, the ability to ingest the prey or the inability to kill bacteria.

Motility defects fall into two major categories: those in which the mechanical machinery for movement is defective, and those in which the cell is not able to respond to chemotactic stimuli. Hypophosphatemia is associated with decreased levels of ATP and impaired motility of the polymorphonuclears. A relative deficiency in 6 nm actin filaments in the cortical zone of the polymorphonuclears has been described in a patient with defective neutrophil motility [7].

Leukotactic defects have only been discovered recently. They fall into two categories: those in which the cell is defective in its ability to respond to the chemotactic stimulus and those in which the humoral factors necessary to induce chemotactism are either absent or inhibited. At least two syndromes are associated with hereditary chemotactic defects: the "lazy leukocyte syndrome" and Chediak-Higashi's disease. In either case the cause of the impaired chemotactic response is unknown. The "lazy leukocyte syndrome" probably covers a group of conditions caused by different pathogenic mechanisms.

The Chediak-Higashi's disease will be described here in some more detail because of the unusual cellular manifestations associated with the disease.

Children afflicted with Chediak-Higashi's disease present a pigmentation defect and are prone to infection, they may die from lymphomatous disease. The disease is inherited as a simple autosomal recessive trait. The absence of melanin pigment is responsible for severe photosensitivity. The hair is light and the skin is pale.

The high sensitivity to infection is associated with the presence of giant granules in neutrophils, eosinophils, lymphocytes and monocytes. The granules are azurophilic and are periodic acid-Schiff-, Sudan black- and peroxidase-positive. Examination of the hair with the electron microscope reveals that the hair is capable of forming melanosomes, but they too are often giant. A common pathogenic mechanism has been proposed which suggests that the primary defect affects the formation of membranes of both melanosomes and lysosomes [98].

A chemotactic defect of unknown origin has been described in patients afflicted with the Job's syndrome which is characterized by "cold" staphylococcal abscesses, chronic eczema and high serum levels of IgE [96].

All interferences with chemotactism are not hereditary, some are acquired. There is a partial chemotactic defect in diabetes mellitus which can be corrected by *in vitro* administration of glucose, potassium and insulin.

The chemotactic response to acute infections varies. In some cases it is increased, in others decreased. The reasons for the difference in responses are not known. The inhibitors of chemotactism include (1) steroidal (corticosteroids and quinoline derivatives) anti-inflammatory agents, (2) increased levels of chemotactic factor inactivator (CFI) which has been observed in patients with Hodgkin's disease.* Other inhibitors have been found, but not well characterized. In cirrhosis, for example, there is still an unidentified serum inhibitor of chemotactism.

As may be anticipated, defects in complement will be associated with defective chemotactism. Defects in C2, C3, C5 and C6 have been identified, but of course those defects that are of greatest consequence for chemotactism affect C3 and C5.

Inasmuch as the activation of C3 is indispensable for opsonification, patients whose serum is unable to activate C3 will be susceptible to recurrent pyogenic

* Patients with α_1 antitrypsin deficiency and pulmonary emphysema have low levels of CFI.

infection. Such defects are sometimes observed in neonates and in patients with sickle cell anemia. Defective opsonic activity probably as a result of low levels of C3, have also been documented in low birth weight infants, in patients with lupus erythematosus, in hepatic cirrhosis, and in glomerulonephritis.

Gross and Histological Appearance of Inflammation

The known molecular and cellular events associated with inflammation have been described. How these fundamental reactions combine to lead to the various types of inflammatory reactions observed grossly and histologically will now be considered. Pathologists group inflammations into three categories: acute, subacute, and chronic. The evolution of one type into another is discussed later.

Acute Inflammation

Depending upon which of the inflammatory events predominate, acute inflammatory processes are categorized as catarrhal, serous, fibrinous, hemorrhagic, and purulent. Catarrhal inflammation affects the mucosa and is characterized by the abundant secretion of mucus. Some examples of catarrhal inflammation are the acute inflammation of the nasal mucosa in the common cold or the reaction of the intestinal mucosa to the ingestion of irritants or the presence of pathogenic bacteria. Grossly, the intestinal mucosa is swollen and congested, and its lumen is filled with sticky mucus. Histologically, the epithelial cells are loaded with mucus, and numerous desquamated cells are found in the lumen mixed with mucus and polymorphonuclears. The chorion contains vasodilated vessels and a polymorphonuclear infiltrate. The connective tissue fibers are dissociated by edematous fluid. If the cause of the inflammation is eliminated or neutralized, the catarrhal inflammation leaves no sequelae and the epithelium is integrally repaired.

In the acute hemorrhagic imflammation, the elementary reaction to the inflammatory agent is no different from that observed in other types of acute inflammation except that blood tends to extravasate. This happens when the pathogenic agent primarily injures the vascular wall or the acute inflammatory process develops in an area of venous stasis. Acute inflammations with hemorrhagic tendencies are often observed in tissues infected with streptococci or in the form of pneumonia caused by the agent of influenza.

In a serous inflammation, edema predominates either in the interstitial tissues (leading to extensive swelling) or in preexisting cavities, such as the pleura, peritoneum, or pericardium. For example, a serous pleurisy or pericarditis is frequently associated with rheumatic fever.

In the fibrinous type of inflammation, the interaction components lead to a special form of coagulation necrosis. Fibrinous inflammation is typical of but not unique to diphtheria. All mucosa constitute favorite breeding grounds for the bacillus of Löffler, but the tonsils and the soft palate are most favorable sites for the infection. The bacillus carrying the appropriate phage (see viral disease) elaborates a toxin that kills the mucosa cells. An inflammatory reaction follows with vasodilation and polymorphonuclear migration as in any typical acute inflammation, but the toxins seem to kill large numbers of polymorphonuclears. The fibrinogen that leaks from the damaged blood vessels forms, after conversion to fibrin, a membrane covering the necrotic bottom. Grossly, at the earlier stages, white spots can be seen on the tonsils and the soft palate. A careful examination reveals a fine reticulum sometimes reminiscent of a spider web. As the bacilli grow and the toxin kills more and more cells in the deeper layers as well as at the periphery, the fibrinous membrane thickens, becomes embedded in the underlying tissue, and invades the larynx and even the bronchial mucosa. The combination of edema and membrane formation leads to obstruction of the respiratory pathways with crouplike respiration.

After the catarrhal, the purulent inflammation is the most common acute inflammation. In purulent inflammation, the offending agents cause tissue necrosis and elicit an inflammatory response. The combination of accumulating bacteria (in bacterial infection) and cellular death elicits an intense chemotactic reaction with a large accumulation of polymorphonuclears, which not only phagocytize the bacteria and die, but, at least in part, help to digest the dead tissue.

The product of necrosis is pus. Its appearance varies with the agent causing the inflammation. Under clinical circumstances, bacteria usually are responsible for purulent inflammation, but purulent inflammation can be caused experimentally by a variety of chemical agents, among which turpentine has been used most frequently. The histological examination of pus reveals, in the midst of liquid, cells at various levels of disintegration and bacterial colonies. The cellular compartment is made primarily of polymorphonuclears, but intact or disintegrated cells from the target tissue, monocytes, lymphocytes, plasmocytes, and red cells are also found. In bacterial infection bacterial colonies can easily be recognized even without special stains. Indeed, the breakdown products of the polymorphonuclears and the host cells plus the extravasated blood and plasma constitute an ideal culture medium for the germs. The gross appearance of the pus varies considerably depending upon the interaction of the various components involved in the inflammatory process—host cells, polymorphonuclears, extravasated blood and plasma, etc.

Agents that cause pus to appear are called pyogenic; the process involved in pus development is called suppuration. Suppuration can appear practically anywhere—in the kidney, brain, liver, and other organs. The most common sites are probably the skin and

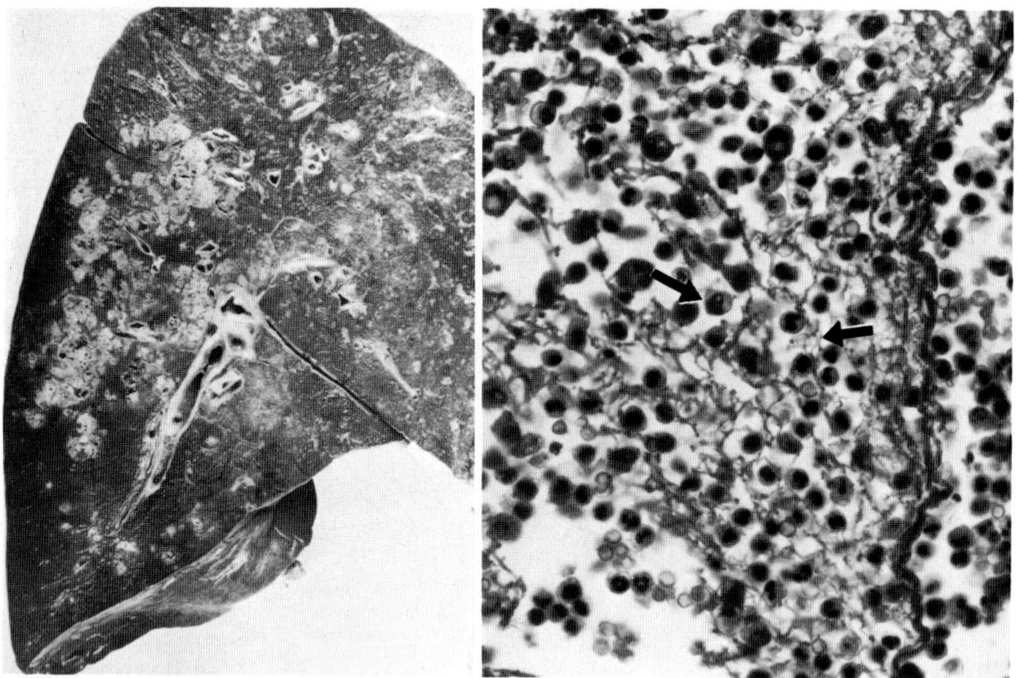

Fig. 13-10. Gross appearance of lung affected with bronchopneumonia showing diffuse foci of inflammation, including necrosis and leukopoietic infiltration (*left*); high-power histological section showing alveoli filled with fibrin and polymorphonuclears (*right*)

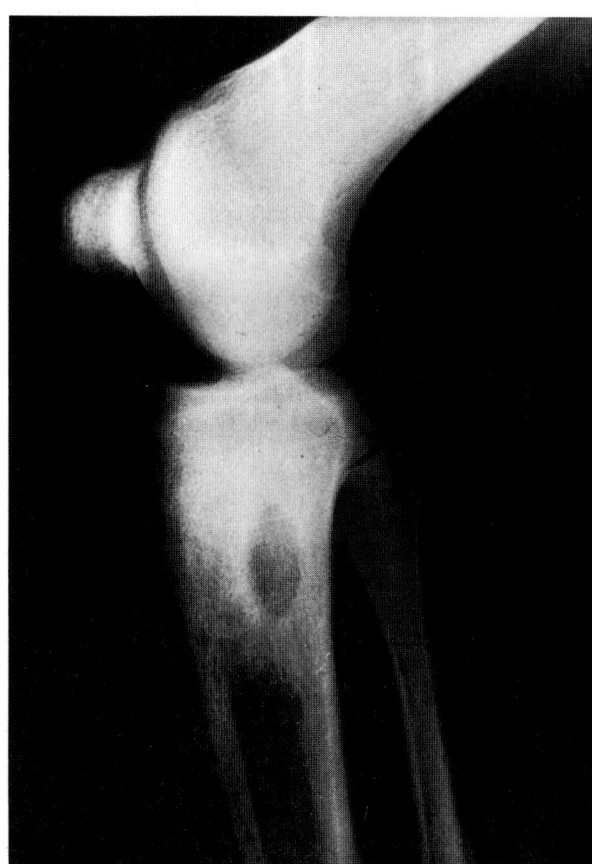

Fig. 13-11. Abscess of long bone (Brodie's abscess)

the superficial mucosa, especially of the oral cavity, the upper respiratory tract and the exterior genitals.

Although one does not wish to belabor a subject with obvious morbid aspects, no respectable textbook on pathology can avoid a description of various kinds of pus. Earlier clinicians were adept at diagnosing the cause of pus and also granted it inherent ethical qualities, speaking of laudable pus, etc.

The pus caused by staphylococci is thick, homogeneous, and creamy yellow. It is (inappropriately) squeezed out of boils. Streptococcal pus is of much poorer quality. It is poorly bound, whitish, with hemorrhagic streaks and flaky yellowish debris. Classic pneumococcal pus is viscous, but more greenish than staphylococcal pus.

The morphological appearance and the evolution of a purulent inflammation also vary depending upon the tissue in which it occurs. A purulent inflammation can arise in practically any part of the body—underneath the skin (pustules), under mucosa, deep in the connective tissues, in the parenchyma of the kidney, liver, or spleen, and in muscles, brain, or bone marrow. In all these purulent acute inflammatory processes, after the inflammatory agent is introduced, the typical vascular and cellular reactions of inflammation occur with invasion by polymorphonuclears, which appear in thick streaks, streaming from the center of the injury—where the pus is found—to the periphery. At some distance from the epicenter, the surrounding tissues organize their own defenses by forming a more or less thick barrier of granulation tissues composed of newly formed capillaries, proliferating fibroblasts, and monocytes. The central collection of pus sur-

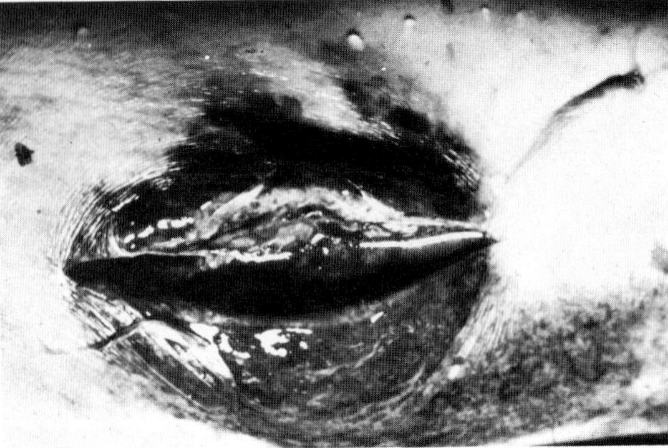

Fig. 13-12. Cellulitis of the subcutaneous tissue of the arm; the acute inflammation is manifested by swelling and reddening of the inflamed area. The inflammatory swelling has been opened by the surgeon with a scalpel

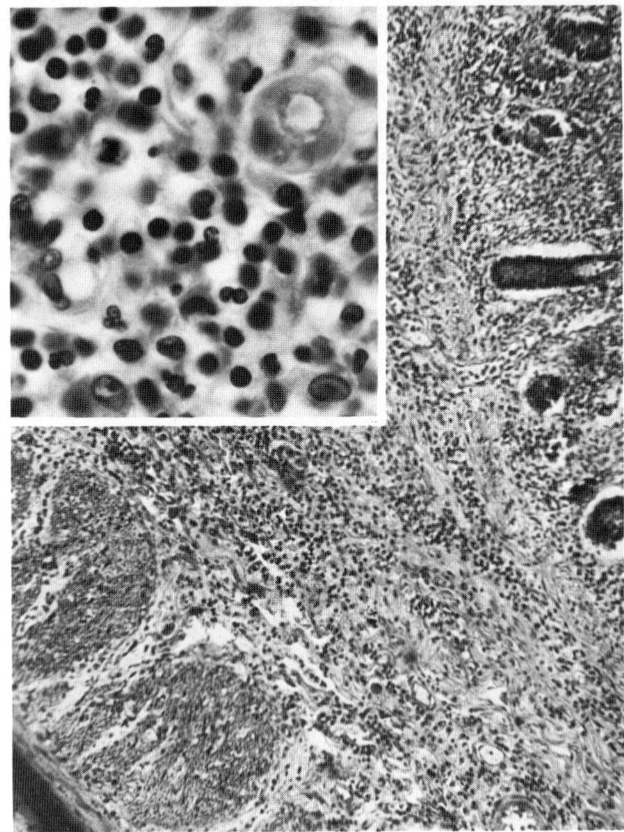

→

Fig. 13-13. Inflammation of the small intestine in a patient with typhoid fever

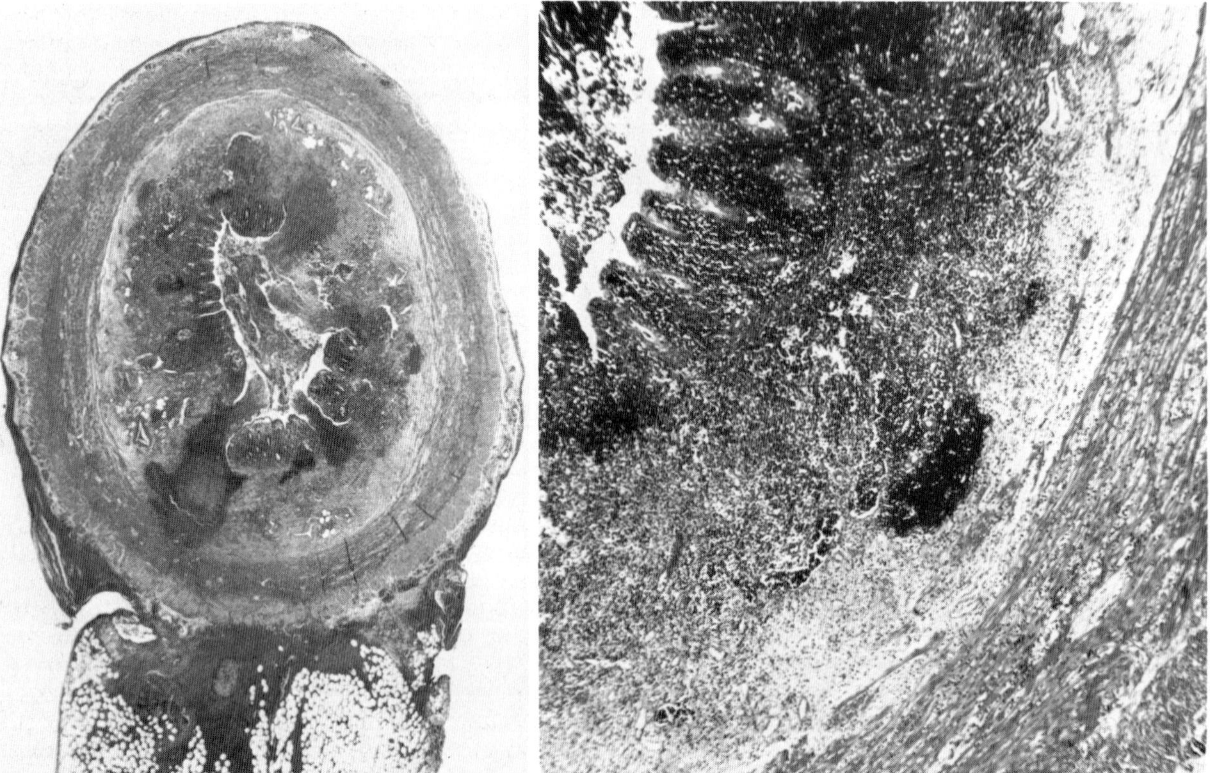

Fig. 13-14. Gross and microscopic appearance of inflamed appendix showing necrosis, fibrin deposition, and leukopoietic infiltration

rounded by granulation tissue forms the pustule when it is located under the skin, the abscess when located anywhere else.

Pustules usually open at the surface of the skin, releasing the necrotic material, and the emptied cavity is then repaired as in any other type of wound healing. The fate of the abscess varies upon whether or not the pus is eliminated spontaneously or surgically. If the purulent content of the abscess is eliminated leaving a sterile barrier, wound healing takes place as in the case of the pustules. But scars remain, varying in depth and extent with the size of the abscess and the ability of the injured tissue to regenerate. However, when an abscess is deeply sequestered in the bone, in the brain, or in the parenchyma, the pus is not evacuated spontaneously. Without surgical intervention, the purulent area is invaded by macrophages, which attempt to digest the remnants of bacterial and cellular necrosis through phagocytosis. If they are successful, a clear liquid left behind may itself be reabsorbed, and ultimately the abscess may collapse leaving only a scar. If the necrotic debris is not digested, it remains entrapped in connective tissue and may become impregnated with calcium.

Occasionally, the purulent inflammation will not collect into a mass referred to as abscess, but will diffuse either between the collagen fibers of connective tissue (as in a phlegmon) or collect in a preexisting cavity, such as in the pleural cavity (empyema). Some examples of the manifestations of acute inflammation are shown in Figures 13-10, 13-11, 13-12, 13-13, and 13-14.

Chronic Inflammation

The basic difference between acute and chronic inflammation resides in the duration of the inflammatory process. An acute inflammation lasts for a week, maybe two, whereas a chronic inflammation lasts for months, sometimes years. These differences in the duration of the inflammatory process are associated with profound differences in histology, gross appearance, and mechanism of production. It is convenient to distinguish two types of chronic inflammation—the regular or nongranulomatous type and the granulomatous type.

If the body's defense mechanisms prove unsuccessful at eliminating or neutralizing the agent causing the acute inflammatory process, the host often chooses to renounce the use of drastic measures and settles for controlled surveillance of the effects of the deleterious agent. No large numbers of chemical mediators are released, no massive mobilization of polymorphonuclears takes place, but the area of inflammation is invaded by monocytes, lymphocytes, and plasmocytes primarily, with only a few polymorphonuclear eosinophils. Necrosis of some of the tissues is inescapable, but it is slow and may be repaired by regeneration of the dead tissue or by active fibrosis. Necrosis, cellular exudate, regeneration, and fibrosis are the hallmarks of chronic inflammation. A case of chronic inflammation in trichinosis is shown in Fig. 13-15.

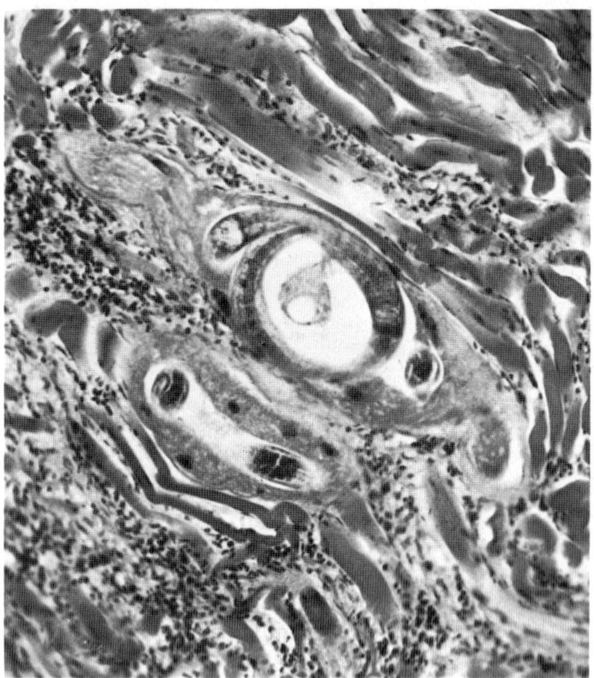

Fig. 13-15. Trichinosis

Necrosis and fibrosis are the main causes of the loss of function. Fibrosis may interfere with the ability of the remaining portion of the organ to function normally. For example, fibrosis following a chronic inflammation in a hollow organ, such as the small intestine, leads to obstruction with all its consequences. A chronic inflammation of parenchymal tissue interferes with function as well. Thus, the chronic hepatitis that follows acute viral hepatitis and results in necrosis, regeneration, and fibrosis typical of cirrhosis (see above) culminates in hepatic failure.

Little is known of the molecular events that trigger the components of chronic inflammation. Whatever brings macrophages, leukocytes, and plasmocytes in an area of chronic inflammation has been discussed either in this chapter or will be reviewed in the chapter on immunopathology.

Whereas the regular chronic inflammation results from diffuse and intermixed infiltration by monocytes, plasmocytes, lymphocytes, etc., in the granulomatous type of inflammation the reactive cells condense in small foci, which may later become visible granular structures and therefore are called granulomas. In granulomas, the various types of reactive cells may be organized to yield a specific histological picture. A granulomatous reaction occurs (1) when undigestible foreign material accumulates (such as lipids, silica, talc, zirconium, unabsorbable sutures, and splinters); (2) in cases of infection by living agents that are not readily digested and disposed of through the regular processes of phagocytosis (such as the mycobacteria in tuberculosis and leprosy, the spirochetes in syphilis, fungi in histoplasmosis, actinomycosis, and sporotrichosis, regular bacteria in brucellosis, and complex parasites in schistosomiasis); (3) in diseases in which hypersensitivity is a causal factor (such as in rheumatoid arthritis and sarcoidosis).

Some of the general features of the granuloma will be described, followed by a brief outline of the macroscopic and microscopic features of the granulomas in tuberculosis, syphilis, and leprosy. The reader is referred to specialized books on pathology or inflammatory diseases for further information on granulomatous infection.

The cells that compose the granuloma include mononuclear cells, macrophages, histiocytes, epithelioid cells, giant cells, lymphocytes, and fibroblasts. The origin and the role of some of these cells in the inflammatory process have already been discussed. The cells that are typical of the granulomatous type of reaction are the epithelioid and the multinucleated giant cells. Under the light microscope the epithelioid cell appears as a plump, polygonal cell with a central nucleus (reminiscent of that of the macrophage) and an eosinophilic cytoplasm. The electron microscope reveals that the epithelioid cell has a well-developed membrane including numerous pseudopods and cups. The pseudopods of one cell may intertwine with those of an adjacent epithelioid cell, but most often two epithelioid cells simply lie close together without any interaction between their membranes. These cells contain numerous mitochondria and a well-endowed endoplasmic reticulum. Vacuoles are often filled with phagocytosed but not yet digested material.

The giant cell is a large, multinucleated cell with a cytoplasm not very different from that of the epithelioid cell. The size of the giant cells varies considerably. The nuclei are numerous; sometimes as many as 100 can be found. They are usually located at the periphery of the cellular body, forming either a crownlike or a horseshoe-shaped structure.

The epithelioid cell is believed to be derived from macrophages, and the giant cells to result from the coalescence of several epithelioid cells.

Very distinct steps are involved in granuloma formation, including immigration of the cells in the inflamed area and transformation of the stem cell into various cellular types (epithelioid, giant cells, etc.). We have already briefly discussed some of the mechanisms of cell migration and questioned whether the mononuclear cells that appear in the chronic inflammatory process migrate at the same time as the polymorphonuclears and proliferate when the polymorphonuclears die, or whether the mononuclear cells are called to the inflammatory area after the polymorphonuclear cells have been eliminated. Transformation of stem cells into other types of inflammatory cells will be discussed in the chapter on immunopathology.

The persistence of the granuloma for long periods of time, sometimes years, is puzzling. Such persistence may be due to extraordinary longevity of the cells involved or to constant repopulation of the granulomatous cells by immigrating cells or by cell division.

The life span of giant cells, epithelioid cells, and macrophages is not known exactly, but it is longer than that of polymorphonuclears. Transfusion of marked cells has shown that every 24 hours about 200,000 circulating mononuclear cells enter the chronic granulomatous lesion caused by the Freund adjuvant. Studies with labeled precursors suggest that macrophages in granulomatous lesions are capable of cell division, but the exact kinetics and rate of macrophage proliferation are not known. The turnover of the cell seems to vary with the type of irritant that is administered. After the administration of a single pulse of [^{3}H]thymidine, the turnover in the carrageen granuloma was low, while it was high in the *Bacillus pertussis* granuloma. The low-turnover granuloma seemed to contain cells with much greater longevity.

Further investigations have established that the high-turnover granuloma tends to become a low-turnover granuloma; therefore, it has been proposed that macrophages with a long life span are gradually selected over those with rapid turnover. Clearly, what will determine whether an irritant persists in the granuloma will depend upon the macrophage's ability to digest it. In that respect, irritants are of three types: digestible, undigestible, and poorly digestible. Although it seems easy to understand why silica or asbestos remains undigested, the reasons why some other types of irritants cannot be digested after phagocytosis are not always clear. There are a number of possibilities: (1) the macrophage population in the granuloma is devoid of enzymes capable of digesting the irritant; (2) only a portion of the irritant is phagocytized; (3) the irritant is picked up by two different cell populations, some containing the enzymic arsenal capable of digesting it, others devoid of it; and (4) the irritant is sequestered inside intracellular vacuoles, which render it inaccessible to enzymic attack.

Tuberculosis is a typical granulomatous inflammation caused by bacteria (the microbacterium of Koch). Laennec was the first to describe the tubercle and its evolution and to introduce a concept of continuity in the process from the tiny tubercle to the massive cavities, a concept that Virchow later vigorously attacked. Thus, Laennec recognized that the tubercle constitutes the unit lesion in tuberculosis. Tubercles are spheric, ovoid masses that are almost colorless, sometimes grayish, with a yellowish center. In Laennec's words, tubercles are the size of *"un grain de millet, ou un grain Seneve."* Histologically, they are composed of three major types of cells usually arranged concentrically within a fine reticulum. One or more multinucleate giant cells occupy the centers. Several layers of epithelial cells are seen in the middle, and a crown of lymphocytes forms the periphery. The cells rest on a fine reticulum that is sometimes difficult to distinguish, but the tubercle is devoid of blood or blood vessels (a significant factor in the therapy for tuberculosis). Special staining (acid fast) reveals the presence of bacilli of Koch in both giant and epithelioid cells in the form of numerous red rodlike structures.

Depending upon the course of the disease, tubercles may be found at the surface of the skin or deeply embedded in the parenchyma, for example, a lung.

In miliary tuberculosis, normal tissues may be seeded with innumerable little granules. More often, several tubercles are confluent and yield larger rounded masses, the centers of which undergo a special form of necrosis referred to as caseation. The combined undigested products of cellular and bacterial death yield a pasty mass called caseum because it has the appearance and the consistency of what Laennec called *fromage mou*. As the lesion ages, the caseum becomes dehydrated, picks up calcium, and acquires a more whitish and chalky appearance. Histologically, caseum appears as a homogeneous, eosinophilic mass. Proper staining almost always demonstrates the presence of Koch's bacilli in caseum. (The bacillus of Koch is an anaerobic bacillus. It is resistant to desiccation, so it remains for a long time even in old lesions.) However, the bacilli may be difficult to identify—especially in the center of the caseous mass, because they often lose their tinctorial properties. Yet, if caseum is injected in guinea pigs, it is certain to transfer tuberculosis. The formation of the tubercles and the large caseus masses is often associated with connective tissue proliferation at the periphery of the inflammatory mass or sometimes infiltrating the mass, especially as the lesion ages. The sclerosing process may be so intense that it is the only component of the tissular reaction that can be recognized radiologically.

As we have seen, three things may happen to caseum: it may stagnate; it may be partially resorbed, dehydrated, and absorb calcium; or it may be eliminated. Caseum is eliminated when the lesion reaches the skin or channels that opens to the exterior through the tracheobronchial, gastrointestinal, or urogenital tract. When a tuberculous lesion opens at the skin, the caseum liquifies, is eliminated, and leaves a typical tuberculous ulcer.

In organs like the lung or kidney, the cavity containing the caseum ultimately opens into a bronchus or a ureter, and the caseum is eliminated in the expectorations or the urine, often becoming a source of infection for others.

In conclusion, the agent of tuberculosis elicits a quick acute inflammatory response followed by mobilization of macrophages which, through a process of selection and differentiation, evolve into three types of cells—giant cells, epithelioids, and lymphocytes—distributed concentrically forming the unit lesion called the tubercle. The tubercles coalesce into larger masses that undergo caseous necrosis. The caseum may be dehydrated and impregnated with calcium, or eliminated directly at the surface of the skin or indirectly through excretory canals. Usually associated with the inflammatory process is a poorly controlled attempt to repair the lost tissue by scarring and fibrosis. These elementary manifestations of tuberculosis are the same in every tissue. However, the ultimate anatomical appearance and functional consequences vary with the anatomy and the physiology of the organ involved. The role that immunology plays in determining the type of tuberculous reaction will be discussed in the chapter on immunopathology. Examples of lung and prostate tuberculosis are shown in Figs. 13-16 and 13-17, respectively.

Probably because it is associated with love making, syphilis has inspired historians and poets more than practically any other disease. Challenging the hypothesis proposing that the disease was brought back from the New World by Spanish conquerors, Fracastorius claimed that syphilis originated from a quarrel between Olympian gods (Jupiter, Saturn, and Mars). As a result, violent interaction between the stars raised from the bottom of the earth and the water unhealthful vapors that spread "the contagious miasma" in the air.* Ingenious as these views may have been, they lacked an essential quality of a good working hypothesis, namely, that it be testable experimentally.

Syphilis is the sum of the reaction of the host to the Treponema invasion. These reactions include cellular injuries, inflammatory and humoral reactions of various types, and attempts to repair damaged tissue. We shall describe here the granulomatous type of reaction involved in syphilis. The syphilitic granuloma, for reasons that will become clear later, is called the gumma. The gumma evolves in four stages: proliferation, softening, ulceration, and repair. Syphilitic gummas may appear anywhere: in the skin, the mucosa, or even the deep viscera. They range in size from small nodules not much larger than a pea to large masses that may compress the surrounding tissue.

Treponema infection elicits a characteristic inflammatory reaction in which cellular infiltration predominates. Infiltrating cells are lymphocytes and plasmocytes; epithelioid cells and giant cells are also seen. A characteristic manifestation of the syphilitic infiltrate is that it tends to surround blood vessels, small arteries, venules, and capillaries, forming typical perivascular cuffs. Although the inflammatory cells may be arranged concentrically—as in the tubercle with giant cells in the center, epithelial cells in the middle, and lymphocytes at the periphery—such cell segregation is less typical in an early syphilitic than in an early tuberculous lesion. In syphilis, the various types of inflammatory cells tend to be intermixed.

The infiltrated area usually becomes necrotic—in part because of the vascular damage, in part because of the hydrolases released by the inflammatory cells. As a result, a whitish, firm, homogeneous mass develops in the center of the lesion. An the earlier stages, grossly the mass resembles the cut surface of a chestnut; histologically, it appears as a homogeneous

---

* Fracastorius' description of the disease does not distinguish between syphilis and gonorrhea. When Hunter inoculated himself with pus of a patient with venereal disease he developed gonorrhea as well as syphilis. The distinction between gonorrhea and syphilis came only in the late 18th century. In 1892 Basedow distinguished the soft chancre of Ducrey from the typical hard chancre of syphilis. In 1903 Mechnikov inoculated syphilis to higher primates. In 1905 F. Hoffman identified *Treponema pallidum*, a spirochete, as the agent of syphilis, and in 1907 Bordet and Wasserman developed the humoral diagnostic test.

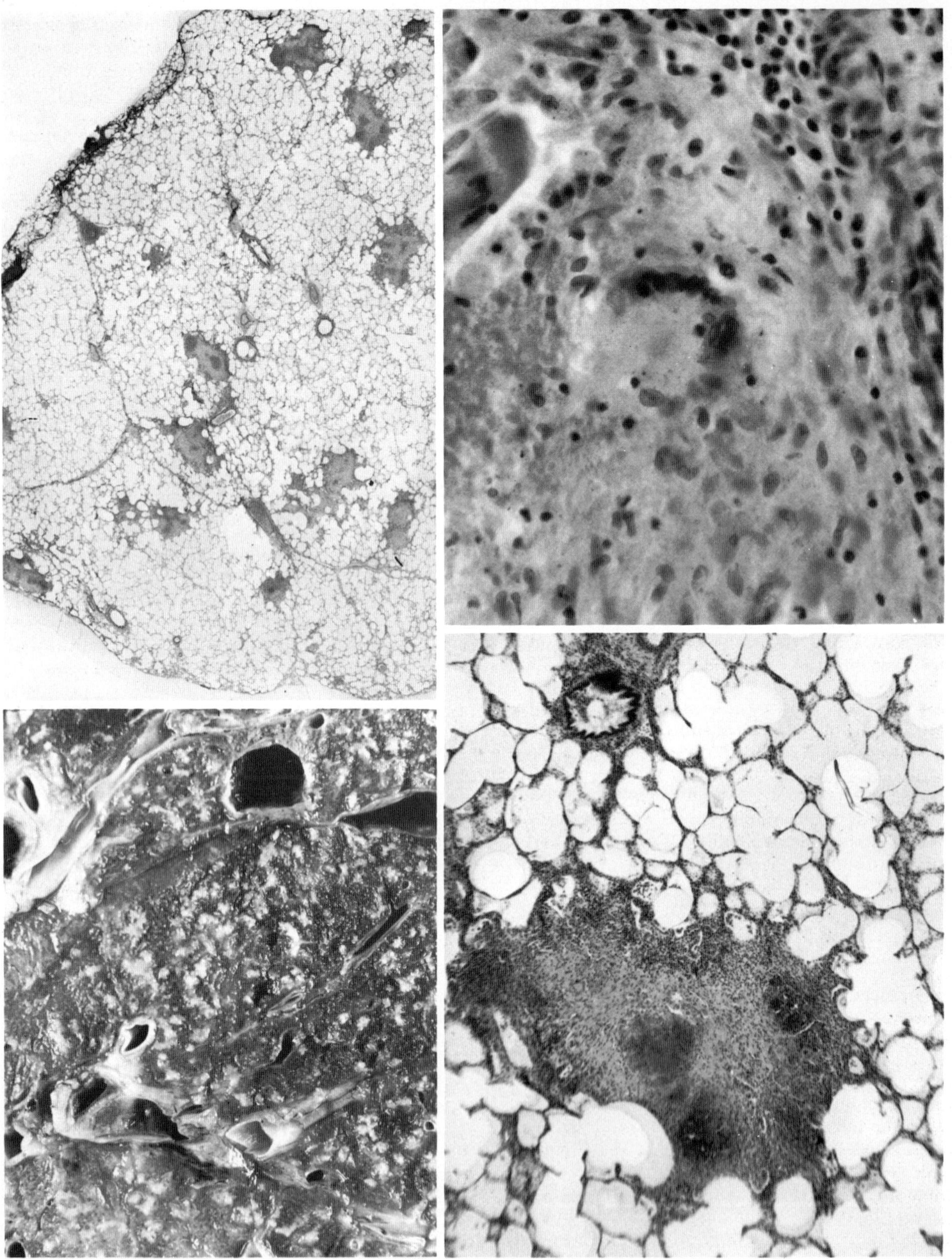

Fig. 13-16. Miliary tuberculosis. Gross appearance of lung (*lower left*); low-power histological appearance showing tubercles *(upper left)*; tubercles at medium- *(lower right)* and high-power *(upper right)* microscopy showing caseous necrosis, giant cells, epitheloid cells, and lymphocytes

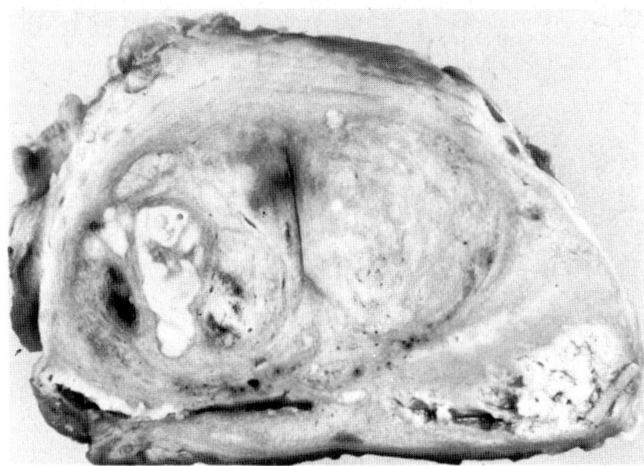

Fig. 13-17. Caseous necrosis, prostate

eosinophilic mass. Later the necrotic material liquifies and appears as a viscous, syrupy, brownish mass with the consistency of a gumma. The gummatous necrotic mass is surrounded by an inflammatory zone, which includes vascular cuffs, epithelioid cells, and giant cells.

If, in spite of the dreadfulness of the disease, writers of poetry and prose have made humorous remarks about syphilis, no one is on record for laughing or even smiling at the earlist signs of leprosy. Leprosy has been known throughout recorded history. An Egyptian papyrus from 4600 B.C. mentions leprosy. The disease seems to have been endemic in Egypt and was brought to Palestine at the time of the exodus of the Israelites through the desert. The Bible (Lev.) mentions leprosy and gives some interesting hygenic advice. In Persia, leprosy must have existed before Herodotus, and it was known to the Persians as the Phoenician disease, suggesting an Asiatic origin. References to leprosy are also found in the Rig-Veda, written in 1400 B.C. It was described in Japan, China, and many other Asian countries.

In Europe, leprosy must have existed for a long time, but it was often confused with other diseases such as elephantiasis, psoriasis, and sometimes syphilis. It appears that Greek physicians did not know about classical lepers. Leprosy appeared in the Roman Empire around 200 B.C. and was introduced there from Egypt by the armies of Pompey. During the Middle Ages leprosy reached its peak in Europe as a result of the Crusades. In spite of the deep religious mysticism of those times, ignorance and intolerance led men to treat lepers as outcasts. Once the disease was discovered, the victim had to wear special clothes, indicate what he wanted with a stick, keep away from public fountains, and never speak in a loud voice. The church pronounced an official burial, and the leper was considered dead. Some charitable monks and nuns instituted leper colonies referred to as lazarettos. The first was established by King Gregory of Tours; King Louis VIII of France established 200 lazarettos. At the end of the Middle Ages, there were 19,000 lazarettos on the continent, 2000 in France alone. Isolating the lepers in the lazarettos helped to eliminate leprosy in the world, and in the 17th century Louis XIV was able to convert lazarettos into regular hospitals. Leprosy still exists in the endemic form in large portions of Asia, the Middle East, and Africa. It is estimated that there are still millions of lepers in the world.

The agent responsible for leprosy is a mycobacterium discovered by Hansen in 1873. As is the case for syphilis, bacterial infection in leprosy is followed by various types of inflammatory reactions. The earliest signs usually appear in the skin and result from the development of a subcutaneous infiltrate of lymphocytes and plasmocytes including lepromatous cells (which will be described later). The development of the inflammatory infiltrate is associated with skin discoloration the pathogenesis of which is not well-understood (except in cases of erythemia). In nonpigmented persons the skin often becomes pigmented, whereas it loses its normal pigmentation in pigmented individuals. At the later stage of tuberculoid leprosy, the infiltrate condenses into irregular round masses of various sizes. The nodules develop practically anywhere—the skin, the lymph nodes, the viscera, etc. These lesions do not have the classical appearance of tubercles; they are composed essentially of lymphocytes, plasmocytes, and the typical lepromatous cell—a large macrophage, swollen and often filled with lipid vacuoles that may become confluent. The cells contain large numbers of bacilli of Hansen. Only in rare cases does leprosy resemble tuberculosis histologically.

References

1. Lewis, T.: Blood vessels of the human skin and their responses. London: Shaw & Sons 1927
2. Bayliss, W.M.: On the origin from the spinal cord of the vaso-dilator fibres of the hind-limb and on the nature of these fibres. J. Physiol. (Lond.) **26**, 173–209 (1901)
3. Bruce, A.N.: Vasodilator axon-reflexes. Quart. J. exp. Physiol. **6**, 339–354 (1913)
4. Luft, J.H.: The ultrastructural basis of capillary permeability. In: The inflammatory process (Zweifach, B.W., Grant, L., and McCluskey, R.T., eds.), p. 121–159. New York: Academic Press 1965
5. Movat, H.Z., Fernando, N.V.P.: Acute inflammation. The earliest fine structural changes at the blood-tissue barrier. Lab. Invest. **12**, 895–910 (1963)
6. Zweifach, B.W.: Microvascular aspects of tissue injury. In: The inflammatory process (Zweifach, B.W., Grant, L., and McCluskey, R.T., eds.), p. 161–196. New York: Academic Press 1965
7. Cochrane, C.G.: Vascular and glomerular inflammation: mechanisms of initiation and mediation. Pathol. Annu. **1**, 22–47 (1966)
8. Schayer, R.W.: Histidine decarboxylase in mast cells. Ann. N.Y. Acad. Sci. **103**, 164–178 (1963)
9. Smith, R.D., Code, C.F.: Histamine formation: histidine decarboxylase determination using carboxyl-^{14}C-labeled histidine. Mayo Clin. Proc. **42**, 105–111 (1967)
10. Rothschild, A.M., Schayer, R.W.: Characterization of histidine decarboxylase from rat peritoneal fluid mast cells. Biochim. biophys. Acta (Amst.) **34**(2), 392–398 (1959)
11. Robinson, B., Shepherd, D.M.: Inhibition of histidine decarboxylases. Biochim. biophys. Acta (Amst.) **53**(2), 431–433 (1961)
12. Fukuda, T.: Induction of histamine forming capacity in canine liver by endotoxin. Nature (Lond.) **214**, 107–108 (1967)
13. Kapeller-Adler, R.: Histamine catabolism *in vitro* and *in vivo*. Fed. Proc. **24**, 757–765 (1965)
14. Snyder, S.H., Axelrod, J.: Tissue metabolism of histamine-C^{14} *in vivo*. Fed. Proc. **24**, 774–776 (1965)
15. Robinson, J.D., Green, J.P.: Evidence for the presence of imidazoleacetic acid riboside and ribotide in rat tissues. Fed. Proc. **24**, 777 (1965)
16. Zeller, E.A.: Identity of histaminase and diamine oxidase. Fed. Proc. **24**, 766–768 (1965)

17. Spector, W.G., Willoughby, D.A.: Chemical mediators. II. In: The inflammatory process (Zweifach, E.W., Grant, L., and McCluskey, R.T., eds.), p. 427–448. New York: Academic Press 1965
18. Green, J.P.: Uptake, storage and release of histamine. Uptake and binding of histamine. Fed. Proc. **26**, 211–218 (1967)
19. Uvnäs, B.: Mode of binding and release of histamine in mast cell granules from the rat. Fed. Proc. **26**, 219–221 (1967)
20. Lichtenstein, L.M., Margolis, S.: Histamine release *in vitro*: inhibition by catecholamines and methylxanthines. Science **161**, 902–903 (1968)
21. Austen, K.F., Bloch, K.J., Baker, A.R., Arnason, B.G.: Immunological histamine release from rat mast cells *in vitro*: effect of age of cell donor. Proc. Soc. exp.Biol. (N.Y.) **120**(2), 542–546 (1965)
22. DeGraw, J.I., Brown, V.H., Ferguson, S.A., Skinner, W.A.: Histamine releasers. II. Synthesis of a trimer in the formaldehyde-p-methoxyphenethylamine series of histamine releasers. J. Med. Chem. **9**, 838–840 (1966)
23. Riley, J.F.: Functional significance of histamine and heparin in tissue mast cells. Ann. N.Y. Acad. Sci. **103**, 151–163 (1963)
24. Benditt, E.P., Holcenberg, H., Luganoff, D.: The role of serotonin (5-hydroxytryptamine) in mast cells. Ann. N.Y. Acad. Sci. **103**, 179–184 (1963)
25. Massart, J., Bordet, C.: Recherches sur l'irritabilité des leucocytes et sur l'intervention de cette irritabilité dans la nutrition des cellules et dans l'inflammation. J. Med. Chir. Pharmacol. (Brussels) **90**, 169–182 (1890)
26. Wilhelm, D.L.: Chemical mediators. I. In: The inflammatory process (Zweifach, B.W., Grant, L., and McCluskey, R.T., eds.), p. 389–425. New York: Academic Press 1965
27. Menkin, V.: Biology of inflammation. Chemical mediators and cellular injury. Science **123**, 527–534 (1956)
28. Kellermeyer, R.W., Graham, R.C., Jr.: Kinins—possible physiologic and pathologic roles in man. New Engl. J. Med. **279**, 754–759, 802–807, 859–866 (1968)
29. Houck, J.C.: Chemistry of inflammation. Ann. N.Y. Acad. Sci. **105**(14), 767–812 (1963)
30. Menkin, V.: Biochemical mechanisms in inflammation, 2nd ed. Springfield, Ill.: Charles C. Thomas Publisher 1956
31. Menkin, V.: Chemical mediators in relation to cytologic constituents in inflammation. Amer. J. Path. **34**(5), 921–941 (1958)
32. Rocha e Silva, M.: The physiological significance of bradykinin. Ann. N.Y. Acad. Sci. **104**, 190–211 (1963)
33. Schacter, M.: Polypeptides which affect smooth muscles and blood vessels (Schacter, M., ed.) Oxford: Pergamon Press 1960
34. Boissonnas, R.A., Guttmann, S., Jaquenoud, P.A., Pless, J., Sandrin, E.: The synthesis of bradykinin and of related peptides. Ann. N.Y. Acad. Sci. **104**, 5–14 (1963)
35. Elliott, D.F.: Bradykinin and its mode of release. Ann. N.Y. Acad. Sci. **104**, 35–46 (1963)
36. Webster, M.E., Pierce, J.V.: The nature of the kallidins released from human plasma by kallikreins and other enzymes. Ann. N.Y. Acad. Sci. **104**, 91–107 (1963)
37. Diniz, C.R., Carvalho, I.F.: A micromethod for determination of bradykininogen under several conditions. Ann. N.Y. Acad. Sci. **104**, 77–89 (1963)
38. Aldrete, J.S., Sheps, S.S., Bernatz, P.E., Didier, E.P.: Vasoactive polypeptides of surgical significance. Mayo Clin. Proc. **41**(6), 399–417 (1966)
39. Wilhelm, D.L.: Kinins in human disease. Annu. Rev. Med. **22**, 63–84 (1971)
40. Hinman, J.W.: Prostaglandins. Annu. Rev. Biochem. **41**, 161–178 (1972)
41. Samuelsson, B.: Biosynthesis of prostaglandins. Fed. Proc. **31**(5), 1442–1450 (1972)
42. Weeks, J.R.: Prostaglandins, introduction. Fed. Proc. **33**(1), 37–38 (1974)
43. McGiff, J.C., Crowshaw, K., Itskovitz, H.D.: Prostaglandins and renal function. Fed. Proc. **33**(1) 39–47 (1974)
44. Brody, M.J., Kadowitz, P.J.: Prostaglandins as modulators of the autonomic nervous system. Fed. Proc. **33**(1), 48–60 (1974)
45. Labhsetwar, A.P.: Prostaglandins and the reproductive cycle. Fed. Proc. **33**(1), 61–77 (1974)
46. Mashiter, K., Field, J.B.: Prostaglandins and the thyroid gland. Fed. Proc. **33**(1), 78–80 (1974)
47. Tashjian, A.H., Jr., Voelkel, E.F., Goldhaber, P., Levine, L.: Prostaglandins, calcium metabolism and cancer. Fed. Proc. **33**(1), 81–86 (1974)
48. Marx, L., Jean, L.: Prostaglandins: mediators of inflammation? Science **177**, 780–781 (1972)
49. Grant, L.: The sticking and emigration of white blood cells in inflammation. In: The inflammatory process (Zweifach, B.W., Grant, L., and McCluskey, R.T., eds.), p. 197–244. New York: Academic Press 1965
50. Harris, H.: Role of chemotaxis in inflammation. Physiol. Rev. **34**, 529–562 (1954)
51. Boyden, S.: Cellular recognition of foreign matter. Int. Rev. exp. Path. **2**, 311–356 (1963)
52. Harris, H.: Mobilization of defensive cells in inflammatory tissue. Bact. Rev. **24**, 3–15 (1960)
53. Marchesi, V.T.: The site of leucocyte emigration during inflammation. Quart. J. exp. Physiol. **46**, 115–118 (1961)
54. Shin, H.S., Snyderman, R., Friedman, E., Mellors, A., Mayer, M.M.: Chemotactic and anaphylatoxic fragment cleaved from the fifth component of guinea pig complement. Science **162**(3851), 361–362 (1968)
55. Adler, J.: Chemotaxis in bacteria. Science **153**, 708–716 (1966)
56. Metchnikoff, E.: Über die phagocytäre Rolle der Tuberkelriesenzellen. Virchows Arch. path. Anat. **113**, 63–84 (1888)
57. Metchnikoff, E.: Lectures on the comparative pathology of inflammation. New York: Dover Publications 1968
58. Metchnikoff, E.: Immunity in infective disease (Binnie, F.G., trans.). New York: Johnson Reprint Corp. 1968
59. Cohn, Z.A.: The metabolism and physiology of the mononuclear phagocytes. In: The inflammatory process (Zweifach, B.W., Grant, L., and McCluskey, R.T., eds.), p. 323–353. New York: Academic Press 1965
60. McRipley, R.J., Selvaraj, R.J., Glovsky, M.M., Sbarra, A.J.: The role of the phagocyte in host-parasite interactions. VI. The phagocytic and bactericidal capabilities of leukocytes from patients undergoing x-irradiation. Radiat. Res. **31**(4), 706–720 (1967)
61. Selvaraj, R.J., McRipley, R.J., Sbarra, A.J.: The metabolic activities of leukocytes from lymphoproliferative and myeloproliferative disorders during phagocytosis. Cancer Res. **27**, 2287–2294 (1967)
62. Wittig, G.: Phagocytosis by blood cells in healthy and diseased caterpillars. II. A consideration of the method of making hemocyte counts. J. Invertebr. Path. **8**(4), 461–477 (1966)
63. Whang-Peng, J., Perry, S., Knutsen, T.: Maturation and phagocytosis by chronic myelogenous leukemia cells *in vitro*. A preliminary report. J. nat. Cancer Inst. **38**, 969–977 (1967)
64. Saba, T.M., Di Luzio, N.R.: Effect of x-irradiation on reticuloendothelial phagocytic function and serum opsonic activity. Amer. J. Physiol. **216**(4), 910–914 (1969)
65. Pisano, J.C., Di Luzio, N.R., Salky, N.K.: Absence of macrophage humoral recognition factor(s) in patients with carcinoma. J. Lab. clin. Med. **76**, 141–150 (1970)
66. McRipley, R.J., Selvaraj, R.J., Glovsky, J.M., Sbarra, A.J.: The role of the phagocyte in host-parasite interactions. V. Phagocytic and bactericidal activities of leukocytes from patients with different neoplastic disorders. Cancer Res. **27**(4), 674–685 (1967)
67. Mouton, H.: Recherches sur la digestion chez les amibes et sur leurs diastase intracellulaire. Ann. Inst. Pasteur Lille **16**, 457–509 (1902)
68. Wright, A.E., Douglas, S.R.: Further observations on the role of the blood fluids in connection with phagocytosis. Proc. roy. Soc. Edinb. B **73**, 128–142 (1904)
69. Lancaster, M.G., Allison, F., Jr.: Studies on the pathogenesis of acute inflammation. VII. The influence of osmolality upon the phagocytic and clumping activity by human leukocytes. Amer. J. Path. **49**, 1185–1200 (1966)
70. Karnovsky, M.L.: Metabolic basis of phagocytic activity. Physiol. Rev. **42**, 143–168 (1962)
71. Karnovsky, M.L.: Metabolic shifts in leukocytes during the phagocytic event. In: Biological activity of the leukocyte (Wolstenholme, G.E.W., and O'Connor, M., eds.), p. 60–78. Boston: Little, Brown and Company 1961
72. Karnovsky, M.L., Shafer, A.W., Cagan, R.H., Graham, R.C., Karnovsky, M.J., Glass, E.A., Saito, K.: Membrane function and metabolism in phagocytic cells. Trans. N.Y. Acad. Sci. **28**, 778–787 (1966)
73. Sbarra, A.J., Karnovsky, M.L.: The biochemical basis of phagocytosis. I. Metabolic changes during the ingestion of particles by polymorphonuclear leukocytes. J. biol. Chem. **234**(6), 1355–1362 (1959)
74. Sastry, P.S., Hokin, L.E.: Studies on the role of phospholipids in phagocytosis. J. biol. Chem. **241**(4), 3354–3361 (1966)
75. Kanfer, J.N., Blume, R.S., Yankee, R.A., Wolff, S.M.: Alteration of sphingolipid metabolism in leukocytes from patients with the Chediak-Higashi syndrome. New Engl. J. Med. **279**(8), 410–413 (1968)
76. Rebuck, J.W., Petz, A.J., Riddle, J.M., Priest, R.J., LoGrippo, G.A.: Human leukocytic functions in the tissues. In: Biological activity of the leukocyte (Wolstenholme, G.E.W., and O'Connor, M., eds.), p. 3–31. Boston: Little, Brown and Company 1961
77. Cline, M.J.: Phagocytosis and synthesis of ribonucleic acid in human granulocytes. Nature (Lond.) **212**, 1431–1433 (1966)
78. Van Lancker, J.L.: Hydrolases and cellular death. In: Metabolic conjugation and hydrolysis (Fishman, W.H., ed.),vol. 1, p. 355–418. New York: Academic Press 1970
79. Bainton, D.F., Farquhar, M.G.: Differences in enzyme content of azurophil and specific granules of polymorphonuclear leukocytes. I. Histochemical staining of bone marrow smears. J. Cell Biol. **39**, 286–298 (1968)
80. Bainton, D.F., Farquhar, M.G.: Differences in enzyme content of azurophil and specific granules of polymorphonuclear leukocytes. II. Cytochemistry and electron microscopy of bone marrow cells. J. Cell Biol. **39**, 299–317 (1968)
81. Zeya, H.I., Spitznagel, J.K.: Antibacterial and enzymic basic proteins from leukocyte lysosomes: separation and identification. Science **142**, 1085–1087 (1963)
82. Hirsch, J.G.: Neutrophil and eosinophil leukocytes. In: The inflammatory process (Zweifach, B.W., Grant, L., and McCluskey, R.T., eds.), p. 245–280. New York: Academic Press 1965
83. Athens, J.W.: Blood: leukocytes. Annu. Rev. Physiol. **25**, 195–212 (1963)
84. Bloom, G.D.: Structural and biochemical characteristics of mast cells. In: The inflammatory process (Zweifach, B.W., Grant, L., and McCluskey, R.T., eds.), p. 355–388. New York: Academic Press 1965
85. Uvnäs, B.: Histamine storage and release. Fed. Proc. **33**, 2172–2176 (1974)

86. Kessler, S., Kuhn, C.: Scanning electron microscopy of mast cell degranulation. Lab. Invest. **32**, 71–77 (1975)
87. Colman, R.W.: Formation of human plasma kinin. New Engl. J. Med. **291**, 509–515 (1974)
88. Fishman, A.P., Pietra, G.G.: Handling of bioactive materials by the lung. New Engl. J. Med. **291**, 953–959 (1974)
89. Lee, J.B.: Perspectives on the prostaglandins. New York: Medcom, Inc. 1973
90. Ward, P.A., Lepow, I.H., Newman, L.J.: Bacterial factors chemotactic for polymorphonuclear leukocytes. Amer. J. Path. **52**, 725–736 (1968)
91. Schiffman, E., Showell, H., Corcoran, B., Smith, E., Ward, P.A., Tempel, T., Becker, E.L.: Isolation and characterization of the bacterial chemotactic factor. Fed. Proc. **33**, 631 (Abstr.) (1974)
92. Keller, H.U., Sorkin, E.: Studies on chemotaxis. V. On the chemotactic effect of bacteria. Int. Arch. Allergy **31**, 505–517 (1967)
93. Ward, P.A.: Leukotaxis and leukotactic disorders. Amer. J. Path. **77**, 520–538 (1974)
94. Spector, W.G.: The macrophage: Its origins and role in pathology. In: Pathobiology annual (Ioachim, H.L., ed.), vol. 4, p. 33–64. New York: Appleton-Century-Crofts 1974
95. Stossel, T.P.: Phagocytosis. New Engl. J. Med. **290**, 833–839 (1974)
96. Hill, H.R., Quie, P.G., Pabst, H.F., Ochs, H.D., Clark, R.A., Klebanoff, S.J., Wedgwood, R.J.: Defect in neutrophil granulocyte chemotaxis in Job's syndrome of recurrent "cold" staphylococcal abscesses. Lancet **1974II**, 617–619
97. Boxer, L.A., Hedley-Whyte, E.T., Stossel, T.P.: Neutrophil actin dysfunction and abnormal neutrophil behavior. New Engl. J. Med. **291**, 1093–1099 (1974)
98. Catacutan-Labay, P., Boyarsky, S.: Bradykinin: Effect on ureteral peristalsis. Science **151**, 78–79 (1966)

Chapter 14

Immunopathology

Introduction 805

Antigens 805

Antibodies 805

Antigen Determinants 808

Theories on Antigen-Antibody Contact 810

Quantitative Aspects of Antigen-Antibody Reactions 810
Secondary Manifestations of Antigen-Antibody Reactions 812
Precipitation 812
Agglutination 812

Activation of Complement 813

Binding and Activation of C1 813
Binding of $C4_b$ 814
Activation of C2 814
Splitting of C3 815
$C3_b$ Peptidase 815

Blood Levels of Antibodies 816

Heredity 816
Age 816
Immunological State of the Host 816
Mode of Administration of Antigens 817

Antibody Synthesis 817

The Cellular Aspects of Immunity 820

Introduction 820
The Lymphatic System 820
Lymphocytes-Properties and Relationship to Lymphatic Organs 821
T Cells 822
B Lymphocytes 824
Lymph Nodes and Antibody Formation 825
Antigen Recognition by B and T Lymphocyte Receptors 825
B and T Cells in Human Peripheral Blood and in Human Diseases 826
Macrophages and the Immune Response 827
T- and B-Cell Interactions 828
Lymphocyte Factors 828
Lymphokinins 829
Immune Tolerance 830

Mode of Action of Humoral Antibodies 832

Cytotropic Antibodies 832
History 832
Pharmacological Mediators and Antigen-Antibody Reactions 832
Cytotoxic Antibodies 833
Hypersensitivity Mediated by Antigen-Antibody Complexes 836

The Arthus Reaction 836
Pathology of the Arthus Reaction · Systemic Arthus Reaction

Cell-Mediated Hypersensitivity, Tuberculin Reactions, and Graft Rejection 837

Antigens in Delayed Hypersensitivity 837
The Fate of Grafted Tissue 838
Immunosuppression 840
Graft-Versus-Host Reaction 840

Blood Groups 840

Introduction 840
ABO (H) System 841
Coombs' Reaction 841
H Gene and the Antigen Structure of the ABO System 842
ABO Incompatibility in the Newborn 843
RH System 843
Erythroblastosis Fetalis 844

Histocompatibility 845

Immunological Response Against Infection by Bacteria, Viruses, and Parasites 848
Immunodeficiency Diseases 852
Third and Fourth Pharyngeal Pouch Syndrome 853
Agammaglobulinemia 853

Immunological Diseases 854

Allergy 854
Allergens · Allergic Rhinitis · Bronchial Asthma · Urticaria · Contact Dermatitis · Atopic Eczema · Miscellaneous Immune Reactions to Drugs · Serum Sickness

Experimental Glomerulonephritis 860
Antigen-Antibody Complexes in Experimental Glomerulonephritis · Anti-Basal Membrane Experimental Glomerulonephritis · Composition of the Basement Membrane

Human Glomerulonephritis 861
Streptococcal Glomerulonephritis · Goodpasture's Syndrome · Glomerulopathy in Renal Transplant · Anatomical Pathology of Glomerulonephritis

Rheumatic Fever and Rheumatic Heart Disease 866
Autoimmune Diseases 869
Autoimmune Hemolytic Anemia · Autoimmune Thyroiditis · Lupus Erythematosus · Rheumatoid Arthritis · Immunological Vasculitis · Polyarteritis Nodosa · Allergic Granulomatous Angiitis · Wegener's Granulomatosis · Hypersensitivity Angiitis · Temporal Arteritis · Takayasu's Disease · Sarcoidosis · Miscellaneous Collagen Diseases

Hyperglobulinemia and Paraglobulinemia 881
Monoclonic Gammaglobulinopathies

Waldenström's Macroglobulinemia 882
Multiple Myeloma 883
Polyclonal Gammopathies 885
Crohn's Disease and Ulcerative Colitis 885
Crohn's Disease · Ulcerative Colitis

References 887

Introduction

Immunology is the study of the host's defenses against foreign material. Immunological reactions include the formation of circulating antibodies and cell-based reactions.

When the mechanism that protects the organism from intrusion by foreign material is absent, excessive or distorted immunological disease develops. Such diseases include; immunodeficiency disease, hypersensitivity, autoimmune disease, and hyperproduction of special classes of antibodies in multiple myeloma.

In this chapter we will review the mechanism of immunological reaction and the pathogenesis of immunological disease.

Two of the most important components in a successful chemical reaction are the compatibility of the reactants and the chance for compatible reactants to meet. Although the laws that govern nonliving and living chemistry are essentially the same, through evolution the living have selected molecules with structures that favor interaction among themselves. This is referred to as specificity. The structures of DNA and RNA, protein synthesis, and the interactions between enzyme and substrate are all examples of specificity, but one of the most remarkable manifestations of biological specificity is the interaction of antibody and antigen. Such interactions guarantee life and also protect it. The secret of such specificity is enshrined in the molecular structures of the antigen and antibody.

Antigens

Antigens are molecules that elicit the elaboration of and combine with antibodies. A detailed description of all known antigens is impossible, and even it if were available, the description would never be complete because any new chemical compound introduced into the environment is a potential antigen. We will describe the antigen in the broadest sense so that the structure of the antibody and the mechanism of antigen-antibody interaction can be described. More details on the structure and properties of antigens will be provided as we review specific immunological reactions.

Antigens are classified in two major groups according to molecular structure: those that act directly without combining with other molecules and those that act in combination with macromolecules, usually proteins. The first group includes proteins and polysaccharides; in the second are lipids, fatty acid, nucleic acid, nucleotides, nucleosides, and a multitude of smaller molecules. When an antigen is incomplete and must be attached to a carrier protein to induce the immunological reaction, that portion of the antigen toward which the antibody is directed is called the haptene. Thus, haptenes are chemicals that elicit antibody formation after complexion with carrier proteins. (A carrier protein is that portion of an antigenic molecule or antigenic complex that determines its immunological specificity. It reacts specifically *in vivo* and *in vitro* with a homologous antibody.)

Exposure to antigens may be noniatrogenic or iatrogenic. Noniatrogenic exposure usually occurs through inhalation, ingestion, or contact with skin. Iatrogenic exposures include injections (serum and drugs), transfusions (blood and plasma), and transplantation.

Antibodies

Antibodies are substances that react specifically with antigens. All known antibodies are proteins categorized as immunoglobulins. Antibodies may circulate freely (humoral antibodies) or be attached to cells (cellular antibodies) [1–20].

When submitted to electrophoresis in an electric field at pH 8.6, immunoglobulins—like other globulins—migrate toward the anode. However, immunoglobulins migrate slower than the two other major groups of proteins in the serum: α- and β-globulins. Because of these electrophoretic properties, Tisselius called immunoglobulins γ-globulins.

At least five major classes of immunoglobulins have been identified in man: immunoglobulins G, A, M, D, and E, which are usually abbreviated IgG, IgA, IgM, IgD, and IgE, respectively. Before we review some of the properties of each of these classes of immunoglobulins, we shall briefly discuss what is known of the molecular structure of IgG.

IgG constitutes one of the most important classes of antibodies. It is composed of at least four groups of proteins referred to as subclasses. They all have a molecular weight of 160,000 and a sedimentation constant of 7. Treatment of a heterogeneous population of IgG molecules with papain yields three polypeptide chains: two with a molecular weight of 52,000 (Fa fragment), and one with a molecular weight of 48,000 (Fc fragment). IgG has two demonstrable biological properties: (1) a special ability to combine with antigens, and (2) the ill-defined abilities of fixing complement, acting with rheumatoid factors, sensitizing human skin, etc. The first of these properties is associated with the Fa fragment, the second with the Fc fragment. Thus, papain hydrolysis of IgG has revealed that the molecule is composed of polypeptide chains that are arranged to form at least three functional units: two antigenic binding sites (Fa fragments) and one Fc fragment that is associated with many other biological properties.

Because Fc fragments readily crystallize, even if they are obtained from a heterogeneous population of IgG molecules, it is clear that the Fc portion of the molecule must be similar in most, if not all, IgG molecules. In contrast, Fa fragments do not crystallize, which suggests that the antigen-binding components are heterogeneous.

Using a different approach to studying the structure of IgG, Edelman [16] and his collaborators demonstrated that the immunoglobulin molecule was made of four different subunits: two large chains, the heavy chain (mol wt 55,000), and one shorter, light chain (mol wt 25,000). These subunits were isolated by treating the immunoglobulin with chemical agents that reduce disulfide bridges and by separating the products of the reaction chromatographically. Thus, each light chain is covalently bound by a disulfide bond to one of the heavy chains. The two heavy chains are bound together by one, two, or possibly three disulfide bonds.

We have already seen that the number of potential antigens is considerable. Therefore, if any immunoglobulin is to combine with the antigen in the fashion of a lock and key, the primary structure of the antigen-binding site must be specific and vary from one immunoglobulin to another. In other words, a population of immunoglobulins is bound to be extremely heterogeneous. This heterogeneity should be reflected in both the heavy and light chains. Such heterogeneity has been demonstrated by studying the antigenic properties of both the heavy and the light chains and by unravelling the amino acid sequences of each type of chain.

When light or heavy chains obtained from human immunoglobulins are injected in another animal, such as a rabbit, they elicit an antibody reaction. An antibody produced by one type of chain can then be cross-reacted with that produced by other types of chains, and the antigenic specificity of each chain can thereby be determined. Such an approach revealed that a homogeneous immunoglobulin (see below) contains two antigenic forms of the light polypeptide chain, referred to as the γ and the λ chain. Thus, even though these chains have similar general physical properties, they differ in antigenic configuration. In contrast, there is only one antigenic configuration for the heavy chain, referred to as γ.

Antigenically speaking, then, an IgG molecule consists of two $\varkappa$ and two λ chains, or two γ and two $\varkappa$ chains. IgG composed of two γ, one $\varkappa$, and one λ has never been found. Those IgG molecules containing the $\varkappa$ chains are referred to as K type, those containing λ chains are referred to as L type.

In contrast to the light chains, which provide a common structural and antigenic unit in all immunoglobulins, the antigenic configuration of the heavy chain is unique for each of its molecular classes; therefore, it represents a unit with distinct antigenic, physical, and functional properties. On the basis of their antigenic properties, heavy chains have been divided into various subclasses referred to as γ_2a, γ_2b, γ_2c, and γ_2d globulins. At least in some cases the difference in antigenicity is associated with functional differences. Thus, whereas γ_2b, γ_2c, and γ_2d globulins can sensitize guinea pig skin and cause anaphylactic reactions, γ_2a cannot.

Clearly, the most direct way to describe the immunoglobulin molecule is to reconstruct the antibody atom by atom. This can be achieved by establishing the amino acid sequence in each of the polypeptide chains. In spite of what to most would appear insurmountable difficulties (*e.g.*, large size of the molecule, heterogeneity of a given preparation of antibodies), Edelman [16] and his collaborators successfully reconstructed the antibody. A critical step in this development was the observation that Bence Jones proteins are, in fact, light chains and that myeloma cells produce one type of immunoglobulin with such predilection that contamination by other immunoglobulins is negligible.

In 1847 an English doctor discovered a peculiar substance in the urine of patients with mollities ossium. When the urine was heated it became turpid, but the cloudiness disappeared with further heating. The substance was shown to be a protein. Knowledge of the origin and structure of the Bence Jones protein, valuable as it might have been for the diagnosis of myeloma, did not come until almost 100 years later when Edelman and Gally [21] heated a solution containing light chains and found that it behaved exactly like the urine containing the Bence Jones protein. Once more, an accident of nature provided the student of biology the necessary substratum of his investigation—in this case, large amounts of light chain immunoglobulins.

Studies of the amino acid composition of Bence Jones proteins in various laboratories soon revealed that no two Bence Jones proteins were alike. Partial sequence studies also showed that the polypeptide chains contained two segments: one that was constant in all Bence Jones proteins and one that was variable. Similar observations were made when the light chains of myeloma γ-globulin were investigated. When the amino acid composition of Bence Jones protein was compared with that of light chains obtained from plasma immunoglobulin of patients with myeloma, similarities between the Bence Jones protein and the light chains were confirmed.

In spite of such remarkable progress, the task of determining the complete amino acid sequence of the immunoglobin was still overwhelming because of the huge size of even the lightest of the two chains. However, the amino acid compositions of H and L chains had revealed that the incidence of methionine residues in both chains was low. If, therefore, breaks could be introduced that were specific for the peptide bond involving methionine residues, then each chain could be split in a number of smaller polypeptides that might be easy to sequence. Cyanogen bromide selectively cleaves polypeptide chains at a position occupied by methionine. Thus, treatments of H and L chains with this reagent yield 7 and 3 polypeptides, respectively. By comparing the sequence of the terminal groups of these polypeptides with that of polypeptides obtained by digestion with proteolytic enzymes, investigators were able to determine the order in which each of the polypeptide chains produced by the cyanogen bromide treatment is inserted into the H or L chain. With these techniques, Edelman and his group deciphered the complete amino acid sequence of γg immunoglobulin.

Although the amino acid sequences of more than 100 human immunoglobulins are now known, rigid structural-functional correlations as are available for hemoglobin and myoglobin (see Chapter 3) are not yet possible for immunoglobulins. A major handicap for a long time was that immunoglobulin could not be crystallized. Without such crystals meaningful X-ray diffraction studies are not possible, and an accurate understanding of the three-dimensional configuration of the molecules cannot be available.

Crystals of intact immunoglobulin obtained from myeloma were obtained by Davies and Edmundson and their associates [14, 22–25]. As a result, the mapping of the molecule by X-ray crystallography has been begun. Physicochemical studies of the molecule have suggested that it is made of roughly three equal parts connected by a flexible zone referred to as the hinge. Such a molecular model was confirmed by electron microscopic studies, which revealed that the molecule is Y shaped.

Analysis of the patterns obtained by X-ray crystallography suggests that the component that forms the immunoglobulin molecule could be assembled in at least four ways, all consistent with the previous model proposed on the basis of physicochemical or electron microscopic studies, but the detailed positions of the atoms—especially those that form the hinge—are not yet available. Moreover, even if they were, it would still be necessary to show that the structure of the myeloma immunoglobulin, which does not combine with antigen, is representative of true antibodies [14, 24, 25]. In spite of the difficulties, the knowledge of the sequence of immunoglobulins has already provided some important clues as to the nature of the combining site of the huge molecule and has raised important questions as to the genetic determination of the antibody.

To avoid confusion, let's review earlier findings on antibody structure. When treated with proteolytic enzymes, the immunoglobulin molecules yield two components, an Fc fraction (a crystallizable fraction that is likely to be a homogeneous fraction) and an Fa fraction that doesn't crystallize, but which is variable in composition and contains the antigenic binding sites. Later, H and L chains were separated by reducing disulfide bonds. Amino acid sequence studies revealed that each chain contained a constant and a variable segment. In each case the constant segment is in the carboxy terminal, the variable segment is in the amino terminal segment. In the variable portion of the light chain, the variable components overlap so that the chains can be grouped in different classes referred to as VK1, VK2, VK3 for the $\varkappa$ chain, and VL1, VL2, VL3, VL4, VL5 for the λ chain.

The amino terminals of all the $\varkappa$ chains (107 residues) are quite variable, and except in inbred strains of mice, no two identical chains have been found.

Within the variable portion of both light and heavy chains, some sequences change relatively little and others are quite variable. These highly variable regions involve residues 24–34, 50–56, and 89–97 for the λ and $\varkappa$ chains, and 31–71 in the heavy chains.

Little is known of the actual antigen-binding sites, but they constitute a small portion of the molecules involving both heavy and light chains. The binding site has been estimated to be the size of a hexapeptide or a hexasaccharide; therefore, the size of the binding site compares with the size of the active site of an enzyme, which is of the order of 15 to 20 amino acid residues. (The analogy between the active site of the antibody and that of an enzyme has brought some to suggest that antibodies are, in fact, degenerated enzymes. Indeed, the enzyme does also bind to the substrate, but after binding it converts the substrate into the product, whereas the antibody simply binds to the antigen without further degrading it.)

Evidence suggests that the variable regions in the light and heavy chains may be brought together by folding of the molecules to contribute to the structure of the binding site. Hydrophobic regions are believed to be adjacent to the combining site. Such hydrophobic regions do not directly bind the antigen but increase the affinity for the antigen [26–28].

Thus, each Ig polypeptide chain is composed of two major amino acid sequences designated as the C region at the carboxy terminal end and the V region at the amino terminal end. It has been proposed and partially substantiated that the amino and carboxy terminals of one chain fold independently into the globular region referred to as "domains" with little affinity for each other, but with marked affinity for homologous domains and a second molecule. Each domain consists of a loop of approximately 100 amino acids linked by disulfide bonds. Optical rotary dispersion studies have revealed that the Ig contains no α-helical structure. A schematic representation of the structure of IgG is presented in Fig. 14-1.

IgG is a glycoprotein containing one or more carbohydrate prosthetic groups. The composition and location of carbohydrate moieties seem to vary widely. In most human IgG molecules, the carbohydrate moiety was found in the Fc fragments, but in some myeloma immunoglobulins, carbohydrate groups

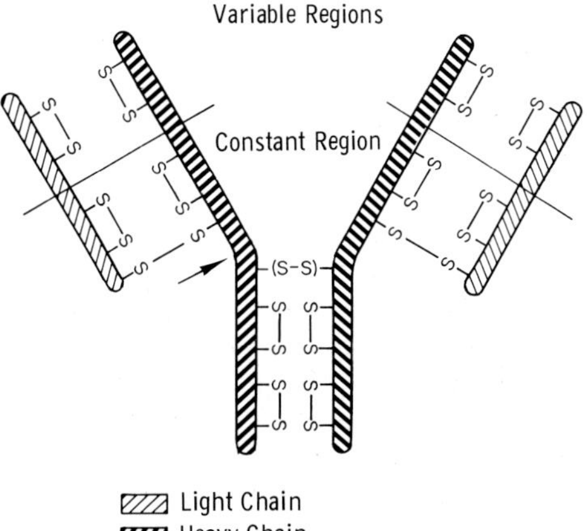

Fig. 14-1. Schematic representation of the molecular structure of IgG

Table 14-1. Characteristics of human immunoglobulins

Characteristics	IgG	IgA[a]	IgM[a]	IgD	IgE
Blood levels (mg/ml)	12–14	2–4	1	0.03	?
Antibody activity	+	+	+	?	+
Structural:					
Molecular weight	150,000	165,000+	900,000	?	?
Sedimentation constant	6.6	7(9,11, 13)	18	7	?
Carbohydrate	2%	10%	10%	?	?
Heavy-chain antigen	γ	α	μ	δ	ε
Light-chain antigen	$\varkappa$ or λ	$\varkappa$ or λ	$\varkappa$ or λ	$\varkappa$ or λ	α
Form polymers	—	+	—	—	—
Functional:					
React with rheumatoid factors	+	–	–	?	?
Active placental transport	+	–	–	?	?
Fix complement	+	–	+	?	?
Sensitize guinea pig skin	+	–	–	–	?
Sensitize human skin	–	–	–	–	+

[a] IgM—the molecule is composed of five subunits referred to as γ Mo (mol wt 180,000). Each subunit is composed of two heavy chains (70,000) and 1 and 2 light chains similar to those of IgG and IgC. Each molecule of IgG has 5 antibody-combining sites.

have been found in both the Fc and the Fab fragments. The structure of the carbohydrate moiety is not known, but complexed branch structures have been described.

In Table 14-1, some characteristics of human immunoglobulin are summarized. From the table, all immunoglobulins appear to be large molecules that may vary in size as a result of polymerization (*e.g.*, IgA) or because they are formed by a number of subunits (*e.g.*, IgM). Monomer or subunits are all composed of a variable heavy chain (IgG=γ, mol wt 55,000; IgA=α, mol wt 65,000; IgM, μ, 20,000; IgD, δ, IgE, ε*) and two light chains of the $\varkappa$ or λ types.

IgG, IgA, and IgM molecules all contain approximately 2% carbohydrate, likely to be bound covalently to the Fc fragment. It is not known whether the polysaccharide moieties are all strung in a single chain or divided in a number of small chains. And nothing is known about the functional role of the carbohydrate moiety.

In conclusion, normal and abnormal immunoglobulins are composed of two light and two heavy polypeptide chains held together by disulfide bonds and strong noncovalent interaction. The two types of light chains are λ and $\varkappa$, and the five types of heavy chains are μ, γ, α, δ, and ε. Each chain is composed of a constant region at the COOH-terminal end (C_L and C_H) and variable regions at the NH_2-terminal (V_L and V_H). The polypeptide chain is believed to fold so that the amino acid sequence of the hypervariable regions of the V_L and the V_H chains interact to form a pocket with a shape complementary to that of the antigen. Thus, the constant regions determine the class of an immunoglobulin. The variable regions determine their specificity.

* The molecular weights of the δ and ε chains are not known.

Antigen Determinants

Whether immunological reactions are nonpathogenic or pathogenic, the process always starts with interaction between antibody and antigen. Surprisingly little is known of the molecular events involved, but three steps can be distinguished: the recognition of the antigen, the binding of antigen and antibody, and the consequences of the apparition antigen-antibody complex [29–34].

Before we discuss the molecular interaction between antigen and antibody, it may be helpful to review briefly the molecular requirements for antigenicity. Studies of the molecular properties of the antigen were initiated by Landsteiner (1868–1943), a young physician who studied chemistry with such famous scientists as Fisher, Hantzsch, and Bamberger. Later Landsteiner became an assistant in the Pathological Anatomical Institute of the University of Vienna, and at the age of 40 he was prosector at the Imperial Wilhelmina Spitaal. After World War I he was invited by Simon Flexner to join the Rockefeller Institute for Medical Research where, as it has often been said, he started a second life at the age of 54.

In the beginning of this chapter, we saw that some relatively small molecular components, haptenes, could act as antigens if they were attached to larger molecules, usually polypeptide chains (carriers). Motivated by his concern to understand disease mechanisms and armed with his knowledge in chemistry, Landsteiner synthesized antigens of known structure. He took advantage of the well-known property of the diazotized aromatic amino acids to combine with amino acid residues of protein (primarily tyrosine residues). The combination of the diazotized amino acid (the haptene) and the polypeptide chain R yielded an antigen (see Fig. 14-2).

The molecular properties of the antigen can be changed at will by modifying either the R or the haptene. Cross-reaction experiments clearly demonstrated that an antiserum is directed primarily toward the haptene and not the carrier. Thus, if one binds haptene A to carrier P and haptene B to carrier P, antibodies to A appear in the serum of the animal injected with the complete antigen. The antibodies are specific for the haptene and not for the protein. As a corollary, if two different animals are injected with a complete antigen composed of the same haptene A but two different carriers, P and P_1, the antibodies that appear in serum of each of the injected animals will cross-react.

Further evidence that the antigen-antibody reaction involves the haptenes is suggested by what is referred to as the haptene reaction. The haptene is not by itself immunogenic, but if injected into an animal containing

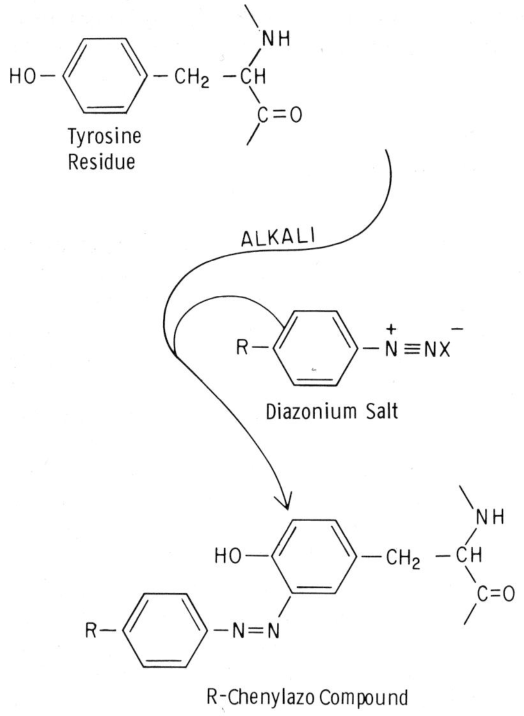

Tyrosine Residue

ALKALI

Diazonium Salt

R-Chenylazo Compound

Fig. 14-2. Landsteiner reaction

antibody directed toward that haptene, the haptene will interfere with further neutralization of the complete antigen. This suggests that the haptene traps the binding site on the antibody and thereby prevents any further reaction with the complete antigen. It must therefore be concluded that the molecular group that determines binding (referred to as the determinant) is located on the haptene.

Additional studies of antigenicity indicate that for the combination of haptene and carrier to be immunogenic, haptene binding must take place at one point of the molecule and must also occur in several areas of the carrier molecule. Therefore, many antigens can be expected to be polyvalent or contain a number of determinants.

The possibility of using synthetic haptenes combined to carriers to stimulate the formation of specific immunoglobulins also has permitted the study of stereochemical restrictions imposed on the antigen-antibody reaction. Maybe one of the most dramatic examples of such restrictions is Landsteiner's experiment using the three forms of tartaric acid discovered earlier by Pasteur (see Fig. 14-3). Thus, stereoisomeric tartaric acids linked to protein by the Landsteiner method yielded three specific antibodies.

Landsteiner's original studies were expanded in many laboratories including those of Pauling and Pressman. For example, all chlorine substitutes of the ortho-, para-, and meta-arsinobenzenes were prepared, and the affinity constant between antigen and specific antibodies was carefully measured. This permitted investigators to map precisely the three-dimensional

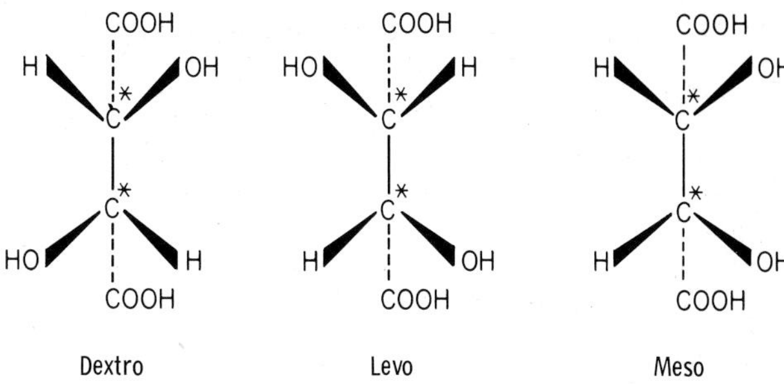

Fig. 14-3. Isomers of tartaric acid

structure of the portion of the antigen determinant that is recognized by the antibody.

A remarkable extension of that observation is the finding that a synthetic polypeptide composed entirely of D-amino acid is not immunogenic, although those made of the corresponding L-amino acid peptides may be [33].

Experiments with haptenes* bound to proteins clearly indicate that the determinant for antibody stimulation is the haptene and that in the haptene-protein combination, the protein moiety contributes relatively little to the antigenicity. Yet, in some cases proteins act as direct antigens. Then what are the conditions for antigenicity? A proteic immunogen is by definition a macromolecule with: a specific amino acid sequence; a definite size; a complex three-dimensional structure; a nebulous distribution of charges, and other characteristics. Which of these properties determines antigenicity? To study the antigenic properties of proteins, investigators have used synthetic polypeptides [34].

For a long time it was believed that only polypeptides with relatively high molecular weights (approximately 10,000 to 15,000) could be antigenic. Recently, copolymers with molecular weights of approximately 4000 have been shown to be antigenic.

D-Amino acid copolymers are nonimmunogenic even when the homologous L-copolymer is. Sayle has synthesized all D and L multichain polyproline polymers, none of which are antigenic. When short peptides composed of L-tyrosine and L-glutamic acid or L-phenylalanine and L-glutamic acid are attached to all D multichain polyproline, the macromolecule becomes immunogenic. In contrast, if all D short peptides are attached to the polyproline, the complex is not immunogenic.

Studies in which the antigenicity of native and denatured ribonuclease was investigated suggested that in addition to possible sequential determinants, conformational determinants exist as well. In the case of conformational determinants, the recognition of the antigen by the antibody is not directly concerned with a specific amino acid sequence but with the three-dimensional structure imparted to the molecule, which, of course, is a consequence of the sequence.

* The haptene must not be attached to a macromolecule to be antigenic. P-Azobenzene arsonate attached to a hexapeptide or a tripeptide of tyrosine can provoke a good immune response in guinea pigs and rabbits.

This concept is further supported by experiments in which a tyrosine-alanine-glutamine sequence is attached to a branched polymer of alanine or to a polymer forming an α-helix; antibodies that form against the branched polymer do not cross-react with those elaborated against the α-helix. Moreover, synthetic polypeptides can be prepared with straight chains or form loops. Again, there is no cross-reaction between antibodies elaborated against these two conformation variants with essentially similar amino acid sequences. A synthetic, collagenlike polypeptide of an ordered sequence was found to cross-react immunologically with collagen, clearly indicating that the triple-helix conformation common to both is the determinant of the antigen-antibody reaction.

This brief, incomplete discussion of the molecular structure of the antigenic determinant could be extended to include polysaccharides, lipoproteins, nucleic acids, and a multitude of antigens. But let us first consider the significance of the data already presented. Clearly, the antibody recognizes precise three-dimensional structural properties of the determinant whether it be the haptene or a portion of an antigenic protein.

Theories on Antigen-Antibody Contact

Studies of the structure of the determinant function of antigen show that the antibody recognizes specific molecular portions of the determinant. Studies of the antibody's structure reveal that the amino acid sequence may vary enough to provide for a multitude of antibodies, each specific for a given antigen. Studies of the equilibrium and kinetics of antigen-antibody reactions indicate that those forces involved in binding antigen to antibody are weak ones, with free energies of the magnitude of those involved in hydrogen, hydrophobic, or van der Waals bonds. Thus, any theory on the antigen-antibody reaction must take into account these two prerequisites: rigid specificity and weak forces.

From the beginning of immunological experimentation, the specificity of the relationship between antigen and antibody was so well recognized that it was used for diagnostic purposes. In 1906 Ehrlich attempted to explain such specificity by proposing a complementarity between the structures of the antigen and antibody, but the details were not known.

In 1940 Pauling provided a plausible model by proposing that the special shape of the antibody, which is complementary to that of the antigen, results from the unique folding of the molecule. However, complementarity does not mean that the surface of the antigen is identical to that of the antibody, but rather that the receptacle on the surface of the antibody molecule, which is destined to "accept" the antigen, is a perfect mold of the surface of the antigen, exactly like a plaster cast molds a face. Thus, for each point at the surface of the antigen there is a complementary point on the surface of the antibody, and joining all the complementary points creates a matrix in which the determinant can comfortably nestle all its parts.

Such complementarity requires close apposition of all parts of the surfaces of the antigen and antibody. This cannot be achieved with one or two strong (*e.g.*, covalant) bonds, but requires a large number of weak bonds the strength of which decreases rapidly with the distance (such as van der Waals forces and hydrogen bonds) [35].

The theory of complementarity, which proposes a close fit between the structure of the determinant and the surface on the antibody, has been compared to the relationship between a lock and key. Although the lock and key hypothesis appears to be the only plausible interpretation for the close interaction between antigen and antibody, it still is nothing more than a hypothesis. Indeed, the details of the molecular arrangement at the surface contact of the antibody with the determinant are not known. Moreover, the hypothesis raises serious questions; for example, what molecular mechanism confers the high specificity of the antibody toward such a great variability of antigens [36–38].

Richards *et al.* attempted to define part of the structure that binds the antibody. These investigators studied the binding of γ-hydroxy vitamin K_1 to immunoglobulin prepared from myeloma (referred to as NEW). Their model proposes that the variable regions of the L chain (L_1, L_2, L_3) and of the H chain (H_1, H_2, H_3) are folded into irregular loops in which the haptene is entrapped like a stone in a ring. These investigators have also proposed that the antigen-antibody–combining sites are polyfunctional. The evidence for polyfunctional activity includes the observation that a myeloma protein called protein 460 binds both menadione and DNP, and that the two binding sites may be inactivated separately [39].

Quantitative Aspects of Antigen-Antibody Reactions

The reaction between antibody and haptene in solution does not in any essential way differ from that of any other bimolecular reaction. Therefore, it obeys the laws of mass action and can be expressed by the equation

$$[\mathrm{Atg}]+[\mathrm{Atb}]\,\frac{K1}{K2}=[\mathrm{Atgb}],$$

in which [Atg], [Atb], and [Atgb] are the concentrations of antigen, antibody, and antigen-antibody complex, respectively, and *K*1 is the forward and *K*2 the reverse reaction constant. At equilibrium,

$$K=\frac{[\mathrm{Atgb}]}{[\mathrm{Atg}]\,[\mathrm{Atb}]}=\frac{K1}{K2}. \qquad (1)$$

Such an equation is valid only if each antibody-combining site on the antibody molecule functions independently of each other. Consequently, the antibody, even if multivalent, may be looked upon as composed of monovalent units.

Equation (1) can be rewritten as follows:

$$\frac{[\mathrm{H-Atb}]}{\mathrm{n}[\mathrm{Atb}]-[\mathrm{H-Atb}][\mathrm{H}]}=K \tag{2}$$

in which H is the concentration of haptene, [H-ATb] is the concentration of haptene bound to antibody, n is the valence of the antibody, and [Atb] is the total antibody concentration.

Equation (2) can be rearranged as follows:

$$[\mathrm{H-Atb}]-(\mathrm{n}[\mathrm{Atb}]-[\mathrm{HAtb}])[\mathrm{H}]K$$

$$[\mathrm{H-Atb}]=\mathrm{n}[\mathrm{Atb}][\mathrm{H}]K-[\mathrm{H}][\mathrm{Atb}]K$$

$$\frac{[\mathrm{HAtb}]}{[\mathrm{Atb}]}=\mathrm{n}[\mathrm{H}]K-\frac{[\mathrm{H-Atb}]}{[\mathrm{Atb}]}[\mathrm{H}]K.$$

If in Equation (3) the concentration of free haptene is replaced by c and the ratio of bound haptene to total antibody by r,

$$\mathrm{r}=\mathrm{nc}K-\mathrm{rc}K, \quad \text{or}$$

$$\frac{\mathrm{r}}{\mathrm{c}}=\mathrm{n}K-\mathrm{r}K. \tag{4}$$

Equation (4) is often referred to as the Scatchard representation of the law of mass action.

$$\frac{1}{\mathrm{c}}=\frac{\mathrm{n}K}{\mathrm{r}}-K, \quad \text{or}$$

$$\frac{1}{\mathrm{r}}=\frac{(1)}{\mathrm{n}K}\frac{(1)}{\mathrm{c}}+\frac{1}{\mathrm{n}}. \tag{5}$$

Equation (5) is referred to as the Langmuir equation.

By plotting r/c against r in (4), one can obtain a straight line, and the valence and equilibrium constant can be evaluated from intercept data. In Equation (5), if 1/r is plotted against 1/c, a straight line is obtained, the slope of which is $1/\mathrm{n}K$.

These equations reveal that to find the value of K, the equilibrium constant, or n, the valance, one needs to know only c, the concentration of free haptene, and the total amount of antibody present.

The concentration of free haptene was measured first by haptene inhibition but later more effectively by equilibrium dialysis.

Ordinarily, antigen-antibody reactions yield complex products that precipitate or agglutinate (see below). These reactions are too complex to be studied accurately by physicochemical methods. However, the simplest common denominator to all these reactions—namely, the binding of the antigen determinant with the antibody-combining site—can be investigated. Even such studies are complicated by the fact that the immunogenic reaction to the antigen is itself complex. For example, when sheep serum, P-azophenyl orsonic acid, is used as an antigen, antibodies develop to: (1) the haptenic group, (2) the protein moiety, and (3) a portion of the antigen including the haptenic group and the adjacent protein moiety.

Thus, to study antigen-antibody reactions quantitatively, one must restrict the studies to noncomplex reactions involving a single antigen-antibody site. This is best achieved by preparing antibodies to one haptene carrier complex and then reacting the antibody only with the haptene. That haptene and antibody form soluble complexes has already been mentioned. The presence of haptene in the solution interferes with the binding of the haptene carrier complex.

In the technique of dialysis equilibrium, the incubation flask is divided into two concentric compartments by a semipermeable membrane that permits the haptene to pass from one compartment to another but contains the antibody or the antibody-haptene complex within the membrane. Thus, all free haptene can readily be dialyzed, and the amount of haptene that binds to the antibody and the concentration of free haptene can be measured.

When such antigen-antibody reactions were investigated even under optimal conditions, the expected straight lines for Equations (4) and (5) were not obtained.

Yet, if we can assume that all haptene molecules are identical and that the binding sites on the antibody show the same affinity for the haptene, we can expect the straight line. However, if the antibody contains binding sites with different affinities for the antigen, a nonlinear response is expected. Therefore, the experimental results indicate that the reaction between haptene and antibody-binding sites is heterogeneous.

Modern knowledge of the structure of antibodies has given some insight on the reasons for such heterogeneity. The types of heterogeneity are classified as class, intrachain, and site heterogeneity. Thus, the same antigen may elicit the elaboration of antibodies of various classes and of antibodies of the same class with different sequences. Moreover, different antigenic sites may appear on the same molecule for different segments of the antigen. Finally, it cannot be excluded that antibody sites which combine with specific determinants do not vary, and it has even been proposed that the haptene itself might not be immutable and may exist in different conformations.

Inasmuch as the decrease in free energy (ΔF) is related to the equilibrium constant according to the following equation

$$\Delta\mathrm{F}=\mathrm{RT}\ln K,$$

the determination of K will permit the calculation of F.

Such measurements revealed that the changes in free energy are small, much smaller than what is needed to form covalent bonds (50 to 100 Cal/mole) and of a magnitude that would permit only hydrogen or van der Waals bonds to be formed.

Thus, the bonds that link antigen to antibody are relatively weak; therefore, they decrease rapidly as the distance between the atoms increases (hydrogen bonds vary as the sixth power of the distance, van der Waals forces as the seventh power of the distance. (Coulombic forces vary inversely as the square of the distance between groups.)

For binding to be tight under such conditions, the surfaces of the antigen and antibody must be closely apposed.

Remember that

$$K = \frac{[\text{Atgb}]}{[\text{Atg}][\text{Atb}]} = \frac{K1}{K2},$$

with $K1$ being the rate constant for the forward reaction and $K2$ the rate of reaction of the reverse reaction. Obviously, by measuring K and either one of the rate constants, the other rate constant can be calculated. Rate constants for antigen-antibody reactions are difficult to measure because (1) the conditions of the reactions are difficult to control, and (2) the reactions are extremely rapid. Ingenious methods have been devised to measure such reaction rates, but these reactions occur in a millionth of a second.

Secondary Manifestations of Antigen-Antibody Reactions

What has been described is the initial reaction between antigen and antibody that is involved in the binding between one monovalent unit of the antibody with one valence of the antigen. This type of reaction is often called the primary reaction, in contrast to subsequent, more complex reactions called secondary reactions.

The binding of the antigen to the antibody yields *in vitro* or *in vivo* a number of visible events, such as precipitation of antigen-antibody complexes, agglutination of particulate antigen carriers (bacteria and viruses), neutralization of toxins, and activation of complement. In fact, depending upon which of these phenomena is elicited by the antigen-antibody reaction, one speaks of precipitins, agglutinins, hemolysins, etc. Such terms are useful only if it is kept in mind that they are not mutually exclusive. Thus, an antibody that may elicit precipitation of complex may also activate complement. Many of these reactions have been modified, sometimes most ingeniously to serve as research or diagnostic tools. Thus, immunodiffusion, radioimmunoassay, and immunoelectrophoresis are techniques based on the ability of the antigen-antibody complex to precipitate.

We will describe here only a few of the basic secondary reactions triggered by the antigen-antibody interaction—namely, precipitation, agglutination, neutralization, and complement activation.

Precipitation

Precipitation reactions have intrigued physical chemists and biochemists ever since attempts were made to understand the biochemistry of life. Precipitation does provide the biochemist with large amounts of biological macromolecules, and as these macromolecules precipitate out of the supernatant, they also concentrate other compounds within the supernatant. Already in 1907 Arrhenius observed that the precipitation of antibodies by antigens did not evolve as expected, especially in that the precipitate redissolved in the presence of excess antigens. The names of many famous immunologists are associated with the elaboration of equations and theories to explain the peculiar behavior of immunological precipitates. The reader is referred to other books for details [1, 40].

When equal amounts of antibody are pipetted in a series of test tubes and increasing amounts of antigen are added keeping the final volume in each tube constant, a precipitate appears in those tubes containing a favorable antigen-antibody ratio. At a high antibody-antigen ratio, no precipitation takes place, but as the proportion of antigen in the tubes increases, precipitation develops and becomes optimal when all antibody sites are combined. When antigen is added in excess of the antibody levels, the precipitate disappears progressively until all components—antigens and antigen-antibody complexes—are again in solution. This peculiar behavior is explained by the interaction between antigen and antibody.

To understand the peculiarities of precipitin reaction, one must keep in mind that antibodies are bivalent and antigens multivalent.

When balanced amounts of antibody and antigen are mixed, each bivalent antibody molecule is attached to antigen determinants. But because the antigen is multivalent it can bind to several antibody molecules, and as a result a complex lattice is formed that readily precipitates. When the amount of antibody molecules exceeds that of the antigen, there are not enough antigen molecules to bind to several antibody molecules; and when the antigen is in excess, there are not enough antibody molecules to form a lattice.

Agglutination

The surfaces of viruses or bacteria are made of protein, lipids, and polysaccharides, compounds that are antigenic. Thus, a patient with pneumonia develops high-titer antibodies in his serum against the surface of the bacteria. If such serum is added to a suspension of pneumococci *in vitro,* the bacteria agglutinate.

Agglutination does not differ essentially from precipitation except that in the former the antigen molecules are at the surface of particles such as viruses or bacteria, and the bivalent antibody molecule reacts with the antigen molecule to form a lattice which traps the cell. In the ordinary antigen-antibody reaction, the attractive and repellent forces between molecules concern the two reactants only. In the agglutination reaction, the cell surface is usually negatively charged so cells repell to bring about agglutination, and the antigen-antibody reaction must overcome this negative force. Therefore, one may expect that the agglutination reaction will depend strongly on changes in pH and ionic strength. Moreover, the greater the affinity of the antibody for the antigen and the more numerous the binding sites on the antibody macromolecular complex, the more effective the agglutination.

For these reasons, only antibodies that exhibit a great affinity for the antigens are able to agglutinate cells, and IgM, which has many more binding sites than IgG, is a more effective agglutinator. Similarly, the incidence and the position of the antigenic determinants on the surface of the cell membrane considerably influence the ability of these cells to be agglutinated by antibody. This has been shown by preparing antibodies to blood group antigens at the red cell surface, where A antigen molecules are 100 times as numerous as B antigen molecules. An antibody against A will agglutinate; an antibody against B won't.

Although it is not clear how great a role precipitation and agglutination have in eliminating foreign antigens *in vivo,* the study of these two reactions has helped us understand the mechanism of antigen-antibody reactions and has also provided useful diagnostic tools that can unfortunately not be discussed here.

One antigen-antibody reaction that has been known for a long time is the neutralization of antitoxin. Some bacterial infections—including diphtheria, tetanus, botulism, cholera, and some staphylococcal and streptococcal infections—are associated with the elaboration of toxin.

Activation of Complement

Serum contains a population of factors (complement) that interact to provide active compounds capable of initiating biological events, such as cellular death, chemotaxis, and opsonization. The activation of complement is triggered by an antigen-antibody reaction. Thus, the interaction between the antigen-antibody complex serves to direct the site of action of complement and to amplify the effect of the antigen-antibody reaction [41–51].

Present knowledge indicates that complement is composed of 11 proteins that react in sequence. The activation step usually involves the splitting of a larger molecule into smaller components, some of which are believed to be lost to the cells' economy, whereas others bind to the cell membrane in small proportions and act either as enzymes (peptidase, esterases) or active pharmacological compounds (*e.g.*, anaphylatoxin).

Safeguards against a chain reaction resulting from the inadvertent activation of all or part of the complement system explain the existence in serum of specific inhibitors of practically every step of the activation sequence. Thus, the pattern of complement activation is reminiscent of that of several other critical functions of blood, such as blood coagulation or activation of the kininogen-kinin system.

We will consider here the steps of the activation one by one, but first the nomenclature usually used in describing complement must be explained. Each component is referred to by a capital C′ with an arabic number, C′1, C′2, C′3, C′4, C′5, C′6, C′7, C′8, and C′9. C1 is a complex of three different proteins, $C1_q$, $C1_r$, $C1_s$, thus accounting for the 11 factors mentioned above. Activators are referred to by placing a bar over the arabic number ($C\bar{1}$, $C\bar{2}$, etc.). Inactivators are indicated by adding the subscript i after the number (*e.g.*, $C3_i$). When a component of complement (*e.g.*, C3) is split into smaller fragments, the origin of the split compound is designated by adding the letters a, b, and c as subscripts to the formula of the parent molecule (*e.g.*, $C3_a$, $C3_b$). The receptor site of complement on a specific antigen-antibody complex is designated SA. Each step of the activation can now be described with these symbols.

The use of such symbolism conveys an aura of mystery to the uninitiated and always frightens the medical student. Someday the molecular structure of each reactant and product of the complement fixation sequence will be describable in precise terms, and, as a matter of fact, much is already known of the molecular properties of the various factors involved in complement fixation (see Table 14-2). In the meantime, we must continue to deal with a symbolism somewhat reminiscent of alchemy.

The sequence of steps in the activation of the complement system has been studied *in vitro* using sheep erythrocytes to which specific rabbit antibodies have been added. The antigen-antibody complex does not by itself trigger hemolysis. Hemolysis occurs only if serum containing complement is added to the sensitized erythrocytes. The event involved in complement activation can be dissected by adding pure compounds one by one. This is possible because to date almost each of the components of complement, except $C1_r$, C6, C7, and C8, have been extensively purified.

Binding and Activation of C1

In the first step of the reaction, C1 binds to antibody molecules already complexed to antigen. IgM and IgG are the only immunoglobulins that can bind C1, and IgM is much better than IgG. Among the molecular variants of IgG, some types are more effective at binding C1 than others. Thus, of the purified myeloma immunoglobulins $\gamma G1$ and $\gamma G3$ have a great affinity and $\gamma G2$ and $\gamma G4$ a low affinity for complement. IgA, IgD, and IgE cannot fix complement.

In contrast to all other components of the complement system, C1 binds spontaneously and reversibly to the immunoglobulin. Once bound, the triple molec-

Table 14-2. Some properties of complement components

	Serum concen- tration mg%	Molecular weight $\times 10^4$	Sedimen- tation constant in S	Electro- phoretic mobility	% $Cn(H_2O)n$ constant	Reactive SH	Function in C′ fixation	Natural inhibitors
C1q	10–20	40	11.1	γ_2	15–17			
r	?	16.5	7	β	?			
s	2.2	8	4	α_2	?		esterase	C1 esterase inhibitor
C4	43	23	10	β_1	14			
a		1.5					lost	
b		21.5					[SAC$\bar{1}$ 4_b]	
C2	<2.5	11.5	5.5	β_2		1 or more		
a		8					[SAC$\bar{1}$ $4_b 2_a$] convertase	
b		3.5					lost	
C3	120	18.5	9.58	β_1	2.7			
a		0.7		γ_2			anaphylatoxin	
b							peptidase	serum inhibitor
C5	7.5		8.7	β	1Q			
a		1.2					anaphylatoxin	
b								
C6			5–6	β_2				
C7			6–7	β_2				
C8		15	8	γ_1				
C9	0.1	7.9	4	α			carboxypeptidase	

ular complex $C1_q$, $C1_r$, and $C1_s$ is activated. The exact mechanism of activation is not known, but $C1_s$ is believed to be a "zymogen," which under the influence of Ca^{++} is converted to an active protease.

$$\left.\begin{matrix}\text{IgM}\\\text{IgB}\end{matrix}\right\rangle + \text{Antigen} \longrightarrow \text{SA}^*$$

$$\text{SA} + \text{C1} \xrightarrow[\text{Ca}^{++}]{} \text{SAC}\bar{1}^{**}.$$

C1 can be activated by a number of proteolytic enzymes, such as thrombin, plasmin, trypsin, and the Hageman factor. The protease (C$\bar{1}$) is inhibited by ε-aminocaproic acid, di-isopropyl fluorophosphate, and a natural inhibitor found in serum.

Binding of $C4_b$

The second component to react with the fixation site is C4 and not C2. The protease C$\bar{1}$ splits C4 into two components, $C4_a$ and $C4_b$. The first is lost to the reaction; the second binds to the fixation site to yield SAC$\bar{1}$ 4_b.

$$\text{C}\bar{1} + \text{C4} \longrightarrow \text{C4}_a + \text{C4}_b$$

$$\text{C4}_a \rightarrow \text{lost}; \quad \text{C4}_b + \text{SAC}\bar{1} \rightarrow \text{SAC}\bar{1}\ 4_b$$

C4 can be inactivated by a number of compounds, including hydrazine, ammonia, diethyl ether, and a factor present in shark serum.

Activation of C2

C2 is the next component to be involved in the sequence of steps leading to complement fixation. In the presence of magnesium, C2 is first bound to the SAC$\bar{1}$ 4_b complex. Then it is split into two fragments—$C2_a$, an enzyme (convertase) involved in the binding of C3, and $C2_b$, which is lost.

Only small amounts of $C2_a$ are bound, even bound $C2_a$ is extremely labile and is degraded to yield $C2_{ai}$ within minutes (half-life 10 minutes). Inasmuch as it contains one or more SH groups indispensable for activity, $C2_a$ is inhibited by p-chloromercuribenzoate and stabilized by iodine.

* An antigen-antibody complex that serves as a specific binding site.

** Esterase is bound to the antigen-antibody complex.

Splitting of C3

As just mentioned, the binding of $C2_a$ to the SAC$\bar{1}$ 4_b complex yields a SAC$\bar{1}$ 4_b2_a complex with "convertase activity." After binding C3 to the complex, the convertase splits native C3 into two fragments: $C3_a$ and $C3_b$. Ten per cent of the $C3_a$ is lost to the cytolytic reaction, but it possesses some pharmacological properties of its own and has therefore been called anaphylatoxin. Of the $C3_b$ originally bound to the activation site, only 10% remains bound, and of that amount a fraction, approximately 10%, is believed to be transferred from the activation site to a specific receptor site on the cell membrane somewhat distant from the site of activation. In any event, the appearance of bound $C3_b$ leads to the appearance of new peptidase activity. The remaining $C3_b$ is rapidly inactivated to yield $C3_{bi}$.

SAC$\bar{1}$ 4_b2_a + C3

(anaphylatoxin) $C3_a$ ← → $C3_b$ Soluble

↓

SAC$\bar{1}$ $4_b2_a3_b$

$C3_b$ Peptidase

$C3_b$ can be inactivated *in vitro* by hydrazine, zymosan, or snake venom as well as by specific inhibitors found in serum. When $C3_b$ binds to the active site, peptidase activity develops that can be demonstrated by cleavage of synthetic dipeptides that contain one aromatic residue (*e.g.*, glycyltyrosine).

When SAC$\bar{1}$ $4_b2_a3_b$ is presented with the next three components of complement—C5, C6, and C7—a highly thermostable complex SAC$\bar{1}$ $4_b2_a3_b5_b6,7$ is formed. The molecular mechanism involved in the formation of the complex is unknown. It appears that during the fixation of C5, C6, and C7, C5 is split into $C5_a$, a potent anaphylatoxin, and $C5_b$.

Except for the fact that the presence of bound $C5_b$ is indispensable for the binding and that C8 must be bound to bind C9, the mode of binding of C8 and C9 is unknown. Neither is it known how membrane damage occurs after the fixation of C9. After that stage, holes detectable with the electron microscope appear in the membrane, and EDTA interferes with membrane damage. The properties of complement components are shown in Table 14-2.

A high molecular weight group of serum proteins called properdin acting together with complement was found to kill some gram-positive or negative bacteria in the absence of antibody or in the presence of small amounts of it. It was later established that the incubation of normal serum with microbes or with polysaccharides derived from other agents such as yeast (zymosan) generate serum enzymes capable of activating C3 and C5 [52–54].

In the classical pathway for complement activation, C1 activates C2, which in turn activates C4 and C3. The properdin pathway differs from the classical pathway in a number of ways, and therefore it is referred to as the alternative pathway. The system is activated in guinea pigs defective in C4 or in humans defective in C2 and is activated spontaneously when the $C3_b$ inactivator (KAF) is absent or neutralized by antibody. As already mentioned, the system does not require the presence of large amounts of antibodies, but is activated by zymosan, bacterial endotoxins, or insulin (in suspension but not in solution). The system requires magnesium rather than calcium for activation, which shows that C1 is not involved.

At least three serum factors distinct from complement are involved in the alternative pathway: properdin, a glycine-rich β-glycoprotein, and a proglycine-rich β-proteinase. Properdin is believed to be composed of two enzymes each made of several subunits; one activates C3, the other C5. Although the properdin enzymes are not identical in structure, they mimick the functions of $C4_b2_a3_b$ complexes. When the properdin system is activated, $C3_b$ is present and an inhibitor of $C3_b$ activator KAF is also found. Although the properdin system can be initiated without C4 and C2, the presence of the full complement system in the blood accelerates the properdin system probably by the formation of $C4_b2_a$, which leads to the generation of $C3_b$. Clearly, too little is known of the factors or the sequence of steps in the alternative pathway for complement activation to be accurately described.

According to Lachmann and his associates, C3 is split to $C3_b$ by the product of the attack on the glycine-rich γ-glycoprotein by the specific proteinase. Thus, the split product of the glycine-rich γ-glycoprotein acts like a "C3 convertase." $C3_b$ is essential for the activity of the glycine-rich glycoprotein proteinase, $C3_b$ is destroyed by the $C3_b$ inactivator (KAF), and thereby its effect on triggering the alternative pathway is restricted. According to this scheme, the alternative pathway is one in which $C3_b$ generates more C3-converting enzyme.

The role of the alternative pathway has not been clarified, but if it can be activated in the absence of antibody, it may represent a mechanism for immune defense when sufficient quantities of antibodies cannot be made. There is also evidence that the system is activated in certain disease processes such as in membranoproliferative glomerulonephritis [55].

Although much remains to be learned about the role of complement in protecting against or causing disease, complement undoubtedly plays a major role in inflammation and hypersensitivity.

Various components of the complement system contribute to inflammation. The release of anaphylatoxins during the C3 and C5 activation steps contribute to vasodilation. The effect of anaphylatoxin can be prevented by administering antihistamines, which indicates that the anaphylatoxins act as histamine releasers. Similarly, C3 and C5 activation leads to the release of chemotactic substances that attract leukocytes to the inflamed area. Enhancement of phagocytosis through opsonization is associated mainly with the C3, and secondarily with the C4, activation step. Complement activation, which ultimately leads to cytolysis of sensitized erythrocytes, may also be involved in the killing of bacteria. If this occurs *in vivo,* only gram-negative bacteria are likely to be sensitive to the cytolytic effect. Indeed, gram-positive bacteria or such infectious agents as Treponema are not killed by complement activation [56–58].

Paroxysmal nocturnal hemoglobinuria occurs during the third or the fourth decade and is associated with hemolytic anemia and hemoglobinuria. The hemoglobinuria develops after sleep. In this disease an alteration of the red cell membrane is unusually sensitive to the third component of complement. The blood contains no antierythrocyte antibodies and therefore the classical pathway for hemolysis (binding of antibody followed by binding of C1, C4, C2) to the cell membrane is not possible. Available evidence shows that the lysis of erythrocytes of patients with paroxysmal nocturnal hemoglobinuria requires the protein component involved in the complement alternative pathway [283].

Clearly, if complement can elicit protective inflammatory reactions, it is also likely to be involved in those diseases in which the immune system is out of gear. For example, there is evidence that complement activation is involved in the pathogenesis of diseases in which antigen-antibody complexes accumulate at the surface of circulating blood components (leukocytes, erythrocytes, platelets), in the basal membranes of glomeruli, or in the walls of blood vessels. Examples of such circumstances will be presented later.

Blood Levels of Antibodies

The levels of antibodies in the blood normally are remarkably constant. Therefore, regulatory mechanisms must control the homeostasis of antibodies. Such mechanisms are likely to include regulation of: (1) the rates of proliferation of antibody-producing cells, (2) the anabolic and catabolic balance, and (3) the relative cell populations in the lymph nodes. A number of factors modulate the blood levels of antibodies, among them are host characteristics (heredity, age, immunological state) and the mode of administration of the antigen.

Heredity

During epidemics, some humans respond to antigenic stimuli better than others. This variation in response to similar antigens among individuals of a single species is, at least in part, determined by heredity. The role of heredity and antibody formation has been well established in experimental animals (we will discuss this point again).

Age

The capacity to form antibodies appears only after birth and decreases after the age of 60. In contrast to the opossum, in which the capacity to form antibodies develops 20 days after the onset of gestation, the mammalian fetus does not respond to antigen stimulation by forming antibodies. Even after birth, all immunoglobulins are not formed at the same time. Moreover, the age at which adult levels of elaboration of the various immunoglobulins are reached varies with the immunoglobulin type. IgA is elaborated 2–3 weeks after birth, and IgB is elaborated 4–6 weeks after birth; they reach adult levels at 12 and 8 weeks, respectively. In contrast, IgM is elaborated during the first few days after birth and reaches adult levels during the second year of age.

Moreover, the various molecular types of antibodies do not usually appear at the same time after antigenic stimulation, but they develop in sequence. When polysaccharides are used as antigens, IgM develops first and IgB follows. Polysaccharides may stimulate IgM production without eliciting IgA elaboration.

Immunological State of the Host

The antibody response varies depending upon whether the antigen is administered to an individual immunologically virgin with respect to antigens, or whether antibodies have been synthesized previously. If the new dose of antigens is administered after all the antibody elicited by the first antigenic exposure has been eliminated, the response to the second dose will be similar to that of the first. A different response occurs when the new dose of antigen is administered before all antibody production elicited by the first dose has ceased. The administration of small amounts of antigens has little effect because the antigen molecules are neutralized by circulating antibodies. The administration of large amounts of antigens leads to neutralization of most, if not all, circulating antibodies, followed by a new burst of antibody formation far exceeding that elicited by the administration of the first dose of antigen. This second, amplified antibody production is referred to as secondary response.

Let's consider these phenomena in molecular terms, albeit they remain unspecific. The first administration of antigen elicits a molecular interaction that dictates the sequence of molecular events that result in antibody formation. The elaboration of antibodies is at first substantial but later slows down and becomes dormant. The second administration of antigens recalls the primary molecular alteration into function, but this time it elicits a much more vigorous antibody elaboration. Because an earlier molecular alteration is recalled into operation even years later, one sometimes speaks of a memory phenomenon. To assume that the immunological memory phenomenon is a macromolecular event in any way comparable to brain memory is premature; nevertheless, such a thought is intriguing.

Mode of Administration of Antigens

The elaboration of antibodies varies depending upon the mode of administration of the antigens and some properties of the host. When a single antigen is administered, the antibody response differs with the dose and the route of administration. Usually a critical amount of antigen is needed to stimulate antibody formation. Levels of antigens below the minimum, although incapable of triggering antibody formation, may maintain production of existing antibodies.

Repeated administration of small doses of antigens are usually more effective in maintaining antibody formation than the administration of single doses. In contrast, the administration of a large excess of antigens may lead to antigenic paralysis or immunological tolerance (see section on allergy).

Depending on the combination of antigens administered, simultaneous administration of antigens may have two opposite effects—competitive or additive. The molecular mechanism by which competition or augmentation is effectuated is not known. However, these phenomena are the reason for administering simultaneously the diphtheria, pertussis, and tetanus antigens.

Antibody response varies considerably depending upon the port of entry of the antigen, because the mode of entrance determines which antibody-forming system is first put in gear. Except for the fetus, the normal route for spontaneous contact with antibodies in humans is the epithelial surface (skin, gastrointestinal and respiratory tracts). In the fetus, antigens must traverse the placental membrane. Sometimes antigens are injected subcutaneously or intravenously, either iatrogenically (*e.g.*, serum injections and blood transfusions) or because of drug addiction.

A new form of iatrogenic administration of antigens has recently been introduced with organ transplantation.

Although they do not increase the initial elaboration of antibodies, a number of substances, called adjuvants, sustain antibody production for longer periods of time. The molecular compositions of adjuvants vary considerably. Freund discovered a classical type of adjuvant made with killed tubercular bacilli mixed with wax and mineral oil. Adjuvants seem to act on some unknown intracellular structure rather than directly at the level of gene expression. Adjuvants are likely to increase antibody production by at least three mechanisms that probably operate in synchrony: (1) attraction of immunologically competent cells at the antigenic site, (2) stimulation of phagocytosis, and (3) activation of lymphocytic proliferation.

The injection of an antigen partially suppresses the immune response to another antigen. The mechanism by which this antigenic competition is expressed is debated. Two hypotheses have been presented; one assumes that the competition is for multipotential stem cells, the other assumes that it is mediated by a humoral factor required by both antigens that becomes enhanced after the first antigen is administered. Available evidence seems to have excluded the first hypothesis [59].

Antibody Synthesis

At first approximation, the biosynthesis of antibodies should not raise any special problems. Because antibodies are polypeptide chains, they should be coded for by a specific DNA sequence that is copied into a messenger RNA molecule, and this molecule is translated after attachment to ribosomes into H and L chains. Once the two chains have been synthesized, because of the proximity of the special noncovalent forces generated by the half molecules, the two halves join. (The immunoglobulin molecules can be split into two exact halves that can be recombined later.)

This panoramic view of antibody synthesis is correct only with respect to chain translation. Translation does occur on ribosomes. The L chain is synthesized first, and it is then believed to become covalently bound to the H chain, possibly before the biosynthesis of that chain is complete.

But the detailed description of the molecular mechanism for storage and transfer of genetic information needed for antibody synthesis and for the triggering of antibody synthesis raises serious questions that will only be touched upon here [60–63].

First, we must consider that antibody elaboration involves two kinds of cells—the macrophage and the lymphocyte. The interaction between the two types of cells will be discussed elsewhere.

Second, the great diversity of the immunoglobulins raises the question of their mode of coding. The first theory to explain the complementarity of the antibody with the antigen was proposed in 1930 by Haurowitz and Brunile. The template theory for determining the antibody structure assumes that the antigen, once it has entered the body, selects the antibody molecule and molds it into complementarity. Early studies on the amino acid compositions of antibody preparations suggested that they are similar, and even the homologies of early partial sequence studies were marshalled in support of the theory. However, we know now that in spite of large zones of homology, antibodies possess discrete areas of variability in amino acid sequence in both chains. Moreover, it has been established that the folding of a protein into a three-dimensional conformation is primarily determined by its amino acid sequence and not by exogenous molecules. For these reasons, despite its early vigor, the template theory succumbed to one that is now considered more plausible: Burnet's [64] selective clonal theory.

As Burnet pointed out, the distinction between the template and the clonal theories is reminiscent of the difference in Lamarck's and Darwin's understanding of evolution. The template theory proposes that the specificity of the antibody is determined by the introduction of free antigen. Similarly, Lamarck believed that environment determines evolution. In contrast, the clonal theory proposes that the specific antibody-forming cells are present and selected because of their ability to react with specific antigen. Darwin proposed that evolution selected species with survival advantages.

Burnet assumes that antibody-forming cells contain within their genome the code for synthesizing one or two antibodies. Without stimulus, little of the information is expressed except for a few antibody molecules that appear at the cell surface. The antigen selects those cells, binds to the antibody, and by some still unknown mechanism (gene derepression?) stimulates the selected cell to produce more antibody and to proliferate.* The cells that are descendants of the cell selected by the antigen form the "clone."

Although the clonal selection theory was vulnerable at first, mainly because it was elaborated before anything was known about the mechanism determining specificity, it did take into account: (1) the fact that antibody elaboration can be recalled even years after exposure to the antigen and (2) the distinction of "self and no-self." Moreover, the clonal selection theory is compatible with the existence of autoimmune diseases. These important facets of the theory will be considered later. At this point we will consider the origin of the codon.

The main unanswered question is whether the theory is compatible with the molecular mechanism of antigen-antibody interaction or with the biosynthesis of specific antibodies. In principle, the theory is not in conflict with the notion of complementarity between antigen and antibody. Indeed, as for all other proteins, the specificity of the molecular structure of an immunoglobulin must be determined by its amino acid sequence. However, the population of immunoglobulins differs from that of other cell proteins in the almost infinite variability of the former.

The genome can store the multitude of cistrons needed to make each antibody by storing the information in the germ cell and through somatic mutation. The genes may all be stored in the germ cell and transferred (like all other genes) to all somatic cells. In most cells these genes are repressed forever, but the antigen can derepress the genes in one or a number of selected cells. Of course, the molecular mechanisms of repression and derepression are not known, and even if they were, it still would be necessary to explain how the antibody cells in the absence of antigen are partly derepressed and produce small amounts of antibodies to cover their surface and become completely derepressed in the presence of antigen. Neither is the stimulus to cell division known. Moreover, is the germ theory for antibody formation compatible with the amount of DNA present in the mammalian cell nucleus? Unfortunately we know too little of the active site of the antibody to be able to answer this question.

The second theory invokes the occurrence of somatic mutation to explain the multitude of antibodies. Unicellular organisms (*e.g.*, bacteria and yeast) mutate spontaneously or under environmental influences. The experimentalist can withdraw these cells from the environment and grow them in a favorable medium or modify the medium so that only the mutated cells can survive. The somatic mutation theory for antibody synthesis proposes that: (1) some cells, including antibody cells, in the mammalian body readily undergo somatic mutation; (2) some of the mutation results in the appearance of at least two cistrons capable of coding for antibody polypeptides; and (3) these cistrons are at least partially derepressed and become further activated in the contact of antigens. The theory is ingenious, but it extends far beyond actual knowledge of molecular biology, so the questions it raises remain unanswered. Is it statistically possible to have enough random mutation for a cell to produce at least two genes that can produce the appropriate antibody? Why is the mutation restricted to these cells, and if it is not, why do other mutated cells remain repressed? Why are the mutations in the antibody-producing cells restricted to a portion of the DNA? Indeed, antibody-producing cells look alike, divide alike, synthesize DNA, RNA, and many proteins in the same way, and produce energy in the same way. Could it be that the short life span of some lymphocytes results from lethal mutation and that only the mutation involving the antibody cistron is viable? But then why are lymphocytes, which at the outset contain a DNA identical in sequence and amount to that of the brain or liver cell, so much more susceptible to expressible mutations? Clearly, these questions will not be answered until we have a better understanding of gene expression in mammalian cells.

Investigators have invoked two mechanisms to explain the high incidence of mutation: point mutation and crossing over. Conclusive evidence for either of these mechanisms is not available.

At present, it is impossible to predict which theory will prevail. In fact, some investigators believe that the genetic mechanism for determining gene specificity is somewhere between these two extremes. The demonstration in several laboratories that some idiotypes (presumably including V genes) are hereditarily transmitted provides strong support for the germ line theory [65].

A third important question raised with respect to the biosynthesis of immunoglobulins is whether or not the same cell can synthesize different immunoglobulins, such as IgA and IgM. Convincing evidence indicates that cell clones can synthesize IgA and IgM, and that a delicate switching mechanism facilitates the passage from the synthesis of one type of immunoglobulin to that of another type [13]. It has been proposed that such switching is controlled by a mechanism in which repressors control the expression of the constant portion of one class of heavy chains (*e.g.*, $C\mu$)

* It is estimated that each cistron is copied into 20×10^3 messenger molecules, which bind to 200×10^3 ribosomes to yield 2×10^3 antibody molecules per minute.

while the expression of the gene coding for the constant segment of the other heavy chains (*e.g.*, $C\gamma$) is derepressed.

However, some investigators have observed that in some myeloma classes, both IgA and IgM are synthesized, but the amounts of IgA formed considerably exceed that of IgM formed. Yet, IgA and IgM messengers are made in similar amounts, which suggests that the control of the off and on switching from one type of immunoglobulin synthesis to another is definitely post-transcriptional.

In the face of these different interpretations, one should keep in mind that myelomas are malignant cells and that during transformation a change in gene expression may result in deviated forms of immunoglobulin assembly.

The synthesis of multiple immunoglobulins by the same cell is related to the differentiation of the immunological cell as indicated by the work of Lawton *et al.* [66]. As we shall see, one can distinguish two stages in immune cell differentiation. The first is clonal development, an event genetically programed and induced by the microenvironment (in the chicken B lymphocytes in the bursa), the second is triggered by the antigen and is typically referred to as the immune response.

In the chicken, clonal development starts with stem cell migration to the bursa. During differentiation in the bursa, IgM is synthesized and most of the IgM antibody is incorporated in the membrane. The IgM-producing cells divide and migrate to other lymphoid tissue, but at some point in the development of the immune system, a few daughter cells switch from IgM synthesis to IgG synthesis. In other words, they switch the pattern of differentiation in that they repress the gene responsible for IgM ($C\mu$) and derepress the gene responsible for IgG synthesis ($C\gamma$).

The cells committed to IgA synthesis are similarly believed to appear as a result of a switch in the expression of $C\gamma$ to $C\alpha$. This stepwise switching in gene expression ($C\mu \rightarrow C\gamma \rightarrow C\alpha$) results in the formation of clones committed to IgM, IgG, and IgA production. Studies of the sequential appearance of antibodies during embryogenesis suggest that a similar mechanism of differentiation may obtain in mammalian cells [67].

A fourth problem concerning the biosynthesis of immunoglobulins is that of the conversion of a monomer into a polymer, as is the case for IgM and IgA.

The molecular weight of IgM of man and other mammals is 900,000. The giant molecule is composed of five similar subunits, each with a molecular weight of 180,000. Each subunit is composed of two light and two heavy chains held together by disulfide bonds. When examined by negative staining techniques in an electron microscope, IgM molecules have a variable spiderlike appearance. A small Δ-chain binds the subunits by disulfide bonds. One mole of Δ-chain is bound to one mole of pentamer.

Two theories have been proposed to explain the role of the γ-chain: the "bracelet" and the "clasp" models. In the bracelet model, the j-chain forms a ring to which each monomer is attached by a disulfide bond. In the clasp model, the j-chain forms disulfide bonds with two monomers and the binding of the j-chain to two adjacent monomers primes the S-S binding between the other monomers. Chapuis and Koshland [68] have provided evidence in favor of the clasp model.

The j-chain (j=joining) was discovered in dimeric or polymeric immunoglobulins. The IgA secretory immunoglobulin is composed of a dimer of IgA, a γ-chain, and a secretory component. The γ-chains of IgA and IgM are identical in molecular weight, electrophoretic mobility, amino acid composition, and antigenic specificity.

The γ-chain is a small glucosamine containing acidic glycopeptides rich in glutamic, aspartic, and cysteine residues. Its molecular weight ranges between 15,000 and 20,000.

The $(IgA)_2$ SC complex is believed to be stabilized by weak but numerous linkages. If disulfide bonds are involved, they are likely to be readily reversible. An exact tridimensional model for $(IgA)_2$ SC is not available [69].

An interesting manifestation of gene expression in the case of immunoglobulins concerns that of the V and C regions of the heavy and light chains. Such expression could take place by at least two different mechanisms: in the first, each immunoglobulin chain is expressed by a single gene coding for both the variable V and the constant C regions. In such a case, a large portion of the DNA would be redundant for C. The second possibility is that even though each constitutes a single polypeptide, the heavy or light chain is coded for by two genes rather than one, one for the V and one for the C region. Available genetic evidence supports the second view [70–75].

The "two genes, one polypeptide" theory raises the question as to how the expression of the C and the V components of the immunoglobulin chain are linked. Are the two polypeptides joined when translation of each segment is completed? Does the joining involve two separate messenger RNA's linked and expressed in a single chain, or does the linkage occur at the level of the DNA? We know little of any of these mechanisms of expression, although linkage after translation seems to be excluded, and the assumption that the linkage occurs at the level of the DNA usually is preferred.

Studies of Williamson and coworkers showing that the whole H chain is encoded on a single nuclear mRNA support the view that the joining of the C and V genes occurs at the DNA level [75].

Thus, two structural genes specify the biosynthesis of a single immunoglobulin L or H chain, one for the C region and one for the V region. The specification of the known population of immunoglobulins requires three different families of genes: one for the $\varkappa$ light chain, one for the λ light chain, and one for various classes and subclasses of heavy chains. These families of genes are also referred to as complex loci.

In the loci, the genes for the C and V regions of a given chain are close together in the same chromosome. But although they are linked in their expression, they may not form contiguous sequences in the DNA. There are usually a large number of V genes and a smaller number of C genes, although no constant ratio between the two types of genes is observed. For example, the mouse $\varkappa$-chain is specified by one C gene and several V genes, whereas the heavy chains of mice, rabbits, and humans are specified by four or more C genes and a large number of V genes.

All somatic cells are diploid. Therefore, the chromosomes are paired, yet the plasmocyte makes only one type of immunoglobulin.

Autosomal allelic exclusion is in keeping with clonal specificity. If the cells could transcribe both paternal and maternal V chains, the principle of one antibody per cell would collapse because the V genes of both parents are likely to be different.

Therefore, in its immune response the plasmocyte must determine: (1) which parental chromosome will be activated, (2) which light chain will be made ($\varkappa$ or λ), (3) and, finally, which class and subclass of heavy chains will be made and what particular set of V genes will be activated. We know little of what determines the selection of genes expressed, but when these problems are clarified, we will undoubtedly learn a great deal about differentiation.

The Cellular Aspects of Immunity

Introduction

Since the days of Pasteur and Metchnikoff, students of the immune response have argued about whether it was primarily a humoral or a cellular event. Although the immunological properties were, in many cases, known to be transferable by serum administration (passive immunity), in other cases, such as the delayed hypersensitivity reaction elicited by tuberculin, the host's immunological state could not be transferred by serum, but it could by injection of intact lymphoid cells.

Because some types of immunity can be passively transferred by serum and other types by injecting cells of the immunized animal, one speaks of humoral and cellular immunity. In reality, the distinction is somewhat artificial because whether the antibodies are released in the serum or remain attached to cells, they are always made by cells; therefore, all immunity is of cellular origin. Yet, some types of immunological challenges lead to the release of the antibody in the serum, whereas others induce the appearance of cells that hold the antibody attached to their surface.

Scientists continue to argue about the level of difference that separates these two types of immunity. One position suggests that humoral and cellular immunity have evolved separately; the other proposes that they are closely related in their development, and that the major difference between the two types is that in one case the antibody is released from the cell surface and in the other it remains attached to it.

It is now established that the lymphoid system is responsible for both types of immunity. Consequently, before dealing with the pathological conditions of the immune system, we should briefly review the key properties of the lymphoid system and its cellular elements. To facilitate the reader's understanding of these complex cellular events, we shall first briefly summarize the status of our knowledge.

First, humoral antibodies are made by plasmocytes, which are derived from a special type of lymphocytes called B cells. Second, cell-mediated antibodies are elaborated by what is usually believed to be a different type of lymphocyte called T cells. Third, although B and T cells play principal roles in their special manifestations of the immunological response, the deployment of the response requires the cooperative action of various cells—B cells, T cells, and even macrophages.

The Lymphatic System

The role of the lymphatic system has eluded physicians ever since Hunter dissected and described it carefully. Only in recent decades was its participation in immunological reactions discovered [76–83].

The lymphatic system collects lymph from all organs in lymph capillaries. For example, the fluids formed in the intestinal lumen are picked up by a fine network of lymphatic capillaries that converge into larger and larger channels, which follow the path of the blood vessels. The lymphatic vessels end by branching out in a lymph node.

Lymph nodes are found throughout the body except the central nervous system. However, they tend to conglomerate in special anatomical regions—for example, the vertebral, axillary, inguinal, and mesenteric regions.

Lymphatic vessels emerge from the node and are collected into larger trunks that finally join to form the bronchomediastinal and thoracic trunks. The thoracic trunk opens in the venous system at the junction of the subclavian and jugular veins. The lymphatic capillaries are lined by a unicellular endothelium with little basement membrane. Although their walls are thinner than those of veins, the lymphatic vessels resemble veins and are composed of three layers. The lymphatic drainage of the intestinal tract is of particular significance because there the fat absorbed by the intestinal mucosa is converted to chylomicrons. After passing through numerous nodes, the chyle enters a lymphatic network around the aorta that ultimately collects in a large lymphatic sac, the cisterna chyli, which is the origin of the thoracic duct.

Lymph nodes are bean-shaped organs of variable sizes. The concave aspect of the organ forms the hilum, which is the point of entry of arteries, veins, and afferent lymphatics. The efferent lymphatics enter the convex portion of the organ. On histological section, cortical and medullar regions can be distinguished. The cortical region contains germinal centers composed of a peripheral crown of small lymphocytes and a central core of larger primitive blast cells. The medulla contains chords of small lymphocytes separated by a dense network of lymphatic sinusoids, lined by reticuloendothelial cells. Thus, the lymph derived from the gastrointestinal tract or from any other portion of the body emerges at the convex portion of the lymph node, circulates through the sinusoids, and is transferred to the afferent vessels, which bring it to the thoracic duct where it ultimately enters the general circulation.

In addition to the lymph nodes, lymphatic tissue is found in a number of other organs: underneath the epithelia of the mouth, the pharynx, and various portions of the intestinal tract, and in the thymus and spleen. In the pharynx, the lymphoid tissue forms a ring at the base of the tongue called the Waldeyer tonsillar ring. In the gastrointestinal tract, it forms the Peyer patches and the appendix. Afferent and efferent lymphatic vessels are indistinguishable in all these structures, and there is no capsule and no separation between cortex and medulla. Thus, these lymphatic structures resemble a collection of lymphocytes with or without active germinal centers.

Lymphocytes—Properties and Relationship to Lymphatic Organs

The morphological characteristics of the lymphocytes are described in the chapter on inflammation. At least two classes of lymphocytes can be distinguished with respect to life span: long- and short-lived lymphocytes. Some long-lived lymphocytes are believed to survive without cell division for as long as 10 years.

Lymphocytes in the lymphoid organs are not stationary; they travel back and forth from the lymphatic to the vascular system. Such movement involves passage from lymph to blood and from blood to lymph. Except for the spleen, no organ permits direct passage of lymphocytes from lymph to blood. Transfer from lymph to blood occurs in the neck where the thoracic duct opens into the jugular vein. From there the lymph follows the path of the venous blood: right side of the heart, lung, left side of the heart, and general circulation.

Lymphocytes are returned to the lymph nodes and the lymphatic channel in a specific anatomical structure of the node, the so-called postcapillary venule, which has a special endothelium. The endothelial cells are so large that in transversal section the venule resembles a glandular acinus. The lymphocyte attaches to the membrane of the endothelial cell, is engulfed in an invagination of the membrane, passes through the cytoplasm of these cells, and reemerges at the opposite surface of the endothelial cell. (One cannot escape being impressed by the molecular gymnastics involved and also by the potential consequences for both the visiting and host cells.)

Most of the recirculating lymphocytes are T cells (80%?), although B lymphocytes have also been shown to recirculate. Moreover, the migration is not random—both T and B cells migrate to their respective anatomical compartments (see below).

Although it is easy to understand why a lymphocyte destined to produce an antibody might need to move to the site of the antigen, the significance of the incessant and massive traffic of lymphocytes continues to elude us.

The lymphocyte that has been programmed in the thymus migrates and makes its home in other specific compartments of the lymphoid tissue called thymus-dependent areas. When a newborn rat is thymectomized, portions of the lymphoid compartment remain depleted, whereas others have their expected population of lymphocytes. The depleted areas are believed to be the thymus dependent, and the populated areas the thymus independent or B-type areas (see Table 14-3).

Table 14-3. Characteristics of immunocompetent lymphocytes

Characteristic	T Lymphocytes	B Lymphocytes
Origin	Bone marrow	Bone marrow
Life span	Months–years	Probably days–weeks
Recirculating pool	Majority (60%)	Minority
Major localization:		
Lymph node	Deep cortical, perifollicular	Subcapsular, medullary, germinal centers
In spleen	Periarteriolar	Peripheral white and red pulp
In Peyer's patch	Perifollicular	Central follicle

Although both B and T cells may circulate, in rodents the majority of recirculating lymphocytes are T cells. Of the lymphocytes in the thoracic duct, 80 to 90% carry the θ antigen, and prolonged thoracic duct drainage depletes those areas of the lymphoid system (lymph node, spleen, and Peyer's patches) where T cells are preferentially lodged. A number of other observations further suggest that an animal does not need to be sensitized for T cells for them to recirculate; indeed, most T cells were found to recirculate in the nonsensitized animal. The T cells' ability to circulate makes them uniquely suited for patrolling tissue and body cavities for foreign intruders, and maybe for cancer cells.

Immunization causes a nonspecific trapping of the lymphocyte in the spleen after intravenous injection and in the draining lymph nodes after subcutaneous and peritoneal injection. The trapped cells are placed in the presence of the antigen and are sensitized; then they proliferate and elaborate the appropriate antibodies. One or two days after conversion, they reappear in the circulation.

It is not known how many B cells circulate, and it is generally believed that most B cells do not recirculate. Yet appreciable numbers of B cells are found in the thoracic duct and it is therefore likely that B cells also recirculate, but in a proportion much lower and at a rate much slower than T cells.

Antigenic stimulation may also induce the migration of lymphoblasts; thus, both B-cell and T-cell blasts appear in the thoracic duct. These blasts do not appear to recirculate, but they migrate to portions of the lymphoid system where T or B cells are preferentially located.

The continuous injection of [^{3}H]thymidine has permitted investigators to measure the life span of lymphocytes by counting the number of unlabeled cells. Estimates of the proportion of labeled cells are unreliable because of isotope reutilization.

After constant infusion of [^{3}H]thymidine, the uptake of the isotope rises sharply, reaches a peak after approximately ten days of infusion, and then drops sharply. Eight per cent of the small lymphocytes remain unlabeled even after 300 days. Cellular life span is defined as the interval between two mitotic divisions, or the time elapsing between the completion of the last division and cellular death. The period of rapid isotope uptake shows that the life span of some cells is short, varying from 5 to 20 days. But those lymphocytes that remain unlabeled for 300 days must be long lived and must have divided before isotope infusion.

At first it was believed that only T cells were long lived because the proportion of long-lived lymphocytes in thymectomized newborn mice decreased sharply. Further evidence showed that B cells can also be long lived. For example, in the nude mice that were deprived of T cells, 70% of the thoracic duct cells were long lived. Thus, both T and B cells contain both short- and long-lived subclasses. The exact delineation of the life span spectrum of B and T cells is not known, but it would appear that more T than B cells tend to live long.

Peripheral lymphocytes can be stimulated to proliferate with unspecific agents, with a specific antibody, or by allogenic lymphocytes. The unspecific agents include plants (phytohemagglutinin, concanavalin A, lentils, wax beans, pockweeds), bacterial liposaccharides (lipid A), staphylococcal enterotoxin B, streptolysin S, and aggregated tuberculin products (PPD). A number of miscellaneous compounds can also stimulate lymphocyte proliferation; these include mitogen, periodate, heavy metals (zinc, mercury, nickel), and proteolytic enzymes such as papain or pronase.

Antibodies specifically stimulate sensitized lymphocytes to proliferate.

When allogenic lymphocytes from genetically unrelated animals are mixed in culture, both types of lymphocytes are stimulated to grow. This process is called the mixed lymphocyte response.

The known molecular events that follow the mitogenic stimulus are described in the chapter on regeneration (Chapter 13). We will briefly review these steps here. It is usually assumed that the mitogen binds to the cell membrane. Clearly, the first interaction of the mitogen with the cell membrane mimicks that of hormones. In fact, insoluble phytohemagglutinin can stimulate mitosis in the lymphocytes, which indicates that entry into the cell is not indispensable. Because of the similarities between mitogens and hormones, it was suspected that a second messenger—namely, cyclic AMP—might be involved.

Although Parker [84] showed that cyclic AMP inhibits phytohemagglutinin-stimulated mitosis and that phytohemagglutinin stimulates adenyl cyclase in lymphocytes, conclusive evidence that cyclic AMP acts as a second messenger in the mitogenic effect is not available [85]. However, one of the earliest changes after mitogenic stimulation (60 seconds after stimulation) is a rise in cyclic AMP. This is followed by a number of membrane changes that include increases in phospholipid synthesis, amino acid uptake, sodium-potassium exchange, and respiration-dependent phagocytosis.

The membrane alterations are followed by or coupled with a number of macromolecular changes. Within 2 hours after stimulation, histone acetylation and nuclear protein phosphorylation increase. The template capacity of DNA for RNA synthesis increases. *In vivo*, an increase in nuclear RNA synthesis can be detected within 30 minutes. An increase in protein synthesis is observed within 4 hours, and DNA is synthesized approximately 24 hours after stimulation.

Finally, microtubules are assembled to form a spindle and the cell divides. Morphologically, during proliferation the chromatin becomes less dense, the cell enlarges, and its cytoplasm becomes more basophilic. Mitoses are apparent although they do not occur in synchrony.

Clearly, we know too little of the sequence of events that trigger lymphocyte mitosis to describe the molecular events. Yet the system provides a unique model for studying cellular proliferation and differentiation. Moreover, stimulation of lymphocyte proliferation may be helpful in stimulating the immune response.

T Cells

Functionally, the lymphatic system consists of three segments: the bone marrow, the central lymphoid organs (thymus, tonsils, Peyer's patches, and appendix), and the peripheral systems (spleen and lymph nodes).

In the adult, all lymphocytes—whether they are immunocompetent or not—originate in the bone marrow. The central lymphoid organs program the lymphocytes for immunocompetence, the thymus for the development of cellular immunity, and the lymphoid tissue associated with the intestinal epithelium for the production of humoral antibody. One distinguishes two types of immunocompetent cells: thymus-dependent (called T lymphocytes or TL cells), and immunoglobulin-producing cells (called plasmocytes or

BL cells because of the role of the bursa in birds; see below).

It is impossible to describe here all the experiments that led to an appreciation of the contribution of the thymus to the development of immunological competence. Some critical observations were made in the chick, which has two major lymphoid organs—the bursa of Fabricius and the thymus. The bursa is a small pouch (found only in birds) attached to the intestine near the cloaca and is named after its discoverer, Fabricius Aquapendente. Excision of the bursa interferes with humoral immunity; in contrast, removal of the thymus interferes with the development of cell-mediated immunity.

The role of the thymus in mammals is not completely known, but in rodents neonatal excision of the thymus interferes with graft rejection and cell-mediated immunity. When it has reached its maximum size, the thymus is a bilobular, triangular organ located in the anterior portion of the upper mediastinum just below the rib cage with its summit directed toward the neck. It is the first lymphoid organ to appear in embryonic life. The thymus originates from bilateral downgrowth of the third bronchial pouches. Obviously, in the fetus it develops in an antigen-free environment. Unlike lymph nodes, the thymus is not involved in handling lymph and does not contain the rich network of lymphatic sinusoids found in the peripheral lymph nodes.

At birth, the ratio of the weight (approximately 10–15 g) of the thymus to that of the body is maximal. The organ grows slowly to reach maximum size at age nine (35–40 g). After that period, the thymus involutes progressively, ultimately assuming a fibroadipose appearance in the adult. Histologically, the unit component of the thymus (of the growing child) is a small, pyramidal-shaped lobule approximately 2 mm in diameter. Two zones can be distinguished in each lobule, the cortex and the medulla. At low power examination, the cortex can be distinguished from the medulla by its darker staining properties, which are due to a dense cellular population. The summit of the pyramidal lobule is directed inward; the base is in contact with a thick, collagenous capsule that projects deep infolds toward the center separating the individual lobules.

Examination at high power reveals that the cortex is made of thickly packed lymphocytes. The medulla is made of lymphocytes entrapped in a reticular system composed of larger chords resting on a basement membrane, made of some eosinophilic cells resembling epithelial cells. These chords are in continuity and form a reticulum that ramifies deeply into the cortex. These cells are believed to secrete a humoral factor that conditions the lymphocytes.

The thymus programs cells derived from the bone marrow to perform cell-mediated immunity, including delayed hypersensitivity, graft rejection, graft-versus-host reaction, and immunosurveillance against foreign organisms and possibly cancer cells. This role of the thymus has been established in a number of species by various methods—prenatal thymus excision, thymus transplant, and others. That the thymus plays a similar role in humans can be concluded from the pattern of symptoms that develop in patients with thymic agenesis.

Three stages can be distinguished in the differentiation of T cells: migration of a multipotential cell to the thymic microenvironment, differentiation of the multipotential cell into a T cell, and T-cell migration to the peripheral tissue.

In the 10–12-day mouse embryo, large basophilic stem cells move from the yolk sac or the embryonic liver into the thymus. Whether these are multipotential or committed cells is not known. In the thymus, the primitive cell is converted into a thymocyte.

When a 14-day-old mouse embryo thymus rudiment is placed in culture, it lives for several days. When it is excised, the thymus rudiment contains only a few stem cells. At the end of 4 days, it is loaded with small lymphocytes most of which carry the θ antigen. Thus, during these 4 days multipotential stem cells differentiate recognizably by morphological changes and acquisition of a surface antigen; in addition, these cells become more sensitive to steroids and X-irradiation. However, the thymus lymphocyte population is not entirely homogeneous. A small fraction has little or no θ antigens and is relatively insensitive to steroids.

Most, if not all, the thymocytes are only transient residents in the thymus. They migrate to peripheral tissues and settle in the areas of the lymphoid organs already described.

When 14-day-old thymic rudiments of CBA mice are transplanted under the renal capsule of thymectomized, X-irradiated AKR mice, thymocytes carrying the donor's θ antigen are found in the peripheral tissue approximately 16 days later, indicating that the thymocytes have migrated from the CBA donor to the recipient's peripheral tissue. Sometimes during the preparation for migration, or during the migration, the T cells differentiate further in that they acquire H_2 antigen.

The stem cells that migrate to the thymus are not self-sustaining. By following chromosome markers in parabiotic animals and in thymic grafts, investigators established that stem cells derived from the bone marrow enter the thymus in postnatal life.

The mechanisms inducing stem cell differentiation into thymic cells are not known. The epithelial cells of the thymus are believed to be involved. Two views prevail: one proposes that direct contact between epithelial cells and stem cells induces the differentiation into thymocytes; the other assumes that the differentiation is induced by a thymic hormone probably secreted by the epithelial cells.

Several thymic extracts have been prepared and tested for their ability to restore T-cell function in T-cell-deprived animals. Hopper and associates [86] have prepared a purified protein, thymosin, made of 108 amino acids (mostly aspartic and glutamic acids) that induces T-lymphocyte maturation.

Thymosin has been shown to correct abnormal DNA synthetic response in NZB mouse thymocytes.

Table 14-4. Physical, chemical and biological properties of some thymus products

Product	Chemical class	Molecular weight	Properties	Activity
Thymosin	Protein	12,000	Heat stable; no lipid, CHO, or polynucleotide	Lymphocytopoiesis; restoration of immunological competence *in vivo* and *in vitro*; enhancement of expression of T-cell characteristics and functions *in vitro* and *in vivo*
Thymopoietin I	Protein	7,000	Heat stable; N-terminus: glycine; C-terminus: lysine	Impairment of neuromuscular transmission *in vivo*; induction of expression of T-cell antigens *in vitro*
Thymopoietin II	Protein	7,000	Same as thymopoietin I	Same as thymopoietin I
Thymic humoral factor (THF)	Polypeptide	< 5,000 > 700	Heat stable	Restoration of immunological competence *in vivo* and *in vitro*; acceleration of generation of specifically committed lymphocytes; prevention of sensitization against self-antigens
Serum thymic activity	Polypeptide	~ 1,000	Heat labile; pH_1 7.5	Induction of expression of T cell antigens *in vitro*, θ-positive cells in nude mice *in vivo*; retardation of growth of Maloney virus-induced tumors *in vivo*
Lymphocyte-stimulating hormone (LSH_h)	Protein	~ 17,000	Heat labile	Relative lymphocytosis; augmented antibody synthesis in newborn mice
Lymphocyte-stimulating hormone (LSH_r)	Protein	~ 80,000	Heat stable	Leukocytosis; lymphocytosis; augmented antibody synthesis in newborn mice
Homeostatic thymus hormone (HTH)	Glycopeptide	1,800–2,500	Heat labile	Antagonizes thyroxine and adrenocorticotropin and thyrotropin in normal resting condition of their target glands; antagonizes gonadotropins; delays puberty; synergistic to growth hormone (lymphocytosis); chemotactic influence on lymphocytes
Thymic hypocalcemic factor (T_1)	Protein	68,000 (100,000)	$pH_1 = 5.65$, 24% CHO	Hypocalcemia
Thymic hypocalcemic factor (T_2)	Protein	57,000 (170,000)	$pH_1 = 5.40$	Hypocalcemia; relative lymphocytosis

These mice progressively lose their T cells during their life span and present a complex symptomatology that resembles lupus erythematosus, Waldenström's macroglobulinemia, and Sjögren's syndrome [87–90]. The extract also induces an increase in the formation of T-cell rosettes when incubated *in vitro* with sheep erythrocytes and lymphocytes obtained from patients with primary immunodeficiency disease [91].

Two thymic polypeptides, thymopoietin I and thymopoietin II, each with a molecular weight of 7000 daltons, have been isolated. The hormones were isolated by following one of their side effects on neuromuscular transmission.

This secondary effect was detected by observing patients with myasthenia gravis who have a typical defect in neuromuscular transmission. Studies of experimental autoimmune thymitis showed that the block in neuromuscular transmission resulted from the presence of thymopoietin. Electrophoretically homogeneous thymopoietin exerts its neuromuscular and maturation effects on prothymocytes. The polypeptide has no effect on B cells. Hematopoietic cells incubated with thymopoietin *in vitro* result in the formation of cells expressing thymus antigen on the cell surface [92–96].

A number of other compounds—such as cyclic AMP, various tissue extracts, polyadenylic and polyuridylic acids, and endotoxin—stimulate prothymocyte maturation. But unlike thymopoietin, they also induce differentiation of B cells, which acquire C3 receptors.

A number of other factors have been extracted from the thymus. Their known properties and their functions are presented in Table 14-4, which was taken from White's paper [96]. For further information on the role of thymus factors in immunity, see Friedman's article [97].

B Lymphocytes

In birds, the surgical or hormonal elimination of the bursa of Fabricius results in a drop in circulating antibodies, but cellular mediated immunity persists. Consequently, a skin allograft transplanted to such a bird will be rejected. It is not known with certainty which lymphoid organ in higher mammals and humans is the equivalent of the bursa.

Like birds, mammals have two types of immunological defenses: serological and cell mediated. Both functions are performed by lymphocytes with relatively long life spans probably elaborated in the bone marrow. The virgin lymphocytes that will be responsible for serological immunity are programmed in birds in the bursa Fabricius and in the lymphoid structures underneath the nasopharyngeal mucosa. The equivalent of the bursa in mammals has not been identified with certainty. Various gastrointestinal lymphoid tissues are suspected—namely, the appendix and the Peyer patches. Studies of spontaneous and induced immunological deficiencies suggest that the TL and BL lymphocytes are in immunocompetent individuals found in different portions of the lymphoid organ, and, as already pointed out, the two types of lymphocytes are further distinguished by their ability to recirculate. Unfortunately, these two types of cells cannot be distinguished morphologically.

There is little doubt that B lymphocytes are the precursors of the antibody-forming cells, the plasmocytes. In a typical experiment, rats were irradiated with doses that deplete the lymphocytic population. They were then injected with an antigenically marked lymphocyte preparation and immunologically challenged. Plasmocytes that produced the antibody carried the markers, thus excluding the possibility that the antibody is produced by radioresistant cells. The circulating antibodies are produced by lymphocytes that later mature into plasmocytes. The use of horseradish peroxidase as an antigen has permitted investigators to identify the cells that produce the antibody and also to locate, with the aid of the electron microscope, their site of synthesis within the cells. In the lymphocyte the antibody synthesis is perinuclear, but as the lymphocytes mature into plasmocytes, most of the antibody is formed inside the membrane of the endoplasmic reticulum. The plasmocyte is not the last representative of its lineage; it can divide, but it continues to elaborate antibodies even during division.

Although the population of lymphocytes is large, few lymphocytes respond by producing antibody to the antigen. This has been demonstrated by selectively eliminating the antibody-producing cells with an antigen so heavily loaded with a radioactive precursor that it kills all cells it specifically binds to. Under those circumstances the lymphocyte population changes little, and all antibodies are formed except those that are produced by the group of cells that have been destroyed.

Although B lymphocytes can sometimes perform alone, in some pneumonia infections they most often need the cooperation of T cells to produce specific antibodies. The significance and the mode of interaction between B and T cells are not clear, but T cells are not precursors of B lymphocytes. There are two major theories about the cooperation between B and T cells. The first assumes that the T-cell response is highly specific and relates to the nature of the antigen. The second proposes that the T-cell response is an unspecific mobilization of the T cell, which responds simply because a group of B cells has been challenged. The matter is far from settled, and evidence for both unspecific and specific B- and T-cell cooperation has been assembled.

Lymph Nodes and Antibody Formation

Two kinds of cells can be distinguished in the lymph nodes with respect of their immunological roles: (1) macrophages, which are capable of phagocytosis and antigen trapping but are not likely to produce antibodies, and (2) antibody-forming cells—reticulum cells, plasmocytes, and lymphocytes. The principal cell types in the lymph nodes can also be classified according to their respective mobilities. The reticuloendothelial cells are fixed, whereas macrophages, lymphocytes, and plasmocytes can migrate from lymph node to blood and *vice versa*.

After a single dose of antigen is administered, the antigen is soon trapped in medullar macrophages of the draining node. Unless the dose of antigen is large or the antigen is exceptionally soluble, the defense mechanism occurs primarily at the site of the draining node and it will suffice to describe the events at that site. As pointed out, macrophages do not produce antibodies, yet they are not passive cells. On the contrary, they are believed to contribute to antibody formation in at least three ways. In some cases they modify the antigen so that it becomes more effective in eliciting antibody production. In other cases, it produces adjuvants. It may also secrete factors that stimulate the proliferation of antibody-producing cells. The molecular composition of these factors is not known with certainty, but it is believed that, at least in some cases, the proliferating factor is a complex between RNA and antigen fragments.

Sometimes after the antigen is introduced and trapped in the draining node, immature cells—hemangioblasts of the germinal center—start to proliferate. These hemangioblasts are precursors of plasmocytes and lymphocytes. It is not clear where these cells come from, but some possibilities are lymphocytes, endothelial cells of capillaries, and reticulum cells.

Plasmoblasts and preplasmocytes appear to be among the most effective antibody-producing cells. Mature plasmocytes continue to secrete antibodies even though they cannot divide.

Antigen Recognition by B and T Lymphocyte Receptors

The search for receptors on the surface of B and T cells was based on the following assumption: the recognition of the antigen by B or T cells must be specific; since immunoglobulin molecules specifically recognize antigens, the surface receptors for antigens are themselves believed to be immunoglobulin [98, 99].

Two types of techniques were used to detect such receptors: direct attempts to isolate the receptors and binding of anti-immunoglobulins. The binding can be followed by using immunofluorescent or ^{135}I-labeled antibodies, antibodies tagged with peroxidase or ferritin, or by following the effects of the antibody on various cellular functions. Of particular interest is the interference of antibody with antigen binding *in vitro*. The details of these techniques cannot be reviewed here, but all of them have serious limitations that have made the identification of surface receptors on B and T cells difficult.

The evidence for detectable cell surface antibodies is compelling only for B cells. The first receptor discovered was a firmly bound IgM molecule. Later, IgG receptors were also demonstrated to exist on B cells. The receptors are believed to be complete immunoglobulin molecules because both $\varkappa$ and λ chains and all heavy-chain determinants are expressed on the B cell surface. B cells are believed to contain as many as 10^4 to 10^6 receptor molecules.

Again, antibody biosynthesis is genetically controlled. Such control leads to the following findings: (1) only one antibody is made per cell, and each antibody-synthesizing cell makes only one light chain ($\varkappa$ or λ); (2) phenotypic expression excludes one of the parental alleles in the genotype; (3) a switch from the biosynthesis of IgM to IgG takes place during cell differentiation. At the present, none of these basic assumptions has been challenged by the study of B-cell receptors. For example, it has been shown that chicken B cells in the bursa contain only IgM. Moreover, immunosuppression by anti-μ antibodies blocks the appearance of IgG and IgA, suggesting that the μ-chain bears IgG precursors. Although the site of maturation of B cells has not been established in mammals, when B cells mature, many of the mouse spleen cells carrying IgG receptors have μ-chains on their surface.

The B-cell receptors are not uniformly distributed on the cell surface, but they are concentrated in so-called hot spots or caps. The life span of the receptor is relatively short, no more than 3 to 10 hours. However, the turnover of the receptor protein does not differ significantly from that of other membrane proteins.

B-cell receptors, immunoglobulin, and their bound antigens are shed from the cells if the helper cells are not present. Thus, the T cell and the macrophage function together to help the B cells produce the antibody. This helping effect is believed to function through chemical mediators, or "helper cells replacing substance."

The addition of such substances to the sensitized B cell prevents the shedding of the surface-bound antigen, and after several days of culture, the antibody-producing cells proliferate. A hypothetical mechanism for B cell activation proposes that the antigens in some way activate T cells, which in turn either directly activate C3 or stimulate B cells to produce activated C3. Activated C3 then attaches to the C3 receptors of B cells. It is believed that the binding of C3 to the B-cell receptors changes the characteristics of the B-cell membrane in such a fashion that the complex "antigen and surface receptors" are engulfed within the cell through endocytosis, thus preventing the shedding of the antigen-receptor complex.

Although most B cells respond positively to antisera with broad specificity, there is evidence that some B cells are deprived of receptors or, in other words, are IgG negative. Such cells are referred to as "null cells."

T cells also are believed to contain surface hemoglobins; however, conclusive evidence of their existence is not available.

The reason why surface immunoglobulins cannot be detected in T cells remains unknown. Different explanations have been proposed: The receptors are few, they belong to a unique class undetectable by available methods, they are buried in the membrane, or they are rapidly shed from the membrane surface.

In conclusion, available evidence indicates that antigen recognition depends on the presence of specific receptors in B and T cells. The receptors are believed to be immunoglobulins. Although there is convincing evidence that IgM and IgG receptors exist on the surface of B cells, the evidence for the existence of receptors on T cells is inconclusive. The B- or T-cell clone that carries the proper receptor recognizes and combines with the antigen. The formation of the antigen-antibody complex triggers proliferation of the clonal cells and their participation in the immune reaction.

Changes in the pattern of surface receptors in malignant lymphocytes have been observed. Thus, leukemic lymphocytes have been found to lack surface immunoglobulin receptors or $C3_b$ receptors. Such findings are not surprising in view of the general distortion in gene expression usually observed in malignancy. However, the observation may be relevant to the immunological deficiences that are observed in patients with leukemia. Whether lymphocytes of patients with nonlymphoid malignancies also have defective receptors is not known. It is important to investigate such a possibility because cancer cell surveillance depends upon lymphocyte immunity; the existence of receptor-deficient lymphocytes could be highly significant.

T-cell receptors have been much harder to identify. Nevertheless, T cells possess a receptor for sheep erythrocytes that helps in their identification. But because the receptor is inactive at 37° C, it is doubtful that it functions at all *in vivo*.

B and T Cells in Human Peripheral Blood and in Human Diseases

We have seen that B lymphocytes can be identified because they contain surface immunoglobulins. Moreover, they contain receptors for aggregated immunoglobulins, the antigen-antibody complexes, antigen, and the third component of complement.

In contrast, T cells contain only small amounts of surface immunoglobulin. In mice, a specific antigen for T cells (the θ antigen) permits their identification. No such antigen has been found in human T cells. However, it has been possible to prepare antisera against fetal thymocytes and to demonstrate that human T cells bind in a rosette formation to uncoated sheep erythrocytes. This method is usually used to identify T cells in humans. Once the rosettes are formed, it is easy to separate T cells from B cells by differential centrifugation. Therefore, it has been possible to establish that 80% of the lymphocytes in the peripheral blood are T cells and 20% are B cells.

With these methods it has also been possible to identify the type of cells involved in some human diseases (see Table 14-5) [100–108].

Table 14-5. Some B- and T-cell diseases

B-cell diseases
Waldenström's macroglobulinemia
Monoclonal B-cell proliferation with normal maturation
Chronic lymphocytic leukemia
Monoclonal B-cell proliferation usually with interference with maturation; occasionally biclonal B-cell proliferation
Well-differentiated lymphoblastic leukemia
Some poorly differentiated lymphomas mixed with lymphocytic histiocytic lymphoma
T-cell diseases
Chronic lymphocytic leukemia (rare)
Sézary's syndrome
Infectious mononucleosis
Some lymphoblastic leukemias
Some poorly differentiated lymphomas (convoluted cell types)

Macrophages and the Immune Response

Although lymphocytes are ultimately responsible for neutralizing the antigen, in some cases neutralization requires the participation of macrophages. In such cases the lymphocyte is believed to attract the macrophage and immobilize it. The factors involved in these reactions will be discussed later.

In some cases the histological site of an immune response reveals proliferation of fixed or free macrophages. The macrophages' role in the immune response is not clear; a number of different theories have been proposed [109]:

1. Macrophages pick up the antigen and then reduce the local concentration and prevent lymphocytes from being overwhelmed. This is sometimes referred to as the sink theory.
2. Macrophages store the antigen and release it when appropriate for stimulation of more lymphocytes.
3. Macrophages process the antigen so that it becomes accessible to the lymphocyte receptors. (When sheep erythrocytes are administered, they are not antigenic until they have been phagocytized by macrophages, but if sonicated sheep erythrocytes are administered, they are antigenic.)
4. Macrophages phagocytize the antigen and elaborate an "informational" RNA, which is then transferred to the lymphocyte. Although the latter view is far from established and often criticized on technical grounds, it has generated so much interest and new work that it deserves some brief consideration.

There can be no doubt that the elaboration of the antibody molecule must be preceded by the synthesis of RNA molecules. Such RNA molecules must certainly include messenger, but possibly ribosomal, transfer RNA, and maybe even an RNA of a kind unknown. Already in 1949, Harris and Harris [110] demonstrated that antibody-forming cells avidly pick up basophilic stains. However, the RNA produced in the macromolecular sequence unexpectedly leads to antibody formation and can, after extraction, serve to transfer the new immunological state to other cells. Even more surprising is that the macrophage elaborates such RNA.

The original experiments were done by Fishman and Adler [111]. Rabbit macrophages incubated *in vitro* were infected with T2 phage. RNA was extracted with phenol. When the extracted RNA was incubated with a culture of normal lymphoid cells, it induced them to produce antibodies against the T2 phage. T2 phage is not antigenic when incubated with the lymphoid cells; therefore, the "immunogenic information" resisted treatment with proteases but was destroyed by ribonuclease.

Only a small portion of the macrophage population is believed to be able to synthesize such informational RNA [112]. The immunological response can be suppressed by adding highly specific antimacrophage globulins to the culture. Similar informational RNA has been extracted from mouse spleen and from livers of rabbits appropriately challenged [113].

If we can, in spite of all the technical difficulties involved and the great possibility of error, assume that the macrophage or any other cell elaborates an RNA which, when transferred to other cells, gives instruction for the biosynthesis of the appropriate antibody, a number of consequences must necessarily follow. First, the macrophage must specifically recognize the antigen if the information it imparts is to be specific; therefore, its membrane should carry specific receptors. Second, if the informational RNA is to be transferred from cell to cell, it must in some way be replicated and its information possibly incorporated into the genome.

Japanese investigators [114] have made some interesting observations in that area. They demonstrated that the biosynthesis of immunogenic RNA in mouse spleen is not affected by actinomycin and therefore does not involve traditional transcription. In the spleen extract, they further identified a replicase that copies informational but not other RNA and a reverse transcriptase that transcribes informational RNA but not other RNA's.

Informational RNA is believed to exert a highly specific stimulatory effect on antibody synthesis. Even if such a specific effect becomes unquestionably established, it must be kept in mind that polynucleotides—including RNA—when administered to cells immunologically challenged, seem to be able to amplify the immunological response, and such amplification is believed to involve cyclic AMP [115–118].

In conclusion, when an animal is challenged with an antigen that will ultimately lead to the appearance of humoral antibodies, the antigen surely binds to specific receptors on the B cell and may or may not bind to specific receptors of the T cell and macrophages. The role of the T cell is unknown. The macrophage has been suspected to elaborate on informational RNA. The specific antibodies are synthesized by small groups of B lymphocytes. However, to reach its optimum, such synthesis requires additional unspecific stimuli that seem to involve the elaboration of cyclic AMP.

The role of the macrophage in the immune response may be related to the close morphological interaction between lymphocytes and macrophages seen on sections. In the germinal centers, the macrophages emit dendritic expansions that interdigitate between the lymphocytes, and antigen uptake by dendrites has been reported.

T- and B-Cell Interactions

The preceding discussion suggests that one of the premises at the basis of our understanding of the immune response is that immune reactions are divided between T and B cells. Although fundamentally true, the concept is an oversimplification because B and T cells interact in many ways. Such interactions vary with the circumstances and often the mechanism regulating them are unknown. The cellular interactions are of three types: T cells enchance the B-cell immunological response, antibody production affects either T- or B-cell response, and T cells inhibit B-cell response.

When normal mice are injected with sheep red blood cells, the B cells of the injected animals secrete antibodies to the red blood cells. Mitchison [119] has shown that the antibody secretion is abolished in thymectomized mice, but it can be restored by injecting T cells.

When mouse spleen cells sensitized with the haptene 4-hydroxy-3-iodo-5-nitrophenyl acetic acid (NIP) combined with chicken γ-globulin are injected in irradiated mice and the mice are challenged later with NIP bound to human serum albumin, the immune response is not stimulated (this phenomenon is referred to as the carrier effect). Yet, if cells primed with the NIP human serum albumin are given at the same time as the cells primed with the NIP γ-globulin, an immune response takes place. Antibodies to NIP serum albumin are ineffective in triggering the immune response. It was further established that the NIP antibodies were made by the cells carrying the NIP γ-globulin antigen (B cells), whereas the NIP serum albumin cells were not making antibody and were T cells. This experiment led to the conclusion that the immunological response in the B cell requires a "helper cell," namely the T cell.

It is not known how T cells help B cells make antibody. A number of assumptions have been made: (1) cooperation requires recognition of the antigen by both types of cells; (2) cooperation involves transfer of genetic information from T to B cells; (3) the immunogenic effect involves antigenic bridging between T and B cells.

Although the last option is often preferred, it is not known whether the bridging involves T and B cells themselves or the release of a T-cell receptor that binds to the B cell. Moreover, the signal the bridging gives to the B cell is unknown.

The allogenic effect discovered by Katz and Benacerraf [120] would seem to militate against the notion that antigenic recognition is indispensable for T- and B-cell cooperation. These investigators showed that a properly timed graft-versus-host response in guinea pigs enhances the secondary response of B cells to a haptene even if the carrier differs from that used in the first haptene exposure. Moreover, when DNA is conjugated to D-glutamic, D-lysine copolymers, it elicits a B-cell response only in the presence of a graft-versus-host reaction. Without a graft-versus-host response, the haptene-loaded copolymer leads to haptene tolerance. Thus, the graft-versus-host response, which is mediated by T cells, influences the B cell, and a signal for tolerance to the haptene is switched to a signal for immunological response. Since the haptene carrier effect is eliminated in these experiments, it is unlikely that this form of cooperation between T and B cells is determined by antigen presentation, and it has been proposed that it may involve membrane-to-membrane interaction.

The immune response of B cells to a number of antigens—for example, the type III pneumococcal polysaccharides or polyvinylpyrrolidone—is enhanced by serum containing anti-T antibodies and is inhibited by injecting syngeneic thymocytes. Thus, T cells can inhibit the B-cell response.

The injection of antibodies may enhance or inhibit antibody production by B cells. In either case, the mechanism modulating antibody production is mysterious.

The injection of antibody or antibody complexes can inhibit or enhance the response of T cells and facilitate tumor growth or retard rejection of allograft. The mechanism of inhibition of T-cell response by antibodies is obscure, but it could involve binding of the antibody to the receptor. Thus, the influence of T on B cells is complex. The best documented effect is a T-B-cell collaboration. The T cells are believed to determine the amount, class, and affinity of the antibody produced by B cells in response to antigen and to regulate the switch from IgM to IgG. A suppression of B-cell responses by T cells has been reported. To explain these conflicting effects of T on B cells, investigators have proposed two hypotheses. Either two types of T cells exist—a stimulator and a suppressor type—or only one type of T cell exists, and under special circumstances it produces suppressor substances.

Lymphocyte Factors

We have seen that the immune response, whether it be the formation of circulating antibodies or cell-mediated immunity, results from the careful orchestration of macromolecular interaction in a number of cells: lymphocytes (B, T, or both) and macrophages. In most cases, the neutralization of the antigen—whether it be a soluble compound or part of living nefarious agents such as viruses, bacteria, parasites, or foreign mammalian cells—usually leads to one or more manifestations of inflammation, vasodilation, chemotactism, phagocytosis, granuloma formation, and cytolysis.

These secondary effects of the immune reaction gain even more significance if we keep in mind that the immune reaction does not always succeed in killing the intruder, and that sometimes it causes more damage than the intruder itself.

Many of these effects are believed to be caused by chemical factors produced by the challenged lymphocytes, some of which have been identified, others of which remain unknown. These factors are called lymphokinins [121–124]. How are these factors studied? Lymphocytes are obtained from individuals sensitized by a specific antigen, and these lymphocytes are believed to carry a specific antibody. These cells are then stimulated *in vitro* by incubating them with the antigens for a given time, approximately 24 hours in most cases. Finally, a cell-free preparation is obtained and its effect is tested *in vitro*.

Although an integral reconstruction or even description of all the molecular events that take place in the immune response is at this time inconceivable, some of the manifestations of these reactions can be identified with specific molecules. Whenever little is known of a molecule to which a specific function can be ascribed, it is called a factor. A number of factors have been identified that can reproduce specific immunological manifestations. We will briefly review some elementary properties of the transfer factor, the migration inhibitory factor, the mitogenic or blastogenic factor, the lymphotoxic factor, and cytophilic antibodies.

The role of these compounds usually is difficult to investigate *in vivo* because they are produced in small amounts by a few sensitized cells. Consequently, their role has been investigated using cultured cells. As a result, the role that these molecules play in the actual *in vivo* immune reaction is not known.

Lymphokinins

Our knowledge of the transfer factor can be traced to an experiment by Landsteiner and Chase. Tuberculin injection sensitizes a human so that a second subcutaneous injection yields what is referred to as a tuberculin reaction (see below). This sensitization can be transferred to another human simply by administering lymphocytes from a sensitized individual. Many years later, it was shown that it was not necessary to inject intact lymphocytes to transfer the immunity, but that extracts of lymphocytes will perform the job. The term transfer factor was coined. The factor was found to be stable in various temperature ranges and to the DNase, RNase, and protease treatments. The molecular weight has been estimated to be of the order of 10,000 by differential dialysis.

Each immunological challenge seems to elicit the appearance of a transfer factor that is released only under conditions that reproduce the original challenge. Thus, if lymphocytes are sensitized with diphtheria toxin and tuberculin, incubation with PPD releases only the tuberculin transfer factor. However, because the transfer factor is found only in human lymphocytes, not much more information is available. Transfer factor can now best be defined as that molecule or complex of molecules, which when extracted from sensitized lymphoid cells confers delayed sensitivity to a normal animal after injection.

According to Dressler and Rosenfeld [282], at least some transfer factors are made in part or in toto of double-stranded RNA.

The migration inhibitory factor (MIF) was discovered by Rich and Lewis nearly 40 years ago. Explants of spleen and lymph nodes from sensitized animals were placed in the presence of specific antigens *in vitro*. The migration of the cells in the explant was found to be inhibited by that procedure. Later, rigid quantitative methods were developed in which the chemotactic movement of cells placed in capillary tubes in the presence of antigen was followed. This approach permitted investigators to measure the distance traveled and count the cells in movement. In addition, it was possible to quantitate the amount of chemotactic agent in the medium.

A factor has been prepared that is stable at 56° for 30 minutes and is nondialyzable. The factor has been partially purified by separation on Sephadex followed by electrophoresis on polyacrylamide gels. The eluted active fraction is then partially degraded by chymotrypsin and neuraminidase. When the degraded product is centrifuged on cesium chloride, it yields an acidic protein with a molecular weight between 35,000 and 55,000.

Two factors with molecular weights of 12,000 and 40,000 have been extracted from tuberculin-sensitized lymphocytes. Each factor binds specifically to antigen, and the factor with the lower molecular weight is cytophilic and can transfer delayed hypersensitivity.

The purified factor seems to affect the stickiness of the macrophages without altering their rate of division. It also modifies the macrophage metabolism in that the glucose consumption is increased four- to eightfold. Most of the glucose is used for oxidation through the hexose monophosphate shunt. Possibly as a result of this stimulation of the bioenergetic pathways, the macrophages increase their phagocytic abilities and exhibit more membrane activity.

Ward has discovered a protein that is chemotactic for macrophages. It has a molecular weight of 35,000 to 55,000 but migrates differently from the classical MIF on the polyacrylamide gel.

Several laboratories have reported the presence of lymphotoxic factors in sensitized lymphocytes. However, little has been accomplished with respect to purifying such factors. Depending upon the laboratories, factors with molecular weights of 35,000, 70,000, 80,000, and 150,000 have been claimed to be responsible for the lymphotoxic effect.

Both growth inhibitory factors and mitogenic or blastogenic factors have been discovered. Valentine and Loren prepared blastogenic factors by stimulating sensitized lymphocytes with specific antigens in culture.

In addition to the various factors already discussed, lymphoid cells derived from human blood elaborate other proteins such as immunoglobulins, the mediators of cellular immunity, and also interferon, fragments of complement and histocompatibility antigens. All these components contribute to the overall immunological reaction, but their interaction with each other, their exact impact, and their place in the sequence of events are not known.

In conclusion, sensitized lymphocytes produce in culture a variety of active "factors" that may conceivably affect the manifestation of the immunological reactions, but little is known of their chemical structure, their mode of action, and their role *in vivo*. It is not even certain whether some of the biological properties described are not effectuated by the same molecule. Needless to say, the elucidation of the molecular events involved in the *in vivo* expression of the immunological reaction could open new avenues in diagnosis (*e.g.*, disease due to missing factors, excessive production of factors) and therapy (*e.g.*, activation of specific factors against specific targets, such as the cancer cell). Some of the most prominent lymphocyte factors are listed in Table 14-6. The molecular identification of each of these factors obviously is of capital importance.

Table 14-6. Some biological effectors extracted from lymphocytes

Transfer factor	Delayed hypersensitivity
Antibodylike factor	Delayed hypersensitivity
Migration inhibition factor (MIF)	Inhibits macrophage migration
Antiproliferative factor	Inhibits DNA synthesis
Lymphotoxin (LT)	Cytolytic for fibroblasts in the absence of C
Mitogenic factor (MF)	Stimulates lymphocytic proliferation
Chemotactic factor	(see Inflammation)

Immune Tolerance

The immune system was devised to protect the organism against foreign proteins and among them, principally those brought into the organism through infection by other living agents such as viruses, bacteria, fungi, and complex parasites. There are two major forms of immunity: humoral and cellular. In both cases the antigen is carried to the lymph nodes where it stimulates lymphocytes: B lymphocytes in the case of humoral, and T lymphocytes in the case of cellular immunity.

The B lymphocytes secrete immunoglobulins that complex with the antigen. The antigen-antibody complex activates a latent group of enzymes, complement. A number of chemical mediators—chemotactic, bactericidal, etc.—are released and, if successful, the source of the antigen is neutralized.

The T cells are sensitized and interact with the cells carrying the antigen; they secrete a group of factors called lymphokinins and, again, if successful, eliminate foreign cells.

Immunity, which may originally have evolved to protect the organism against infectious agents, also affects foreign cells introduced in the form of organ transplants obtained from other species or even from the same species but from organisms genetically unrelated. Except for lymphocyte transplants, the type of immunity involved in graft rejection is of the cellular type. Cancer cells can, at least under some circumstances, be recognized as foreign. Because of the therapeutic value of transplantation, it is critical to find ways to prevent immunological reactions against transplanted tissue. This can be achieved by administering physical or chemical agents that more or less selectively destroy the immune cells.

However, in some physiological situations, the symbiosis of the self and nonself is possible. Although the prototype of immunological tolerance is the symbiotic relationship between mother and fetus, immunological protection exists in so-called privilege sites; for example, the anterior chamber of the eye, the brain in mammals in general, and the cheek pouch of the hamster.

To understand the relationship between mother and fetus, we should review the steps involved in conception: a haploid spermatozoon penetrates a haploid ovum, and the chromosomes of the father are intimately blended with those of the mother. This fertilized egg divides and yields a cystic structure, the blastocyst, which directly contacts the columnar epithelium of the endometrium. The stroma of the endometrium differentiates and proliferates, yielding a new type of tissue called the decidua. The blastocyst proliferates at the point of contact to form the trophoblast, which penetrates inside the endometrium, thus grafting the embryo to the mother's tissues. Later the placenta and the embryo develop at the site of contact. Clearly half the genes of the embryo are of paternal origin. They will carry the genes for histocompatibility antigens. Therefore, the fetus is a graft and the mother is a host. Yet, the mother does not reject the fetus. This special relationship between host and graft does not result from the fact that half of the genetic material is stored by the mother and fetus because blastocysts collected in a different mother and transplanted will not be rejected.

Cows occasionally produce dizygotic twins. In such cases each fetus is derived from a different fertilized ovum and the twins are genetically different. Yet, during fetal life their circulation is common and, therefore, each fetus is continuously exposed to blood cells and proteins derived from the other. The twins survive, indicating that they "tolerate" each others' antigens during fetal life. Moreover, the pair will permanently accept skin grafts from each other [125].

In humans, mutual tolerance does not occur in dizygotic twins but only with uniovular or genetically identical twins. But occasionally nonidentical human twins have double blood groups.

Burnet and Fenner [126] injected fetuses of one strain of mice with spleen cells of another strain.

The adult recipient accepts through its life span skin grafts of the donor, but it continues to reject grafts from other strains. These findings reveal that fetal tolerance involves T as well as B cells and also that it is specific.

However, tolerance is not restricted to fetal life. Under special circumstances individuals endowed with a fully responsive immune system develop tolerance to nonself antigens. In 1927 Schieman and Casper demonstrated that the intravenous injection in guinea pigs of high doses of diphtheria toxoid or pneumococcal polysaccharides suppressed the immune reaction normally elicited with smaller doses. Thus, the injected animals developed a state of acquired tolerance or of immunological unresponsiveness. Further experiments of the same vein established that the tolerance is specific for the antigen [127–129].

Tolerance cannot be simply established with any antigen under any circumstances. A number of special requirements must be fulfilled. First, there seems to be an inverse relationship between the immunogenicity of the antigen and its ability to establish tolerance. Tolerance is difficult to induce with highly immunogenic antigens without simultaneously applying immunosuppressive measures. In contrast, weak antigens, like foreign serum protein, are more effective toleragens. Tolerance can, in fact, be established by administering nonimmunogenic polypeptides. The capsule of *Bacillus anthracis* contains a homopolymer of D-glutamic acid with a molecular weight of approximately 33,000. The homopolymer is not antigenic by itself but will elicit an immunological response if mixed with Freund adjuvant. The administration of large doses of the homopolymer induces tolerance against the homopolymer mixed with the adjuvant.

Reduction in the size or chemical alteration of the antigen may modify its ability to act as a toleragen *in vivo*. Although aggregates of γ-globulin are primarily immunogenic, soluble γ-globulins can act as toleragens. The monomeric form of flagellin (mol wt 18,000), which is the flagellar protein of *Salmonella adelaide*, is a more potent toleragen and a weaker immunogen than the polymeric form. Diener and Feldmann [127] found the reverse in a study of the effect of flagellin on antibody cells "*in vitro*." The monomer was less toleragenic than the polymer of flagellin. Depolymerization of polyvinylpyrrolidone improves its potential as a toleragen. The acetylation of flagellin by diketenes eliminates its immunogenic and enhances its toleragenic potential.

Tolerance is specific for the antigen determinant used to induce it. We have already seen that it is true for T-cell tolerance. Mice of strain A rendered tolerant to cells of strain B reject grafts from strains C, D, or E. Similarly, the induction of tolerance to one humoral antigen does not prevent a humoral response against other types of antigens.

Tolerance to B and T cells seems to require the continuous presence of antigens. Animals made tolerant to allogeneic tissues by lymphocyte injection remain tolerant all their lives because of the persistence of the donor's histocompatibility antigen. A similar situation obtains with soluble antigens. The longer the antigen persists in the host, the longer the tolerance. Thus, rapidly metabolizable antigens are less toleragenic than nonmetabolizable antigens. If the antigen is rapidly metabolized or eliminated, repeated administration is required to maintain tolerance.

The transfer of cells rendered tolerant to a specific antigen to an irradiated animal restores immunopotency, and it also establishes tolerance in the host for the donor's toleragen.

The fate of the toleragen during tolerance is not known—it is not certain where and in what form it is stored—but tolerance induced with a specific haptene reduces the tolerance for the antihaptene immunoglobulin. Whether tolerance specifically eliminates the clone of cells that carry the haptene receptor or whether the receptors are blocked by the toleragen is unknown. The fate of the irreversibly suppressed antigen-coated cells is unclear. They are believed to be eliminated by phagocytosis.

Tolerance can be broken in a number of ways. Since residual antigen is required to maintain tolerance, tolerance can be broken by administering antibody specific for the toleragen. Tolerance to a given haptene can also be broken by challenge with an antigen containing the same haptene on a different carrier. This is explained by assuming that the haptene contains several determinants and that tolerance is directed only at one of them. This is illustrated by an experiment of Taussig, who showed that ten times more IgG is required to obtain tolerance to the Fc than the Fab determinants [128]. Similarly, the administration of cross-reacting antigens structurally related to the toleragen breaks tolerance. Tolerance established with bovine serum albumin is broken by administering human serum albumin. The transfer of cells sensitized against a specific antigen to an animal tolerant for that antigen breaks the tolerance temporarily until the host has destroyed the sensitized cells in a host-versus-graft reaction. Tolerance can be broken by X-irradiation or other immunosuppressors. The exact mechanism involved is not known, but the killed cells are believed to include most of the tolerant cells. Later, when cellular restoration takes place, the tolerant cells are either not reproduced or are overwhelmingly outnumbered by immunogenic cells.

Large doses of the toleragen were believed to be needed to induce immunological tolerance. The need for large doses is a major handicap to attempts to render an animal or a human tolerant to transplantation antigen. Mitchison [129] disclosed that tolerance to bovine serum albumin could be established in mice by the repeated administration of subimmunogenic doses. Low doses of flagellin can also produce tolerance. To distinguish between the forms of tolerance induced with low doses and high doses of toleragen, one speaks of "low-zone" and "high-zone" tolerance. A low zone of tolerance cannot be produced with all antigens. Thus, highly immunogenic antigens cannot induce tolerance at low doses, and even human serum albumin, a relatively weak immunogen, does not produce low-zone tolerance.

The two tolerance zones are separated by a medium concentration of the foreign substance that induces an immunogenic response.

The molecular mechanisms responsible for tolerance are hypothetical. In a normal immunogenic response, the antigen binds to receptors and the available receptors migrate at one pole of the cell to form clusters of antigen-receptor complexes. This phenomenon is called "capping," and it is immediately followed by the formation of more surface receptors. The surface changes convey a signal to the cell that triggers the immunological response (proliferation, antibody formation, etc.).

The molecular mechanism of tolerance induction has been deduced from *in vitro* experiments. The toleragen is assumed to contain several determinants that bind to cell surface receptors. With large doses, there is extensive cross-linking of the toleragen molecules and the surface of the lymphocyte is frozen, incapable of giving the signal that triggers the immunogenic response.

Mode of Action of Humoral Antibodies

The ultimate purpose of antibody production by the B cell is to neutralize living organisms (viruses, bacteria, parasites), foreign macromolecules (mainly proteins and polysaccharides), or even small chemicals that could otherwise be toxic. Under normal conditions, the nefarious agent is neutralized with minimal damage to the host. Sometimes the immune response is out of proportion with the threat to the host, and immunological disease develops. Before we consider the manifestation of immunopathology in humans, we will review briefly the mechanism by which humoral antibodies react with cells and antigens to injure the host [130–142].

Soluble antibodies can cause injuries by three basic mechanisms: (1) the so-called cytotropic antibodies may adhere to tissue mast cells and lymphocytes and initiate a sequence of events that culminate in the release of chemical mediators; (2) the cytolytic or cytotoxic antibodies may specifically bind to cell-bound antigens and kill the cell carrying the antigen; (3) the antibodies may form antigen-antibody complexes that may accumulate in the kidney or reticuloendothelial cell and cause acute or chronic injury.

Cytotropic Antibodies

The experimental prototypes of situations in which cytotropic antibodies play the central role are anaphylaxis and the Prausnitz-Küstner reaction.

History

To produce anaphylaxis in an experimental animal, the investigator must first sensitize the animal to an antigen. The same antigen is injected intravenously within two or three days. The animal develops a catastrophic systemic reaction that may lead to death. Although the reaction is generalized, the prominent manifestations vary from one animal to another. In guinea pigs, bronchiolar spasm causes acute emphysema and respiratory distress. Platelet leukocyte thrombi obstruct the pulmonary capillaries of rabbits, whereas in dogs engorgement of the viscera (liver, spleen, intestine) and lung hemorrhage are the most obvious gross and histological pathological findings.

In the Prausnitz-Küstner reaction, serum obtained from a sensitized (allergic, see below) individual (Küstner in this instance) is injected under the skin of unsensitized individuals (Prausnitz in this instance). When the previously unsensitized individual is again exposed to the sensitizing agents (fish proteins in the original Prausnitz-Küstner reaction), a localized wheal and flare reaction develops at the challenged site. Thus, experimental anaphylaxis and the Prausnitz-Küstner reaction are examples of generalized and localized immunological responses to antigens involving cytotropic antibodies. In humans, this response is elicited by the IgE class, also called reagin. The IgE unspecifically adheres to unsensitized lymphocytes and mast cells through a specific configuration of the Fc fragment. The antigen-antibody reaction that takes place at the cell surface culminates in the release of chemical mediators of inflammation and the slow reacting substance of polymorphonuclears.

Pharmacological Mediators and Antigen-Antibody Reactions

The mechanism whereby an antigen-antibody reaction can lead to the release of a pharmacological mediator is, for the large part, unknown. The fixation of antibody to mast cells and leukocytes has been studied both *in vivo* and *in vitro*. The adsorption of cytotropic antibody is reversible and partly dependent upon diffusion. Temperature and pH are also important: optimal fixation occurs at 37° and at a pH of 7.4. *In vitro* sensitization of human leukocytes by homocytotropic antibodies is enhanced by EDTA, which chelates calcium ions. The removal of calcium ions from the cell surface reveals antibody-binding sites. However, both calcium and magnesium are necessary for subsequent antigen-induced histamine release. Heparin can act synergistically with EDTA to further enhance antibody fixation. Nonspecific γ-globulin can interfere with the rate, although not the extent, of specific antibody fixation.

Histamine release from mast cells and leukocytes follows the reaction of antigen with the fixed antibody. The degree of release is exponentially proportional to antigen concentration. Using human leukocytes sensitized passively *in vitro* with homocytotropic antibody to ragweed antigen, investigators have calculated that each molecule of antigen can trigger the release of 10^6 or more histamine molecules. High concentrations of antigen, however, can inhibit histamine release. A lag of up to approximately 20 minutes, depending upon the amount of antigen added to the sensitized leukocytes, is observed between the addition of antigen and histamine release. Histamine release is sensitive to pH (optimal 7.3–7.8) and ionic strength. Adequate levels of calcium and magnesium are required. Histamine release is enhanced by normal human serum. This is apparently not due to the presence of complement in normal serum, although it has not been completely ruled out that no component of complement is involved.

The biochemical basis of antigen-induced release of histamine, or any other mediator, has not yet been elucidated. In histamine release in antibody-fixed lung slices of guinea pigs, the addition of antigen was found to activate a tissue enzyme precursor from an inactive state. This precursor, which was heat labile, was transformed in the presence of calcium into a short-lived enzyme responsible for somehow releasing histamine from mast cell granules. The catalytic properties of the enzyme, or enzymes, involved are still unknown, although a serine esterase and a chymotrypsin have been implicated.

The release of histamine from mast cells is not necessarily associated with cell damage or death. Histamine release is a secretory process apparently involving a number of steps and requiring metabolically active cells. Along with heparin, histamine is contained within the granules of mast cells and basophils. These granules are discharged during histamine release in a process called degranulation. Some assays for cytotropic antibody use as their end point the degree of mast cell degranulation.

Substances such as bradykinin, slow-releasing substance (SRS-A), the prostaglandins, and serotonin may also be involved in anaphylaxis in man, but the evidence for this does not warrant detailed discussion here. As mentioned earlier, serotonin is often referred to as the rodent histamine, but this is probably not completely accurate.

In any event, the lack of any real beneficial effect of antihistaminic drugs on many cases of immediate-type allergy suggests that other mediators may be extremely important in anaphylaxis. Histamine has received the most attention by clinicians and experimentalists, and therefore it may seem to play a greater role in allergy than in fact it does.

Allergic reactions are frequently characterized by blood and tissue eosinophilia. This is of diagnostic significance, but the role of eosinophils in immediate hypersensitivity is not yet known.

Histamine itself, β-adrenergic catecholamines, and certain prostaglandins can modulate: (1) the release of histamine and other mediators; (2) the ability of sensitized lymphocytes to kill allogenic cells; and (3) the release of antibody from lymphocytes mediated by IgE. The molecular mechanism by which such modulation takes place is unknown. But it is believed that the modulator (*e.g.,* histamine, which blocks its own release) binds to specific receptors, activates adenyl cyclase, and leads to increased intracellular cyclic AMP concentrations that then inhibit the release of mediators by basophils and antigens by B cells and allogenic responsive T cells [143].

A number of human diseases resemble the generalized or localized reaction that develops as a result of the appearance of the IgE-type cytophilic antibodies. All the intricacies of the pathogenesis of such diseases are not always understood because all aspects of the experimental reaction are not known and because in humans the antigenic challenge is often multiple; therefore, the antibody response is more complex than in simpler experimental conditions. The human disease is believed to be caused, at least in part, by IgE cytotropic antibodies and includes generalized anaphylaxis reaction and atopic reactions such as some forms of urticaria, hay fever, and bronchial asthma. The diseases will be decribed in more detail later. The steps involved in the anaphylactic and the Prausnitz-Küstner reactions are summarized in Fig. 14-4A and B.

Cytotoxic Antibodies

Cytotoxic antibodies specifically bind to cellular antigen and cause cell death. In a prototypic experiment, sheep red cells, leukocytes, or platelets are administered to a rabbit. The rabbit forms antibodies against antigens that are present at the surface of these cells. The chemical nature of such antigens will be discussed later; remember that the antibodies are elaborated by B cells and almost always are of the IgG type (except cold hemagglutinins, which are of the IgM type). In contrast to the cytotropic antibodies that bind to cells unspecifically, the cytotoxic antibody binds to the cellular antigen through its specific antigenic site in the Fab portion of the antibody. Once the cell is coated with the antibody it is doomed. It may die immediately (intravascular death), or it may survive long enough to reach the spleen, the liver, or the lungs where it is spotted by the reticuloendothelial cells and phagocytized. The mechanism by which the cells are killed is not known in detail, but it does involve activation of complement components fixed to antibody-coated cell membranes.

The primary event in extravascular cytolysis is believed to result from modification of the membrane

A. ANAPHYLAXIS

1. Intravenous injection of antigen.
2. Intravenous challenge with antigen.

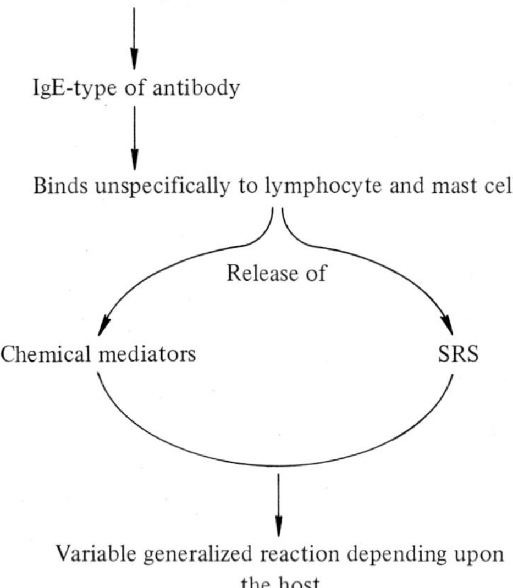

B. PRAUSNITZ-KÜSTNER REACTION

1. Localized sensitization with sensitized serum
2. Localized or systemic challenge

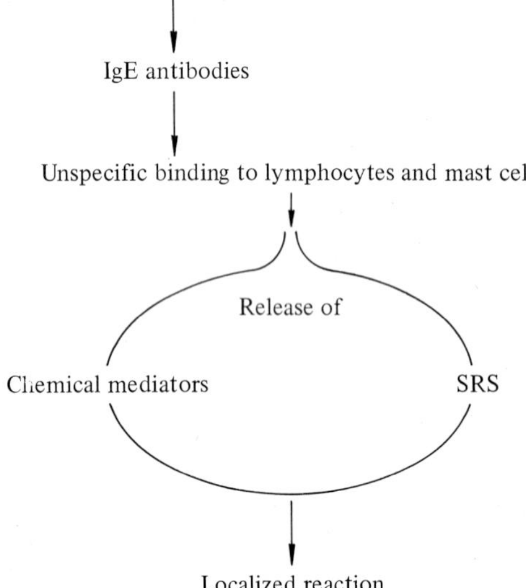

Fig. 14-4. (A) Schematic representation of mode of action of cytotropic antibodies (B) Prausnitz-Küstner reaction

permeability. In the lesser instances, the membrane is capable of retaining macromolecules but is unable to retain smaller molecules; as a result, the cell swells and explodes in osmotic shock. In the more severe cases, the cell membrane is unable to retain hemoglobin, which leaks out in the plasma. The consequences of osmotic and nonosmotic hemolysis have already been discussed.

If the cells do not die within the blood vessels, the cells coated with antibody to which C3 is attached

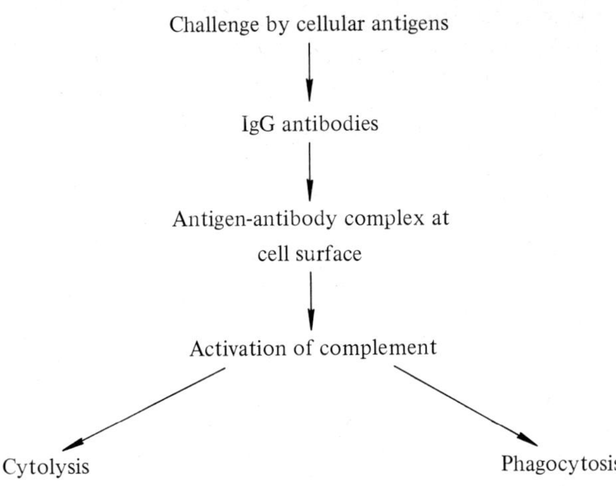

Fig. 14-5. Schematic representation of mode of action of cytolytic immune response

are spotted by the reticuloendothelial cells of the spleen, liver, and lungs and are phagocytized. Some of what is known of the mechanism of phagocytosis is discussed in the chapter on inflammation. (The site of sequestration appears to depend on the amounts of antibody that coat the cell; heavily coated cells are phagocytized by the liver, lightly coated cells by the spleen. The reason for this difference is not clear, and the anatomical and physiological arguments used to explain it are not compelling.) The mode of action of the cytolytic immune response is presented in Fig. 14-5. The effects of the exposure of a human lymphocyte to allogenic antibodies and complement are shown in Fig. 14-6. Compare these effects with those of a lymphocyte exposed to normal serum (see Fig. 14-7).

A number of diseases in humans are likely to evoke a cytotoxic immune response. Most involve circulating blood cells (see Table 14-7), but it cannot be excluded that other types of cellular immunological executions result from coating with cytotoxic antibodies and rejection of homograph, and antitissue immune injuries may be a causal point.

Table 14-7. Diseases evoking cytotoxic responses

Blood elements
Red cells
Hemolytic anemia of the newborn
Autoimmune hemolytic anemia
Blood transfusion reaction
White cells
Leukopenia
Platelets
Thrombocytopenia
Other cell types
Homologous graft rejection
Antitissue antibodies
Goodpasture's syndrome

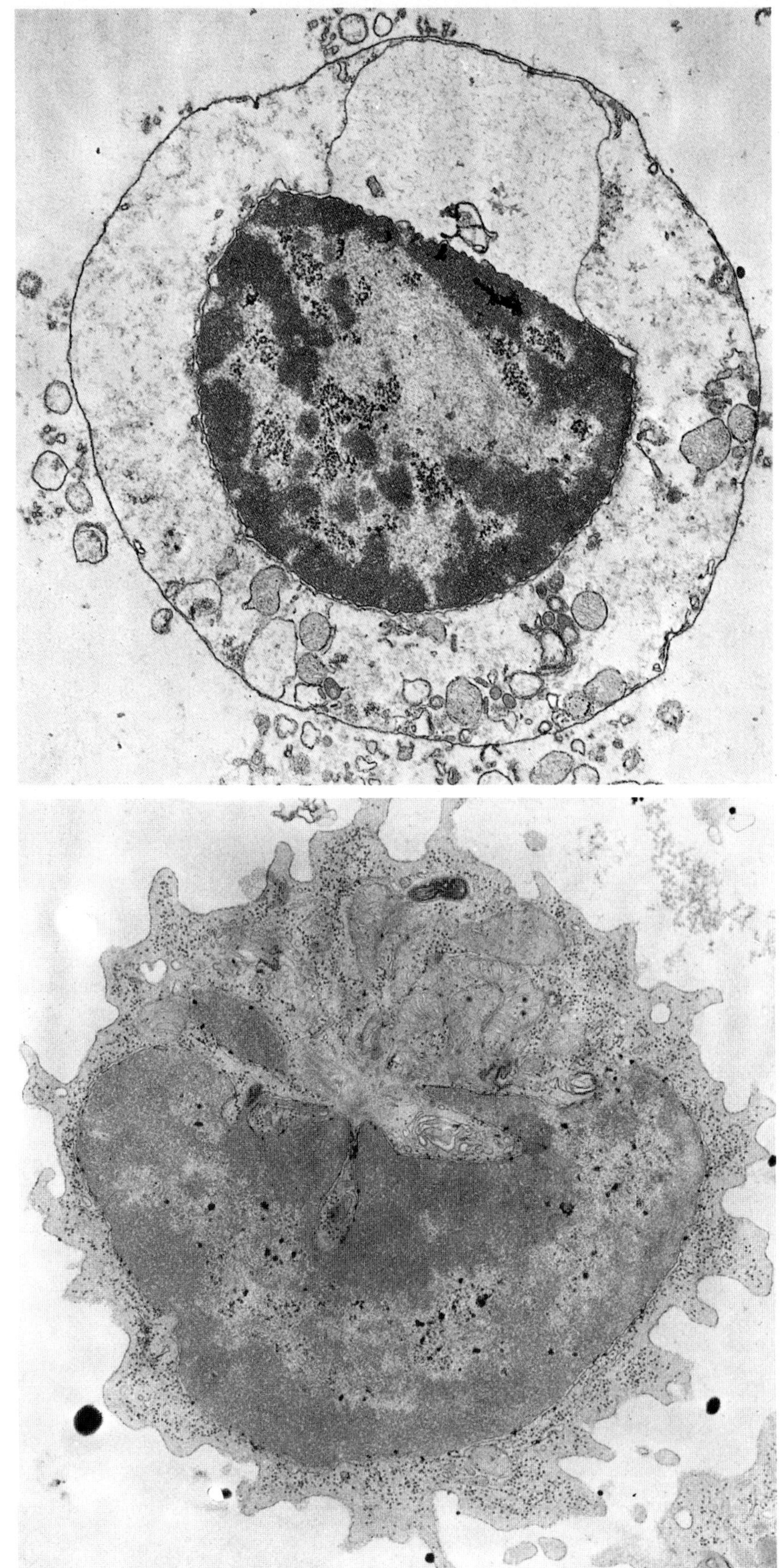

Fig. 14-6. Necrosis caused by antiserum; effects of exposure of human lymphocytes to allogenic antibodies and complement for 90 minutes. Comparison with Fig. 14-7 shows that the cytoplasm has become rounded and lost the pseudopods. Some of them have probably been pinched off to form the free vesicles outside the cell. Ribosomes have disappeared; mitochondria have fragmented into spherical forms. Cytoplasmic vesicles and endoplasmic reticulum have become swollen sacs. The pyknotic nucleus shows pronounced peripheral margination of the chromatin and clumping of interchromatin granules. The great expansion of the nuclear envelope at the top is unusual in other types of necrosis and seems to be a relatively specific reaction to antiserum. Lysosomes seem to play little or no part in this type of cell death. (Electron micrograph; ×18,000.) (From H. Latta)

Fig. 14-7. Normal human lymphocyte exposed to normal serum for 90 minutes and used as a control for the reaction shown in Fig. 14-6. Mitochondria, Golgi membranes, and a centriole lie together on one side of the nucleus. Monoribosomes and a few small profiles of endoplasmic reticulum are scattered through the cytoplasm. The large, dark masses in the nucleus represent precipitate of the lead hydroxide stain. (Electron micrograph; ×23,000.) (From H. Latta)

Hypersensitivity Mediated by Antigen-Antibody Complexes

Soluble antigens complex with humoral antibodies produced by B cells to form soluble-insoluble complexes. Normally, those complexes are rapidly cleared by the kidney or by the cells of the reticuloendothelial system. Sometimes because the antigen persists in excess of the amount of antibody formed, soluble complexes of intermediate size appear and are not phagocytized. Then these complexes accumulate in the glomeruli because they are not filtered or in blood vessel walls because the endothelial permeability is increased. The experimental prototypes of injuries caused by soluble complexes are the Arthus reaction and serum sickness.

Contrary to what might be expected, the antigens involved in immune complex disease are not in any way unique. In fact, the antibodies produced determine whether active, disease-producing complexes are formed. For example, although rabbit, human, and guinea pig antibodies can form active complexes, bovine, chicken and horse antibodies cannot. The antibody involved in complex formation can be either IgM or IgG globulin, although complexes are more common with the latter. The antigen-antibody complex, as well as the antibody portion of it, has special affinities for certain tissues and can also react with complement, properties necessary to induce disease. The Fc portion of the antibody molecule determines both the affinity for tissues and the ability to react with complement.

The reaction of antibody with antigen to form an active complex is accompanied by a change in the optic rotation of the immunoglobulin, suggesting that the role of the antigen in immune complex disease is to bring about a necessary configurational change in the antibody molecule. Heat and chemical aggregation also bring about configurational changes of γ-globulin molecules. Aggregates formed in this way may fix complement and induce some form of immune complex disease.

Active complexes are formed in slight antigen excess, so the complexes are soluble and can circulate. Very small complexes may circulate for a long time. Large complexes are removed by the reticuloendothelial systems. Disease results when moderately large complexes become localized in the tissues and trigger an inflammatory response. The localization and distribution of the complexes in the tissue depend on anatomic or physiologic factors and not, apparently, on immunological ones. The pathology of immune complex disease arises from the inflammatory response to the deposited complexes and the processes of healing accompanying it, as well as from the disposition of the complexes.

The Arthus Reaction

Although the basis of immune complex disease is only now being elucidated, examples of this type of hypersensitivity have been known for some time. The use of antiserum therapy (horse antitoxins) in the early part of this century frequently resulted in the development of hypersensitivity to the foreign serum protein. The manifestations of this hypersensitivity appear in the so-called Arthus reaction and in serum sickness. Recent experimental studies of these reactions indicate that they are immune complex diseases.

The Arthus reaction was first described by Arthus as a progressively necrotizing lesion developing from repeated subcutaneous or intradermal injections of antigen into unsensitized rabbits at 6-day intervals. Although the first injection is innocuous, as the injections are repeated, erythema, then edema, and finally necrosis develop at the injection site. A new site can be used for each injection. It is now clear that the Arthus reaction stems from the precipitation of antigen-antibody complexes in the vascular tissue at the site of antigen injection. As the number of antigen injections is increased, the amount of antigen-antibody complexes increases, leading to progressively more severe lesions.

The lesions can be elicited in any tissue of the body, not only in the skin. The phenomenon can also be produced passively by either injecting antigen locally and antibody intravenously, or by injecting antibody locally and the antigen intravenously (reverse sensitive reaction). In the passive situation, the reaction appears immediately upon injection of both components of the complex. No latent period is necessary as with cytophilic antibodies because the mechanism of production of injury by the antibody in the Arthus reaction does not involve sensitization of cells. The most important property of antibody in this reaction is its ability to precipitate antigen. Nonprecipitating antibody will not induce an Arthus response.

The injurious agent in the Arthus reaction is an antigen-antibody precipitate capable of fixing complement (C′); thus, in guinea pig the α_1 antibodies, which do not fix complement, do not elicit an Arthus reaction in contrast to α_2 antibodies which can fix C′. The antibodies involved in the Arthus reaction are of the IgM and IgG types.

Pathology of the Arthus Reaction

Within 30 minutes of the injection, the injection site reddens and swells. Erythema and edema are followed within hours by hemorrhage and necrosis. Thus, the reaction is a typical inflammatory reaction followed by necrosis.

Histologically, all the signs of inflammation (vasodilatation, endothelial swelling, leukocytic margination, polymorphonuclear exudation) and later of cellular death are seen. In addition, using immunofluorescent techniques, one can demonstrate antigen-antibody complexes in the vessel walls.

The mechanism of the necrosis that develops in an Arthus reaction includes the following steps: deposition of an antigen-antibody complex, fixation of C′, degradation of complement, release of special and potent chemotactic agents, polymorphonuclear migration, phagocytosis of the antigen-antibody complex, and polymorphonuclear death with release of acid hydrolases.

It is clear from the description of the pathogenesis of the disease that antihistaminics cannot prevent the Arthus reaction since plasma cell degranulation does not occur.

Of particular interest, however, is the formation of the antigen-antibody complex and the mechanism of complement activation (see above).

Systemic Arthus Reaction

If a specific antigen is injected in a guinea pig under conditions that secure slow absorption and if the animal's serum contains high titers of the antibody, the animal often dies in circulatory failure within a matter of hours. Although the events are reminiscent of anaphylaxis, the symptoms are different and cannot be relieved by antihistaminics. For these reasons, the antigen-antibody reaction in these cases is believed to elicit a different pathogenic sequence, which is again believed to involve the deposition of antigen-antibody complexes with complement fixation. Because of the similitude between the systemic Arthus reaction and anaphylaxis, the systemic Arthus reaction is often referred to as protracted anaphylaxis.

The injection of serum, vaccine, or antibiotics may result in an Arthus reaction in man and lead to tissue necrosis at the injection site. Other forms of the Arthus reaction in humans are probably acute glomerulonephritis, systemic lupus erythematosus, polyarteritis nodosa, and pigeon breeder disease.

Cell-Mediated Hypersensitivity, Tuberculin Reactions, and Graft Rejection

Fascinating as it may be, a review of the historical steps that led to the discovery of cell-mediated hypersensitivity or a description of why the term "delayed hypersensitivity" is in most cases used to refer to cellular hypersensitivity would be long and confusing. The reader who seeks further information on either of these aspects of cellular hypersensitivity is referred to the excellent article of Benacerraf and Green [144].

Humoral immunity is necessarily of low effectiveness against those agents that can survive intracellularly; namely, some bacteria, viruses, and protozoa. To deal with nefarious agents, organisms elaborated a different type of defense through evolution—namely, cellular immunity.

Thus, some immunological reactions, instead of being mediated through circulating antigens, are mediated by antigens "fixed" to migrating T lymphocytes. This cell-mediated type of sensitivity—which is responsible for the tuberculin reaction, contact dermatitis, and graft rejection—is often called "delayed hypersensitivity" because the reaction to antigen-antibody combination usually does not appear for several hours. Delayed hypersensitivity reactions develop slowly, but they persist for a long time.

Antigens in Delayed Hypersensitivity

The antigens that can cause delayed hypersensitivity vary greatly, but all have a protein component, although some may contain a protein and polysaccharide component. Some forms of delayed sensitivities, for example, contact dermatitis, are initiated by haptenes that *in vivo* are conjugated with proteins. Typical examples are the allergens of contact dermatitis that combine with skin protein. The antigens in question are a mixture of three substituted catechols. Some skin proteins seem to be particularly apt to combine with such haptenes. This may explain why sensitization occurs when the haptene is applied to the skin, but not when it is given by other routes.

Because the duration of the immunological reaction depends on the presence of the antigen, one property of the antigen relevant to the clinical manifestations is its survival in the host. For example, whereas the tuberculin antigen is rapidly destroyed, other antigens seem to persist for long periods of time. Thus, the reaction ceases with the disposition of the antigen, but it persists for long times if the antigen is not destroyed. Some of the granulomatous reactions observed in autoimmune diseases are believed to be the hallmark of a persistent antigen-antibody reaction.

As already mentioned, in delayed hypersensitivity the antibody is not a circulating one, but it is probably produced by lymphocytes and carried by them to the antigen. Lymphocytes are not the only cell type involved in the delayed hypersensitivity reaction, macrophages intervene as well. Thus, in delayed hypersensitivity not only is the antigen-antibody reaction complicated, but it elicits unusual cellular interaction. Before we attempt to analyze the individual factors involved, it may be worthwhile to take a synoptic view of delayed hypersensitivity as it is understood to develop at this time.

The antigen sensitizes circulating lymphocytes. The sensitized lymphocyte reacts with the antigen, and as it does, it releases a factor (macrophage inhibitory factor or MIF, see above) that *in vivo* or *in vitro* exhibits a number of properties: it inhibits the movement of circulating monocytes, which adhere to the adjacent endothelium and pass through the vessel walls. The cellular necrosis in the area is caused, at least in part, by (1) the lymphocyte factors, which kill fibroblasts and target cells holding the antigen, and (2) macrophages, which may attack adjacent parenchymal cells after simple proliferation without activation or after activation by cytophilic antibodies elaborated by lymphocytes.

One prototype for the cellular hypersensitivity reaction is the cutaneous tuberculin reaction. When tuberculin is injected subcutaneously it takes 6 to 12 hours for he skin to react. Then a visible, indurated, and slightly painful inflammatory reaction is seen, which reaches its peak 24 hours after the injection. The intensity of the inflammatory reaction ranges from mild induration and erythema to substantial necrosis depending upon the patient's sensitivity; the more sensitive he is, the more severe the reaction. The most striking histological feature is the abundance of lymphocyte and macrophages in the injected area; many of the lymphocytes are large and have a blastlike appearance.

Tuberculin sensitivity cannot be transferred with serum, but if lymphoid cells of tuberculous guinea pigs are injected intravenously or intraperitoneally in a normal guinea pig, the recipient becomes sensitized to tuberculin and develops a typical tuberculin reaction after subcutaneous injection. However, such positive transfer can be effectuated only with lymphocytes obtained from animals of the same species. Moreover, the administration of antilymphocyte serum or X-irradiation before transferring the lymphocytes from a tuberculous host to a virgin recipient makes the recipient unreactive probably by eliminating the lymphocytes and macrophages of the recipient that are indispensable for the reaction.

Inasmuch as lymphocytes obtained from the thoracic duct can transfer hypersensitivity, it seems established that only lymphocytes are required from the donor to transfer sensitivity.

The lymphocytes involved in delayed hypersensitivity are small, spheric cells with little endoplasmic reticulum and few polyribosomes. This is in contrast to plasmocytes, which are rich in endoplasmic reticulum. This observation suggests that if lymphocytes are involved in protein synthesis, the amount of proteins that they synthesize must be restricted.

The Fate of Grafted Tissue

Except for special situations to be described later, graft rejection by the host results from cellular hypersensitivity. This conclusion was reached by Lawrence in 1957 because of the similarities between graft rejection and other forms of delayed hypersensitivity. The similarities included the "latent period" (10–12 days), the absence of detectable circulating antibodies, and the inability to transfer the "sensitivity" with serum. Studies of thymectomized and bursectomized birds by Miller [145] and Good and his associates [146] established that T rather than B cells were involved.

Before we discuss graft rejection in detail, it would be wise to define the vocabulary. In an autograft, the tissue is obtained from the recipient himself and transplanted in a different area. An isograft is provided by a donor of the same species with a genetic background that is identical or nearly identical to that of the recipient (identical twins or inbred animals). An allograft is provided by a donor genetically similar to and of the same species as the recipient. A xenograft is provided by a donor of a different species than the recipient.

Although the legend of Saint Damien, who apparently had lost his leg, tells us that two kind angels came in the night and replaced the lost limb with a black leg that became functional, few successful allografts or xenografts have been reported in medical history. There is, however, documented evidence that the surgeons of ancient India performed autografts to replace facial appendages lost in battle. In fact, it is said that because excising the nose was a form of punishment for minor crimes in some parts of India, executioners were requested to burn the precious appendage in fear that the culprit might retrieve it and have a skillful Indian surgeon regraft it.

Reverdin in 1870 was apparently the first to transplant pinched skin autografts in extensive granulating wounds. Dr. Hoffacker (1787–1844) from the University of Heidelberg repaired, mainly through autografting, the mutilated faces of 20,000 victims of duels.

Even though skin allografts are certain to be rejected, they are somewhat successful in patients with extensive burns because the allograft may persist long enough to allow partial repair of the skin of the burned individual, thereby preventing the massive fluid loss that causes death in these patients.

Observing burned patients in World War II, Medawar concluded that allograft rejection resulted from a systemic reaction that was probably immunological in origin. A burned patient received soon after admission one autograft and two allografts. To further accelerate healing, surgeons administered two more allografts approximately 2 weeks later. All grafts healed and were integrated within the patient's normal skin. However, after 4 weeks, all allografts were rejected at once, but the autograft survived. If the cause of allograft rejection was some kind of local genetic incompatibility, as was believed at the time, the first set of allografts should have been rejected first and the second set 2 weeks later. But the fact that they were all rejected at the same time suggested that the first set of allografts had ellicited an immune reaction involving the formation of antibodies, which was fully expressed 4 weeks later for all the allogenic tissue. Yet no antibodies against the allograft could be found in the serum; therefore, the immunological response to the allograft had to involve a type of immunity different from the traditional humoral immunity, which was the only one known at that time.

The systematic study of the fate of the allograft was long impeded because inbred strains of animals were not available for such studies. Only after investigators had access to such strains of animals did allografting become possibile.

In 1943 Gibson and Medawar, using an inbred strain of mice, confirmed the notion of systemic graft rejection. When a second set of grafts obtained from the same donor was transplanted to the host, it was quickly rejected. Medawar and his associates further demonstrated that lymphocytes carried at least some of the antigens that ultimately led to the rejection of the skin grafts. Thus, if an animal was first injected with spleen lymphocytes, the response to a first skin graft was similar to that expected in a second set of grafts.

Later, Medawar proposed that specific genes—now known as histocompatibility genes—control the elaboration of the cell factors that elicit the immune reaction after transplantation.

Maybe the easiest way to understand the fate of allografts is to consider first the fate of autografts, which is uncomplicated by immunological reactions. If a piece of skin is transplanted from one area to another area of an individual's body, the graft becomes edematous soon after grafting and for a period of time is primarily nourished by diffusion of fluids from the graft bed. The presence of the graft elicits an inflammatory reaction in the graft bed. Although some of the inflammatory cells may infiltrate the graft, inflammation is minimal and has little consequence for the survival of the graft. In a second step, the small vessels of the host bed and those of the grafted skin grow independently and anastomose. Approximately 3 days after grafting, the graft becomes pinkish as effective blood circulation is reestablished in the grafted area. Lymphatic circulation and invasion by growing nerves follow the reestablishment of the blood circulation, and the grafted area becomes permanently and fully integrated with the host's surrounding tissues.

Isografts behave much like autografts.

Similarly, allografts in inbred strains, provided that the animals are of the same sex, behave similarly to the autografts. But the graft may be rejected in animals of different sexes. Thus, females may reject a graft obtained from a male because of histocompatibility antigens determined by the male Y chromosomes. For example, females of the C57 black strain regularly reject skin grafts of males of the same strain.

The fate of a full thickness of rejected skin allograft is as follows: At first, the allograft is accepted in a manner resembling autograft acceptance, but soon the allograft is infiltrated—especially in the perivascular and perifollicular areas and at its periphery—by a large number of lymphocytes, macrophages, and plasma cells. Within a week, the allograft becomes edematous, partly because of poor vascularization, and hardens and thickens because of lymphoid infiltration. At that stage, focal necrosis may develop, but within 10 days blood flow is completely occluded by thrombi; hemorrhage occurs and the entire grafted tissue is rejected.

All the details involved in the immunological response to graft rejection are unknown. It seems certain that large amounts of antigens are released from the graft in the first few hours after grafting. The antigens are immediately drained to the local nodes, which then mount the immune response. Thus, cells from the local node are much more effective than cells from distant nodes in transferring immunity. The allograft immune response involves a modification of the population of the node in that large polymorphic cells appear, and reticuloendothelial cells—usually with increased phagocytic ability—proliferate.

It is not really known which antigens are involved in graft rejection (see below), but investigators usually assume that most of the antigens are part of the cellular structure. However, the release of soluble antigens cannot be excluded. Most of the antigens probably are located at the cell surface, and a panel of antigens responsible for allograft rejection has been more or less identified. These are referred to as the transplantation antigens. Although certain cell types, such as lymphocytes, seem to contain an abundance of most if not all the important transplantation antigens, other cells (like the kidney) have much less. By comparing inbred animals, investigators have been able to identify the genetic loci of some of these antigens. Their chemical structures are in general not known, although it is believed that the H_2 (histocompatibility) antigens of the mouse system are lipoproteins found at the cell surface.

In most cases, the immunological reaction elicited by the transplantation antigen is of the cell-mediated type. Therefore, it cannot be transferred by serum, but it can be transferred by lymphocytes of a recipient of an allograft to a virgin host who will reject the allograft from the same donor.

However, graft rejection may evoke both humoral and cellular immunity. An immune response can occur within 2 or 3 hours after the allograft is transplanted, and it is partially due to the elaboration of specific humoral antibodies to soluble antigens of the graft. Often the implantation of the second allograft may follow a course similar to that of the first allograft for 2 or 3 days, but then it suddenly becomes ischemic because of interruption of the vascularization.* This response is believed to result from the combined development of humoral cytotoxic antibodies and cellular immunity. In conclusion, it would appear that cellular immunity is primarily involved in the rejection of primary allografts, whereas both humoral and cellular immunity can be involved in the rejection of secondary allografts.

Even before much was known about cell-mediated immunity, it was established that some tissues were easier to graft than others. For example, allografts of cartilage survive more effectively than many other forms of allografts. The cartilage cells are believed to be protected by sialomucins, which prevent contact with cell-mediated antibodies.

Similarly, some areas of the body constitute privileged sites for allografting. Extensive studies were made with grafts placed in the cornea and in the ante-

* A case at point is the rejection of kidney allografts in patients subjected to a second or third kidney transplant. In such patients, rejection is associated with the development of circulating antibodies toward the histocompatibility antigens. Even the rejection of the first graft in patients receiving immunosuppressive therapy may result from the formation of antigen-antibody complexes. These are cases of allograft rejection in which the basal membrane of the glomeruli is thickened and the vascular walls exhibit fibrinoid necrosis. This form of rejection is not to be confused with the rejection that occurs immediately after implantation usually as a result of ABO incompatibility. In such cases, the kidney is seeded with small thrombi and areas of cortical necrosis.

rior chamber of the eye; the success of such allografting is due to the avascularity of these portions of the organism. Grafts can be successfully transplanted in the brain because of its lack of lymphoid tissue and the presence of the brain-blood barrier, which prevents the extrusion of transplantation antigen and the penetration of immune cells. The hamster cheek pouch is a favorite experimental site for grafting because: (1) it has no lymphatic drainage, so the antigen is not normally drained to the lymph nodes; and (2) it seems to be protected by a special fibrinoid barrier that prevents the penetration of immune cells.

Immunosuppression

When we discuss immunodeficiency disease, it will become obvious that in several natural states humoral or cellular immunity is abolished and, therefore, graft rejection is prevented, at least in cases of deficiencies in cellular immunity. Such immunosuppressive states can be induced by destroying the lymphoid system with cortisone, X-irradiation, or some immunosuppressive chemicals, or, more specifically, with antilymphocyte globulin. Naturally, such agents are used to prolong allograft survival under therapeutic conditions [147–151].

Graft-Versus-Host Reaction

We described an interaction between host and graft in which the immune system of the host plays the major role and ultimately eliminates the graft. But sometimes the immune response of the host is successfully suppressed or is naturally absent, and then the immunocompetent cells of the graft may take over and attack the host; this is called graft-versus-host reaction. Thus, an immunologically immature individual, an older individual with an immunological deficiency, or an adult receiving immunosuppressive therapy may be severely injured by immunologically competent cells of the graft and develop what is sometimes referred to as "secondary disease" or "wasting disease." In this type of disease, the immunocompetent cells of the graft colonize the host and recognize the histocompatibility antigens of the host. The principal targets are organs rich in lymphoid tissues—thymus, bone marrow, spleen, and lymph nodes.

Thus, if rats from two different inbred strains are mated, the first generation will possess all the transplantation antigens of both mother and father; consequently, the hybrids will accept grafts from each other. But lymphocytes from one parent of the first-generation litter that are injected in an F_1 hybrid will recognize the transplantation antigen of the other parent and trigger an immune response against the host. The host then wastes away and is ultimately killed by the lymphocytes (graft) of his own parent.

The killing of susceptible cells by T lymphocytes is the common denominator in all forms of cellular hypersensitivity. Little is known of the molecular or morphological events that take place in cytolysis.

It has been observed that cytochalasin B and prostaglandins inhibit the cytolysis of DBA/2 mastocytoma cells by sensitized T lymphocytes. It would appear, therefore, that cytolysis occurs in discrete steps: one involving cation binding and preceding changes in membrane permeability, another that occurs later and involves molecular events more complex than cation binding [152].

Even when extremely sophisticated morphological studies give little information on the molecular changes that take place in the deployment of biological events, they are still helpful because in addition to providing a panoramic view of the events, they often uncover the most significant changes.

A case at point is the study of lymphocyte target cell interaction *in vitro* by Able, Lee, and Rosenau [153]. These authors sensitized the lymphocytes of one strain of mice to cells of another strain of mice by inoculating the latter intraperitoneally. Then they observed the interaction of the target cell (the inoculated one) with sensitized lymphocytes obtained from inoculated animals and nonsensitized lymphocytes. They found that all lymphocytes moved in the field in what appeared to be an undirected, randomized fashion, but ultimately the sensitized lymphocytes attached to the target cell. Electron microscopy revealed that although at first this attachment involved simple cell-to-cell contact, later true interdigitation between the two cell membranes developed. After a certain time, the target cell swells, rounds up, and finally lyses, releasing its intracellular components in the medium. This victory of the lymphocytes over the target cell is a Pyrrhic victory because ultimately the sensitized lymphocytes die. In contrast, when nonsensitized cells are used, attachment is rare and never do the lymphocytes or the target cells die.

Such morphological events clearly illustrate how sensitization has provided the lymphocyte with the power of inflicting on the target cell the kiss of death. The hope that someday lymphocytes can be sensitized to kill cancer cells has generated a great deal of work in that field; and if this can be achieved, perhaps a factor or factors capable of curing cancer may become available.

Blood Groups

Introduction

The membrane of the red cell is made of a mosaic of glycoproteins, lipoproteins, proteins with catalytic activities, receptors, and other proteins. At least some surface components of each of these proteins are potentially antigenic. The mosaic varies with the individual phenotype. Therefore, the population of surface antigens on the red cell varies considerably. Some membrane components may be expected to be more antigenic than others and thus may be more important in the immunological reaction elicited by red cell administration. This antigenic property of the red cell has so long prevented the therapeutic use of blood transfusions. Consequently, the probability that an incompatible transfusion will lead to hemolysis depends on: (1) the frequency of a particular blood group antigen in a population considered, and (2) the potency of the antigens.

We will principally consider the ABO and Rh systems [154, 155].

Although blood transfusions were attempted in the 16th and 17th centuries, the response of patients to early blood transfusions was unpredictable. Rarely did the patients benefit from the transfusion; in most cases the host reacted to the donor's red cells by killing them. An immunological reaction toward the red cells was suspected. In 1900 Landsteiner discovered by testing red blood cells of one individual against the serum of others that the red cell carried an antigen A or an antigen B. Those carrying A had no antibodies to A in their serum but carried antibodies to B. A third group had neither antigens nor antibodies and were called O. In a fourth group, the red cells carried antigens A and B, but no antibodies were found in the serum. Although these are the major red cell antigens, other groups of antigens were found in the red cells—namely, the MN and the P group and the Rh group.

When rhesus red cells are injected into a rabbit, the rabbit makes antibodies against a special antigen in the rhesus red cell, now called the Rh antigen. When such anti-Rh serum was put in the presence of human red cells, the red cells of 85% of the individuals tested reacted with the antibody; such individuals are known as Rh-positive, the others are referred to as Rh-negative. In 1939 Levine and Stetson investigated the pathogenesis of a fetal death in a woman who had received a blood transfusion from her husband. He found that that woman's serum contained an antiserum that agglutinated her husband's red cells. When the woman's serum was tested against the red cells of a number of other individuals compatible with respect to the ABO system, it was found to agglutinate 80% of the red cells.

ABO(H) System

Three allelic genes determine the appearance of the ABO antigenic pattern at the surface of the red cell. I^A for antigen A, I^B for antigen B, and i for antigen O; I^A and I^B are apparently dominant to i. Thus, as Table 14-8 shows, six genotypes are possible, but only four phenotypes are detectable.

As mentioned, the serum contains the reciprocal antibody. The exact reason for the appearance of the antibody is not clear. The antibodies are absent during fetal life or at birth except for those that are contributed by contamination by the mother's blood. Such transfer is more common when the mother's phenotype is O.

Table 14-8. Genotypes and phenotypes of the ABO system

Genotype	Phenotype	
	Antigen in red cell	Antibody in plasma
I^AI^A [a]	A [a]	Anti-B
I^Ai		
I^BI^B	B	Anti-A
I^Bi		
I^AI^B	AB	None
ii	O (none)	Anti-A, anti-B

[a] A number of subclasses of the A antigen have been ignored for the sake of simplicity.

The antibody appears first at approximately 3 to 6 months of age, increases through adolescence, and then slowly decreases. These antibodies are usually of the IgM or IgG type (IgA antibodies have been described in the ABO system), and are therefore capable of fixing complement—a property indispensable for intravascular hemolysis.

Coombs' Reaction

Normally, when red cells are suspended in a saline solution, they are repelled by the negative surface charges and the ζ potential, the cloud of positive ions that surround each cell. To agglutinate cells, the antibody must span the gap between the cells or reduce it. IgM is large enough to span the cells. But for IgG to secure agglutination, the force of the ζ potential must be dissipated with polyvinylpyrrolidone, which generates an anisotropic medium, or be overcome by centrifugation. Such procedures are not rigidly specific or highly sensitive, especially in detecting Rh antigens. The Coombs' reaction deals with this problem in a different way, mainly by adding serum-containing antibodies prepared against the antibodies found at the red cell surface.

The test had been used before, but Coombs, Mourant, and Race rediscovered it and markedly improved upon it. Their finding is a landmark in immunology and immunopathology, and few discoveries have proved as effective in saving lives. They developed the test because a more sensitive method of detecting Rh antibodies was needed. Human serum is injected in a rabbit, and the rabbit builds antibodies to each of the antigenic proteins in the serum, including the globulins, thus including Rh or other antibodies. By reacting the red cell with antihuman antibody, the red cells absorb the antibodies at their surface; therefore, it is possible to determine what antibodies are at the red cell surface. The test can also be used against the patient's serum. The direct Coombs' reaction uses red cells, the indirect Coombs' reaction uses serum.

The direct test is thus used to detect antibodies that coat the patient's red cells, as in some hemolytic anemias of the newborn in which coating by maternal antibodies takes place *in utero*. The presence of the antibody can then be detected at birth on the red cells of cord blood.

The indirect test is used to detect special antibodies in the serum of transfusion recipients or of pregnant women.

H Gene and the Antigen Structure of the ABO System

In addition to the gene needed to express the A, B, and O phenotypes, the A, B, O systems require another gene for expression called the H gene. The H gene is needed because it provides the molecular scaffold on which either A or B antigenic determinants can be added. Thus, without H genes there can be no A or B antigens, and one may expect to find anti-H antibodies in the serum. The antigen was discovered by studying the red cells of O-type individuals. The red cell surface was found to contain an antigen related to the fact that these individuals were of the group O and the amount of the antigen was inversely proportional to the levels of A or B antigen.

The mode of inheritance of H genes is different from, and thus independent of, that of A, B, or O genes. Most of the world's population is homozygous for H, so their genotype is HH. The H gene produced is expressed in the phenotype, and no anti-H antibodies are found in the serum.

Some individuals, usually descendants of a high inbred group, lack the ABO(H) antigens altogether. They are usually referred to as the "Bombay type" because such types were first discovered among the Mahari-speaking people of India. Typical immunological reactions are (1) absence of A or B antigens; (2) lack of reaction of their red cells with anti-H antibody (which excludes the possibility of an O type); (3) high titers of anti-A, anti-B, and anti-H antibodies. (Clearly, only the blood of one Bombay type can be compatible with that of another Bombay type.) For these reasons, it was concluded that Bombay-type individuals lack the H gene and that their genotype is therefore hh.

On the basis of chemical studies of ABO(H) antigens, investigators developed a theory for the interrelationship between the I^A, I^B, ii, and H genes. The antigens are believed to be globosides (see Chapter 3), proteins, or lipoproteins to which oligosaccharides are attached. The oligosaccharides are believed to be tetrasaccharides composed of N-acetylgalactosamine, D-galactose, N-acetylglucosamine, and D-galactose.

The H gene codes for a fucosyl transferase, which places a DL-fucose residue on the terminal D-galactose of the globoside. The I^A gene codes for an N-acetylgalactosamine transferase, which places an additional N-galactosamine on the terminal D-galactose. The I^B gene instead produces a galactose transferase, which places an additional D-galactose on the terminal galactose (see Fig. 14-8).

Because they are gene products, one expects the ABO(H) blood types to remain constant throughout an individual's life. Yet occasionally blood type may change: A types may acquire B-type properties, and in some cases the ABO(H) system is weakened or lost. The former occurs when intestinal permeability is modified to permit the absorption of *E. coli* polysaccharides, which cross-react with the B antigen. The bacterial antigen is absorbed at the surface of the red cell and reacts with anti-B as well as anti-A sera.

The second instance has been observed in leukemic patients. The ABO(H) system is not restricted to red cells and we shall see later that sometimes the conversion of a normal into a cancer cell is associated with loss of ABO antigenicity.

It is also sometimes difficult to determine the red cell type of some patients with cancer of the stomach or pancreas. In these cases, the red cell is antigenic, but excessive amounts of antigen are released in the serum, which neutralizes the antiserum used in the test.

At least two pathological manifestations are associated with the existence of the ABO system: the transfusion reaction and immunization to ABO in the newborn [156].

When a patient with phenotype A is given blood from a patient with phenotype B, the recipient usually develops chills with fever, nausea, and vomiting. The donor's anti-A antibody reacts with the A antigen of the recipient's red cells. The antigen-antibody complex fixes complement, and vasoactive amines are released, and intravascular hemolysis takes place, usually resulting in a transient hemolytic anemia and oliguric state.

Of particular significance is the reaction sometimes observed when blood from an O, Rh-negative donor is given to recipients with phenotypes of the ABO group.

For a long time, O donors were considered universal donors and their blood was administered to any patient

Gene	*Product*
	Protein-N-acetylgalactosamine–D-galactose-N-acetylglucosamine–D-galactose (globoside)
H gene	Protein-N-acetylgalactosamine–D-galactose-N-acetylglucosamine–D-galactose/L-fucose/
I^A gene	Protein-N-acetylgalactosamine–D-galactose-N-acetylglucosamine–D-galactose/L-fucose-N-galactosamine/
I^B gene	Protein-N-acetylgalactosamine–D-galactose-N-acetylglucosamine–D-galactose/L-fucose–D-galactose

Fig. 14-8. H, I^A, and I^B genes coding for red cell antigen polysaccharide moieties

in an emergency. The principles behind such procedures were that the donor's red cells did not contain antigen and would therefore not be hemolyzed by the isoantibodies of the donor. These isoantibodies would be so diluted by the recipient's blood that their titer would be too low to yield a significant immunological reaction.

In practice, the administration of O blood to patients with high titers of anti-A or anti-B antibodies has resulted in intravascular hemolysis and sometimes in intravascular coagulation followed by fibrinogen, platelet, prothrombin, and factors V and VIII depletion. In these accidents due to "dangerous universal donors," the recipient's red cells are slowly and progressively destroyed.

ABO Incompatibility in the Newborn

Although the incidence of ABO incompatibility between mother and fetus is of the order of 20%, hemolytic disease attributable to such incompatibility occurs only in 0.5 to 3% of pregnancies. The antibodies elaborated against fetal antigens must be small enough to cross the placental barrier and must be able to fix complement to bring about isoimmunization of the newborn. Therefore, IgG types of antibodies are usually those involved in hemolytic anemia due to ABO incompatibility. It is therefore of interest that the anti-A and anti-B activities in the O group are due to 7S antibodies, whereas those of the B or A groups are of the IgM type and thus are too large to cross the placental barrier [157]. Consequently, if the mother's serum contains anti-A or anti-B antibodies (group O type) and the fetus' phenotype is A or B and the antibodies cross the placenta, the red cells of the fetus will be destroyed primarily through an extravascular process with a concomitant hemolytic anemia.

The trophoblast constitutes the main immunological barrier between mother and fetus. Because it is antigenically inert and therefore cannot be destroyed by the mother's antibodies, it is, indeed, deprived of histocompatibility and A, B, and (H) antigens. The endothelium of the blood vessels of the chorion and the chord seems to contain only H antigens [158].

RH System

After Levine and Stetson's observation, a study of the blood groups of individuals in New York City revealed that 85% were Rh positive.* In other words, their red cells were agglutinated by the serum of a rabbit to which red cells of rhesus monkeys had been injected. The antigen on the red cell was referred to as the D antigen.

* It is now established that 15% of the population of Europe and the United States is Rh negative. The remainder is Rh positive, and 50% of them are homozygous for the Rh positive gene and 50% heterozygous.

It was further established that women who had recently delivered babies with erythroblastosis fetalis had anti-Rh antibodies (anti-D) in their sera. However, anti-D antibodies were not found in all women whose infants had hemolytic disease. Thanks to the development of more sensitive tests to detect antibodies by adding 22% albumin to the serum (which presumably dissipates the zeta potential), and later the Coombs' test, other antibodies were found which gave reactions similar but not identical to anti-D. The blood that reacted was Rh positive, but not D positive, and it reacted with 70% of the population. The new antibody was called anti-C.

Similarly, an anti-C antibody that agglutinates red cells of Rh-negative and D-negative individuals was discovered and was called anti-c. Later, two other antibodies were found, anti-E and anti-e.

The chemical structure of the Rh antigen remains unknown, but it is assumed that the antigen sites at the surface of the red cell are numerous (approximately 30,000 D sites for each cell).

To explain the mode of inheritance of the Rh factor, the Fisher-Race theory proposes that the Rh locus is made of a cluster of three closely associated genes referred to as Cc, Dd, and Ee (in at least one type of nomenclature). The three loci that carry the Rh antigen are so closely linked that they never separate during mitosis and meiosis and are therefore transferred "*en bloc*" from one generation to another. Theoretically, crossing over could occur during meiosis and be at the source of new combinations, but there is no evidence that this occurs with the Rh system. This is why one speaks of the "Rh complex." Thus, if one of the chromosomes of the pair carries DCc and the other dcc, the progeny will inherit either DCC or dcc from one parent, but no other combination.

Each locus will code for one gene, for example, C or its allele, c. Since the offspring inherits two chromosomes, the individual may be homozygous for the gene of a given locus (CC or cc) or heterozygous (Cc).

As we shall see, in histocompatibility antigens, some loci may have many alleles. In the Rh system, according to the Fisher-Race theory, there are few alleles on each loci. For example, for the locus of D, the alleles are D, d, and D^u. D^u is a variant of the D antigen, fairly common among blacks, yet not rare in whites. Similarly, the alleles for the C locus are C, c, C^W. The last is a variant of C. If we neglect the existence of D^u and C^w, eight different gene complexes can be possible theoretically; DCc, Dcc, DcE, DCE, dce, dCe, dcE, and dCE.

In contrast to what was observed with the ABO group, there is no dominance and each allele codes for its own antigen. Five antibodies have been found; anti-D, anti-C, anti-c, anti-E, and anti-e. Anti-D agglutinates only Rh-positive cells; anti-c agglutinates Rh-negative cells. The phenotype of D does not have C antigen and is designated as cD. In contrast, phenotype c has no D antigen and is designated as Cd. However, no antiserum will agglutinate d cells.

Two other antibodies directed toward the alleles E and e antigens have also been discovered. Since these basic antigenic systems—Cc, D, and Ee—are always inherited together in fixed combinations, they must, as already pointed out, be alleles of a single gene. The Rh locus is believed to consist of a cluster of three closely associated genes, Cc, Dd, and Ee. Of course, other nomenclatures are also in use.

Thus, according to the Fisher-Race theory, the antigenic properties of the red cells can be predicted as in Table 14-9.

Table 14-9. Antigenic properties of red cells

Gene complex	Antigen	Gene complex	Antigen
Dcc	DCc	dcc[a]	cc
DCc	Dcc	dCc	Cc
DcE	DcE	dCE	CE
DCE	DCE		

[a] Thus, the gene for d is not expressed in the phenotype and is therefore an "amorph."

Weiner has proposed a different genetic mechanism to explain the Rh phenotype. In his view, instead of three linked genes, only one gene on each locus of the chromosome determines the Rh phenotype. Of course, the two genes are alike in the homozygous and differ in the heterozygous. Each gene is represented by multiple alleles. The eight major ones are referred to as R^0, R^1, R^2, R^3, r, r^1, r^2, and rY. Each allele can code for a specific antigen.

Clearly, we are dealing here with a complex mode of gene expression in mammalian cells in which the appearance of one gene in the phenotype is linked to that of others by molecular mechanisms still unknown. Whether any of the theories proposed above will survive a detailed description of the molecular events in gene expression is hard to predict because in each one a structure of the genotype is extrapolated by observing the phenotype. Yet, the genetic models have proved most useful in detecting Rh positive and Rh negative blood types; therefore, the models continue to be needed. The identification of Rh positive–Rh negative individuals is, indeed, of considerable practical significance in preventing erythroblastosis fetalis and transfusion accidents.

A genetic model for Rh blood group systems based on the operon theory has been proposed. It is, however, too early to evaluate its meaning [159].

As will become obvious, the identification of the Rh type is of capital significance for predicting and preventing erythroblastosis fetalis. For the purpose of identifying the Rh genotype, one first determines whether the type is Rh positive or negative.

This is achieved with anti-D serum since a woman who is deficient in D antigen will most frequently have blood that contains high titers of anti-D antibody. Similarly, an Rh-negative recipient who receives Rh-positive blood will most often produce anti-D antibodies.

In a second step, the father's genotype must be determined so that the couple's chance of having an Rh-negative baby can be estimated.

In an Rh-negative individual (D-negative), both inherited Rh chromosomes code for the d gene, and the individual must be homozygous. If he is Rh positive, both chromosomes carry the D gene or one carries the D and the other d. If the father is DD and the mother dd, the father can transmit only a D gene and all his descendants will be Rh positive. If, in contrast, he is heterozygous, there is a 50% chance that the fetus will receive d chromosomes from both the father and mother.

In addition to those of the ABO and the Rh systems, a large number of other antigens can cause transfusion accidents or isoimmunization in the fetus. They won't be reviewed here because the principles of the pathogenesis of those types of diseases are clearly illustrated by outlining the risk involved with the ABO and the Rh systems.

Erythroblastosis Fetalis

The actual incidence of erythroblastosis is about 10% of what could be expected on the basis of calculations. Twenty per cent of the potential cases of erythroblastosis are cancelled out because of ABO protection.

Ordinarily, ABO incompatibility occurs only when the mother has anti-A or anti-B immunoglobulins of the IgG type and the offspring is A_1 or B type. The mother is usually of the O type because the incidence of IgG-type immunoglobulins is more frequent among the O type but the ABO system does in some ways protect against autosensitization of the mother against the fetal red cells. Thus, if A or B fetal red cells cross the placental barrier and enter the mother's blood even in large amounts and the mother is of the opposite type (B or A), she will have anti-A or anti-B antibodies that will neutralize the fetal red cells. Sometimes this protective mechanism breaks down. If the red cells of the fetus are of the same ABO group as the mother or of the O group, then they are not destroyed by the mother's anti-A or anti-B antibodies. They may survive or be sequestered in the spleen, an immunocompetent organ, and become antigenic in other ways—especially if the mother is Rh negative (Rh^-) and the fetus is Rh positive (Rh^+).

Protection by the ABO system is not the only mechanism by which potential erythroblastosis is cancelled out. Some Rh mothers do not make antibodies against the Rh^+ red cells of the fetus, or the amount they make is too little to cause disease of the fetus.

The time at which the red cells of the fetus enter the maternal blood is still debated [160]. At first it was believed that it occurred primarily during parturition. But only a small number of mothers whose infants have erythroblastosis have massive hemorrhage at delivery, so it cannot be excluded that transplacental hemorrhages during the earlier stages of pregnancy might also be responsible for the isoimmunization of the mother. Moreover, 1 ml of blood is enough to induce isoimmunization.

The leaking of the Rh^+ antigen in the blood of an Rh^- mother, either during pregnancy or during delivery, results in the building up of anti Rh^+ antibodies (IgG) in the mother. Such antibodies are harmless for the first born, but if a second Rh^+ fetus is conceived, the mother will cause the red cells of the fetus to hemolyze, and severe hemolytic anemia develops when the antibody binds to the red cell antigen unless the blood of the fetus is withdrawn and replaced by other compatible blood not containing the Rh^+ antibodies (exsanguination transfusion).

For a generation the therapy for Rh babies has been based on exsanguination transfusion. More recently, the incidence of erythroblastosis fetalis has been reduced markedly by the administration of small amounts of incomplete anti-D γ-globulins [161, 162].

In conclusion, erythroblastosis fetalis is a form of host-versus-graft reaction. Antigens from the Rh^+ fetus pass the placental barrier and immunize the Rh^- mother, who elaborates anti-Rh^+ IgG. These immunoglobulins are returned to the fetus, where they combine with red cell antigens and cause hemolysis. For further information on Rh immunization and its prevention read Woodrow [163]. The pathogenesis of erythroblastosis fetalis is shown in Fig. 14-9.

We have restricted this discussion on neonatal isoimmunization to that against red blood cell antigens, but isoimmunization—especially in the newborn—has been described against leukocytes causing neutropenia with sepsis and platelets causing blood coagulation defects [163].

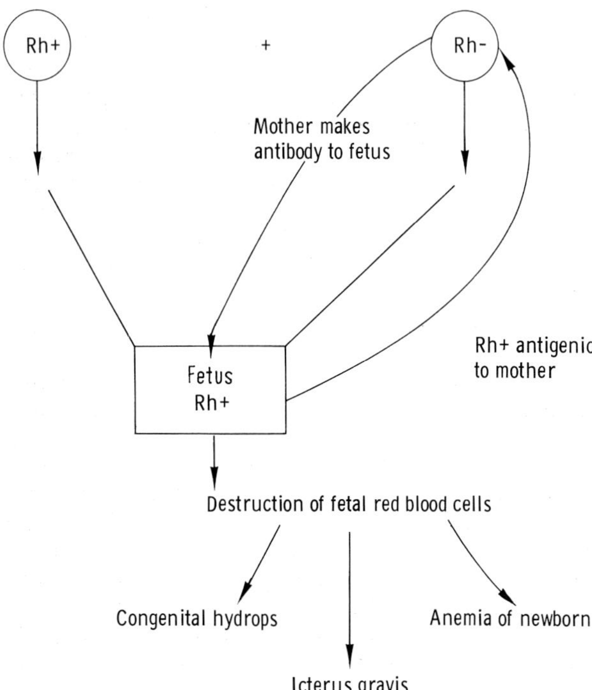

Fig. 14-9. Pathogenesis of erythroblastosis fetalis

Histocompatibility

Clearly, the immune reaction of the host versus the graft is aimed at antigens carried by the graft cells. Most of these antigens are believed to exist at the cell surface. Little is known of these antigens in the normal cellular state because whatever has been extracted has been done so with such drastic methods (sonication, protease treatment, etc.) that it is not certain that the antigenic preparation is representative of the *in vivo* cellular components. Nevertheless, some of these antigens are known to contain lipids, proteins, and carbohydrates, and it seems established that the major determinants are proteins. It is also likely that *in vivo* these antigenic components constitute important functional complexes of the cell membrane, for example, in cell transport.

Antigens are products of cell metabolism. The lipid and polysaccharide structures are determined by the cell's enzyme mosaic, which is a function of gene expression, and obviously all proteins are directly coded for by the DNA and mRNA of these cells. Therefore, it seems obvious that (1) the distribution of the antigens will follow the mendelian laws of genetics, and (2) variation of the antigenic profile will be less in related than in unrelated individuals.

But even if the antigen's molecular structure is unknown, it should be possible to determine how these antigens are inherited, provided that adequate tests for antigenicity are available. Empirical experiments in skin grafting and transplantation in humans and animals suggested that a combination of antigens that existed at the surface of the transplant itself or on lymphocytes must be considerable because only isogenic grafts or autografts would succeed. Such observations can theoretically be interpreted in two ways: each antigen is dictated by a single gene located on a different chromosome or at some variable distance on the chromosome, or histocompatibility is determined by a few genes existing in many allelic forms, as in the ABO and Rh blood group systems [164–172].

By controlled inbreeding, one can obtain strains of mice that differ by only one gene. Such mice are called coisogenic. If that gene codes for an antigen recognized as foreign by the lymphocytes of the other inbred strain, grafts between individuals of coisogenic strains will be rejected. Thus, lymphocyte injections, skin grafts, and even organ transplants in inbred mice have permitted investigators to define the genetic makeup of the histocompatibility antigen. In mice, it was discovered that the loci were indeed numerous—they totalled 15 and 2 of them were related to the sex chromosome, so they are referred to as H_1 to H_{13}, and H_Y and H_X. The H stands for histocompatibility. But during these studies it became obvious that some histocompatibility genes coded for antigens capable of eliciting much more powerful immunological responses than antigens coded by other histocompatibility genes; therefore, a distinction was made between major and minor histocompatibility genes. It was further discovered that the immune response elicited by antigens coded for by minor loci was much easier to suppress by immunosuppressive agents.

Mouse germ cells contain one major histocompatibility locus, the H_2 locus. Thus, an individual mouse inherits an H_2 locus from each parent, and these loci are codominant. In other words, the antigens coded for by the individual locus inherited from each parent will be expressed in the progeny. However, it is not unusual for a locus to code for a number of different polypeptides that are mutually exclusive (see ABO and Rh systems). Such polymorphism of the H_2 system is at the source of multiple antigenic combinations.

In all species studied, the major histocompatibility antigens are coded for by a small region of an autosomal chromosome. The loci are called AgB in the rat, SL-A in the pig, DL-A in the dog, Rh L-A in the rhesus monkey and HL-A in man.

In humans, inbreeding cannot be practiced at will, so the typing of cellular antigens has to be based on a different approach. The fetus inherits some histocompatibility antigens from the father and others from the mother. Any antigen the fetus possesses that is different from that which exists on the mother's cells elicits an immunological response in the mother. Therefore, the blood of a multiparous mother contains antibodies to several histocompatibility antigens present on the cells, including lymphocytes of her different children. Now, if one exposes this serum to lymphocytes of a broad panel of individuals, ultimately all antibodies found in the mother's blood will react with the proper antigen.

One can imagine that with the appropriate detective approach, it is possible to prepare monospecific sera that will react with only one of the antigens in the leukocytes of some of the offspring. Similarly, antibodies to the histocompatibility antigens will be found in the sera of persons who have received multiple transfusions. At present, much of the sera used is prepared by deliberately immunizing the donor against specific antigens.

For a long time only cumbersome biological tests were available to type the lymphocytes of various human individuals. But once specific antisera became available, two major types of assays were used: one involved leukoagglutination and proved to be easy but unspecific and therefore unreliable, and another involved lymphocytotoxicity. After it was miniaturized by Terasaki and McClelland [173], the latter assay became the test of choice. In this test, the target cell reacts with specific cytotoxic antibodies, complement is added, and cellular death is determined by uptake of vital dyes, release of fluorescent material, changes in cell morphology, or release of radiolabel from target cells.

Workers in laboratories around the world attempted to type human histocompatibility antigens. After a period of confusion, some clarification was achieved. This effort was an impressive illustration of what worldwide scientific communication and cooperation (in exchanging sera) can achieve to improve basic knowledge indispensable for the advance of medicine. After such consultations and exchanges, at least 30 antigens were identified.

In humans as in mice there are several histocompatibility systems: a major HL-A system and several minor systems. Fifteen to twenty identifiable antigens have been found in the HL-A system (see Fig. 14-10). The genes coding for this antigen are located on an autosomal chromosome in two different loci. Each locus codes for several mutually exclusive alleles. Consequently, since the somatic cell contains two chromosomes (one from the father and one from the mother) and since the expression of the gene coded for by each locus is codominant, each individual expresses at the most four antigens in the phenotype (see Figs. 14-11 and 14-12).

Individual antigens of the H_2 system have been isolated from papain-solubilized plasma membrane fractions. They have molecular weights of approximately 65,000, and the glycoproteins contain 3–5% neutral sugar, 1–4% glucosamine, 1–2% sialic acid. Inasmuch as further proteolytic digestion of the isolated antigen abolishes its antigenicity, the protein is believed to play a key role in antigenic determination. In contrast, most of the sialic acid, 70% of the galactose, and 25% of the galactosamine can be removed without affecting antigenicity.

Human HL-A antigens obtained by papain solubilization of spleen cell membrane yield glycoproteins. Immunological studies suggest that the carbohydrate moiety is indispensable for antigenicity.

So much work has been done on histocompatibility antigens in mice and men that only highlights can be mentioned here. Suffice to emphasize 3 major points that were learned from these studies: (1) there is cross-reactivity between the HL-A antigens and some antigens in bacteria, some antigens obtained from different species, and among the histocompatibility antigens of the same individual; (2) a correlation exists

FIRST LOCUS	HL-Al, HL-A2 (Mac), HL-A3, HL-A9, HL-A10, HL-A11, W 28 (Da 15, Ba), W 19 (Da 22, CE 33, Ao 77, Da 25, Ao 28, Lc 26-1)
SECOND LOCUS	HL-A5, HL-A7, HL-A8, HL-A12, HL-A13, W 5 (Da 20, R), W 10 (BB, Te 60), W14 W 14 (Da 18, Maki), W 15 (Da 23, LND), W 17 (Mapi, Orl.), W 18 (Te 58), W 22 (AA, Bt 22), Da 24, Da 30, Da 31

Fig. 14-10. HL-A system in humans

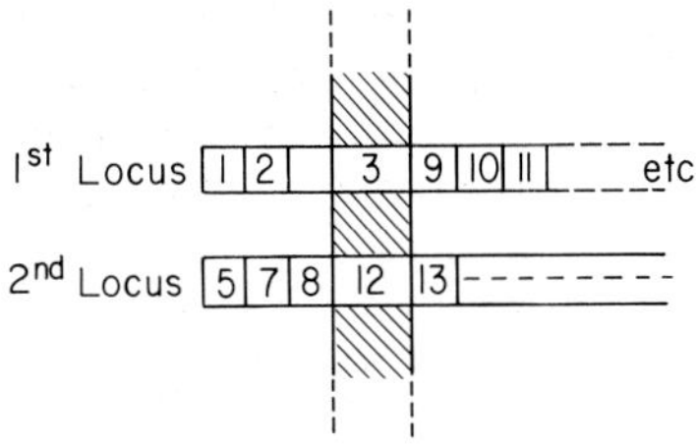

Fig. 14-11. Segments of a chromosome containing the 2 HL-A loci, which can be conceived of as 2 separate slots on the chromosome. A rule carrying a number of different genes represented by a number that is assigned to the allelic HL-A antigen can be slid through the slot. Clearly, although there is a wide choice of numbers for filling each slot, only 1 can fill each slot in a given chromosome. Therefore, in spite of the many allelic genes, only 2 per chromosome (4 per individual) can be expressed in the phenotype. But since there are so many alleles (at least 30), so many choices on the rule, the total antigenic combination is enormous (10,000)

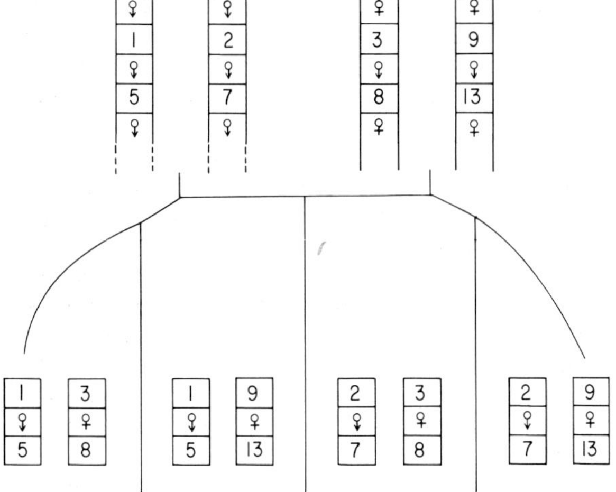

Fig. 14-12. Transfer of the parents' genotypes to the siblings

between the presence of HL-A antigens and the lymphocytes of the donor and graft rejection by the host; (3) some HL-A genetic patterns are more frequently associated with disease than others.

Cross-reactivity with antigens on bacteria indicates that man and bacteria may, under some circumstances, share the same antigen. If this is the only strong antigen carried by the bacteria or the parasite, the invader's survival is favored because it will be unable to elicit a proper immunological reaction. Therefore, the wide polymorphism of HL-A systems in humans may in some way have protected the race against bacterial destruction.

The study of cross-reactions between humans and other species may tell us about the phylogenic development of the HL-A system, but, more important, it will reveal which animals carry specific antisera that otherwise can be obtained only from human volunteers and are indispensable for leukocyte typing.

Most important of all is the relationship between the HL-A antigens and the transplantation antigens. Terasaki and Singal [164] have reviewed this correlation and have established that although takes are possible with unmatched individuals, the chances of take are better and the histological damage is reduced when the donor and the recipient are matched for the HL-A antigens. The typing of HL-A antigens on leukocytes or even kidney cells has become imperative as a preparative procedure for organ transplantation; the kidneys function better and the chances of survival are significantly increased. The original observations were confirmed in cases of both renal and bone marrow transplantation [174–181].

Walford and his colleagues [182] have summarized the medical application of blood typing. They include (1) typing of leukocytes for leukocyte transfusion; (2) typing of platelets for platelet transfusion; (3) attempts to correlate disease incidence—such as that of acute leukemia, chronic glomerulonephritis, sterility in man, and choriocarcinoma—with the antigenic cell type; (4) exclusion of paternity on the basis of cell types rather than on the basis of red blood cell antigenic groups.

The observation that some HL-A antigens are more frequently associated with disease has stimulated a great deal of interest [183–188]. In mice, it was observed that the histocompatibility pattern not only determined the immune response, but also correlated with the strain's susceptibility to leukemogenic viruses (see Table 14-10).

The findings made in rodents stimulated investigators to define the phenotype of patients with Hodgkin's disease or diseases with a suspected autoimmune pathogenesis; in some cases an unquestionable correlation between a prevalent phenotypic pattern and the incidence of the disease was established. The significance of the relationship between HL-A patterns and the incidence of a disease is not obvious. One possibility is that genes other than the HL-A gene, which in some way renders the individual more susceptible to that disease, are closely linked to a specific HL-A gene. A second possibility is that the presence of the antigen at the surface of some cells directly makes them more susceptible to the disease, in some cases by facilitating the binding of a virus, in others by facilitating viral infection because of cross-reaction between the HL-A and the viral antigen.

Table 14-10. HL-A specificity associated with some diseases

Celiac disease	HL-A1/HL-A8
Chronic autoimmune hepatitis	HL-A1/HL-A8
Childhood asthma	HL-A1/HL-A8
Hay fever	HL-A1/HL-A8
Herpetic dermatitis	HL-A1/HL-A8
Hodgkin's disease	HL-A1/HL-A8
SLE with dermatitis	HL-A8
Ankylosing spondylitis	HL-A27
Psoriasis	HL-A13, HL-A17
Myasthenia gravis	
in males with thymoma	HL-A3
in females with follicular lymphoid hyperplasia	HL-A8

Similarly, in celiac disease, it has been proposed that the presence of certain HL-A antigens on the cell surface facilitates the binding of gluten to cells that are then damaged as a result; or the antigens prevent the deployment of an immune response against gluten, which is left free to attack the cells because of cross-reaction between HL-A and gluten determinants.

HL-A antigens can be detected because they elicit the elaboration of specific antibodies in the serum. However, some histocompatibility antigens could trigger a cellular rather than a humoral immune response. The mixing of lymphocytes from unrelated individuals mutually stimulates each to grow. Such mutual stimulation does not occur if the lymphocytes are obtained from identical twins. On the basis of this finding, a team of Wisconsin investigators devised a new test called the mixed-lymphocyte culture test, which will provide a more sensitive measure of histocompatibility in man. The test can be used to detect siblings whose lymphocytes do not, when mixed, stimulate each other to divide.

Immunological Response Against Infection by Bacteria, Viruses, and Parasites

Before we consider immunological disease, it might be appropriate to view panoramically the mechanisms the human organism devises to protect itself against infections by bacteria, viruses, and parasites. The first line of defense is the tegumenta of the skin and the gastrointestinal, respiratory, and genitourinary tracts. Those epithelia protect the organism through the continuity of their cellular structures and also through their secretions, the movement of cilia, and other mechanisms. For example, the skin harbors a number of bacteria, some of which may be lodged deep in the glandular structures. However, the skin is protected against bacterial growth by its low pH (3.5–5.8), which is caused by the lactic acid of sweat and the organic acids elaborated by bacteria. The mucosa of the gastrointestinal and the respiratory tracts secretes IgA antibodies, which contribute to the local defense against bacterial invasion. Phagocytes may appear at some mucosal surfaces. They may digest the bacteria, but occasionally they are unable to kill them and carry the bacteria inside the tissues. Urinary pH and the constant flushing of the bladder prevent bacterial growth in the urine below the ureterovesical junction (urine is sterile above that junction). The eyes are protected against bacterial growth through the secretion of tears, which contain several antibacterial substances including lysozymes.

When these barriers fail, bacteria, viruses, or parasites enter the tissues and many additional defense mechanisms are put in gear. Many of these defenses have been described in detail, including: (1) inflammation, (2) elaboration of humoral antibodies, and (3) cellular immunity. We will consider here only the immunological defense mechanisms.

Immunological defenses against bacteria* consist of neutralization of toxins, elaboration of antimicrobacterial antibodies that combine with complement, opsonization, and production of cellular immunity. Several bacteria—such as streptococci and those that cause diphtheria and tetanus—produce toxins (see Chapter 16). Usually, these toxins are proteins, so they can mount immunological reactions. The toxin is then neutralized by direct combination with the antibody. By altering the toxin so that it is no longer toxic but is still immunogenic, the antibody confers active immunity against the toxin to the organism.

Gram-negative bacteria are destroyed by an antibody-complement reaction that damages the bacterial wall. The most effective antibodies are of the IgM type, although a complement-antibody reaction can also occur with IgA and IgG. Opsonins are antibodies that coat bacteria and facilitate their phagocytosis.

The role that delayed hypersensitivity plays in bacterial infection is not clear. Tuberculosis is a good example of the problem. Protection against the spreading of tuberculosis involves the formation of humoral antibodies, the transformation of the appropriate cell type into epithelioid and giant cells to form the granuloma, and cellular immunity. Only the last is considered here.

The role of cellular immunity in protection against chronic bacterial infections, especially tuberculosis, although under investigation for many years is still not clarified. Tuberculosis differs from many bacterial infections in that the bacteria proliferate and disperse slowly (except maybe in newborn children who are exposed to parent tuberculosis). It has been estimated that tuberculous bacilli reproduce in 1 day, whereas the typhoid bacillus reproduces in only 30 minutes. The structure of the wall of Koch's mycobacterium is also somewhat special in that instead of being made of polysaccharides and proteins, it is composed of a waxy substance that is much less antigenic than the typical polysaccharide-protein complexes. This waxy structure renders the bacteria somewhat resistant to phagocytosis and slows the diffusion of food within the bacterial cells.

Two observations demonstrate the ability of the organism to mount an immune defense reaction against tuberculosis. Koch found that guinea pigs infected with the mycobacteria exhibit a much more violent local reaction than noninfected animals to tuberculous bacilli administered intradermally. However, the second infection does not spread and the local lesion rapidly heals. In the past, a large number of children developed a small focus of pulmonary tuberculosis with concomitant infection of the mediastinal node; frequently, this first infection healed leaving a stellate scar in the lung and a calcified node in the mediastinum. The combination is called the Ghon complex.

---

* The mode of immunity established against bacteria is often not clearly understood. A case at point is gonorrhea, which elicits the elaboration of IgA antibodies in the urethral mucosa, the formation of serum antibodies, and, in gonorrheic patients exposed to *Neisseria gonorrhoeae*, blastogenesis of the lymphocytes. Still this immune response cannot effectively prevent reinfection [189].

Although the tuberculous bacilli might be sequestered in the scars, reinfection was rare.

A major question raised by the protection against tuberculosis is whether bacterial proliferation is prevented by humoral or cellular immunity. Clearly, the response to tuberculin injection invokes cellular immunity, but it is not certain that this reaction to tuberculin is beneficial to the host (see below). Moreover, there is some evidence that cellular immunity is not required to establish resistance to tuberculosis. Thus, already in 1925 Negra and Bouquet demonstrated that a methanol extract of tuberculous bacilli confers resistance without delayed sensitivity, and later it was shown that the injection of some bacillar extracts could lead to tuberculin reactivity without resistance.

Although these experiments suggest that cellular immunity is not indispensable for resistance against tuberculosis, they do not exclude the possibility that it may play a role. In support of such a notion is the fact that macrophages prepared from the peritoneal cavity of tuberculous animals are much more effective in destroying the infectious organism than macrophages from noninfected animals. But the macrophages' enhanced phagocytic ability is not restricted to tuberculous bacilli and therefore is not specific. Nevertheless, it is believed that the macrophages do not develop an enhanced phagocytic ability unless a highly specific cellular immune response has taken place before the macrophages are activated. Thus, it would appear that lymphocytes are first sensitized to tuberculin and then in some way the lymphocyte communicates with macrophages and brings them to proliferate and to increase their ability to phagocytize bacteria in general (possibly by activating the digestive enzymes in the cytoplasm).

Also, to what degree is the cellular immunity mounted against tuberculin responsible for cellular damage? When tuberculous bacilli are administered to two different strains of mice—one with high resistance and high tuberculin sensitivity, and the other with low resistance and low tuberculin sensitivity—only mice from the strain with high tuberculin sensitivity develop necrosis and inflammation. On the basis of these and similar experiments, investigators generally assume that the tuberculin reaction is largely responsible for the inflammatory reaction, excluding, of course, the granulomatous reaction, which seems to be elicited by the special properties of the bacteria.

Leprosy is another condition that illustrates the complexity of the immune response to bacterial infection. In the chapter on inflammation, we discussed the two forms of leprosy—tuberculoid and lepromatous. In the tuberculoid form, humoral antibodies are high and delayed sensitivity to lepronin is low; the reverse is true for the lepromatous form [190].

The barriers against bacteria also work against viruses [191, 192]. For example, the keratin layer of the skin needs to be intercepted to permit viral entry. Interference with mucus secretion or ciliary movement in the respiratory tract facilitates respiratory infection by viruses. A unique feature of the virus is that it must bind to surface receptors before entering the cell. If such surface receptors are missing, infection will not occur. Mice are not susceptible to the poliomyelitis virus because they do not have, in contrast to man, specific receptors to bind the virus to the cell surface.

The second line of defense against viral infection involves the macrophages, which act by their phagocytic and digestive properties. The first attack on the virus is believed to be mounted by local macrophages, such as those of the lung or the peritoneal cavity. Once the capacity of the local macrophage contingent is exhausted, the macrophages of the liver and spleen take over. If the macrophages kill the virus, antigens are released that permit successful immunization against a further attack. But sometimes the virus replicates in macrophages, and, as a result, the virus spreads to other tissues. Under such circumstances, if antibodies are elaborated against viral proteins, antigen-antibody complexes form, as in Aleutian mink disease (see below).

The third line of defense is the formation of mucosal and humoral antibodies. The oral administration of live polio vaccine elicits the appearance of IgA in the intestinal mucosa. The antibodies prevent viral penetration through the mucosa. In contrast, if dead vaccine is administered by inoculation, humoral antibodies—IgM and IgG—appear and primarily interfere with the spreading of the virus. Humoral antibodies prevent viremia: (1) directly by neutralizing the virus or (2) indirectly by killing the infected cells, probably by inducing the formation of antigen-antibody complexes that activate complement. The antigen-antibody complexes can in turn cause vasculitis and glomerulonephritis.

The immune response can also kill viruses indirectly by destroying the infected cells. However, the host may destroy itself in the process. When mice are infected with choriomeningitis virus [193, 194], the infection is not apparent until the sixth day, which is also when the immune response is elicited. That the damage is caused essentially by the immune response is demonstrated in an experiment in which animals are irradiated before infection. Whereas nonirradiated, infected animals have symptoms of choriomeningitis, the irradiated immunosuppressed animals do not. It is believed that by attaching to the cell membrane, the virus modifies its structure and makes it antigenic. As a result, the T-lymphoid cells mount an immune response against the infected cells, which are ultimately destroyed. Experiments in tissue cultures with mumps and choriomeningitis viruses support these assumptions. If virus-infected cells are put in the presence of lymphocytes obtained from an animal immunized against that virus, the lymphocytes destroy the infected cells.

In many viral infections, a cellular immunity response is elicited against the host cell, as in a host-versus-graft reaction; but the mechanism by which this autoimmune response is elicited is not clear. A number of possibilities can be considered, among them: (1) viral modification of the cell membrane's

Table 14-11. Immunodeficiency diseases

Name	Synonyms	Mode of inheritance	Onset	Cell-mediated immunity	Humoral immunity
Reticular dysgenesis	DeVaal and Seynhaeve syndromes	Unknown			
Third and fourth pharyngeal pouch syndrome	Digeorge's syndrome			Markedly reduced	Normal
Thymic hypoplasia and hypothyroidism				Defective	
Thymic aplasia and lymphopenia (2 types)	1. X-linked lymphoplasia 2. Swisstype agammaglobulinemia	1. X-linked occurs only in women 2. Autosomal recessive		Defective	All γ-globulins reduced
Thymic dysplasia		Autosomal recessive		Diminished	Normal immunoglobulin
Immunological deficiencies	Nezelof's syndrome when associated with thymic dysplasia, lymphopenia and agammaglobulinemia			Variable pattern of immunodeficiencies; may resemble recessive form of thymic aplasia with lymphopenia and agammaglobulinemia or predominantly cell-mediated immunity defect	
Combined IgA and IgG deficiency	Dysgammaglobulinemia type 1			Normal	IgA and IgG low or absent; IgM increased
Combined IgA and IgM deficiency	Dysgammaglobulinemia type 2	Sex-linked recessive, thus seen in men only	Infancy	Normal	IgA and IgM decreased IgG normal
IgA-IgM deficiency with nodular lymphoid hypoplasia				Normal	IgM and IgA decreased
Selected IgA deficiency				Normal	Low IgA
Selected IgG deficiency				Normal	Low IgG
Selected IgM deficiency	Wiskott-Aldrich syndrome	Sex-linked recessive	At birth	Normal	Low IgM

Blood lymphocytes	Phytohemagglutinin stimulation	Sensitivity to infection	Other	Pathology	Pathogenesis
				Absence of lymphoid tissue	Agenesis of the anlage of white cell
Normal	Reduced		Parathyroid agenesis ↓ Hypoparathyroidism ↓ Hypocalcemia		Defect in development of the third and fourth pharyngeal pouches
			Hypothyroidism; antithyroglobulin antibodies		Defect in the embryonic development of the second and third pharyngeal pouches; thymic hypoplasia with secondary destruction of thyroid through autoimmune process
Low	Reduced	Fail to thrive from birth; sensitive to infections	Hemolytic anemia; uremic syndrome	Thymic aplasia with absence of Hassall's corpuscles	
		Miscellaneous; terminal event is often a wasting disease similar to that seen in neonatally thymectomized mice		No lymphocyte in lymphoid tissue; normal plasma cells; small thymus difficult to identify; no corticomedullary differentiation; no Hassall's bodies	
			Fine hair, lost early; erythroderma; ichthyosis; short-limbed dwarfism; ectodermal dysplasia		
		Susceptible to respiratory infections	Lymphadenopathy, hepatosplenomegaly	Plasma cell "normal," but IgM-containing plasma cells predominate	
		Increased sensitivity to infection			
			Spruelike symptoms	Lymphoid hyperplasia with enlarged lymphoid follicles within the lamina propria	Lymphoid hyperplasia may result from overcompensation
			Malabsorption; IgA deficiency may exist in association with ataxia telangiectasia	Less numerous lymphoid follicles and germinal centers in peripheral lymphoid tissue; reduction in IgA-producing plasma cells	
Cyclic leukopenia		Increased susceptibility to infection	May be associated with Down's syndrome		
Lymphopenia		Increased susceptibility to infection	High incidence of lymphoreticular malignancies, eczema, thrombocytopenia; causes bleeding and splenomegaly	Depletion of small lymphocytes in thymus, lymph nodes; plasma cell normal	

Table 14-11 (continued)

Name	Synonyms	Mode of inheritance	Onset	Cell-mediated immunity	Humoral immunity
Ataxia telangiectasia		Autosomal recessive	Not known whether they exist at birth or develop after birth; children usually normal during first year	Diminish response to DNCB; persistence of skin homograft	Varies considerably from patient to patient; 80% have low IgA, low IgE, low or normal IgG, normal IgM
Primary agammaglobulinemia (2 types)	1. Bruton's type 2. Acquired	1. X-linked recessive 2. Unknown but likely autosomal recessive	1. First 2 years 2. Adult	Normal, including allograft rejection	Deficiency in all immunoglobulins (IgG, IgA, IgE, IgM, IgD)

permeability, and release of antigen that is otherwise inaccessible to the immune response; (2) viral modification of the cell membrane's antigenic properties—as a result, the cell membrane becomes antigenic to its own lymphocytes; (3) cross-reaction between viral and cell membrane antigens, so that the antibodies produced attack the normal tissues; (4) viral induction of an abnormal immune response of T lymphocytes, which become unable to recognize the self.

Clearly, the immunological reaction mounted against the virus can be deleterious to the host. A typical example of such a reaction is Aleutian mink disease [195]. The disease is caused by a virus which, although it proliferates rapidly, persists for a long time and causes slow, progressive pathological manifestations. The infected animal develops plasmacytosis with monoclonal gammopathy. The accumulating gammaglobulins are believed to be antibodies to some viral antigen. A circulating virus is found in the form of an antigen-antibody complex. The complex accumulates in the blood vessel, activates complement, causes vasculitis on the surface of the glomerular membrane, and causes glomerulonephritis. For reasons unknown, intrahepatic bile ducts frequently proliferate.

The role that immune reactions mounted against viral infections play in the pathogenesis of human diseases is not known. Such a pathogenic mechanism has been suspected in serum hepatitis and a number of autoimmune diseases, such as rheumatoid arthritis and lupus erythematosus.

Various examples of the interactions between the immune system and viruses are described in other chapters.

On the basis of what has been said about the immunological reactions mounted against bacterial and viral infections, it is almost a "La Palissade" to say that little is known about the immune reaction mounted against more complex parasites. Fascinating as the molecular properties of parasites may be, we must resist describing them here; the reader is referred to specialized texts on the matter [196]. Suffice it to point out that animal parasites are often multicellular organisms with complicated cellular architecture, unique metabolism, and a life cycle during which material is often shed or secreted. Hence, the antigenic population of parasites far exceeds that of bacteria and viruses; consequently, one may anticipate that the immunological reaction will also be complex. It will involve the formation of cytophilic antibodies, humoral antibodies, and macrophage immunity.

Immunodeficiency Diseases

The immune response results from the elaboration of a number of complex molecules (antibodies, factors, complement, etc.) that interact closely and are formed in a variety of cells whose cooperation is often needed to elaborate one or many macromolecules. Any tampering by nature or man with the delicate interaction distorts the immune response, often causing disease.

Immunopathology includes the study of: immunodeficiency diseases; overreactions or undesirable reactions referred to as immediate and delayed hypersensitivity; diseases in which the distinction between self and non-self has been lost (autoimmune diseases); and the uncontrolled hyperplasia of antibody-producing diseases, such as myelomas of hypergammaglobulinemia [197–201].

The immunodeficiency diseases are of two major types: inherited, or primary, and acquired, or secondary, immunodeficiency. The hereditary immunodeficiencies may exist in isolation or may be associated with other congenital anomalies, such as absence of the thyroid, telangiectasia, and thrombocytopenia.

The clinical and anatomicopathological manifestations are usually determined by the type of deficiency. Defects that primarily concern the thymus abol-

Table 14-11 (continued)

Blood lymphocytes	Phytohemagglutinin stimulation	Sensitivity to infection	Other	Pathology	Pathogenesis
	Reduced	Repeated bacterial infection of the respiratory tract	Progressive ataxia observable when the child first walks; telangiectasia of conjunctiva, face (butterfly area), ears, neck; gonadal dysgenesis	*Thymus*—small thymus, lymphodeficiency, absence of Hassall's bodies; poorly developed lymphoid tissue with decreased plasma cells, increased stromal cells; *Brain*—degeneration of Purkinje cells, increased tortuosity of cerebral vessels; *Skin*—dilated veins with telangiectasia	Failure of mesenchymal tissue development
Cyclic leukopenia		Low titer of antibodies after infection; high susceptibility to all kinds of infection	Association with autoimmune disease in adult form	Absence of germinal centers and plasma cells even after antigenic challenge; normal thymus	

ish cellular immunity. The patient cannot be sensitized with contact antigens such as dinitrobenzene, he is not able to reject allographs, and he is unusually susceptible to fungus infections.

Defects in the lymphoid system programming for immunoglobulin synthesis lead to the absence of one or more immunoglobulins, which may be associated with lymphoid tissue hypertrophy. In IgG and IgM deficiencies, the victim is usually highly sensitive to infection. Defects restricted to IgA do not necessarily lead to severe clinical symptoms except for steatorrhea in some cases. The lipid malabsorption is believed to result from the immunoglobulin defects.

A detailed description of all types and anatomicopathological manifestations of immunological deficiences is beyond the scope of this book. We shall present two typical defects—one resulting from the absence of the thymus, the other from the inability to synthesize immunoglobulin. The other characteristics of immunological deficiences are summarized in Table 14-11.

Third and Fourth Pharyngeal Pouch Syndrome

Third and fourth pharyngeal pouch syndrome results from a defect in the development of the embryonic anlage of the thymus and the parathyroid glands—the third and fourth pharyngeal cleft pouches. The disease manifests itself by an immunological defect and hypoparathyroidism. Only the immunological defects will be discussed.

Clinical manifestations include reduced delayed hypersensitivity and an inability to transform or stimulate lymphocytes *in vitro*. The lymphocyte count in the blood and the immunoglobulin levels in the serum are usually normal. Yet patients respond inadequately to antigenic stimulation. The pathogenesis of the disease is not known.

The immunological defects of third and fourth pharyngeal pouch syndrome can be corrected by thymus transplantation. After transplantation, the patient who was insensitive to the NFB antigens quickly becomes sensitive, and close examination of the responding cells demonstrates that they carry the donor's chromosome markers (for example, male). It has therefore been proposed that the defect is not in recognition or processing of antigen, but in the cell-mediated immune response.

An understanding of the pathogenesis of the Digeorge syndrome is further complicated by its association with other congenital anomalies, including a characteristic facies—low-set ears, shortened vertical groove of the median portion of the upper lip, small lower jaw, and cleft in the nose. Such patients also often have congenital anomalies of the heart and the great vessels.

Agammaglobulinemia

Primary agammaglobulinemia constitutes a family of immunodeficiency syndromes characterized by an absence of all major immunoglobulins (IgA, IgM, IgD, and IgE). Three factors modulate the clinical type: the mode of inheritance, the age of onset, and the coexistence of autoimmune disease. Two patterns of inheritance have been observed in patients with agammaglobulinemia, a sex-linked type (Bruton-type agammaglobulinemia) and an autosomal type. The sex-linked type usually is apparent at an early age; the autosomal may develop later, even in adulthood [202, 203]. (Because one can develop agammaglobulinemia at different ages, investigators distinguished a primary and acquired type of agammaglobulinemia. It is now believed that genetic defects are responsible for both types. But the reasons for late development in the adult type are unclear.)

In Bruton-type agammaglobulinemia, the patient, normal during the first month of age, becomes prone to a wide variety of infections as soon as the antibody reserves transferred from the mother are metabolized. Infections common to children (otitis, mastoiditis, etc.) occur repeatedly among children with agammaglobulinemia because they do not develop effective immunity. Infections that are rare in normal individuals occur more frequently in agammaglobulinemic individuals. For example, pneumocytosis carinii has been described among patients with agammaglobulinemia. Smallpox in these patients may lead to extensive and even gangrenous lesions. Vaccination against smallpox is often ineffective and may lead to serious complications, even death.

Nevertheless, the victim is not deprived completely of the ability to synthesize γ-globulin, despite the absence of the electrophoretic peak. More sensitive methods (immunological techniques) have demonstrated that about 1% of the total amount of antibodies synthesized in normal individuals is synthesized in patients with agammaglobulinemia.

The histological differences are few except for absence of plasma cells in all tissues and a reduced level of lymphocytes in the blood. Furthermore, the lymph nodes and spleen lose their ability to develop secondary follicles after antigen administration. Reticulum cells proliferate, probably as part of a compensatory mechanism. Insofar as agammaglobulinemic patients are acceptable recipients of homographs, the homotransplantation of lymphatic tissue was attempted and resulted in an increased rate of γ-globulin synthesis. The disease is best controlled by the administration of large doses of γ-globulin (especially during periods of epidemics) and by antibiotic therapy when infection has developed.

In agammaglobulinemia the immunoglobulin levels are low (less than 200 mg/ml), and there is a significant decrease in all immunoglobulin classes. However, cell-mediated immunity including allograft rejection is usually intact. The characteristics of some immunodeficiency diseases are summarized in Table 14-11.

Immunological Diseases

Allergy

In a previous section of this chapter, we described a number of experimental conditions in animals and humans that were typical of a mode of antigen-antibody reaction. These conditions included response to: homocytotropic antibodies, cytolytic antibodies, antigen-antibody complexes, and cell-mediated immunity. A large number of diseases, called hypersensitivity diseases, in humans result from the activation of one or more of these immunological types of reactions. However, because of the complexity of the antigenic stimulus in humans, a pure form of one type of reaction rarely develops; therefore, one must in each form of hypersensitivity attempt to separate the major form from the minor manifestations of the immunological reactions.

The term allergy was introduced by von Pirket, who studied reactions to repeated injections of antisera for diphtheria and scarlet fever. The word allergy comes from the two Greek words *αλλος εργον* and means changed activity. Therefore, generically the word should cover all forms of abnormal immunological responses. In practice, the word allergy primarily refers to those conditions in which specially sensitized individuals react to special antigens primarily by an acute inflammatory process usually of the catarrhal type. The reaction may occur in the skin (urticaria), in the respiratory mucosa (allergic rhinitis and bronchial asthma), or in the gastrointestinal tract.

In 1923 Coca and Cook coined the term atopic allergy to designate a group of diseases in which sensitization by the Prausnitz-Küstner reaction depended upon heredity rather than upon unusual (compared with that in nonsensitive individuals) exposure to the antigen. Coca listed the following characteristics for the disease: it appears spontaneously in the absence of a known sensitizing event; the disease is genetically determined; it is peculiar to the human species; and the skin of nonallergic recipients can be sensitized locally with the serum of affected individuals.

As knowledge of the mechanism of atopic disease developed, it became clear that the immune response is not spontaneous and that a sensitizing event must take place.

The antibodies involved in the reaction (as we have pointed out) are cytophilic antibodies (referred to as reagins) and are of the IgE type. However, not all atopic reactions are elicited by IgE types of immunoglobulins. Some involve the IgG class antibodies, and they are therefore classified as immune complex diseases. Urticaria, angiodermatitis, and gastrointestinal allergic reactions are probably immune complex diseases [204–206].

Allergens

The special antigens, called allergens, that induce immediate hypersensitivity are found in a wide variety of chemical forms. To date, no special molecular characteristics of allergens that distinguish them from other types of antigens have been discovered. The chemical characterization of allergens is difficult because allergens can be identified only by measuring their ability to cause an anaphylactic response. In allergic patients, antibodies can be found that react with several components of the allergenic substances. But as will be seen later, not all such antibodies are involved in the hypersensitive reaction. Those antibodies that are involved are difficult to assay *in vitro,* so the *in vitro* techniques are not effective for testing or isolating allergens. A common technique for testing allergens is skin testing, in which a small amount of the test substance is injected into the skin of an allergic patient. If he develops urticaria, this indicates the presence of the allergy. Although skin testing is the most popular method of testing allergens, it is costly and in some cases endangers the patient's health. When a complex chemical substance proves to be allergic, it is sometimes difficult to determine whether the reaction results from the presence of a chemical actually in the substance or from the metabolic conversion of one of the substances.

Pollen from ragweed and grass has been found to contain at least two and probably more allergens. The major allergenic component is a protein with a molecular weight of approximately 32,000–37,500. Traces of carbohydrates are associated with this protein, but apparently they do not contribute to the substance's allergenic activity. A minor allergenic component of pollen is a small molecule (mol wt 10,000). The allergens from grass pollen are extremely stable and withstand heat (100° C), treatment with acid bases (pH 3–10), and freeze drying. In contrast, ragweed allergens are stable only at pH 6–8.5 and are inactivated by freeze drying. As we shall see later, the responses of allergic patients to these two types of allergens vary considerably.

Before eliciting the vascular and cellular reactions that characterize an allergic reaction, allergens must penetrate the mucous membrane. The exact mechanism by which such large molecules (mol wt 32,000) can penetrate these membranes is not known, but two hypotheses have been postulated. One proposes that the molecules are broken down to smaller fractions before entering the mucous cell; the other suggests that the mucous membranes of allergic persons have permeability properties different from those of normal individuals.

Some allergens are haptenes (including many drugs or their chemically reactive derivatives). These are low molecular weight substances incapable of inducing an allergic response unless covalently bound to a host protein whose nature is often unknown.

Benzylpenicillin (penicillin G) [207] is one of the drugs studied extensively for hypersensitivity reactions. After penicillin G is administered, at least three haptenes appear, two of which have been identified (benzylpenicilloyl and benzylpenalmadic acids). Benzylpenicilloyl acid is a major haptenic determinant. It is attached to proteins through an amino group, and approximately 95% of the benzylpenicillin that reacts with tissue protein is conjugated in this fashion. A minor haptenic determinant, benzylpenalmadic acid, forms mixed disulfide groups that are attached to proteins via sulfhydryl groups.

Studies in patients allergic to penicillin have helped to determine which haptenes are important in penicillin allergy. The reaction measured by skin tests appears to be directed against the minor determinants rather than by BPO. Using a number of methods for testing antibodies in the sera of allergic patients, investigators discovered that both IgG and IgM classes of antibodies against BPO can be detected. Conclusive evidence that IgE antibodies against BPO develop is not available. This is significant because neither IgG nor IgM but only IgE is believed to be involved in anaphylactic hypersensitivity. In fact, the presence of excessive IgG or IgM may compete for antigens with IgE antibodies and block the skin test reaction. There is, however, evidence that some late-developing allergic response to benzylpenicillin might be due to a drop in titer of blocking anti-BPO antibodies with the emergence of skin-synthesizing antibodies of BPO specificity.

Haptenic determinants of drugs other than penicillin have not been identified. Many drugs probably are rendered allergenic by metabolic conversion *in vivo* to compounds reacting chemically with proteins. Thus, metabolic conversions leading to the formation of high reactive quinones, epoxides, thiols, and aldehydes have all led to the production of haptenes.

Allergic Rhinitis

Clinically, allergic rhinitis is characterized by itching of the nose, sneezing, nonpurulent rhinorrhea, and nasal stuffiness. This may or may not be associated with itching of the palate, pharynx, ear, and eyes [208, 209].

Some of the most common complications of rhinitis are headaches, principally over the bridge of the nose as a result of accompanying frontal sinusitis, and acute and chronic infections that may even involve the eustachian tubes and lead to chronic otitis with serious loss of hearing.

Whether allergic rhinitis is related to sinusitis and the development of nasal polyps has never been convincingly established, but polyps in patients with allergic rhinitis further obstruct the nasal passages, thus increasing the symptoms and the incidence of complications. In acute rhinitis, the local antigen-antibody reaction is believed to lead to the release of histamine or histaminelike factors that modify capillary permeability. Inasmuch as the submucosa of the nasal epithelium has a loose texture, fluid accumulation is prominent. Vasodilatation and edema are thus the hallmarks of allergic rhinitis. Histological examination of PAS-stained submucosa reveals a loss of stainability of the fundamental substance and the basal membranes.

In allergic rhinitis, the mucous and seromucous glands are distended, enlarged, and sometimes hyperplastic. Although there is no massive polymorphonuclear invasion, the presence of eosinophils is characteristic.

In addition to its olfactive role, the nasal mucosa heats, cleans, and humidifies inspired air. Air is heated primarily by transfer of heat from the blood circulating in the submucosal capillaries to the inspired air. The heating process is so effective that cold air inspired at 0° reaches the pharynx with a temperature between 36° and 37°. The water needed to humidify the air is derived primarily from circulating blood and secondarily from the mucus. Cleansing involves trapping of the larger particles by the coarse and stiff hairs of the nostrils and trapping of smaller particles in the mucus that coats the nasal passages.

Mucus is continuously drained from the nostrils into the pharynx because of the constant movement of the cilia at the surface of the epithelial cells. Bacteria are often killed in the mucus because of the low mucosal pH or because their walls are digested by lysozymes. In allergic rhinitis, the edema fluid of the mucosa dilutes the mucus, impairs the movement of the cilia, and therefore interferes with the cleansing function of the nasal mucosa. Such interference with the physiology of the nasal mucosa may well be responsible for the higher susceptibility to infection that is frequently observed in patients with allergic rhinitis.

Bronchial Asthma

The air that reaches the pharynx travels down the trachea and the smaller bronchi [209–211]. The tracheobronchial tree is lined with a pseudostratified epithelium composed of at least four types of cells: (1) tall, ciliated, columnar cells (270 cilia per cell); (2) groups of isolated goblet cells dispersed among the ciliate cells and secreting mucus; (3) ciliated serous cells between the goblet cells (electron microscopy reveals that the serous cells form close cytoplasmic contacts with the goblet cells, suggesting metabolic interaction between the two types of cells); and (4) short, basal cells that line a basement membrane.

Concentric with the epithelium are four layers: (1) a basal membrane composed of reticulum and collagen fibers; (2) a layer of collagenous tissue containing capillaries, lymphatics, and fine ramifications of nerves; (3) a mesh of smooth muscle cells that is distributed around the bronchial wall without forming a concentric ring; and (4) cartilage. Between the muscle and cartilaginous layers are deep bronchial mucus glands. From the larger bronchi to the bronchioles, the complexity of the epithelium is reduced. The smaller bronchioles are made of a columnar lining of cuboidal cells with few goblet cells or mucus-producing glands.

The air that flows from the pharynx down the trachea and the bronchial tree is not entirely free of particles. Whether such particles reach the smaller bronchioles depends on a number of physical properties of the environment, including the viscosity of the mucus and the density and the nature of the particles. In some cases, the particle is eliminated through phagocytosis by macrophages. In others, the particles are insoluble and remain in the lung for long periods or forever (see Table 14-12).

If the particles contain allergens, they may, in susceptible individuals, elicit bronchial asthma. Bronchial asthma results from airway obstruction due to constriction of the bronchioles associated with viscous mucus secretion. At first, airway obstruction leads to the distortion of some of the pulmonary physiology; this may be followed by anatomical changes in the

Table 14-12. Classes of allergens causing rhinitis or bronchial asthma

Seasonal	Pollens	Ragweed
		Trees
		Grass
	Spores	Molds
Perennial	House dust	
	Feathers	
	Danders	
	Bacteria ?[a]	
Occupational		
Dusts	Flour	
	Cottonseed	
	Flaxseed	
	Castor bean	
	Coffee bean	
	Grains	
Chemicals	Formaldehyde	

[a] The role of bacteria in triggering allergic rhinitis and asthma is disputed. Although no reagins (IgE antibodies) to bacteria have ever been detected, a simple vaccination or inhalation of bacterial aerosols can trigger an asthma crisis.

lung. We will describe the symptomatology of asthma, the respiratory changes in bronchial asthma, and the anatomical changes in bronchial asthma.

In the beginning of a crisis, asthmatics have no trouble inspiring air. The difficulty is with expiration. In a typical crisis, the patient sits with his trunk forward and arms elevated to shoulder level and expectorates blood-free sputum. The expiratory phase is prolonged, and this is associated with sibilant rales. The respiratory rate is usually close to normal, or only slightly accelerated, but if the crisis worsens the patient may have trouble inspiring air as well. Usually an asthma attack starts while the patient is at rest; he has a feeling of chest tightness and dizziness and starts sneezing, coughing, and sometimes expectorating sputum. In severe attacks, the chest is distended conspicuously and the patient may even become cyanotic. The patient often feels perfectly normal between attacks, but auscultation reveals sonorous, sibilant rales. The attack may last from a few minutes to an hour and sometimes days. At the end of an attack, some patients cough vigorously and expectorate viscous mucus. Anxiety or intensive work may exacerbate the wheezing, dyspnea, and cough.

On inspiration, the bronchi dilate and the thorax expands, thus generating a hypoatmospheric pressure on the alveoli and facilitating air flow. On expiration the bronchi contract slightly, and elastic recoil of the lungs forces the air from the alveoli into the trachea. Thus, air flows continuously from trachea to alveoli and from alveoli to trachea. Because the bronchi constrict, even in normal expiration, and because the thoracic muscles that contract during expiration are less powerful than those that work during inspiration, the difficulty in patients with bronchial constriction rests mainly with expiration. In other words, since the bronchi dilate during inspiration, there is little interference with air intake in the asthma attack, but because of increased constriction during expiration, resistance to flow develops during expiration and the patient traps some of the inspired air.

At the end of a normal expiration, all the air contained in the lungs is not expired, and the lung volume reaches what is called the resting respiratory level. Part of the air in the lung at the resting respiratory level can be exhaled by forced expiration, and another portion cannot be removed. The volume of the air exhaled after forced expiration is called the expiratory reserve volume. That portion that stays in the lungs is called the residual volume. As may be expected from what we said about the pathogenesis of asthma, the residual volume can be expected to be increased during an asthma attack.

At rest, a normal individual inhales 300–500 ml of air per inspiration. This is referred to as the tidal volume. But if one is forced to inspire to maximal lung capacity, he can inspire much more air. The total volume of air inspired under forced inspiration is called the vital capacity. The difference between the vital capacity and the tidal volume constitutes the inspiratory reserve volume. During an asthma attack, the vital capacity is reduced.

Both the vital capacity and the residual volume return to normal as the patient recovers from his attack spontaneously or as a result of therapy, provided, of course, that no anatomical complications have set in.

After inspiration is completed, a normal person exhales 83% of the exhalable air during the first second, and 94% and 97% during the second and third seconds, respectively. In patients with asthma, the time needed to exhale similar amounts of exhalable air is markedly increased. As the residual volume increases, CO_2 tension in the alveoli increases as well; therefore, the CO_2 dissolved in the plasma increases, leading to respiratory acidosis, which may be compensated for by hyperventilation.

The increased intra-alveolar pressure associated with the bronchial obstruction is also believed to cause the pulmonary hypertension sometimes observed in patients with asthma.

Blood gases are usually normal in asthmatics except during severe attacks. In such cases, bronchial obstruction leaves portions of the lungs unventilated, and as a result the CO_2 level drops. However, CO_2 retention with hypercapnia is rare because the asthmatic tends to hyperventilate and exhale the excess CO_2. Marked CO_2 retention in an asthmatic uncomplicated by emphysema suggests that the patient has massive obstruction of the bronchi and that death may be imminent.

There seems to be little doubt that bronchial asthma, like allergic rhinitis, involves the participation of antibodies of the IgE type aimed at the allergen. The antibodies are homocytotropic, so they are expected to bind to cells and release chemical mediators including histamine. The serum levels of IgE are significantly increased in 65% of asthma patients in whom an extrinsic cause of the asthma is clearly identified.

Although immune mechanisms are believed to play a role in the pathogenesis of bronchial asthma, other factors—such as heredity, the individual's emotional status, and the incidence of infection—are important in precipitating the crisis and in influencing its severity and duration. It has also been proposed that the bronchial constriction that develops during the crisis results in part from an increased sensitivity of the bronchial neuromusculature to the chemical mediators, and possibly from partial insensitivity of the β-adrenergic receptors in the patient's mucosal glands, smooth muscles, and blood vessels.

Patients who die from uncomplicated bronchial asthma have pale and distended lungs with viscous mucus in the small and middle-sized bronchi.

In a classical status asthmaticus, the main changes take place in the capillary layer and in the bronchial lumina. The capillaries are dilated and their endothelia are swollen. The lumina of the small and medial bronchi are filled with a combination of mucus, fibrin, and cellular debris—mainly eosinophils and desquamated epithelial cells. Neutrophils are rare in uncomplicated cases of asthma. Except for submucosal edema and small foci of metaplasia, the bronchiolar walls are normal. Large bronchi may be congested and reveal prominent goblet cells. The mucous glands of the deeper layers are often hypertrophied with a preponderance of serosal-type glands. The submucosa is edematous and usually contains a cellular exudate made of eosinophils, lymphocytes, and plasma cells. This feature aids in differentiating asthma from chronic bronchitis, in which the mucous type is prominent. The bronchi may contain corkscrewlike, twisted mucus accumulations referred to as Curschmann's spirals. Crystal structures, the Charcot-Leyden crystals, are also seen (two six-sided pyramids placed base to base, hexagonal in transversal cuts).

If the patient dies, the lungs remain distended and do not collapse when the thorax is opened. On section, viscous mucus plugs can be seen; these can be expressed from the bronchioles. These plugs may cause the small areas of atelectasis, which appear as collapsed, dry areas on the lung surface.

Urticaria

The typical lesion in urticaria is the formation of the urticaria wheal, which is often—but not always—associated with pruritis. The wheal is characterized by vasodilatation with increased vascular permeability leading to subcutaneous edema. Mast cells are found in the skin, liver, spleen, bone marrow, and enteric nodes. The lesions may be localized, as in bee stings or after direct contact with poison ivy, or generalized, as in food intoxication. Chemical mediators—in particular but not exclusively, histamine—are primarily responsible for the vascular reaction in urticaria. Histamine can be released in at least two ways: directly by the substance administered or indirectly through an immunological response involving cytophilic (IgE) antibodies [212, 213].

The nonimmunological release in man includes urticaria developing after the administration of opium alkaloids, especially codeine, tubocurarine, polymyxin B, thiamine, and sodium dehydrochloride. Allergic types include allergy to penicillin, tetracycline and its derivatives, sulfanilamides, chlorothiazide, and tolbutamides.

Although foods may cause urticaria through an immunological response, it is believed that urticaria caused by shellfish, strawberries, and citrus fruits is due to potent histamine-releasing substances.

Generalized urticaria provoked by heat can be reproduced by the intradermal injection of cholinergic drugs. Thus, this form is often referred to as cholinergic urticaria.

Intracellular or extracellular parasites, such as those that cause helminthiasis, schistosomiasis, ascariasis, trichomoniasis, or even malaria, may cause urticaria probably through an immunological reaction to foreign proteins.

A special type of nonallergic urticaria, urticaria pigmentosa, is characterized by infiltration of the dermis with mast cells. It begins early in life with the development of wheals at any site of the body, but principally over the trunk. The wheals leave pigmented macules or nodules that vary in diameter from a few millimeters to several centimeters.

The immunological pathogenesis of urticaria caused by cold is not clear. Sometimes, but not always, urticaria is associated with cryoglobulinemia, cryofibrinogenemia, or strokes.

Urticaria must be distinguished from angioedema, or so-called hereditary angioneurotic edema, in which the edematous process is not restricted to the immediate subcutaneous tissue but involves the dermis and may lead to large areas of edema. The edema usually develops as a result of exhaustion, extreme cold or heat, or extreme emotional upset and lasts for 24 hours. The edema may be associated with abdominal pain and occasionally with laryngeal edema, which may cause death by suffocation. The pathogenesis of angioedema is not allergic; the disease results from an inherent defect in the inhibitors of the enzyme C1 esterase.

Contact Dermatitis

Contact dermatitis is a chronic (erosion, scaling, crusting, and lichenification) or acute (vesiculation, exudation of fluid, and localized dermal edema) dermatitis not in any essential way different from other types of dermatitis caused by direct contact with usually small molecular chemicals. Characteristically, contact dermatitis develops approximately 48 hours after exposure. Artificial interruption of the lymphatic circulation between the skin and the draining local lymph nodes interferes with the development of the hypersensitive reaction.

Contact dermatitis has all the features of delayed hypersensitivity, and it is believed that the allergens in part bind to the local tissue and in part are carried to the lymph nodes. There the allergens stimulate the proliferation of a special clone, which is attracted to the site of contact and causes the injuries. Contact dermatitis, therefore, resembles the tuberculin reaction. However, in contrast to the ease with which the tuberculin reaction is transferred by lymphocytes, contact dermatitis is not readily transferred by lymphocytes.

Atopic Eczema

The pathogenesis of atopic eczema is discussed here primarily because the disease, which occurs mainly in children, affects those patients who later develop typical atopic reactions, such as hay fever, rhinitis, and bronchial asthma. (Atopic eczema must be distinguished from contact dermatitis, which is a form of cell-mediated sensitivity.) The manifestations of atopic eczema illustrate the complexities involved in the pathophysiology of allergic diseases. Although allergic factors may be involved (albeit they have not been identified), other factors are also involved, such as infection and seborrhea. In fact, in patients with eczema, treating the disease's nonallergic components may be the most effective management [214].

Except for the report that skin extracts of patients with atopic eczema can induce blast cell formation in the lymphocytes of sensitized animals but not in normal lymphocytes, at present little evidence for direct immune involvement in atopic eczema is available. The primary event in eczema is capillary and other small blood vessel vasodilation, which results first in the development of erythema and later in the appearance of intraepithelial edema. At first, the edema is limited to small areas and papules form, but later the papules become confluent. The edema fluid lifts up the superficial layers of the skin, breaks the intracellular bridges, and leads to vesicle formation. The vesicles break and serum is lost at the surface of the skin, as occurs in patients with burns. It has been reported that in some cases the serum loss is marked enough to lead to a drop in the blood protein levels.

These primary lesions—vasodilation and edema—are followed by more complex reactions. Principal among these are superimposed infection and parakeratotic and hyperkeratotic reactions of the epithelium. The sweat glands may be obstructed by keratin, but, contrary to earlier beliefs, sweat retention is not likely to play a key role in the pathogenesis of atopic eczema. Similarly, seborrheic glands may be abnormal, but they certainly are not overactive. Therefore, the practice of prescribing a low-fat diet for eczematous children to reduce sebum secretion is of little value.

Although an immunological reaction could play a primary or secondary role in atopic eczema, a fundamental distortion of the skin physiology must be involved as well.

Whether the clue to the pathogenesis of atopic eczema is linked with an abnormal response of the epithelial vasculature remains to be seen. Hitting the eczematous skin with a blunt instrument, instead of yielding erythema and a flare with wheal formation (as in normal skin), results in the formation of a white ring; blanching and whealing never take place. The injection of acetylcholine in normal individuals produces vasodilatation. In patients with eczema, 5 to 30 minutes after acetylcholine is injected, blanching develops and is maintained for 10 minutes. Finally, patients with eczema have abnormally low temperatures in their fingers and toes after chilling. Thus, patients with allergic eczema appear to have an abnormal tendency toward epithelial vasoconstriction, and it has been proposed that this results from abnormal binding of epinephrine to the skin. Whether all these findings are primary or secondary to an immunological reaction of the skin remains to be seen, but similar findings have been made in other forms of dermatosis.

Miscellaneous Immune Reactions to Drugs

All drug reactions do not involve reagin type of antigens, as is the case for penicillin. Penicillin elicits a variety of immunological reactions, including the drug-induced sensitization of blood cells. At least three different mechanisms have been described: the haptene, the innocent bystander, and the α-methyldopa. Penicillin is typical of the haptene mechanism. Penicillin binds to erythrocytes in detectable amounts, acts as an antigen, and induces the formation of a specific IgG antibody [215, 216].

A number of drugs—and prominent among them are quinidine, hydantoin, acetophenetidin, and p-aminosalicylic acid—induce an immunological reaction and may cause hemolytic anemia and thrombocytopenia. Yet, attachment of the drug to cell membranes cannot be demonstrated. The combined presence of the patient's serum, complement, and the drug is needed to demonstrate cellular injury. It is assumed that in such cases an antibody—IgM in thrombocytopenia, IgG (the reason for IgG formation in one case and IgM in the other is not known) in hemolytic anemia—is formed and complexes with the drug. The complex binds to the cell membrane and activates complement, which remains attached to the membrane while the complex is freed and thereby able to attach to new cells.

One argument in support of this view is that the anticomplement Coombs' test is positive. In this model the red cell does not trigger the immune reaction, so it is said to be an innocent bystander and victim of an immunological reaction triggered by the drug-antibody complexes.

Methyldopa is one of the many drugs used to treat hypertension. Often (in approximately 40% of the cases) after 6–12 months of treatment and provided that the dose is sufficient, the patient develops a positive IgG Coombs' test. The antibody is directed toward the Rh antigen. These findings have been interpreted by assuming that methyldopa modifies the structure of the cell membrane during erythrocyte maturation. For reasons unknown, only 1% of the patients with positive Coombs' tests develop overt hemolytic anemia.

Immunological disturbances have been observed among a relatively small number of hypertensive patients. They include a high incidence of antinuclear antibodies and a positive Coombs' test.

An intriguing form of asthma is caused by aspirin intake in patients who suffer from nasal polyps, eosinophilia, and intrinsic asthma. Aspirin (acetylaminosalicylic acid), but not salicylic acid, triggers increasingly severe asthma crises. The mechanism by which this occurs is not known. It has been related to the ability of aspirin (but not salicylic acid) to acetylate proteins.

Serum Sickness

Before chemicals and antibiotics were available to combat infections, large doses of antibodies were injected to neutralize nefarious antigens, such as snake venom and those causing cholera, tetanus, botulism, etc. To prepare such antibodies, investigators injected antigens in a large animal, usually a horse, whose serum was collected and injected in the infected patient. The first serum injection was in most cases innocuous, but the second often elicited a dramatic reaction. Von Pirket and Schmidt were the first to describe this reaction in man, which is now known to be a form of anaphylactoid shock.

The classical victim of serum sickness has received a previous injection of horse serum. When he is subjected to a second, inadvertent injection, depending upon the dose administered, a dramatic reaction develops within 1–3 days after the serum is administered.

The symptoms of serum sickness include fever, generalized swelling of the lymph nodes, splenomegaly, urticaria, arthralgia, dyspnea, and wheezing; a small number of patients develop peripheral neuritis. Serum sickness rarely is fatal, and the severity of the disease depends upon the dose administered, its purity, the route of administration, and the "sensitivity" of the individual. The symptoms may recede after a few days, but sometimes they persist for weeks. Complications include neuritis of the brachial plexus, Guillain-Barré syndrome, optic neuritis, carditis, nephritis, and periarteritis nodosa. It has been estimated that with 100 ml of serum, 90%, and with 10 ml of serum, 10% of individuals would develop serum sickness. Purification of some of the antitoxins, such as the tetanus antitoxin, permits the administration of large doses of antitoxin (1500 units in as little as 0.5 ml of serum).

Although there are great similarities, one cannot expect the pathogenesis of serum sickness to mimick exactly that of anaphylactic shock or the Arthus reaction. Horse serum contains at least 15 to 20 antigens; therefore, one may expect horse serum injection to elicit a multiple antibody response with complex antigen-antibody reactions.

Because of the multiple antibody response, it has not been possible to identify those antibodies that are specifically responsible for the development of serum sickness. Evidence available at the present suggests that various types of antigen-antibody reactions are involved in serum sickness. Thus, urticaria is believed to be induced by homocytotropic antibodies of the IgE type. Also, some of these cytotropic antigens could bind to other tissues, for example, nerves, because skin and nerves are derived from the ectoderm. (However, it cannot be excluded that the damage to the nerves is secondary to the vasculitis that develops in serum sickness.) Thus, some believe that the binding of the antibody to the nerve tissue induces edema of the perineural tissues, which then compress the nerves. In contrast, the vascular lesions, which resemble those observed in the Arthus reaction, and the glomerulonephritis associated with serum sickness result from the formation of antigen-antibody complexes [137, 217–219].

Experimental Glomerulonephritis

Acute glomerulonephritis is an inflammatory reaction of the glomeruli, usually of immunological origin. Our knowledge of the pathogenesis of acute glomerulonephritis in man can best be understood by first reviewing the pathogenesis of experimental glomerulonephritis.

Acute glomerulonephritis can be produced in animals by two major immunological mechanisms: the accumulation of antigen-antibody complexes, as in serum sickness, and the development of antibodies against the glomerular basal membrane. The two types of experimental glomerulonephritis have their counterparts in human diseases.

Dixon, whose laboratory has contributed much to our understanding of the pathogenesis of acute glomerulonephritis, has reviewed some of the experimental data [220]. The reader is also referred to the reviews of Merrill [221–223] and to other literature.

Antigen-Antibody Complexes in Experimental Glomerulonephritis

The typical experiment in producing acute glomerulonephritis was modeled after the classical production of serum sickness. The experimenters injected a single dose of serum and then determined antigen-antibody titers in the serum. They found that over a period of several days the antigen-antibody complex increases in the serum, and this increase is associated with a drop in the levels of circulating complement, suggesting complement fixation. At autopsy, lesions similar to those found in an Arthus-type reaction are found in the kidney, heart, blood vessels, and joints. Antigen-antibody complexes can be demonstrated in the lesions with the aid of immunofluorescent techniques. Further evidence indicating that acute serum sickness results from the accumulation of antigen-antibody complexes became available when it was demonstrated that direct injection of antigen-antibody complexes prepared *in vitro* could elicit similar lesions.

When small amounts of foreign sera are injected daily, circulating complexes are maintained at low levels, but for long periods of time. In such experiments under appropriate conditions, the complexes accumulate in the kidney and lead to chronic glomerulonephritis. The study of this extended or chronic form of serum sickness has permitted investigators to identify some of the variables involved in the development of the disease.

Of course, the antigen must evoke an antibody response. If the animals are spontaneously or artificially rendered nonimmunoresponsive, then no antibody appears and no complex forms.

The quantitative relationship between the levels of antigen and antibody is also important. If the antigen is in large excess of the antibody, only small amounts of complex form. Moreover, the complex is of small size (one or two antigen molecules per antibody) and is not deposited on the filtering membranes of the glomeruli. Conversely, if the antibody level largely exceeds that of antigen, a large complex is formed. If the aggregates are of the size of particles that are readily phagocytized and a good phagocytic response is possible, no disease develops.

At some intermediate ratio of circulating antigen-antibody complexes, intermediate aggregates are formed that are too large to be filtered, yet too small to be phagocytized. These are the kinds of aggregates that are deposited on filtering membranes.

It is believed that injuries caused by viruses and the pathological features of some autoimmune diseases develop according to a similar pathologic scheme.

Anti-Basal Membrane Experimental Glomerulonephritis

When antirat kidney serum prepared in rabbits is injected in rats, the anti-glomerular basement membrane antibody can be detected by immunofluorescence at the inner aspect of the basal membrane soon after injection. The accumulation of the antibody detaches the membrane from the epithelium, which, under the electron microscope, appears as a subendothelial electron-dense deposit. But no further injury takes place until complement fixation is followed by complement degradation and polymorphonuclear exudation. The formation of the antigen-antibody complex can also be triggered and yield the same results simply by immunizing the animals with their heterologous glomerular basement membranes. Although the first experiments were done by injecting antisera to an animal sensitized against glomerular basement membranes of other animals, it was later shown that the disease could be produced by immunization with heterologous, homologous, or even autologous glomerular basal membranes. The pathogeneses of both types of experimental glomerulonephritis are shown in Figs. 14-13 and 14-14.

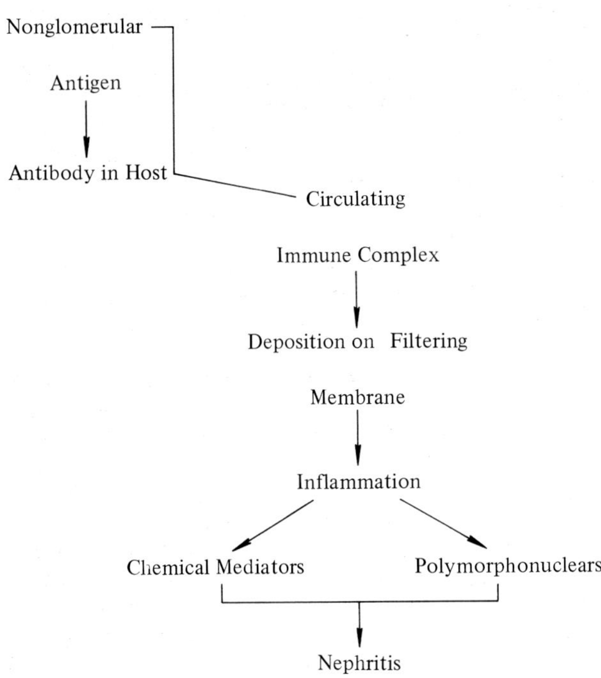

Fig. 14-13. Pathogenesis of experimental glomerulonephritis. May be exogenous, as in streptococcal infection, or endogenous, as in lupus

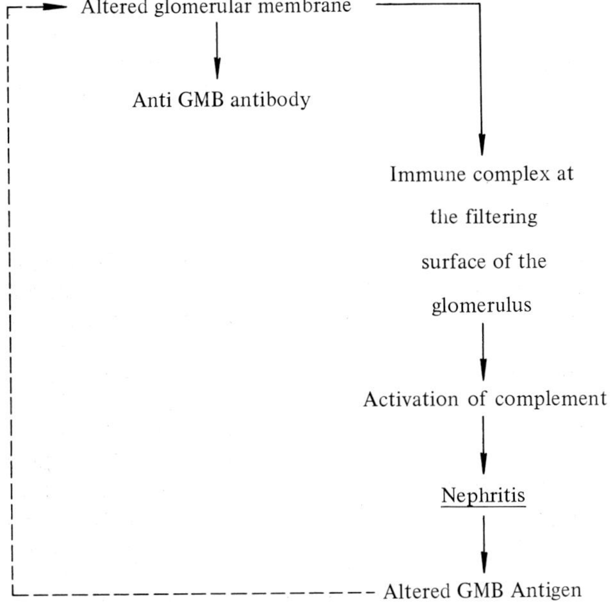

Fig. 14-14. Pathogenesis of anti-GBM glomerulonephritis

Composition of the Basement Membrane

Kopf and Bowman recognized the basement membranes in a variety of tissues as early as 1848. Basement membranes are a specialized form of connective tissue the components of which are elaborated by cells of mesenchymal origin (Descemet's membrane) or of ectodermic origin (the basement membrane of the lens).

Ultrastructurally, the basement membrane is composed of an amorphous matrix in which a fine, partially oriented fibrous network can be distinguished. The fibers are 30–40 A in diameter.

Like collagen, basement membranes are water insoluble. Therefore, their exact chemical compositions are sometimes in doubt, but they are significant because such membranes are known to be antigenic. The chemical compositions of basement membranes have been investigated with material derived from kidney, Descemet's membrane, and the lens. Although the amino acid sequences and carbohydrate composition of the three types of membranes differ, the membranes show qualitative similarities. They all contain a low molecular weight glycoprotein (200,000) and collagen. The collagen resembles that of cartilage more than that of connective tissues; it is formed of α_1 chains, is rich in hydroxylysine, and contains half-cysteines and 10–12% carbohydrates. All three proteins are antigenic, but it would appear that, at least in the antiglomerular membrane antibodies, the principal antigenic component is one or both of the noncollagenous proteins.

Solubility studies in 8 M urea and experiments in which sulfhydryl bonds are reduced or alkylated suggest that the interaction between the three types of macromolecules involves hydrogen and disulfide bonds. However, the exact three-dimensional arrangement of the macromolecules is not known [224].

Studies on laboratory animals have established that tubular nephritis can be produced by injecting crude preparations of rabbit tubular membranes incorporated in Freund's adjuvant to guinea pigs [225]. These findings have been extended to rats. The lesions are associated with focal deposition of IgG and β_1C. A similar immunologically mediated tubular and interstitial disease is believed to occur in man either in association with immune glomerulonephritis or in isolation [226]. Methicillin-associated interstitial nephritis is an example. In some cases methicillin administration causes fever, rash, eosinophilia, and proteinuria. Antitubular basement membrane antibodies were detected in patients with severe renal failure. On biopsy, IgG, C3, and dimethoxyphenylpenicilloyl were found in a linear pattern along the tubular basement membrane. The antigenic component of the drug, the dimethoxyphenylpenicilloyl, forms a haptene protein conjugate that elicits an immune response with the formation of antitubular membrane antibodies [227].

Human Glomerulonephritis

Immune human glomerulonephritis is either primary, in which the disease is restricted to the kidney, or secondary, in which the renal lesions are part of broader immunological syndromes, such as lupus erythematosus, periarteritis nodosa, cryoglobulinemia, and anaphylactoid purpura. Secondary glomerulonephritis is discussed in other sections of this chapter. The forms of primary glomerulonephritis are further classified as: (1) those caused by the precipitation of antigen-antibody complexes as a result of bacterial or viral infections (streptococcal, staphylococcal, pneumococcal, bacterial endocarditis, secondary syphilis, and hepatitis B); (2) the antiglomerular membrane antibody diseases (Goodpasture's syndrome, some forms of rapidly progressive and chronic glomerulonephritis); and (3) glomerular diseases of unknown etiology (membranous glomerulonephritis, membranoproliferative glomerulonephritis, IgA, IgG nephropathy).

We will discuss streptococcal glomerulonephritis, Goodpasture's syndrome, and the glomerulopathy associated with renal transplants as examples and will then describe the pathological findings associated with glomerulonephritis.

Streptococcal Glomerulonephritis

Ninety per cent of cases of glomerulonephritis are preceded by a streptococcal A infection (usually of the throat, more rarely affecting the respiratory tract, skin, or ear) with an interval of approximately 10 days between the onset of the streptococcal infection and that of the nephritis.

Streptococcal infections are not always followed by the onset of glomerulonephritis, and bacteriologists have been able to identify those strains that are most prone to elicit glomerulonephritis. Among the antigenic substances that have been identified from streptococci, a group of antigens is referred to as the M-type antigen. Some streptococci carrying certain types of M antigens are more apt to generate antigen-antibody complexes than others (*e.g.*, M_4, M_{12}, M_{29}, M_{45}).

The typical patient with streptococcal glomerulonephritis is young (but since the advent of renal biopsies, it has become obvious that the disease can also affect older people) and has an established history of streptococcal infection. He has malaise, headaches, hypertension, an increased sedimentation rate, and sometimes puffiness of the eyes and face, swelling of feet and hands, and tenderness in the region of the loins.

The urine is usually reduced in amount and may be dark brown, or even red, as a result of hemoglobinuria. Examination of the urine reveals proteinuria, microscopic hematuria, and the presence of various types of casts, mainly red cell and hyalin casts.

Renal functions are impaired, and this is manifested by a decrease in the glomerular filtration rate and an increase in BUN and creatinine levels. If a renal biopsy is obtained when the disease has reached its peak, the histological features include a diffuse increase of cellularity in the glomeruli, resulting from proliferation of the endothelial cells of the glomerular capillaries, and increased migration of leukocytes, mainly polymorphonuclears.

The combination of cellular proliferation, swelling of the endothelial cells, and polymorphonuclear accumulation obstructs the blood flow of the capillaries, giving them a bloodless appearance, and resulting in a combination of increased permeability to red cells and proteins and a reduced glomerular filtration rate.

If immunofluorescent antibodies are prepared, either against immunoglobulin (IgG) or against complement, most of the fluorescence is localized in the immediate proximity of the basal membrane, but in a discontinuous fashion, giving a granular appearance to the distribution of the fluorescent antibody. The presence of antigen-antibody complexes has been confirmed by electron microscopic examination of the kidney; indeed, electron-dense deposits are visible at the epithelial site of the basement membrane. Moreover, the use of ferritin-labeled antibodies prepared against streptococcal components demonstrates that such antibodies are localized in areas where immunoglobulin and complement antibodies are found. The nature of the streptococcal antigen involved is not certain, but cell wall components have been suspected.

However, some investigators believe that the pathogenesis of the disease does not directly involve streptococcal antigens, but that either the streptococci modify the basal membrane, which becomes autoantigenic, or that the cross-reactivity between the streptococcal antigen and the basal membrane is so effective that antibasement membrane antibodies accumulate.

Blood Immunology. In a typical case of streptococcal glomerulonephritis, one may be able to detect at least two types of immunological changes: the appearance of antibodies against streptococcal components, and a decrease in blood level complement. The antistreptococcal antibodies are of two types: (1) antibodies against cellular M antigens, which are believed to provide specific immunity and prevent reinfection by the same strain; and (2) antibodies against extracellular antigens—namely, streptolysine (ASO antibody)—which are unrelated to the immediate pathogenic mechanism but can serve as a prognostic gauge. There is an inverse relationship between the incidence of acute glomerulonephritis and the blood titers of ASO antigens. Thus, patients with the highest ASO titers appear to heal completely.

Although the course of streptococcal glomerulonephritis was unclear for a long time, the performance of biopsies has somewhat clarified the potential fate of patients with acute glomerulonephritis. With respect to the disease course, patients with acute glomerulonephritis have four possibilities: (1) recover completely; (2) progress into a subacute type of glomerulonephritis and die within 6–18 months after onset of the disease; (3) slowly evolve toward chronic nephritis; and (4) appear well but develop renal insufficiency several years later. The incidence of complete recoveries, depending upon the study, varies in pediatric groups from 50–100%. In adults, the incidence of progressive disease seems to be much higher. The pathogenesis of human streptococcal glomerulonephritis is summarized in Fig. 14-15.

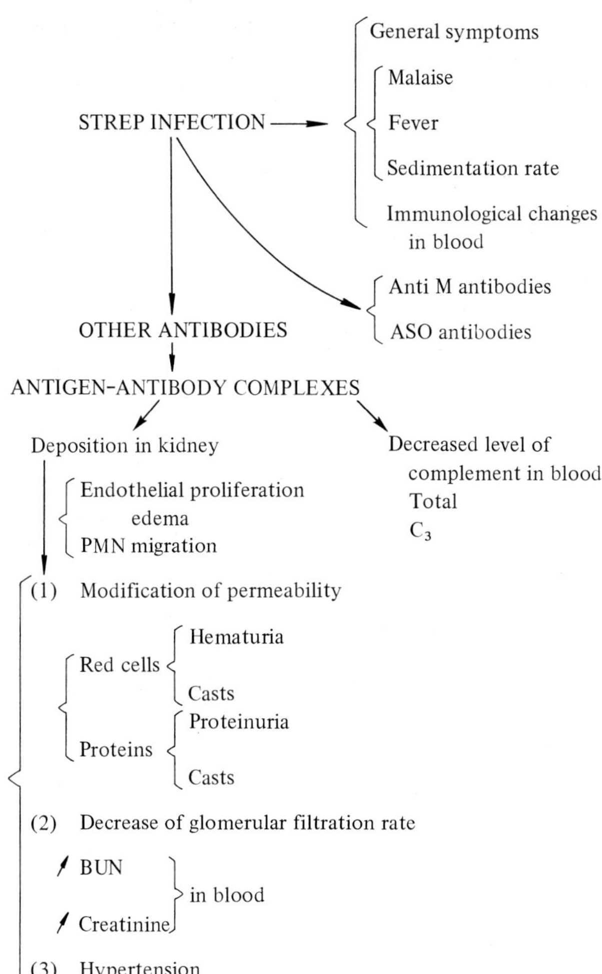

Fig. 14-15. Pathogenesis of streptococcal glomerulonephritis

Goodpasture's Syndrome

Goodpasture's syndrome consists of severe acute glomerulonephritis believed to result from deposition of antiglomerular basment membrane antibodies associated with massive lung hemorrhage. The typical patient is a young boy, over 16 years old, who has hemoptysis associated with rapidly progressing renal failure.

The glomerulonephritis is diffuse and histologically cannot be distinguished readily from the streptococcal counterpart; but immunofluorescent techniques have demonstrated that the antibodies that accumulate at the epithelial site of the basement membrane are antibasement membrane antibodies, although IgG and C3 deposits have also been demonstrated. The cause of the lung damage is not entirely clear; but it has been proposed that the structures of the basement membrane of the lung and that of the glomeruli are so closely related that they cross-react antigenically.

Glomerulopathy in Renal Transplant

Glomerulopathy may develop in the transplanted kidney either as a recurrence of the original disease or because the host forms antibodies against the donor's glomerular membrane.

In 1955 Hume and his associates [228] reported the results of transplanting a cadaver kidney in a patient with fatal renal failure due to polyarteritis nodosa. The kidney never functioned normally, and when the patient died the autopsy revealed that the donor's kidney looked exactly like that of the patient before transplantation.

Several reports of recurrence of glomerulonephritis detectable by immunofluorescence and electron microscopy in the donor's kidney have since been described.

That in some cases the disease is unlikely to be caused by a host-versus-graft reaction is indicated by the high incidence of glomerulopathies in kidneys obtained from identical twins. The course of the disease in the donor's kidney sometimes mimicks the pattern in the diseased host kidney. Lerner and associates [229] have clearly established that such recurrence of the original disease may also take place in allografts.

A patient underwent nephrectomy for glomerulonephropathy, and a complete immunological study of the diseased host kidney revealed that the glomerular basement membrane contained IgG. When the antibodies were taken from the diseased kidney and injected in a squirrel monkey, glomerulopathy was induced.

After nephrectomy, IgG antibodies (suspected to be antiglomerular basement membrane antibodies) appeared in the blood. After a period of dialysis, a new kidney allograft was transplanted and the immunological status of the host was carefully reviewed. First, the circulating IgG disappeared as soon as an adequate anastomosis was established between the vasculature of the host and the donated kidney. Second, the patient exhibited proteinuria within hours, indicating that glomerulopathy was established in the allograft almost immediately after transplantation; and, third, when a biopsy of the transplanted kidney was made, a linear deposition of immunoglobulin along the basal membrane was clearly demonstrated by immunofluorescence and electron microscopy.

Although some forms of glomerulopathy undoubtedly result from recurrence of the original disease, this is believed to be rare, and allografts develop glomerulopathy more as a result of a host-versus-graft reaction rather than from a recurrence of disease. Maybe the most impressive evidence supporting such a view is the development of glomerulopathy in a patient in which kidney disease was absent. The patient had a single ectopic kidney that was removed by mistake, and a kidney allograft was made. The patient developed nephropathy 1 year after implantation and progressed to typical glomerulonephritis with renal failure. Since then, large numbers of rejected allografts have been studied, and a high incidence of glomerulopathy has been observed.

Moreover, the phenomenon has been observed under experimental conditions; thus, when allografts between two different strains of rats result in glomerulopathy in the donated kidney, the stimulus to the immunological reaction is not known [230]. At least four possibilities have been contemplated: (1) development of antibodies against renal transplantation antigens (this view is challenged by Dixon and coworkers [231], who claim that there is no cross-reaction between glomerular basement membrane and that histocompatibility antigens do not cross-react); (2) the antibodies are directed toward the antilymphocyte serum, which is prepared in horses and used to maintain immunosuppression; (3) immunosuppressive therapy results in new types of kidney infections (*e.g.*, with cytomegalovirus) that provide the antigenic stimulus; (4) the antibodies are directed against the glomerular basement membranes of the donated kidney.

Some of the arguments in support of the fourth view have already been discussed, but they will be briefly summarized here.

First, when levels of GBM antibodies were measured in the serum of patients suffering from subacute glomerulonephritis before and after bilateral nephrectomy and renal transplantation, the GBM antibodies absent before nephrectomy appeared after nephrectomy, persisted during the entire period of preparation for transplantation, and disappeared again 24 hours after transplantation. Second, renal biopsies taken from patients subjected to transplantation because of chronic glomerulonephritis demonstrated that the GBM antibodies accumulate in the basement membranes of the new kidney. Third, if for some reason the transplanted kidney of such a patient is removed and the antibody elicited by transplantation is injected in squirrel monkeys, the monkeys will develop acute proliferative glomerulonephritis.

Although GBM antibodies clearly can produce glomerulonephritis in man, the stimulus to the antibody production remains to be discovered. The stimulating antigen could be of exogenous or endogenous origin. If heterologous, the antigen must exist in the environment and be introduced in the victim's body, where, because of cross-reaction with GBM, it induces the formation of antibodies against that membrane. There is no evidence that such an exogenous antigen exists. If endogenous, the antigen should be found in sera or urine, or both.

Such basal membrane antigens have been found in the urine of most individuals. The antigens are the breakdown products of basement membranes of various origins—lung, arteries, kidney, and other organs. The antibodies induced against them will complex with antigens derived from membranes of various origins. Although much progress has been made in our understanding of the pathogenesis of this form of glomerulonephritis, many questions remain unanswered. For example, why do the antibodies complex selectively with the glomerular basement membrane, and why does the complex accumulate only in some individuals and not in others?

In conclusion, in a first type of pathogenic mechanism, the antigen and the antibody complex in the circulating blood, and the antibody is not specific for the GBM, but the antigen-antibody complex accumulates in the GBM in the kidney. In most of these cases (70 to 75%), it is not known which antigen-antibody complexes are involved. In the second pathogenic mechanism of glomerulonephritis, the circulating antibody reaches the kidney, where it complexes with the specific antigen in the GBM.

The differentiation of the two different pathogenic forms of glomerulonephritis depends in part on the distribution of immunofluorescent material in the kidney. When the globulin deposited is anti-GBM, it is neatly and linearly distributed along the basement membrane, as if it were part of that membrane. When circulating complexes are trapped, the deposits appear as granular, lumpy masses in the walls of the glomerular capillaries.

Our search for an understanding of the pathogenesis of a disease is often motivated by our desire to improve therapy. In acute glomerulonephritis, although we have made much progress in understanding its mechanisms of development, little progress has been made in therapy. Only tentative results are available. They include interference with antibody development using immunosuppressive drugs, interference with complement activation using cobra venom, and minimization of polymorphonuclear participation and release of vasoactive amines.

Anatomical Pathology of Glomerulonephritis

We have discussed three types of glomerulonephritis: one is due to the accumulation of antigen-antibody complexes, another results from the formation of anti-GBM antibodies, and a third may involve antigen-antibody complexes or the accumulation of anti-GBM antibodies. The first type is acute and usually disappears without causing permanent damage; but in a few cases the clinical pattern of the disease evolves into a subacute or chronic phase. The second type of glomerulonephritis progresses to renal failure in a matter of weeks or months. The third type may evolve slowly and take years to culminate in renal insufficiency.

Many patients are seen with rapidly progressive glomerulonephritis or chronic glomerulonephritis of unknown etiology. Therefore, an etiological classification of the disease is often impossible, and glomerulonephritis must be classified on the basis of clinical course and histological features. Even though most patients with glomerulonephritis are now subjected to renal biopsies, a great deal of confusion in the nomenclature of glomerulonephritis continues to exist.

In all glomerular lesions, the fundamental injuries are endothelial, epithelial, and mesangial proliferation associated with necrosis, thrombosis, exudation of polymorphonuclears and sometimes lymphocytes, hyalinization, and fibrosis. The ultimate histological and clinical pictures vary depending upon the interaction between the host and the injurious agent, which may be exogeneous or endogeneous.

Two types of pathological glomerulonephritis can be distinguished on the basis of the distribution of the lesions: diffuse (90–100% of glomeruli are involved), and focal (only some glomeruli are involved).

Diffuse proliferative and exudative glomerulonephritis is characteristic of streptococcal nephritis. There is proliferation of mesangial cells and endothelial cells with infiltration by polymorphonuclears, and swelling of the endothelium. The epithelial cells of the Bowman's capsule only occasionally participate in forming crescents. As a result of the cellular proliferation, capillary lumens are occluded by the pressure of proliferating swollen cells.

Malignant rapidly progressive glomerulonephritis, sometimes called subacute glomerulonephritis, is uniformly fatal in a period of weeks or months and is characterized by multiplication of the cells of the Bowman's capsule with the formation of large crescents and compression of capillary tufts. Mesangial and endothelial cell proliferation is usually less conspicuous. Malignant glomerulonephritis is associated with a variety of syndromes, such as Goodpasture's syndrome or polyarteritis nodosa.

Chronic glomerulonephritis evolves into slow, progressive destruction and obliteration of the glomeruli by hyalin and fibrous material and is ultimately associated with tubular atrophy, interstitial fibrosis, and arterial sclerosis. Special forms of chronic glomerulonephritis include globular glomerulonephritis and membranous glomerulonephritis. In the first, mesangial cell involvement predominates, and renal failure develops in a few years; in the second, basement membrane thickening can be demonstrated by periodic acid–silver metanamine stain. Such a procedure demonstrates a thick epithelial membrane with short, silver-positive, mushroom-shaped projections.

In focal glomerulonephritis, at least initially, only segments of glomeruli are involved by necrosis and thrombosis. It is not known whether focal glomerulonephritis may evolve into a diffuse form.

We will not describe in detail the anatomical pathology of all types of glomerulonephritis. Streptococcal glomerulonephritis will be an example. For further information, see the works of Golden and Maher [232] and Kashgarian and associates [233].

Acute Streptococcal Glomerulonephritis. In acute streptococcal glomerulonephritis, the kidneys are usually enlarged and swollen. The capsule is dense, smooth, and is easily removed from the parenchymal surface. The color of the kidney depends upon the degree of vascularization and ranges from deep red to gray. On section, the cortex is swollen and the pyramids are congested and clearly distinguishable. Sometimes the surface of the kidney contains many small red dots; in more advanced cases, the individual glomeruli can be recognized as small gray dots.

Most of the damage is in the glomeruli, which are swollen and hypercellular. Hypercellularity results from the proliferation of endothelial cells, epithelial cells, and sometimes even mesangial cells. Numerous polymorphonuclears may be found in the glomerular tufts, either within the capillary lumen or between the cells (see Fig. 14-16). Occasionally, small masses of fibrinoid material can be identified at the external aspect of the basal membrane. Such lesions may be associated with necrosis of the capsule and active epithelial proliferation, yielding the typical crescent-shaped formation. A significant feature of streptococcal glomerulonephritis is that all glomeruli seem to be affected and appear to be at the same stage of alteration. Yet, in a given patient, the histological features of the lesions may vary and may range from primarily proliferative lesions to primarily exudative

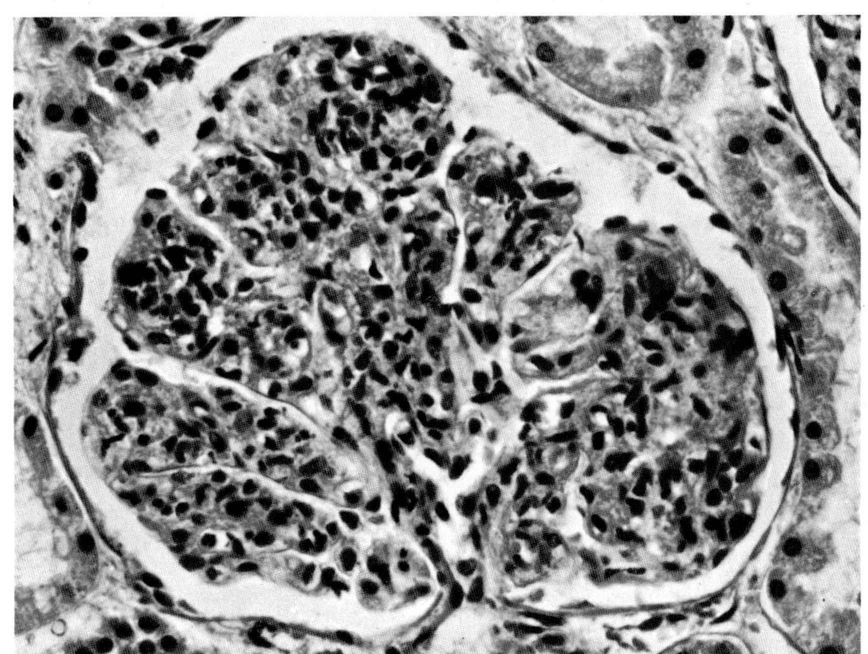

Fig. 14-16. Streptococcal glomerulonephritis; the lumina of the glomerular capillaries have been obliterated by an influx of polymorphonuclear neutrophils from the blood and by swelling and proliferation of axial (mesangial and endothelial) cells. This 10-year-old boy died 3 weeks after the onset of symptoms. (H+E stain; ×420; from Harrison Latta, M.D.)

lesions. The tubules usually are not affected, except for the presence of casts.

Subacute Glomerulonephritis. If the acute lesion does not heal and progresses to subacute glomerulonephritis, the kidneys become enlarged, soft, and pale, and the capsule becomes somewhat thickened and may be adherent at spots. The cortex is wider than normal, pale, and glassy. Severe damage to the glomeruli is visible microscopically and consists of active endocapillary proliferation, fibrinoid necrosis of the capillary walls and of the epithelial cells, and marked cellular epithelial proliferation forming crescents around the base of the glomeruli. The crescents encroach on the tufts and compress them.

Chronic Glomerulonephritis. One-fifth of the cases of chronic glomerulonephritis are preceded by a well-established acute process 1 or 2 years before the onset of proteinuria and gradual renal failure that is associated with chronic glomerulonephritis. The kidney is small with a finely granular surface and a capsule that is often firmly attached to the underlying parenchyma. When one attempts to pull the capsule off, portions of parenchyma remain attached to the capsule. The weight of the kidney may be half of what it is normally (70 g instead of 140 g). The normal radial pattern of the cortex with the pyramids and the columns of Bertin is replaced by a grayish-red line reduced in width and poorly separated from the medulla.

The histological appearance ranges from normal glomeruli to glomeruli that are entirely replaced by hyalin masses. Intermediary lesions may reveal discrete proliferation (primarily between the capillaries) or moderate proliferation, in which the center of each glomerulus is occupied by a voluminous hypercellular nodule that with time becomes hyalinized. This latter form of lesion is referred to as lobular glomerulopathy. Finally, extensive proliferation may take place, and this thickening and enlargement of the endothelial cell cytoplasm and the accumulation of a hyalin substance bring the capillaries in close contact with Bowman's capsule. This type of glomerulopathy is often called membranoproliferative or parietoproliferative.

Goodpasture's Syndrome. In Goodpasture's syndrome the glomerular lesions are focal. They may be proliferative, but often there is fibrinoid necrosis followed by focal hyalinization. The hyalin material is often spread to the periphery and becomes attached to Bowman's capsule. The lungs are heavy and have multiple foci of hemorrhage with massive hemosiderosis. There are no arterial lesions reminiscent of those seen in polyarteritis nodosa.

Rheumatic Fever and Rheumatic Heart Disease

There seems to be little doubt that rheumatic fever, like some forms of glomerulonephritis, is a poststreptococcal disease. (In some rare cases, a virus infection—coxsackie-virus B—has been suspected.) Rheumatic fever is a generalized inflammatory disease with associated pancarditis. The most prominent symptoms are associated with the lesions of the valves of the left chamber of the heart, primarily the mitral valve [234–237].

The relationship between rheumatic fever and streptococcal infections, especially those of throat and upper respiratory tract, has been established by following the incidence of rheumatic fever after infectious epidemics in schools and military camps. Moreover, there is a correlation between the incidence of scarlet fever and rheumatic fever (a fact well established by epidemiological studies in the United States training camps during World War II).

The advent of sulfonamides first and penicillin later has markedly reduced the incidence of poststreptococcal rheumatic fever. The mechanism by which streptococci influence the development of rheumatic fever is unknown. Attempts to recover bacteria from the principal sites of injury have been notoriously unsuccessful. In the absence of direct bacterial invasion, two other pathogenic mechanisms have been proposed: the elaboration of a cardiotoxin, and the deployment of an unfavorable immunological response to some streptococcal component.

Although streptococci elaborate several extracellular toxins, such toxins are unlikely to be significant in the pathogenesis of rheumatic fever for two reasons. First, there is no correlation between the intensity of the streptococcal infection and the incidence of rheumatic fever, as would be expected if a toxin played a key role. Second, if a toxin were responsible for the tissue damage, it would act immediately and there would be no latent period between the onset of the infection and the development of cardiopathy. One is therefore left with the alternative of an unfavorable immunological response. However, evidence in support of an immunological mechanism is meager and circumstantial.

When rabbits are infected with streptococci A, they produce antisera against the bacteria. If immunofluorescent antirabbit antibodies are prepared, they are found to bind to cardiac muscle. Thus, a streptococcal antigen, now known to be widely distributed among streptococcal strains, appears to induce the formation of antibodies that cross-react with some component of the heart muscle. The specificity is not rigid, and the toxin may bind to cardiac, skeletal, and arteriolar smooth muscle.

Little is known of the streptococcal antigen that binds to the muscle; bacterial wall, bacterial membrane, and intracellular antigens have been suspected. Whether these streptococcal antigens cross-reacting with heart muscles play any role in the pathogenesis of rheumatic heart disease remains to be established. However, the blood of patients with rheumatic heart disease contains twice as many heart-reactive antibodies as that of normal individuals. The titers decrease after the acute attack and disappear completely 3 years after the onset of the disease. Moreover, the heart antibodies of reactive patients can be absorbed by streptococcal cell membranes, whereas those of normal individuals cannot.

Thus, an argument often invoked in favor of an autoimmune pathogenesis of rheumatic fever is the finding of heart-reactive antibodies in patients with rheumatic fever. But Tag and McGiven have shown that these antibodies play no role in the pathogenesis of the disease.

The pathological manifestations of rheumatic fever include carditis, arthritis, chorea, erythema marginatum, and subcutaneous nodules. The arthritis of rheumatic fever is usually a form of polyarthritis. The affected joints are tender and later swell and become reddened. The knees and ankles are the sites of predilection, but other joints of the long bones are often affected (elbow, hip, wrist), and joint movement becomes limited. The chorea of rheumatic fever results from neurological involvement and is characterized by spasmodic, purposeless involuntary motion of the muscles of the face, tongue, and sometimes of the limbs and trunk (Sydenham's chorea; this is not to be confused with Huntington's chorea, which is hereditary).

The erythema is nonpruritic and is characterized by circular or serpiginous reddened areas with a pale center on the trunk or at the proximal end of the limbs, but never on the face.

Painless, colorless, firm masses 1–2 cm in diameter form the subcutaneous nodules; they are usually at the extensor surfaces of joints (elbow, knee).

The symptoms associated with carditis will become obvious when we discuss the pathology of the rheumatic heart; the major complication of rheumatic fever is heart disease. A patient may exhibit all or several of the signs described. If the streptococcal infection is treated properly, no heart disease develops; even if the infection is not treated, only a small portion of individuals with rheumatic fever develop cardiac complications. It is not known why some individuals are more susceptible to these complications than others.

In discussing the pathogenesis of rheumatic heart disease, one must distinguish between acute and chronic events.

The acute events are characterized by pancarditis. Thus, the pericardium, myocardium, and endocardium are all involved. The major chronic event is valvular injury with stenosis.

Rheumatic fever involves the valves of the heart with predilection. Some valves are preferentially affected: the mitral valve is the most frequently and the most severely involved, followed by the aortic valve. Combined damage of the aortic and the mitral valves is the next most frequent occurrence. The tricuspid valve is often involved but is seldom severely affected. The pulmonic valve is rarely damaged.

In summary, the left side of the heart is more frequently and more severely damaged than the right in rheumatic fever. There is no scientific evidence available to explain this selectivity, but it has been proposed that the higher mechanical strain that prevails in the left side of the heart increases the incidence of local trauma.

The primary injury is believed to be located in the endocardium (an erosion or an ulceration?). The discontinuity in the endocardial lining leads to the formation of thrombi made essentially of agglutinated platelets.

However, there is no myocardial defect or hypertension, hence the blood flow washes the endocardial wall with its normal force. Consequently, no large thrombi form, and the valves have ample time to react to the injury. Soon the thrombi are surrounded by fibrous deposits that become hyalinized by an unknown biochemical transformation.

At this time, the "verruca" is formed by a central core of thrombotic material surrounded by a dense hyalin capsule. The verruca is firm, translucent, and adherent to the valvular structure. Its base is pushed back at the connective tissue stroma of the valve. Occasionally, a palisading lining of the fibroblast may be seen at the junction of this nodule and its valvular support. This fibroblastic reaction is the fence preventing future invasion of the leaflet, and it is also the front line of the valvular tissue's reaction to injury.

Thus, fibroblasts invade the nodule from the base to the periphery. The nodule becomes cellular first and fibrous later as collagen fibers are formed. It loses its translucency and becomes opaque and gray. Associated with the fibroblastic reaction is a moderate capillary reaction; an occasional Anitschkow's myocyte and a few lymphocytes and eosinophils are also present. The damaged portion of the valve is often impregnated with calcium.

Rheumatic fever is a chronic, recurrent disease, so some clusters or groups of nodules heal while others blossom. Often all degrees of damage from the small, thrombuslike lesion to the hard, calcified nodule may be found on the same valve. As a result of this process, the valves lose their elasticity and become thickened and irregular; consequently, their size, shape, and consistency are altered. Such extensive valvular damage greatly affects the heart's function; and the result of this local injury—with its extensive reaction, hyalinization, fibrosis, and calcification—is the pathological complex known as mitral or aortic stenosis.

Mitral stenosis is almost always of rheumatic origin. Healed mitral endocarditis rarely leads to stenosis primarily because bacterial endocarditis heals integrally when treated. If it is not treated or is not responsive to treatment, it is often fatal. Among the types of bacterial endocarditis that cause mitral stenosis, gonococcic endocarditis has been incriminated more frequently than others. (A condition of unknown origin, calcific annular fibrosis, can also cause mitral stenosis. This disease may be associated either with rheumatic fever or arteriosclerosis.)

The gross changes of mitral stenosis will, of course, vary greatly depending upon the extensiveness of the reaction described above. In classical severe lesions, the surfaces of the leaflets become uneven and nodular, and the closing edges are thickened and hardened by fibrosis. The leaflets are fused along the edges, and instead of two separate leaflets, there is a single circular membrane. For normal functioning, the distance from the ring of the valve to its line of closure must equal *r*, the radius of the valvular orifice.

The valvular leaflets have only one line of attachment in the horizontal plane—namely, the ring. The center of the valve is free. Hence, after valvular scarring no tension is exerted outside the valve. The valve simply retracts, and this retraction prevents valve closure in the middle, and the new distance from the ring of the valve to the line of closure (x) is smaller than *r*.

A similar phenomenom occurs in the vertical plane. Free, normal valve leaflets would be forced into the atrium if it weren't for the chordae tendineae, which hold back the valve; of course, the valve closes properly only if the chordae tendineae are long enough to allow closure. If the inflammatory process and its reaction described above also involve the chordae tendineae, they retract and the thickened valve is pulled downward.

The fusion of the leaflets, the thickening and retraction of the valve, and the retraction of the chordae tendineae lead to the replacement of the functional mitral valve with a thick, firm, and rigid diaphragm with a central hole referred to as a "buttonhole" or "fish mouth."

These valvular changes by necessity affect the function of the circulatory system. The blood brought from the lungs through the pulmonary arteries is trapped in the left atrium, which becomes distended. The atrium is sometimes as big as an orange and may contain as much as 100 cc of blood. The left atrial pressure rises as high as 35 mm Hg. The atrial wall is hypertrophied, its myocardium is thickened, and enlarged nuclei and scarring can be found upon microscopic examination. The endocardium becomes roughened, grayish, and thickened. Sometimes these endocardial changes are more apparent in areas about 1–1.5 cm above the valvular ring. These areas of grayish endocardial thickening are often called MacCallum's patches.

The atrium's marked enlargement predisposes it to fibrillation. As a matter of fact, atrial fibrillation is exceedingly common in rheumatic heart disease when heart failure begins.

Nevertheless, the atrial changes progress slowly for the following reason. Normally, during diastole the blood rushes from the atrium to the ventricle, and only one-third of the diastolic time is required to empty the left atrium and fill the left ventricle. When mitral stenosis sets in, the rate of flow from the atrium to the ventricle is decreased, and the transfer spans the entire diastole. Consequently, the ventricle is full and the atrium is empty when systole starts, and only in the presence of severe stenosis is the atrium unable to compensate for the reduced flow.

The endocardial changes and the modification in the rate of blood flow in the left atrium may also promote the formation of thrombi, occasionally ball thrombi. Not infrequently, the thrombi become the source of emboli.

The increased left atrial pressure sooner or later affects the pulmonary arteries and their branches. However, there is a wide margin of safety before pulmonary edema occurs because edema appears only if the hydrostatic pressure in the pulmonary capillaries (normally 5 mm Hg) is higher than the colloid osmotic pressure (25 mm Hg).

Five millimeters of mercury for the pulmonary capillaries is a mean value; in fact, the hydrostatic pressure is higher in the lower than in the upper parts of the lungs. Exudation therefore is more common at the base than at the apex. (Pulmonary congestion is, of course, exacerbated when the patient lies down because the blood shifts from the systemic circulation to the pulmonary circulation and the abdominal viscera press the diaphragm cranially. This explains why a patient with mitral stenosis often can breathe normally when standing but not when lying down.)

If fluid leaks into the lungs, the alveolar membranes swell and the alveoli may even be filled. As a result, oxygen transfer through the alveolar membranes is greatly diminished and the patient dies in anoxemia. Bacteria find a perfect culture medium in this poorly aerated portion of the lung, and the patient often develops so-called hypostatic pneumonia. This occurs in aortic as well as in mitral stenosis.

How do the changes in the left heart chamber in mitral stenosis influence the right side of the heart? There is no adaptive system in the lung capable of increasing the resistance of the pulmonary vessels to an increased pressure in the left atrium. Therefore, the increase in hydrostatic pressure in the left atrium is transmitted integrally to the pulmonary artery. For instance, if the left atrial pressure increases from 4 to 20 mm Hg, the left pulmonary hydrostatic pressure increases from 13 to 27 mm Hg, or twice its normal pressure. This implies that the right side of the heart has to increase its input to overcome this pressure. The normal right side of the heart can stand a load of twice the normal size, but if the load is too large or if the right side of the heart is weakened, it fails. The increased pressure then is transferred from the left to the right side to the heart and to the systemic venous circulation. The right ventricle enlarges, the tricuspid ring becomes distended, the right atrium dilates, and generalized pressure congestion follows.

Aortic stenosis is another frequent finding in rheumatic heart disease. Although Mönckeberg thought that such aortic stenosis was always a consequence of arteriosclerosis, the presence of rheumatic stigma has frequently been found in association with aortic stenosis. Therefore, it is recognized that at least some forms of aortic stenosis are rheumatic in origin. (Other rare cases of aortic stenosis result from healed bacterial endocarditis and congenital bicuspid aortic valve.) Aortic stenosis is often associated with mitral stenosis, but the aortic valve alone is involved more commonly in men than in women.

A process similar to that described in mitral stenosis progressively alters the structure of the aortic valve and the flexible cusps, the free borders of which can normally be pulled together tightly to seal the valve or be pushed against the arterial wall to allow free blood flow. In aortic stenosis, the cusps are rigid and irregular. The bases of the cusp are reinforced by "buttresses" of calcified material; the valvular ring is often calcified, and nodules may be found in the sinuses of Valsava. Because blood flow is impeded at the level of the aortic valve, blood accumulates above the obstruction and the output is reduced.

In aortic stenosis, the left ventricle cannot pump all the blood from the chamber into the aorta during systole. The blood entering the left side of the heart during diastole is added to the blood remaining in the ventricle at the end of systole. The cardiac chamber adapts to the overload through myocardial hypertrophy; the size of the heart and the intracardial pressure increase considerably (pressure may reach 450 mm Hg).

In moderate stenosis, the blood pressure in the aorta remains normal while the heart adapts to the overload.

The left side of the heart fails if the stenosis progresses until only a slitlike opening is left for the passage of the blood or if the myocardium is injured. In those cases, the heart does not hypertrophy, it dilates and becomes enormous.

At this stage the aortic pressure drops, and, as a result, the coronary blood pressure decreases. Thus, a vicious circle is installed. The damage to the failing myocardium is increased further because of an inadequate oxygen supply; consequently, angina pectoris is common among patients with aortic stenosis.

Once the ventricle has failed, the blood is pulled into the left atrium; the left atrial pressure may rise to 170 mm Hg. The increase in intra-atrial pressure is transmitted to all the vessels of the lung, and pulmonary congestion results. The patient usually dies in ventricular failure or ventricular fibrillation after a slight exertion.

The arthritis in acute rheumatic fever consists of an unspecific diffuse synovitis resulting from edema. The edema fluid is rich in fibrin, and the synovial membrane is infiltrated with lymphocytes and plasmocytes. Aschoff bodies are usually absent.

The subcutaneous nodules, sometimes referred to as the subcutaneous nodules of Minet, have a center of fibrinoid necrosis surrounded by histiocytes, lymphocytes, and plasmocytes.

The pericarditis associated with rheumatic fever is usually sterile, fibrinoid pericarditis. Thus, the epicardium and pericardium are covered with a layer of fibrin, which, depending upon its extensiveness, may give these layers a velvety or bread and butter appearance. Histologically, there is capillary vasodilatation of the epicardium with leukocytic and histiocytic infiltration. During diastole, the fibrin-covered pericardium comes in contact with the epicardium, and the two leaflets are separated during systole. In patients with rheumatic fever, dense fibrin adhesions may form between the epicardial and pericardial surfaces as a result of the heartbeats. Typical Aschoff bodies can be found in the subepicardial tissues. Usually, the fluid from pericardial effusions is completely resorbed, leaving an occasional fibrous patch and sometimes fibrous adhesions, but these seldom have functional significance.

The typical myocardial lesion is the Aschoff body. Two weeks after the onset of rheumatic fever, some collagen fibers (usually those found around small arteries) swell. Consequently, the fibers lose their typical staining properties and progressively undergo a form of necrosis referred to as fibrinoid necrosis. Once the necrosis is established, first neutrophilic and then lymphocytic exudation appears at the periphery of the necrotic cells. Later, macrophages invade the area and become the most numerous cell type. In addition, multinucleated cells may appear, but their origin is not known. Long ago they were assumed to be of muscular origin, but the existence of antimyoglobin has never been established convincingly. In the final stage of development, the nodular area is invaded by fibroblasts that soon elaborate collagen, leaving a microscopic scar.

Aschoff bodies are widespread in patients with rheumatic fever, but they are typically found in the myocardium. They are usually more numerous under the pericardium, where they may compress the heart's conducting system. For unknown reasons, the left side of the heart and the posterior wall of the left atrium are more frequently involved. Sometimes several Aschoff bodies become confluent, forming the so-called MacCallum patches.

Autoimmune Diseases

A perfect immune system should cause minimal damage to the host while neutralizing the foreign antigen, and it should never confuse self with nonself. In many cases immune reactions overshoot the target and cause hypersensitivity through promoting cytophilic antibody formation, precipitating antigen-antibody complexes, or triggering a nefarious cellular immunity reaction. In glomerulonephritis, antibodies are formed against the basal membrane of the glomeruli. Investigators do not always know whether this occurs as a result of: cross-reaction between the antigens of membrane and infectious agent; modification of the basal membranes, making it immunogenic; or the formation of a clone of cells that mistakenly recognize the basal membrane as foreign.

Many diseases are characterized by alterations of humoral and cellular immunity and tissue damage of various kinds, all of which are suspected to be autoimmune. In other words, in these diseases the immune system is believed to deploy the immunological reaction against its own tissue. In none of these diseases are the reasons for the aberration understood. One hypothesis proposes that the clone of lymphocytes emerges from a mutated cell that recognizes the individual's tissues as foreign. But, as in glomerulonephritis, modification of cellular membranes and cross-reaction with viral bacterial antigens have not been excluded.

A number of findings can be expected in autoimmune disease. First, the antigen must be accessible to the antibody-forming system, and the antibody-forming system must respond to the antigenic stimulus; antigen-antibody reactions must lead to the death of the cell that contains the antigen. Thus, the sequence of events is likely to be associated with the presence of the antigen in the circulation, the formation of specific antibodies, the migration of cells carrying the antibodies to the source of the antigen, and the deposition of the antigen-antibody complex.

Histological features of the site of the affected organ include lymphocytic, plasmocytic, and macrophage infiltration and cellular necrosis followed by regeneration. The combination of cellular infiltration, necrosis, and regeneration varies with each tissue depending upon its vascularization and its regeneration capacity (of both connective tissue and parenchyma).

Autoimmune Hemolytic Anemia

Autoimmune hemolytic anemia constitutes a group of diseases in which the individual builds antibodies against its own red blood cells. The disease is the first in which autoimmunity was recognized as the cause of the pathology; and, as such, it remains typical of autoimmune diseases. Depending upon the temperature at which they interact with the antigen, the circulating antibodies that will cause the hemolysis may be warm or cold agglutinins. The disease may be primary (50 to 70% of cases) or secondary, and then it is associated with another autoimmune disease such as SLE, a viral infection, or lymphoma.

Obviously, a major question raised by the pathogenesis of these diseases is the mechanism by which antibody elaboration is stimulated. It is believed that in most cases either drugs (see drug sensitivity, *e.g.*, α-methyldopa) or viruses change the erythrocyte membrane, resulting in the development of new surface antigens that then are recognized by the victim's immune system. Because of the high incidence of autoimmune hemolytic anemia among patients with thymoma or lymphoreticular malignancies, some investigators have proposed that the primary defect is not in the red cell membrane, but in the immunogenic system itself. Thus, a lymphocyte, which may later proliferate, as a result of a mutation becomes unable to distinguish the self from the nonself and elaborates antibodies against its own erythrocytes. If such a theory were to obtain, it would tend to negate theoretical differences between at least some forms of cancer and autoimmunity. Indeed, both conditions would be the result of somatic mutations, and both would be manifested by distortions of gene expression.

A variety of immunological findings can be associated with autoimmune hemolytic anemia (AIHA). Those anemias caused by warm antibodies (reacting with the target cells at 37°) can be due to the elaboration of IgG, IgG and complement, and complement alone, with prior sensitization of the red cell by IgM and IgG. In most cases of AIHA, the antigen against which the antibody is directed has not been identified. They are believed to be "panantibodies" reacting with universal antigen.

In AIHA resulting from the development of cold antibody, red cells are agglutinated at a low t° of 1–20° C, and this is reversed by warming. The antibodies are IgM globulins and have properties of cryoglobulins. There are two major types: idiopathic and secondary. Both involve IgM antibodies; these react with the I antigen blood group in the first case, the non-I antigens in the second. The first has $\varkappa$ light chains, the second $\varkappa$ or λ light chains. The main manifestation of AIHA is intravascular agglutination in superficial blood vessels that are exposed to cold.

A number of isoimmunological reactions against blood components other than red cells have been described. They are at the origin of immunological neutropenia, thrombocytopenia, and coagulation defects. Immunological neutropenia occurs either primarily as a result of the appearance of antileukocyte antibodies, or secondarily in association with other immunological disorders. Immunological thrombocytic purpura develops after transfusion or drug administration, or in association with other immune disorders. Circulating anticoagulants are a component of acquired hemophilia, and they may appear in normal individuals or in association with immune disorders [156].

Autoimmune Thyroiditis

Autoimmune thyroiditis, also known as Hashimoto's disease or lymphoid goiter (see Chapter 8), was for long thought to be the prototype of autoimmune disease [238].

Autoimmune thyroiditis has a predilection for middle-aged women. The disease progresses slowly but seldom evolves into myxedema. The main gross feature is enlargement of the thyroid, usually without compression. The thyroid becomes hard and rubbery (usually weighing 60–130 g) with slight nodularity.

Histologically, the normal thyroid structure is replaced by lymphoplasmocytic infiltration (see Fig. 14-17). The follicles are atrophied with loss of colloid, and large cells appear with eosinophilic cytoplasm, Askanazy cells, and variable degrees of collagen infiltration. The patient's serum has elevated α-globulin levels. Rose and Witebsky [239] suspected and Roth and his associates established that the immune system becomes incapable of distinguishing self from nonself in Hashimoto's disease.

The clinical findings found support from animal experiments. Thyroid-specific antibodies were produced in rabbits and dogs by injecting thyroid extracts of various species; and the injection of rabbit thyroid extracts in rabbits, dogs, and guinea pigs

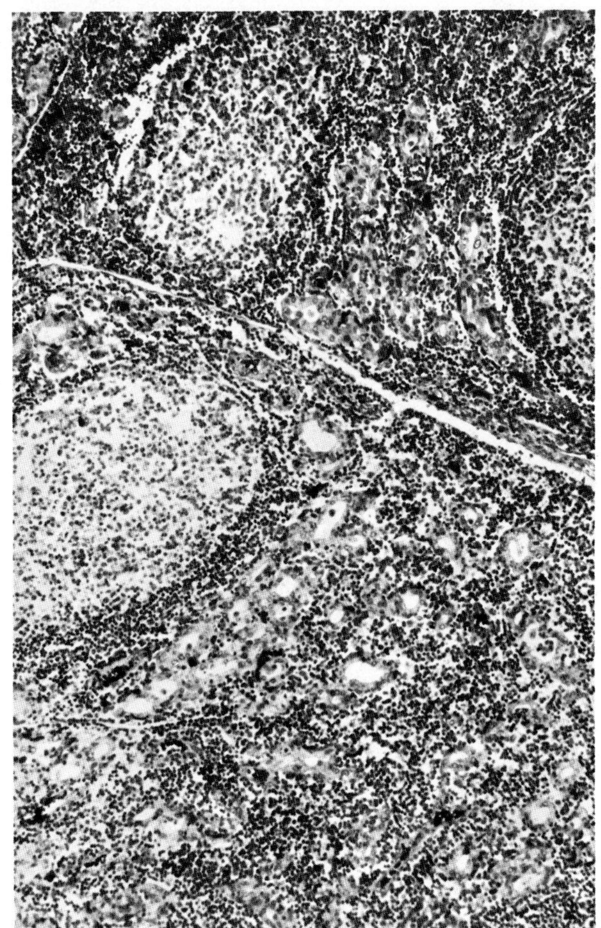

Fig. 14-17. Histological appearance of the thyroid in Hashimoto's disease

resulted in the development of antithyroid antibodies that could induce histological changes in the thyroid reminiscent of the lesions found in the human disease.

The immunologic origin of autoimmune thyroiditis is based on the detection of an antithyroid antibody in the serum and the reaction of immunofluorescent antithyroid antibody with the diseased gland. There are several antithyroid antibodies, including antithyroglobulin antibodies, antibodies against the noniodinated component of colloid, antimicrosomal antibodies, and long-acting thyroid stimulator (LATS). These antibodies are mainly of the IgG type, rarely of the IgA type (20%), and never of the IgM type.

Although little is known about the antibodies that develop against the noniodinated component of colloid, these antibodies may play a pathogenic role in some types of Hashimoto's diseases in which the antithyroglobulin antibodies are missing. The immunofluorescent antibody reacts with the diseased organ, but the pattern of distribution of the fluorescence is different from that of the antithyroglobulin antibody.

Immunofluorescent techniques have led to the discovery of antibodies that react with the cytoplasmic microsomes; they are IgG immunoglobulins. Their role in the pathogenesis of thyroid disease is not known.

We have already discussed the significance of LATS, an IgG immunoglobulin suspected to affect the pathogenesis of Graves' disease.

One of the major questions that arises during a discussion of autoimmune thyroiditis concerns how the immune mechanism is stimulated to work against the thyroid. The earliest theory proposed that the thyroid components, normally inaccessible to the immune system, leak out of the cellular shell and are recognized as foreign antigens. Conditions that cause the thyroid components to be released are infection and other forms of injury. If such a hypothesis is correct, one would expect the antithyroid antibody titer to rise after surgery or radiation therapy, but this is not the case. Moreover, there is little correlation between antithyroid antibody titer and immune thyroiditis. In fact, minute amounts of antithyroid antibody are found in normal individuals, and in some cases of so-called autoimmune thyroiditis no antibodies are found. The theory is therefore shaky, and the discovery that experimental thyroiditis can be transferred with lymphocytes has led to the assumption that the thyroiditis results primarily from cellular hypersensitivity [240].

Lupus Erythematosus

Lupus erythematosus* is one of the most intriguing immunological diseases. Even its name inspires fear. The name lupus comes from the Latin noun for wolf. Medieval physicians used *lupus* to describe a facial ulceration that assumed the shape of a wolf bite. The word is still used to refer to a special form of tuberculosis of the skin (lupus vulgaris) and to the immunological disease systemic lupus erythematosus (SLE). SLE was first suspected to be caused by toxins of the bacillus of Koch and later by streptococcal infection.

Rich associated lupus, rheumatic fever, and rheumatoid arthritis with hypersensitivity; and in 1942 Klemperer classified several diseases—namely, lupus, polyarteritis nodosa, scleroderma, dermatomyositis, rheumatoid arthritis, rheumatic fever, and thrombocytic pupura—under the generic name of "collagen disease." Admittedly, all these diseases were of unknown origin, but fibrinoid necrosis was characteristic of each of them. The name collagen disease should be avoided because of its anatomical connotations, which are not necessarily representative of all the diseases.

Natural History. To describe the natural history of lupus erythematosus is a challenge because of the great variety in the pattern and the intensity of the symptoms.

One can distinguish between severe and mild forms of lupus and between spontaneous and acquired lupus. Thus, a number of drugs (diphenylhydantoin, isonia-

* In French, *lupus* means "loup." The word is also used to designate the mask worn on Mardi Gras to protect the wearer from wrongdoings, such as robbery and rape. One can't escape the comparison between the feats of a masked villain and the insidious undermining of every organ by lupus erythematosus.

zid, hydralazine, and procainamide) are known to cause lupus. However, the symptoms usually subside after drug therapy is withdrawn.

Victims of spontaneous lupus are usually between 20 and 40 years old; women are much more frequently affected than men. (This is true only for spontaneous lupus; in drug-produced lupus, there is no sex difference. The incidence of the disease is for some unknown reason influenced by childbirth and increases a few weeks after delivery.

In what used to be assumed the classic picture of lupus, the patient has a severe systemic illness characterized by a skin rash, high fever, polyarteritis, effusion in the serosal cavities (pleura, pericardium, peritoneum), and sometimes central nervous system disturbances. The disease is rapidly fatal. In the last decade, it has become obvious that lupus is much more common than was previously assumed and may exist in a mild, slowly progessive form.

Among 641 patients with lupus followed by various authors, these symptoms were seen with the following incidence (see Table 14-13).

Table 14-13. Incidence of lesions in systemic lupus erythematosus

Manifestation	Mean %
Fever	88.7
LE cell test	88.0
Arthralgia	87.3
Skin lesions	67.5
Renal lesions	65.5
Heart lesions	46.0
Pleurisy	43.0
Lymphadenopathy	38.0
Enlarged liver	34.8
Pericarditis	27.5
Pulmonary infiltrates	25.7
Enlarged spleen	25.0
Gastrointestinal lesions	22.0
Raynaud's disease	15.3

The most common symptoms are febrile episodes, arthralgia, and skin and renal lesions. Various patients have different combinations of symptoms, for example: facial rash, nephrosis, arthritis, hemolytic anemia, and grand mal seizures. Moreover, the pattern may change so that whereas nephritis or myopathy may predominate at some time in the course of the disease, hemolytic anemia may dominate at others. In spite of this apparently confusing and sometimes deceptive symptomatology, the diagnosis of SLE is not out of reach. Clearly, SLE is a remitting febrile noninfectious illness of young women that is sooner or later associated with kidney disease, arthralgia, and sometimes rash. If the patient's immunological status is carefully investigated (see below), the diagnosis is often conclusive.

Clinical Immunology. Before the pathological manifestations in the various organs of patients with lupus are described, it may be helpful to review the immunological alterations associated with lupus erythematosus [241–247].

One can't escape the feeling that in lupus the barrier that separates self from nonself has been destroyed. Changes may take place in the macromolecular constituents of the cell, making them antigenic (afferent limb theory), or clones of forbidden lymphocytes (as Macfarlane Burnet proposed) may for some reason—possibly as a result of somatic mutation—lose their ability to discriminate self from nonself and recognize normal macromolecular complexes as antigens.

Thus, in lupus, a population of macromolecules or macromolecular complexes becomes antigenic. Common among them are DNA and DNA-protein complexes.

Free-circulating DNA is found in the sera of patients with lupus. Moreover, DNA antibodies have been detected in sera and joint fluids of patients with lupus by a variety of methods, including agar diffusion and complement fixation. In some cases, the appearance of free-circulating DNA reduces the antibody titer in the serum, suggesting that antigen-antibody complexes form. These antigen-antibody complexes are believed to be important to the pathogenesis of the disease.

The presence of free-circulating DNA and DNA antibodies raises a number of important questions. Is circulating DNA unique to lupus? Is the DNA of exogenous or endogenous origin? Is it necessary for the DNA to be specifically altered to elicit an antigen-antibody reaction? Do the DNA-antibody complexes play a role in the pathogenesis of the lesions observed in lupus?

DNA can be detected in the sera of patients with other massively destructive diseases, such as hepatitis, metastatic carcinoma, and miliary tuberculosis. However, in most cases the DNA is not antigenic. The DNA in sera of patients with lupus could be exogenous; for example, from bacteria or viruses. One can then assume that the immune response is dictated by the differences in the base sequence of such DNA and that of the host DNA. Nevertheless, investigators believe that the DNA that circulates in lupus is of endogenous origin and is derived from destroyed cells in the skin and joints. Such DNA could, as we have already mentioned, be recognized as antigenic by a clone or by regular lymphocytes because it carries some anomalies.

The fact that the symptoms of lupus may be aggravated by exposure to ultraviolet light may be significant. Although no direct evidence is available, the presence of base alterations (in exposure to UV light, the formation of thymine dimers) might elicit or enhance the antigenic properties of the DNA. And it is not inconceivable that inability to repair DNA may in part or *in toto* be responsible for the immunological symptoms. When rabbits are immunized with UV-irradiated DNA, they elaborate an antibody specific for UV-irradiated DNA.

There is convincing evidence that the formation of DNA-antibody complexes is essential in the development of lupus nephritis. Schur and Sandson [243] have shown that there is no correlation between the presence of antibodies to DNA in the serum and the incidence of nephritis, but that there is a good correlation between the presence of high titers of complement-fixing antibodies to DNA and low complement levels in the serum. The low complement levels suggest that antigen-antibody complexes are formed that are capable of fixing complement. Furthermore, as these authors pointed out, high titers of antinuclear factors and complement-fixing antibody to nuclear proteins have been detected in normal individuals.

In contrast, there is no correlation between anti-RNA antibodies and either complement fixation or nephritis. Therefore, patients with high anti-RNA titers appear to have a better prognosis than patients with high anti-DNA titers.

At least two other antibodies have been found in patients with SLE—an antinuclear protein antibody and a so-called anti-Sm antibody. Precipitation in agar gel has shown that antibodies to soluble nuclear proteins are present in 50% of patients with SLE. The antigenic determinant of the nuclear histone has not been identified. In addition, an antibody directed toward a ribosomal component—the so-called Sm antigen—has been detected in the sera of 75% of patients with SLE in the acute stage. However, similar antibodies have been found in patients with other autoimmune diseases (*e.g.*, scleroderma, dermatomyositis) and in patients with various lymphoreticular malignancies. In addition to this classical pattern of immunological disturbances, a number of other antibodies may be found in patients with SLE—such as the rheumatoid factor, a positive Coombs' test (if autoimmune hemolytic anemia exists), and antibodies against neutrophils, platelets, and blood-coagulating factors.

Cold antilymphocytic antibodies have been found in the sera of patients with SLE. They react with another person's and the patient's lymphocytes, and they are likely to be directed against some histocompatibility antigens. Such antilymphocyte cytotoxins are not unique to lupus; they occur in allogenic immunization (pregnancy and transfusion), infectious diseases (*e.g.*, rubella, rubeola, infectious mononucleosis), and autoimmune diseases (SLE and rheumatoid arthritis). The role of the antilymphocyte antibodies in the pathogenesis of any of these diseases is unknown. However, repressed lymphocytes (B, T, or both) are suspected of playing a key role in determining the symptomatology in these patients.

Antinucleolar antibodies, most frequently of a single class of IgG, have been found in SLE and also in rheumatoid arthritis. The chance of detecting such antibodies is three times as great in SLE as in rheumatoid arthritis.

Pathology. The skin lesions of lupus erythematosus are on the face and assume the shape of butterfly wings. They may extend to the ears and the scalp. Typically, the lesions are erythematous and hyperkeratotic. Histological changes occur both in the epithelium and the chorion. The basal and malpighian layers are markedly atrophic. In contrast, the keratin layer is thickened and hyperkeratosis is obvious.

Keratin cells may penetrate deeper in the chorion and fill sweat glands and hair follicles. The chorion shows minimal edema and vasodilatation, but marked lymphocytic infiltration. Frequently, one can find small areas of eosinophilic necrosis of the capillaries, which contain numerous nuclei undergoing karyorrhexis. The lesion is by no means pathognomonic and histologically resembles those of several other skin diseases. Occasionally, especially in the more acute stages, fibrinoid necrosis of the dermis can be detected, and the basal membrane and the vascular walls stain deeply with PAS. The muscles usually contain small, discrete inflammatory lesions with occasional areas of fibrinoid necrosis.

Two types of renal lesions have been described in lupus. The classical lesion is a focal glomerulonephritis with fibrinoid necrosis, proliferative changes, and wire loop basement membrane thickening of the glomeruli. Immunofluorescent techniques reveal granular antigen-antibody complexes and electron microscopy shows coarse, electron-dense deposits on both sides of the basement membrane (see Figs. 14-18–14-20). Collagen degeneration and elastic tissue proliferation are apparent in the dermis. Sometimes lupus is also associated with a diffuse glomerulonephritis usually of the membranous type (see above). Renal lesions are found in 70% of patients with disseminated lupus erythematosus. Renal lesions constitute the major cause of death.

In the spleen, there is frequently periarterial fibrosis surrounding the central arteries of the malpighian bodies; this is often referred to as "onion skin" arteriolar sclerosis. Similar lesions can be found in the lymph nodes and in the tonsils.

Lupus may be associated with vasculitis, and cases with diffuse, devastating vasculitis have been described. The vasculitis then causes thrombosis, which leads to other complications, such as mesenteric occlusion and necrosis of the femoral head.

One of the characteristic histological manifestations of lupus is the accumulation of lymphocytes and plasma cells in affected tissues; these form perivascular tufts or genuine granulomas. Although articular symptoms (arthralgia, joint swelling, stiffness, and redness) are common in lupus, they are seldom associated with bone destruction. Frequently affected joints are the phalangeal, carpal, and wrist joints.

Lupus may be associated with various coagulation defects: neutropenia, thrombocytopenic purpura, and hemolytic anemia.

The most typical cardiac lesion of lupus is the localized endocarditis of Libman-Sacks, which occurs in 30% of the cases. It usually involves the inferior aspect of any valve cup, but it is seldom associated with valvular impairment except for a distinct cardiac murmur.

More significant to the course of the disease are the vascular lesions that may lead to such complications as thrombotic occlusion of arteries and arterioles,

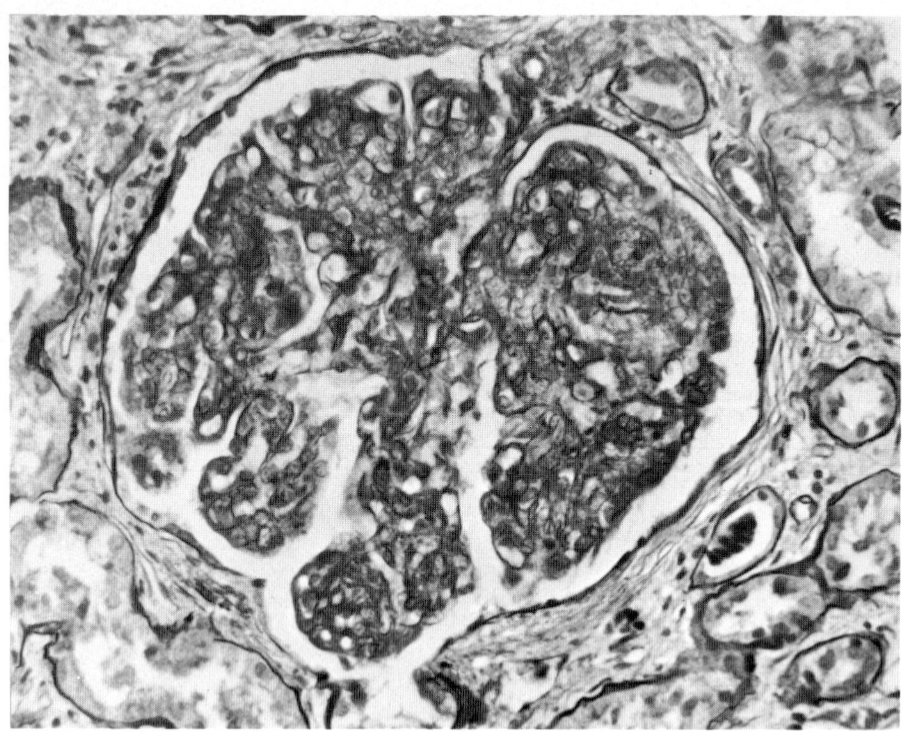

Fig. 14-18. Lupus glomerulonephritis (1965), proliferation of mesangial and endothelial cells in the glomerulus of a 17-year-old boy who has had nephritis due to SLE for 4 months. (PAS stain; ×400; from Smith, F., Litman, N. and Latta, H.: Am. J. Dis. Child. Vol. 110: **3**, 302–308 1965)

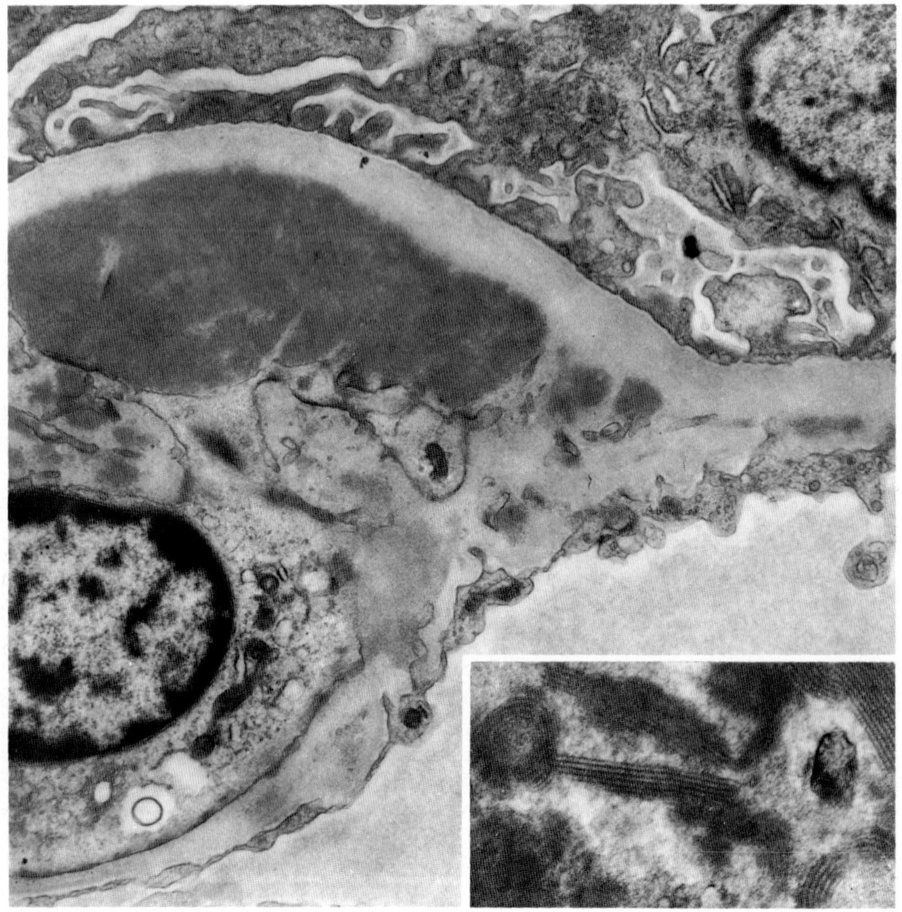

Fig. 14-19. Electron micrographs of immune complex deposits in glomerulus of patient with SLE. (×11,600; ×33,800; from Zamboni, M.D.)

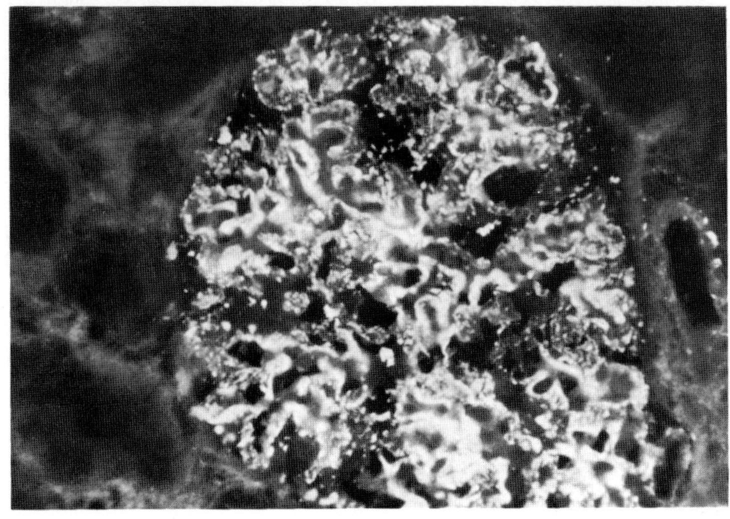

Fig. 14-20. Nodular deposits of immune complexes in the glomerular capillary walls of a patient with nephritis due to SLE. Deposits were stained with fluorescent-conjugated anti-human IgG. (×300; from Richard Glassock, M.D.)

recurrent thrombophlebitis, and Raynaud's syndrome.

Polyserositis involving the pericardium, the pleura, and the peritoneal cavities is frequently seen in lupus erythematosus.

Involvement of the central nervous system is not unusual. It is associated with convulsive disorders, aberrant mental function, and cranial neuropathies. It may evolve into more complex symptoms, such as hemiplegia, disorder of movements, and impaired hypothalamic function. These lesions probably result from vasculitis. Retinopathy and corneal involvement are also common in lupus. Indeed, 90% of patients with SLE have abnormal staining of the cornea with fluorescein.

Two morphological observations are of diagnostic value in lupus: the hematoxylin bodies and the LE phenomena. The hematoxylin bodies are swollen cell nuclei devoid of cytoplasm and coated with γ-globulin. Hematoxylin bodies can be found in the lymph nodes, kidney, lung, and spleen of SLE patients. They stain purple with hematoxylin and may exist in isolation or in the form of aggregates (most frequently found in lymph nodes). However, they are not always easy to detect in the skin (where they are rare) or even in the kidney.

Hematoxylin bodies are the *in vivo* counterpart of the LE cell phenomenon. Their incidence in SLE varies, and they are believed to be primarily a feature of acute disease; therefore, they are not expected to be detected in the milder form of lupus or in cortisone-treated diseases.

In 1948 Hargraves and his associates [248] described a peculiar polymorphonuclear that contained large cytoplasmic basophilic inclusion bodies adjacent and sometimes compressing the nucleus. These cells, which were found in patients with lupus erythematosus, were called LE cells. They are polymorphonuclears that phagocytize nuclear material previously reacted with nuclear antibodies. LE cells can be found occasionally *in vivo* in circulating blood or at necropsy.

The LE phenomenon can also be produced *in vitro*. Usually it is best demonstrated *in vitro* by bringing together polymorphonuclears, damaged lymphocytes, and sera of patients with lupus erythematosus. A factor in serum is known to precipitate the LE phenomenon. They are nuclear antibodies (7-S γ-globulin, mol wt approximately 160,000) that attack susceptible nuclei of the damaged lymphocytes and thereby lead to their phagocytosis by polymorphonuclears. Whether complement is involved in the reaction is not certain. The LE phenomenon is considered to have a greater diagnostic value than the demonstrations of antinuclear antibodies by either immunofluorescence or serological techniques. However, the LE phenomenon is not pathognomonic for lupus and may be seen in patients with rheumatoid arthritis, chronic active liver disease, chronic ulcerative colitis, or leprosy.

In conclusion, lupus erythematosus is an immunological disease characterized by the elaboration of antibodies against macromolecules. Prominent among the antigenic macromolecules are DNA and nuclear proteins. Whether the immunological reaction results from alteration of the DNA (afferent limb theory) or from an autoimmune reaction (efferent limb theory) remains to be established, although the association of lupus erythematosus with other immune diseases favors the latter hypothesis. Yet, lupus erythematosus can be produced experimentally by the administration of drugs.

Circulating DNA or circulating antibodies to DNA do not cause damage directly. The cellular and tissular insults are much more likely to result from the elaboration of antigen-antibody complexes that react with complement and precipitate at some preferential sites in the organism [249].

Rheumatoid Arthritis

Rheumatoid arthritis is an inflammatory connective tissue disease of unknown etiology that is manifested clinically primarily by inflammation of the joints and periarticular tissues. Sir Alexander Garod coined the name rheumatoid arthritis a little more than a century ago to distinguish it from other types of acute or subacute arthritis. Although in most cases rheumatoid arthritis is characterized by joint lesions, the disease is widespread; the joint lesions may be the first to appear and may dominate the clinical picture [250–257].

Incidence. Because of the difficulties involved in identifying the milder forms of rheumatoid arthritis, the exact incidence of the disease is not known, but, in general, it is estimated that 2% of the population is affected. Women are two to three times more susceptible to the disease than men. The disease may occur at any age and has been observed in young people, but it usually appears between the third and fifth decades. There have been poorly substantiated claims that the disease is hereditary.

Clinical Symptoms. In a typical case of rheumatoid arthritis, a 40-year-old woman experiences fatigability, anorexia, weight loss, and even fever for a period of time, and she complains of symmetrical swelling, stiffness, and limitation of movement in the joints of her hands and knees. For example, the proximal interphalangeal and the metacarpophalangeal joints of the fingers and toes are involved. The wrist, knee, and elbow joints may also be inflamed. The swelling is usually moderate, but in some cases it may be extensive enough to lead to fusiform deformities and to the accumulation of large amounts of fluid in the joint. At this stage of acute or subacute inflammation, radiological examination reveals narrowing of the joint space and periarticular swelling.

Although there may be remission, rheumatoid arthritis is usually progressive. The repeated inflammatory bouts lead to destruction of the synovia, scarring of the tendons, and limitation of movement, which in turn leads to muscle wasting. The pathological changes culminate in joint distortion, which includes ulnar deviation, swan neck deformities, and even subluxation. At these more advanced stages, the radiological picture reveals loss of articular space with frank erosion of the bone surface. Sometimes small cystic areas are seen in the bone underneath the cartilage. Ultimately, complete ankylosis takes place and osteoporosis also develops, probably as a consequence of restricted activity.

Although the hand and knee joints are most frequently involved, no joint is spared in rheumatoid arthritis. In fact, one of the characteristics of the disease is its migratory tendency—it jumps from one set of joints to another.

The limitation of function depends upon the severity and location of the disease. For example, involvement of the temporomandibular joint impairs mastication, whereas involvement of the cricoarytenoid joint may lead to hoarseness. Progressive disease in the spine may result in compression of the cord, especially in the cervical region. In addition to the articular manifestations of rheumatoid arthritis, neuromuscular and cutaneous changes are also seen.

Polymyositis is often a part of the syndrome and is characterized by muscle aching, tenderness, and stiffness especially in the morning. Restriction of movement and direct nerve involvement or nerve compression also contribute to muscle atrophy.

Changes in the skin include: (1) erythema of the inflamed area, which may be especially marked near the hypothenar; (2) excessive sweating of the palms; (3) a dry, shiny appearance of the skin covering the affected joint, probably a consequence of poor nutrition due to vasculitis; (4) hemorrhagic infarcts at the base of the nails or in the finger pulp; (5) subcutaneous nodules.

The last skin change deserves further consideration. Firm, nontender, round subcutaneous masses ranging from 2 mm to 2 cm are found in the subcutaneous tissue in approximately 25% of the patients with rheumatoid arthritis, usually those with severe disease. A preferred location for these lesions is the posterior aspect of the forearm just below the elbow. Clearly, such nodules should be distinguished from those seen in gout, xanthomatosis, or scleroderma.

Because rheumatoid arthritis is a generalized disease (with preference for joints), a panoply of other associated symptoms is sometimes observed, such as pleurisy, pulmonary interstitial fibrosis (giving the lung a honeycomb appearance radiologically), and polyneuritis.

The pathogenesis of these various manifestations is not always clear, but perivasculitis is likely to contribute to many of the symptoms.

Pathogenesis. A discussion of the pathogenesis of rheumatoid arthritis brings to mind two critical questions: what is the primary event triggering the inflammatory process, and why is the inflammatory process located principally in the joints? The pathogenesis of rheumatoid arthritis is not known. The mechanisms that have been proposed include: (1) a viral or bacterial infection; (2) a primary defect in the connective tissue; and (3) an autoimmune reaction. Viral infection with special tropism for the joints could explain both types of symptoms, but so could an autoimmune process. Although viruses and bacteria have indeed been found in joints of patients with rheumatoid arthritis, their pathogenic role has never been demonstrated convincingly [254].

Whatever the pathogenic mechanism may be, rheumatoid arthritis is almost always associated with serum and cellular immunological changes. Most typical of the immunological alterations is the appearance of the rheumatoid factor—a macroglobulin (19 S, mol wt about 1,000,000) found in the sera of 95% of patients with rheumatoid arthritis that can agglutinate particles coated with human 7-S γ-globulin (IgG). Any particle (*e.g.*, bacteria, sheep and human erythrocytes, latex, bentonite) coated with the IgG is agglutinated. Although often of diagnostic value, the presence of the rheumatoid factor in serum is not always indicative of rheumatoid arthritis because it is found in many other diseases, including lupus erythematosus (30%

of the cases) and other autoimmune diseases. But the factor is also found in the sera of patients with such clear-cut inflammatory diseases as leprosy and syphilis, or even in individuals subjected to multiple vaccinations. Therefore, the incidence of false-positive diagnoses is high in rheumatoid arthritis.

The biological role of the rheumatoid factor is not known, but a number of recent findings are relevant. A 22-S complex has been found in the sera of some patients with rheumatoid arthritis. The complex can be split into the 10-S rheumatic factor and a 7-S component, IgG, indicating that the rheumatoid factor does complex with IgG *in vivo*. Further studies have shown that the rheumatoid factor reacts with the Fc portion of the γ-globulin molecule. This explains why the rheumatoid factor doesn't react with IgM and IgA, which have different Fc portions.

Thus, the rheumatoid factor found in serum and synovium could be considered a humoral immune response toward IgG immunoglobulins. Circular dichroism studies have suggested that conformationally altered IgG molecules can be found in sera of patients with rheumatoid arthritis. Johnson and coworkers proposed that the altered IgG elicits an immunogenic response from competent B cells that carry the proper membrane Fc receptors [258].

It has also been shown that the rheumatoid factor-IgG complex can fix human complement, and that the largest levels of complement fixation occur in joints.

Although none of these observations conclusively demonstrates that the rheumatoid factor plays a central role in the pathogenesis of rheumatoid arthritis, they indicate that rheumatoid arthritis and the rheumatoid factor go hand in hand. Even if the coincidence does not prove that the rheumatoid factor acts as an autoimmune antibody, there is sufficient evidence to contemplate a working hypothesis.

What seems certain is that an immune complex forms in the synovial fluids or in the synovia itself, activates complement, and thereby releases chemotactic agents for polymorphonuclears, which are in turn killed after they have phagocytized the immune complex and complement. The dead polymorphonuclears release enzymes that progressively destroy collagen, synovial cells, and even cartilage [259, 260].

The necrotic process is followed by the classic attempt to repair the lesion through the formation of granulation tissues and fibrosis. Whether the immunological sequence is triggered by an autoimmune reaction against some component of the synovial cell or the synovial fluid remains to be seen.

Pathology. The pathological manifestations of rheumatoid arthritis affect mainly the joints, the muscles, and the connective tissues. Rarely are the heart and lungs also involved. The early joint lesions consist of vasodilatation with increased vascular permeability and the development of a cellular exudate that is composed mainly of polymorphonuclears, lymphocytes, and plasmocytes. None of these events is unique to rheumatoid arthritis, and they can be observed in any form of joint trauma or infection.

As the lesions develop, the increased vascular permeability allows fluids to accumulate in the joint cavities, and the lymphocytic-plasmocytic accumulations may become large enough to repel the synovia, giving it a villous appearance. The synovia may react by promoting synovial cell proliferation. With the proper immunofluorescent technique, investigators have been able to demonstrate that some of the exudative cells contain the rheumatoid factor. The presence of the rheumatoid factor, IgG complexes, IgG-complement complexes, and C3 and C4 components has also been demonstrated by immunofluorescent techniques.

As rheumatoid arthritis progresses, necrosis of the synovia and cartilaginous tissue becomes more extensive, and the lost tissues are replaced by a granulation tissue referred to as a panus, which is composed of neoformate capillaries, young fibroblasts, and exudative cells. Soon the two articular surfaces are joined by fibrous adhesions, leading to ankylosis with severe limitation of movement, muscular atrophy, and osteoporosis. In fact, in some cases the granulation tissue penetrates so deep in the bone that it destroys the bone, and cystic formation can be detected radiologically.

Arteritis is common but not necessarily characteristic or typical in rheumatoid arthritis, and sometimes severe necrotizing vasculitis is seen.

The subcutaneous nodules are quite characteristic. They are formed by a center of fibrinoid necrosis, surrounded by young connective tissue and a ring of granulation tissue infiltrated with lymphocytes and plasmocytes. The mechanism by which these nodules form is not known, but it is suspected that the primary lesion consists of an acute vasculitis; patients with subcutaneous nodules are more apt to develop widespread systemic arteritis.

Associated lesions include valvular lesions (reminiscent of those seen in rheumatic heart disease), fibrous pneumonia, pleurisy, enlargement of the spleen, and, in 20% of the cases, amyloidosis.

The synovial fluid is turbid with reduced viscosity and low levels of mucin. Cytological examination reveals a large number of polymorphonuclear leukocytes (10,000–50,000 cu mm). In addition to the appearance of the rheumatoid factor, other clinical laboratory changes are often observed in patients with rheumatoid arthritis. For example, the levels of total serum immunoglobulins of the polyclonal type are often elevated. However, there is no correlation between the immunoglobulin levels and the severity of the disease. Serum complement levels are usually normal or slightly elevated in patients with rheumatoid arthritis, except in those patients with a juvenile, widespread, malignant form. Sedimentation rates are increased. Patients with rheumatoid arthritis often develop a normocytic, hypochromic anemia of unknown origin that is usually unresponsive to treatment with iron, vitamin B_{12}, folic acid, and other agents.

In most cases there is a slight leukocytosis, but sometimes lymphopenia with splenomegaly is observed. In the muscles, nonspecific mononuclear infiltrates usually with a perivascular distribution have been observed. However, frank necrotizing arteritis is seldom seen.

That the chronic inflammation of the synovia, which ultimately erodes the cartilage, can be induced by the injection of lysosomal contents—a potpourri of hydrolases—is hardly surprising. Whether such experiments prove that the release of the lysosomal contents, as a result of a change in the permeability of the lysosomal membrane, constitutes a primary injury in rheumatoid arthritis is debatable. Hydrocortisone reduces the inflammatory reaction, supposedly by stabilizing the lysosomal membrane. A direct action of hydrocortisone on the lysosomal membrane has been shown in isolated lysosomes, and stabilization of lysosomal membranes has been demonstrated in tissue slices.

Nevertheless, it is not established that in patients with rheumatoid arthritis hydrocortisone acts directly by stabilizing lysosomal membranes, and the primary effect of hydrocortisone could occur at an early step in a chain of events that ultimately prevent cell death and alter cell membrane permeability.

Whatever the pathogenic mechanism of rheumatoid arthritis and the mechanism of action of hydrocortisone in retarding the disease, an interesting working hypothesis has been proposed. As a result of an imbalance of the redox potential in the cytoplasm (measured by —SH/—S—S ratio), the permeability of the lysosomal membrane is altered and lysosomes become leaky. Hydrocortisone depresses type 2 hydrogen production (see Chapter 6) from NADPH, which normally is channeled in the biosynthetic pathway. This depression results in a decrease in the redox imbalance, which, according to the hypothesis, causes the disease.

Certainly, the beneficial effects of steroids on inflammatory processes are not restricted to lysosomes. In psoriatic patients, topical steroids reduce 5-nucleotidase activity in the dermal papillae and the small capillaries, and they reduce cellular and extracellular edema. These effects are believed to be due to a direct action of steroids on plasma membrane permeability. Corticosteroid also inhibits fibroblast growth *in vivo* and *in vitro* and interferes with collagen synthesis by preventing the formation of the appropriate precursors.

Immunological Vasculitis

The prominent injury in the Arthus phenomenon and in experimental serum sickness is vasculitis. In humans a number of diseases are characterized primarily by vasculitis that affects large or small arteries (angiitis) and even veins.

The prototype of these diseases is polyarteritis nodosa, which is primarily a nonsuppurative arteritis. A number of diseases with other components (*e.g.*, nonperivascular granulomatous lesions) as well as vasculitis are also included in that group: namely, allergic granulomatous angiitis, Wegener's granulomatosis, hypersensitivity angiitis, temporal arteritis, and Takayashu's disease.

Whether these are various manifestations of the same disease or whether they are similar morphological reactions to different pathogenic stimuli is not clear. However, arteries can react to injuries in limited ways, so different insults may result in similar morphological manifestations.

In addition to the fact that these diseases present some morphological similarities to the Arthus phenomenon, circumstantial evidence suggests an immunological etiology for the diseases, although a consistent pattern of clinical immunological symptoms is not present in any.

But γ-globulin and immunoglobulins have been found in the affected vessels by immunofluorescence, and these diseases are sometimes associated with polyclonal hyperglobulinemia and occasionally with the rheumatoid factor. Moreover, at least some of the diseases are often associated with hypersensitivity syndromes, such as bronchial asthma.

But what triggers these immunological changes is not known. Autoimmune reactions and reactions to foreign antigens (such as drugs and bacterial antigens, as seems to be the case for hypersensitivity angiitis) have been incriminated.

Polyarteritis Nodosa

Polyarteritis nodosa is a nonsuppurative inflammatory arthritis affecting short lengths of the small- and medium-sized vessels (200–500 μ in diameter) of almost any organ and causing localized vascular obstruction [261].

The disease is rather uncommon, and—in contrast to SLE, which is more prevalent in women than in men—polyarteritis nodosa is three to four times more common in men than in women. It may affect people of any age but is usually seen in adults.

Prodromic Factors. Polyarteritis nodosa is often preceded by a recent streptococcal or respiratory infection. The early histological manifestations are usually fibrinoid necrosis of the media (see Fig. 14-21), followed by infiltration first with polymorphonuclears and a few eosinophils and later by lymphocytes and plasmacytes (see Fig. 14-22). The lesions spread from the media to all layers of the arterial wall and may heal by fibrosis. When the lesions reach the endothelium, thrombosis develops causing ischemia and infarction. Occasionally, the weakened wall allows aneurysm formation. Fluorescein-labeled antihuman fibrin was used to investigate the nature of the hyalin material, and the findings suggest that it is composed primarily of fibrin although γ-globulins and albumins may also be found.

The larger and smaller arteries of the kidneys are involved in 75% of the cases. Typical glomerulonephri-

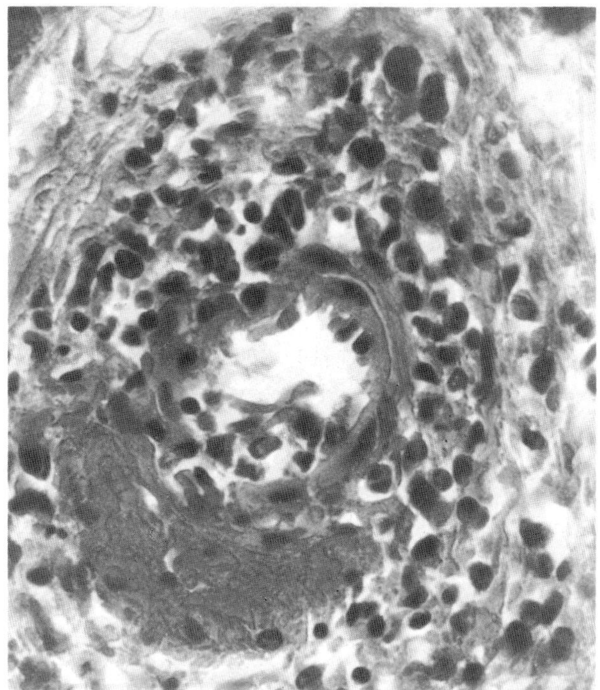

Fig. 14-21. Fibrinoid necrosis in polyarteritis nodosa

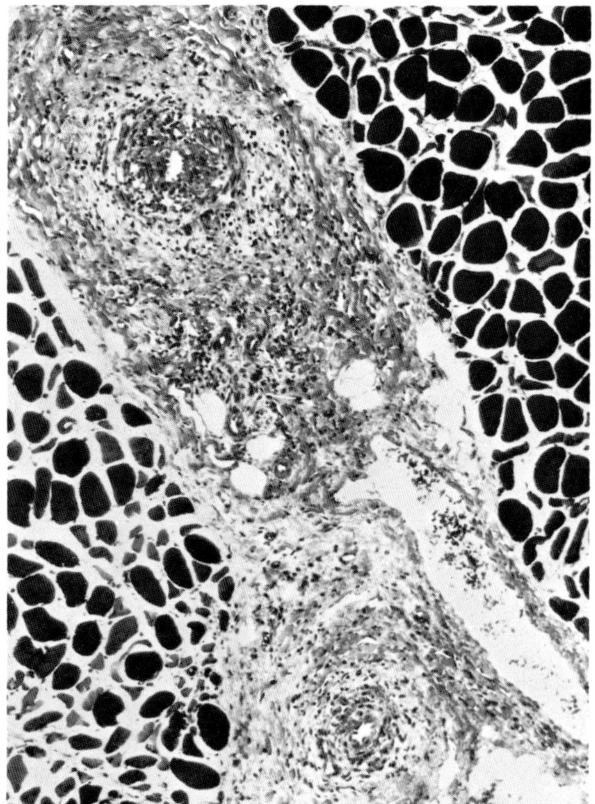

Fig. 14-22. Leukocytic infiltration of arterial wall in polyarteritis nodosa

tis may follow. Focal fibrinoid necrosis* appears in the glomerular tufts and is associated with early and marked capsular proliferation. Polyarteritis nodosa is almost always associated with hypertension.

Vascular involvement in the joints causes arthralgia, but true arthritis is rare. In muscles the vascular lesions cause myalgia, and in the gastrointestinal tract they may be responsible for symptoms simulating various acute conditions, such as acute pancreatitis, acute appendicitis, and perforated ulcers.

Vascular lesions of the lung result in 50% of the cases in infarction or pneumonitis. In contrast to SLE, in which central neurological involvement is known to occur, in polyarteritis nodosa the peripheral nerves are affected. The patient often complains of paresthesia, muscle weakness, and pain. Sometimes the coronary arteries are affected, causing a disease that resembles classical coronary heart disease; but more frequently the heart disease evolves into slowly progressive myocardial failure. Subcutaneous nodules of the skin, along the arteries, are frequently found.

Allergic Granulomatous Angiitis

Allergic granulomatous angiitis resembles polyarteritis nodosa in most ways except that the former is associated with severe respiratory disease, which is manifested histologically by extravascular granulomatous lesions. Patients with allergic granulomatous angiitis usually have a history of severe asthma.

Wegener's Granulomatosis

Wegener's granulomatosis is a necrotizing granulomatous disease of the upper and lower respiratory tracts associated with glomerulitis. The patient usually has a history of rhinitis, sinusitis, fever, cutaneous vasculitis, arthralgia, and peripheral neuropathy, but asthma is rare. Increased concentrations of IgA and C3 have been found in the sera of some patients with Wegener's granulomatosis [262].

Hypersensitivity Angiitis

Hypersensitivity angiitis is an arteritis of small vessels, usually those of the extremities (foot and hand). It follows drug administration or bacterial infections and results in ischemic lesions of the tips of the fingers and toes.

* The term *fibrinoid necrosis* was coined in 1880 by Neumann, who observed material with staining properties of fibrin in connective tissue. It was long argued whether the fibrinoid material was a product of degeneration or resulted from the deposition of substances elaborated by inflammatory cells. Although it is now generally accepted that the accumulation of fibrinoid material results, at least in part, from degeneration, the exact origin is not certain. Degradation products of collagen, ground substance, smooth muscles, and nuclear proteins have all been incriminated as has the accumulation of altered plasma proteins.

Temporal Arteritis

Temporal arteritis may involve one or more branches of the carotid artery.

Takayasu's Disease

Takayasu's disease is an arteritis of the aortic arch and its branches.

Sarcoidosis

Sarcoidosis is a systemic chronic granulomatous disease of unknown origin that may involve any organ but is most often seen in skin, lungs, and lymph nodes; the disease is associated with a more or less consistent pattern of immunological disturbances.

The geographic distribution of sarcoidosis is peculiar. It is more common in northern Europe, the eastern United States, Australia, and New Zealand than in other parts of the world. In the United States, the racial distribution is of interest. A study in New York City suggests that the incidence of sarcoidosis is ten times greater among blacks than among whites. The tendency of the disease to be geographically concentrated and racially restricted suggests that its etiology might include, among other factors, epidemiological and hereditary components [263, 264].

Although sarcoidosis is predominantly a disease of adults, it has been reported in children [265].

A number of infectious agents—tuberculous microbacteria, pine pollen, and, more recently, "anonymous" microbacteria—have been incriminated as the potential causal agents in sarcoidosis. But there is little convincing evidence for any of these pathogenic mechanisms. (Some clinicians have suggested that sarcoidosis does not constitute a special disease entity but is a uniform response to these various types of infections, and, if efforts are made, a definitive diagnosis can be reached [266]. Increased sensitivity to infection has never been convincingly established in sarcoidosis.)

Microscopically, the lesion of sarcoidosis is typical but not pathognomonic. At the florid stage, the lesion is a noncaseous granuloma composed primarily of a peripheral crown of lymphocytes with a central core of epithelioid cells. Giant cells are sometimes found, but they are rare.

Sarcoidosis may be difficult to distinguish from tuberculosis, toxoplasmosis, berylliosis, leprosy, brucellosis, histoplasmosis, or even Hodgkin's disease. Diagnostic clues include the absence of caseation, the large size of epithelioid cells, the low incidence of giant cells, and the tendency of the granulomas to remain separate rather than fuse into one another. Granulomas may disappear completely or may leave a fibrotic or hyaline scar. Sometimes healing and granulomatous proliferation occur at the same time, so that as some granulomas heal, new ones develop. As a result, much organ tissue is destroyed, causing fibrosis and loss of function. This course often prevails in the lungs.

Schaumann described special intracytoplasmic structures in the multinucleated cells of the sarcoid granulomas. These structures, referred to as Schaumann's bodies, are rounded, laminated bodies 20–50 μ in diameter that stain with hematoxylin, are double refractive, and may contain iron. The presence of these inclusions is not pathognomonic—they are absent in some cases of sarcoidosis and are seen in other granulomatous lesions.

The organs most frequently affected are the lymph nodes, spleen, liver, and lungs. The lymph nodes are moderately enlarged. On cut surface, small, gray-yellow, usually sharply delineated foci stand out against the normal background of the lymph nodes. The number of granulomas varies from a few to almost a confluent mass that may replace the entire surface of the node.

Similar lesions are found in the spleen and liver; the spleen may be enlarged and weigh from 200–1000 g and, in advanced cases, may be hard and fibrous and contain mature and healing granulomas. Granulomas may involve the lungs, heart, stomach, and even meninges and brain.

Obviously, the symptomatology of sarcoidosis is varied. To identify the disease, clinicians look for a pattern of associated symptoms. In most patients, the predominant symptoms are isolated hilar lymphadenopathy, pulmonary fibrosis, uveoparotid fever, erythema nodosum, and hypercalcemia.

The lung pathology often dominates the clinical picture. Patients complain of dyspnea or coughing that may be reflected in the X-ray picture. In classical cases, mediastinal adenopathy and pulmonary fibrosis are detectable. The fibrosis results from healing of the granuloma. Sometimes granulomas become confluent in the lung parenchyma, and punched out, dense masses can be found. Hyperventilation may cause focal or generalized emphysema. Pleural effusions are rare. In some patients the lung symptoms evolve progressively into incapacitating dyspnea and cor pulmonale. Acute granulomatous uveitis causes corneal and lenticular opacities and sometimes glaucoma. Involvement of the lacrymal and salivary glands may compress the excretory channels and result in enlargement of the glands.

The cause of hypercalcemia is not clear; only 10% of patients with sarcoidosis have punched out bone lesions. Renal insufficiency is, however, a common complication of hypercalcemia. Seldom does a sarcoidosis granuloma cause renal insufficiency.

Nevertheless, renal disease in sarcoidosis may be more common than previously anticipated. Autopsies of patients with sarcoidosis revealed that many presented variable types of glomerulonephritis [267]. The lesions were diffuse or focal, proliferative or membranous, or a combination of various types.

A number of immunological distortions have been observed in sarcoidosis, including polyclonal α-globulinemia, false-positive Wassermann reaction, marked reduction in the manifestation of cell-mediated immunity (negative tuberculin test and the test becomes positive after BCG injection but does not remain positive for long). Studies of homograft rejection have not been reported in detail in sarcoidosis.

Kviem discovered that the intracutaneous injection of a heat-sterilized suspension of sarcoid spleen or lymph nodes yields within 4 to 6 weeks a papular skin reaction that contains lymphocytes and epithelioid cells. There are few false-positive tests, but there are many false-negative tests, especially in advanced cases. Moreover, stable standardized test material is difficult to obtain.

Miscellaneous Collagen Diseases

Scleroderma. Scleroderma, the most typical collagen disease, is characterized by sclerosis that is restricted to the skin or involves the connective tissue of every organ; the latter form of scleroderma is known as progressive systemic sclerosis. Cases have been reported in which only the visceral organs are involved. Scleroderma usually affects people between the ages of 20 and 50 and, like SLE, is more common among women than men (3 to 1).

Pathologically, the main feature of scleroderma is proliferation of collagen fibers leading to fibrosis and sclerosis as the fibers become more densely packed. In general, little if any inflammatory reaction is associated with the process, although the histological pattern of the disease may vary in that in some cases sclerosis predominates whereas in others inflammation is prominent.

Usually the lesions are associated with epithelial atrophy of the organs involved.

A sort of chronic vasculitis is often observed in most tissues involved. The vascular lesion is characterized by fibrosis and sclerosis of all layers of the vascular wall with endothelial proliferation. The lesions are found in skin, lungs, kidneys, gastrointestinal tract, skeletal muscles and the heart.

Like that of SLE, the symptomatology of scleroderma varies considerably depending upon the location of the disease. The skin changes include early swelling of the digits and reddish discoloration. This is followed by sclerosis of the corium with atrophy of the epithelium with destruction of the hair follicles and the sweat glands. The skin becomes tight, shiny, and nonelastic and cannot be moved over the subcutaneous layer. As a result, movement may be limited; the face, for example, becomes immobile and expressionless. As the lesion progresses, discoloration becomes more severe as a result of focal pigmentation, areas of depigmentation, and telangiectasia. Calcium may even be deposited under the surface of the skin.

Renal lesions primarily affect the interlobular arteries and the glomeruli, which may show fibrinoid necrosis and hyperplasia. The ultimate result is often diffuse glomerular basement membrane thickening of the wire loop type. Arterial obstruction leads to small kidney infarcts and ultimately to tubular degeneration. The kidney changes ultimately cause renal failure, which may develop with or without hypertension.

Restriction of the arterial blood flow in the extremities is often responsible for Raynaud's syndrome, which may be the first symptom of scleroderma.

In the lungs, the arterial walls are usually thickened and interstitial fibrosis may lead to focal emphysema with cystic formation. Fibrotic tissue may become impregnated with calcium visible on X-rays. Pulmonary symptoms are not uncommon. They usually start with dyspnea and coughing, which worsen as the fibrosis progresses and ultimately result in right-sided heart failure.

A typical radiological feature is the marked thickening of the periodontal membrane due to sclerosis. The membrane may be two to four times its normal thickness. Histological examination reveals that the membrane is widened and the normal arrangement of the collagen bundle is lost.

Alarcón-Segovia and associates have found antibodies to single-stranded RNA in sera of patients with scleroderma. The antibodies were specific for uracil bases and were different from the anti-RNA antibodies found in SLE [268].

Polymyositis. Polymyositis is a generalized acidophilic degeneration of the muscle fibers associated with lymphocytic infiltration. Histological examination of the muscle reveals, in addition to necrosis of the muscle fibers, a chronic inflammatory exudate that is often perivascular. As the necrosis progresses, the muscle fibers might be replaced by collagen in the process of fibrosis. Occasionally, some of the muscle fibers regenerate, which is indicated by the presence of large nuclei.

The muscle lesions in polymyositis must be distinguished from those observed in periarteritis nodosa (in which the changes are secondary to vasculitis) and from those observed in SLE, rheumatoid arthritis, scleroderma, and rheumatic fever (in which the inflammatory process is the prominant histological feature).

Polymyositis may exist alone (approximately 35% of the cases) or in association with other diseases. Sometimes the disease is associated with inflammatory skin lesions (35% of the cases) and is then often called dermatomyositis. Polymyositis may also occur in genuine collagen vascular diseases—such as SLE, scleroderma, rheumatic fever, and Sjögren's syndrome (approximately 10% of the cases)—or in malignancies, such as primarily carcinomas of the lungs, breast, stomach, and female pelvic organs.

Hyperglobulinemia and Paraglobulinemia

In a number of diseases, fragments, intact immunoglobulins, or even polymeric forms of immunoglobulins are produced. Such diseases may be distinguished on the basis of the protein elaborated; in some cases, primarily a single type of protein is elaborated (monoclonic), whereas in others a population of immunoglobulins (polyclonic) is elaborated.

The diseases can also be classified according to the type of hypercellularity that prevails (*e.g.*, plasmocytes in myeloma, lymphocytes in Waldenström's disease). In this discussion, we will describe the simplest of these diseases first and progress toward the more complex. However, such an approach does not reflect the incidence or the gravity of the disease. Myeloma is prominent in this group of diseases because of its relatively high incidence as well as its relentless progress to death.

Monoclonic Gammaglobulinopathies

Light-Chain Disease. Light-chain discasc is characterized by the disproportionate production and urinary excretion of light chains. The disease can exist in isolation or be associated with the excretion of other γ-globulins (see myeloma). Only the isolated form is discussed here.

We have already stated that the Bence Jones proteins found in the urine are light-chain proteins; therefore, light-chain disease is associated with the presence of the Bence Jones proteins and a monoclonic protein peak in the urine. The serum is usually hypogammaglobulinemic, and no light chains are detected at least until renal failure has begun. At that stage, a monoclonic peak of light chains can be detected electrophoretically. The renal failure results from an overload of the tubules by light chains. The tubules are involved in catabolizing as well as in excreting the light chains [269–271].

Heavy-Chain Disease. Like the names of many diseases, the term *heavy-chain disease* is inappropriate because what accumulates is not heavy chains, but immunoglobulin fragments (mol wt 55,000) of the Fc type with antigenic properties similar to those of the γ-, α-, and μ-chains. Heavy-chain disease is rare [272, 273].

The defects may affect the constant or the variable components. For example, some of the γ-chains contain $C\gamma 2$ and $C\gamma 3$, but lack $C\gamma 1$. Others have amino-terminal sequences similar to that of V_H, but segments on either side of the V-C junction are missing. Many heavy chains prepared from sera of patients with heavy-chain disease have heterogeneous sequences at their NH_2-terminal. This finding has been interpreted two ways: either the chains consist of different sequences that have been split off the rest of the molecule, or the V_H sequence (which is located at the amino terminal site of the molecule) has undergone partial hydrolysis [274].

Seligman and his associates found an abnormal α-chain that contains the entire Fc fragment of IgA but has a molecular weight 30% lower than IgA. These findings suggest that the immunoglobulins underwent postsynthetic proteolysis [275].

Further studies by Wolfenstein-Todel and associates have shown that at least in some cases the proteolysis is associated with a molecular defect. Their proteins have a heterogeneous NH_2-terminal resulting from proteolysis of the variable region, but they are also defective in several amino acids in the $C_H 1$ region [276].

The patient with heavy-chain disease complains of repeated infection, and examination reveals a painful lymphadenopathy and enlarged liver and spleen. Blood examination often reveals pancytopenia (anemia, leukopenia, thrombocytopenia) except for eventual eosinophilia associated with hyperuricemia and azotemia, probably due to renal failure. Electrophoresis of both urine and serum reveals monoclonic peaks of γ-globulin. The use of anti-Fc sera demonstrates Fc fragments. Examination of the bone marrow shows infiltration of a population of cells normally associated with immunocompetence—namely, plasma cells, lymphocytoid cells, reticulum cells, and lymphocytes. Therefore, the histological picture may be confused with that of Hodgkin's disease; sometimes heavy-chain disease is associated with a true lymphoma without bone involvement. The pathogenesis of this restricted distortion of gene expression remains unknown [277].

Waldenström's Macroglobulinemia

Waldenström's macroglobulinemia is more common in men (three to four times) than in women, it usually occurs after the fifth decade, and it is characterized by the appearance in the serum of a 19-S immunoglobulin of the IgM type. The symptoms resemble those of lymphoma, and there are no osteolytic lesions [278].

A patient with Waldenström's macroglobulinemia may be asymptomatic for years, but in progressive cases the disease is usually detected because the patient complains of fatigue, weakness, weight loss, nosebleeds, and bleeding of the mouth. An examination of the blood reveals a moderate to severe monochromic anemia, an unusually high sedimentation rate, normal or high lymphocyte levels with a differential favoring the lymphocytic series. The lymph nodes, liver, and spleen may be enlarged, but marked splenomegaly is rare. Serum electrophoresis reveals a marked monoclonic hyperglobulinemia of the IgM class. Both 7-S and 19-S IgM are found, but the proportion of the monomer to the polymer is increased, suggesting that the primary defect in the disease consists of an inability to polymerize the 7-S into 19-S units.

Whatever the primary mechanism, the globulin levels are so high that there is marked hyperviscosity of the blood, and this is largely responsible for the symptomatology. The hyperviscosity is clearly responsible for the high sedimentation rate and the "rouleau" formation of the red cells. Whereas blood viscosity normally is 1.65 that of water, the blood of patients with Waldenström's macroglobulinemia may be six or more times as viscous as water. When the blood becomes eight to ten times as viscous as water, the following symptoms develop: (1) hemorrhage (nose and mouth bleeding, but no purpura) due to chelation of blood factors, capillary stasis, and reduced platelet

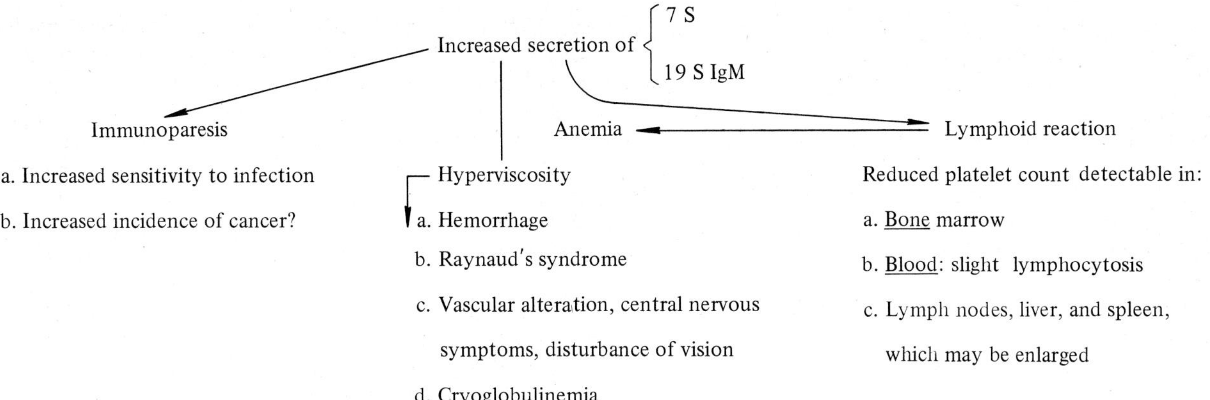

Fig. 14-23. Pathogenesis of Waldenström's disease

formation of unknown origin; (2) Raynaud's syndrome because of slowing of circulation in the extremities and the appearance of cryoglobulins in the blood.

The high levels of globulins in the blood ultimately result in vascular lesions, which may cause blurred vision and central nervous system symptoms (confusion, depression, and even delirium). The pathogenesis of Waldenström's disease is summarized in Fig. 14-23.

Waldenström's macroglobulinemia is associated with the proliferation of small, round cells, called lymphocytoid cells, which are intermediate between plasmocytes and lymphocytes. These cells have scarce cytoplasm, and budding of the membrane is common with abnormally large amounts of endoplasmic reticulum. The cells may contain PAS-positive inclusions, probably reflecting the presence of abnormal globulins. In addition to lymphocytes and plasmocytes, the lymphocytic infiltration of the marrow may be marked enough to make the disease difficult to differentiate from lymphoma.

The normal immunological response is impaired in macroglobulinemia. This impairment is responsible for the increased sensitivity to infection and perhaps also for the suspected increased incidence of cancer in these patients. Treatment of Waldenström's disease includes plasmapheresis and the administration of chlorambucyl and cyclophosphamide.

Multiple Myeloma

Multiple myeloma is a true neoplasm resulting from the uncontrolled proliferation of a clone of plasmocytes,* the accumulation of monoclonic globulins (usually IgG or IgA, rarely IgD or IgM) in the serum and sometimes urinary excretion of Bence Jones proteins.

The appearance of globulin in the sera of patients with myeloma raises the question of how these proteins are released from the plasma cells. Such mechanisms are not known for certain; holocrine secretion has been proposed, but it is generally accepted that release occurs through "clasmatosis"—a shedding of portions of the cytoplasm.

Multiple myeloma occurs spontaneously in at least certains strains of mice (*e.g.*, C-3H) and can be induced by injecting Freund adjuvants, mineral oil, or plastics in BALB/C. But the relevance of observations in animals to the pathogenesis of myeloma in humans is not understood. As in other neoplasms, viruses have been incriminated as the cause of myeloma, and 30- to 50-A particles have been detected in the cytoplasm of bone marrow cells of myeloma patients.

Plasmocytes were discovered by Cajal, and Wright associated them with myeloma in 1894. The pathognomonic feature is the increased level of plasmocytes in the bone marrow (see Fig. 14-24). Plasmocytes are not always easy to demonstrate in the marrow because the accumulations may be patchy. Therefore, several bone marrow aspirations may be needed to establish the histological diagnosis. Attempts have been made to correlate the symptoms of multiple myeloma with the type of plasma cells found in the marrow. It is said that myeloma associated with hypergammaglobulinemia in the serum, without Bence Jones proteins in the urine, is due to mature plasmocytes (AC cells) with eccentric nuclei containing condensed chromatin and large nucleoli. The cytoplasmic RNA is peripherally distributed, leaving a perinuclear clear zone; the endoplasmic reticulum is well developed and contains γ-globulins detectable by immunofluorescence.

In contrast, when the myeloma is associated with the excretion of Bence Jones proteins without hypergammaglobulinemia in the plasma, the plasma cells appear more immature (B cells) with large, less eccentric nuclei, evenly distributed chromatin, conspicuous nucleoli, and randomly distributed cytoplasmic RNA. Intermediate cytological features are found in cases of myeloma in which both Bence Jones proteins and hypergammaglobulinemia are seen. These findings are taken to indicate that the more mature plasmocyte

* Multiple myeloma with monoclonic production of IgE and IgD has been reported, as has as double myeloma with the production of IgG and IgA λ-type chains.

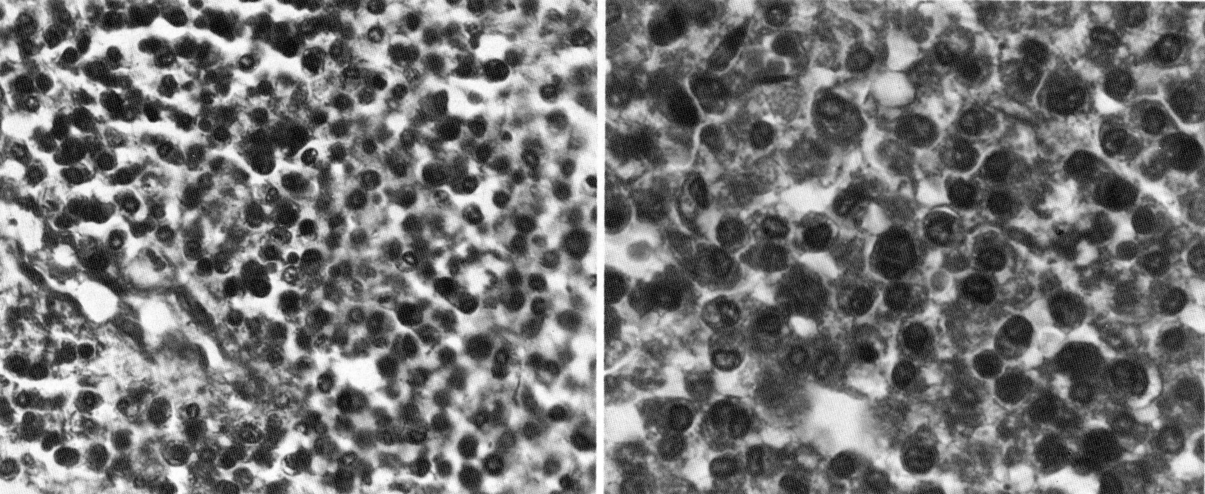

Fig. 14-24. Low- and high-power views of plasmocytic infiltration of bone marrow in patient with myeloma

is needed to assemble a complete γ-globulin. Interesting as the conclusion may be, one must doubt the reality of the correlation because myeloma cells, in general, are pleomorphic and usually contain mature, immature, and intermediate plasmocytes.

Electron microscopy reveals that the plasma cells in myeloma often contain distended cisternae of the endoplasmic reticulum. However, there seems to be no correlation between the electron microscopic appearance and the type of γ-globulin formed. Two special types of cells, "flame cells" and thesaurocytes, are believed to be predominant in some myelomas. These are storage cells whose endoplasmic reticulum cisternae are filled with Russell's bodies (large round or oval PAS-positive inclusions that stain eosinophilic with Giemsa-containing gammaglobulin, as shown by immunofluorescence) and acid phosphatase-positive vacuolated structures [279].

The plasma cell proliferation is so intense that it results in the replacement of bone tissue by plasma cells. This causes osteolytic destruction of bone, which may be manifested by generalized osteoporosis (20% of cases) or, more frequently, by the development of punched out lesions in the long bones, vertebrae, ribs, skull, and other bones. Diffuse or localized bone pains are often the first complaints of patients with myelomas.

The vertebrae or the ribs and sometimes other bones are the site of pathological fractures. Vertebral collapse may lead to compression of the spinal cord with paraplegia. Bone resorption results in hypercalcemia and hypercalciuria, which contribute to the renal insufficiency often seen in myeloma. The gross appearance of the skull and vertebrae in myeloma is shown in Fig. 14-25.

As was the case in Waldenström's disease, hypergammaglobulinemia in myeloma causes hyperviscosity of the blood with its consequences, and it may be associated with cryoglobulinemia. A combination of plasmocytes and amyloid infiltration may be the source of the polyneuropathy that is sometimes seen in myeloma patients.

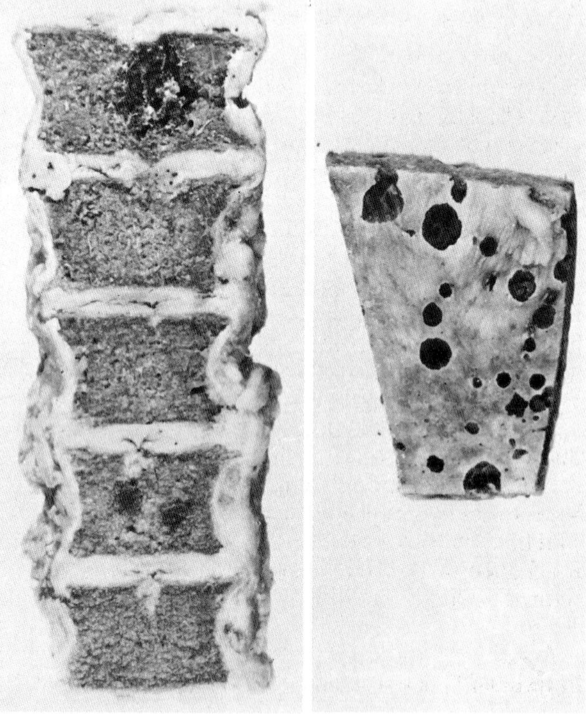

Fig. 14-25. Multiple myeloma; typical punched out areas of bone in the vertebrae (*left*) and skull (right)

In myeloma, patients develop immunoparesis with increased sensitivity to infection, which may include pyoderma, pyelonephritis, pneumonia, and even septicemia.

For unknown reasons (see Chapter 10), amyloidosis is frequently associated with myeloma.

Renal insufficiency is a frequent complication of myeloma; it may be a direct consequence of the pro-

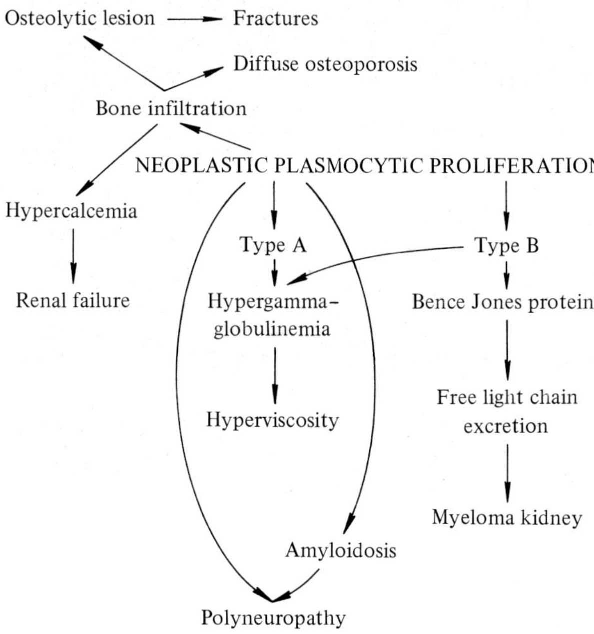

Fig. 14-26. Pathogenesis of myeloma

duction of γ-globulins, or it may have a multiple etiology. The free light chains in the urine may produce what is referred to as the myeloma kidney, with accumulations of light chains in the cytoplasm of tubular cells (demonstrated by immunofluorescence) and albumin, γ-globulin, and fibrinogen casts in the tubular lumen in association with tubular degeneration. However, there is no correlation between the amount of light chains excreted and renal insufficiency. A combination of factors, such as hyperviscosity, hypercalcemia, hyperuricemia, and amyloidosis may also result in renal insufficiency.

As we have pointed out already, it is not certain that the γ-globulins of myeloma can act as antibodies or are even normal proteins. But these γ-globulins do have antibody properties to Fc fragments of IgG, serum lipoproteins, pneumococcal polysaccharides, and 2,4-dinitrophenol. The pathogenesis of myeloma is summarized in Fig. 14-26.

Polyclonal Gammopathies

Polyclonal gammopathies occur in a number of conditions including collagen vascular diseases, autoimmune diseases, some neoplasms, lipid storage disease, sarcoidosis, mongolism, infectious diseases, and liver diseases. We will consider only a few of these here.

Infectious diseases associated with polyclonal gammopathies include chronic bacterial (lung abcess, osteomyelitis) and parasitic infections (*e.g.*, trypanosomiasis). IgG predominates in the bacterial, IgM in the parasitic infections.

The cause of the gammopathy (increased IgG and IgA in alcoholic cirrhosis and IgM in biliary cirrhosis) is not known.

Waldenström described an interesting polyclonic gammopathy that consists of the accumulation of 9-S and 15-S gammaglobulins in the serum and necrosis of the vascular wall; the disease is manifested by purpura. The development of purpura can be triggered by a number of factors, including unusual physical strain (*e.g.*, protracted dancing), strenuous sitting (*e.g.*, in a plane), or excessive pressure on the skin (tight belts, tight garments).

Crohn's Disease and Ulcerative Colitis

We will describe briefly two gastrointestinal diseases that are suspected, but not proven, to be of immunological origin [280, 281].

Crohn's Disease

Crohn's disease (regional enteritis, terminal ileitis, regional jejunitis, ileocolitis, segmental colitis) is a nonspecific granulomatous disease that usually involves the terminal ileum but may also affect the colon, the jejunum, or the rectum. Crohn's disease rarely affects the stomach or the duodenum. It may occur at all ages, but half of the cases are found in the third decade and the remainder are found in the fourth and fifth decades. The incidence is slightly higher in men than in women; the disease is believed to be more common among Jews than among other races.

The cause of Crohn's disease is unknown. Infection, trauma, and psychological disturbances have all been incriminated.

Autopsy examination reveals that a segment of the intestine is thick and hard (this segment has been said to resemble a hose). Closer examination of the surface of the serosa covering the diseased portion of the intestine reveals fibrosis with adhesions to the surrounding loops of the intestine. Sometimes the serosa is covered with small white spots that resemble those seen in miliary tuberculosis. The intestinal lumen is narrowed, and, as a result, there is hypertrophy of the bowel above the constriction. In the intestinal mucosa, areas of ulceration alternate with nodular elevations of the mucosa. This varied pattern of injury leads to what is often referred to as the cobblestone appearance of the mucosal surface. Fissures are often found between the nodules (they are the source of the fistulas that will be described below). The lymph nodes are enlarged but soft in consistency, in contrast to lymph nodes containing metastatic carcinoma.

When Crohn's disease affects the small intestine, it is usually restricted to approximately 30 cm of the terminal ileum, which stops abruptly at the ileocecal valve. A single stricture is rare; more often multiple strictures are separated by areas of healthy intestine approximately 2 cm or less in length. These healthy areas are referred to as skip areas.

Similarly, in the large intestine there may be single or multiple lesions. Crohn's disease of the large intestine is sometimes difficult to distinguish from ulcerative colitis.

The histological unit of the lesion in Crohn's disease is a noncaseating tuberculoid focus formed of clusters of epithelioid cells and giant cells with small nuclei. The granuloma is often infiltrated with lymphocytes and plasmocytes. There is associated edema and fibrosis.

The chronic granulomatous inflammatory reaction that primarily involves the Peyer's patches leads to enlargement of the lymphoid structure. This results in a number of complications, including lymphatic obstruction with edema, inflammatory infiltration along the lymphatics, lymphatic dilatation, and involvement of all layers of the intestinal wall leading to fibrosis, fistula formation, and ulceration of the mucosa.

The anatomical complication most often associated with Crohn's disease is the formation of fistulas between the intestinal loops (20% of the cases) or of the ileal, ileocolic or ileorectal type. Enterocutaneous as well as anal fistulas are also seen. The second obvious anatomical complication of Crohn's disease is obstruction. Functionally, the disease is associated with slow but progressive malabsorption of fats, proteins, and vitamins. The degree of malabsorption usually does not correlate with the extensiveness of the intestinal involvement.

Crohn's disease may be difficult to differentiate from ulcerative colitis (see below) and from other diseases that cause granulomatous lesions, such as tuberculosis, syphilis, lymphogranuloma inguinale, and sarcoid and fungal infections. Tuberculosis rarely affects the large intestine, and if tuberculosis is seen in the large intestine, it is usually associated with pulmonary tuberculosis. Moreover, the tubercular granulomas are usually caseated. Similarly, in syphilis the center of the granuloma is necrotic; moreover, gummas of the rectum or the intestine are rare. Lymphogranuloma inguinale occurs predominantly in women, involves primarily the rectum and the pelvic colon, and leads to the formation of fistulas and condylomas. It can be readily distinguished from Crohn's disease by comparing the histological appearances of the lesions and by performing Frei's test. Actinomycosis of the cecum associated with actinomycosis of the appendix has been described. The histological appearances of the lesions and the presence of fungi readily distinguish actinomycosis from Crohn's disease.

Ulcerative Colitis

Ulcerative colitis is an acute or chronic inflammatory reaction of the intestinal mucosa of unknown origin. Various causes have been incriminated, including psychological factors, hypersensitivity, and autoimmunity. The incidence of ulcerative colitis is equal in both sexes, and the disease may occur at any age.

Autopsy examination of a patient with ulcerative colitis reveals shortening of the bowel segment involved with thickening of the wall and loss of haustration. The subserosal blood vessels are congested. The intestinal wall, which is usually very friable, resembles rotten leather. There is hemorrhagic sluffing of the mucosa with superficial ulceration, edema, and vasodilation of the submucosa, and a certain degree of muscular hypertrophy of unknown origin. But even the unulcerated portions of the mucosa found throughout the affected bowel are not normal. They may be reddened and, even if not congested, are usually thickened and velvety and have lost the bright sheen of the normal mucosa.

Histologically, the typical findings include vasodilation with cellular infiltration and edema of the mucosa and submucosa. The typical lesion, the crypt abscess, results from the blocking of the opening of the gland of Lieberkühn with mucous stagnation, secondary infection by bacteria, and polymorphonuclear invasion.

The crypt abscess may evolve in two ways: it may discharge the products of the infection at the surface, or it may open into and infiltrate the submucosa. When the mucosa is sluffed off, it leaves an infected, ulcerated surface. Fibrosis is usually minimal and occurs only in the form of patches and scars at the site of the healing ulcers. Occasionally, thromboses are seen in the intestinal wall.

The two phases of ulcerative colitis are the acute and quiescent. During the quiescent phase, lymphocytic infiltration and attempts to repair of the epithelial surface predominate. The anatomical complications include multiple perforations of the colon that lead to peritonitis, the formation of perineal abscesses with fistulas and anal stenosis, and the development of carcinoma.

The incidence of carcinoma of the colon in patients with ulcerative colitis is not clear, and the reported figures range from 5–11%. There is usually a latent period of 10 years between the onset of ulcerative colitis and the development of the colonic cancer, and cancer in these patients usually occurs in the fourth decade. Cancer may be multiple and often resembles the diffuse scirrhous carcinoma of the stomach. The tumors appear as flat, inflated masses with ill-defined edges. Carcinomas that develop in patients with ulcerative colitis are usually highly malignant.

The two major gastrointestinal diseases that may be confused with ulcerative colitis are chronic bacillary dysentery and Crohn's disease. Indeed, one-third of the patients with ulcerative colitis have ileal involvement, and in one-quarter of the patients with Crohn's disease, the disease occurs in the colon. Both diseases occur most often in people 30 years old, and both diseases affect men and women. Table 14-14 lists some of the criteria usually used to make the differential diagnosis.

In patients with ulcerative colitis, the number of IgG-containing plasma cells is greatly increased. Moreover, the connective tissue of the rectal mucosa stains with immunofluorescent IgG antisera. These findings suggest that ulcerative colitis is associated with the triggering of an immunological reaction. Also,

Table 14-14. Differential diagnosis of ulcerative colitis and Crohn's disease

	Ulcerative colitis	Crohn's disease
Gross appearance		
Ulceration	Diffuse	More sharply demarcated
Skip area	No skip area; mucosa is abnormal even between ulceration	Skip areas detectable with X-rays
Cobblestone appearance	None	Visible
Fistulas	Low incidence	High incidence
Cancer	High incidence	Low incidence
Lymph nodes	Not prominent	Enlarged
Microscopic features		
Granulomatous infiltration	None	In 76%
Leukocytic infiltration	Some	In 100%
Fibrosis	Rare except in scar zones	In 100%
Fissure ulcer	None	In 59%
Crypt abscesses	Common, with crypt degeneration beginning anywhere	Crypt degeneration limited to base, abscess rare
Degree of penetration	Primarily mucosal, no serositis	Submucosal muscular serositis causing adhesions

the presence of complement in the connective tissue suggests that the immunological response may be associated with cytotoxicity, which may be at the origin of the mucosal ulceration.

References

1. Talmage, D.W., Cann, J.R.: The chemistry of immunity in health and disease. Springfield, Ill.: Charles C. Thomas Publisher 1961
2. Cohen, S.: The structure of antibody. In: Immunological diseases (Samter, M., and Alexander, H.L., eds.), p. 32–51. Boston: Little, Brown and Company 1965
3. Smithies, O.: Antibody variability. Science **157**, 267–273 (1967)
4. Nisonoff, A.: Molecules of immunity. Hosp. Pract. **2**, 19–27 (1967)
5. Putnam, F.W.: Immunoglobulin structure: Variability and homology. Science **163**, 633–644 (1969)
6. Merler, E., Rosen, F.S.: The gamma globulins. I. The structure and synthesis of the immunoglobulins. New Engl. J. Med. **275**, 480–486, 536–542 (1966)
7. Day, E.D.: Foundations of immunochemistry. Baltimore: Williams & Wilkins Co. 1966
8. Janeway, C.A., Rosen, F.S.: The gamma globulins. IV. Therapeutic uses of gamma globulin. New Engl. J. Med. **275**, 826–831 (1966)
9. Ishizaka, K.: The identification and significance of gamma E. Hosp. Pract. **4**, 70–81 (1969)
10. Haurowitz, F.: The molecular basis of immunity. Ann. N.Y. Acad. Sci. **169**, 11–22 (1970)
11. Tomasi, T.B., Jr.: Structure and function of mucosal antibodies. Annu. Rev. Med. **21**, 281–298 (1970)
12. Finger, H., Seeliger, H.P.R.: The origin, development, and significance of immunoglobulins. In: Research in immunochemistry and immunobiology (Kivapinski, J.B.G., ed.), vol. 1, p. 3–70. Baltimore: University Park Press 1972
13. Nisonoff, A., Wilson, S.K., Wang, A.C., Fudenberg, H.H., Hopper, J.E.: Genetic control of the biosynthesis of IgG and IgM. In: Progress in immunology (Amos, B., ed.), p. 61–70. New York: Academic Press 1971
14. Davies, D.R., Sarma, V.R., Labaw, L.W., Silverton, E.W., Terry, W.D.: Three-dimensional structure of immunoglobulins. In: Progress in immunology (Amos, B., ed.), p. 25–32. New York: Academic Press 1971
15. Porter, R.R.: Structural studies of immunoglobulins. Science **180**, 713–716 (1973)
16. Edelman, G.M.: Antibody structure and molecular immunology. Science **180**, 830–839 (1973)
17. Gally, J.A.: Structure of immunoglobulins. In: The antigens (Sela, M., ed.), vol. I, p. 161–298. New York: Academic Press 1973
18. Smith, G.P., Hood, L., Fich, W.M.: Antibody diversity. Annu. Rev. Biochem. **40**, 969–1013 (1971)
19. Jerne, N.K.: The immune system. Sci. Amer. **229**, 52–60 (1973)
20. Franklin, E.C.: Structure of antibodies. In: Textbook of immunopathology (Miescher, P.A., and Muller-Eberhard, H.J., eds.), vol. 1, chap. 3, p. 25–32. New York: Grune & Stratton 1968
21. Edelman, G.M., Gally, J.A.: A model for the 7S antibody molecule. Proc. nat. Acad. Sci. (Wash.) **51**, 846–853 (1964)
22. Svehag, S.-E., Bloth, B.: Ultrastructure of secretory and high-polymer serum immunoglobulin A of human and rabbit origin. Science **168**, 847–849 (1970)
23. Valentine, R.C., Green, N.M.: Electron microscopy of an antibody-hapten complex. J. molec. Biol. **27**, 615–617 (1967)
24. Edmundson, A.B., Wood, M.K., Schiffer, M., Hardman, K.R., et al.: A crystallographic investigation of a human IgG immunoglobulin. J. biol. Chem. **245**, 2763–2764 (1970)
25. Sarma, V.R., Davies, D.R., Labaw, L.W., Silverton, E.W., Terry, W.D.: Crystal structure of an immunoglobulin molecule by X-ray diffraction and electron microscopy. Cold Spr. Harb. Symp. quant. Biol. **36**, 413–419 (1972)
26. Paul, C., Shimizu, A., Köhler, H., Putnam, F.W.: Structure of the hinge region of the mu heavy chain of human IgM immunoglobulins. Science **172**, 69–72 (1971)
27. Shimizu, A., Paul, C., Köhler, H., Shinoda, T., Putnam, F.W.: Variation and homology in the mu and gamma heavy chains of human immunoglobulins. Science **173**, 629–633 (1971)
28. Putnam, F.W., Florent, G., Paul, C., Shinoda, T., Shimizu, A.: Complete amino acid sequence of the mu heavy chain of a human IgM immunoglobulin. Science **182**, 287–291 (1973)
29. Sela, M., Fuch, S.: On the role of charge and optical configuration in antigenicity. In: Molecular and cellular basis of antibody formation (Šterzl, J., Hahn, P., Rudinger, J., et al., eds.), p. 43–56. New York: Academic Press 1965
30. Haurowitz, F.: The molecular basis of immunity. Part I. The molecular basis of immunology. Ann. N.Y. Acad. Sci. **169**, 11–22 (1970)
31. Eisen, H.M.: The immune response to a simple antigenic determinant. Harvey Lecture Series 60, p. 1–34. New York: Academic Press 1966
32. Sela, M.: Structure and specificity of synthetic polypeptide antigens. Ann. N.Y. Acad. Sci. **169**, 23–35 (1970)
33. Sela, M.: Antigen design and immune response. Harvey Lecture Series 67, p. 213–246. New York: Academic Press 1971
34. Crumpton, J.H.: Protein antigens: The molecular bases of antigenicity and immunogenicity. In: The antigens (Sela, M., ed.), vol. II, p. 1–78. New York: Academic Press 1974
35. Pressman, D.: Molecular complementariness in antigen-antibody systems. In: Molecular structure and biological specificity (Pauling, L., and Itano, H.A., eds.), Publ. #2, p. 1–17. Washington, D.C.: American Institute for Biological Sciences 1957
36. Schlossman, S.F.: The immune response, some unifying concepts. New Engl. J. Med. **277**, 1355–1361 (1967)
37. Singer, S.J., Doolittle, R.F.: Antibody active sites and immunoglobulin molecules. Science **153**, 13–25 (1966)
38. Capra, J.D., Kehoe, J.M.: The antibody combining site. In: Fractions; News of Biochemical Instrumentation, No. 1, p. 1. Palo Alto, Calif.: Beckman Instruments, Inc. 1972
39. Richards, F.F., Konigsberg, W.H., Rosenstein, R.W., Varga, J.M.: On the specificity of antibodies. Science **187**, 130–136 (1975)
40. Weiser, R.S., Myrvik, Q.M., Pearsall, N.N. (eds.): Fundamentals of immunology. Philadelphia: Lea & Febiger 1970
41. Yachin, S.: Functions and mechanism of action of complement. New Engl. J. Med. **274**, 140–144 (1966)
42. Ward, P.A.: A plasmin-split fragment of C′3 as a new chemotactic factor. J. exp. Med. **126**, 189–206 (1967)
43. Gewurz, H.: The immunologic role of complement. Hosp. Prac. **2**, 45–56 (1967)
44. Burkholder, P.M., Littleton, C.E.: Immunobiology of complement. In: Pathobiology annual (Ioachim, H.L., ed.), vol. 1, p. 215–239. New York: Appleton-Century-Crofts 1971
45. Ruddy, S., Gigli, I., Austen, K.F.: The complement system of man. New Engl. J. Med. **287**, 489–495, 545–549 (1972)
46. Ruddy, S., Gigli, I., Austen, K.F.: The complement system of man. New Engl. J. Med. **287**, 590–596, 642–648 (1972)
47. Ward, P.A., Hill, J.H.: Biologic role of complement products. J. Immunol. **108**, 1137–1145 (1972)
48. Lachmann, P.J.: Complement. In: Defence and recognition. MTP international review of science (Porter, R.R., ed.), Biochemistry series 1, vol. 10, p. 361–397. London: Butterworth and Co., Ltd., 1973
49. Mayer, M.M.: The complement system. Sci. Amer. **229**, 54–66 (1973)

50. Müller-Eberhard, H.J.: The serum complement system. In: Textbook of immunopathology (Miescher, P.A., and Müller-Eberhard, H.J., eds.), vol. I, chap. 4, p. 33–47. New York: Grune & Stratton 1968
51. Müller-Eberhard, H.J.: The molecular basis of the biological activities of complement. Harvey Lecture Series **66**, 75–104 (1971)
52. Pillemer, L., Schoenberg, M.D., Blum, L., Wurz, L.: Properdin system and immunity. II. Interaction of the properdin system with polysaccharides. Science **122**, 545–549 (1955)
53. Götze, O., Müller-Eberhard, H.J.: The role of properdin in the alternate pathway of complement activation. J. exp. Med. **139**, 44–47 (1974)
54. Lachmann, P.J., Nicol, P.: Reaction mechanism of the alternative pathway of complement fixation. Lancet **1973 I**, 465–467
55. Ruley, E.J., Forristal, J., Davis, N.C., Andres, C., West, C.D.: Hypocomplementemia of membranoproliferative nephritis. Dependence of the nephritic factor reaction on properdin factor B. J. clin. Invest. **52**, 896–904 (1973)
56. Ward, P.A., Cochrane, C.G., Müller-Eberhard, H.J.: The role of serum complement in chemotaxis of leukocytes *in vitro*. J. exp. Med. **122**, 327–346 (1965)
57. Ward, P.A., Cochrane, C.G.: Bound complement and immunologic injury of blood vessels. J. exp. Med. **121**, 215–234 (1965)
58. Simson, J.V., Spicer, S.S.: Activities of specific cell constituents in phagocytosis (endocytosis). Int. Rev. exp. Path. **12**, 79–118 (1973)
59. Radovich, J., Talmage, D.W.: Antigenic competition: Cellular or humoral. Science **158**, 512–514 (1967)
60. Buxbaum, J.N.: The biosynthesis, assembly and secretion of immunoglobulins. Semin. Hemat. **10**, 33–52 (1973)
61. Baumal, R., Bargellesi, A., Buxbaum, J., Scharff, M.: Mechanisms of antibody assembly. 3rd Intl. Convocation on Immunology, Buffalo, June 1972. Basel: Karger 1972
62. Williamson, A.R.: Biosynthesis of immunoglobulins. In: Defence and recognition. MTP international review of science (Porter, R.R., ed.), Biochemistry series 1, vol. 10, p. 229–256. London: Butterworth and Co., Ltd. 1973
63. Milstein, C., Munro, A.J.: Genetics of immunoglobulins and of the immune response. In: Defence and recognition. MTP international review of science (Porter, R.R., ed.). Biochemistry Series 1, vol. 10, p. 199–228. London: Butterworth and Co., Ltd. 1973
64. Burnet, F.M.: The clonal selection theory of acquired immunity. London: Cambridge University Press 1959
65. Eichmann, K.: Idiotypic identity of antibodies to streptococcal carbohydrate in inbred mice. J. Immunol. **2**, 301–307 (1972)
66. Lawton, A.R., Kincade, P.W., Cooper, M.D.: Sequential expression of germ line genes in development of immunoglobulin class diversity. Fed. Proc. **34**, 33–39 (1975)
67. Potter, M.: Gene regulation in differentiation and development. Introductory remarks. Fed. Proc. **34**, 21–23 (1975)
68. Chapuis, R.M., Koshland, M.W.: Mechanism of IgM polymerization. Proc. nat. Acad. Sci. (Wash.) **71**, 657–661 (1974)
69. Baenziger, J., Kornfeld, S.: Structure of the carbohydrate units of IgA_1 immunoglobulin. II. Structure of the O-glycosidically linked oligosaccharide units. J. biol. Chem. **249**, 7260–7269 (1974)
70. Shreffler, D.C.: Molecular aspects of immunogenetics. Annu. Rev. Genet. **1**, 163–184 (1967)
71. Milstein, C., Munro, A.J.: The genetic basis of antibody specificity. Annu. Rev. Microbiol. **24**, 335–358 (1970)
72. Hood, L.E.: Two genes, one polypeptide chain—fact or fiction? Fed. Proc. **31**, 177–209 (1972)
73. Hood, L., Talmage, D.W.: Mechanism of antibody diversity: Germ line basis for variability. Science **168**, 325–334 (1970)
74. McDevitt, H.O.: Genetic control of the antibody response. Hosp. Prac. **8**, 61–74 (1973)
75. Williamson, A.R., Premkumar, E., Shoyab, M.: Germ line basis for antibody diversity. Fed. Proc. **34**, 28–32 (1975)
76. Owen, J.J.T.: Anatomy of the lymphoid system. In: Defence and recognition. MTP international review of science (Porter, R.R., ed.). Biochemistry series 1, vol. 10, p. 35–64. London: Butterworth and Co., Ltd. 1973
77. Zacharski, L.R., Hill, R.W., Maldonado, J.E.: The lymphocyte. Mayo Clin. Proc. **42**, 431–451 (1967)
78. Craddock, C.G., Longmire, R., McMillan, R.: Lymphocytes and the immune response, part I. New Engl. J. Med. **285**, 324–331 (1971)
79. Craddock, C.G., Longmire, R., McMillan, R.: Lymphocytes and the immune response, part II. New Engl. J. Med. **285**, 378–384 (1971)
80. Nossal, G.J.V., Ada, G.L.: Antigens, lymphoid cells and the immune response. New York: Academic Press 1971
81. Editorial: The lymphocyte. Lancet **1973 I**, 409–410
82. Ford, W.L.: The cellular basis of immune response. In: Defence and recognition. MTP international review of science (Porter, R.R., ed.), series 1, vol. 10, p. 65–102. London: Butterworth and Co., Ltd. 1973
83. Greaves, M.F., Owen, J.J.T., Raff, M.C.: T and B lymphocytes: Origins, properties and roles in immune responses. Amsterdam: Excerpta Medica 1974
84. Parker, C.W.: Complexities in the study of the role of cyclic nucleotides in lymphocyte responses to mitogens. In: Cyclic AMP, cell growth, and the immune response (Braun, W., Lichtenstein, L.M., and Parker, C.W., eds.), p. 35–44. Berlin-Heidelberg-New York: Springer 1974
85. Hirschhorn, R.: The effect of exogenous nucleotides on the response of lymphocytes to PHA, PWM, and CON A. In: Cyclic AMP, cell growth, and the immune response (Braun, W., Lichtenstein, L.M., and Parker, C.W., eds.), p. 45–54. Berlin-Heidelberg-New York: Springer 1974
86. Hooper, J.A., McDaniel, M.C., Thurman, G.B., Cohen, G.H., Schulof, R.S., Goldstein, A.L.: Purification and properties of bovine thymosin. Ann. N.Y. Acad. Sci. **249**, 125–144 (1975)
87. Howie, J.B., Helyer, B.J.: The immunology and pathology of NZB mice. In: Advances in immunology (Dixon, F.J., Jr., and Kunkel, H.G., eds.), vol. 9, p. 215–266. New York: Academic Press 1968
88. Mellors, R.C.: Autoimmune and immunoproliferative diseases of NZB / Bl mice and hybrids. In: International review of experimental pathology (Richter, G.W., and Epstein, M.A., eds.), vol. 5, p. 217–252. New York: Academic Press 1966
89. Talal, N.: Autoimmunity and lymphoid malignancy in New Zealand black mice. In: Progress in clinical immunology (Schwartz, R.S., ed.), vol. 2, p. 101–120. New York: Grune & Stratton 1974
90. Sugai, S., Pillarisetty, R.J., Talal, N.: Monoclonal macroglobulinemia in NZB/NZW F_1 mice. J. exp. Med. **138**, 989–1002 (1973)
91. Wara, D.W., Goldstein, A.L., Doyle, N.E., Ammann, A.J.: Thymosin activity in patients with cellular immunodeficiency. New Engl. J. Med. **292**, 70–74 (1975)
92. Basch, R.S., Goldstein, G.: Induction of T-cell differentiation *in vitro* by thymin, a purified polypeptide hormone of the thymus. Proc. nat. Acad. Sci. (Wash.) **71**, 1474–1478 (1974)
93. Miller, J.F.A.P.: T-cell regulation of immune responsiveness. Ann. N.Y. Acad. Sci. **249**, 9–26 (1975)
94. Davies, A.J.S.: Thymic hormones? Ann. N.Y. Acad. Sci. **249**, 61–67 (1975)
95. Miller, J.F.A.P.: Endocrine function of the thymus. New Engl. J. Med. **290**, 1255–1256 (1974)
96. White, A.: Nature and biological activities of thymus hormones. Prospects for the future. Ann. N.Y. Acad. Sci. **249**, 523–530 (1975)
97. Friedman, H. (ed.): Thymus factors in immunity, vol. 249. Annals of the New York Academy of Sciences (Boland, B., and Hasher, J., eds.), New York: The New York Academy of Sciences 1975
98. Wigzell, H., Andersson, B.: Isolation of lymphoid cells with active surface receptor sites. Annu. Rev. Microbiol. **25**, 291–308 (1971)
99. Roelants, G.: Antigen recognition by B and T lymphocytes. In: Current topics in microbiology and immunology (Arber, W., Braun, W., and Haas, R., et al., eds), vol. 59, p. 135–166. Berlin-Heidelberg-New York: Springer 1972
100. Stein, H., Lennert, K., Parwaresch, M.R.: Malignant lymphomas of B-cell type. Lancet **1972 II**, 855–857
101. Wybran, J., Chantler, S., Fudenberg, H.H.: Isolation of normal T cells in chronic lymphatic leukaemia. Lancet **1973 I**, 126–129
102. Dwyer, J.M., Bullock, W.E., Fields, J.P.: Disturbance of the blood T:B lymphocyte ratio in lepromatous leprosy. New Engl. J. Med. **288**, 1036–1039 (1973)
103. Lisowska-Bernstein, B., Rinuy, A., Vassalli, P.: Absence of detectable IgM in enzymatically or biosynthetically labeled thymus-derived lymphocytes. Proc. nat. Acad. Sci. (Wash.) **70**, 2879–2883 (1973)
104. Sell, S., Sheppard, H.W., Jr.: Rabbit blood lymphocytes may be T cells with surface immunoglobulins. Science **182**, 586–587 (1973)
105. Kersey, J.H., Sabad, A., Gajl-Peczalska, K.: Acute lymphoblastic leukemic cells with T (thymus-derived) lymphocyte markers. Science **182**, 1355–1356 (1973)
106. Kaur, J., Catovsky, D., Spiers, A.S.D., Galton, D.A.G.: Increase of T lymphocytes in the spleen in chronic granulocytic leukaemia. Lancet **1974 I**, 834–836
107. Sandilands, G.P., Gray, K., Cooney, A., Browning, J.D., Grant, R.M., et al.: Lymphocytes with T and B cell properties in a lymphoproliferative disorder. Lancet **1974 I**, 903–904
108. Seligmann, M.: B-cell and T-cell markers in lymphoid proliferations. New Engl. J. Med. **290**, 1483–1484 (1974)
109. Carr, I.: The macrophage. A review of ultrastructure and function. London: Academic Press 1973
110. Harris, T.N., Harris, S.: Histochemical changes in lymphocytes during the production of antibodies in lymph nodes of rabbits. J. exp. Med. **90**, 169–179 (1949)
111. Fishman, M., Adler, F.L.: Antibody formation *in vitro*. II. Antibody synthesis in X-irradiated recipients of diffusion chambers containing nucleic acid derived from macrophages incubated with antigen. J. exp. Med. **117**, 595–602 (1963)
112. Fishman, M., Adler, F.L., Rice, S.G.: Macrophage RNA in the *in vitro* immune response to phage. Ann. N.Y. Acad. Sci. **207**, 73–82 (1973)
113. Herscowitz, H.B., Stelos, P.: Immunogenicity of mouse spleen RNA. Ann. N.Y. Acad. Sci. **207**, 104–121 (1973)
114. Mitsuhashi, S., Saito, K., Kurashige, S.: The role of RNA as amplifier in the immune response. Ann. N.Y. Acad. Sci. **207**, 160–171 (1973)
115. Braun, W.: RNAs as amplifiers of specific signals in immunity. Ann. N.Y. Acad. Sci. **207**, 17–28 (1973)
116. Duke, L.J., Miller, C., Harshman, S.: *In vitro* induction of antibody formation with immunogenic RNA. Ann. N.Y. Acad. Sci. **207**, 145–159 (1973)

117. Miller, J.F.A.P., Basten, A., Sprent, J., Cheers, C.: Interaction between lymphocytes in immune responses. Cell. Immunol. **2**, 469–495 (1971)
118. Playfair, J.H.L.: Cell cooperation in the immune response. Clin. exp. Immunol. **8**, 839–856 (1971)
119. Mitchison, N.A.: The carrier effect in the secondary response to hapten-protein conjugates. V. Use of antilymphocyte serum to deplete animals of helper cells. Europ. J. Immunol. **1**, 68–75 (1971)
120. Katz, D.H., Benacerraf, B.: The regulatory influence of activated T cells on B cell responses to antigen. In: Advances in immunology (Dixon, F.J., and Kunkel, H.G., eds.), vol. 15, p. 1–94. New York: Academic Press 1972
121. Glade, P.R.: Products of lymphoid cells in continuous culture. Amer. J. Path. **69**, 483–492 (1970)
122. Lawrence, H.S., Valentine, F.T.: Transfer factor and other mediators of cellular immunity, President's Symposium. Amer. J. Path. **60**, 437–452 (1970)
123. Sherwood, L.M., Parris, E.E.: Transfer factor and cellular immune deficiency disease. New Engl. J. Med. **283**, 411–419 (1970)
124. Fudenberg, H.H., Levin, A.S., Spitler, L.E., Wybran, J., Byers, V.: Therapeutic uses of transfer factor. Hosp. Prac. **9**, 95–104 (1974)
125. Owen, R.D.: Immunogenetic consequences of vascular anastomoses between bovine twins. Science **102**, 400–401 (1945)
126. Burnet, F.M., Fenner, F.: The production of antibodies. Melbourne: MacMillan & Co., Ltd. 1949
127. Diener, E., Feldmann, M.: Relationship between antigen and antibody-induced suppression of immunity. Transplant. Rev. **8**, 76–103 (1972)
128. Taussig, M.J.: Studies on the induction of immunological tolerance. The inhibition of tolerance-induction by antiserum: Split tolerance and the time-course of tolerance induction. Europ. J. Immunol. **1**, 367–371 (1971)
129. Mitchison, N.A.: Induction of immunological paralysis in two zones of dosage. Proc. roy. Soc. B **161**, 275–292 (1964)
130. Ishizaka, K.: Experimental anaphylaxis. In: Immunological diseases (Samter, M., and Alexander, H.L., eds.), chap. 10, p. 131–145. Boston: Little, Brown and Company 1965
131. McKay, D.G.: A partial synthesis of the generalized Schwartzman reaction. Fed. Proc. **22**, 1373–1379 (1963)
132. Raffel, S.: Delayed (cellular) hypersensitivity. In: Immunological diseases (Samter, M., and Alexander, H.L., eds.), chap. 11, p. 146–160. Boston: Little, Brown and Company 1965
133. Dixon, F.J.: Experimental serum sickness. In: Immunological diseases (Samter, M., and Alexander, H.L., eds.), chap. 12, p. 161–171. Boston: Little, Brown and Company 1965
134. Austen, K.F.: Histamine and other mediators of allergic reactions. In: Immunological diseases (Samter, M., and Alexander, H.L., eds.) chap. 15, p. 211–225. Boston: Little, Brown and Company 1965
135. Orange, R.P., Austin, K.F.: Chemical mediators of immediate hypersensitivity. In: Immunobiology (Good, R.A., and Fisher, D.W., eds.), chap. 12, p. 115–122. Stamford, Conn.: Sinauer Associates, Publishers 1971
136. David, J.R.: Lymphocytic factors in cellular hypersensitivity. In: Immunobiology (Good, R.A., and Fisher, D.W., eds.), chap. 15, p. 146–160. Stamford, Conn.: Sinauer Associates, Publishers 1971
137. Dixon, F.J.: Mechanisms of immunologic injury. In: Immunobiology (Good, R.A., and Fisher, D.W., eds.), chap. 16, p. 161–166. Stamford, Conn.: Sinauer Associates, Publishers 1971
138. Waksman, B.H.: Delayed hypersensitivity: Immunologic and clinical aspects. In: Immunobiology (Good, R.A., and Fisher, D.W., eds.), chap. 3, p. 28–36. Stamford, Conn.: Sinauer Associates, Publishers 1971
139. David, J.R.: Lymphocyte mediators and cellular hypersensitivity. New Engl. J. Med. **288**, 143–149 (1973)
140. David, J.R.: Lymphocytic factors in cellular hypersensitivity. Hosp. Prac. **6**, 79–94 (1971)
141. Wiener, J.: Ultrastructural aspects of delayed hypersensitivity. In: Current topics in pathology (Altmann, H.-W., Benirschke, K., and Bohle, A., et al., eds.), vol. 52, p. 143–208. Berlin-Heidelberg-New York: Springer 1970
142. Müller-Eberhard, H.J., Polley, M.H., Nilsson, U.R.: Molecular events during immune cytolysis. In: Immunopathology (Grabar, P., and Miescher, P.A., eds.). IVth Intl. Symp., February 1965, Monte Carlo, p. 421–432. New York: Grune & Stratton 1965
143. Lichtenstein, L.M.: The role of the cyclic AMP system in inflammation: An introduction. In: Cyclic AMP, cell growth, and the immune response (Braun, W., Lichtenstein, L.M., and Parker, C.W., eds.), p. 147–162. Berlin-Heidelberg-New York: Springer 1974
144. Benacerraf, B., Green, I.: Cellular hypersensitivity. Annu. Rev. Med. **20**, 141–155 (1969)
145. Miller, J.F.A.P.: Immunological function of the thymus. Lancet **1961 II**, 748–749
146. Good, R.A., Dalmasso, A.P., Martinez, C., Archer, O.K., Pierce, J.C., Papermaster, B.W.: The role of the thymus in development of immunologic capacity in rabbits and mice. J. exp. Med. **116**, 773–796 (1962)
147. Rowley, D.A., Fitch, F.W., Stuart, F.P., Köhler, H., Cosenza, H.: Specific suppression of immune responses. Science **181**, 1133–1140 (1973)
148. Skinner, M.D., Schwartz, R.S.: Immunosuppressive therapy, part 1; Renal disease. New Engl. J. Med. **287**, 221–226 (1972)
149. Skinner, M.D., Schwartz, R.S.: Immunosuppressive therapy, part 2; Renal disease. New Engl. J. Med. **287**, 281–286 (1972)
150. Kaplan, S.R., Calabresi, P.: Immunosuppressive agents, part 2; Purine antimetabolites. New Engl. J. Med. **289**, 1234–1236 (1973)
151. Swanson, M.A., Schwartz, R.S.: Immunosuppressive therapy. The relation between clinical response and immunologic competence. New Engl. J. Med. **277**, 163–170 (1967)
152. Bloom, B.R.: *In vitro* approaches to the mechanism of cell-mediated immune reactions. Advanc. Immunol. **13**, 101–208 (1971)
153. Able, M.E., Lee, J.C., Rosenau, W.: Lymphocyte-target cell interaction *in vitro*. Ultrastructural and cinematographic studies. Amer. J. Path. **60**, 421–427 (1970)
154. Marcus, D.M.: The AB0 and Lewis blood-group system. New Engl. J. Med. **280**, 994–1006 (1969)
155. Hakomori, S-i, Kobata, A.: Blood group antigens. In: The antigens (Sela, M., ed.), vol. II, p. 80–141. New York: Academic Press 1974
156. Swisher, S.N.: Immune hemolysis. Annu. Rev. Med. **15**, 1–22 (1964)
157. Oski, F.A., Naiman, J.L.: Erythroblastosis Fetalis. In: Hematologic problems in the newborn, vol. 4, chap. 6, p. 136–172. Philadelphia: W.B. Saunders Co. 1966
158. Szulman, A.E.: The A, B and H blood-group antigens in human placenta. New Engl. J. Med. **286**, 1028–1031 (1972)
159. Rosenfield, R.E., Allen, F.H., Jr., Rubinstein, P.: Genetic model for the Rh blood-group system. Proc. nat. Acad. Sci. (Wash.) **70**, 1303–1307 (1973)
160. Lee, R.E., Vazquez, J.J.: Immunocytochemical evidence for transplacental passage of erythrocytes. Lab. Invest. **11**, 580–584 (1962)
161. Clarke, C.A.: The prevention of Rh isoimmunization. Hosp. Prac. **8**, 77–84 (1973)
162. Clarke, C.A.: Prevention of Rh-haemolytic disease. Brit. med. J. **4**, 5570, 7–12 (1967)
163. Woodrow, J.C.: Rh immunization and its prevention. In: Pathobiology annual (Ioachim, H.L., ed.), vol. 4, p. 65–86. New York: Appleton-Century-Crofts 1974
164. Terasaki, P.I., Singal, D.P.: Human histocompatibility antigens of leukocytes. Annu. Rev. Med. **20**, 175–188 (1969)
165. Walford, R.L.: The isoantigenic systems of human leukocytes: Medical and biological significance, series haematologica, II, 2 (Jensen, K.G., and Killmann, S.-A., eds.). Copenhagen: Munksgaard 1969
166. Joysey, V.C.: Tissue typing in relation to transplantation. Int. Rev. exp. Path. **9**, 233–285 (1970)
167. Mann, D.L., Fahey, J.L.: Histocompatibility antigens. Annu. Rev. Microbiol. **25**, 679–703 (1971)
168. Ramseier, H.: Antibodies to receptors recognizing histocompatibility antigens. In: Current topics in microbiology and immunology (Arber, W., Braun, W., et al., eds.), vol. 60, p. 31–78. Berlin-Heidelberg-New York: Springer 1973
169. Reisfeld, R.A., Kahan, B.D.: Histocompatibility antigens, Part 1, A chemical approach to transplantation antigens. In: Defence and recognition. MTP international review of science (Porter, R.R., ed.). Biochemistry series 1, vol. 10, p. 257–294. London: Butterworth and Co., Ltd. 1973
170. Bodmer, W.F.: Histocompatibility antigens, Part 2, Genetics of the HL-A and H-2 major histocompatibility systems. In: Defence and recognition. MTP international review of science (Porter, R.R., ed.). Biochemistry series1, vol. 10, p. 295–328. London: Butterworth and Co., Ltd. 1973
171. Bach, M.L., Bach, F.H.: The genetics of histocompatibility. Hosp. Prac. **5**, 33–44 (1970)
172. McDevitt, H.O., Bodmer, W.F.: HL-A, immune-response genes, and disease. Lancet **1974 I**, 1269–1274
173. Terasaki, P.I., McClelland, J.D.: Microdroplet assay of human serum cytotoxins. Nature (Lond.) **204**, 998–1000 (1964)
174. Wonham, V.A., Winn, H.J., Russell, P.S.: Serotyping and genetic analysis in the selection of related and renal-allograft donors. New Engl. J. Med. **284**, 509–513 (1971)
175. van Hooff, J.P., Schippers, H.M.A., Hendriks, G.F.J., van Rood, J.J.: Influence of possible HL-A haploidentity on renal-graft survival in eurotransplant. Lancet **1974 I**, 1130–1132
176. Terasaki, P.I., Mickey, M.R., Singal, D.P., Mittal, K.K., Patel, R.: Serotyping for homotransplantation. XX. Selection of recipients for cadaver donor transplants. New Engl. J. Med. **279**, 1101–1103 (1968)
177. Belzer, F.O., Fortmann, J.L., Salvatierra, O., Perkins, H.A., Kountz, S.L., Cochrum, K.C., Payne, R.: Is HL-A typing of clinical significance in cadaver renal transplantation? Lancet **1974 I**, 744–777
178. Meuwissen, H.J., Gatti, R.A., Terasaki, P.I., Hong, R., Good, R.A.: Treatment of lymphopenic hypogammaglobulinemia and bone-marrow aplasia by transplantation of allogeneic marrow; crucial role of histocompatibility matching. New Engl. J. Med. **281**, 691–697 (1969)
179. Dausset, J., Hors, J., Busson, M., Festenstein, H., et al.: Serologically defined HL-A antigens and long-term survival of cadaver kidney transplants. A joint analysis of 918 cases performed by the France-transplant and the London-transplant group. New Engl. J. Med. **290**, 979–984 (1974)
180. Braun, W.E., Murphy, J.J.: Histocompatibility testing in human renal allografts. I. Evidence for a strong and a weak HL-A sublocus in recipients of allografts from living related donors. Cleveland clin. Quart. **37**, 13–21 (1970)

181. Morris, P.J.: Histocompatibility in organ transplantation in man. In: Pathobiology annual (Ioachim, H.L., ed.), vol. 3, p. 1–26. New York: Appleton-Century-Crofts 1973
182. Walford, R.L., Waters, H., Smith, G.S.: Human transplantation antigens. Fed. Proc. **29**, 2011–2017 (1970)
183. Stokes, P.L., Asquith, P., Holmes, G.K.T., MacIntosh, P., Cooke, W.T.: Histocompatibility antigens associated with adult coeliac disease. Lancet **1972 II**, 162–164
184. Russell, T.J., Schultes, L.M., Kuban, D.J.: Histocompatibility (HL-A) antigens associated with psoriasis. New Engl. J. Med. **287**, 738–740 (1972)
185. Katz, D.H., Hamaoka, T., Dorf, M.E., Benacerraf, B.: Cell interactions between histoincompatible T and B lymphocytes. The H-2 gene complex determines successful physiologic lymphocyte interactions. Proc. nat. Acad. Sci. (Wash.) **70**, 2624–2628 (1973)
186. Copenhagen Study Group of Immunodeficiencies: Bone-marrow transplantation from an HL-A non-identical but mixed-lymphocyte-culture identical donor. Lancet **1973 I**, 1146–1150
187. Brewerton, D.A., Caffrey, M., Nicholls, A., Walters, D., James, D.C.O.: HL-A 27 and arthropathies associated with ulcerative colitis and psoriasis. Lancet **1974 I**, 956–958
188. Fritze, D., Herrman, C., Jr., Naeim, F., Smith, G.S., Walford, R.L.: HL-A antigens in myasthenia gravis. Lancet **1974 I**, 240–243
189. Kearns, D.H., Seibert, G.B., O'Reilly, R.O., Lee, L., Logan, L.: Paradox of the immune response to uncomplicated gonococcal urethritis. New Engl. J. Med. **289**, 1170–1174 (1973)
190. Bullock, W.E.: Studies of immune mechanisms in leprosy. I. Depression of delayed allergic response to skin test antigens. New Engl. J. Med. **278**, 298–304 (1968)
191. Porter, D.D.: Destruction of virus-infected cells by immunological mechanisms. Annu. Rev. Microbiol. **25**, 283–290 (1971)
192. Merigan, T.C.: Host defenses against viral disease. New Engl. J. Med. **290**, 323–329 (1974)
193. Oldstone, M.B.A., Dixon, F.J.: Tissue injury in lymphocytic choriomeningitis viral infection virus-induced immunologically specific release of a cytotoxic factor from immune lymphoid cells. Virology **42**, 805–813 (1970)
194. Hanaoka, M., Suzuki, S., Hotchin, J.: Thymus-dependent lymphocytes: Destruction by lymphocytic choriomeningitis virus. Science **163**, 1216–1218 (1969)
195. Porter, D.D., Larsen, A.E., Porter, H.G.: The pathogenesis of Aleutian disease of mink. III. Immune complex arteritis. Amer. J. Path. **71**, 331–343 (1973)
196. von Brand, T.: Biochemistry of parasites, 2nd ed. New York: Academic Press 1973
197. Good, R.A., Peterson, R.D.A., Gabrielsen, A.E.: The thymus and immunological deficiency disease. In: Immunological diseases (Samter, M., and Alexander, H.L., eds.), p. 344–352. Boston: Little, Brown and Company 1965
198. Weigle, W.O.: Immunologic unresponsiveness. Hosp. Prac. **6**, 121–136 (1971)
199. Symp. of American Society for Experimental Pathology: 56th Annu. Meeting of the Fed. of Am. Societies for Exp. Biol., Atlantic City, April 10, 1972. Immunodeficiencies and pathogenesis of disease. Amer. J. Path. **69**, 484–540 (1972)
200. Good, R.A.: Disorders of the immune system. Hosp. Prac. **2**, 39–53 (1967)
201. Shuster, J.: Immunologic deficiency disorders. In: Clinical immunology (Freedman, S.O., ed.), p. 342–371. New York: Harper & Row Publishers 1971
202. Rosen, F.S., Janeway, C.A.: The gamma globulins. III. The antibody deficiency syndromes. New Engl. J. Med. **275**, 709–715 (1966)
203. Rosen, F.S., Janeway, C.A.: The gamma globulins. III. The antibody deficiency syndromes. New Engl. J. Med. **275**, 769–775 (1966)
204. Patterson, R. (ed.): Modern concepts in clinical allergy. New York: Medcom Press 1972
205. Becker, E.L.: Cellular mechanisms and involvement in acute allergic reactions, Introduction, Immunology Society Symposium. Fed. Proc. **28**, 1702–1703 (1969)
206. Norman, P.S.: Antigens that cause atopic disease. In: Immunological diseases (Samter, M., and Alexander, H.L., eds.), p. 511–518. Boston: Little, Brown and Company 1965
207. Levine, B.B.: Immunologic mechanisms of penicillin allergy. New Engl. J. Med. **275**, 1115–1124 (1966)
208. Rappaport, B.Z.: Physiology of the nose and pathophysiology of allergic rhinitis. In: Immunological diseases (Samter, M., and Alexander, H.L., eds.), p. 562–568. Boston: Little, Brown and Company 1965
209. Freedman, S.O.: Clinical immunology of the nose and bronchi (allergic rhinitis and bronchial asthma). In: Clinical immunology (Freedman, S.O., ed.), p. 79–99. New York: Harper & Row, Publishers 1971
210. Middleton, E., Jr.: Physiology and pathology of bronchial asthma. In: Immunological diseases (Samter, M., and Alexander, H.L., eds.), p. 578–586. Boston: Little, Brown and Company 1965
211. Seebohm, P.M.: Respiratory changes in bronchial asthma. In: Immunological diseases (Samter, M., and Alexander, H.L., eds.), p. 587–592. Boston: Little, Brown and Company 1965
212. Sherman, W.B.: The atopic diseases. In: Immunological diseases (Samter, M., and Alexander, H.L., eds.), p. 503–505. Boston: Little, Brown and Company 1965
213. Freedman, S.O.: Clinical immunology of the skin. In: Clinical immunology (Freedman, S.O., ed.), p. 121–151. New York: Harper & Row Publishers 1971
214. Rostenberg, A., Jr., Bogdonoff, D.R.: Atopic dermatitis and infantile eczema. In: Immunological diseases (Samter, M., and Alexander, H.L., eds.), p. 635–645. Boston: Little, Brown and Company 1965
215. Parker, C.W.: Drug allergy. Part 1. New Engl. J. Med. **292**, 511–514 (1975)
216. Parker, C.W.: Drug allergy. Part 2. New Engl. J. Med. **292**, 732–736 (1975)
217. Parker, C.W.: Drug reactions. In: Immunological diseases (Samter, M., and Alexander, H.L., eds.), p. 663–681. Boston: Little, Brown and Company 1965
218. Freedman, S.O.: Human anaphylaxis and serum sickness. In: Clinical immunology (Freedman, S.O., ed.), p. 59–78. New York: Harper & Row Publishers 1971
219. Dixon, F.J., Vazquez, J.J., Weigle, W.O., Cochrane, C.G.: Pathogenesis of serum sickness. Arch. Path. **65**, 18–28 (1958)
220. Dixon, F.J.: Glomerulonephritis and immunopathology. In: Immunobiology (Good, R.A., and Fisher, D.W., eds.), p. 167–174. Stamford, Conn.: Sinauer Associates, Publishers 1971
221. Merrill, J.P.: Glomerulonephritis. Part 1. New Engl. J. Med. **290**, 257–262 (1974)
222. Merrill, J.P.: Glomerulonephritis. Part 2. New Engl. J.Med. **290**, 313–319 (1974)
223. Merrill, J.P.: Glomerulonephritis. Part 3. New Engl. J. Med. **290**, 374–381 (1974)
224. Kefalides, N.A.: Chemical properties of basement membranes. Int. Rev. exp. Path. **10**, 1–39 (1971)
225. Steblay, R.W., Rudofsky, U.: Renal tubular disease and autoantibodies against tubular basement membrane induced in guinea pigs. J. Immunol. **107**, 589–594 (1971)
226. McCluskey, R.T., Klassen, J.: Immunologically mediated glomerular, tubular and interstitial renal disease. New Engl. J. Med. **288**, 564–570 (1973)
227. Border, W.A., Lehman, D.H., Egan, J.D., Sass, H.J., Glode, J.E., Wilson, C.B.: Antitubular basement-membrane antibodies in methicillin-associated interstitial nephritis. New Engl. J. Med. **291**, 381–384 (1974)
228. Hume, D.M., Merrill, J.P., Miller, B.F., Thorn, G.W.: Experiences with renal homotransplantation in the human: report of nine cases. J. clin. Invest. **34**, 327–382 (1955)
229. Lerner, F.A., Glassock, R.J., Dixon, F.J.: The role of antiglomerular basement membrane antibody in the pathogenesis of human glomerulonephritis. J. exp. Med. **126**, 989–1004 (1967)
230. White, E., Hildemann, W.H., Mullen, Y.: Chronic kidney allograft reactions in rats. Transplantation **8**, 602–617 (1969)
231. Dixon, F.J., McPhaul, J.J., Jr., Lerner, R.: Recurrence of glomerulonephritis in the transplanted kidney. Arch. intern. Med. **123**, 554–557 (1969)
232. Golden, A., Maher, J.F.: Structure and function in disease. Monograph series, "The kidney". Baltimore: Williams & Wilkins Co. 1971
233. Kashgarian, M., Hayslett, J.P., Spargo, B.H.: Renal disease. Kalamazoo, Mich.: The Upjohn Company 1974
234. Feinstein, A.R.: A new look at rheumatic fever. Hosp. Prac. **3**, 71–75 (1968)
235. Markowitz, M., Kuttner, A.G., Gordis, L.: Rheumatic fever diagnosis, management and prevention, vol. II., In: Major problems in clinical pediatrics. Philadelphia: W.B. Saunders Co. 1965
236. Tagg, J.R., McGiven, A.R.: Some possible autoimmune mechanisms in rheumatic carditis. Lancet **1972 II**, 686–688
237. Cluff, L.E., Johnson, J.E., III: Poststreptococcal disease. In: Immunological diseases (Samter, M., and Alexander, H.L., eds.), p. 418–429. Boston: Little, Brown and Company 1965
238. Weigle, W.O.: Experimental autoimmune thyroiditis. In: Pathology annual (Sommers, S.C., ed.), vol. 8, p. 329–347. New York: Appleton-Century-Crofts 1973
239. Witebsky, E., Rose, N.R.: Studies on organ specificity. IV. Production of rabbit thyroid antibodies in the rabbit. J. Immunol. **76**, 408–416 (1956)
240. McMaster, P.R.B., Lerner, E.M., II, Exum, E.D.: The relationship of delayed hypersensitivity and circulating antibody to experimental allergic thyroiditis in inbred guinea pigs. J. exp. Med. **113**, 611–624 (1961)
241. Holman, H.R.: The L.E. cell phenomenon. Annu. Rev. Med. **11**, 231–242 (1960)
242. Vaughan, J.H., Barnett, E.V., Leddy, J.P.: Immunologic and pathogenetic concepts in lupus erythematosus, rheumatoid arthritis and hemolytic anemia. New Engl. J. Med. **275**, 1426–1432 (1966)
243. Schur, P.H., Sandson, J.: Immunologic factors and clinical activity in systemic lupus erythematosus. New Engl. J. Med. **278**, 533–538 (1968)
244. Koffler, D., Schur, P.H., Kunkel, H.G.: Immunological studies concerning the nephritis of systemic lupus erythematosus. J. exp. Med. **126**, 607–624 (1967)
245. Ritchie, R.F.: Antinucleolar antibodies. New Engl. J. Med. **282**, 1174–1178 (1970)

246. Terasaki, P.I., Mottironi, V.C., Barnett, E.V.: Cytotoxins in disease: autocytotoxins in lupus. New Engl. J. Med. **283**, 724–728 (1970)
247. Koffler, D.: Immunopathogenesis of systemic lupus erythematosus. Annu. Rev. Med. **25**, 149–164 (1974)
248. Hargraves, M.M., Richmond, H., Morton, R.: Presentation of two bone marrow elements: the "tart" cell and the "L.E." cell. Mayo Clin. Proc. **23**, 25–28 (1948)
249. Peltier, A.P., Estes, D.: Antinuclear antibodies. In: Pathology annual (Ioachim, H.L., ed.), vol. 2, p. 77–110. New York: Appleton-Century-Crofts 1972
250. Christian, C.L.: Rheumatoid arthritis. In: Immunological diseases (Samter, M., and Alexander, H.L., eds.), p. 725–736. Boston: Little, Brown and Company 1965
251. Dodson, W.H., Hollingsworth, J.W.: Pleural effusion in rheumatoid arthritis. New Engl. J. Med. **275**, 1337–1342 (1966)
252. Bartfeld, H., Epstein, W.V. (consulting eds.): Rheumatoid factors and their biological significance. Ann. N.Y. Acad. Sci. **168**, 1–207 (1969)
253. Cathcart, E.S., O'Sullivan, J.B.: Rheumatoid arthritis in a New England town. New Engl. J.Med. **282**, 421–424 (1970)
254. Sharp, J.T.: Infectious agents in the arthritides: Current status. Hosp. Prac. **6**, 142–151 (1971)
255. Ziff, M.: Pathophysiology of rheumatoid arthritis. Fed. Proc. **32**, 131–133 (1973)
256. Crocker, J.F.S., Ghose, T., Rozee, K., Woodbury, J., Stevenson, B.: Arthritis, deformities and runting in C5-deficient mice injected with human rheumatoid arthritis synovium. J. clin. Path. **27**, 122–124 (1974)
257. Calabro, J.J.: The three faces of juvenile rheumatoid arthritis. Hosp. Pract. **9**, 61–68 (1974)
258. Johnson, P.M., Watkins, J., Holborow, E.J.: Antiglobulin production to altered IgG in rheumatoid arthritis. Lancet **1975 I**, 611–614
259. Bacon, P.A., Cracchiolo, A., Bluestone, R., Goldberg, L.S.: Cell-mediated immunity to synovial antigens in rheumatoid arthritis. Lancet **1973 II**, 699–702
260. Huth, F., Soren, A., Klein, W.: Structure of synovial membrane in rheumatoid arthritis. In: Current topics in pathology (Altmann, H.W., Benirschke, K., and Bohle, A., et al., eds.), vol. 56, p. 55–78. Berlin-Heidelberg-New York: Springer 1972
261. Rose, G.A.: Polyarteritis nodosa. In: Immunological diseases (Samter, M., and Alexander, H.L., eds.), p. 749–757. Boston: Little, Brown and Company 1965
262. Shillitoe, E.J., Lehner, T., Lessof, M.H., Harrison, D.F.N.: Immunological features of Wegener's granulomatosis. Lancet **1974 I**, 281–284
263. Israel, H.L.: Sarcoidosis. In: Immunological diseases (Samter, M., and Alexander, H.L., eds.), p. 406–417. Boston: Little, Brown and Company 1965
264. DeRemee, R.A., Andersen, H.A.: Sarcoidosis. A correlation of dyspnea with roentgenographic stage and pulmonary function changes. Mayo Clin. Proc. **49**, 742–745 (1974)
265. Siltzbach, L.E., Greenberg, G.M.: Childhood sarcoidosis—a study of 18 patients. New Engl. J. Med. **279**, 1239–1245 (1968)
266. Kent, D.C., Houk, V.N., Elliott, R.C., Sokolowski, J.W., Jr., et al.: The definitive evaluation of sarcoidosis. Amer. Rev. resp. Dis. **101**, 721–727 (1970)
267. McCoy, R.C., Tisher, C.C.: Glomerulonephritis associated with sarcoidosis. Amer. J. Path. **68**, 339–358 (1972)
268. Alarcón-Segovia, D., Fishbein, E., García-Ortigoza, E., Estrada-Parra, S.: Uracil-specific anti-R.N.A. antibodies in scleroderma. Lancet **1975 I**, 363–366
269. Seligmann, M., Mihaesco, E., Hurez, D., Mihaesco, C., Preud'homme, J.-L., Rambaud, J.C.: Immunochemical studies in four cases of alpha chain disease. J. clin. Invest. **48**, 2374–2389 (1969)
270. Zawadzki, Z.A., Benedek, T.G., Ein, D., Easton, J.M.: Rheumatoid arthritis terminating in heavy-chain disease. Ann. intern. Med. **70**, 335–347 (1969)
271. Clyne, D.H., Brendstrup, L., First, M.R., Pesce, A.J., Finkel, P.N., et al.: Renal effects of intraperitoneal kappa chain injection. Induction of crystals in renal tubular cells. Lab. Invest. **31**, 131–142 (1974)
272. Ellman, L.L., Bloch, K.J.: Heavy-chain disease. New Engl. J. Med. **278**, 1195–1201 (1968)
273. Buxbaum, J.N., Preud'homme, J.-L.: Alpha and gamma heavy chain diseases in man: Intracellular origin of the aberrant polypeptides. J. Immunol. **109**, 1131–1137 (1972)
274. Mage, R., Lieberman, R., Potter, M., Terry, W.D.: Immunoglobulin allotypes. In: The antigens (Sela, M., ed.), vol. I, p. 299–376. New York: Academic Press 1973
275. Seligmann, M., Danon, F., Hurez, D., Mihaesco, E., Preud'homme, J.-L.: Alpha-chain disease: A new immunoglobulin abnormality. Science **162**, 1396–1397 (1968)
276. Wolfenstein-Todel, C., Mihaesco, E., Frangione, B.: "Alpha chain disease" protein def: Internal deletion of a human immunoglobulin A_1 heavy chain. Proc. nat. Acad. Sci. (Wash.) **71**, 974–978 (1974)
277. Lebreton, J.-P., Rivat, C., Rivat, L., Guillemot, L., Roparty, C.: Une immunoglobulinopathie méconnue: La maladie des chaines lourdes. Presse méd. **75**, 2251–2254 (1967)
278. Waldenström, J.: Macroglobulinemia. In: Immunological diseases (Samter, M., and Alexander, H.L., eds.), p. 364–371. Boston: Little, Brown and Company 1965
279. Osserman, E.F.: Multiple myeloma. In: Immunological diseases (Samter, M., and Alexander, H.L., eds.), p. 353–363. Boston: Little, Brown and Company 1965
280. Zetzel, L.: Granulomatous (ileo)colitis. New Engl. J. Med. **282**, 600–605 (1970)
281. Glotzer, D.J., Gardner, R.C., Goldman, H., Hinrichs, H.R., et al.: Comparative features and course of ulcerative and granulomatous colitis. New Engl. J. Med. **280**, 582–587 (1970)
282. Dressler, D., Rosenfeld, S.: On the chemical nature of transfer factor. Proc. nat. Acad. Sci. (Wash.) **71**, 4429–4434 (1974)
283. May, J.E., Rosse, W., Frank, M.M.: Paroxysmal nocturnal hemoglobinuria. New Engl. J. Med. **289**, 705–709 (1973)

Chapter 15

Regeneration, Hypertrophy, and Wound Healing

Regeneration 895

- Tail Regeneration 895
- Limb Regeneration in Amphibians 896
- Lens Regeneration 897
- Reproductive and Adaptive Growth in Mammalian Tissues 897
- Cellular Hyperplasia: Liver Regeneration 898
  - Parenchymal Restoration: Morphological Changes
  - Bioenergetic and Storage Pathways
  - Protein Synthesis
  - RNA Synthesis in Regenerating Liver
  - Nucleotide Pools
  - Regulation of Gene Expression in Regenerating Liver
  - Regulation of RNA Synthesis in Regenerating Liver
  - Regulation of DNA Synthesis in Regenerating Liver
- Polyamines in Liver Regeneration 913
- Triggering of Liver Regeneration 914
- Regeneration of Other Organs 916
  - Kidney Regeneration
  - Pancreas Regeneration
  - Cell Division in Stimulated Lymphocytes
  - Cell Division in Salivary Gland
  - Cardiac Hypertrophy
  - Miscellaneous Types of Regeneration

Wound Healing 920

- Causes and Purposes of Wound Healing 920
- Healing of Skin Wounds 921
  - Wound Healing in Amphibians
  - Wound Healing in Mammals
- Biochemistry of Wound Healing 924
  - Cell Proliferation
  - Collagen Formation
  - Architecture of the Collagen Molecule
  - Elastin
  - Basement Membranes
  - Lathyrism and Cross Links
  - Collagen Biosynthesis
  - Collagen Breakdown
  - Molecular Diseases of Collagen
- Ground Substance 934
- Factors Affecting Wound Healing 936
- Miscellaneous Enzyme Changes in Wound Healing 937
- Epitheliomesenchymal Interactions 938
- Mucopolysaccharidosis 938

References 939

Living beings have a major advantage over the inanimate. The living can respond to stress and injury by adapting their growth rate, regenerating lost tissue, and healing wounds. Damage to the robot is hopelessly permanent without human intervention; machines that repair themselves appear only in the imaginations of science fiction writers.

Living beings repair their tissue losses either by cellular proliferation (hyperplasia) or by cellular enlargement (hypertrophy). Cellular proliferation may result in the integral anatomical restoration of the preexisting organ (regeneration) or in the growth of the remaining structures by increasing the number of cells (hyperplasia). Wound healing is a combination of reactions to injury that protect the internal milieu of the organ by preventing hemorrhage and infection and partially restore the anatomical integrity through hyperplasia or hypertrophy of the intact tissues.

Reparative and adaptive growth are the subjects of this chapter [1]. The tissues' ability to repair their losses by growth varies considerably with species and organs. Lower vertebrates can regenerate an amputated limb or an excised lens. These regenerative capacities were lost in the process of evolution, and mammals respond to limb amputation only by wound healing. The selection during evolution in favor of species with lower regenerative capacities suggests that extensive regenerating abilities are incompatible with other evolved functions, which provide greater advantages for survival. For example, the evolutionary development of warm-blooded animals might have been associated with the loss of regenerative abilities. A cold-blooded animal can survive for long periods of time (long enough to regenerate a limb) on small amounts of food. The warm-blooded animal needs relatively large amounts of food for homeostasis. If the food restrictions were maintained for the period required for integral restoration of an amputated limb, the animal would starve to death. For these reasons, evolution is assumed to have selected in favor of those species that would heal the wound without regeneration of the amputated limb. As appealing as such reasoning may be, it could also be argued that evolution could have produced warm-blooded animals capable of regenerating their limbs rapidly, or a species strong enough to find food and regenerate a limb at the same time.

Although limb and lens regeneration do not occur in higher animals, the study of these phenomena is of considerable significance. The elucidation of the mechanism that controls these regenerative processes could shed light on the mechanism controlling morphogenesis in higher animals. A comprehensive discussion of limb and lens regeneration can be found in specialized books. Only a few critical points will be covered here [2, 3].

Regeneration

Tail Regeneration

Salamanders can regenerate their amputated tails. This integral anatomical restoration involves morphogenesis of the spinal cord, the vertebrae, and the bilateral muscle masses. Tail regeneration is the most complete regenerative process occurring in vertebrates because the entire axial system regenerates. Although the regeneration of the salamander's tail does not repeat ontogenesis exactly, the similarities between embryonic growth and regeneration of the tail involve the origin and differentiation of the cells and the induction and organization of the tissues. During the first few days after a 30–35-mm amputation of the tail of the salamander larva, two major alterations in the stump are observed: (1) migration of the wound's epithelial and ependymal cells, and (2) widespread dissolution of the myofibrillar material.

Within a few hours of tail amputation, the surface of the wound is covered by cells that migrate from the surface epithelium. Few or no mitotic figures are found among the migrating cells. The spinal cord is sealed by the migration of cells of the ependymal layers. Within 24 hours after amputation, the muscles of the trunk become acidophilic. Then from the second through the fourth day after amputation, the muscle is invaded by leukocytes and macrophages that appear to phagocytize the muscle fibrils, leaving a hyalin-honeycombed sarcoplasmic shell. The degenerate muscle cells then seem to extrude their nuclei. The nuclei of the degenerated muscle fibers are surrounded by a shallow cytoplasmic ring. The nuclei and their adherent cytoplasm are assumed to be the origin of the blastema cells, which appear first in the area of degenerated muscle, in an area cranial to the plane of amputation.

The blastema cells then migrate caudally. On the sixth day after amputation, the spinal cord elongates and the dividing mesenchymal blastema cells proliferate caudally. On the eighth day, some of the blastema cells differentiate into procartilaginous cells, which aggregate to form a rod located ventrally but well separated from the spinal cord's surface. Cranially, the cartilage cells abut on the surface of the notochord. Gradually, cartilaginous cell proliferation tapers off. During tail regeneration, the procartilaginous rod plays the role that the notochord plays during the embryonic development of the axial structures.

The tail regenerates further by elongation of the spinal cord, differentiation and segmentation of the procartilaginous rod into a cartilaginous skeleton, and differentiation of the blastema cells into muscle cells.

Holtzer's excision and transplantation experiments have clearly established the spinal cord's central role during embryological and regenerative development of the salamander's tail. In the regenerating tail, the spinal cord is necessary for (1) differentiation of mesodermal cells into cartilaginous cells, (2) morphogenesis and general architecture of the vertebrae, and (3) tail axiation. Differentiation of mesenchymal into cartilaginous cells appears to be induced by substances or neurological impulses that originate in the motor half of the spinal cord and are transmissible through the mesenchymal layer that separates the procartilaginous rods derived from the blastema cells.

Limb Regeneration in Amphibians

Regeneration of the amphibian limb results from a complex sequence of cellular reactions, including migration, histolysis, proliferation, and differentiation.

One day after amputation, the amphibian's wound is covered by a new epidermis, and phagocytosis and new tissue formation begin. The epithelial layer that covers the clot forms through epithelial cell migration rather than cell division. The cells migrate even in the presence of antimitotic agents. The epithelial cells start to migrate 15 minutes after amputation, and this persists for 72 hours.

As the wound is slowly covered by new epithelium, the tissues underlying the wound surface are actively phagocytized by macrophages and replaced by fibrocellular elements. Again, there is no recognizable mitosis in the tissue underlying the wound surface, and the accumulation of the fibrocellular elements is not arrested by the administration of antimitotic agents. Therefore, "scar tissue" is assumed to form through mesenchymal cell migration.

This early "wound healing phase," which may not be completed for 5 days, is followed by a "phase of cellular dedifferentiation." During this phase, the tissues of the stump continue to break down, but the breakdown is associated with the appearance of blastema cells. The blastema cells are long, undifferentiated cells that resemble the mesenchymal cells of the embryo. In the beginning, blastema cells are scattered among the "debris" of the stump tissue, but later they are thickly packed together to form a cellular interphase between the surface epithelium and the intact portion of the stump.

The origin of the blastema cells is still debated. They could originate from distant organs or from the stump itself. Irradiation studies of the regenerating limb suggest that the old stump is the sole source of the blastema cells. The limb fails to regenerate only if a narrow band of the limb, including the amputation plane, is irradiated. In contrast, limb regeneration is normal and the inhibitory effect of irradiation is completely offset by implantation of bone or epithelial fragments in the irradiated stump or after shielding the amputation plane in an animal whose body is irradiated.

The blastema cells could be derived from a single type of mesenchymal cell, like a fibroblast, with multiple potentialities; or they may be a scrambled population of dedifferentiated cells of multiple origin (osteocytes, chondrocytes, fibrocytes, etc.). During regeneration, these dedifferentiated cells find their proper place in the stump and redifferentiate into the "original patterns."

Tissue culture studies in which cells of various origins are scrambled after trypsin dissociation suggest that blastema cells could well have a multicellular origin. It appears, however, that the bulk of the new tissue forming the regenerating limb is derived from muscle and nerve sheath cells [98]. The epithelial cells do not influence blastema formation. Similarly, electron microscopy and radioautography [99] have shown that muscle cells are transformed in blastema cells. The possibility that chondrocytes may also become blastema cells is, however, not excluded.

Although the morphological observation of the formation of the blastema and its progressive differentiation is a fascinating experience, the molecular changes that dictate cellular "dedifferentiation" and differentiation and histological and anatomical organization are not less intriguing (see section on gene expression and differentiation).

What determines the conversion of a myoblast, a fibroblast or a chondrocyte into a blastema cell? Why does a blastema cell differentiate into an osteocyte or a myocyte? Why are all myocytes associated with muscles and all osteocytes with bone? What determines the position of the flexor or the extensor muscles? If all these questions could be answered, the molecular mechanism of most biological problems (except the origin of life) would be known. Studies of the molecular events in tail, limb, and organ regeneration may partially answer these questions, but today little is known of these molecular changes.

After the blastema forms, the stump develops into a new limb by a combination of cellular proliferation, cellular differentiation, and tissular organization; and nerves play a vital role in these processes.

Denervation of the stump at amputation prevents regeneration, and only wound healing takes place. Nerves are indispensable for regeneration throughout blastema formation. Denervation of the limb after blastema formation is followed by cellular differentiation and tissular organization, which yields a small limb that grows in length but not in volume. The nerve may influence limb regeneration in various ways. The anatomical development of the nerve could provide a guideline for the histological arrangement of the blastema cells. The nerve might be the source of the blastema cell, or it could elaborate substances (neurohormones, acetylcholine) that influence the differentiation of the blastema cells. The mode of action of the nerve in limb regeneration is still speculative.

In addition to their role in limb regeneration, nervous influences have also been described in regeneration of the tail (spinal cord) and lens (retina). Loss of the ability to regenerate limbs during phylogenesis seems to be associated with a decrease in the number of nerve fibers per unit volume. Singer has counted the nerve fibers in amphibian leg and in the rat leg. By implanting nerve fibers in the stump of mammalian amputated rat limbs, Singer was able to induce a beginning of limb regeneration [4].

Although the regenerative process restores a lost limb or tail, the biological events involved do not often, if ever, integrally repeat those events that take place during embryological development of the limb or tail. Therefore, different gene sets must be placed in gear in regeneration and embryological development.

Lens Regeneration

Calucei observed in 1891 that the excised lens of a Triturus newt regenerates from epithelial cells along the free margin of the dorsal iris. Although lens regeneration after lentectomy occurs only in a few amphibians and is not observed in vertebrates, it provides a disarmingly simple tool for the study of regeneration.

Lentectomy is followed by a latent period that precedes a thickening of the dorsal aspect of the iris close to the margin of the pupil. The thickening involves the pigmented cells of the outer layers of the iris. It results from cellular swelling and is associated with depigmentation. Electron microscopists have studied depigmentation. Ameboid cells migrate between the epithelial cells of the iris, and the iris epithelial cells emit pseudopods containing the pigment granule. The ameboid cells touch the pseudopods, and the pigment granules are engulfed in the ameboid cells where they disintegrate. Iris cell dedifferentiation is followed first by a period of active RNA and protein synthesis, and later by an increased rate of mitotic activity. The presence of normal lens tissue prevents lens regeneration after lentectomy. Therefore, it has been postulated that the lens elaborates inhibitory substances that prevent lens regeneration. When both lens and retina are excised, lens regeneration is slower than after simple lentectomy. Thus, the retina is thought to influence lens regeneration, possibly by elaborating stimulating substances. Although the retina may influence lens regeneration, the lens regenerates in the absence of retina. If the pigmented cell layers of the iris are eliminated in eyes in which both the retina and lens have been excised, the lens may regenerate even though retinal regeneration is impaired.

If the iris is excised and regrafted inside out, a new lens is formed with normal polarity and fiber poles directed toward the neural retina. As a result of such experiments, the determination of polarity of the lens fiber has been ascribed to retinal influences. But the other parts of the eye may also be involved. However, the polarity of the lens fiber, an example of histological organization, undoubtedly is determined in part by environmental factors.

The lens contains a number of specific proteins: α-, β-, and γ-crystallins. These proteins can be purified (some have been crystallized, and antibodies and antisera antigenic for specific lens proteins can be prepared). The effect of antisera on regeneration can be tested *in vivo* by injecting the antiserum; the localization of the specific protein in the various components of the embryo during development can be tested by immunoelectrophoretic or immunofluorescence techniques. Lens development during embryonic life and regeneration after lentectomy provide an exceptional tool for studying differentiation at a molecular level.

In the chick lens, proteins can be detected during embryonic development when the optic vesicle contacts the portion of the ectoderm from which the lens cells will later develop. A specific lens protein appears before morphological differentiation takes place. This observation provides a striking illustration in support of a concept ennounced before, which states that morphological differentiation stems from the assemblage of specific proteins and, consequently, that proteins constitute units of specificity.

Lens antiserum blocks lens regeneration in larvae of the newt incubated in antiserum provided that the newt's cornea is slit to permit the antiserum to reach the iris. Furthermore, regeneration is inhibited only if the antiserum reaches the iris when the iris is making the antigen. Thus, lens regeneration is not inhibited if the newt is immersed in antiserum before lentectomy because only after lentectomy does the newt iris acquire detectable amounts of lens antigen (between 5 and 15 days after lentectomy).

Reproductive and Adaptive Growth in Mammalian Tissues

Mammalian tissues can be grouped into three classes with respect to their ability to proliferate: the renewing, the expanding, and the static cell populations.

In renewing cell populations, a stem cell proliferates by cell division, and the new cells differentiate into a highly specialized cell structure that is ultimately eliminated by secretion (sperm, holocrine secretion), degeneration (red blood cell), or exfoliation (epithelia of the intestine or mucosa).

The differentiated cell produced in these renewing systems normally is incapable of cell division and has a relatively short life span. In normal individuals, the turnover of the cells of renewing systems is rigidly scheduled, and new mature cells are provided as the organism needs them. (Interference with cell renewal will be more appropriately discussed in the sections devoted to the effect of x-irradiation and cancer cells.) Under normal conditions, the energy of the expanding tissue is used for functions rather than for proliferation. Without dividing, these tissues secrete polypeptides, protein or steroid hormones, enzymes, mucopolysaccharides, and other substances and perform numerous metabolic functions (urea synthesis, fatty acid oxidation and synthesis, detoxification). Yet the ability to divide is not lost in the expanding cell population. These tissues can readily repair their losses by rapid cellular proliferation.

When lost, the cells of the brain cannot be replaced. During their lifetime, these cells are all business: they have sacrificed proliferation for the sake of function. The cells storing the information so painfully acquired by the medical student have forsaken all desires of dividing for the sake of promoting memory. Slow death, however, is the sad price we have to pay for such security. The life of static cells is not indefinite, and brain cells die as one ages. These cells can never be replaced; and our brains addle until finally we succumb to an inexorable fate.

However, nature has provided the static cell with some means of adapting to increased functional demand. The nerve cell can regenerate dendrites or emit more dendrites; the striated muscle cell can increase in size. A given cell population can respond to injuries that decrease the cell population by: accelerating a preexisting high level of cellular proliferation, triggering cell division in a tissue in which mitoses are rare, and enlarging the size of remaining cells. In hyperplasia, cells divide; in hypertrophy, cells increase in size to compensate for the loss in mass or function.

Cellular Hyperplasia: Liver Regeneration

The liver, the pancreas, the kidney, and many of the endocrine glands repair their losses, at least in part, by hyperplasia. This discussion of hyperplasia is centered on restoration of liver tissue after partial hepatectomy.

When a portion of liver is excised, hyperplasia of the remainder of the organ occurs until the original weight of the liver is restored. This phenomenon is often referred to as liver regeneration. Yet, regeneration means that the integral anatomical structure of the organ is restored, as in the limbs, lenses, and tails of amphibians. After partial hepatectomy, however, the liver regains its original weight, but not its original structure. When three of the lobes of the liver are excised in a rat, the remaining lobe grows in size by hyperplasia, but no new lobes are formed. Therefore, the liver restoration observed after hepatectomy should be referred to as hyperplasia rather than regeneration. Nevertheless, the term liver regeneration is so well entrenched that it is useless to attempt to rename the phenomenon.

For all practical purposes, regeneration involves one type of cell, and the metabolic events occur in a rigidly scheduled sequence. (To be sure, the liver is composed of more than one cell type, and all cells ultimately participate in the regenerative process.) During the first 24 hours after hepatectomy, 95% of the cells that participate in the regeneration are hepatic cells, and a typical sequence of metabolic and morphologic events takes place. Consider first the changes in the hepatic cell.

Parenchymal Restoration: Morphological Changes

For a long time, investigators debated whether the individual lobules increase in size during liver regeneration. It seems now well established that after partial hepatectomy, the number of the lobules, rather than the size, increases. Lobular proliferation is assumed to result from budding of the preexisting cords along the branches of the bile ducts and the hepatic veins.

But even the term hyperplasia does not describe exactly what happens after partial hepatectomy. The cellular events occur during a period of cellular hypertrophy and one of mitosis. Immediately after partial hepatectomy, the size of the liver cells increases. Six hours later, the volume of the parenchymal cells of the regenerating liver is 2.6 times that of the normal liver cells. There seems to be some disagreement about when the enlargement starts and reaches its maximum, and about the extent of the enlargement. The maximum cellular enlargement generally is assumed to precede or accompany the maximum rate of mitosis.

In resting cells, the ratio of cytoplasmic to nuclear volume is constant. If the cytoplasmic volume is increased, the nuclear-cytoplasmic ratio is maintained by cellular division or by a proportionate increase in the size of the nucleus. Although some investigators have claimed results to the contrary, it is generally agreed that the size of the nucleus is temporarily increased in the regenerating liver cells, but it is not clear whether the enlargement of the nucleus accompanies, precedes, or follows the increase in cytoplasmic volume. That reputed morphologists have arrived at such a widespread range of interpretation of their results may seem puzzling, yet it should be kept in mind that although regeneration is a constant observation after partial hepatectomy, the time sequence and the rate of the various regenerative processes are influenced by many different factors; therefore, the different results could be due to different experimental conditions.

Many investigators have attempted to count the number of mitoses in the normal liver. The results vary considerably, ranging between 0.005% and 0.05%. Since the organ's total cell population does not increase, the liver cells must turnover at a rather slow rate. The average life span of a liver cell has been calculated to be at least 150 days—five times that of a red cell. In regenerating liver, the incidence of mitosis increases sharply 24 hours after partial hepatectomy and reaches a peak 4 hours later, to fall during the following days. At 28 hours after partial hepatectomy, 4–5% of the hepatic cells are in mitosis (mitotic time is 8 hours). Some cells that have gone through the stages of hypertrophy, DNA synthesis, and chromosome duplication never divide. In normal liver, 70–80% of the hepatic cells are tetraploid, and 1–2% are octaploid. The incidence of octaploids is increased 50%, and that of the tetraploids 10%.

Although mitosis peaks 28 hours after the operation, the mitotic rate is increased from 10–15 days after partial hepatectomy. In fact, some investigators have claimed that the high incidence of mitosis observed 28 hours after partial hepatectomy is followed by a second mitotic wave 72 hours after partial hepatectomy. The second peak of mitosis is said to involve nonhepatic cells.

Bioenergetic and Storage Pathways

It is generally accepted that growth after hepatectomy is completed 3 days postoperatively. Although there are striking quantitative differences, depending upon the author, with respect to the time and the actual value of the maximum mitotic rate, there is general agreement that mitoses in regenerating liver are preceded by a lag period during which important molecular changes occur.

Morphologically, cell division is preceded by a doubling of: the volume of the endoplasmic reticulum, the number of mitochondria and other cellular organelles, and the chromosome complement. Physiologically, liver regeneration involves an integral restoration of function. In oversimplified terms, liver regeneration results in replacement of the macromolecules that were withdrawn during the partial hepatectomy (phospholipids, lipoprotein, proteins, and nucleic acids). Chemical energy is required for the *de novo* synthesis of the macromolecules, and liver regeneration is therefore likely to be associated with changes in the storage pathways (glycogen and lipids), and with shifts in the pathways involved with ATP synthesis.

Little is known of the source of the chemical energy needed for the macromolecular biosynthesis in liver regeneration. Whether one or more of the pathways involved in ATP synthesis (glycolysis, hexose monophosphate shunt, Krebs cycle, glucuronic pathway) are modified during liver regeneration has not been established. Neither is it known if the rate of ATP synthesis is increased by the formation of new enzymes or by increasing the efficiency of the already existing multiple-enzyme pathways (by removal of inhibitory mechanisms or by direct activation of the enzyme). Also, the amount of ATP synthesized could be unchanged after partial hepatectomy, and regeneration could involve a redistribution of ATP for usage in biosynthesis.

The lipid content of all the hepatic cells increases rapidly after partial hepatectomy, reaching a maximum 24 hours after operation. Two days postoperatively the lipid inclusion tends to disappear, and the lipid content of the hepatic cell is negligible the fourth day after partial hepatectomy. The lipid accumulation in the hepatic cell could result from decreased fatty acid oxidation, increased triglyceride synthesis, or from mobilization of lipids from other tissues.

An increase in the ability of mitochondria to produce ATP has been described in 36 hour regenerating liver [100]. The increased respiratory activity develops only after regeneration is almost completed and therefore, its role in the regenerative process is not clear.

To our knowledge, fatty acid oxidation has not been investigated, but there is no indication that fatty acid synthesis is increased after partial hepatectomy. In contrast, studies of the incorporation of acetate into fatty acids show that it decreases 18 hours after partial hepatectomy. This decrease is maintained during the second day after partial hepatectomy. The incorporation of acetate into cholesterol of 18-hour regenerating liver is increased. That most of the lipids that accumulate in liver cells after partial hepatectomy are derived from mobilization of fats found in other tissue is suggested by the following observation: fatty infiltration does not occur in regenerating liver after chordotomy and adrenalectomy procedures which depress fat mobilization. Most of the lipids that accumulate in the regenerating liver are neutral fat, and the esterification of the lipids to yield triglycerides is increased 18 hours after partial hepatectomy.

The rate of cephalin and lecithin synthesis is increased as early as 6 hours after partial hepatectomy, as indicated by acetate incorporation into these compounds.

It is not known whether the lipids accumulate as a result of injury, or whether they are stored in the liver for use as a source of chemical energy or as precursors for new lipid synthesis. The fact that new membranes of the endoplasmic reticulum containing lecithin, phospholipids, and neutral lipids have to be synthesized suggests that the lipids accumulate in the regenerating liver to provide precursors for this new cell structure. Yet it cannot be excluded that the lipids accumulate as a result of injury. Indeed, if injury caused by partial hepatectomy were to block protein synthesis selectively, lipids could accumulate in the hepatic cell exactly as they do in carbon tetrachloride intoxication. It is therefore interesting that the levels of polyunsaturated fatty acids are decreased in the regenerating liver.

While the lipids increase during liver regeneration, glycogen decreases, especially in dividing cells. It is therefore assumed that glycogen is used as an energy source during mitosis. This assumption must be reconciled with the concept that lipids provide the source of chemical energy during cellular division. It is of interest (although the observation is sometimes difficult to interpret) that intranuclear glycogen is increased in regenerating livers. A correlation between an increase in fat or a decrease in glycogen when the mitotic rate is highest does not necessarily imply that fat or glycogen provides a source of energy for mitosis.

Protein Synthesis

When the liver grows after partial hepatectomy, the total nitrogen levels increase proportionately with the weight of the organ, so that the nitrogen content per gram of liver remains practically unchanged during regeneration. Similarly, the specific activity of many enzymes is unchanged, or only slightly increased, after partial hepatectomy. The increase in nitrogen results from an increase in proteins and nucleic acids. Since the increase in protein occurs before mitosis, the amount of protein synthesized per cell must be increased in regenerating liver. This increase probably starts 10 hours after partial hepatectomy and reaches a peak at later stages after the operation.

If the nitrogen content of regenerating liver is expressed as a percentage of the nitrogen in the normal liver (100%), the values increase 35–45% between 10 and 24 hours after partial hepatectomy, and from 45–60% during the next 48 hours. This increase in liver nitrogen levels indicates that acid-precipitable compounds have been synthesized (including RNA, DNA, and protein) and that the maximum rate of synthesis occurs between 10 and 24 hours after partial hepatectomy (see Fig. 15-1). After partial hepatectomy, the liver continues to degrade protein and form urea. The amount of urea formed in partially hepatectomized rats is the same as that in normal rats. Consequently, the amount of urea formed per gram of liver is increased after liver regeneration. Harkness [5] found that the amino acid content of the regenerating liver increases 6 hours after partial hepatectomy. He thinks that this increase results not from an increased rate of protein synthesis, but from increased urea formation per unit cell (glutamine, glutamic acid, lysine, aspartic acid, glutathione).

It seems that an increase in the rate of protein synthesis and the determination of the peak of protein synthesis after partial hepatectomy could easily be established by studies with labeled amino acids. Such studies, however, meet with considerable difficulty. The labeled amino acid injected in the liver is drowned in a pool of free amino acids, which may be considerably altered in regenerating livers compared to those in normal livers.

Normal or regenerating livers synthesize a large number of proteins. It is unlikely that the rates of synthesis and breakdown, and consequently the turnover rates, of these proteins are identical. As a result, curves expressing the rate of incorporation of labeled amino acid in the total protein population provide only a distorted view of the rate of protein synthesis in regenerating liver. Despite these limitations, isotopic studies have been useful in establishing which cell fraction most rapidly incorporates the amino acid and when maximum incorporation takes place in different protein populations.

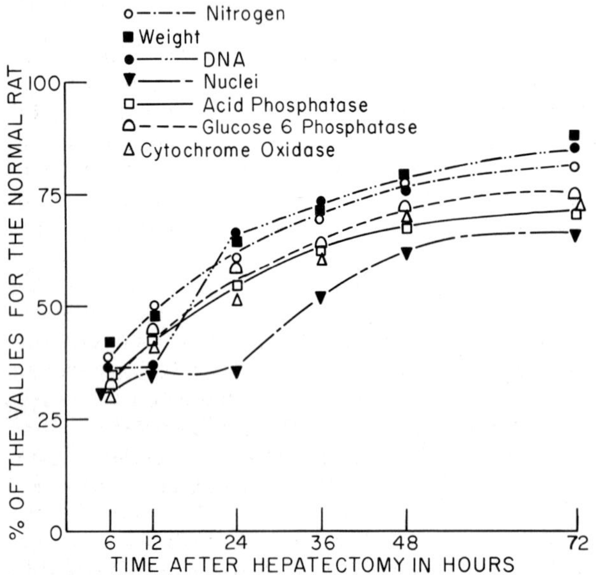

Fig. 15-1. Protein synthesis in regenerating liver. (From Van Lancker and Sempoux [6])

The cytoplasmic proteins are more rapidly labeled than the nuclear proteins, and in each case a double peak is observed. Studies of [^{15}N]glycine incorporation showed that the radioactivity of the cytoplasmic protein reaches a small peak 26 hours after partial hepatectomy, and a second larger peak 40 hours after partial hepatectomy. Among the cytoplasmic proteins, the microsomes are not only the first to be labeled, but the specific activity of their proteins is much higher than that of proteins prepared from other cell fractions. The first peak in the rise of radioactivity of the nuclear proteins coincides with the first peak in the cytoplasmic protein; the second peak in the nuclei occurs much later (56 hours after partial hepatectomy).

The population of proteins formed in the cytoplasm of regenerating liver can be divided into two main classes: specific liver proteins and blood proteins. Immediately after partial hepatectomy, the plasma protein levels drop to values below normal. These low levels are maintained for several days. Consequently, it appears that the liver first rebuilds its own protein and then proceeds to elaborate plasma proteins only 48 to 72 hours after operation.

These observations probably explain the two peaks found for the rate of incorporation of amino acid precursors in regenerating liver protein. The first peak (26 hours after hepatectomy) coincides with the formation of liver protein; the second peak coincides with the formation of both liver and blood proteins. The distinction between these two stages in protein synthesis is of vital importance for the understanding of the regulation of regeneration after partial hepatectomy.

Because liver function and liver regeneration are related, a comparative study of the rate of synthesis of specific liver proteins and specific blood proteins could shed some light on that relationship. Such a study could be achieved by comparing the rate of amino acid incorporation in specific enzymes (β-glucuronidase and glucose-6-phosphatase) and specific blood proteins (fibrinogen or albumin).

The rate of protein synthesis could be stimulated by: (1) increased activation of the amino acid; (2) accelerated transfer of the amino acid from RNA to the ribosome; (3) increased efficiency of the ribosomes in lining up the amino acids; (4) an increase in the number of active ribosomes; (5) an increased amount of mRNA. Several of these factors seem to be modified in regenerating liver. Hultin and his associates studied the incorporation of [^{14}C]leucine in the microsomes of regenerating liver and found that the rate of incorporation is doubled 24 hours and quadrupled 40 hours after partial hepatectomy. The specific activity of the microsomal proteins drops rapidly when the microsomes are obtained from livers of animals sacrificed more than 40 hours after partial hepatectomy. Using the *in vitro* system, Hultin and coworkers further observed an increase in the activity of the amino acid-activating enzyme and an above normal ability of the microsomes to incorporate [^{14}C]leucine into microsomal proteins.

If microsomes of regenerating livers are more active than those of normal livers in stimulating incorporation of labeled amino acids into their proteins, is this capability attributable to increased efficiency of each ribosomal particle or to an increase in the ribosomal population? Studies by Mueller and his associates suggest that the increased efficiency of the microsomal preparation results from the increase in the number of ribosomes.

Scornik [101] has studied protein synthesis in regenerating livers either after flooding the leucine pool with massive doses of radioactive leucine (rendering changes in the endogenous pool of leucine negligible) or by labeling nascent chains with trace or massive amounts of radioactive leucine and measuring the time needed for the release of the chains in normal and 36 hour regenerating livers. These studies revealed that 36 hours after partial hepatectomy the total number of ribosomes had increased 30%. The concentration of ribosomes per unit weight and probably per cell was not increased and the proportion of ribosomes converted to polyribosomes was only increased 10%. The relationship of these findings to liver growth is difficult to understand. The results are in contradiction with the *in vitro* studies. The discrepancies may result from differences in the rate of regeneration that are often observed in different laboratories.

Anderson et al. [102] studied the electrophoretic properties of ribosomal proteins of the ribosomal 60 and 40 S subunits at various times after partial hepatectomy. Although no changes were seen in the 60 S units, changes were found in 40 S units early after hepatectomy. Two hours after regeneration, one protein (protein S_6) had disappeared and was replaced by a new protein spot more negatively charged. This alteration persisted for 70 hours. Another protein (protein S_2) which normally migrates as a single spot after partial hepatectomy migrates in two spots for periods lasting between 2 and 4 and 8 and 18 hours. The electrophoretic pattern is normal between these periods. It is not known how these changes in ribosomal protein pattern relate to increased protein synthesis in regenerating liver.

In Chapter 2 it was shown that the incorporation of amino acids into proteins during protein synthesis requires messenger RNA, ribosomes, aminoacyl-tRNA, GTP and various transfer, initiation and termination factors. A soluble system for the incorporation of some amino acids into proteins, not requiring GTP, ribosomes or template nucleotides has been described. Its performance requires a source of energy and aminoacyl-tRNA as the amino acid donor. The soluble system adds, by the formation of a peptide bond, one amino acid to the free amino group of a polypeptide chain preformed in the conventional way. Only one amino acid is added at the acceptor site and no further elongation of the chain takes place. The incorporation of amino acid into proteins by the soluble system is inhibited by cycloheximide and puromycin. The soluble system has been found in bacteria, rat liver, ascites cells and other tissues. The biological significance of the soluble amino acid incorporating system is not known. Yet, it is of interest that the activity of the system is increased 2 to 3 times in regenerating liver [103].

Liver regeneration is associated with such drastic metabolic changes that enzyme activities are bound to be modified. The activity of some enzymes is increased (for example, thymidylic kinase), but that of others may be decreased. However, changes in enzyme activities are difficult to interpret because they may result from so many different factors: (1) change in the concentration of cofactors; (2) change in the concentration of inhibitors; (3) release of a bound inactive form into a soluble active form; (4) activation of an antagonistic enzyme system (for example, increase of catabolism versus anabolism); (5) shift in intracellular enzyme distribution; (6) accelerated breakdown or synthesis of the enzyme molecule; and (7) direct activation or inactivation of the enzyme molecule (see metabolic regulation). Only rarely can it be decided which factor determines the changes in enzyme activity during liver regeneration. (An example of such studies will be presented in the case of thymidylic kinase.)

The activity of many enzymes decreases during the first 6 hours after partial hepatectomy and rises between the 12th and 24th hours. Potter and Novikoff found that the activities of succinoxidase, malic dehydrogenase, cytochrome reductase, and oxaloacetic oxidase are markedly reduced during the first hours after partial hepatectomy, remain low for the first 2 days, and then rise 48 hours after partial hepatectomy. Others found that the rhodanese, ATPase, and amino oxidase activities are reduced after partial hepatectomy.

On the basis of these findings, the rate of mitochondrial enzyme regeneration appears to be slowed down after partial hepatectomy. In contrast, the activity of glutamic aspartic transaminase, an enzyme found mainly in the liver supernatant, is restored faster than is the weight of the liver. Similarly, the activity of glucose-6-phosphatase increases rapidly after partial hepatectomy.

These findings suggest that microsomal and supernatant enzymes regenerate before mitochondrial enzymes. But, as mentioned previously, these enzyme studies are difficult to interpret because the experimental conditions vary considerably; and when the regeneration rates of three markers (acid phosphatase for lysosomes, cytochrome oxidase for mitochondria, and glucose-6-phosphatase for microsomes) were studied in the same animals, the rates of reappearance of the activities of the three enzymes closely followed the rate of restoration of nitrogen levels and liver weight.

These studies were done in my laboratory in cooperation with Sempoux [6]. We interpreted the results to mean that all cytoplasmic organelles regenerate at the same time. This was a somewhat sweeping generalization, which, although not in contradiction with available evidence, was not quite justified considering the limited observations that we had made. But, when the intracellular distributions of nitrogen, RNA, cytochrome oxidase, catalase, acid phosphatase, and β-glucuronidase were compared in cytoplasmic pellets obtained from normal and regenerating liver, the similarity of the distribution spectra of these various components was striking. These were elaborate tissue fractionation experiments in which the cytoplasmic fraction was divided into eight different pellets, which were sedimented by gradually increasing the centrifugal forces. The results of these tissue fractionation studies confirmed our impression that the regenerating liver reconstitutes, in an orderly fashion, its entire population of the various cellular organelles simultaneously.

The only significant difference between the intracellular distribution of biochemical components in normal and regenerating liver was that in regenerating liver, all components tended to be associated with cellular structures smaller than those with which they were associated in normal liver.

For example, a greater portion of the two acid hydrolases studied was found in the microsomal pellet. These experiments raised the question of the origin of the enzymes found in cellular structures other than the endoplasmic reticulum. In the light of available knowledge of the mechanism of protein synthesis, one is tempted to conclude that most, if not all, proteins are synthesized in the endoplasmic reticulum. But because amino acids are incorporated in nuclei and mitochondria *in vitro*, the source of nuclear and mitochondrial protein is still debated.

The site of synthesis of β-glucuronidase and glutamic dehydrogenase was also studied. β-Glucuronidase was purified from the mitochondria, lysosomes, supernatant, and microsomes obtained from 24-hour regenerating livers of partially hepatectomized rats. Labeled leucine or [^{14}C]valine was injected 30 minutes before sacrifice. The results were clear-cut—only the microsomal enzyme was labeled; the lysosomal enzyme remained cold, indicating that it is made in the endoplasmic reticulum. (The transfer of β-glucuronidase from ER to lysosomes is discussed elsewhere.) An astute reader could argue that the β-glucuronidase found in microsomes does not necessarily have molecular properties identical to those of the β-glucuronidase found in the lysosomes. This is a valid criticism and is difficult to refute irrevocably. This possibility was investigated as best as possible with the small amount of purified enzyme available by comparing a battery of properties of samples of enzymes purified from lysosomal, microsomal, and other cell fractions.

The mobility properties of lysosomal and microsomal β-glucuronidase were studied by starch-gel and disc electrophoresis. The mobilities of lysosomal and microsomal enzyme were identical. Furthermore, the curves for pH optimum, thermoactivation, thermoinactivation, and the Lineweaver-Burk plot for the purified lysosomal and microsomal enzymes were identical. Although it now seems well established that the enzyme in lysosomes is synthesized in the microsomes, the mode of transfer of the enzyme from microsomes to lysosomes remains unknown. Cell biologists have often proposed that lysosomes are developed by a mechanism similar to that which causes the formation of the zymogen granules. For example, acid phosphatase is synthesized in the endoplasmic reticulum, concentrated in the Golgi apparatus, and from there transferred to lysosomes. The evidence is essentially histochemical, via methods that do not distinguish between various phosphatases with widely different molecular properties. Even the determination of acid phosphatase activity in an isolated Golgi apparatus does not permit us to conclude that the low phosphatase activity detected in the Golgi is due to enzymes with molecular properties identical to those of the enzyme found in the endoplasmic reticulum and the lysosomes, since activities of other phosphatases are found in the Golgi apparatus. Therefore, direct transfer of the enzyme from endoplasmic reticulum to lysosomes can not be excluded.

Although certainly β-glucuronidase and possibly all lysosomal enzymes are synthesized in the endoplasmic reticulum, the origin of the mitochondrial enzymes is still not clear. Cytochromes and glutamic dehydrogenase are known to be synthesized in the endoplasmic reticulum and later transferred to mitochondria, but the mode of enzyme transfer remains unknown. The structural proteins found in mitochondria are likely to be synthesized in that organelle (see Chapter 1).

After partial hepatectomy, new proteins and enzymes related to DNA synthesis, and possibly mitosis, appear. Their biosynthesis will be best discussed when we consider DNA synthesis in regenerating liver.

RNA Synthesis in Regenerating Liver

A net gain in protein must involve an increased rate of synthesis. To increase the amount of proteins it synthesizes, the cell must increase the efficiency with which it uses its machinery for protein synthesis, or it must amplify that machinery. Amplification of the cytoplasmic machinery for protein synthesis demands that new RNA be made. Since all cellular RNA, except for a small fraction of mRNA, is made on DNA templates, changes in nRNA metabolism are likely to take place after partial hepatectomy.

In fact, studies on the incorporation of labeled precursors into regenerating liver RNA preceded our knowledge of the pathways for protein synthesis. Some of the earliest studies were done in the laboratories of Barnum, Potter, and Rush with ^{32}P or orotic acid as a precursor.

These early experiments clearly established that the uptake of the precursor in liver RNA was increased after partial hepatectomy. Moreover, the rise in isotope uptake was greater in nuclear than in cytoplasmic

RNA. Although the significance of these findings has often been challenged because of the quantitative differences reported in different laboratories and because the studies did not include analyses of the nucleotide pools, the findings are in keeping with the net increases in cytoplasmic and nuclear RNA, the appearance of new templates, and the activation of protein synthesis that take place after partial hepatectomy. Moreover, interference with DNA or protein synthesis by X-irradiation or antimetabolites is paralleled by a reduction of the incorporation of precursors in nuclear RNA.

As one may expect, all the newly synthesized RNA is not likely to be retained. Some may be degraded; consequently, the net increase in RNA will not coincide and not even be proportional to the incorporation of the precursors into regenerating liver RNA. Thus, increases in net RNA occur late and are relatively small. The total RNA content of the liver increases to approximately 20% above normal 12 hours after partial hepatectomy and reaches 60% 20 hours after operation. Since only the hepatic cells participate in hypertrophy and hyperplasia during that time, the increase in RNA per participating cell is likely to be more than 60%.

Using competitive hybridization techniques, McCarthy and his associates [7] showed that a new template pattern developed after partial hepatectomy. Although such results were to be anticipated, the significance of the hybridization experiment is beclouded by the fact that the template pattern detected in regenerating liver resembled that found in embryonic liver, an organ stuffed with immature hematopoietic cells. The similarities between the nucleotide sequences of regenerating liver and those of embryonic liver RNA are, therefore, likely to result not so much from the similarity of a few structural templates as from the occurrence of redundant sequences in both tissues. The temptation is to propose that growing tissues elaborate a new kind of RNA that has frequently repeated sequences and may be involved in regulating gene expression.

The cell contains various populations of RNA that can be distinguished on the basis of their intracellular location or their molecular weights.

At 6 hours after partial hepatectomy, incorporation of precursors into nucleolar RNA is five times greater than incorporation in chromatin RNA. This is in contrast to normal liver, in which the rate of precursor incorporation into chromatin RNA is twice that in nucleolar RNA. The meaning of this observation is not obvious. All RNA is believed to be synthesized on DNA. Thus, in normal liver the chromosome must acquire new molecules of tRNA and ribosomal, messenger, and possibly regulating RNA molecules of the kind described by Bonner and postulated by Britten and Khone (see gene expression).

All RNA, except the "regulating RNA," is released from the chromatin and stored in the nucleolus before it enters the cytoplasm. The only way to explain a greater incorporation of the isotope into nucleolar RNA in regenerating liver is to propose that the molecules of transfer, messenger, and ribosomal RNA are not only synthesized on chromatin at an accelerated rate, but are also transferred faster to the nucleolus, thereby activating the machinery for protein synthesis.

These observations concur with studies on the incorporation of [^{14}C]orotic acid into nuclear and cytoplasmic RNA prepared by phenol extraction after differential centrifugation of regenerating liver homogenates. After partial hepatectomy, the specific activity of the phenol-extracted nRNA increases for the first 6 hours and from the 12th to the 24th hour, but remains unchanged between 6 and 12 hours after the operation.

The specific activity of the cytoplasmic RNA increases 6 hours after partial hepatectomy, reaches a maximum at 12 hours, and decreases thereafter. RNA fractions of 4S, 18S, and 28S were separated by sedimentation on sucrose gradients. After orotic acid injection, 4S RNA is labeled first, followed by the labeling of 18S and 28S RNA. Orotic acid is incorporated into 4S from two processes: (1) elaboration of the polynucleotide chain on the DNA template, and (2) lengthening of the chain in the cytoplasm. Inasmuch as no efforts were made to distinguish between these two processes, interpretation of incorporation of precursor in 4S RNA is difficult.

The incorporation of the precursor is increased in both 18S and 38S RNA after partial hepatectomy. The highest specific activity is reached at 12 hours for 18S RNA and at 24 hours for 28S RNA. The rate at which 18S and 28S RNA are made changes in regenerating liver. In normal liver, the specific activity of 18S RNA is greater than that of 28S RNA. The ratio of the specific activities equals 0.4. This ratio increases up to 18 hours after partial hepatectomy, when it reaches 0.8. The ratio of the specific activities remains unchanged between 18 and 24 hours after operation.

It is not certain what 28S and 18S RNA are; but for the sake of argument, consider for a moment that 18S RNA contains the messenger fraction, and 28S, the ribosomal fraction. These experiments clearly demonstrate that both types of RNA turn over in normal and regenerating liver, and that the turnover rate is increased in regenerating liver. Moreover, in both normal and regenerating liver, rRNA (28S) is more stable than 18S RNA.

In the absence of changes in nucleotide pools (and when the investigations were made after partial hepatectomy, no such change took place) and in the presence of a net increase in RNA, an increased specific activity must mean increased rates of synthesis. Although RNA must be synthesized, the kinetics of this synthesis are not revealed by measurements of specific activities because the rates of breakdown of various types of RNA are not known.

In any event, it seems safe to conclude that the rates of messenger and ribosomal, and possibly transfer, RNA synthesis are increased in regenerating liver. Most of the new mRNA is likely to have reached the cytoplasm 12 hours after partial hepatectomy, whereas rRNA continues to accumulate at least until 18 hours after partial hepatectomy.

The appearance of messenger RNA in the cytoplasm follows the first peak of uptake of RNA precursor in the nucleus (6 hours).

The significance of the second peak of nuclear uptake (at 24 hours) remains obscure. However, it suggests that some of the rRNA made after partial hepatectomy remains associated with the nucleus, a conclusion in agreement with hybridization studies, which indicate that after partial hepatectomy a class of newly made RNA remains associated with the nucleus. The acceleration in messenger and ribosomal RNA synthesis precedes the biosynthesis of new proteins in regenerating liver.

The addition of regenerating liver RNA to an incubation mixture containing *E. coli* ribosome, pH 5 enzyme, and all other ingredients necessary for the incorporation of labeled amino acids into proteins stimulates the incorporation of the precursor into the acid-insoluble fraction.

The level of stimulation is independent of the stage the cell has reached in the generation cycle. Thus, equal amounts of RNA prepared from nuclei of normal liver or of 6–12-, 18-, and 24-hour regenerating liver stimulate amino acid incorporation equally. If it can be assumed that the RNA which stimulates the amino acid incorporation is mRNA, then equal quantities of normal and regenerating liver RNA appear to contain equal proportions of mRNA.

If such is true, two consequences must follow: (1) in regenerating liver, new RNA's are synthesized in equal proportions, and these relative proportions are the same as those in normal liver; and (2) the increase in the rate of protein synthesis results from a proportionate increase in RNA, rather than from a selective rise in messenger or ribosomal RNA.

Inasmuch as the ratio of the specific activity of the ribosomal RNA versus that of messenger RNA increases with time, one must also conclude that a large amount of the new messenger is likely to be rapidly degraded in regenerating liver, while the rRNA is much more stable. Consequently, if all or most of the ribosomes are engaged in protein synthesis, a large portion must form polysomes with stable templates.

Nucleotide Pools

Although studies on orotic acid incorporation into RNA allow us to distinguish the direction of the incorporation and to compare relative changes in one type of RNA to those in another type of RNA, exact rates of RNA synthesis cannot be calculated without measuring the nucleotide pools. We shall now briefly describe the fate of orotic acid in liver.

Orotic acid is a pyrimidine with a carboxyl group in position 4. Since the late 1940's, orotic acid has been known to be a good precursor of pyrimidine nucleotides in bacterial and mammalian tissues. Yet, the conversion of the aglycon into the riboside remained mysterious until Kornberg and his associates discovered the PRPP reaction. Orotidylic pyrophosphorylase is the enzyme responsible for converting orotic acid to orotidylic acid. The enzyme has been purified 20 times from yeast and has also been found in liver. The reaction catalyzed by the phosphorylase is reversible, and the equilibrium constant equals 20. The purified enzyme exhibits absolute specificity for orotic acid.

The conversion of OMP to UMP in the presence of a decarboxylase has already been discussed. UMP is apparently converted to CMP after the UMP has been phosphorylated to UTP in the presence of UMP kinase. The kinase requires magnesium for activity. Studies on HeLa cells and other mammalian tissues have shown that glutamine is the amino donor. Asparagine or ammonia cannot replace glutamine.

UTP and CTP are the immediate precursors of nRNA. However, these precursors can also engage in numerous metabolic pathways, including coenzyme biosynthesis (*e.g.*, UDPG). Little is known of the properties and the intracellular distribution of the enzymes involved in breaking down these nucleotides, but the nucleotides at various levels of phosphorylation can be attacked by specific or unspecific pyrophosphatases, phosphatases, and deaminases. The nucleotides can be converted into the base and sugar; hydrogenation and opening of the ring of the base yield simple carbon or nitrogen compounds (see pyrimidine metabolism).

Because of the number of pathways involved in the conversion of orotic acid, it seems unlikely that the pools of the immediate pyrimidine precursors of RNA would be constant at all times. In fact, the composition of the pool can be expected to change with time after the precursor is injected and after partial hepatectomy. If the amounts of UTP and CTP available for RNA synthesis vary, the concentration of the label will vary also; and differences in specific activities of UTP and CTP at different times after partial hepatectomy will not necessarily reflect the rate of conversion of the precursor; such changes may also result from contraction or expansion of the individual pools of UTP and CTP.

No sophisticated analysis of the nucleotide pools was undertaken until the study of Bucher and her associate [8]. Even then, interpretation of these results is restricted because rigid kinetic studies were not possible. Bucher's results clearly established a fluctuation in the specific activity of the nucleotide pools after orotic acid injection. The fluctuation depends on the time elapsing between injection and sacrifice and the duration of regeneration.

The labeling of UTP and CTP were followed 5, 10, and 15 minutes after an intravenous injection of 0.5 μCi of [^{14}C]orotic acid. The UTP pool was labeled rapidly. The labeling reached its peak at 5 minutes, then the specific activity of the pool started to fall. The fall may have resulted from diluting the pool with newly synthesized UTP or from the usage of UTP. The labeling of the pool of CTP lags behind that of

UTP, and during the first 2 minutes after orotic acid injection, practically no labeling appears in the CTP. This is not surprising. The time lapse probably measures the time necessary for the conversion of UTP to CTP. After 2 minutes the CTP pool becomes rapidly labeled, as was the case for the UTP. The specific activity of CTP peaks 5 minutes after the isotope is injected and then drops. A rapid contraction of the CTP pool is unlikely, and, therefore, the increase in the labeling in the CTP pool probably results from the conversion of UTP to CTP. Consequently, it may be concluded that the conversion of UTP to CTP starts 2 minutes after injection of the isotope and proceeds rapidly between 2 and 5 minutes. However, the exact amounts of UTP converted to CTP cannot be determined by looking at the labeling of CTP because at every moment after injection, small and different amounts of labeled UTP and CTP are withdrawn from the pool for breakdown or synthesis of RNA and DNA nucleotides. Thus, the specific activity of the nucleotide pool changes constantly.

The label in the CTP and UTP pools drops between 5 and 10 minutes after injection. Since in the normal animal the rates of synthesis and breakdown of UTP and CTP presumably are constant, one must conclude that after 5 minutes the nucleotides are rapidly used and replaced by newly synthesized nucleotides. In other words, the turnover of these two nucleotides is very rapid.

In view of these rapid changes in the pools, Bucher and her associates felt that the most reliable data on specific activity would be obtained early after the isotopes were injected. Their study on the changes in specific activity of UTP and CTP at various times after partial hepatectomy (5 and 30 minutes after injection of the precursor) are of particular interest. If the specific activities of UTP and CTP (ordinate) are plotted versus the time after hepatectomy (abscissa) on the same graph, the values used in the ordinate must be modified. Thus, the specific activity of CTP is always 10 times lower than that of UTP. Although the specific activity of UTP practically doubles between 0 and 45 minutes, this is the only time after partial hepatectomy when the specific activity is much higher than normal. Between 45 minutes and 3 hours, the specific activity of the UTP slowly returns to normal and it reaches normal value around 13 hours after partial hepatectomy. In contrast to what happens to the specific activity of UTP, the specific activity of CTP drops between 0 and 45 minutes after partial hepatectomy. It remains below normal between 1 and 6 hours and then rises slightly above normal between 6 and 12 hours after partial hepatectomy.

When the animals are killed 45 minutes after partial hepatectomy and 30 minutes after isotope injection, the specific activity of the UTP pool reaches highest values. The specific activity of the UTP pool decreases from 45 minutes to 4 hours and remains low but constant from 6 to 24 hours after partial hepatectomy.

In contrast, in animals killed 30 minutes after isotope injection, the specific activity of the CTP pool is 10 times lower than that of the UTP pool, and it rises slowly from 0 to 24 hours after partial hepatectomy. In fact, 20 hours after hepatectomy the specific activity of the CTP is twice that observed at time 0.

In the face of such data on the pools, can an interpretation of the incorporation of precursors into various kinds of RNA be valid? Clearly, no quantitative measurements are possible with a changing pool unless the kinetics of the pool change and the incorporation of orotic acid into RNA are known. Yet, is it possible to compare the incorporation of one type of RNA with that of another type? Only if there is a single pool from which the nucleotides are drawn for synthesis of all RNA types. But even if the pool were compartmentalized, rapid equilibration between compartments would probably take place. Consequently, one can safely compare the specific activity of one kind of RNA with that of another provided that the specific activity is measured at various times after the isotope is injected. Is it then possible to compare meaningfully RNA specific activities at various times after partial hepatectomy? Yes, but only if the pool remains constant, and we have seen that the UTP pool is stable between 6 and 24 hours after partial hepatectomy. CTP levels rise constantly, but participation of the CTP pool in RNA synthesis is negligible compared with that of UTP since the specific activity of CTP is 10 times less than that of UTP. Thus, specific activities of RNA can be compared between 6 and 24 hours after partial hepatectomy, but comparisons are meaningless before 6 hours after partial hepatectomy.

Origins of Deoxyribonucleotides and Nucleotide Conversion. The demonstration that the pool of deoxynucleotides (dTMP, dGMP, dCMP, and dAMP) was rapidly labeled after the administration of labeled precursors further suggested that deoxynucleotides were made in regenerating liver.

Normal DNA synthesis starts at least with the formation of four deoxynucleotides (dTMP, dCMP, dGMP, and dAMP) and terminates with the exact duplication of the existing DNA molecules. Deoxynucleotide usage for DNA synthesis occurs in at least two steps—phosphorylation of the monophosphate to yield the triphosphate, and polymerization of the triphosphates in the presence of primer DNA. The origin of the deoxyribose remains to be demonstrated. Early experiments using ^{14}C-labeled glucose were difficult to interpret because of the many pathways in which glucose can engage.

Yet these early results suggested that a triose was preferentially used for deoxyribose biosynthesis. Later it was suspected that in regenerating liver, deoxyribose was synthesized through the deoxyribose aldolase reaction, which Racker discovered. The aldolase catalyzes the reversible cleavage of deoxyribose-5-phosphate to acetaldehyde and glyceride-3-phosphate and is found in many bacterial and mammalian tissues. Further evidence did not support the early findings.

Although the possibility of several different pathways for deoxyribose formation in regenerating liver cannot be excluded, available evidence indicates that at least part, if not all, of the deoxyribose is formed by direct reduction of the ribonucleotide.

The early work of Reichard [9] and that of Moore and Hurlbert [10] on the CDP-reductase has already been described. Studies by Larsen in which ^{32}P and uniformly labeled cytidine were used simultaneously to label both DNA and RNA of regenerating liver, although limited in their interpretation, suggested that the DNA deoxyribose was derived from the direct reduction of the ribose.

A reductase capable of reducing CDP to dCDP appears in regenerating liver 18 hours after partial hepatectomy. Reductase activity is undetectable in normal liver. The new enzyme activity is likely to result from *de novo* synthesis since elaboration of new activity is inhibited by X-irradiation and actinomycin D.

The incorporation of randomly labeled adenosine into DNA and the reduction of ADP to dADP was studied in regenerating liver at various times after partial hepatectomy [104]. Adenosine incorporation peaks at 24 hours and drops to lowest levels at 42 hours after partial hepatectomy. The conversion of ADP to dADP starts at 18 hours, peaks at 24 hours and drops between 24 and 36 hours after hepatectomy. This is in contrast to CDP reduction which continues to rise at least up to 48 hours after hepatectomy (Fig. 15-2).

The activity of ADP reductase is like that of CDP reductase inhibited by hydroxyurea. The development of both ADP and CDP reductase rises after partial hepatectomy, but while the activity of CDP reductase drops to 7% of normal, that of ADP reductase is only reduced 50%.

Thus, except for the fact that dGTP, rather than dATP, is required for activity, the properties of CDP and ADP reductases are similar; but although the activities of both enzymes rise prior to the onset of DNA synthesis 24 hours after hepatectomy, the pattern of development of activity of CDP and ADP reductases is different. While that of CDP reductase continues to increase, that of ADP reductase decreases. Yet, the incorporation of both uniformly labeled cytosine and adenosine reach a maximum at the peak of DNA synthesis and drop afterwards.

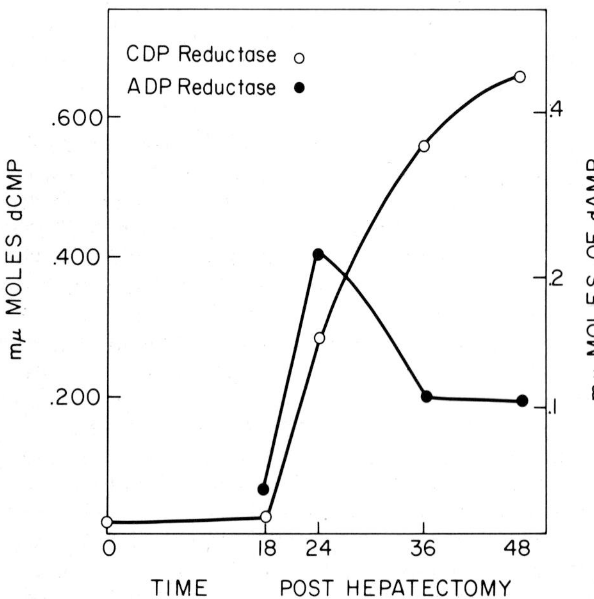

Fig. 15-2. CDP/ADP reductase activity after partial hepatectomy

The difference in the pattern of incorporation of the precursor and that of the enzyme, especially CDP reductase activity, may be explainable by the variation in the nucleotide pools. Söderhall *et al.* [105] have shown that the concentration of all deoxynucleotides is low in normal liver and that they reach a peak between 20 and 30 hours after partial hepatectomy to drop back to low values after that time. Pyrimidine deoxynucleotide triphosphates achieve the highest concentration, first dCTP, then dTTP. For example, at 24 hours after partial hepatectomy, a time which coincides with the peak of DNA synthesis, the concentrations of dCTP, dTTP, dATP, dGTP are 4.8, 2.4, 3.2, 1.1 p moles per μg of DNA. At 30 hours, when mitoses reach their peak, these values are 2.3, 2.3, 2.0, 0.8. The concentrations of dGTP are the lowest at all times. Therefore, dGTP concentrations are believed to be rate limiting for DNA synthesis. In normal liver the amounts of dGTP present are so low that they won't allow for more than 30 seconds of DNA synthesis, assuming that the S phase is 8 hours long and that the newly synthesized DNA is not catabolized.

Between 24 and 30 hours after hepatectomy there is a drop in the levels of the sum of both pyrimidine and both purine nucleotides with a drop of the ratio of dCTP/dTTP from 4.4 to 2.3, but no significant drop (2.9 to 2.5) in the ratio of dATP/dGTP.

In summary, the results of measurement of the CDP and ADP reductase activity in regenerating liver reveal that CDP activity continues to increase after the peak of incorporation of the pyrimidine precursors into DNA, while the activity of ADP reductase parallels that of the incorporation of the precursor into DNA. Moreover, between 24 and 30 hours after hepatectomy there is a drop in the levels of reduced pyrimidine nucleotides and a switch from the reduction of CDP to that of TTP. During the same period there is a drop in the reduction of purine nucleotide, but the ratio of dATP/dGTP remains approximately the same. These findings suggest complex regulation of the activity of the nucleotide reductase(s) in regenerating liver.

Nothing is known of the molecular properties of the regenerating liver enzyme and therefore the exact mechanism of regulation of the liver reductase remains to be clarified.

In bacteria two enzyme systems are involved in the conversion of ribose to deoxyribose nucleotides, thioredoxin and ribonucleotide reductase. In the first reaction the primary donor of hydrogen is NADPH and the ultimate donor reduced thioredoxin (Fig. 15-3). The ribonucleotide reductase catalyzes the reduction of a variety of ribonucleotide diphosphates, but is without effect on mono or triphosphates. The activity of

1. Thioredoxin Reductase

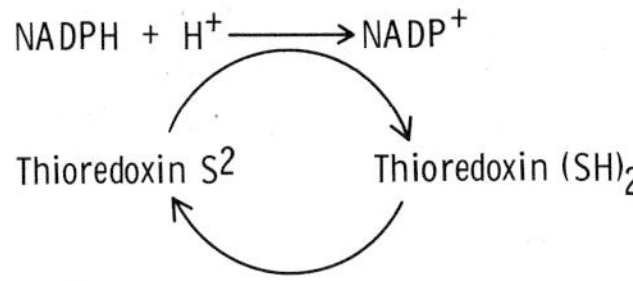

2. Ribonucleotide Reductase

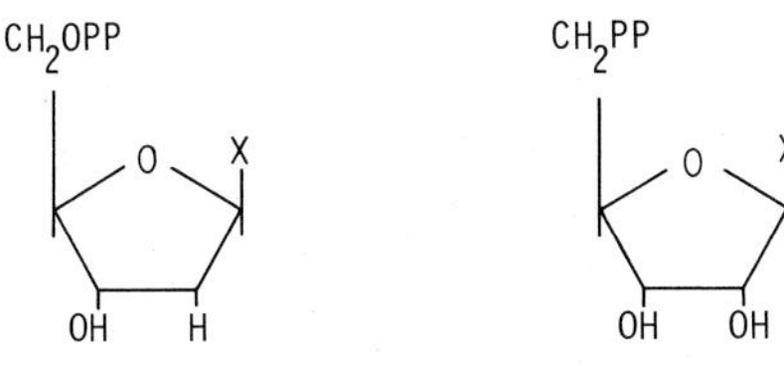

X = Base

Fig. 15-3. Enzymic mechanism of ribonucleotide reduction. (After Reichard)

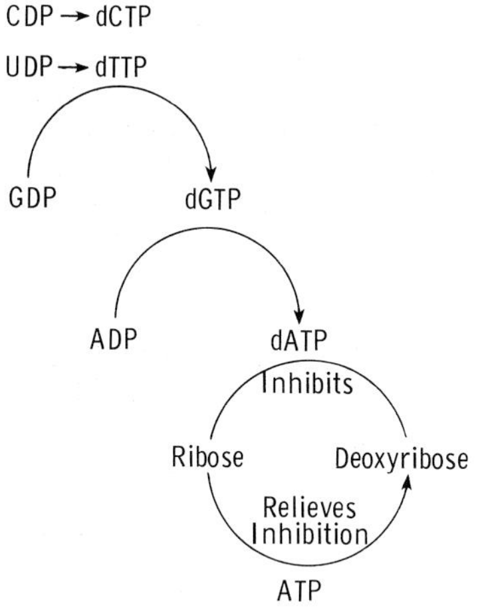

Fig. 15-4. Sequence of steps in nucleotide reduction

the enzyme is allosterically regulated in various ways by different nucleotide triphosphates [101, 106]. ATP stimulates the reduction of pyrimidine, but not of purine nucleotides, dGTP enhances the reduction of ADP to dADP and dTTP, that of GDP to dGDP. It is believed that the sequence starts with the reduction of UDP which yields dTTP, which in turn effectuates the reduction of GDP yielding dGTP indispensable for the conversion of ADP to dADP. dATP inhibits the enzyme, the inhibition is relieved by ATP and therefore, the level of enzyme activity is regulated by the ratio of ATP to dATP (Fig. 15-4).

Finally, the combination of dTTP and ATP inhibits the reduction of pyrimidine nucleotides and thus converts the pyrimidine nucleotide reductase into a purine nucleotide reductase.

The bacterial enzyme is a molecular complex formed by equimolecular amounts of two subunits: B_1 (200,000 daltons) and B_2 (78,000 daltons); each subunit is a dimer made of two identical polypeptide chains [108]. On the basis of these observations, it has been assumed that the molecular complex contains two catalytic sites probably located at the point where the two subunits are united and four effector sites all located on the B_1 unit: two of which bind ATP, dATP, dTTP and dGTP and two of which bind dATP or ATP [109].

The binding affinity of the effector sites varies with the nucleotide and therefore, the composition of the nucleotide pools is critical, not only in determining the level of activity of the enzyme, but also the specificity of its catalytic reduction. For example, binding of ATP, dTTP, or dATP induces changes in configuration which will favor respectively the reduction of CDP and UDP, GDP and ADP.

Thymidylic synthetase activity starts to appear 18 hours and reaches a maximum 30 hours after hepatectomy; then the activity of thymidylic synthetase returns to normal.

We mentioned that dUMP is the precursor of dTMP. The amount of TMP formed could conceivably be accelerated by increasing the amount of dUMP available. dUMP can be derived from dCMP or from UMP. The enzyme dCMP deaminase removes the NH_2 group of the CMP to yield UMP. The activity of that enzyme is, again, barely detectable in normal liver; it rises after 1 hour and reaches its maximum at 48 and 72 hours after partial hepatectomy. The pyrimidine nucleotide UMP is synthesized in regenerating liver through a pathway already described in detail.

It is believed that although the biosynthesis of pyrimidines is increased in regenerating liver, their breakdown is slowed. Because of the conflicting results reported, pyrimidine metabolism in regenerating liver must be reexamined before any definite conclusion can be reached.

TMP can also be derived through a salvage pathway, namely, direct phosphorylation of thymidine under the influence of thymidine kinase. Thymidine kinase activity is low in normal liver, increases between 12 and 18 hours after partial hepatectomy, and reaches highest values between 48 and 70 hours after operation.

Last Steps of DNA Synthesis. TMP kinase and DNA polymerase activities in regenerating liver have been investigated in many laboratories; we studied them in collaboration with Dr. Fausto. Low levels of TMP kinase activity are present in normal liver; the activity doubles between 12 and 24 hours after partial hepatectomy and reaches a maximum between 48 and 96 hours. DNA polymerase activity is present in normal liver, and it changes little after partial hepatectomy (see Fig. 15-5).

If the changes in the activities of the enzymes involved in DNA synthesis in regenerating liver are viewed panoramically, it can be concluded that: (1) the activities of many of the enzymes involved in DNA synthesis increase after partial hepatectomy; (2) the increase starts before DNA is synthesized and reaches a maximum after the peak of DNA synthesis has been reached. Thus, the peak activity of these enzymes

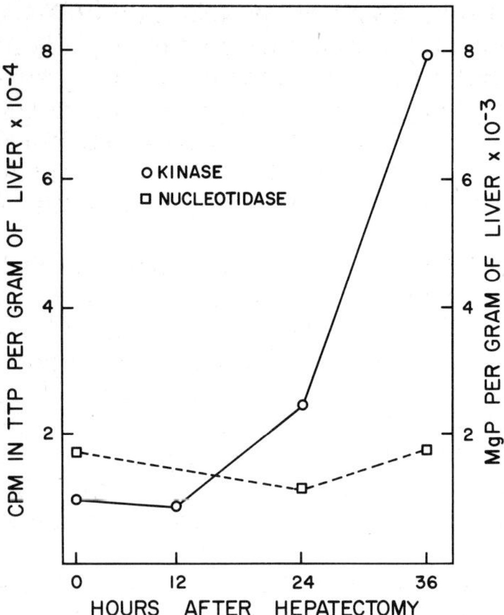

Fig. 15-5. Thymidylic kinase and deoxynucleotidase activities in regenerating liver. (From Van Lancker and Fausto, J. Biol. Chem. **240**, 1247–1255, 1965)

occurs when DNA synthesis *in vivo* has practically fallen to zero. The significance of these findings with respect to the control of DNA synthesis will be discussed later.

These increased enzyme activities result from one or more of a number of possible changes: (1) synthesis of new enzyme molecules; (2) activation of latent molecules either by shift in the intracellular distribution or by unknown activators (coenzymes, metals, etc.); (3) removal of inhibitors. These various possibilities have been investigated in thymidylic kinase and DNA polymerase. After establishing the optimal conditions (of pH and magnesium, ATP, and substrate concentrations) for the reaction, we studied the intracellular distribution of thymidylic kinase and found that in normal liver, large amounts of TMP kinase are associated with particles.

When enzyme activities are tested in various cell fractions, the recovery of the enzyme activities is calculated by summing the activities in each cell fraction. These calculated recoveries can then be compared with the enzyme activity measured in the original homogenate. For most enzymes, the activities in the homogenate are higher than the calculated activity. This results from loss of activity during fractionation.

Occasionally, the calculated recovery is higher than the activity measured in the homogenate, suggesting that the homogenate contains latent enzyme activity that is revealed after differential centrifugation of the cell fraction. Various mechanisms can repress the enzyme activity in the homogenate: (1) the enzyme may be surrounded by membranes that separate substrate from active center (amylase in zymogen granules); (2) the structure of the enzyme molecule may lock the active centers (chymotrypsinogen, trypsinogen); (3) cofactors or activators (*e.g.*, metals) are necessary for enzyme activity but are dispersed in the homogenate, and the relative concentrations of activators to enzyme molecules do not favor maximum activity; (4) the homogenate may contain antagonistic pathways or inhibitors that are separated from the enzyme or inactivated during differential centrifugation.

In normal liver, the recovery values for TMP kinase were 74% higher than the actual activity measured in the homogenate. Release of particulate enzymes could not account for all the latent activity.

Whether the increased activity results from modifications of the catalytic properties of the thymidylic kinase molecule due to increased availability of activators or elimination of inhibitors after homogenization is not known.

Two possible mechanisms of interference with thymidylic kinase activity were, however, eliminated: (1) competition between TMP kinase and TMP 5′-nucleotidase (the enzyme which splits the phosphate group of TMP to yield thymidine), and (2) an inhibitory effect of microsomes on TMP kinase activity. Latent TMP kinase is found only in normal liver; in 24-hour regenerating liver, the recovery values for TMP kinase were identical to the activities measured in the homogenate.

Moreover, in regenerating liver, almost none of the TMP kinase is particulate, whereas 30% of TMP kinase is recovered with the mitochondrial and microsomal fractions in the normal liver.

The increase in thymidylic kinase observed between 12 and 24 hours after partial hepatectomy clearly occurs as a result of *de novo* synthesis, because after a single injection of actinomycin D to partially hepatectomized rats, the thymidylic kinase activity 24 hours after the operation was the same as in normal liver.

Although these studies establish that thymidylic kinase activity increases in the liver cell population by *de novo* synthesis, they do not reveal which cells participate in the synthesis. Are these hepatic cells which already contain a stock of TMP kinase, or does the new TMP kinase appear in cells that originally did not contain the enzyme? Only histochemical methods for determining TMP kinase activity can answer these questions.

If these studies on thymidylic kinase fall short of explaining the mechanism that triggers or stops the regenerative process or even the mechanism of regulation of thymidylic kinase activity in normal and regenerating livers, they nonetheless call attention to the many variables that may affect such a regulation.

Regulation of Gene Expression in Regenerating Liver

The molecular events of liver regeneration, like the cellular events, occur in two major periods: hypertrophy and hyperplasia. During hypertrophy, the cell not only maintains its existing molecular structure, but it also doubles most, and possibly all, its cytoplasmic components in preparation for cellular division. During hypertrophy, the activities of at least three enzymes are increased: UMP phosphorylase, RNA polymerase, and orotidine decarboxylase. UMP phosphorylase and orotidine decarboxylase are formed early during hypertrophy; RNA polymerase is synthesized later.

At 24 hours after partial hepatectomy, the activities of several enzymes expressed per nucleus have doubled. This finding suggests that the cellular content has doubled within 24 hours after partial hepatectomy in preparation for cellular division. Hypertrophy probably lasts for approximately 24 hours after the operation. While hypertrophy is still going on, hyperplasia also starts, beginning with the formation of deoxyribonucleotides and ending with cellular division. During that period, the biosynthesis of messenger RNA is markedly accelerated, and several new enzymes involved in DNA synthesis (TMP kinase, TMP synthetase, cytidylic deaminase, etc.) are synthesized *de novo*. Several unknown proteins involved in DNA synthesis and mitosis probably are synthesized also during that period.

The molecular changes that accompany hypertrophy are not astounding, but the questions about the mechanisms that trigger them—such as the number of triggering mechanisms, their site of action, the molecular chain of events, and the origin of the triggering substance—are among the most perplexing in biology.

A single mechanism could trigger a sequence of events leading to hypertrophy and hyperplasia. Yet the mechanism is likely to be complex; and different triggering mechanisms might exist for hyperplasia and hypertrophy, particularly since hypertrophy occurs independently of hyperplasia in some tissues. Furthermore, the period of hyperplasia can be divided into two segments, one of DNA synthesis and one of mitosis. The mechanism that triggers DNA synthesis is not necessarily the same as that which triggers mitosis because DNA often is synthesized in hepatic cells without mitosis, thus leading to polyploidy.

Before the nature of the trigger or triggers (and we shall see that little is known about them) can be discussed, it may be helpful to attempt to identify their site of action in the cell.

The common denominator in hypertrophy, DNA synthesis, and mitosis is the acceleration of the rate of synthesis of some specific proteins for RNA synthesis, DNA synthesis, or mitosis. Thus, the central event in liver regeneration, as in differentiation and embryonic development (see Chapter 4), is a rearrangement of the phenotype; in other words, a reassortment of the types of genes that are expressed. The protein mosaic of a cell, whether the proteins are structural or catalytic, can be modified by various mechanisms that may involve changes in breakdown and biosynthetic pathways.

We shall briefly examine the regulation of these two aspects of protein metabolism. In regenerating liver, the change in the protein mosaic is associated with an overall increase in protein synthesis. Even if a slowing down of the activities of the breakdown pathways contributed to increasing the protein level observed in regenerating liver, it could not by itself explain the marked increase that occurs. Indeed, even early after partial hepatectomy, amino acid incorporation into protein steadily increases and new enzyme molecules (*e.g.*, β-glucuronidase) are made. Thus, the overall increase in the intracellular level must result from *de novo* synthesis.

An increase of the level of protein the genes of which were already expressed in the normal liver may result from acceleration of translation, acceleration of transcription of the depressed gene, or from transcription of redundant genes that were repressed in normal liver and became derepressed in regenerating liver. New or accelerated transcription would require that new messenger be formed. We have seen that this probably takes place even during the early stages after partial hepatectomy.

Is it possible to distinguish acceleration of transcription of the gene repressed in normal liver from new transcription of the gene repressed in normal and derepressed in regenerating liver? We shall see later that X-irradiation affects only the latter. Since there is no interference with protein synthesis during the early phases of liver regeneration, acceleration of transcription appears to be responsible for the increased protein synthesis at that stage. Now, if it is kept in mind that the effectiveness of the RNA templates on a weight basis is not modified by partial hepatectomy and that new ribosomal RNA is made, the silhouette can be drawn of the macromolecular changes associated with the acceleration of synthesis in regenerating liver of proteins usually made in normal liver.

After partial hepatectomy, the hepatic cell expands both its nuclear and cytoplasmic machinery for protein synthesis, probably until it is doubled in each cell that will divide. Although available data do not allow a quantitative evaluation of the events, they do suggest that the expansion occurs by a proportionate acceleration of synthesis of new templates, new ribosomes, and probably new transfer RNA. The new templates are formed by activation of the rate of transcription of a gene that was derepressed in normal liver.

Once the messenger and ribosomal RNA molecules have reached the cytoplasm, they are organized into functional polyribosomal units. Of course, it is not excluded that especially during the early hours after partial hepatectomy, stimulation of new protein synthesis is effectuated by activating dormant RNA, which may combine with preexisting or new ribosomes. Control at the translational level has been demonstrated in stimulation of carboxylase activity with growth hormone and suggested for ornithie decarboxylase in regenerating liver.

In regenerating liver, when new proteins not found in normal liver are made, the cytoplasmic events are the same as those that occur for the biosynthesis of other proteins, but the mechanism of gene expression is likely to be different. Since the hepatocyte remains in G_0 for extremely long periods of time, it seems unlikely that it would store and keep dormant the templates of those proteins that are indispensable for regeneration (*e.g.*, proteins involved in the last steps of DNA synthesis). Thus, activation of translation is almost excluded in the case of the biosynthesis of those proteins. But even if activation of translation were to take place for that special class of proteins, it is definitely not the only regulatory process; moreover, it is not likely to be able to provide for the extensive expansion of the cellular stocks of these proteins. The biosynthesis of many, if not all, of the proteins involved in the last steps of DNA synthesis is blocked by actinomycin, indicating that the biosynthesis of these proteins involves transcription. X-Irradiation blocks the biosynthesis of these proteins and, since in regenerating liver X-irradiation damage is lasting only when the DNA is irradiated while repressed, the transcription of this special class of protein must involve derepression of DNA repressed in normal liver.

Regulation of RNA Synthesis in Regenerating Liver

The biosynthesis of all types of RNA molecules (messenger, transfer, and ribosomal) must play a key role in hypertrophy and possibly in hyperplasia. Surely the biosynthesis of new messenger RNA is indispensable for DNA synthesis. All cellular RNA is synthesized on DNA templates. What is known of the steps involved in RNA synthesis (see determination of specificity) and the regulation of RNA synthesis (see Chapter 16) is discussed elsewhere. We shall consider here only the regulation of the formation of the precursors needed for RNA synthesis.

At some time after partial hepatectomy, the steady state of the cell must be altered, and a new steady state with increased rates of RNA synthesis develops. This transition from normal levels to accelerated levels of RNA synthesis could constitute the first event in regeneration.

RNA synthesis could be regulated at two levels, the template or the precursor. Let's examine first a hypothetical regulatory mechanism that acts by controlling the availability of precursor. The availability of precursors could be increased by reducing the breakdown pathway (and the breakdown of uracil has been claimed to be decreased in regenerating liver) or by increasing the activity of the enzymes involved in ribonucleotide biosynthesis.

Bresnick [11] studied the incorporation of [^{14}C]carbamyl aspartate in liver RNA and the breakdown of carbamyl aspartate in liver at various times after partial hepatectomy. The incorporation of the precursor is doubled in the acid-soluble fraction within 2 hours after partial hepatectomy, and it increases steadily until 12 hours after operation. An increase of the incorporation of carbamyl aspartate in RNA is detected first between 6 and 8 hours and reaches a peak at 12 hours after hepatectomy.

The increased incorporation of carbamyl aspartate into UMP found in the acid-soluble fraction precedes the increase of its incorporation into RNA and CMP by many hours. At 2 hours after partial hepatectomy, the incorporation of carbamyl aspartate into UMP is four times that in normal liver. This high rate of incorporation is maintained until approximately 6 hours after hepatectomy, and it drops later. In contrast to the early rise of the specific activity of the precursor, the specific activity of the total liver RNA is not increased until 6 hours after partial hepatectomy. Incorporation into RNA rises rapidly between 6 and 12 hours after operation, then it starts to drop.

Bresnick measured the conversion of carbamyl aspartate to CO_2 in normal and 2-, 4-, 6-, 8-, and 24-hour regenerating liver. The rate of conversion to CO_2 was the same in all cases. Bresnick also found that during the first 6 hours after partial hepatectomy, the activities of carbamyl aspartate synthetase, carbamyl phosphate synthetase, aspartic transcarbamylase, dehydroorotic acid dehydrogenase, and uridine kinase were unchanged. Consequently, this increased utilization of the precursor for nRNA synthesis cannot be explained by reduced breakdown of the precursor (carbamyl aspartate) or by the increase in the activities of the enzymes listed above. However, two more enzymes are needed to convert carbamyl phosphate into UMP. The activities of these two enzymes are increased (180% of normal) within 2 hours after partial hepatectomy, and the increase can be prevented by the administration of actinomycin D.

Thus, Bresnick's experiments suggest that an increase in the rate of transcription of messenger for biosynthetic enzymes, rather than a decrease of precursor breakdown, is responsible for the acceleration of RNA synthesis.

Since Fausto [12] has shown that the development of OMP phosphorylase is not affected by X-irradiation, it would seem that the activation of transcription does not require gene derepression.

The increase in OMP phosphorylase occurs early and could constitute the early enzymic event in liver regeneration. If that were the case, acceleration of transcription of the messenger for OMP phosphorylase would occur even earlier in liver regeneration.

Acceleration of transcription could result from *de novo* synthesis of RNA polymerase. RNA polymerase activity does not change much in the first few hours after partial hepatectomy. Significant changes are observed between 12 and 24 hours after hepatectomy, and the major rise in RNA polymerase activity occurs after 24 hours.

Such findings suggest that at least in the early hours after partial hepatectomy, RNA polymerase activity is not rate limiting for RNA synthesis. One is thus led to conclude that a transcription site on the gene is the target of the trigger for regeneration. The trigger cannot be endogenous cellular precursor because in the steady state the level of precursor is constant, and a change in the steady state would require OMP phosphorylase synthesis, which itself requires new RNA synthesis.

Therefore, the trigger must act in a specific way on RNA transcription, either by specific activation of RNA polymerase of the kind observed in bacteria (see factors in regulation of gene expression) or by modulation of regulatory genes.

Regulation of DNA Synthesis in Regenerating Liver

Because DNA plays a key role in determining cellular specificity, it is essential that it be copied integrally and that the copy be transferred to the daughter cell. Therefore, regulation of DNA synthesis is one of the most important functions of the cell.

When faced with the necessity of duplicating its macromolecular components, the hepatic cell rearranges its pattern for protein synthesis by reducing the rate of synthesis of some proteins and increasing that of others. In addition, the regenerating liver makes new proteins that are not found in the normal liver. Among those are the proteins involved in the last steps of DNA synthesis, such as cytidylic reductase, thymidylic kinase, histones, probably acidic proteins and, to a lesser degree, DNA polymerase.

This panoramic description of the macromolecular events that precede DNA synthesis immediately raises two important questions: (1) what causes these proteins involved in the last steps of DNA synthesis to appear between 18 and 24 hours after partial hepatectomy, and (2) what triggers, maintains, and stops DNA synthesis in regenerating liver?

In regenerating liver, DNA synthesis is preceded by the appearance of proteins indispensable for the process. The appearance of new proteins could result from the triggering of a translational or a transcriptional event. Triggering of translation by activating a latent mRNA is unlikely since it would require that the cell retain stocks of dormant messenger.

Activation of a transcriptional event is more plausible because the appearance of cytidylic reductase or thymidylic kinase is interrupted by actinomycin. A transcriptional event could be modified in two ways: acceleration of preexisting or triggering of new template synthesis. The appearance of proteins indispensable for DNA synthesis after partial hepatectomy cannot simply result from acceleration of transcription, because at least some of the proteins needed for DNA synthesis are not made in normal liver. Consequently, the development of those proteins in regenerating liver must involve the formation of new templates after derepression, following partial hepatectomy of a DNA that is repressed in normal liver. This conclusion is in agreement with studies of the incorporation of precursor into nRNA and with the fact that X-irradiation interferes with the incorporation of rapidly labeled nRNA and 18S cytoplasmic RNA and with biosynthesis of proteins indispensable for DNA synthesis (PIDS).

Therefore, a critical event in determining DNA synthesis is the conversion of repressed to derepressed DNA; and, reciprocally, a critical event stopping regeneration is repression of some special DNA molecules that have become derepressed after partial hepatectomy.

We do not know what causes DNA to be repressed, but whatever the substance is, it appears to sensitize DNA or prevent repair of DNA after X-irradiation.

This conclusion was strongly suggested by the fact that irradiation of normal liver interferes with the appearance of thymidylic kinase after partial hepatectomy. Experiments in which rats were submitted to two consecutive hepatectomies and irradiated at various times after the first partial hepatectomy provide further evidence for a selective injury of the repressed DNA. Rats were partially hepatectomized and irradiated (800 R) 6 hours, 18 hours, and 7 days after the operation. At the end of the seventh day, they were partially hepatectomized a second time, injected with [^{3}H]thymidine 23 hours after the second operation, and killed 1 hour later. At 6 hours or 7 days after partial hepatectomy, there is no *de novo* synthesis of cytidylic reductase or thymidylic kinase. Consequently, it seems safe to state that the DNA which dictates PIDS biosynthesis is repressed. In contrast, at 18 hours after the first operation, both PIDS and DNA are synthesized. Therefore, the DNA that dictates biosynthesis of proteins indispensable for DNA synthesis must be derepressed. The findings were conclusive. When the DNA coding for PIDS is repressed, irradiation markedly interferes with the incorporation of thymidine after the second hepatectomy (50% reduction). In contrast, when the DNA coding for PIDS is derepressed, irradiation has no effect on the incorporation of [^{3}H]thymidine into DNA after the second partial hepatectomy.

At first approximation, it would appear logical to assume that the mechanism that derepresses DNA might well regulate DNA synthesis, since derepression would lead to the appearance of the enzymes involved in DNA synthesis. However, such reasoning is difficult to reconcile with the fate of the enzymes involved in DNA synthesis. Some of these enzymes are present in normal liver and increase only slightly (DNA polymerase) at the peak of DNA synthesis; others are absent or have low activities in normal liver and are synthesized actively (cytidylic reductase and thymidylic kinase) between 18 and 24 hours after partial hepatectomy. However, except for that of ADP reductase, the activities of all of the enzymes involved in DNA synthesis continue to rise after the peak of DNA synthesis has been reached. Determination of the incorporation of ^{3}H-labeled thymidine into TMP and TTP in normal and regenerating liver confirms the measurement of enzyme activities in liver cytosol of partially hepatectomized animals (see Fig. 15-6).

The *in vivo* studies clearly established that [^{3}H]thymidine is incorporated into TTP (a measure of the activity of TMP kinase *in vivo*) in normal liver, even though nDNA is not synthesized. The possibility that TMP kinase activity in normal liver is entirely associated with mitochondria cannot be excluded, but it is unlikely. In normal liver, as in regenerating liver, a major fraction of the TMP kinase activity is found

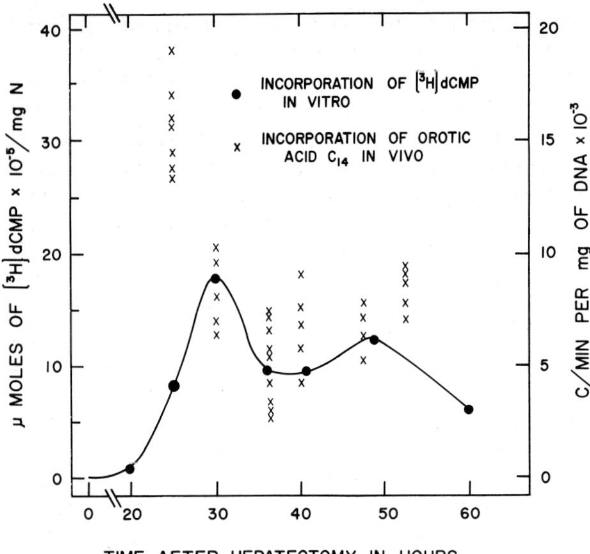

Fig. 15-6. DNA synthesis after partial hepatectomy measured by [^{14}C] orotic acid incorporation into DNA *in vivo* is compared to combined assays for nucleotide kinase and DNA *in vivo* is compared to combined assays for nucleotide kinase and DNA polymerase activities measured by following the incorporation of [^{3}H]dCMP *in vitro*. (From Van Lancker, Fed. Proc. **21**, 1118–1123, 1962)

in the cytosol. Measurements of TMP kinase activity *in vivo* also established that the activity of the enzyme was greater at 36 hours (low DNA synthesis) than at 24 hours (maximal DNA synthesis) after partial hepatectomy.

In conclusion, measurements of activities of enzymes involved in the last steps of DNA synthesis indicate that although these enzymes are indispensable for DNA synthesis, they are not likely to regulate the rates of DNA synthesis once it has started or when it stops.

Could the development of the activity of any of the enzymes just discussed trigger DNA synthesis? Cytidylic reductase activity is undetectable in normal liver, but is clearly developed in regenerating liver. Therefore, the appearance of deoxyribonucleotides could in some way unleash DNA synthesis. If this were the case, however, one would have to explain why DNA synthesis stops 36 hours after partial hepatectomy in spite of even greater cytidylic reductase activity.

In addition to the reductase, kinase, and polymerase, primer DNA and unknown protein or proteins are also needed for DNA synthesis. If the enzymes involved in the last steps of DNA synthesis do not trigger, regulate, or stop the process, then DNA synthesis must be controlled by DNA, the unknown protein, or both.

Exact quantitative reproduction of DNA is so vital to cellular integrity that it is difficult to conceive of a regulatory mechanism far removed from the DNA molecule itself. Therefore, it seems logical to assume that the DNA molecule is involved in regulating its own synthesis. One mechanism by which DNA could do this is by modifying its ability to act as a template for deoxynucleotide polymerization. Therefore, it is relevant that changes in the priming ability of the DNA have been reported after partial hepatectomy. Studies of changes in activities of the enzymes involved in the last step of DNA synthesis in regenerating liver or in spleen before and after X-irradiation suggest that proteins other than the enzymes involved in the last step of DNA synthesis are necessary for the process.

If a protein is involved in converting resting to priming DNA, it can be a DNA polymerase or a special DNA-activating protein. DNA polymerase activity is present in normal liver and after partial hepatectomy, and therefore it is not likely to activate the conversion of resting into priming DNA. In fact, at 48 hours after partial hepatectomy, the DNA polymerase activity is five times as great as its activity at 24 hours after partial hepatectomy—the time of maximal DNA synthesis.

Therefore, one must conclude that in regenerating liver a new protein appears either just before or at the time of DNA synthesis and converts resting into primer DNA.

Although we have no knowledge of the molecular structure of the "X protein" that is involved in DNA synthesis, available data lead to speculation on its nature. Such a protein is likely to appear at 18 hours after partial hepatectomy; it must have a great affinity for double-stranded DNA and must facilitate the attack on DNA by DNA polymerase. When the cellular DNA contingent has been duplicated, the protein must be inactivated.

A key role of such a protein is its effect on the DNA molecule in preparing it for semiconservative replication in the presence of DNA polymerase. So little is known of the mode of action of regenerating liver DNA polymerase that any interpretation of its effects can be only speculative and based on knowledge acquired on the bacterial enzyme. One thing is certain: mammalian polymerase, like the bacterial, must bind to the DNA and the triphosphate nucleotide. If the protein modifies the binding of enzyme to primer, it must act on the primer or the enzyme.

The "X protein" is not likely to modify the binding properties of the polymerase by acting directly on the enzyme molecule because even the enzyme obtained from liver in which little or no DNA is synthesized can catalyze deoxynucleotide polymerization *in vitro*.

Consequently, it would seem more logical to assume that the "X protein" must act on the DNA molecule itself and make it suitable for binding and attack by the polymerase. Binding could be facilitated by uncovering the DNA from the accompanying histones, uncoiling the double DNA strands, or by other unknown mechanisms.

Modulation of gene expression in rat liver is associated with changes in the properties of chromatin. Those changes will be reviewed in the section on gene expression in Chapter 16.

In conclusion, the problem of hyperplasia is raised by the exact duplication of the cellular macromolecular population, the specificity of which is ultimately enshrined in the DNA molecule. DNA can be divided into units the activities of which are regulated by a dual mechanism: an off and on switch, which converts a repressed into a derepressed (transcribing DNA), and a fine regulatory switch, which regulates the rate of transcription of derepressed DNA.

When the cell passes from interphase into the stage of hypertrophy in the early hours after partial hepatectomy, it resets its regulatory switches and, as a result, accelerates the rate of transcription or translation of some proteins and may slow down that of others. Whether this resetting is indispensable for DNA synthesis is not certain.

Between 12 and 18 hours after partial hepatectomy, some DNA switched off in normal liver is switched on in the regenerating liver, and new templates—those templates needed for the biosynthesis of proteins involved in the last steps of DNA synthesis—are transcribed. When regeneration is completed, that special DNA is switched off again. Whether DNA coding for other proteins is also switched off and on, either at earlier or later stages after partial hepatectomy, is not known.

The newly made proteins include the enzymes involved in the last steps of DNA synthesis (*e.g.*, cytidylic reductase, thymidylic kinase, DNA polymerase, histones, and possibly other unknown proteins). Although indispensable for DNA synthesis, the enzymes are not likely to trigger or stop DNA synthesis or regulate its rates.

The triggering and stopping of DNA synthesis are likely to be a combined property of DNA and some unknown protein or proteins that are synthesized either before or simultaneously with DNA.

Polyamines in Liver Regeneration

The polyamines putrescine 1,4-diaminobutane), spermidine, and spermine are aliphatic, nonprotein nitrogenous substances. Anton van Leuwenhoek is credited for having made the first observation of polyamines. He recognized crystals in semen which are believed to have been spermine phosphates. Polyamines have been found in microorganisms, plants and various mammalian tissues. In bacteria the principal polyamine is spermine, in animals both spermine and spermidine are found. In animals it seems that those tissues actively synthesizing proteins are richest in polyamines. Large amounts of polyamines are found in the prostate, the bone marrow and the pancreas. The biosynthesis of polyamines has been investigated in bacteria, chicken embryo and rat liver.

The biological role of polyamines still eludes us. Herbst and Snell demonstrated that they were essential for bacterial growth [111]. In mammalian cells they have been shown to prevent denaturation and enzymic degradation of DNA and RNA and to stimulate RNA polymerase activity and RNA synthesis. Large amounts of polyamines are associated with, and exert a stabilizing effect on, ribosomes. Polyamines are also believed to stimulate amino acid incorporation into protein. The data are, however, controversial.

Present findings suggest that polyamines play a role in gene expression and in regulating growth [112]. The activity of ornithine decarboxylase could play an important role in regulating the synthesis of polyamines. The activity of the enzyme was measured in regenerating liver either by determining the formation of putrescine or by decarboxylation of ornithine [113].

The biosynthesis of polyamines starts with the decarboxylation of ornithine to yield putrescine.

$$\underset{\text{L-ornithine}}{H_2N{-}CH_2{-}CH_2{-}CH_2{-}\underset{COOH}{\underset{|}{CH}}{-}NH_2} \xrightarrow[\text{decarboxylase}]{\text{Ornithine}} \underset{\text{Diaminobutane (putrescine)}}{NH_2CH_2CH_2CH_2CH_2NH_2}$$

Methionine, after conversion to S-adenosyl methionine and the decarboxylation of the latter, provides the amino propyl unit of spermidine. The enzyme catalyzing the reaction is spermidine synthetase.

Spermine synthetase catalyzes the condensation of another aminopropyl group with spermidine to yield spermine and methylthioadenosine. Although the decarboxylated adenosylmethionine has been shown to be a free intermediate in bacteria, it has not been isolated in mammalian tissues and one single enzyme is believed to catalyze the decarboxylation of S-adenosylmethionine and the condensation of the aminopropyl moiety and the diaminomethane. Putrescine stimulates the decarboxylation of S-adenosylmethionine.

Little is known of the fate of polyamines. A diamino oxidase catalyzes the oxidative deamination of putrescine. The activity of the diamino oxidase decreases with age and its blood levels are increased 400 to 600 times in the plasma of pregnant women.

$$\text{(adenine)}{-}CH(CHOH)_2\underset{CH_3}{\underset{|}{C}}HCH_2SCH_2CH_2CH_2NH_2 + NH_2CH_2CH_2CH_2CH_2NH_2 \rightarrow NH_2CH_2CH_2CH_2NHCH_2CH_2CH_2NH_2 + \text{(adenine)}{-}CH(CHOH)_2CHCH_2SCH_3$$

Decarboxylated adenosylmethionine + Diaminobutane → spermidine + Methylthioadenosine

Ornithine decarboxylase activity rises early (three times the normal level) after partial hepatectomy. The activity continues to rise up to 16 hours after partial hepatectomy (25 times the activity in controls) and then drops slowly. At 96 hours after partial hepatectomy the activity is still three times greater than in controls. The activity of other amino acid decarboxylases remains unchanged after partial hepatectomy. The rise in enzyme activity results from *de novo* synthesis, partly regulated at the level of transcription and at the level of translation. Actinomycin D administered immediately after partial hepatectomy interferes with the development of new activity in ornithine decarboxylase, but does not abolish it completely. Complete interference with the development of ornithine decarboxylase in regenerating liver can only be achieved by further addition of cycloheximide and puromycin which interfere with translation (see Chapter 2).

Protein inhibitors have been used to determine the half life of ornithine decarboxylase compared to other hepatic enzymes. It is surprisingly short (11 to 20 minutes). Other liver enzymes whose turnover has been determined have half lives between one hour and five days.

Factors which modulate the rate of mitosis in regenerating liver also affect the development of ornithine decarboxylase; hypophysectomy reduces the activity, the administration of growth hormone increases it. The increase in ornithine decarboxylase is associated with an increase in polyamines which parallels the activation of RNA synthesis. The molecular effect of polyamine on cellular hypertrophy is speculative, it could derepress repressed genes or it could stabilize messenger and ribosomal RNA [114].

Ornithine is also an important intermediate in the urea cycle (see Chapter 9). In presence of CO_2 and NH_2, carbamylphosphate synthetase yields carbamylphosphate.

$$CO_2 + NH_2 \xrightarrow[\text{Carbamylphosphate synthetase}]{} \text{Carbamylphosphate}$$

Ornithine is in presence of carbamylphosphate converted to citrulline. Carbamylphosphate is also a precursor of pyrimidines (see Chapter 3), thus carbamylphosphate condenses with aspartate to yield carbamylaspartate, a precursor of dehydroorotate.

After partial hepatectomy the ammonia levels in blood do not increase, therefore the remaining cells must increase the activity of the urea cycle and this probably explains the increased concentrations of ornithine in the regenerating liver. There is, however, no evidence that the ornithine is channelled toward the polyamine pathway.

If, however, after partial hepatectomy the liver is overloaded by the exogenous administration of ammonia, there is an increase in both ornithine decarboxylase and orotic acid in the liver. Orotic acid by itself has no effect on the levels of ornithine decarboxylase, but dehydroorotic acid, a precursor of pyrimidines, increases the enzyme activity. These findings suggest that in regenerating liver, the polyamine, urea and pyrimidine pathways interact [115]. The relation of these interactions with cellular hypertrophy are not clear, but it would seem that clarification of the mechanism regulating such interaction might help our understanding of the early molecular events associated with hypertrophy.

Triggering of Liver Regeneration

Although at first approximation it seems inconceivable that a biological event as complex as liver regeneration could be triggered by a single substance, the existence of specific growth factors justifies the search for a substance which specifically stimulates liver cell hyperplasia.

Unspecific and specific growth substances are presently known.

Unspecific growth substances—such as growth hormone—have been known for a long time. We can describe the growth hormone in great detail since its full amino acid sequence is known. Such knowledge does not preclude a molecular description of the hormone's mode of action, as is indicated in the case of insulin, the amino acid sequence of which has been known for more than 15 years.

A number of specific growth factors have been identified in the recent years. The molecular structures of some are known whereas those of others are guessed at. Specific substances that have proven effective in cell proliferation in various systems include: erythropoietin, which stimulates the growth of bone marrow cells (see iron metabolism); phytohemagglutinin, which induces cell division in dormant lymphocytes; and isoproterenol, which stimulates DNA synthesis and mitosis in the salivary glands. A mouse-transplantable lymphoma produces a mitogenic factor different from erythropoietin, which acts specifically on spleen lymphocytes. Factors stimulating lymphocytic proliferation have been extracted from autologous lymphocytes. A nondialyzable thermolabile factor is produced in, and released from, chick embryo cells infected with Rous's sarcoma virus. An epidermal growth factor has been isolated from the salivary gland and found to act specifically on epidermic cells *in vivo* and *in vitro*.

Levi-Montalcini [13] has reviewed her work on a nerve growth factor isolated from salivary gland.

The factor enhances growth of peripheral sensory and sympathetic nerves in embryos and *in vitro* induces the production of dendrites.

The factor was purified and its amino acid sequence determined. It is a polypeptide made of 118 amino acids whose sequence resembles that of insulin. Like insulin the polypeptide specifically binds to nervous cell receptors [116, 117]. The properties of binding are similar to those of insulin to fat and liver cells, and the binding of nerve growth factor is inhibited by insulin.

In the stimulation of dendrite formation one of the earliest effects of the nerve growth factor is the induction of microfilaments and microtubules (see Chapter 1). The nerve growth factor was found to have a high affinity for tubulin, the protein unit of the microtubules [118]. The increased tubular formation is accompanied by increased colchicine binding to the differentiating neuroblasts [119], suggesting *de novo* synthesis of tubulin units.

Neuroblasts in culture differentiate and the addition of nerve growth factors promotes the production of dendrites. A special protein also appears, called protein 14-3-2. Once the cells have stopped dividing and begun differentiation, the production of that protein is not affected by the nervous growth factor.

Except for the nerve growth factor, the molecular structures of all these factors are unknown, but they are suspected to be proteins. Moreover, the actions of the Rous sarcoma factor, the nerve factor, and the epidermal factor seem to be mimicked by proteolytic enzymes, so these factors might be peptidases. The role of these factors in embryogenesis and morphogenesis is not known [14].

One epidermal growth factor has been isolated from the submaxillary gland of male mouse. It is a single-chain polypeptide with asparagine and arginine with NH_2 and COOH terminals. Its complete amino acid sequence has been established [15].

Puck and his associates [16] have discovered in calf serum a purified α-globulin, fetuin, that stimulates mammalian cell growth in culture. Although the compound can be separated by treatment with ammonium sulfate, the final preparation is far from homogeneous. Electrophoresis on polyacrylamide gel yields one major (a glycoprotein, mol wt 45,000) and six or seven minor bands. Fetuin antibodies have been prepared which, when added to the culture medium, block the stimulatory effect of fetuin on growth.

The existence of specific growth factors raises the important question of their site of action in the cell cycle. Clues to the mechanism of action of the growth substances in mammalian tissue may come from studies on plants. In 1892 Wiesner proposed the existence of substances that stimulate plant growth. Since then many laboratories have shown that plant extracts stimulate growth, but the breakthrough came in 1955 when a group of investigators working in Skoog and Strong's laboratories demonstrated that old or heated DNA stimulated plant growth. The investigators characterized the active substance as an N-6 substituted adenine and it was found that 6-furfuryl amino purine or 6-benzylamino purine had an effect similar to that of the original product. Only in 1964 was the active substance associated with the DNA identified: 6-(4-hydroxy-3-methyl-trans-2-butenyl-amino) purine. The component, often referred to as zeatin, has been found in RNA hydrolysates of corn, peas, and spinach [17–20].

RNA hydrolysis from various sources has yielded compounds related to zeatin which are also effective in stimulating plant growth: dihydrozeatin and 6-(γ,γ-dimethylaelyl-amino) purine. Although nothing is known of the mode of action of these compounds, their effect on the plant economy is probably not simple because many aspects of plant life are affected by these substances. In addition to stimulating cellular proliferation in some parts of the plant, zeatin-related compounds also regulate branching, flowering, and other functions. It would thus seem that this compound, instead of simply stimulating mitosis, also regulates harmonious growth in all aspects of plant life. Consequently, the effect of the growth regulator varies with the location of the cell in the anatomical structure of the plant. For example, in peas, kinetin interferes with root growth while it stimulates cell division in mature tissues. The inhibition of root growth would result, according to Van't Hof [20], from impairment of G_1 events associated with DNA synthesis.

Liver regeneration is much more complex than stimulation of lymphocytes, erythrocytes, nerve cells, or salivary gland cells. In the liver, stimulation involves a great variety of cells the proliferation of which, although it may not be simultaneous, must ultimately restore histological relationships close to those of the original organ.

Therefore, several triggering substances may be needed to deploy the well-orchestrated events of liver regeneration. For example, the mechanism triggering hypertrophy may differ from that which triggers cell division (see above). Whether they appear simultaneously or in sequence, whether one single mechanism suffices to release them all or whether they are released one by one are matters of speculation. Most of the investigations on humoral factors in liver regeneration have been concerned with hepatic cell stimulation.

Many investigators have attempted to demonstrate the existence of specific or unspecific humoral factors capable of stimulating liver growth. These experiments were done with parabiotic rats or after injection of serum or whole blood of partially hepatectomized animals. The proliferating activity of the liver was measured by counting mitoses or by measuring the incorporation of precursors such as orotic acid or thymidine into DNA. Parabiotic triplets or even quadruplets have even been prepared. In some experiments, 1, 2, or 3 of the parabionts were hepatectomized, and the rate of mitosis correlated with the amount of liver excised. Furthermore, experiments with orotic acid in parabiotic animals demonstrate that partial hepatectomy of one of the parabionts stimulates the incorporation of [^{14}C]orotic acid into the liver of the nonhepatectomized parabiont. (The carbamyl phosphate-aspartic transcarbamylase activity is doubled in the normal liver of rats paired with a partially hepatectomized parabiont.)

Transfusion of the blood of an 18-hour partially hepatectomized rat to an exsanguinated nonhepatectomized rat stimulates thymidine incorporation in the liver of the transfused animal. In these experiments the blood of the hepatectomized rat had no effect on the incorporation of thymidine into tissues other than the liver. Cross-circulation between partially hepatectomized and nonhepatectomized rats has been reported to stimulate mitosis and DNA synthesis in the hepatic cells of the nonhepatectomized animals [21–30].

These studies all included a statistical analysis of the data. However, similar experiments were done in other laboratories, including that of E. Fisher, and analysis of the results failed to demonstrate the existence of a humoral factor stimulating hepatic cell proliferation. These discrepancies probably result from the difficulty in controlling regeneration. The rate and the time sequence of the biological changes can be influenced by a multitude of variables. Although it is impossible to define which of these variables determine the appearance of positive results, several careful investigators have observed a trend positive enough to encourage further research.

Conclusive evidence for the existence of a humoral factor that stimulates liver regeneration can come only from purification of substances that stimulate liver growth. This is at present a nearly impossible task because even in those experiments that deal with positive results, the response to serum or whole blood of hepatectomized animals is so variable that large numbers of animals need to be injected. The purification from blood or any other source of a substance that stimulates liver growth requires a sensitive response; for example, rapid proliferation of liver cells in tissue culture, or the sudden marked increase in enzyme activity in the liver. Therefore, it is interesting that an organ-specific factor has been found in the blood of 24-hour and 48-hour partially hepatectomized hamsters. The factor stimulates the growth of explants of embryonic liver and facilitates the growth of liver cells in tissue culture.

If little is known about what triggers regeneration, even less is known of the mechanism that stops cellular proliferation and hypertrophy. A simple postulation is that as soon as the biosynthesis of the new compound is completed, the machinery responsible for activating the enzymes involved in synthesizing that compound is cut off. For example, when RNA synthesis reaches a peak, RNA polymerase reaches a peak; and when RNA synthesis returns to normal, RNA polymerase activity returns to normal. Similarly, when DNA synthesis reaches a peak, the activities of DNA polymerase and TMP kinase reach specific peaks; and when the DNA synthesis is completed, the activities of these two enzymes return to normal. We have seen already that there is in fact no coincidence between the incorporation of orotic acid or [^{3}H]TDR into the DNA of regenerating liver and the activities of TMP kinase and DNA polymerase.

Triggering of cell division in regenerating liver or other tissues could result from the elimination of tissue-specific substances that block mitosis. Bullough [31] has described such a group of substances and has called them "chalones" from the Greek χαλαω, to loosen. For example, an epidermal-specific chalone has been found in the skin.

A 3 mm piece of epidermal tissue was removed from the anterior aspect of the earlobe of a mouse. Mitoses were counted after the administration of Colcemid in the epithelium adjacent to the wound and also in the epithelium at the back side of the ear. A peak of mitosis was not only observed at the site opposite the edge of the wound but also at the site opposite the center of the wound. This suggested to Bullough and Laurence [120] that the removal of the epidermis had also eliminated an inhibitory substance which could no longer diffuse through the thin mouse ear and inhibit mitosis at the opposite site. Chalones are believed to be tissue specific, but not species specific. The epidermal chalone was partially purified from pig skin and is believed to be a water soluble glycoprotein, sensitive to trypsin, but not pepsin, with a molecular weight between 30,000 and 40,000 daltons. The isoelectric point ranges between pH 5.2 and 6.0. At 38° the protein is active for at least 10 hours.

Chalones are believed to block mitosis. A tissue specific factor that blocks DNA synthesis in epidermis, with a molecular weight of 100,000, has been described by Marks [121].

The findings suggest that during the steady state tissue specific substances are present which inhibit the processes of mitosis and DNA synthesis. After removal of tissue the amount of inhibitor in the remaining tissue is inadequate to maintain the inhibition and DNA synthesis and mitoses take place. Chalones for erythrocytes (molecular weight 2,000 to 4,000), for granulocytes (molecular weight 4,000), for lens cells (molecular weight 20,000 to 30,000), for lymphocytes (molecular weight 30,000 to 50,000), for melanocytes (molecular weight 2,000) and for fibroblasts (molecular weight 30,000 to 50,000) have been described.

Verly and his associates measured the incorporation of [^{3}H]thymidine *in vitro* in rat liver slices and claimed to have inhibited incorporation with a partially purified liver chalone with a molecular weight of 1,000. The block is believed to occur sometime between the Gl and S phases of the cycle. The liver chalone is without effect on intestinal villi or tongue epithelial cells [32, 122].

Liver cell homogenate contains a number of enzymes which once solubilized will interfere with mitosis (*e.g.*, arginase) or with the incorporation of [^{3}H]thymidine (*e.g.*, thymidine hydrolase) in cells in culture.

Regeneration of Other Organs

Kidney Regeneration

Although few, if any, organs have been investigated as extensively as liver, regeneration occurs in many other organs, some of which were not (like the skeletal muscle) suspected of being capable of hyperplasia.

Compensatory growth of the kidney has been known to occur for a long time. This fact is of considerable practical importance to those who have lost one kidney. Within a day after unilateral nephrectomy, the weight of the remaining kidney starts to increase and this continues for several weeks, until the remaining kidney has reached a mass equal to approximately 80–90% of the total kidney mass before nephrectomy.

The sequence of events in kidney compensatory growth resembles that observed in liver, except that growth is much slower and tends to be restricted to the tubular portion of the nephron.

According to Malt [33], the earliest event consists of a modification of the rate of synthesis of heterodispersed rapidly labeled nRNA. This event precedes net increase in RNA and accumulation of new proteins. The increase in the rate of protein synthesis is biphasic. The first peak develops between approximately 14 and 24 hours after nephrectomy, the second between 48 and 72 hours. The net gain in proteins is always small and never exceeds 10% between 14 and 24 hours after nephrectomy. The changes in protein levels are paralleled by increases in the activities of enzymes normally found in kidney. In addition, thymidylic kinase and DNA polymerase have been reported to appear in the remaining kidney before DNA synthesis.

The peak of DNA synthesis occurs within 2 days after nephrectomy, but the peak never reaches levels comparable to those seen in liver after partial hepatectomy. After the peak has been reached, low levels of DNA synthesis are sustained in the remaining kidney for 2 weeks.

At approximately 40 hours after nephrectomy, a peak of mitosis develops. The absolute number of mitoses is small, but most mitoses occur in the proximal tubules where the incidence is five times the normal. A small number of mitoses also occur in the ascending limbs of the collecting ducts.

In addition to bringing up all the problems raised by liver regeneration, kidney regeneration suggests new ones, such as the reason for slow and selective growth. An example of kidney hypertrophy is given in Fig. 15-7.

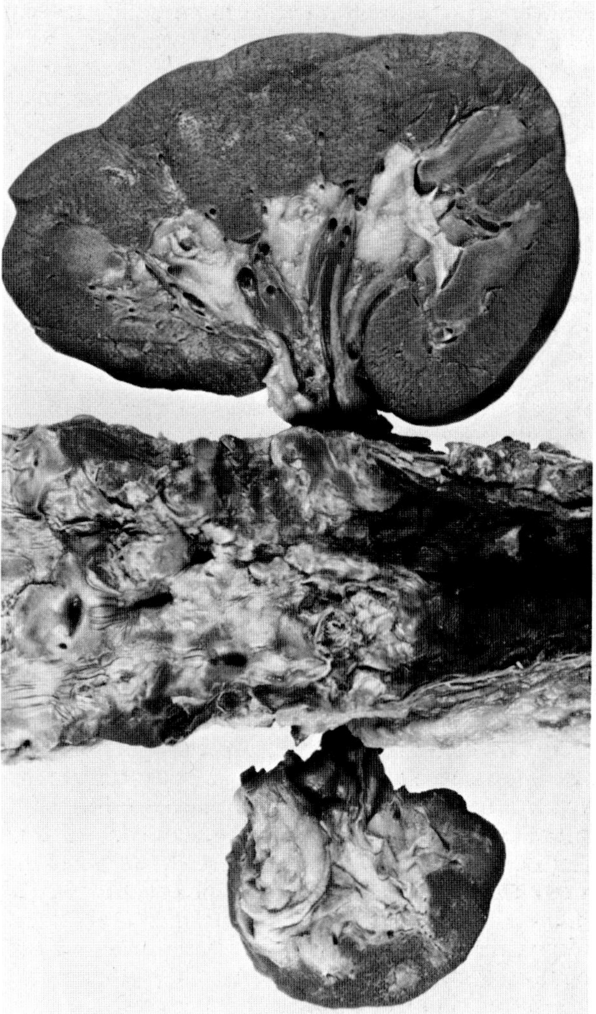

Fig. 15-7. Compensatory hypertrophy of the right kidney

Pancreas Regeneration

The adult exocrine pancreas is a well-differentiated organ in which mitoses are rare. The main function of the pancreas is to elaborate digestive enzymes that are stored in zymogen granules and excreted in the intestines. The regenerative capacity of the pancreas was believed to be low, and no systemic study had been carried out until Fitzgerald and his associates reported a series of laborious and well-conceived experiments using light and electron microscopy, thymidine radioautography, and enzyme biochemistry of the pancreas [34–39].

These investigators demonstrated that the pancreas was able to restore most of its weight and its cellular integrity after both partial pancreatectomy and destruction of the acinar component by ethionine.

When the splenic and gastric segments of rat pancreas are resected, the weight of the residual parabiliary and duodenal portions (44% of the total weight) increases slowly until, after 9 to 12 months, the total pancreatic mass is 66% of normal.

Radioautographic studies after [^{3}H]thymidine injection demonstrate DNA synthesis in the acinar cells during restoration. The peak of DNA synthesis is at 36 hours after the operation, when the incidence of labeled acinar cells is three times normal. After 12 months, the levels of amylase and chymotrypsinogen per milligram of nitrogen are the same as in controls.

These results are most intriguing because they clearly establish the ability of the acinar pancreas to regenerate. Yet pancreatic regeneration, as compared to that of liver or even kidney and adrenal, is extremely slow. Moreover, regeneration is far from complete; the remnant portion of the pancreas (44% of the total mass) restores only 50% of its own mass, so that after pancreatectomy the weight of the restored pancreas is never more than 66% of normal.

Inasmuch as the main function of the pancreas is excretion of digestive enzymes, the critical event in restoration is not total mass or total cell number but ability to elaborate the needed contingent of enzyme molecules. This ability is not integrally restored either, since 12 months after operation the enzyme activity in the total pancreas is the same per milligram of nitrogen, or only 66% of normal.

If it is difficult to understand why liver regeneration stops when the total mass of the organ is restored, it seems even more difficult to understand why pancreatic restoration stops at two-thirds of the total mass. Thus, as Fitzgerald suggested, comparison of regenerative processes in pancreas and liver could give new clues as to the mechanism regulating organ regeneration.

Pancreatic restoration after the administration of ethionine is not less intriguing than restoration after surgical resection. Combined administration of ethionine and a protein-free diet to rats for 10 days leads to extensive cellular degeneration. In fact, experiments were designed in which 90% of the pancreatic acinar cell mass was destroyed. If the rats fed a protein-free diet supplemented with ethionine are fed a regular stock diet, the weight of the pancreas returns to the pre-ethionine level in a matter of weeks, and the cellular and histological structures are integrally restored.

The sequence of steps in the restoration includes DNA and enzyme synthesis. DNA synthesis in duct and intestinal cells increases within 2 days after restoration of the stock diet, reaches a peak 3 days later, and slowly drops to normal for 2 weeks.

The enzymic elaboration is also restored, but not at the same time for all enzymes studied. Chymotrypsinogen is the first to return to a normal level (5 days after the administration of a stock diet), but it takes 7 more days for the lipase and 21 more days for amylase to return to pre-ethionine levels of activity.

The pancreatic model is most unusual because the organ's restorative abilities vary with the injury. Restoration is slow and incomplete after surgical excision; it occurs relatively fast and is complete after the administration of ethionine and a protein-free diet. Moreover, during restoration, the reappearance of the three digestive enzymes studied is not in phase. Yet these enzymes are ultimately found in the same organelles.

To explain the rise in DNA synthesis, Fitzgerald and his colleagues have proposed that during the period of ethionine administration, protein synthesis falls to a low level. Not only is the cell unable to elaborate enzymes needed for DNA synthesis, but it also fails to synthesize repressors of DNA synthesis. When the stock diet is administered, protein synthesis is restored in a stepwise fashion; first for the enzymes involved in DNA synthesis, and later for the repressor.

The pancreatic model has been pursued one step further. A number of investigators have shown that the embryonic rudiment of mammalian pancreas can be explanted in culture medium. The explant grows and differentiates. Histogenesis and cytodifferentiation are essentially identical in embryonic pancreas *in utero* and in culture. Moreover, similar patterns of DNA synthesis and digestive enzyme appearance have been observed in embryonic pancreata *in utero* and in explant. Similarly, incorporation of [^{3}H]leucine detected by radioautography is the same in both types of embryonic pancreata. The greatest amounts of labeled leucine are found in the nucleus at first. Later, when the ergastoplasm develops and the zymogen granules form, more leucine is found in the cytoplasm than in the nucleus. The function of the nuclear protein is not known. As Fitzgerald and his colleagues suggested, this population of proteins could include repressors for DNA synthesis and effectors for differentiation.

Indeed, the organ culture technique provides a unique model for investigating the passage from one type of gene expression—DNA synthesis and mitosis during the proliferative period—to another—elaboration of enzymes with concomitant formation of endoplasmic reticulum and zymogen granules.

For these reasons, it is of interest that Fitzgerald and his group discovered that the withdrawal of methionine from the incubation mixture allows proliferation but interferes with differentiation. The role of methionine in differentiation remains to be understood.

Cell Division in Stimulated Lymphocytes

Lymphocytes circulate in peripheral blood for long periods of time in a seemingly "hibernating" state. They function with minimal metabolic requirements until an appropriate immunological stimulus recalls the cells' ability to divide.

The biological significance of this event will not be discussed here (see Chapter 14); we shall be concerned only with the fact that DNA synthesis and mitosis can be initiated *in vitro* simply by adding antigen, antisera, or even unspecific substances such as phytohemagglutinin to a culture medium containing lymphocytes. Phytohemagglutinin brings 50–90% of the cells in the medium to enter DNA synthesis and mitosis [40, 41].

DNA synthesis begins 20 hours after the stimulus reaches a peak (between 48 and 72 hours). The peak of DNA synthesis is rapidly followed by a peak of mitosis.

Before DNA is synthesized, incorporation of labeled precursor is accelerated in polydispersed and 45-S RNA (precursor of rRNA). The increase in specific activity of 45-S RNA, but not that of polydispersed RNA, is blocked by inhibitors of protein synthesis. Quantitative analyses of the various kinds of RNA indicate that the increased synthesis of 45-S RNA is proportionally greater than the increase in polydispersed RNA. The fact that rRNA synthesis is proportionally greater and cannot take place without protein synthesis suggests that in the stimulated lymphocyte, rRNA synthesis is regulated independently of mRNA synthesis.

45-S RNA is the precursor of 28-S cytoplasmic RNA, and 32-S nRNA is an intermediate. Although 45-S RNA synthesis increases, at least during the first

20 hours after stimulation, the conversion of 45- to 32-S RNA is not accelerated until later, suggesting that the transfer of RNA from nucleus to cytoplasm is carefully controlled.

The possible relationship between rRNA and DNA synthesis in stimulated lymphocytes is suggested by the following experiment. Low doses of actinomycin block the biosynthesis of new rRNA and DNA without blocking all cytoplasmic protein synthesis.

The situation in lymphocytes suggests the following sequence of events: antigenic stimulation initiates new messenger synthesis, which is followed by new protein synthesis, which in turn is indispensable for 45-S RNA synthesis. The conversion of 45-S to 32-S RNA is accelerated, and rRNA accumulates in the cytoplasm. The increase in rRNA in the cytoplasm is followed by DNA synthesis.

What regulates this sequence is not known, but as Cooper suggested, two control points seem likely: triggering of 45-S RNA synthesis and conversion of 45-S to 32-S RNA. Whether DNA synthesis is triggered as the result of the achievement of a critical concentration of ribosomes in the cytoplasm remains to be seen.

The mechanism of gene activation in the lymphocyte* has not yet been discovered, but Allfrey and his associates have shown that in phytohemagglutinin-stimulated lymphocytes, acetylation of arginine-rich histones and phosphorylation of phosphoproteins associated with chromatin precede the increase in nRNA synthesis. The relationship of these events to gene activation is not known [42].

Cell Division in Salivary Gland

When rats are injected for several months with isoproterenol, their salivary glands are markedly enlarged. The enlargement results from cellular proliferation, and a single injection of isoproterenol will induce 60–80% of the cells of the parotid gland to divide. Other salivary glands also respond to isoproterenol injection, but fewer cells enter mitosis [43, 44].

Baserga [45, 46] has demonstrated that it is isoproterenol and not its metabolites (3-methoxyisoproterenol, isoproterenol glucuronide, and 3-methoxyisoproterenol glucuronide) which causes the cell hyperplasia. The hyperplasia is preceded by a period of DNA synthesis which begins 20 hours after injection, reaches a peak 8 hours later, and subsides within 48 hours after injection. DNA synthesis is dependent upon protein elaboration. Inhibitors of RNA or protein synthesis block DNA synthesis as well.

Careful time sequence studies by Baserga and his associates on the inhibition of DNA synthesis by cycloheximide have permitted the conclusion that the protein indispensable for DNA synthesis is made during the first hour after stimulation on a relatively labile template.

* In human lymphocytes cultured in the presence of phytohemagglutinin, DNA polymerase activity is markedly stimulated. The increase in activity parallels the cell's ability to incorporate thymidine into DNA. Moreover, native DNA that has been maximally activated with pancreatic deoxyribonuclease is the most effectively used primer for the phytohemagglutinin polymerase.

Cardiac Hypertrophy

Cardiac hypertrophy is of particular interest, not only because it is a frequent clinical occurrence, but also because function is the stimulus, and the muscle fiber's response stops short of cell division.

The cardiac muscle hypertrophies when the heart is overworked as a result of: a local pathological change (*e.g.*, valvular stenosis), interference with pulmonary circulation, resistance in general circulation (hypertension; see Fig. 15-8), increased oxygen requirements (athletes, anoxemia, anemia), or increased blood volume (beer drinker's heart). Depending upon the type of overload, the hypertrophy may involve one or more chambers or the entire heart. The degree of hypertrophy is determined by the extent of the overload. The link between function and hypertrophy is not clear. What is certain is that the hypertrophy results from enlargement of the muscle fiber, rather than from an increase in the number of muscle fibers. A number of different methods have been used to produce cardiac hypertrophy experimentally in dogs and rodents. Some methods result in rapid enlargement of the heart (*e.g.*, constriction of aorta or pulmo-

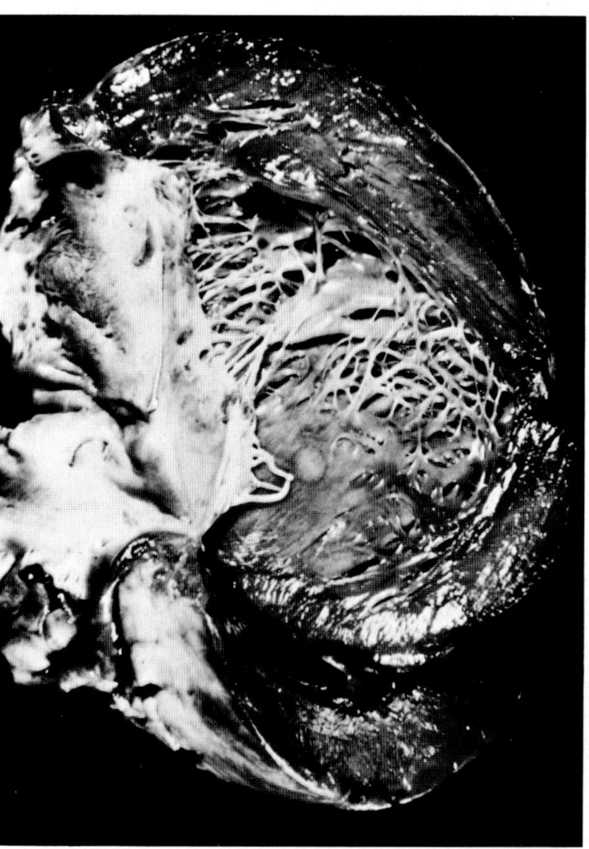

Fig. 15-8. Cardiac hypertrophy and dilation in a case of hypertension

nary artery, unilateral nephrectomy with renal artery ligation); others induce slow, progressive cardiac enlargement (hypoxia, production of anemia, injection of thyroxine, etc.).

Electron microscopic studies of the enlarged heart reveal that the hypertrophy results from the formation of new myofibrils, which, in general appearance and size, are identical to those seen in normal hearts. Other findings, the significance of which is unclear, are the presence of enlarged, swollen mitochondria with disarranged or fragmented crystae, widening of the pores of the nuclear membrane, and distension of the sarcotubular system.

The study of the bioenergetic pathway of the hypertrophied heart has not revealed any surprising evidence. Oxidative phosphorylation is unimpaired, the Krebs cycle functions normally, and fatty acid (palmitate) is used preferentially to glucose in hypertrophied as in normal hearts. Two alterations may be significant: increased glucose uptake and usage and activation of the hexose monophosphate shunt.

Glucose oxidation through the shunt pathway, which is almost nonexistent in the normal heart, becomes appreciable in the hypertrophied heart. Whether this shift in glucose pathways is related to greater need for reduced nucleotides or to the elaboration of ribonucleotides is not certain.

Uridine nucleotide pools are increased 50% in hearts obtained 2 days after aortic constriction has been induced experimentally. Clearly, the important event in cardiac hypertrophy is the elaboration of new muscle protein.

Does the increased level of protein synthesis result from: acceleration of translation on already active templates by awakening dormant templates, or does it result from activation of transcription and formation of new RNA templates? Two pieces of evidence indicate that transcription is necessary for hypertrophy to take place. Experimental cardiac hypertrophy is blocked after the administration of actinomycin. Also, incorporation studies with radioactive precursors suggest that, in addition to rRNA, other kinds of RNA—which must include mRNA—are formed in the nucleus. In fact, hybridization experiments using RNA and DNA from dog heart after aortic constriction established that new templates are likely to be formed.

Certainly, ribosomes are needed to carry on the new protein synthesis; but must new ribosomes be made during hypertrophy, or is the muscle cell stocked with enough ribosomes to carry on in the presence of new templates? In hypertrophied hearts, new RNA is made in the nucleus, the largest proportion of which (70–80%) is rRNA. An increase of ribosomes has been found in the hypertrophied heart, and the proportion of ribosomes that are engaged in polyribosome formation is also increased.

Ribosome synthesis itself requires protein synthesis, and the appearance of ribosomes in the hypertrophied heart is inhibited by puromycin. Curiously, the protein needed for ribosome formation develops early after the installment of aortic constriction in the rat. Puromycin administration within the first hour prevented rRNA formation.

Maybe the most intriguing molecular event in myocardial hypertrophy is that the hypertrophying muscle cell, although it synthesizes DNA, remains locked in polyploidy instead of entering mitosis. When the heart hypertrophies, enzymes involved in DNA synthesis appear and the incidence of polyploidy increases, but the cells do not enter mitosis. Mitoses occur, however, in the fibroblasts of hypertrophying heart. The reasons for this uncoupling between DNA synthesis and mitosis remain unknown.

DNA synthesis is not obviously necessary and it does not normally take place in adult myocardial fibers. Of course, heart muscle fibers synthesize DNA during embryonic life and even for a few months after birth. After that, the degree of polyploidy and the total number of cells remains unchanged, even though the heart doubles in size.

Miscellaneous Types of Regeneration

Function, and to some extent gross, microscopic, and ultrastructural morphology, are not restored only in the biological systems just described, but restoration occurs also in a large number of other tissues [47].

The skin, intestinal mucosa, spleen, bone marrow, and even the gonads regenerate after most of their cell population is destroyed by X-irradiation or antimetabolites. The endothelial wall of blood vessels and even smooth muscle cells divide after trauma. The adrenal cortex regenerates after enucleation by active cellular division.

Each restorative process raises its own questions regarding the extent of the participation and influence of mesenchymal cells, the origin of the restorative cells, etc. Yet, in each case, the restorative event is the consequence of modulation of the cell's machinery for gene expression and involves programmed macromolecular synthesis. The modalities of these other forms of regeneration are touched upon in other chapters.

Wound Healing

In this discussion of regeneration and hypertrophy, we have emphasized cellular changes and have not considered the multicellular interactions in such events. The complexity of these interactions is best illustrated by wound healing in mammals.

Regeneration of liver and pancreas and compensatory growth of kidney are primarily experimental models and are seldom observed in patients. Wound healing is the most frequently encountered form of repair.

Causes and Purposes of Wound Healing

The circumstances under which wounds heal are much the same as those resulting in necrosis and inflammation. They include massive mechanical trauma (concussions, cuts, gun wounds); anoxemia (infarcts, decubital ulcers); burns (by infrared or ultraviolet light); total or local exposure to ionizing radiation; application, ingestion, or endogenous production of toxins; viral, bacterial, and fungal infections; and introduction of foreign bodies.

Wound healing follows necrosis and inflammation, and it is often impossible to determine where inflammation stops and repair starts. Thus, although sometimes (*e.g.*, an acute abscess) it is relatively easy to distinguish between the periods of acute inflammation and repair through scar formation; in others (*e.g.*, cirrhosis) the processes of necrosis, regeneration, and fibrosis seem to occur simultaneously.

Consequently, in some pathological situations wound healing, necrosis, and inflammation remain closely interwoven. Whether necrosis is clearly followed by repair, and whether repair constitutes the terminal event in the sequence of changes that follow the insult to the tissues depend upon whether the injurious agent has been removed from the environment while no new deleterious agent has been introduced.

The wound caused by the surgeon's aseptic scalpel illustrates an injury in which the deleterious agent is immediately and integrally removed. If there is no added infection and the wound is not dehiscent, wound healing takes place without interference; this is known as healing by first intention. In contrast, if, as a result of infection or because large segments of tissue are lost, the wound remains dehiscent, repair is complicated; this is called healing by second intention.

In some cases, repair does not take place because the blood supply is shut off, the exposed wound is repeatedly reinfected, or fluid constantly drains from a deep wound through a fistula at the surface of the skin.

The most essential effect of wound healing is the preservation of homeostasis. A panoramic review of the economy of the mammalian organism will permit us to appreciate the significance of wound healing in biology and pathology.

A mammal can be regarded as a living organism with its own specific internal milieu separated from the surrounding medium by the epithelia of the skin and the mucosa of the respiratory, gastrointestinal, and genitourinary tracts.

The epithelial envelopes protect five essential systems: (1) a rigid, soft skeleton on which contractible elements are attached allowing independent movement; (2) a complex texture of nerves securing response to stimuli; (3) a number of parenchymal organs responsible for elaboration, secretion, and excretion of various biochemicals; (4) a rich arborization of blood and lymph vessels; and (5) the reproductive organs. Adequate function of any portion of the specialized organism requires building blocks to replace losses and a supply of energy for conduction, contraction, and chemical modifications.

Thus, for survival the animal depends on the intake of oxygen and food provided by the environment and on the elimination of waste products in the environment. The integrity of function and structure of every portion of the mammalian organism is preserved in a well-defined chemical environment, which is not allowed to vary extensively or suddenly. Homeostasis is essential to survival.

Consequently, intake and elimination of gas, fluid, and solid must be delicately regulated, and this is achieved by selective absorption and excretion by epithelia. Interruption of the epithelial surface, be it skin or mucosa, if not rapidly corrected will drastically disturb homeostasis. In addition to restoring function and structure of the injured segment of the body, wound healing also restores homeostasis to the entire organism. A dramatic example of the loss of homeostatic control that follows destruction of the epithelial surface is the massive loss of body fluid that occurs after extensive burns.

Superficial wounds interrupt epithelia and the underlying connective tissue; deeper wounds may destroy parenchyma, bone, muscle, or nerve tissue. The efficiency of the repair depends on the organ's ability to recall into function the mechanisms that operate during morphogenesis of the organ. We have already seen that this ability is limited in mammals. Restoration of intact limbs is impossible and, although function in damaged parenchyma and muscle can be partially restored through hyperplasia or hypertrophy, the central nervous system cannot be restored.

Healing of Skin Wounds

We shall focus this discussion of wound healing on skin wounds. In the absence of infection, an injury which breaks the skin and underlying connective tissue is immediately followed by the formation of a clot, which secures homeostasis, and by a mild inflammatory reaction, which eliminates necrotic tissue. Actual restoration of continuity of the superficial envelope involves migration and proliferation of epithelial cells and fibroblasts, and deposition of new collagen fibers. After healing, the restored skin and connective tissue should be identical to the preexisting tissues. Obviously, integral restoration is possible only if healing of epithelia and connective tissues is perfectly correlated, and, therefore, epitheliomesenchymal interaction is of particular significance in wound healing [48, 49].

Wound Healing in Amphibians

Much information on the mechanism of wound healing has been obtained by observing the process in amphibian larvae, because the histology of larval skin is less complicated than it is in mammals [50]. The skin of amphibian larvae is composed of three layers of epidermal cells resting on a basement membrane made of collagen fibers. Between basement membrane and epithelium is an intermediary zone made of a carbohydrate-rich fundamental substance in which lipid or lipoprotein granules seem to be trapped. The inner aspects of the epithelial cells are attached to the cement by adhesive discs shaped like bobbins. A cut of the skin is quickly followed by clot formation, retraction, and exudation.

The epithelial cells become detached and migrate and divide to restore epithelial continuity. After injury, the cement swells and the bobbins which link the cell to the cement are detached. A wave of detachment spreads from the site of the injury deep into the healthy epithelium, and the loose epithelial cells move on the surface of the basement membrane.

Once they are detached, the cells start to migrate (using the fibrin threads of the clot as a guide) to fill the epithelial gap. During this migration, the epithelial cells can dispose of cell debris or fibrin fragments that might interfere with their orderly progress by phagocytizing and digesting them intracellularly. When cells have migrated far enough to restore the epithelial continuity, they divide and the multilayered epithelial structure is reconstructed.

For movement, the cell requires energy in the form of ATP, and movement is readily inhibited by classical metabolic inhibitors. The locomotion of the cell is also guided by the texture and orientation of the collagen fibers of the wound matrix. Experiments of White and Barber illustrate this point. The pH at which fibrin is coagulated determines the orientation of the fibers; thus, fibrin coagulated at a low pH forms coarser and better oriented meshes than fibrin coagulated at a high pH. The movement of the cell is slowest in the clot containing disoriented fibers.

Wound Healing in Mammals

In mammals, after the injury, the cells which were attached by desmosomes become detached. They migrate and phagocytize as they move, dividing and differentiating to reconstruct the original epithelial layer.

In normal skin and epithelia lining internal cavities and ducts, dead surface cells are constantly eliminated and replaced by new cells as a result of cell division in the basal layers of the skin (*e.g.*, crypt cells in the gastrointestinal tract).

In the normal individual, the rate of cell replacement is so delicately regulated that thickness and appearance of the skin do not change. After a wound has been inflicted, this pattern of replacement is temporarily distorted, but it is restored to normal after healing. The temporary distortion includes block of mitosis, cell migration, and acceleration of the rate of mitosis. Thus, apart from the mechanism of migration, the problem of epithelial repair after wound healing centers on the regulation of mitosis.

Clearly, among the major biological questions raised by wound healing are those of the mechanisms triggering and stopping cell division. (Cell migration and locomotion will be discussed in the section devoted to invasiveness in cancer.) Few conclusive data have been assembled on the subject of cell division in wound healing. Bullough [31] has studied extensively mitotic responses to wounding. Mitosis is blocked during cell migration, but it is accelerated once epithelial continuity is reestablished. The greatest mitotic activity is at the wound edge from which a falling gradient of activity extends toward the healthy epithelium to about 1 mm of the edge. In the wounded mouse skin, the incidence of dividing cells rises from 0.2 to 4%.

To explain the rise in mitotic activity, Bullough has postulated the existence of mitotic inhibitors called chalones. The concentration of such inhibitors is believed to decrease after wound healing.

"Contact inhibition" is also believed to participate in regulating the rate of mitosis. As we shall see in more detail later, the concept of contact inhibition was developed by Abercrombie, who believes that short feedback loops link the genes which trigger DNA synthesis to the cell membrane. When cells are in contact, the signal to those genes is to stop their expression. When cells become separated, those genes are activated. Thus, when all epithelial layers are reconstructed and all cells except the death cells of the surface and the cells of the basal layer are surrounded and in close contact with other epithelial cells, the rate of mitosis is expected to drop, except in the basal cells. Although contact inhibition has been demonstrated *in vitro*, its role *in vivo* and thus in wound healing remains to be established.

Toward the end of the inflammatory reaction and about the same time as epithelialization occurs, fibroblasts appear in the wounded area and begin to elaborate collagen fibers. The origin of these fibroblasts is not known with certainty. They may be derived from proliferation of local connective tissue, metaplasia of wandering cells, or even, according to some, from metaplasia of the endothelial cells of the capillaries. Little is known of the factors stimulating fibroblast proliferation in the healing wound, although many substances—especially products of cell necrosis—are claimed to be effective in stimulating fibroblast proliferation.

The fibroblasts that enter the wound have moderately developed endoplasmic reticula and large numbers of unattached ribosomes. As these fibroblasts begin to elaborate collagen, the membranes of the Golgi complex become more abundant, the endoplasmic reticulum develops further, free ribosomes are organized to form polyribosomes, and filaments 50 to 60 A in diameter are found near the surface of the cell. Ross [51] has reviewed the morphological features of fibrogenesis. A collagen precursor is believed to be formed on the polyribosomes of the rough endoplasmic reticulum and is then secreted into the extracellular space without passing through the Golgi apparatus. The secretion may involve either the formation of vesicles, which coalesce with the cell membrane before extruding their content, or simply the transport of the precursor through channels that link the ER to the plasma membrane.

The intracellular fate of the collagen precursor seems to be different from that of the new proteins involved in forming protein-polysaccharide complexes. After sequestration within the cisternae of the endoplasmic reticulum, those proteins are enclosed in small vesicles that fuse with membranes of the Golgi apparatus.

The direction and the amount of collagen fibers formed determine the properties of the scar tissue. The direction of the fibrous tissues affects the tensile strength of the wound, and distorted patterns of fibrous tissue deposition also affect the distribution of blood vessels, lymphatics, and nerves; consequently, this deposition may contribute to the discoloration, pain, and edema observed in scars.

Thus, wound healing involves much more than restoration of continuity of the gaping edges. It also involves restoration of tensile strength of the wound.

The skin is an elastic envelope that adapts to movement and distension of subcellular tissue or internal cavities and can be depressed without rupturing under considerable pressure. Biophysicists distinguish two major mechanical characteristics of the skin: its natural tension and its extensibility. Both characteristics vary considerably. The variation depends upon hereditary and environmental factors, age, and disease (*e.g.*, natural tension is nonexistent in scrotum and eyelids but is considerable in other parts of the body; it decreases with age, but it increases in the skin of the abdomen during pregnancy). When the skin is stretched, the extensibility increases with the load; rapidly at first, slowly later. Extensibility is low in scalp skin, high in eyelid skin.

Surgeons are well aware of these properties of skin because incisions that oppose these natural forces might prove difficult to heal. At least four structural factors are known to affect the mechanical properties of skin: (1) the molecular structure of collagen; (2) the orientation of the fibers; (3) the thickness of the tissues; and (4) the type and amount of interfibrillar substance.

As we shall see later, the collagen molecule is composed of three polypeptide chains each with the shape of an α-helix. These three chains are wound around each other in a suprahelical conformation. The collagen fibers are aggregates of a large and variable number of these individual collagen molecules, or fibrils. The arrangement of the amino acids in the collagen chains to form an α-helix and the intertwining of the three chains to form a supercoil provide a fibril with unique mechanical properties. The fibril can be extended, and after extension it recovers its original length by a springlike recoil. It can be bent in every direction without breaking.

In the skin, each collagen fiber is long, unbranched, and free of other fibers, but it is surrounded by a mucopolysaccharide sheath that separates each fiber from the other and from the surrounding environment. A number of molecular properties may influence the tensile properties of the collagen fibers, but the formation of covalent cross-links (see below) is important in determining the tensile strength. The administration to animals of the lathyrogen aminoacetonitrile prevents the formation of cross-links, and, as a result, the collagen fibers that are formed have poor tensile strength. Similarly, when collagen fibers are reconstituted from solution, they are not cross-linked and have poor tensile strength. However, if covalent cross-links are introduced—for example, by tanning with formaldehyde—tensile strength is markedly increased.

In the dermis, the collagen network is composed of unconnected collagen fibers distributed randomly. The thickness of the fibers varies, depending upon the depth relative to the skin. Those closest to the epithelium are thinner, whereas those closest to the subcutaneous tissue are thicker than the fibers that form the bulk of the subcutaneous tissue. When the skin is extended in any direction, all the fibers orient themselves parallel to the direction of the applied force (except the thin subepithelial fibers). This arrangement of the fibers into a random network in which all fibers can align with the direction of the tensile force provides unique resistance to stretch and unique ability for the skin to return to its original size after it has been stretched.

Scar collagen is brittle, primarily because of inadequate morphogenesis at the fiber and network level. Free fibrils not properly intertwined to form fibers are often seen in scar tissue and, as a result, a random network capable of orienting old fibers parallel to the direction of the stress does not form in scar tissue and tensile strength is reduced.

Breakage of collagen fibers does not result from the rupture of covalent bonds. This would require forces not usually available. The fibers are disrupted by the sliding of fibrils over each other. The fibrils are apparently held together by a glycoproteic cement, the strength of which influences the mechanical properties of the fibers. If the glycoprotein that surrounds each fibril is removed by chemical or enzymic methods, the tensile strength of the fiber is markedly reduced. When under tension, the collagen fibers are displaced from a random network to form parallel fascicles; the interstitial fluid in which the fibers are bathed is extruded. The mechanical properties of collagen are affected by the amount of interstitial fluid present. This explains why a fresh wound flap is easy to manipulate, in contrast to the stiff edematous flap that develops within hours after wounding. In the latter case, the fluid accumulation in the mesh of the collagen network prevents the alignment of the fibers.

As was the case for regeneration of limbs and tails in amphibians, wound healing in the mammal raises the intriguing question of the origin of the various types of cells that participate in the process. In spite of many histological and ultrastructural studies, this important matter is far from settled.

The conclusions of the investigators in the field fall into two major categories. Whereas some believe that at least some of the differentiated cells are derived from the same pluripotential cell, others believe that such pluripotential cells do not exist and that preexisting fibroblasts, endothelial cells, and monocytes yield, by proliferation, the respective fully differentiated cells that appear in the healing wound.

If there is no doubt that most macrophages in the healing wound are derived from circulating monocytes, that most fibroblasts appear because of the proliferation of the fibroblasts of the connective tissue found at the edge of the wound, and that the terminal portion of severed capillaries is at the origin of the newly formed capillaries, the possibility that multipotential cells also contribute to restoring the cellular population of the wound cannot be excluded.

Ross and Benditt [52] have claimed that fibroblasts may arise from a multipotential cell of hematogenous origin. Others have observed primitive mesenchymal cells with few intracytoplasmic organelles in the healing wound. Traditional macrophages were seen also. They differed from multipotential cells in that they contained many cytoplasmic granules. The primitive mesenchymal cell formed cuffs around newly formed capillaries, became embedded in the vascular basement membrane, and differentiated into pericytes—perivascular cells that are associated with the capillaries of many tissues [53].

Biochemistry of Wound Healing

Several laboratories have investigated the biochemical changes that take place in wound healing or in the formation of granulation tissue. Such studies are difficult because they examine heterogeneous material. However, the biochemistry of wound healing can be understood if one attempts to catalog the events that take place: cellular proliferation and elaboration of extracellular fibers (collagen, elastic and reticulin fibers) and elaboration of ground substance.

Cell Proliferation

Little is known of the biochemistry of cellular proliferation. We have already described the sequence of metabolic events in hyperplasia. Whether what is observed in proliferating tissue, such as regenerating liver, can be extrapolated to restoration of epithelial or mesenchymal cells remains to be seen. Crude as they may be, the results suggest that indeed a common pattern of events does exist in most, if not all, proliferating tissues.

We have already seen that in wound healing, mitosis (and consequently DNA synthesis) is 10 to 20 times the normal level. In normal skin, DNA is synthesized only in the basal layer; however, RNA transcription takes place even in highly keratinized cells. In skin, differentiation consists primarily in the elaboration of a specific sulfur-rich protein, keratin.

There would be no point in describing here the special enzyme mosaic found in epithelial skin because usually skin biochemistry and function cannot be correlated. Suffice it to point out that at the end of its journey, the epithelial cell, which started as a multipotential basal cell, becomes an envelope filled with keratin, which progressively loses enzymes involved in biosynthetic and bioenergetic pathways, and even loses its entire nucleus. Hydrolases are among the last biochemicals to survive the slow metamorphosis of the multipotential cells into a keratinous scale. In fact, high acid phosphatase activity is believed to be correlated with nuclear disapperance. In wound healing, the process of differentiation is not altered in essential ways; it is simply accelerated.

Collagen Formation

Before discussing collagen biosynthesis, we will review collagen structure.

Architecture of the Collagen Molecule

The collagens are a population of fibrous proteins found in connective tissue. Their major role is structural, yet collagens are also believed to influence mitosis, differentiation, and blood coagulation, and they certainly play a key role in mineralization. As Piez [54] pointed out, collagen is one of the most successful proteins; it has survived with few alterations through evolution from sponge to man. Its molecular structure is unusually well fitted for its function, and its biological stability is remarkable—collagen exists in some tissues for many years with little or no turnover. Collagen is found in the form of connective tissue in every organ of the body. It also constitutes the major molecular component of tendons, fasciae, ligaments, cartilage, bone, and dentin. Leather is primarily dermis collagen in which new cross-links have been introduced between the polypeptide chains by tanning. Tanning of hide involves three consecutive steps: depilation, solubilization of keratin by cleavage of the dithio bonds, and tanning—usually with tannic acid.

All the details of collagen's molecular structure are not known. The molecule is indeed difficult to solubilize; in fact, most of the early studies on the properties of collagen were done on gelatin, which is an irreversible denaturation product of collagen obtained by heat or chemical treatment of connective tissue.

In 1948 Bowes and Kenten [55, 56], and later other workers, succeeded in extracting collagen using water and sodium chloride at room temperature. After purification, collagen was hydrolyzed and its amino acid composition was analyzed.

Some common features were found in most collagen. In contrast to keratin, collagen does not contain sulfur amino acids. The proportion of glycine is high in all collagen; glycine accounts for up to one-third of the total amino acid residues. Another third of the amino acid residues is made of proline and hydroxyproline. In human collagen, the remaining amino acid residues are represented by all other amino acids except cysteine, cystine, and tryptophan. In human collagen, the sum of aspartic and glutamic residues is 129, and that of arginine, lysine, hydroxylysine, and histidine is 101 moles per 10^5 g protein.

Because of the arithmetical relationship between the total number of glycine, proline (plus hydroxyproline), and all other amino acids, Astbury [57] suggested that a tripeptide formed the unit sequence of collagen: Gly-Pro-X or Gly-Hyp-X, where X is any other amino acid except cysteine or tryptophan. Thus, according to this hypothesis, the entire sequence of collagen could be written [Gly-Pro- (or Hyp)X]^n. Grassman and Riedel [58] isolated the tripeptide Lys-Pro-Gly, thus providing indirect evidence for the hypothesis. The concept of a strictly homogeneous sequence collapsed, however, in the following decades when investigators isolated a number of polypeptides with sequences that contradicted the theory.

Work done in Grassman's laboratory was at the origin of modern concepts on the amino acid sequence of collagen. After treating purified collagen with proteolytic enzymes, the investigators isolated six polypeptides of various lengths (from 39 to 79 residues), and the following findings were made: (1) the amino acid composition was different for each polypeptide, and (2) sequences of polar amino acids were separated from sequences of nonpolar amino acids. Thus, segments of the sequence rich in proline and devoid of polar residues were obtained. The first of these observations proved that the sequence was far from regular; the second provided, as we shall see later, an explanation for the peculiar electron microscopic appearance of the collagen fiber, namely, the cross-striation. These original findings were confirmed and extended in other laboratories.

It is now believed that the apolar sequences of collagen are composed of regular sequences (Gly-Pro-R, where R is Pro, Ala, Gly, Glu, Arg, Phe, Thr, or Ser) and represent 50–60% of the molecule.

Glutamyl residues are located in the polar sequences within the molecules; aspartic residues are found at the carboxyl end of the chain and within the polypeptide, but close to the carboxy terminal. Terminal and intramolecular aspartyl residues serve to link one chain to another by forming a bond between their carboxyl (α-carboxyl for terminal aspartyl, and β-carboxyl for intramolecular aspartyl) and an unknown alcohol function.

Thus, in his model, ordered segments (Gly-Pro-R)^n alternate with unstructured amorphous segments containing the polar groups. Under the electron microscope, the polar groups appear as bands; the nonpolar groups as interbands [59, 60].

As we shall see later, collagen is made of a number of different polypeptide chains referred to as α_1, α_2, etc. Although the complete sequence of the α_1 or α_2 chain is not yet available, the sequences of large segments of α_1 (see Table 15-1) and even α_2 are known, and it is only a matter of time before the complete primary structure of collagen will be described. The new findings have already confirmed some of the general principles discovered in the earlier sequence studies, namely: (1) the preponderance throughout the chain, except in the amino terminals, of repeated triplets of the kind Gly-Pro-X/Gly-X-Hyp, and Gly-X-Y-; (2) the triads form apolar regions separated by polar regions containing clusters of basic and acidic amino acids.

Once the amino acid composition and the electron microscopic and X-ray diffraction properties of collagen were known, attempts were made to build molecular models. Pauling and Corey [61, 62] were among the first to propose such a model. They assumed that in the macromolecule, the bond length and angles would not vary markedly from their value in the amino acid. They also proposed that all the atoms involved in the formation of the peptide bond fit in a single plane because of the resonance between the

$$—C—NH—(C{=}O)—C— \quad \text{and}$$
$$—C—NH+{=}C—O—$$

groupings. Finally, it was proposed that every —CO— and —NH— group was involved in the formation of intramolecular or intermolecular hydrogen bonds. The parameters of the hydrogen bond are also defined: its length is 2.72 A, and a 30° angle is described between the O—N hydrogen bond and the vector of the NH— bond. The collagen wide-angle X-ray diffraction pattern reveals a fiber axis repeat at 2.86 A, which is increased to 3.1 when the fiber is stretched. In addition, there are two meridional diffractions; a constant one at 4.6 A and one that varies between 10 and 17 A,

Table 15-1. Collagen α_1 chain – rat skin (fragments)

	5 10 15 20 25
1	Gly-Tyr-Asp-Glu-Lys-Ser-Ala-Gly-Val-Ser-Val-Pro-Gly-Pro-Met-Gly-Pro-Ser-Gly-Pro-Arg-Gly-Leu-Pro-Gly-Pro-Pro-Gly-Ala-
30	Pro-Gly-Pro-Gln-Gly-Phe-Gln-Gly-Pro-Pro-Gly-Glu-Pro-Gly-Glu-Pro-Gly-Ala-Ser-Gly-Pro-Met-Gly-Pro-Arg-Gly-Pro-Pro-
58	Gly-Pro-Pro-Gly-Lys-Asn-Gly-Asp-Asp-Gly-Glu-Ala-Gly-Lys-Pro-Gly-Arg-Pro-Gly-Gln-Arg-Gly-Pro-Pro-Gly-Pro-Gln-Gly-
86	Ala-Arg-Gly-Leu-Pro-Gly-Thr-Ala-Gly-Leu-Pro-Gly-Met-Lys-Gly-His-Arg-Gly-Phe-Ser-Gly-Leu-Asp-Gly-Ala-Lys-Gly-Asn-
114	Thr-Gly-Pro-Ala-Gly-Pro-Lys-Gly-Glu-Pro-Gly-Ser-Pro-Gly-Glu-Asn-Gly-Ala-Pro-Gly-Gln-Met-Gly-Ala-Asx-Gly-Ala-Pro-
142	Gly-Ala-Pro-Gly-Ala-Ile-Gly-Phe-Pro-Gly-Ala-Arg-Met-Gly-Phe-Pro-Gly-Pro-Gly-Asn-Asn-Gly-Ala-Pro-Gly-Asx-Asx-Gly-Ala-
171	Lys-Gly-Ala-Pro-Gly-Ala-Ser-Gly-Glx-Pro-Gly-Thr-Glx-Gly-Ala-Asx-Gly-Leu-Pro-Gly-Met

depending upon the degree of hydration of the molecule.

The diffraction pattern was interpreted to display helical characteristics. However, when attempts were made to fit a polypeptide chain (dry or at various degrees of hydration) of the amino acid composition of collagen within a helix with parameters defined by X-ray diffraction, it proved impossible to insert an integral number of amino acids per turn of the helix, even when both *cis* and *trans* forms of the amino acid were incorporated in the molecule.

Ramachandran [63] suggested that the peptide occurs only in the *trans* form and showed, with the aid of infrared spectroscopy, that both the NH and CO bonds were nearly at right angles to the fiber axis. When these notions were integrated with the fact that one-third of the amino acid residues are glycine and that the structure must accomodate proline and hydroxyproline, amino acids with a rigid five-membered ring, a triple helical structure was proposed for collagen. Thus, three separate helical polypeptide chains were assumed to be wound around each other to form a suprahelix. The stability of this new type of helix is secured by intermolecular hydrogen bonds, unlike the monomolecular helix, in which all hydrogen bonds are intramolecular.

Rich and Crick improved the model, and it is now believed that the collagen molecule is composed of three polypeptides wound around each other in a suprahelical conformation. The individual polypeptides are referred to as chains. In bone dermis, tendon, and dentin, two types of α chains can be separated—α_1 and α_2.

Rich and Crick [64] proposed two collagen models that are compatible with the results of X-ray diffraction and infrared spectroscopy data obtained on the purified molecules, as well as with the physicochemical properties and chemical composition of the molecule. The models are referred to as collagen I and II. Both form tripolypeptide supercoils; the individual chains are believed to be twisted into left-handed coils because such coils would best accomodate the proline residues.

In such a structure, one must distinguish between the pitch of the individual chains and that of the supercoil. When individual amino acids are arranged in sequence along the thread of the screw formed by the helix, each residue is displaced by an angle of 120° with respect to the other one. The distance which separates two residues in the direction of the axis of the fibers is 3A. The number of residues per turn is 3. Now, if three such chains are wound around each other like the individual threads of a rope, but are also kept 5A apart from each other, a new left-handed helix develops with its axis located in the middle of the horizontal plane occupied by the three polypeptide chains. The suprahelix has a pitch of 28.6A.

The structure is stabilized by hydrogen bonds. One (Rich and Crick model) or two (Ramachandran model) hydrogen bonds link every third residue of one chain with every third residue of one of the parallel chains: —N—CO—. The trihelical structure is further stabilized by the involvement of the side chains of the amino acids in the formation of hydrogen bonds.

The proline residues may be inserted into this model in two different positions. In the first, the OH group faces inward (collagen I); in the second, the OH group may extend radially from the periphery of the chain (collagen II). The collagen II model is preferred because in this model the OH groups of hydroxyproline can form hydrogen bonds with C=O groups of adjacent individual molecules of the trihelical structure. Moreover, the collagen II model is in agreement with the thermal transition temperature studies [65].

Soluble collagen, or tropocollagen, is now believed to be a macromolecule composed of three polypeptide chains. Various combinations of chains have been found.

The composition of tropocollagen varies with the tissue. In bone dermis, tendon, and dentin, α_1 and α_2 are found in the ratio of 2 to 1. The chain composition is expressed by the formula α_1(I) α_2(II). In cartilage tropocollagen is composed of three identical chains, the chains have an amino acid composition different for α_1 or α_2 and are referred to as αIII and thus the structure of cartilage collagen is represented by the formula $(\alpha\text{III})_3$. Another genetically distinct collagen $(\alpha1\text{III})_3$ has been solubilized from the dermis, the aorta, and leiomyoma of the uterus, and an (αIV) chain has been found in basement membranes. Thus there exist several different genes coding for the biosynthesis of collagen [123-125]. A schematic representation of tropocollagen is presented in Fig. 15-9.

Piez and his collaborators [66, 67] have contributed much to our knowledge of collagen. This information was obtained by chromatographic analysis on carboxymethyl-cellulose of the denaturation products of soluble collagen. When denatured collagen is extracted with salt in the cold and analyzed chromatographically, two major peaks appear in the eluent. The first polypeptide is α_1, the second α_2. The amount of α_2 is approximately half that of α_1. When collagen is extracted with acid, four distinct peaks appear in the chromatogram. The first and the last, under the condition of the experiment, correspond to α_1 and α_2. Of the two others, one is a dimer of α_1, referred to as $\beta_{1,1}$, and the other is a complex of α_1 and α_2 ($\beta_{1,2}$).

The conclusions concerning the composition of $\beta_{1,1}$ and $\beta_{1,2}$ were reached on the basis of measurements of molecular weights and analyses of amino acid compositions. Although the exact values reported for the molecular weights of collagen are sometimes debated, it seems well accepted that the molecular weight of $\beta_{1,1}$ and $\beta_{1,2}$ ($196{,}000 \pm 10{,}000$) is twice that of α_1 and α_2, which were found to have identical molecular weights.

The amino acid compositions of α_1 and α_2 are very different. That of $\beta_{1,1}$ is double that of α_1, and that of $\beta_{1,2}$ is intermediate between that of α_1 and α_2.

The molecular weight of collagen—calculated on the basis of the length of the molecule (3000A), the distance between residues (2.86A), and the average molecular weight of each residue [91]—is 286,000. This

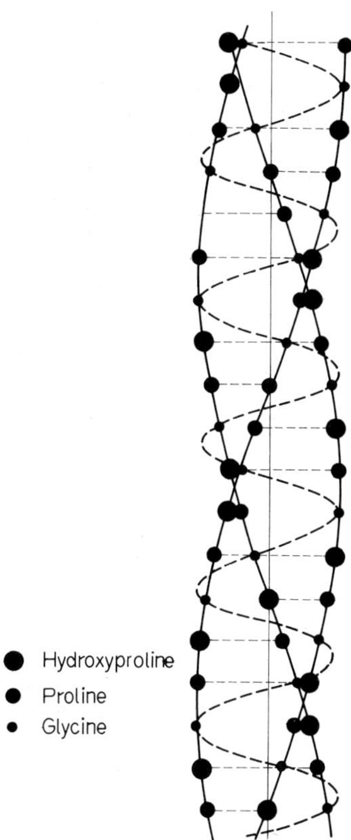

Fig. 15-9. Schematic representation of tropocollagen

value would agree with the expected molecular weight of 294,000 for a molecule composed of two α_1 and one α_2 polypeptides. Measured molecular weights of 345,000 and 310,000 have been reported.

Confirmation of tripolypeptide structure was obtained by isolation from the connective tissue of dogfish of a so-called γ component, which could be separated by chromatography and had an amino acid composition compatible with α_1 α_2 composition.

Reasoning that known properties of connective tissue require, in addition to the intramolecular cross-links just described, intermolecular cross-links, Piez and his coworkers attempted to study the polypeptide composition of collagen, which had resisted salt and acid extraction. Collagen extracted with 5 M guanidine yielded a dimer of the $\alpha_2(\beta_{2,2})$ type, suggesting that intermolecular cross-linking occurs since only one α_2 is found per collagen molecule.

On the basis of these findings, the workers of the National Dental Institute proposed that during collagen elaboration, three non-cross-linked strands are formed first, two identical α_1's and one α_2. Then intramolecular cross-links are formed to join the individual polypeptide chains into a molecule of tropocollagen. Finally, additional cross-linking produces larger aggregates. These may be end-to-end cross-links. This important work reveals the significance of cross-linking in the elaboration of the collagen molecule [68–70].

Three polypeptides form a molecule, and aggregation of molecules forms connective tissue fibers. The fibers are sturdy under pressure and are not very extensible. Therefore, covalent bonds must link individual peptides and individual molecules. Moreover, there is evidence that the structure of the polypeptide chain is itself stabilized by intramolecular cross-links. Consequently, on the basis of the type of structural elements that are united, three types of cross-links can be distinguished in connective tissue: intrachain, intramolecular (or interchain), and intermolecular cross-links. We shall see later that maturation and development of cross-links are closely correlated at various levels of organization. In fact, the formation of cross-links has been implicated in aging.

A breakthrough in the knowledge of cross-link chemistry came when Rojkind and his associates [71] discovered, isolated, and characterized a peptide that contained an aldehyde group. (The amino aldehydes were not isolated, as such, but were isolated in the form of alcohol after collagen was reduced with tritiated $NaBoH_4$, sodium borohydride.) The collagen had been obtained from the carp swim bladder, and the peptide was released from the bulk of the protein by treatment with collagenase.

The peptide is composed of 30 amino acids. It contains a β-hydroxyaldehyde, which by dehydration would yield an α-β unsaturated aldehyde. No amino terminal residue could be detected in the peptide, suggesting that the aldehyde group must be located close to the N-terminal residue of the peptide. Inasmuch as aldehyde groups are usually quite reactive, it was suspected that the aldehyde peptide was involved in the formation of cross-links.

A second breakthrough came from the laboratory of Piez, who isolated and characterized a peptide containing the cross-link. Piez prepared α_1 and α_2 chains, and the cross-linked $\beta_{1,2}$ (composed of α_1 and α_2) dipeptides were dismembered into a number of smaller peptides. The method of cleavage involved breaking a methionyl residue with cyanogen bromide. The authors had reasoned that since the α_1 chain contains only eight methionine residues, cleavage of these would yield a number of peptides small enough to permit complete separation.

The peptide mixture obtained from the cleavage of α_1, α_2, and $\beta_{1,2}$ peptides was resolved by chromatography. The following critical observations were made: (1) the digest of $\beta_{1,2}$ contained a double-chain peptide that was absent from the digest of α_1 and α_2; (2) the digests of α_1 and α_2 each contained one peptide (a pentadecapeptide for α_1 and a tetradecapeptide for α_2) that was not found in the digest of $\beta_{1,2}$; and (3) the amino acid composition of the cross-linked double chain was the 'ame as that of the sum of the amino acids found in the peptides of the α_1 and α_2 digests that were missing in the $\beta_{1,2}$ digest.

This finding indicated that one interchain cross-link existed, and that that segment of the α_1 and α_2 chains containing the cross-link could be isolated from the digest of $\beta_{1,2}$. The amino acid sequence of these segments contains only one lysine residue, and in the segments of the α_1 and α_2 chain, the amino acid

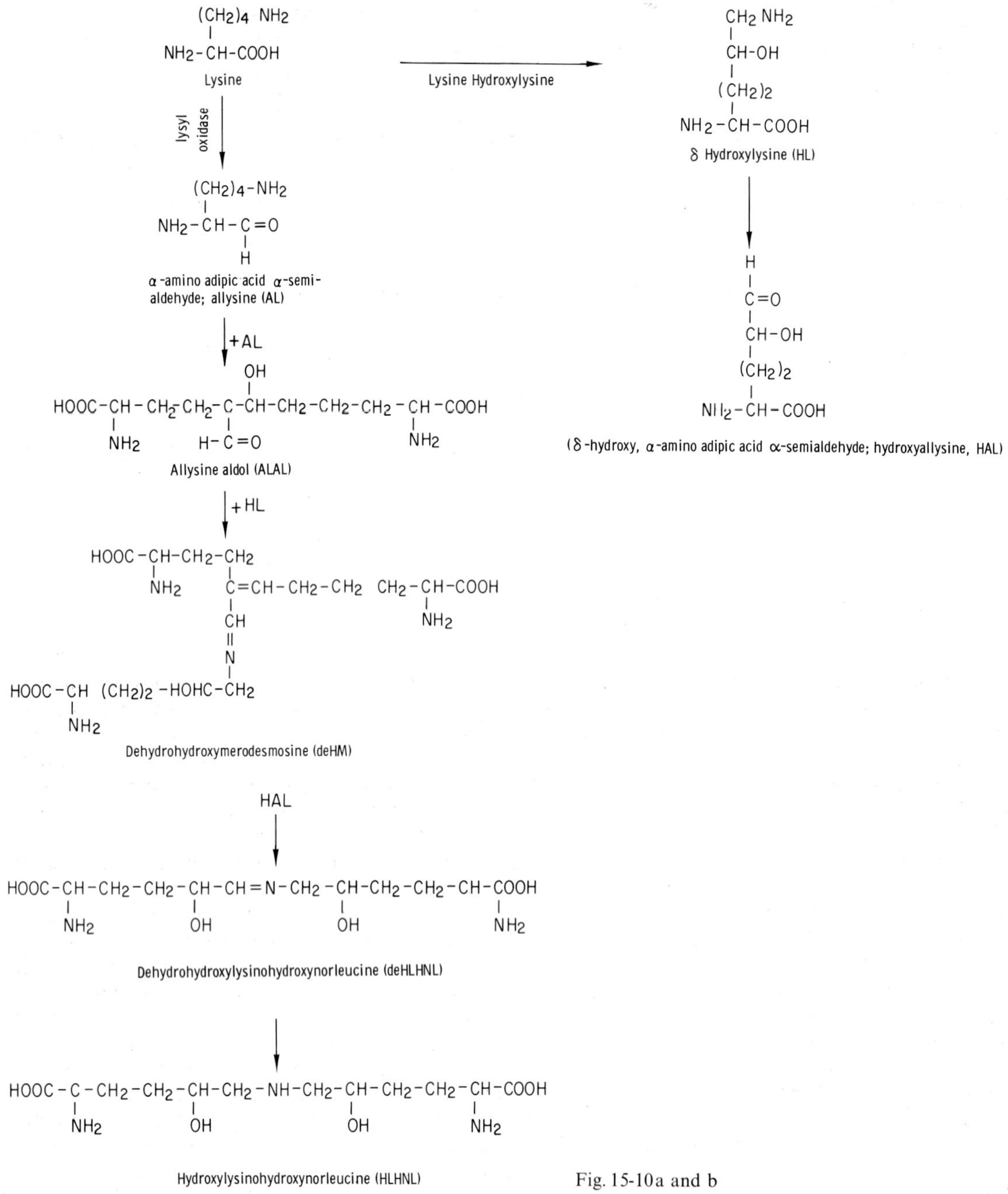

$(CH_2)_4NH_2$ — NH_2-CH-COOH

Lysine

Lysine Hydroxylysine

CH_2NH_2 — CH-OH — $(CH_2)_2$ — NH_2-CH-COOH

δ Hydroxylysine (HL)

lysyl oxidase

$(CH_2)_4$-NH_2 — NH_2-CH-C=O — H

α-amino adipic acid α-semi-aldehyde; allysine (AL)

H — C=O — CH-OH — $(CH_2)_2$ — NH_2-CH-COOH

(δ-hydroxy, α-amino adipic acid α-semialdehyde; hydroxyallysine, HAL)

+AL

HOOC-CH(NH_2)-CH_2-CH_2-C(OH)(H-C=O)-CH-CH_2-CH_2-CH_2-CH(NH_2)-COOH

Allysine aldol (ALAL)

+HL

HOOC-CH(NH_2)-CH_2-CH_2-C(=CH-CH_2-CH_2 CH_2-CH(NH_2)-COOH)-CH=N-CH_2-CHOH-$(CH_2)_2$ CH(NH_2)-COOH

Dehydrohydroxymerodesmosine (deHM)

HAL

HOOC-CH(NH_2)-CH_2-CH_2-CH(OH)-CH=N-CH_2-CH(OH)-CH_2-CH_2-CH(NH_2)-COOH

Dehydrohydroxylysinohydroxynorleucine (deHLHNL)

HOOC-C(NH_2)-CH_2-CH_2-CH(OH)-CH_2-NH-CH_2-CH(OH)-CH_2-CH_2-CH(NH_2)-COOH

Hydroxylysinohydroxynorleucine (HLHNL)

Fig. 15-10a and b

sequence is heterologous with glycine residues dispersed throughout the peptide sequence, rather than regularly distributed every other three amino acids. Thus, the sequence is located in the nonhelical portion of the collagen molecule, and it has also been shown to be part of the N-terminal sequence.

A large number of different types of cross-links have now been chemically identified in collagen and elastin. Although some types of cross-links are believed to be precursors of more complex forms of covalent binding, the exact relationship between one type of cross-link and another is still unknown. What seems certain is that most cross-links involve lysine or hydroxylysine residues, which after oxidation are converted to a more reactive aldehyde form that reacts with other amino acid residues to form aldimines (Schiff bases), or other types of condensation products. Further oxidation or reduction of the original covalent bonding between lysine and the other residue leads to the formation of different types of cross-links. A hypothetical scheme for cross-link formation in collagen thus involves as a first step either the hydroxylation of the δ-methylene group of lysine to yield hydroxylysine (HL), or the oxidative deamination of lysine at the ε-amino group

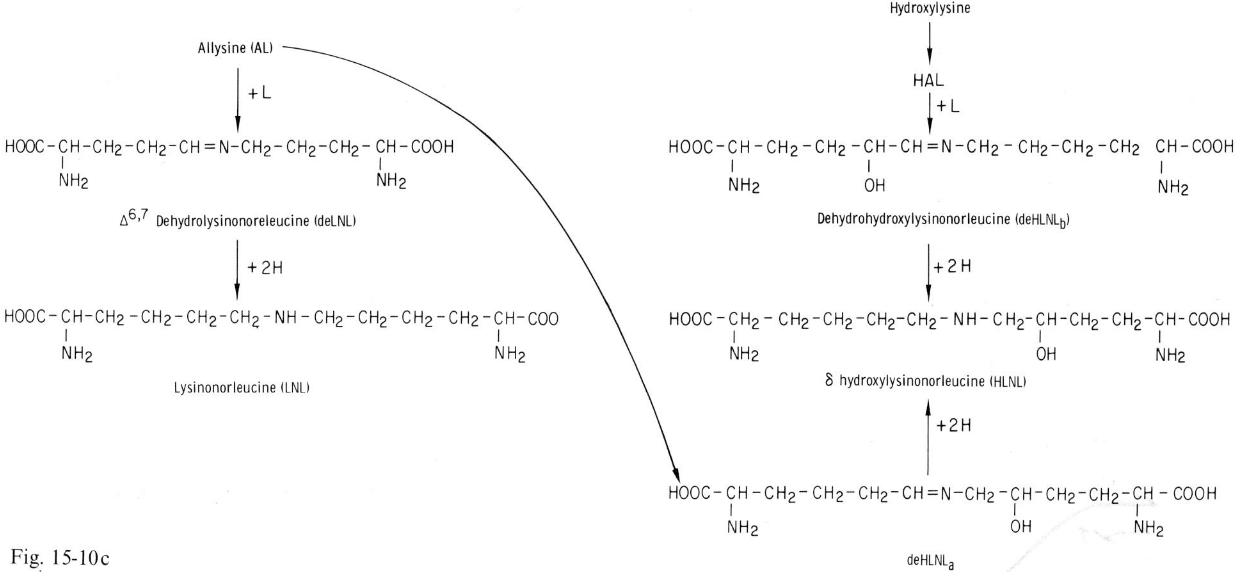

Fig. 15-10c

to yield α-amino adipic acid α-semialdehyde (AL). The oxidative deamination of lysine or hydroxylysine is catalyzed by a copper-requiring enzyme and pyridoxal phosphate. Therefore, one may anticipate that cross-linking may be inhibited in copper and pyridoxal deficiency. Moreover, penicillamine inhibits the enzyme by reacting with the AL residue to form thiazolidine derivatives. AL seems to have a triple fate: it may form (1) the "allysine aldol," or ALAL, by aldol condensation of two AL residues (by further condensation with hydroxylysine, ALAL may yield dehydrohydroxymerodesmosine, or deHM); (2) the dehydrohydroxylysinorleucine (deHLNL), the aldimine of AL and HL, which may be reduction be converted to hydroxylysinorleucine (HLNL); (3) lysinorleucine (LNL) by condensation with lysine. Similarly, HAL will yield deHLHNL by condensation with lysine and HLHNL by consideration with hydroxylysine (see Fig. 15-10).

Complicated as this scheme may appear, it is believed to be far from completed. One can anticipate that the profile of cross-linking will vary from one type of collagen to another. When the sequence of each polypeptide chain and the exact sites and type of cross-linking have been mapped for each tissue, it is likely that we will have some understanding of the function of collagen.

Although little is known of other types of cross-links in collagen, it cannot be excluded that collagen fibers are in part cross-linked by ionic or covalent bonds of types different from those just described. Little is known of these other forms of cross-linking. β-Mercaptoethylamine and penicillamine solubilize collagen by cleaving recently formed intermolecular cross-linking. Their effect on collagen is reversible. In contrast to BAPN, β-mercaptoethylamine and penicillamine do not affect the intramolecular cross-links. It is postulated that these compounds act by blocking aldehyde groups.

Elastin

Like collagen, elastin is an insoluble protein. This is because the polypeptide chains that form elastin molecules are covalently bound into a tight network by the so-called cross-links. We have seen that the first step in the formation of cross-links is the oxidation of lysine and that the lysyl oxidase is a copper-dependent enzyme. When young pigs are raised on a copper-deficient diet, the wall of the aorta is so weak that it bulges to form aneurysms under the pressure of the circulating blood. Careful morphological studies of distorted aortic wall revealed that the lesions probably resulted from abnormal maturation of elastin. Carnes and Sandberg [72] and their associates took advantage of this observation to prepare non-cross-linked soluble elastin, or tropoelastin, and succeeded in establishing the amino acid composition of the product. Tropoelastin has an amino acid composition similar to that of the insoluble compound in that it contains no detectable residues of cystine, threonine, or histidine. It differs from the insoluble compound in that it has a relatively larger lysine content. The exact size of the molecule is still not known. Tropoelastin is believed to be made of various components ranging from 30,000 to 100,000 daltons.

At least one of the modes of cross-links in elastin has been studied in some detail. It has been known for some time that elastin contains a compound, desmosine, which is likely to be involved in cross-link formation, since the difficulties in isolating elastin increase with the amount of desmosine present in the molecule. Desmosine is a molecule likely to be derived from the condensation of four lysine molecules. More recently, it was discovered that elastin contains two other amino acids, lysinorleucine and nerodesmosine, which could be derived from the condensation of two or three lysine residues, respectively.

On the basis of these observations and investigations into the incorporation of labeled precursors into the lysine and lysine derivatives of elastin, a hypothetical pathway for the formation of cross-links in elastin was proposed. First, one or more lysine residues included in the polypeptide chain are converted to the d-semialdehyde of the α-amino adipic acid with, of course, elimination of the ε-amino group of lysine. The conversion of several intrapeptide lysine residues to the cross-linking desmosine is believed to involve a sequence of condensation and dehydration steps, as well as oxidation (see Fig. 15-11).

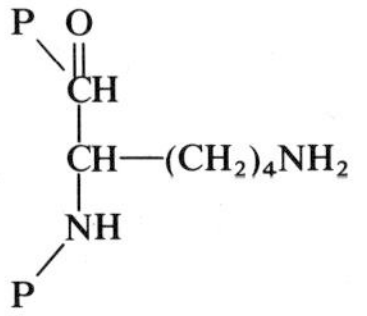

P–C(=O)–CH–(CH$_2$)$_4$NH$_2$ with NH–P (Lysine)

P–C(=O)–CH–(CH$_2$)$_3$–CHO with NH–P (β-Semialdehyde of α-amino adipic acid)

Lysine

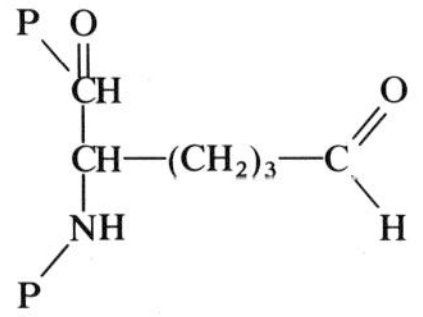

β-Semialdehyde of α-amino adipic acid

The cells that elaborate elastin (the fibroblast in tendons and skin, the smooth muscle cell in the arteries) are, like those that elaborate collagen, faced with the problem of transporting from their cytoplasm to the outside a molecule that is ultimately insoluble. The cellular approach in facing this problem is somewhat different from that for collagen elaboration. Elastin's immediate precursor is believed to be tropoelastin, a molecule mainly composed of hydrophobic amino acid and charged lysine residues. Because of this amino acid composition, the elastin molecule is believed to be folded into a globular structure with a hydrophobic core and a charged surface (lysine). As tropoelastin is converted to insoluble elastin, the charged lysine residues disappear through the formation of cross-links. This results in the elaboration of a continuous network of insoluble hydrophobic corpuscles held together by cross-links, just as the springs of a mattress are held together by wires or rope [73].

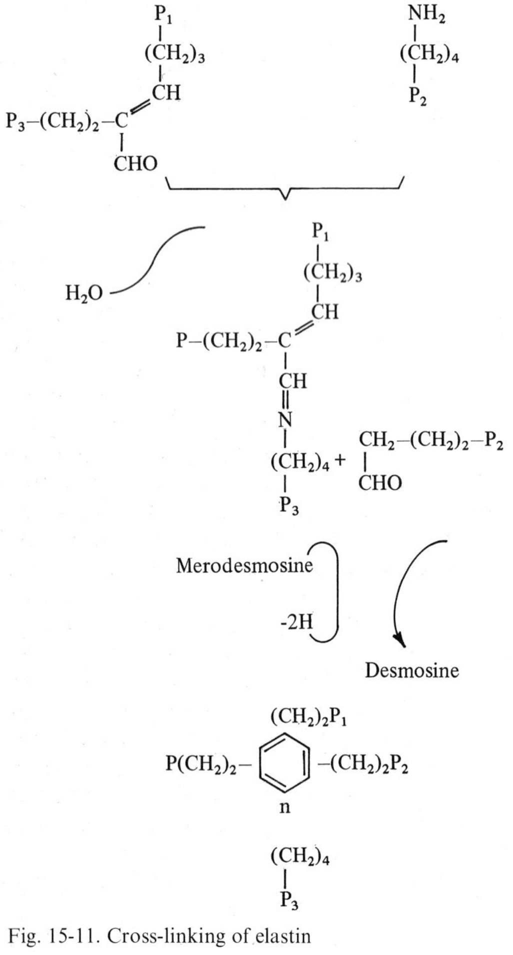

P$_1$–(CH$_2$)$_3$–CH=C(CHO)–(CH$_2$)$_2$–P$_3$ + NH$_2$–(CH$_2$)$_4$–P$_2$

H$_2$O

P$_1$–(CH$_2$)$_3$–CH=C[–(CH$_2$)$_2$–P]–CH=N–(CH$_2$)$_4$–P$_3$ + CH$_2$–(CH$_2$)$_2$–P$_2$ (CHO)

Merodesmosine

-2H

Desmosine

P(CH$_2$)$_2$–, (CH$_2$)$_2$P$_1$, –(CH$_2$)$_2$P$_2$, n, (CH$_2$)$_4$–P$_3$

Fig. 15-11. Cross-linking of elastin

Basement Membranes

A number of epithelia, including the capillary endothelia, are lined with a thin fibrous membrane that provides support and sometimes functions as a filter for substances passing from the intraepithelial lumen to the extracellular space, and *vice versa*. These membranes are called basement membranes; they are made of glycoproteins and therefore exhibit a strong periodic acid-Schiff reaction (PAS positive). Basement membranes form the lining of the capillaries, the kidney tubules, the pulmonary alveoli, the thyroid acini, the lens capsule, and Descemet's membrane. Basement membranes are made of polypeptide chains that are similar, but not identical, to the α-chains of collagen. However, the chains are not connected by covalent bonds, possibly as a result of interference with cross-linking by glycosylation of the hydroxylysine residues.

A large number of hexoses have been found in association with the basement membrane proteins. They include glucose, galactose, sialic acid, and hexosamine, but the most common are glucose, galactose and a disaccharide, galactoglucoside. The exact mechanism by which these glycosylated derivatives are formed is not clear, but glucose and galactose transferases have been found in basement membranes and are believed to affect the attachment of the hexose residues [74].

Lathyrism and Cross-Links

In humans, continuous and almost exclusive feeding of *Lathyrus sativus* causes a progressive spastic paraplegia known as lathyrism. In animals, severe skeletal deformities and aortic aneurysms are prominent. Whether the human and animal diseases are related is unknown. The administration of a diet of sweet peas to rats induces scoliosis, dissecting aneurysm, hernias, and gross disturbances in endochondral and bone formation. Lathyrism obviously results from damage to connective and elastic tissue. Of considerable importance for the interpretation of the pathogenesis of lathyrism is Ponsetti's observation, which established that the dissecting aneurysm and other manifestations of lathyrism could be induced only in young rats. When a diet of sweet peas is administered to pregnant rats, all elastic fibers appear in fragments rather than in network. The isolation of the active agent permitted further investigation of the toxin's mode of action [75, 76].

Lathyrism may be one of the most interesting examples of cross-fertilization between pathology and biochemistry. Although rare, the disease has been known for a long time. Lathyrism was observed in India and sometimes in Spain during famines. In those times, the people fed mainly on the sweet pea *Lathyrus sativus*. Efforts to isolate the active agent from the *Lathyrus sativus* failed, but the toxic factor was isolated from the garden variety, *Lathyrus odoratus*. β-Aminopropionitrile (BAPN) was found to be the active agent.

It was observed that collagen was easier to extract from lathyritic than from normal rats. The fact that the proportion of soluble collagen was increased suggested that BAPN interfered with collagen cross-linking. Since BAPN affects collagen only during development and is without effect on mature collagen, cleavage of existing cross-links appears to be excluded. As Levine [77] suggested, interference with cross-link formation could result from blocking of the aldehyde through binding, interference with aldehyde synthesis, or disruption of the collagen fiber.

Studies in which labeled BAPN were used eliminated the possibility of direct binding of the toxin to aldehyde groups. Available evidence suggests that BAPN acts by preventing the formation of the aldehyde. The levels of aldehyde found in collagen are decreased in lathyritic rats.

In collagen of lathyritic rats, α_1 chains have half the aldehyde content of collagen from normal rats. In contrast, the aldehyde content of α_2 chains was unchanged. Similarly, elastin extracted from lathyritic animals has an increased level of lysine and decreased levels of aldehyde and desmosine. BAPN thus seems to act by preventing the participation of lysine in cross-linking.

Collagen Biosynthesis

The elaboration of collagen in the fibroblast involves at least four steps: formation of a tropocollagen precursor, procollagen, splitting of the extended polypeptide to yield tropocollagen, assembly of tropocollagen into collagen fibrils, and collagen cross-linking.

Inasmuch as various types of collagen chains exist, the cell must first select the proper gene for the synthesis of a given chain. It is not known whether or not a single cell can synthesize different types of collagen.

In the intact animal a specialized cell, the fibroblast, is responsible for collagen elaboration *in vivo*.

The synthesis of procollagen starts with the elaboration of pro α chains through conventional processes of protein synthesis. A messenger RNA binds to polysomes and is translated into proteins with the aid of tRNA.

Rich and his collaborator [64] have demonstrated two differences between collagen synthesis and other forms of protein synthesis. The polysomes that synthesize collagen are larger than those that synthesize other proteins, and collagen synthesis is relatively resistant to ribonuclease attack. Because hemoglobin synthesis requires five ribosomes, Rich calculated that the mRNA (mol wt 17,000) of the pro α_1 chain binds 30 to 40 ribosomes. In fact, the sedimentation characteristics of the polysome population which synthesizes collagen are greater that those anticipated for a chain of 30 to 40 ribosomes. The reasons for this high sedimentation rate are not known. Complexing of the nascent strand with strands of adjacent polysomes, the existence of a polycistronic mRNA, or a unique affinity of collagen-synthesizing polysomes for the endoplasmic reticulum could be the causes. Studies in which the polysome preparation was treated with deoxycholate have eliminated the last possibility.

Careful studies of the kinetics of collagen synthesis have permitted investigators to estimate the rate at which the α_1 chain is elaborated. The rate of translation of the RNA for one collagen chain is believed to be 209 residues per minute. Thus, it would take 6 minutes to synthesize a pro-α chain of 1250 residues.

There are two peculiarities with respect to tRNA's in the fibroblast. As may be anticipated, the concentrations of tRNA for proline and glycine are twice that in other cells and in spite of the high levels of hydroxyproline and hydroxylysine associated with the collagen molecule, there are no tRNA's for these amino acids in the fibroblast, suggesting that the hydroxylation is posttranslational.

Like many excreted proteins, collagen is initially synthesized as a larger precursor which is later modified by proteolysis [126–128].

The formation of procollagen as soluble precursor of collagen has been demonstrated in numerous systems. The body of procollagen has the triple helical structure, but the NH_2 terminus (or in some cases the COOH terminus) portion of each chain differs in conformation and the extended portions of the chains contain disulfide bonds linking the chains. Denaturation of procollagen yields a pro α chain with a molecular weight that is 15 to 25% greater than that of normal α chains. The extended portion of the chain does not contain the high glycine content and is rich in aspartic acid, glutamic acid, serine and contains higher contents of histidine and tyrosine than the regular portion of the chain. Limited proteolysis by pepsin or chymotrypsin converts procollagen into collagen. The reason for the elaboration of an extended molecule is not known. It has been proposed that the extended portion of the molecule facilitates the formation of the helical conformation and the association of the various chains. Others believe that the extended portion is involved in the transport of the collagen molecule.

Although the enzyme has not been purified, the conversion of procollagen to collagen is believed to be catalyzed *in vivo* by a special neutral peptidase: procollagen peptidase. The enzyme is missing in cattle afflicted with dermatosparaxis. The proteolysis of procollagen may occur partly intracellularly and partly extracellularly.

Ten percent of the amino acid residues of the chain is composed of hydroxyproline. However, during the elaboration of the chain on ribosomes, proline is used to form the peptide bond. Therefore, hydroxylation of proline and lysine are post-translation events.

The hydroxylations of the two amino acids occur while the chain is still attached to the ribosomes and are catalyzed by two different enzymes; a peptidyl proline hydroxylase and a peptidyl lysine hydroxylase. The proline hydroxylase has been purified to homogeneity in the ultracentrifuge and on polyacrylamide gel. The lysine hydroxylase has only been partially purified. Both enzymes require molecular oxygen, iron, α ketoglutarate and ascorbic acid. The iron may serve as a binding site for the oxygen, the α ketoglutarate is an absolute requirement and its decarboxylation is stoichiometrically linked to the hydroxylation of proline. Ascorbic acid serves as the reducing agent, or as a cofactor necessary for the conversion of inactive to active hydroxylase. The exact intracellular location of the enzyme is debated, while tissue fractionation has shown enzyme activity in both microsomes and supernatant. Electron microscopy with tagged antibodies suggests that most, if not all, the enzyme is found in the cisternae of the ER.

When hydroxylation is prevented by the addition of a metal chelate, collagen chains are made, but stable triple helical structures are not formed. Therefore it appears that hydroxylation is indispensable for the stabilization of the triple helix and in absence of hydroxylation unstable collagen accumulates in the cell because when hydroxylation is incomplete, protein folding is inadequate.

The extent of the hydroxylation is not identical in all chains. $\alpha 1$(I), $\alpha 1$(II) and $\alpha 2$ contain 100 hydroxyproline residues while $\alpha 1$(IV) contains 140. The proportion of hydroxylysine residues is much smaller than that of hydroxyproline residues in the collagen chains.

Collagen molecules contain covalently bound galactose and glucosylgalactose. The mono and disaccharides are bound to the hydroxylysine through a O-glycosidic linkage. The reactions are catalyzed by two microsomal transferases: a peptidyl galactosyl hydroxylysine transferase and a peptidyl glucosyl galactosyl hydroxylysine transferase.

The role of carbohydrate moieties is not known, but the number of hydroxylysine and carbohydrate groups in the α chains correlate.

Electron microscopic studies have settled the argument concerning the site of biosynthesis of collagen which started with Schwann, who thought that it was intracellular, and Virchow, who thought it was extracellular. It is clear that collagen is secreted in the cells. There is, however, debate as to whether or not the Golgi is involved [129].

In conclusion, the biosynthesis of collagen takes place in mesenchymal cells, principally fibroblasts, but also chondroblasts, odontoblasts, osteoblasts, etc. The process starts by conventional transcription of an extended chain coded for by a typical messenger RNA. The NH_2 terminal extended portion forms interchain S—S bonds which facilitate the formation of the triple helical structure. The procollagen is made of the three chains and their extended NH_2 fragments are partially hydroxylated in the cisternae and glycosylated possibly in the Golgi or, according to others, close to the cell membrane. The mechanism of transport of the procollagen fibers from the interior of the cells to the periphery requires energy and an intact tubular system. Colcemid blocks the transport. Cytochalasin B, which interferes with the actin filaments and prevents membrane movements, does not interfere with the extrusion of collagen. The proteolysis of the procollagen to tropocollagen occurs intracellularly near the membrane and possibly partly extracellularly. Tropocollagen is ultimately cross-linked in the extracellular fluid. The steps involved in the biosynthesis of collagen are shown in Fig. 15-12.

Collagen Breakdown

Although normal collagen turns over slowly, more or less extensive breakdown of collagen takes place under physiological (bone and uterus resorption) and pathological conditions (e.g., destruction of joints in patients with rheumatoid arthritis). In contrast to most other proteins, collagen, because of the triple helical structure, is relatively protected against other proteases, and large concentrations of trypsin or chymotrypsin are needed to cause partial cleavage. Consequently, effective cleavage requires a specific enzyme: collagenase. Collagenases have been prepared from various sources and the enzymes vary in their properties [130–132].

We shall only describe briefly the steps believed to be involved when pure mammalian collagenase is used. The enzyme makes one cut in the triple helical tropocollagen fibril (e.g., $(\alpha 1)_2\alpha 2$). The cut occurs at the C terminal site and yields an N terminal fragment with a molecular weight that is 75% of the normal $(\alpha 1)_2\alpha 2$ chain. The cleaved fragments are then either degraded by endopeptidases found in the extracellular fluid (such endopeptidases have been found in the culture media of joint synovia or in culture of two rheumatoid nodules), or they are phagocytized and degraded inside of macrophages.

In some cases, as in the case of resorption of the uterus, special collagenases attach several fibrils of the collagen network yielding a large segment of the network which is then phagocytized by macrophages. Although much has been learned about collagenases, their exact role remains unknown.

Molecular Diseases of Collagen

Many inherited diseases have been suspected to involve connective tissue. In none of them was the molecular

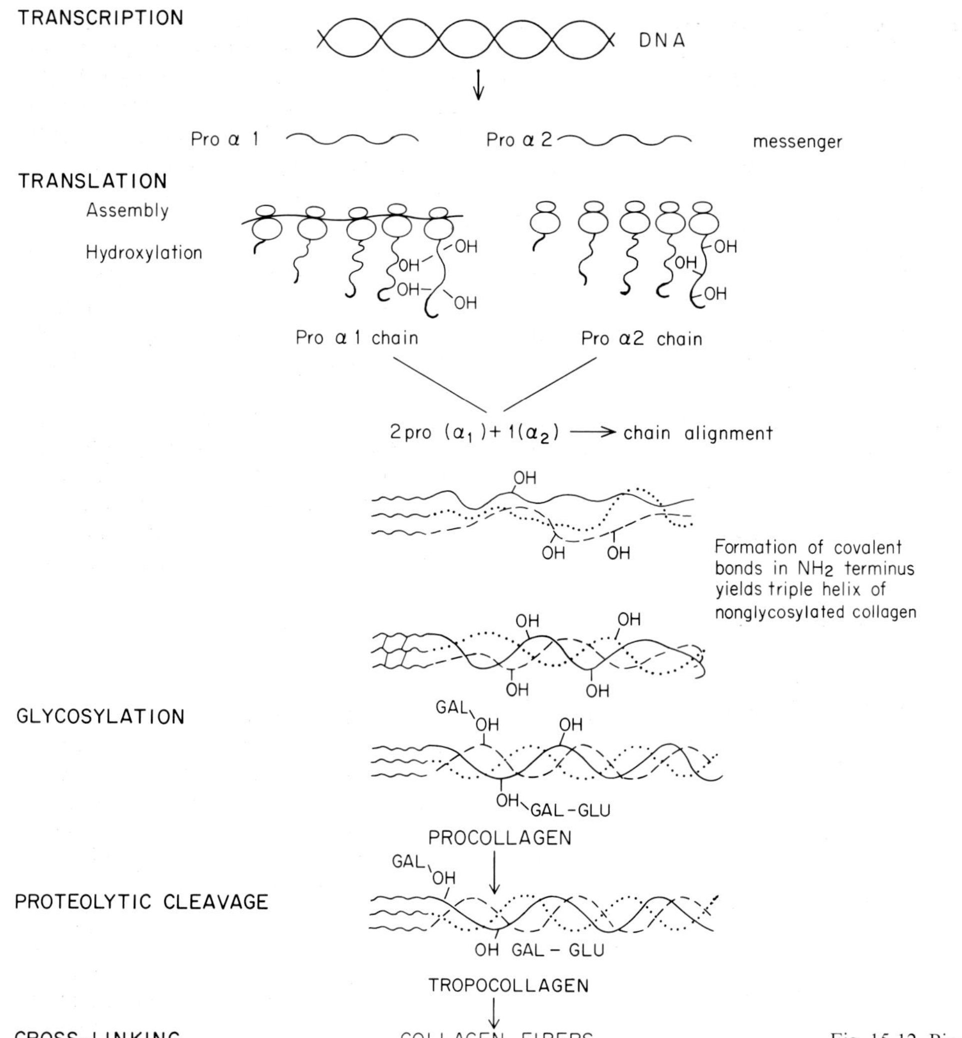

Fig. 15-12. Biosynthesis of collagen

pathogenic mechanism known until recently. No structural mutations of the collagen chains have, however, been reported [133–139].

Dermatosparaxis is a disease of cattle characterized by the extreme fragility of the skin and the laxity of the articular ligaments. The procollagen peptidase has been demonstrated to be missing in the diseased animals. As a result the collagen chains of the dermis do not interact properly to form fibers, but instead clump into irregular bundles that can be recognized under the electron microscope. This distortion of collagen structure is believed to be responsible for the unusual fragility of the skin. A disease similar to dermatoparaxis exists in sheep, but has not been observed in man [138].

A hydrolysine deficiency as a result of lysine hydroxylase deficiency (demonstrated in fibroblast culture) has been described in two young sisters who presented severe kyphoscoliosis from birth with marked joint laxity and a tendency to bruise easily in absence of a clotting defect. The collagen also contained low levels of carbohydrates. The hypothetical pathogenesis of the bleeding tendency is of interest. Two mechanisms have been proposed: vascular hyperelasticity causes the blood vessel wall to gape, and adhesion of platelets to collagen is impaired. The latter mechanism implies that the hydroxylysines are involved in the adhesion process. Platelets have been found to contain two glycosyl transferases that are specific for hydroxylysine. Thus, the initial step in hemostasis would involve the recognition of collagen hydroxylysine by the platelet glycosyl transferase [133].

A defect of lysine oxidase has also been suspected in osteogenesis imperfecta, a hereditary bone disease transmitted as a dominant trait. The disease may become manifest immediately after birth, but more often develops during childhood. The cortical bone is greatly reduced in amount and does not develop lamellar structures. Instead it presents a spongy network of nonlamellar bone. The bones are very soft and friable and as a result the child develops multiple fractures. Attempts to repair the fractures cause cartilaginous calluses to appear. Histologically the collagen fibers are thin. The hydroxylysine content is increased, but glycosylation is reduced. An inability to form normal cross-links is believed to be at the origin of the symptoms.

Ehlers-Danlos syndrome, or cutis hyperelastica, is a hereditary disease transmitted and characterized by excessive elasticity of the skin and laxity of the joints. The skin is readily bruised, and pseudotumors, referred to as "raisin tumors," may develop at the site of injury. The laxity of the joint causes recurrent dislocation. The collagen fibers are thinner than normal and have much less tendency to form an interwoven network.

Hydroxylysinorleucine and hydroxyalanine accumulate without being involved in the formation of cross-links. New cross-links appear, but their nature is unknown. Some miscellaneous acquired lesions of collagen metabolism are listed in Table 15-2.

Table 15-2. Acquired lesions involving collagen metabolism

Increased proline hydroxylase activity
Scleroderma
Pseudoxanthoma elasticum
Atherosclerosis
Aorta of hypertensive rats
Alcoholic cirrhosis
Decreased proline hydroxylase activity
Chronic inflammation
Chronic iron deficiency?
Ascorbic acid deficiency?
Increased glycosyl transferase
In kidney of alloxan diabetic rat
Increased soluble collagen
Dermatomyositis
Scleroderma
Lupus erythematosus
Decreased soluble collagen
Uremia
Pellagra

Ground Substance

Fibroblasts, collagen, elastin, and reticulum fibers bathe in gels of varying consistencies, depending upon the tissue. These gels, referred to as ground substance, are made up of protein-polysaccharide complexes. If we know little about the ground substance, we know even less about the role it plays in metabolism. Yet the ground substance is more than a bathing fluid; it is alive and, in part, composed of complex molecules. To ignore its existence and its importance would be naive. Therefore, we should be familiar with the fundamentals of what is known about its molecular composition.

Much of the work on polysaccharides was done in Meyer's laboratory [79–81]. Meyer was the first to propose a classification for this group of macromolecules. A class of simple polysaccharides was distinguished from a class of complex polysaccharides. The simple ones include hyaluronic acid and chondroitin; the complex polysaccharides include the chondroitin sulfates (A, B, and C), keratosulfate, and heparin sulfate. Except for keratosulfate, most polysaccharides are nonbranched polymers in which hexouridine groups alternate with N-acetylhexosaminidic groups. In keratosulfate, the D-galactose residue replaces the uridinic group.

Hyaluronic acid is a ubiquitous linear unbranched polymer. The repeating dissaccharide unit is glucuronic acid and acetylglucosamine linked in a 1–3 linkage. A 1–4 linkage forms the bond between two adjacent dissaccharide repeating units.

Three groups of chondroitin sulfates can be distinguished on the basis of their optical rotation, solubility, and enzyme hydrolysis. One example is chondroitin sulfate B. In contrast to chondroitin sulfates A and C, the B form is relatively resistant to hydrolysis with testicular hyaluronidase. Resistance to hydrolysis is probably a consequence of the fact that chondroitin sulfate B contains a uronic acid different from the one found in the A and C types. Studies of the colorimetric reactions and isolation of sugar derivatives in the crystal form have shown that chondroitin sulfate B contains the 5 epimer of glucuronic acid, namely, iduronic acid.

Chondroitin sulfates are found in varying amounts in tissues. Cartilage and bone are among the best sources of chondroitin sulfates, but these polysaccharides are also found in other tissues, such as the aorta, tendons, and the ligaments. For example, chondroitin sulfate C is especially abundant in tendons, umbilical cord, nucleus pulposus, and osteosarcomas. Chondroitin sulfate B has been found in skin and in heart valves. The proportions of the various types of chondroitin sulfates change with age. Examples have already been cited for the aorta. In the skin, the amount of the B type is large in the embryonic skin but decreases with age. The significance of the differences in polysaccharide content of the various tissues with respect to function and structure remains to be established.

The cornea is somewhat unique in its polysaccharide composition. In addition to chondroitin sulfates A and B, it contains large amounts of keratosulfates. Keratosulfates are also found in bones and aorta of patients who have died from Marfan's syndrome.

The repeating units of the various polysaccharides are presented in Fig. 15-13. It is clear that the disaccharide moieties of chondroitin sulfates A and C and of hyaluronic acid are the same. The only difference between chondroitin sulfates A and C is that the sulfate is in the position 4 of the N-acetylglucosamine in A, and in the position 6 in C. In chondroitin sulfate B, the sulfate is in the same position as in chondroitin sulfate A.

Polysaccharides, as we have described them, are artifacts of preparation because in tissue they form complexes with proteins. A three-dimensional reconstruction of the molecular structure of the ground substance requires that the details of these interactions between proteins and polysaccharides be known.

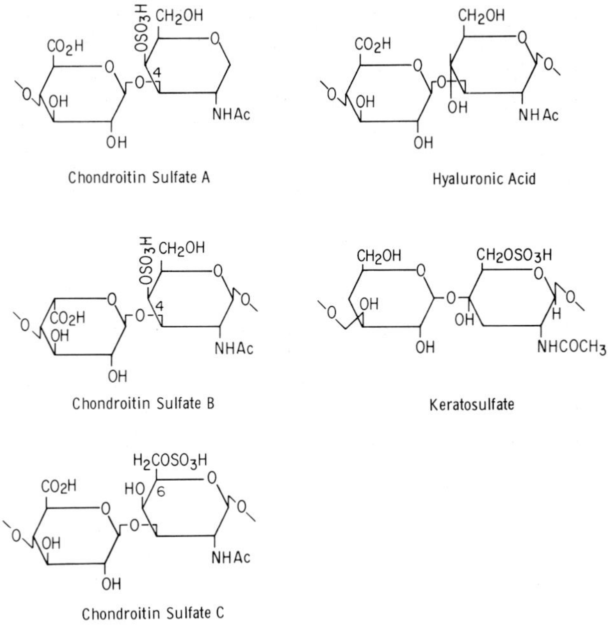

Fig. 15-13. Repeating units of various polysaccharides

In fact, little is known of the proteins of the ground substance except that they form covalent complexes with the polysaccharide and the type of linkage involved in forming the complex has been identified. Thus, the ground substance contains a special kind of glycoprotein in which the carbohydrate chain is unusually long. Therefore, structural similarities can be expected between the properties of the protein polysaccharides and those of the other glycoproteins.

Helen Maher has reviewed the development of knowledge of the protein-polysaccharide complex. The mode of extraction of the polysaccharides suggested binding to protein. Much of our knowledge of the structure of the protein-polysaccharide complexes is derived from studies made in complexes extracted from cartilage. At first, cartilage was extracted with alkaline solutions. Alkaline extracts contain good yields of chondroitin sulfate, a fact which was in 1925 interpreted to indicate that in cartilage the polysaccharide was linked to a protein by an ester-type bond, which readily could be split by alkali. Extraction with neutral calcium chloride yields a viscous solution made of a polydispersed population of macromolecules from which the polysaccharide cannot be extracted.

Addition of papain to the viscous solution markedly reduced the viscosity of the calcium chloride extract.

High-speed homogenization of cartilage followed by differential centrifugation has yielded two major fractions, which can be distinguished by their sedimentation rates and protein content. The fraction that sediments the quicker contains 50% protein, whereas that which sediments the slower contains only 15%. The lighter fraction is often referred to as protein polysaccharide light, or PPL fraction. PPL was at first believed to be a pure form of the chondroitin-4-sulfate protein complex. It is now clear that PPL prepared from human costal cartilage is, in fact, a mixture of at least two or possibly three protein-polysaccharide complexes—namely, keratosulfate and chondroitin. In these extracts, polysaccharides and protein could be separated by bringing the solution to pH 12.5. All these findings strongly supported the notion of a protein-polysaccharide complex. Light-scattering studies of a solution of chondroitin-4-sulfate obtained from the cartilage of the pig nasal septum led Mathews and Lzaityte to propose that the complex was made of a protein core to which several carbohydrate chains were attached.

Guided by these findings, several laboratories attempted to identify the type of linkage involved in the formation of the protein-polysaccharide complex and to build molecular models of the ground substance. The details of these studies can be found in the "Chemical Physiology of Polysaccharides."

It is now clear that the common polysaccharides (chondroitin sulfates A, B, and C, heparin, and heparin sulfate) and protein linkage is covalent and involves a serine residue. In asmuch as the linking sequence is formed by a galactose, xylose serine, it is clear that the linkage sequence is different from the repeating unit of the polysaccharide. Studies on protein-polysaccharide complexes of cornea cartilage and intervertebal discs revealed that the keratins also exist in the form of protein-polysaccharide complexes. However, as we shall see later, the keratinosulfate and the chondroitin sulfate complexes differ with respect to the amount of protein in the complex and the mode of linkage between protein and polysaccharide. There is relatively more protein in the keratinosulfates than in the chondroitin sulfate complex. In keratinosulfate, the protein-polysaccharide linkage may involve serine, threonine, or asparagine on the protein side; or N-acetylgalactosamine on the polysaccharide side. (The asparagine linkage has been found only in keratinosulfate-protein complexes extracted from the cornea.) It is not known if xylose is involved in the linkage. Several investigators have reported finding a keratinosulfate and chondroitin peptide in the urine of patients with Marquio-Ullrich disease; therefore, it has been suggested that the disease may result from increased proteolysis or from the formation of an abnormal polypeptide moiety in the keratinosulfate protein-polysaccharide macromolecule. The type of polypeptide linkage occurring in the hyaluronic acid-protein complex is not known.

Researchers needed to determine whether the polysaccharide attaches to the protein by one or more binding sites. A polysaccharide that binds to the protein by more than one binding site should form loops. Controlled treatment of such a protein-polysaccharide complex with hyaluronidase should release new reducing ends. Since this is not the case, it is believed that the polysaccharide, at least in the chondroitin-protein complex, is attached only by one bond at one site.

Little is known of the amino acid composition and nothing is known of the amino acid sequence of the proteins involved in the formation of protein-polysaccharide complexes. Nevertheless, some evidence indicates that the binding of chondroitin sulfate to protein involves serine residues, and that an alkali-labile xylosyl-serine bond is formed between the serine and the glucuronosyl-galactosyl-galactosyl-xylosyl polysaccharide chain. However, the discovery of this alkali-labile mode of binding does not exclude the possibility that other forms of protein-polysaccharide modes of binding also exist.

Several steps must be distinguished in the biosynthesis of polysaccharide proteins: (1) biosynthesis of the monosaccharide and the hexosamine; (2) elaboration of the polysaccharide chain; (3) sulfation of the polysaccharide; (4) formation of the polysaccharide-protein linkage; (5) introduction in the polysaccharide chain of the galactose-xylose unit, which links protein and polysaccharides.

The biosynthesis of the building blocks of the polysaccharide chain has been discussed in other chapters of this book. The mechanism of polymerization remains unknown. Particularly intriguing is the fact that the sugar units alternate in the polysaccharide structure. To explain the special sequence in the polysaccharide chain, it was once proposed that the polymer was built on an RNA template, but no evidence has been assembled in support of that hypothesis. A more plausible explanation is that the polymer is built from prefabricated smaller units; but again, evidence in support of this interpretation is lacking. The specificity of the sequence may result from the enzyme's special properties, which catalyze the reaction. For example, a three-point attachment mechanism has been proposed to explain the alternation of the building blocks in the polysaccharide chain. 3-Phosphoadenosine-5-phosphosulfate is the sulfur donor in the sulfation of the polysaccharide. The enzyme responsible for the reaction is found in the smooth endoplasmic reticulum and possibly in the Golgi apparatus, but the evidence for the latter location is weak.*

A microsomal preparation obtained from chick embryo epiphyseal cartilage has been used successfully to synthesize chondroitin, using UDP-[^{14}C]glucuronic acid and UDP-M-[^{3}H]acetylgalactosamine as precursors. The reaction requires a primer and probably a polymerizing enzyme, both of which seem to be present in the microsomal preparation. The newly synthesized protein polysaccharide can serve as acceptor for sulfates [82–85].

To form the polysaccharide-protein linkage, an enzyme found in the endoplasmic reticulum catalyzes the binding of xylose to serine, and a galactose molecule is then introduced to join the polysaccharide and the xylosylated protein [82–87].

Protein polysaccharides are found in two major forms: as constituents of the ground substance and as secretions [88]. In the former, they are part of the mesenchymal tissue to which they contribute structure and possibly function. Although polysaccharide proteins undoubtedly are important in determining consistency, elasticity, and other properties peculiar to the various kinds of mesenchymal tissues, the exact molecular interaction between collagen and the polysaccharide protein is still hypothetical. Models for the connective tissue-polysaccharide interaction in cartilage have been proposed by Schubert [89] and Mathews [90].

In Mathews' model, the chondroitin sulfate protein molecule is composed of a protein core (4000 A) to which chondroitin sulfate chains (1000 A long) are attached perpendicularly to the long axis of the protein molecules. In cartilage, the chondroitin sulfate protein macromolecules are believed to be aligned parallel to collagen fibrils, to which they are connected by electrostatic linkages. Of course, variation in composition and structure of the polysaccharide-protein molecules may determine the extensiveness of the interactions with the connective tissue, the degree of hydration, the exclusion of other macromolecules, and possibly the seeding of mineral crystals during mineralization [91].

Factors Affecting Wound Healing

The healing wound is a microcosm of pathology. Wound healing recapitulates most responses to injury—inflammation, hyperplasia and hypertrophy—and therefore the molecular events that take place in these cellular reactions must be called into action during wound healing. The biochemistry of wound healing is unique, not so much because it involves special types of molecular reactions, but because of the special sequence of events and the way one form of cellular reaction, such as inflammation, affects another, such as hyperplasia. Therefore, any factor which disturbs this constellation of events interferes with adequate wound healing. Although each molecular event is important in wound healing, some events are more important than others because they determine the effectiveness of the repair (e.g., cross-links). Thus, rather than redescribing all the biochemical events associated with inflammation, hyperplasia, hypertrophy, and elaboration of collagen fibers and mucopolysaccharide-protein ground substance, I will briefly discuss factors that modify the biochemistry of wound healing.

We have already mentioned that wounds can heal in two major ways—by primary and secondary intention. A classical example of wound healing by primary intention is that of the wound of the skin and dermis caused by the sharp cut of a surgeon's scalpel. Such wounds heal optimally and are devoid of secondary infection. However, the healing of most accidental wounds is not that simple. Cuts are irregular, and many blood vessels are torn and cannot readily be brought together. Blows may destroy large pieces of skin and connective tissue with massive areas of hemorrhage and ischemia. Penetrating foreign bodies, such

* The sulfation of heparin is preceeded by N-acetylation. The mechanism by which N-acetyl is replaced by sulfate in the presence of 3-phosphoadenosine 5-phosphosulfate is not known.

as bullets or stones, tear the skin and the connective tissue and bring infection into the body. Thus, most wounds contain areas of necrosis and inflammation. How much inflammation and necrosis are necessary for adequate healing has never been determined. Clearly, massive infection with local formation of abscesses and phlegmons (and, consequently, high fever and leukocytosis) are to be avoided. But experimentation also suggests that even mild superinfection of wounds interferes with optimal healing.

Burke's studies have shown that blocking of cell-mediated immunity facilitates wound healing by preventing the inflammatory sequence (accumulation of polymorphonuclears, release of vasodilators, etc.) that usually follows cell-mediated immune responses. Thus, as Dumphy pointed out, asepsis continues to be the best guarantee for optimal healing. When bacterial infection is unavoidable, modification of immune responses and inflammatory reactions may improve healing conditions.

Drugs that inhibit cellular hyperplasia (such as the nitrogen mustards) or X-irradiation also retards wound healing when administered before or during repair.

The deficiency of cofactors indispensable for some of the biochemical reactions involved in wound healing slows down repair and may even be responsible for imperfect closure. A classical example is the effect of ascorbic acid deficiency on wound healing. The role of ascorbic acid in the hydroxylation of proline has been discussed in the chapter devoted to vitamins.

As pointed out already, collagen cross-linking is of particular significance in wound healing because this molecular reaction, more than any other, helps to build a network with unique, resilient tensile strength normally found in connective tissues. β-Aminopropionitrile, which prevents cross-links, interferes with adequate wound healing. Some drugs used frequently for patients with massive wounds—*e.g.*, penicillin and isonicotinic acid hydrazide—interfere with repair, possibly by preventing cross-links. Penicillin is believed to act by conversion to penicillamine, which then chelates copper and possibly other metals indispensable for the cross-link reaction. It is also believed, on the basis of little evidence, that isonicotinic acid hydrazide acts by preventing cross-link formation. Nevertheless, the possibility that the drug acts on collagen synthesis has not been excluded.

Surgeons have always known that a patient's nutrition determines his ability to heal his wounds. Two dietary components seem to play a key role in wound healing, proteins and ascorbic acid. Low-protein diets retard wound healing, but although the administration of most essential amino acids is of little value in reverting the effect of a low-protein diet, the administration of methionine and cysteine has been claimed to be beneficial. Yet the two amino acids are not exactly equivalent, even though methionine is known to be converted into cysteine. According to Williamson and Frome, wound tissues pass through two stages of sulfur amino acid content. In the early stage, more methionine than cysteine is retained; in the later stage, more cysteine is retained. Such findings suggest that methionine-rich protein is synthesized in the early stages, while cysteine-rich protein is synthesized later.

At the same time that uptake is increased, there seems to be an increased breakdown of sulfur amino acid in the wounded rat. In the wounded animal, sulfur excretion is increased and the animal becomes protein depleted. Further studies on methionine metabolism in liver, kidney, and plasma suggest that an animal put on a protein-free diet withdraws sulfur amino acids from other tissues to reuse the amino acid for protein biosynthesis in the healing wound.

These interactions between protein diet and wound healing further illustrate the sophistication of the homeostatic mechanism. Yet, a full appreciation of their significance requires that the elementary components of healing, proliferation of different cell types, and elaboration of fibrous tissue be studied separately.

It was long ago concluded that the delay in wound healing observed in scorbutic individuals resulted from the inability of fibroblasts to form connective tissue fibers. In the discussion of vitamin C, its role in wound healing, in general, and in converting proline and lysine to hydroxyproline and hydroxylysine, in particular, have been discussed.

Miscellaneous Enzyme Changes in Wound Healing

Numerous enzyme changes have been observed either histochemically or biochemically in healing wounds. In choosing the enzyme to be studied, investigators are guided by techniques available or by predictable metabolic changes. As usual, hydrolases have been studied quite extensively. Alkaline phosphatase is believed to increase in two steps, a first associated with leukocytic infiltration and a second with fibroblastic differentiation. Whatever the significance of the findings, it seems clear that granulation tissue is unusually rich in alkaline phosphatase. It has also been claimed that epithelial proliferation is associated with a decrease in acid phosphatase and an increase in β-glucuronidase activities, a finding somewhat surprising since both enzymes are assumed to be found in the same granule. However, it is not excluded that β-glucuronidase is increased in the endoplasmic reticulum, and that the change in enzyme patterns results from a shift in cell population. Increase in hydrolase activities associated with a relative decrease in respiratory enzymes have been described in areas of inflammation. Aminopeptidase activity was found to increase in wound healing, and the increased level in healing tissue paralleled the levels in plasma.

An increase in enzyme activities in mucopolysaccharide and protein synthesis has been reported in wound healing, but unless the selective contribution of each cellular-type change can be related to the change in enzyme activity, the interpretation of the finding will remain obscure. It would seem that studies on wound healing will benefit from the development of accurate enzymic determination in single cells.

Although cell proliferation and connective tissue elaboration may be easier to investigate in other systems, the healing wound offers a unique opportunity for studying the interaction between epithelial and mesenchymal tissues.

Epitheliomesenchymal Interactions

In this discussion, we have usually examined the hyperplasia of one type of cell, ignoring the interaction between parenchymal or epithelial cells and the mesenchymal tissues. This gross oversimplification is helpful for didactic puposes, but it does not reflect reality *in vivo*.

The proliferative stages of regeneration and wound healing evolve from a well-orchestrated sequence of cellular events, which, in wound healing, includes proliferation of epithelial and mesenchymal tissues. These two processes of hyperplasia do not occur independently—they influence each other. Although examples of mesenchymal-epithelial interaction are described in other chapters, it seems appropriate to consider briefly some of the knowledge relative to this interaction.

Among the most remarkable experiments on epitheliomesenchymal interaction are those of Grobstein with the salivary glands. Relatively simple techniques for the culture of embryonic tissue *in vitro* are now available. Samples of the tissues are suspended in a plasma clot and incubated in Eagle's medium with 10% horse serum and 3% embryo extract. The culture is carried out in an apparatus made of a ring of plexiglass to which a millipore membrane has been cemented. Mesenchymal and epithelial tissue can be separated in the salivary gland, or in most other cultured organs, by treating the embryo with trypsin. Mesenchymal and glandular tissue can then be cultured either together or one on each side of the millipore membrane. When embryonic salivary glands are cultured in such fashion they differentiate, and one aspect of the differentiation process is the development of acinar structures by epithelial branching. Glandular epithelium separated from its mesenchymal tissue does not differentiate unless a salivary gland mesenchyma is cultured at the other side of the millipore membrane. To stimulate salivary gland differentiation, the mesenchyma must be of salivary gland origin and must be alive.

Similar findings were made with mammary gland tissue and mesenchyma. The branching pattern in embryonic mammary tissue differs from that of salivary glands. Nevertheless, when mammary cells are cultured with salivary mesenchyma, they develop a branching pattern which resembles that of the salivary gland. In fact, the skin, which is part of the mammary gland explants, appears to be influenced by the mesenchyma in that it does not keratinize but acquires, instead, properties of a secretory cell. The exact mechanism by which mesenchyma influences morphogenesis is not clear, but collagen seems to play a role. Indeed, treatment of the mesenchyma with collagenase interferes with its morphogenetic effects.

The role of collagen in epithelial morphogenesis has been further amplified by the experiments of Grobstein. Grobstein cultured epithelium and collagen, each at one side of the millipore filter, and found that collagen fibers appeared at the epithelial side. It was established that the collagen that appeared at the epithelial side was derived from the mesenchymal cells and was transferred through the filter in a soluble form. Treatment of the mesenchymal preparation with collagenase prevented differentiation of the epithelial cell. Grobstein found that the epithelium seems to elaborate a mucopolysaccharide that is susceptible to the action of hyaluronidase and affects the formation of collagen fibrils. This latter finding suggests that the interaction between mesenchyma and epithelium in morphogenesis is a two-way road.

The role of the dermis in epithelial morphogenesis has been investigated by somewhat different methods in the laboratory of Billingham, who took pig epithelium obtained at one site, combined it with dermis from another site, and transplanted the combined graft to another host. For example, when mucosal epithelium was combined with dermis obtained from the trunk, it acquired the morphological properties of trunk epidermis. Canscott was able to grow adult epithelial cells on a glass surface and, after 2 or 3 weeks, the cells developed several layers resembling those seen in normal skin. The cells of the bottom layer, those in contact with the surface of the glass, are actively dividing; the top cells in contact with the nutrient undergo progressive keratinization. However, complete keratinization with the development of a stratum corneum and the formation of keratohyalin granules did not take place in the absence of connective tissue.

We shall see later that these epitheliomesenchymal interactions are not only of considerable importance in understanding the intricacies of wound healing, but are also relevant to our understanding of the pathogenesis of metastasis.

Mucopolysaccharidosis

A number of diseases are characterized by the deposition of acid mucopolysaccharides—dermatan and heparin sulfate—in tissues rich in those substances and excretion of the mucopolysaccharides in the urine. Hunter was the first to describe such a condition in 1917; two years later Hurler described a similar disease. The major difference between Hunter's and Hurler's syndromes is that the former is transferred as an autosomal recessive trait, and the latter is linked to the X chromosome. Two other milder forms of mucopolysaccharidosis have been described; they are referred to as the Sanfilippo syndrome and syndrome S.

In a typical case of Hurler's or Hunter's syndrome, the patient develops grotesque facial features with an enlarged head when he is 2 years old. Hydrocephalus results from interference with the flow of the intraventricular fluids. The eyes are widely spread, the ears are set low, the lips are enlarged and thick, the bridge of the nose is depressed, and the feet are widely spaced and peglike. Deformities of the thorax and of the spine are common. Because of the enlargement of the liver and spleen, the abdomen protrudes. The cornea often shows diffuse or spotty cloudiness. For reasons that are not quite clear, the disease is associated with growth retardation, which leads to dwarfism, and severe and progressive mental retardation. Mucopolysaccharide deposition in the valves, the myocardium, and pericardium leads to cardiac failure, which is a frequent cause of death. Another major cause of death is respiratory infection.

In Hurler's and Hunter's syndromes, mucopolysaccharides accumulate in abnormal amounts in tissues normally rich in these substances; for example, the dermis, the heart valves, and Bowman's layer of the cornea.

Although much work has been done to determine the pathogenesis of mucopolysaccharidosis, in most cases the cause of the disease has not been identified. Three theories have been proposed: abnormal binding of the polysaccharide moiety to protein, excessive production of polysaccharides, and defective breakdown of polysaccharides.

Available data favor the third hypothesis. Among the enzymes that have been incriminated is β-galactosidase. Low β-galactosidase activity in fibroblasts and livers of patients with both Hunter's and Hurler's syndromes has been shown. In some cases, a specific isoenzyme of β-galactosidase is missing. The absence of β-galactosidase could explain the accumulation of gangliosides frequently observed in the brain neurons of patients with Hurler's disease.

Other enzyme defects that have been found are deficiencies in: sulfiduronate sulfatase, β-glucosamidase, heparin sulfate sulfatase, and β-glucuronidase [92]. A defect in β-galactosidase has also been described. Although defects in the first four enzymes could explain the accumulation of polysaccharides, a defect in β-galactosidase is not likely to cause the accumulation of the polymer. Indeed, polysaccharides do not accumulate in other storage diseases, such as generalized gangliosidosis, in which galactosidase is deficient.

Kent and his associates have therefore reexamined the pathogenic mechanism of the β-galactosidase defect in mucopolysaccharidosis. They have shown that: first, β-galactosidase activity is decreased, but the decrease in activity results from the covalent binding of the β-galactosidase to the accumulated mucopolysaccharides. They assume that the binding occurs through the two galactose residues at the reducing end of the carbohydrate chain with the active center of the enzyme, thus causing competitive inhibition. Second, Kent and his coworkers have shown that other lysosome enzyme activities are increased in the cell in which the mucopolysaccharides accumulate. Electrophoretic studies of these enzymes again suggest that they are bound to mucopolysaccharides. Consequently, binding of the polymer to the enzyme molecules would increase their total number in the cell and thus increase their activity by preventing normal enzyme catabolism.

Studies performed with fibroblast cultures obtained from patients with various kinds of mucopolysaccharidoses have helped to clarify the pathogenesis of the disease, and they have also contributed to improved differential diagnosis. If fibroblasts obtained from patients with Hurler's syndrome are mixed in culture with normal fibroblasts, the accumulation of polysaccharides in the Hurler cells disappears. The mixing of cells obtained from patients with Hurler's and Hunter's syndromes again abolishes the accumulation of polysaccharides, which suggests that the factor missing in each case is different. The missing factor is known to be a thermolabile compound that is proteic in nature [93]. Similar "corrective factors" have been found in other mucopolysaccharidoses, and attempts have been made to identify their function.

The Hurler corrective factor is a protein with a molecular weight of 87,000, which is distinct from known lysosomal enzymes including galactosidase [94]. The Hunter corrective factor is believed to be a sulfiduronate sulfatase [95]. The Sanfilippo corrective factor is suspected to be a heparin sulfatase [96], or an α-acetylglucosamidase [97]. In conclusion, there exists a family of diseases in which mucopolysaccharides accumulate in various tissues; although there is in some cases indirect evidence as to the enzyme defect, in most cases conclusive evidence is not available.

References

1. Goss, R.J.: Adaptive growth. In: Lens regeneration, p. 96–117. London: Logos Press 1964
2. Bucher, N.L.R.: Regeneration of mammalian liver. Int. Rev. Cytol. **15**, 245–300 (1963)
3. Abell, C.W., Kamp, C.W., Johnson, L.D.: Effects of phytohemagglutinin and isoproterenol on DNA synthesis in lymphocytes from normal donors and patients with chronic lymphocytic leukemia. Cancer Res. **30**, 717–723 (1970)
4. Singer, M.: Nervous mechanisms in the regeneration of body parts in vertebrates. In: Developing cell systems and their control (Rudnick, D., ed.), p. 115–133, New York: Ronald Press 1960
5. Harkness, R.D.: Changes in the liver of the rat after partial hepatectomy. J. Physiol. (Lond.) **117**, 267–277 (1952)
6. Van Lancker, J.L., Sempoux, D.G.: Incorporation of orotic acid-C^{14} in rat liver DNA after partial hepatectomy of one partner of a parabiotic pair. Arch. Biochem. Biophys. **80**, 337–345 (1959)
7. Church, R., McCarthy, G.J.: Changes in nuclear and cytoplasmic RNA in regenerating mouse liver, Proc. nat. Acad. Sci. (Wash.) **58**, 1548–1555 (1967)
8. Bucher, N.L.R., Swaffield, M.N.: Rate of incorporation of [6-C^{14}] orotic acid into uridine 5′-triphosphate and cytidine 5′-triphosphate and nuclear ribonucleic acid in regenerating rat liver. Biochim. biophys. Acta (Amst.) **108**, 551–567 (1965)
9. Reichard, P.: Control of deoxyribonucleotide synthesis in vitro and in vivo. In: Advances in enzyme regulation (Weber, G., ed.), vol. 10, p. 3–16, Fairview Park, N.Y.: Pergamon Press 1972
10. Moore, E.C., Hurlbert, R.B.: Regulation of mammalian deoxyribonucleotide biosynthesis by nucleotides as activators and inhibitors. J. biol. Chem. **241**, 4802–4809 (1966)
11. Bresnick, E.: Early changes in pyrimidine biosynthesis after partial hepatectomy. J. biol. Chem. **240**, 2550–2556 (1965)
12. Fausto, N.: The control of RNA synthesis during liver regeneration. OMP pyrophosphorylase and decarboxylase activities in normal and regenerating liver. Biochim. biophys. Acta (Amst.) **182**, 66–75 (1969)
13. Levi-Montalcini, R.: The nerve growth factor: its mode of action on sensory and sympathetic nerve cells. Harvey Lecture Series **60**, 217–259 (1965)

14. Schenkein, I., Levy, M., Bueker, E.D., Tokarsky, E.: Nerve growth factor of very high yield and specific activity. Science **159**, 640–643 (1968)
15. Savage, C.R., Jr., Inagami, T., Cohen, S.: The primary structure of epidermal growth factor. J. biol. Chem. **247**, 7612–7621 (1972)
16. Puck, T.T., Waldren, C.A., Jones, C.: Mammalian cell growth proteins. I. Growth stimulation by fetuin. Proc. nat. Acad. Sci. (Wash.) **59**, 192–199 (1968)
17. Khan, A.A.: Cytokinins: permissive role in seed germination. Science **171**, 853–859 (1971)
18. Galston, A.W., Davies, P.J.: Hormonal regulation in higher plants. Science **163**, 1288–1297 (1969)
19. Fredrick, J.F.: Plant growth regulators. Ann. N.Y. Acad. Sci. **144** (Art. 1), 1–382 (1967)
20. Van't Hof, J.: The action of IAA and kinetin on the mitotic cycle of proliferative and stationary phase excised root meristems. Exp. Cell Res. **51**, 167–176 (1968)
21. Glinos, A.D.: Mechanism of growth control in liver regeneration. Science **123** (Abstracts Annu. Meet.), 673–674 (1956)
22. Ogawa, K., Nowinski, W.W.: Mitosis stimulating factor in serum of unilaterally nephrectomized rats. Proc. Soc. exp. Biol. (N.Y.) **99**, 350–354 (1958)
23. Davis, J.C., Hyde, T.A.: The effect of corticosteroids and altered adrenal function on liver regeneration following chemical necrosis and partial hepatectomy. Cancer Res. **26**, 217–220 (1965)
24. Moolten, F.L., Bucher, N.L.R.: Regeneration of rat liver: transfer of humoral agent by cross circulation. Science **158**, 272–273 (1967)
25. Moskowitz, M., Schenck, D.M.: Growth promoting activity for mammalian cells in fractions of tissue extracts. Exp. Cell Res. **38**, 523–535 (1965)
26. Gentile, J.M., Grace, J.T., Jr.: A cell growth stimulating factor in partially hepatectomized rat serum. Surg. Forum **19**, 62–63 (1968)
27. Telepneva, S.I.: Action of humoral factors controlling cell division during the first hours of liver regeneration. Bull. exp. Biol. Med. **65**, 446–448 (1968)
28. Grisham, J.W.: Hepatocytic proliferation in normal rats after multiple exchange transfusions with blood from partially hepatectomized rats. Cell Tiss. Kinet. **2**, 277–282 (1969)
29. Loeper, J., Compere, R.: L'action d'un extrait total de foie sur la régénération hépatique, Soc. Biol. (Paris) **163**, 1346–1350 (1969)
30. Van Lancker, J.L., Borison, H.L.: Incorporation of tritium-labelled thymidine into rat-liver deoxyribonucleic acid after exchange transfusion with blood from partially-hepatectomized rats. Biochim. biophys. Acta (Amst.) **51**, 171–172 (1961)
31. Bullough, W.S.: Epithelial repair, in Repair and Regeneration. The scientific basis for surgical practice (Dunphy, J.E., and Van Winkle, W., Jr., eds.), p. 35–46, New York: McGraw-Hill Book Company 1969
32. Forscher, B.K., Hovck, J.L. (eds.): Chalones, concepts and current researches. Natl. Cancer Inst. Monogr. No. 38, Bethesda 1973
33. Malt, R.A.: Compensatory growth of the kidney. New Engl. J. Med. **280**, 1446–1459 (1969)
34. Marsh, W.H., Goldsmith, S., Crocco, J., Fitzgerald, P.J.: Pancreatic acinar cell regeneration. II. Enzymatic, nucleic acid, and protein changes. Amer. J. Path. **52**, 1013–1037 (1968)
35. Fitzgerald, P.J., Vinijchaikul, K., Carol, B., Rosenstock, L.: Pancreatic acinar cell regeneration. III. DNA synthesis of pancreas nuclei as indicated by thymidine-H^3 autoradiography. Amer. J. Path. **52**, 1039–1065 (1968)
36. Lehv, M., Fitzgerald, P.J.: Pancreatic acinar cell regeneration. IV. Regeneration after surgical resection, Amer. J. Path. **53**, 513–535 (1968)
37. Fitzgerald, P.J., Carol, B., Lipkin, L., Rosenstock, L.: Pancreatic acinar cell regeneration. V. Analysis of variance of the autoradiographic labeling index (thymidine-H^3). Amer. J. Path. **53**, 953–970 (1968)
38. Carol, B., Fitzgerald, P.J.: Pancreatic acinar cell regeneration. VI. Estimation of error of the autoradiographic labeling index (thymidine-H^3)—maximum possible error (MPRE) and sensitivity (S). Amer. J. Path. **53**, 971–987 (1968)
39. Marsh, W.H., Ord, M., Stocken, L., Fitzgerald, P.J.: Pancreas acinar cell regeneration. VII. Phosphate content of nuclear histones during pancreas degeneration and regeneration, Fed. Proc. **29**, 1433–1438 (1970)
40. Cooper, H.L.: Alterations in RNA metabolism in lymphocytes during the shift from resting state to active growth. In: Biochemistry of cell division (Baserga, R., ed.), p. 91–112. Springfield, Ill.: Charles C. Thomas, Publisher 1969
41. Hashem, N.: Mitosis: induction by cultures of human peripheral lymphocytes. Science **150**, 1460–1462 (1965)
42. Allfrey, V.G.: The role of chromosomal proteins in gene activation. In: Biochemistry of cell division (Baserga, R., ed.), p. 179–205. Springfield, Ill.: Charles C. Thomas, Publisher 1969
43. Barka, T.: Induced cell proliferation: the effect of isoproterenol. Exp. Cell Res. **37**, 662–679 (1965)
44. Barka, T: Stimulation of protein and ribonucleic acid synthesis in rat submaxillary gland by isoproterenol. Lab. Invest. **18**, 38–41 (1968)
45. Baserga, R., Sasaki, T., Whitlock, J.P., Jr.: The prereplicative phase of isoproterenol-stimulated DNA synthesis. In: Biochemistry of cell division (Baserga, R., ed.), p. 77–90. Springfield, Ill.: Charles C. Thomas, Publisher 1969
46. Baserga, R.: Induction of DNA synthesis by a purified chemical compound, Fed. Proc. **29**, 1443–1446 (1970)
47. Fisher, E.R.: Repair by regeneration. Path. Annu. **4**, 89–126 (1969)
48. Dumont, A.E.: Fibroplasia: a sequel to lymphocyte exudation. In: The inflammatory process (Zweifach, B.W., Grant, L., and McCluskey, R.T., eds.), p. 535–557. New York: Academic Press 1965
49. Zarafonetis, C.J.D.: The treatment of scleroderma: results of potassium and para-aminobenzoate therapy in 104 cases. In: Inflammation and diseases of connective tissues (Mills, L.C., and Moyer, J.H., eds.), p. 688–696. Philadelphia: W.B. Saunders 1961
50. Patterson, W.B.: Wound healing and tissue repair. Chicago: University of Chicago Press 1959
51. Ross, R.: The fibroblast and wound repair. Biol. Rev. **43**, 51–96 (1968)
52. Ross, R., Benditt, E.P.: Wound healing and collagen formation. I. Sequential changes in components of guinea pig skin wounds observed in the electron microscope. J. biophys. biochem. Cytol. **11**, 677–700 (1961)
53. Ross, R.: Wound healing. Sci. Amer. **220**, 40–50 (1969)
54. Piez, K.A.: Cross-linking of collagen and elastin. Annu. Rev. Biochem. **37**, 547–570 (1962)
55. Bowes, J.H., Kenten, R.H.: Some observations on the amino-acid distribution of collagen, elastin and reticular tissue from different sources. Biochem. J. **45**, 281–285 (1949)
56. Bowes, J.H., Kenten, R.H.: The amino acid composition and titration curve of collagen. Biochem. J. **43**, 358–365 (1948)
57. Astbury, W.T.: The molecular structure of the fibres of the collagen group. J. Int. Soc. Leath. Trades Chem. **24**, 69 (1940)
58. Grassman, W., Hannig, K., Endres, H., Riedel, A.: I. Mitt.: Aminosäuresequenzen des Kollagens. Zur Bindungsweise des Prolins und Hydroxyprolins. Hoppe Seylers Z. physiol. Chem. **306**, 123–131 (1956)
59. Hannig, K., Nordwig, A.: General sequence studies on collagen. In: Structure and function of connective and skeletal tissues (Fitton Jackson, S., Harkness, R.D., Partridge, S.M., Tristram, G.R., eds.), p. 7–16. London: Butterworth and Co., Ltd. 1965
60. Piez, K.A., Bornstein, P., Lewis, M.S., Martin, G.R.: The preparation and properties of single and cross-linked chains from vertebrate collagens. In: Structure and function of connective and skeletal tissues (Fitton Jackson, S., Harkness, R.D., Partridge, S.M., Tristram, g.R., eds.), p. 16–21, London: Butterworth and Co., Ltd. 1965
61. Corey, R.B., Pauling, L.: Fundamental dimensions of polypeptide chains. Proc. roy. Soc. B **141**, 10–20 (1953)
62. Pauling, L., Corey, R.B.: Stable configurations of polypeptide chains. Proc. roy. Soc. Lond. B **141**, 21–33 (1953)
63. Ramachandran, G.N.: Structure of fibrous proteins and polypeptides. In: Collagen (Ramanathan, N., ed.), p. 3–35, New York: Interscience Publishers 1962
64. Rich, A., Crick, F.H.C.: The structure of collagen. Nature (Lond.) **176**, 915–916 (1955)
65. Gustavson, K.H.: Hydroxyproline and stability of collagens. Acta chem. scand. **8**, 1298–1299 (1954)
66. Piez, K.A., Lewis, M.S., Martin, G.R., Gross, J.: Subunits of the collagen molecule. Biochim. biophys. Acta (Amst.) **53**, 596–598 (1961)
67. Bornstein, P., Piez, K.A.: The nature of the intramolecular cross-links in collagen. The separation and characterization of peptides from the cross-link region of rat skin collagen. Biochemistry **5**, 3460–3473 (1966)
68. Martin, G.R., Gross, J., Piez, K.A., Lewis, M.S.: On the intramolecular cross-linking of collagen in lathyritic rats. Biochim. biophys. Acta (Amst.) **53**, 599–601 (1961)
69. Bornstein, P.: Cross-linking of collagen chains. Fed. Proc. **25**, 1004–1009 (1966)
70. Bornstein, P.: The cross-linking of collagen and elastin. In: Repair and regeneration. The scientific basis for surgical practice (Dunphy, J.E., Van Winkle, W., Jr., eds.), p. 137–149. New York: McGraw Hill Book Company 1969
71. Rojkind, M., Blumenfeld, O.O., Gallop, P.M.: Localization and partial characterization of an aldehydic component in tropocollagen. J. biol. Chem. **241**, 1530–1536 (1966)
72. Sandberg, L.B., Weissman, N., Smith, D.W.: The purification and partial characterization of a soluble elastin-like protein from copper-deficient porcine aorta. Biochemistry **8**, 2940–2945 (1969)
73. Ross, R., Bornstein, P.: Elastic fibers in the body. Sci. Amer. **224**, 44–52 (1971)
74. Kefalides, N.A.: Chemical properties of basement membranes. Int. Rev. exp. Path. **10**, 1–39 (1971)
75. Peacock, E.E., Jr., Madden, J.W., Smith, H.C.: Some applications of lathyrism to clinical medicine. In: Repair and regeneration. The scientific basis for surgical practice (Dunphy, J.E., and Van Winkle, W., Jr., eds.), p. 287–307. New York: McGraw Hill Book Company 1969
76. Rojkind, M., Juarez, H.: The nature of the collagen defect in lathyrism. Biochem. biophys. Res. Commun. **25**, 481–486 (1966)
77. Levine, C.I.: Collagen in experimental osteolathyrism. Fed. Proc. **22**, 1386–1388 (1963)
78. Grant, M.E., Prockop, D.J.: The biosynthesis of collagen. New Engl. J. Med. **286** (I) 194–199, (II) 242–249, (III) 291–300 (1972)
79. Meyer, K., Hoffman, P., Linker, A.: Chemistry of ground substances in connective tissue, thrombosis and atherosclerosis (Page, I.H., ed.), p. 181–191. New York: Academic Press (1959)
80. Meyer, K., Anderson, B., Seno, N., Hoffman, P.: Peptide complexes of chondroitin sulphates and keratosulphates. In: Structure and function of connective and skeletal tissues (Fitton Jackson, S., Harkness, R.D.,

Partridge, S.M., Tristram, G.R., eds.), p. 164–168. London: Butterworth and Co., Ltd. 1965

81. Meyer, K.: Introduction to biochemistry and biosynthesis of mucopolysaccharides in connective tissue: Intercellular macromolecules. Proc. Symp. N. Y. Heart Assoc., p. 117–118. Boston: Little, Brown and Company 1964
82. Dorfman, A.: The biosynthesis of acid mucopolysaccharides. In: Structure and function of connective and skeletal tissues (Fitton Jackson, S., Harkness, R.D., Partridge, S.M., and Tristram, G.R., eds.), p. 297–302. London: Butterworth and Co., Ltd. 1965
83. Richmond, M.E., DeLuca, S., Silbert, J.E.: Biosynthesis of chondroitin sulfate. Assembly of chondroitin in microsomal primers. Biochemistry **12**, 3904–3910 (1973)
84. Richmond, M.E., DeLuca, S., Silbert, J.E.: Biosynthesis of chondroitin sulfate. Sulfation of the polysaccharide chain. Biochemistry **12**, 3911–3915 (1973)
85. Richmond, M.E., DeLuca, S., Silbert, J.E.: Biosynthesis of chondroitin sulfate. Microsomal acceptors of sulfate, glucuronic acid, and N-acetylgalactosamine. Biochemistry **12**, 3989–3903 (1973)
86. Ginsburg, V., Neufeld, E.F.: Complex heterosaccharides of animals. Annu. Rev. Biochem. **38**, 371–388 (1969)
87. Rogers, H.J.: Very high molecular weight mucopolysaccharides and mucopolysaccharide-protein complexes. How far can we extrapolate? Fed. Proc. **25**, 1035–1036 (1966)
88. Jakowska, S.: Mucous secretions. Ann. N. Y. Acad. Sci. **106**, 157–809 (1963)
89. Schubert, M.: Structure of connective tissues, a chemical point of view. Fed. Proc. **25**, 1047–1052 (1966)
90. Mathews, M.B.: The macromolecular organization of connective tissue. In: The Chemical physiology of mucopolysaccharides (Quintarelli, G., ed.), p. 189–197. Boston: Little, Brown and company 1968
91. Laurent, T.C.: The exclusion of macromolecules from polysaccharide media. In: The chemical physiology of mucopolysaccharides (Quintarelli, G., ed.), p. 153–170. Boston: Little, Brown and Company 1968
92. Hall, C.W., Cantz, M., Neufeld, E.F.: A β-glucuronidase deficiency mucopolysaccharidosis: studies in cultured fibroblasts. Arch. Biochem. Biophys. **155**, 32–38 (1973)
93. Kint, J.A., Dacremont, G., Carton, D., Orye, E., Hooft, C.: Mucopolysaccharidosis: secondarily induced abnormal distribution of lysosomal isoenzymes. Science **181**, 352–354 (1973)
94. Barton, R.W., Neufeld, E.F.: The Hurler corrective factor. Purification and some properties. J. biol. Chem. **246**, 7773–7779 (1971)
95. Bach, G., Eisenberg, F., Jr., Cantz, M., Neufeld, E.F.: The defect in the Hunter syndrome: deficiency of sulfoiduronate sulfatase. Proc. nat. Acad. Sci. (Wash.) **70**, 2134–2138 (1973)
96. Kresse, H., Neufeld, E.F.: The Sanfilippo A corrective factor. Purification and mode of action. J. biol. Chem. **247**, 2164–2170 (1972)
97. O'Brien, J.S., Miller, A.L., Loverde, A.W., Veath, M.L.: Sanfilippo disease type B: enzyme replacement and metabolic correction in cultured fibroblasts. Science **181**, 753–755 (1973)
98. Chalkley, D.T.: The cellular basis of limb regeneration. In: Vertebrate regeneration (Thornton, C.S., and Bromley, S.C., eds.), Chapt. 2, p. 24–48. Stroudsburg, Pennsylvania: Dowden, Hutchinson & Ross, Inc. 1973
99. Hay, E.D.: Electron microscopic observations of muscle dedifferentiation in regenerating amblystoma limbs. In: Vertebrate regeneration (Thornton, C.S., and Bromley, S.C., eds.), chapt. 3, p. 49–79. Stroudsburg, Pennsylvania: Dowden, Hutchinson & Ross, Inc. 1973
100. Choi, S.C., Hall, J.C.: A study of respiration and oxidative phosphorylation of mitochondria from regenerating liver of normal and diabetic rats. Canad. Res. **34**, 2351–2357 (1974)
101. Scornik, O.A.: *In vivo* rate of translation by ribosomes of normal and regenerating liver. J. biol. Chem. **249**, 3876–3883 (1974)
102. Anderson, W.M., Grundholm, A., Sells, B.H.: Modification of ribosomal proteins during liver regeneration. Biochem. biophys. Res. Commun. **62**, 669–676 (1975)
103. Tanaka, Y., Kaji, H.: Incorporation of arginine by soluble extracts of ascites tumor cells and regenerating rat liver. Canad. Res. **34**, 2204–2208 (1974)
104. Collins, T., David, F., Van Lancker, J.L.: CDP and ADP reductases in rat regenerating liver. Fed. Proc. **31**, 641 (1972)
105. Söderhall, S.S., Larsson, A., Skoog, K.L.: Deoxyribonucleotide pools during liver regeneration. Europ. J. Biochem. **33**, 36–39 (1973)
106. Larsson, A., Reichard, P.: Enzymatic synthesis of deoxyribonucleotides. X. Purification of purine ribonucleotides; allosteric behavior and substrate specificity of the enzyme system from *Escherichia coli B*. J. biol. Chem. **241**, 2540–2549 (1966)
107. Brown, N.C., Reichard, P.: Role of effector grinding in allosteric control of ribonucleoside diphosphate reductase. J. molec. Biol. **46**, 25–39 (1969)
108. Brown, N.C., Canellakis, Z.N., Lundin, B., Reichard, P., Thelander, L.: Ribonucleoside diphosphate reductase. Purification of the two subunits, proteins B1 and B2. Europ. J. Biochem. **9**, 561–573 (1969)
109. Reichard, P.: The biosynthesis of deoxyribonucleotides. Europ. J. Biochem. **3**, 259–266 (1968)
110. Thelander, L.: Physicochemical characterization of ribonucleoside diphosphate reductase from *Escherichia coli*. J. biol. Chem. **248**, 4591–4601 (1973)
111. Herbst, E.J., Snell, E.E.: Putrescine and related compounds as growth factors for hemophilus parainfluenzae 7901. J. biol. Chem. **181**, 47–54 (1949)
112. Kremzner, L.T.: Polyamines, Introductory Remarks, Pharmacology Society Symposium. Fed. Proc. **29**, 1560–1562 (1970)
113. Snyder, S.H., Russell, D.H.: Polyamine synthesis in rapidly growing tissues. Fed. Proc. **29**, 1575–1582 (1970)
114. Raina, A., Jänne, J.: Polyamines and the accumulation of RNA in mammalian systems. Fed. Proc. **29**, 1568–1574 (1970)
115. Fausto, N., Brandt, J.T., Kesner, L.: Interrelationships between the urea cycle, pyrimidine and polyamine synthesis during liver regeneration. In: Liver regeneration after experimental injury (Lesch, R., ed.). Stratton Intercontinental Medical Book Corp. (In press 1975)
116. Marx, J.L.: Nerve growth factor: Regulatory role examined. Science **185**, 930–972 (1974)
117. Frazier, W.A., Boyd, L.F., Bradshaw, R.A.: Properties of the specific binding of ^{125}I-nerve growth factor to responsive peripheral neurons. J. biol. Chem. **71**, 5513–5519 (1974)
118. Calissano, P., Cozzari, C.: Interaction of nerve growth factor with the mouse-brain neurotubule protein(s). Proc. nat. Acad. Sci. (Wash.) **71**, 2131–2135 (1974)
119. Kolber, A.R., Goldstein, M.N., Moore, B.W.: Effect of nerve growth factor on the expression of colchicine-binding activity and 14-3-2 protein in an established line of human neuroblastoma. Proc. nat. Acad. Sci. (Wash.) **71**, 4203–4207 (1974)
120. Bullough, W.S., Laurence, E.B.: The control of epidermal mitotic activity in the mouse. Proc. roy. Soc. B **151**, 517–519 (1960)
121. Marks, F.: A tissue-specific factor inhibiting DNA synthesis in mouse epidermis. Nat. Cancer Inst. Monogr. **38**, 79–89 (1973)
122. Simard, A., Corneille, L., Deschamps, Y., Verly, W.G.: Inhibition of cell proliferation in the livers of hepatectomized rats by a rabbit hepatic chalone. Proc. nat. Acad. Sci. (Wash.) **71**, 1763–1766 (1974)
123. Chung, E., Miller, E.J.: Collagen polymorphism: Characterization of molecules with the chain composition $[\alpha 1(\mathrm{III})]_3$ in human tissues. Science **183**, 1200–1201 (1974)
124. Bradley, K., McConnell-Breul, S., Crystal, R.G.: Lung collagen heterogeneity. Proc. nat. Acad. Sci. (Wash.) **71**, 2828–2832 (1974)
125. Bradley, K.H., McConnell, S.D., Crystal, R.G.: Lung collagen composition and synthesis. Characterization and changes with age. J. biol. Chem. **249**, 2674–2683 (1974)
126. Church, R.L., Pfeiffer, S.E., Tanzer, M.L.: Collagen biosynthesis: synthesis and secretion of a high molecular weight collagen precursor (procollagen). Proc. nat. Acad. Sci. (Wash.) **68**, 2638–2642 (1971)
127. Bornstein, P.: The biosynthesis of collagen. Ann. Rev. Biochem. **42**, 567–619 (1974)
128. Miller, E.J., Matukas, V.J.: Biosynthesis of collagen. Fed. Proc. **33**, 1197–1203 (1974)
129. Weinstock, M., Leblond, C.P.: Formation of collagen. Fed. Proc. **33**, 1205–1218 (1974)
130. Harris, E.D., Jr., Krane, S.M.: Collagenases, part 1. New Engl. J. Med. **291**, 557–563 (1974)
131. Harris, E.D., Jr., Krane, S.M.: Collagenases, part 2. New Engl. J. Med. **291**, 605–609 (1974)
132. Harris, E.D., Jr., Krane, S.M.: Collagenases, part 3. New Engl. J. Med. **291**, 652–660 (1974)
133. Pinnell, S.R., Krane, S.M., Kenzora, J.E., Glimcher, M.J.: A heritable disorder of connective tissue. Hydroxylysine-deficient collagen disease. New Engl. J. Med. **286**, 1013–1020 (1972)
134. Veillard, A., Borel, J.-P.: La biosynthese du collagene et sa pathologie. Path. et Biol. **21**, 1024–1036 (1973)
135. Lichtenstein, J.R., Martin, G.R., Kohn, L.D., Byers, P.H., McKusick, V.A.: Defect in conversion of procollagen to collagen in a form of Ehlers-Danlos syndrome. Science **182**, 298–300 (1973)
136. Herbert, C.M., Lindberg, K.A., Jayson, M.I.V., Bailey, A.J.: Biosynthesis and maturation of skin collagen in scleroderma, and effect of D-penicillamine. Lancet **1974 I**, 187–192
137. Ooshima, A., Fuller, G.C., Cardinale, G.J., Spector, S., Udenfriend, S.: Increased collagen synthesis in blood vessels of hypertensive rats and its reversal by antihypertensive agents. Proc. nat. Acad. Sci. (Wash.) **71**, 3019–3023 (1974)
138. Fjolstad, M., Helle, O.: A hereditary dysplasia of collagen tissues in sheep. J. Path. **112**, 183–188 (1974)
139. Nimni, M., Deshmukh, K.: Differences in collagen metabolism between normal and osteoarthritic human articular cartilage. Science **181**, 751–752 (1973)

Chapter 16

Cancer

Introduction 947

Benign and Malignant Tumors 947

Benign Tumors 947
Malignant Tumors 948

Cancer and Heredity 955

In Animals 955
In Humans 956
Chromosomes in Cancer 957

Hormones and Cancer 959

Breast Cancer 959
Carcinoma of the Cervix 962
Cancer of the Body of the Uterus 962
Other Uterine Tumors
Ovarian Tumors 963
Cancer of the Adrenals 964
Cancer of the Hypophysis 964
Tumors of the Prostate 965
Tumors of the Testicles 966
Effect of Hormones on Cancer in Other Tissues 966
Transplacental Cancer 967
Some Biochemical Effects of Endocrine Cancer 967

Carcinogens, Their Metabolism and Mode of Action 970

Polycyclic Hydrocarbons 970
Azo Derivatives 977
Fluorene Derivatives 979
Aflatoxin and Cycasin 983
Aniline Derivatives 983
Urethane 984
Polymers 984
Mechanism of Chemical Carcinogenesis 985
Two-Stage Carcinogenesis 986
Chemical Transformation in Vitro 988
Chemical Carcinogenesis and DNA Repair 990
Carcinogenesis and Mutations 990
Carcinogens in Humans 991

Viruses and Cancer Viruses 996

Introduction 996
Viruses 996
Introduction to the Molecular Biology of Viruses
Types of Injuries Caused by Viruses
Antiviral Vaccination
Antiviral Chemotherapy
Viral Toxins and Lysogeny

Slow Virus Disease
Viroids

Viral Carcinogenesis 1010
Experimental Viral Carcinogenesis 1010

Avian Leukosis Viruses
Shope Papilloma Virus
Bittner Virus
Murine Leukemia Viruses
Polyoma Virus

Morphological Characteristics of Tumor Viruses 1014
Factors Modulating Viral Carcinogenesis in Vivo 1015
Antigenic Properties of Viruses 1017
Biochemistry of Tumor Viruses 1018

Viral Replication 1019

Transformation 1022

Cancer and Viruses in Humans 1024
Hypothesis on the Mechanism of Viral Carcinogenesis 1027

Metabolic Pathways in the Cancer Cell 1027

Introduction 1027
Glycolysis in Cancer 1028
Other Bioenergetic Pathways in Cancer 1029
Oxidative Phosphorylation in Tumors 1032
Amino Acid Metabolism in Cancer 1034
Amino Acid Incorporation in Tumor Proteins 1035
Incorporation of Nucleic Acid Precursors in Tumors 1036
Growth Rate of Tumors 1038
DNA Content, Properties, and Metabolism in Cancer 1039
RNA in Cancer 1040

Metabolic Regulation and the Malignant State 1041

Control of Glycolysis 1042
Pasteur Effect 1043
Crabtree Effect 1044
Hexokinase Regulation 1044
Gluconeogenesis 1045

Properties of the Enzymes Involved in Gluconeogenesis
Regulation of Gluconeogenesis

Control of Glycogen Metabolism 1049
Regulation of Cholesterol Metabolism 1050
Coenzymes and Metabolic Regulation 1051
Metabolic Regulation in Cancer Cells 1051

Regulation of Gene Expression and Differentiation 1052

Gene Expression and Regulation of Cell Division 1062
Reversion of Gene Expression in the Cancer Cell 1065

The Cell Membrane and the Malignant State 1065

Function of the Plasma Membrane 1066

Transport
Movement
Contact Inhibition
Adhesion
Cellular Communication
Regulation of Cellular Metabolism

Molecular Composition of the Cell Membrane 1072
Molecular Organization of the Cell Membrane 1075

Biosynthesis of the Cell Membrane 1077
Cancer and Cell Membranes 1078
Conclusion 1081

Metabolic Regulation in Minimal Deviation Hepatomas 1081

Minimal Deviation Hepatomas 1082
Glycolysis in Minimal Deviation Hepatomas 1084
Amino Acid Pools in Minimal Deviation Hepatomas 1085
Enzyme Induction in Minimal Deviation Hepatomas 1085
Isozymes in Cancer 1086

Invasion, Metastasis, and Host Reactions 1088

Invasion 1088
Metastasis 1089
Membrane Alteration in Invasion and Metastasis

Tumor Host Relationships 1096

Ectopic Hormones 1096
Cancer and the Host's Nutrition 1097

Miscellaneous Alterations in Cancer Patients 1097

Anemia 1097
Degeneration 1097
Uric Acid Accumulation 1097
Angiogenesis in Tumors 1098

Cancer Immunity 1098

Introduction 1098
Animal Experiments 1100
Immunosurveillance 1103
General Conclusions 1104

References 1105

Introduction

Cancer is a new growth of cells that have become autonomous with one or more of the control mechanisms that regulate normal growth and differentiation. Although cancer can be produced by a gamut of agents ranging from pure chemicals to parasites, its pathogenesis remains one of the most irreducible challenges of this scientific era. Cancer must have plagued the living universe from before the beginning of recorded history. It has been observed in plants and animals alike. X-Rays of the bones of mummies of the Vth dynasty of Egypt demonstrate the existence of osteosarcoma. Democedes, a Greek physician of the city of Creton, claims that he cured Atossa, the wife of Darius I and the daughter of Cyrus the Great, from cancer of the breast by burning her tumor with a hot iron.

The disease is repeatedly referred to in the Ebers papyrus (1500 B.C.) and in the Rig-Veda. Hippocrates gave the name *καρκινοσ* to malignant tumors because he was impressed by the congested veins, in some tumors radiating from the center to the periphery, which reminded him of the many-legged crab. The Germans have not adopted the Greek terminology but have accepted the analogy and refer to cancer by the word *krebs*, which in their language means crab. Gallen thought cancer resulted from an accumulation of "atrabilia" (black bile). The Arab Avicenna discovered the first chemotherapeutic agent against cancer, arsenic.

The modern era of cancer biology rests on three observations that were made in about 150 years. First, Sir Percivall Pott observed (1774–1788) that cancer of the scrotum in chimney sweepers resulted from the injurious effect of accumulated tar. About 100 years later, the research of two Japanese investigators Yamagiwa and Itchikawa culminated in the production of the first experimental cancer induced by chemical carcinogens. In the meantime, Raspail and later Virchow had recognized that cancer consists of an accumulation of cells, an observation that administered the final blow to the theory that "atrabilia" accumulation caused cancer.

Practically every tissue of the body may degenerate into a cancerous growth. The cancer in turn may show various degrees of differentiation; therefore, the nomenclature of tumors is quite complex. In this chapter, the names of the various tumors will be defined as the tumors are described.

Benign and Malignant Tumors

Tumor is a generic term which at first extended to all abnormal swelling—whether it resulted from fluid accumulation, an inflammatory reaction, or cellular proliferation.

But as concepts in pathology have evolved and inflammatory reactions have become clearly distinguished from cellular proliferation, the word *tumor* has, by convention, been restricted to swellings resulting from cellular proliferation. In this restricted sense, most tumors can be defined as abnormal masses composed of new cells and cellular products.

In rare cases, a segment or a major portion of the tumor mass is made of fluids; those tumors are referred to as cystic. Depending upon their impact on the host's health, tumors are categorized as benign or malignant. The former are usually compatible with prolonged survival of the victim; the latter lead to sure death unless treated.

Benign Tumors

Benign tumors result from cellular proliferation. Each cell of the mass usually is a faithful copy of the cell of origin. Although benign tumors escape those control mechanisms that normally maintain cellular proliferation within the rigid boundaries expressed by the normal histological structure, they are not autonomous enough to invade surrounding tissues or to release cell clusters that colonize distant organs. Consequently, benign tumors afflict their host primarily by compressing the surrounding tissue. Benign tumors have histological features closely resembling those of normal tissues, but they are characteristically surrounded by a fibrous capsule, which is believed to be derived in part from a reaction of the surrounding tissue, and in part from condensation of the tumors' connective stroma.

When the proliferating cells composing a benign tumor are of glandular origin, they may continue to secrete their normal exocrine or endocrine products. Since the secretion product usually cannot escape, fluids accumulate inside the cavities and lead to the formation of cysts. Such cysts may develop in benign proliferations of sweat glands, sebaceous glands, breast, and other glands. Sometimes benign proliferations of epithelia, which do not normally secrete large amounts of fluid, may do so and lead to the formation of multiloculated cysts (*e.g.*, multilocular cysts of the ovaries).

The important questions to be asked about benign tumors are their origin and their relation to malignancy.

Little is known of the mechanism of benign tumor production. In fact, investigators have notoriously neglected benign tumors. According to their origin, benign tumors can be classified as congenital and acquired. Common congenital examples are benign tumors of the vascular tree (hemangiomas and lymphangiomas), pigmented skin tumors (nevi), skeletal tumors (chondromas and osteomas), tumors of the muscle (rhabdomyomas), and tumors of the nerve sheaths (neurofibromas).

Acquired benign tumors may develop practically anywhere in the body. Classical examples include lipomas, fibromas (*e.g.*, of the uterus), and osteomas. An interesting benign tumor is the dermoid cyst.

Examples of the gross appearances of some benign tumors are shown in Figs. 16-1, 16-2, and 16-3.

If untreated, most benign tumors continue to grow and sometimes will reach fantastic proportions, as is the case in some neurofibromas and lipomas. Such tumors damage surrounding tissues through the action of their mass. If the tumor grows in compact parenchyma like the liver or kidney, the surrounding tissues are destroyed by compression. In contrast, if the tumor grows in a hollow organ such as the esophagus or urethra, the normal flow is obstructed. When treated, a benign tumor rarely recurs.

Some, fortunately few, benign tumors tend to develop into malignant tumors. This is the case of intestinal polyps, pigmented nevi, and chondromas. The change from benignity to malignancy illustrates the need for the cancerologist to be thoroughly familiar with the "biological properties of tumors"; indeed, eradication of a potential cancer may prevent much misery.

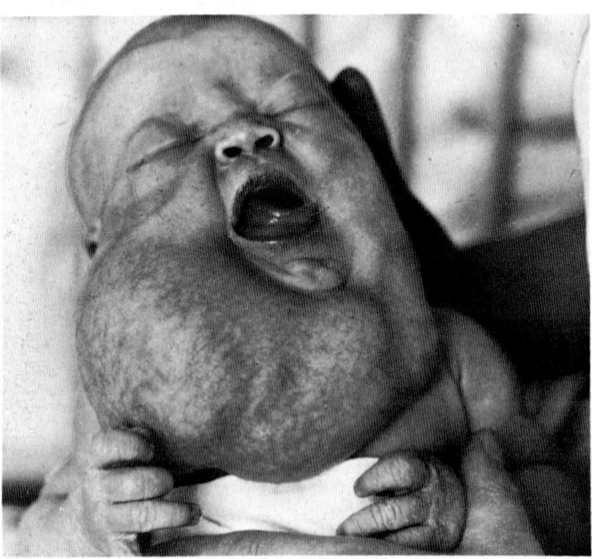

Fig. 16-1. Lymphangioma in a 3-month-old child; a benign tumor is developing at the expense of the lymphatics

Malignant Tumors

A typical florid malignant tumor can best be defined as a growing population of cells escaping the mechanisms that control cellular proliferation, cellular differentiation, and interaction between cells and surrounding tissues. This definition applies only to cancer that has evolved to exhibit all manifestations of malignancy, and no alteration *per se* is pathognomonic of malignancy.

What can we expect to see in a florid cancer? Both local and systemic changes take place. We shall de-

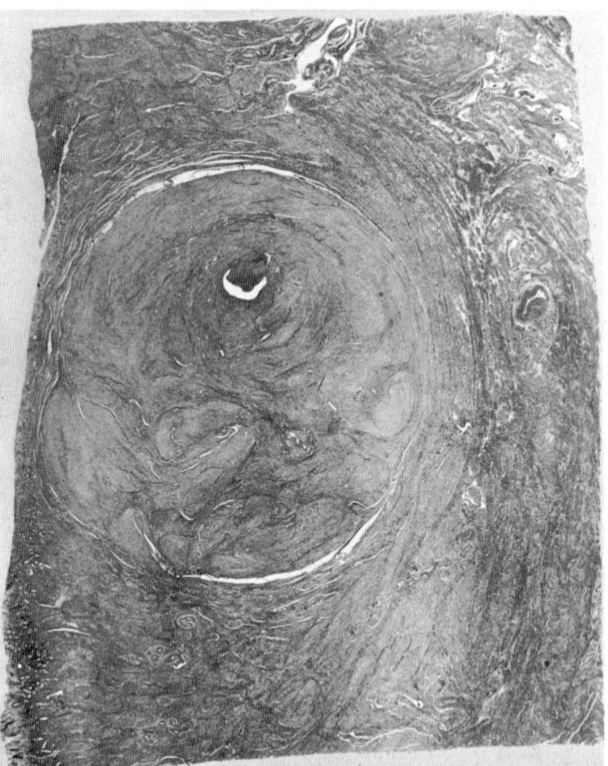

Fig. 16-3. Low-power microscopic view of fibroadenoma of the uterus. Note delineation of the tumoral mass from the surrounding tissues

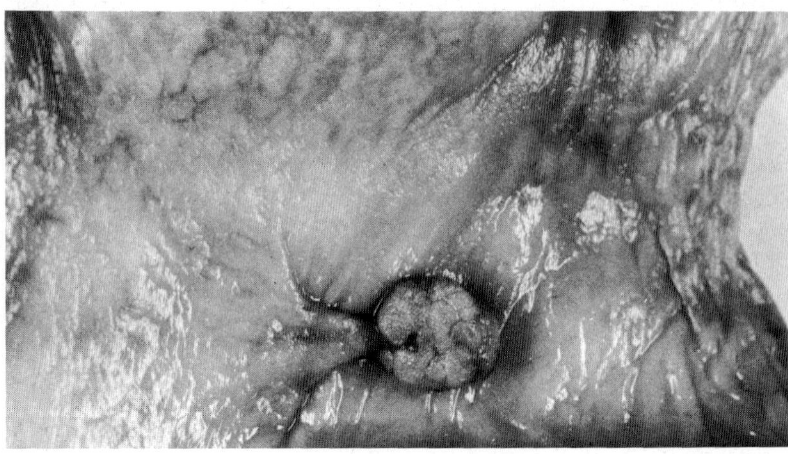

Fig. 16-2. Sessile-type intestinal polyp bulges at the epithelial surface without invading it

scribe successively the changes as they occur in the cell, in the tissue, at a distance from the primary tumor, and in the entire body.

Both the nucleus and the cytoplasm of malignant cells change. Nuclei are enlarged, irregular in shape and size, usually hyperchromatic, and often contain several nucleoli. When mitoses takes place, they are abnormal. Instead of forming bipolar spindles, the cancer cell may have no spindle at all, or it may form multipolar spindles with several equatorial plaques within a single nucleus. Instead of becoming clearly distinct from each other during prophase, chromosomes may remain hooked together or may fragment and reassociate, sometimes resulting in chromosomal anomalies. In some cells, chromosomes duplicate but do not separate, leading to polyteny and hyperchromatism. When the chromosomes separate after metaphase, they are often distributed unequally to the daughter cells, resulting in anaploidy and heteroploidy. Telophase may or may not be complete. Nuclei do not separate completely, and the normal chromosome number per nuclei may double or become a multiple of two (polyploidy). If the cells are not separated by two distinct membranes, some cells may contain two or more nuclei. Such cells are often called giant cells. Giant cells appear with predilection in some types of tumors, such as myeloplax tumors and chorioepitheliomas.

Cytoplasmic abnormalities may be seen as: (1) changes in size; (2) changes in staining properties; and (3) modifications of the maturation process. The ratio between the volume of the nucleus and that of

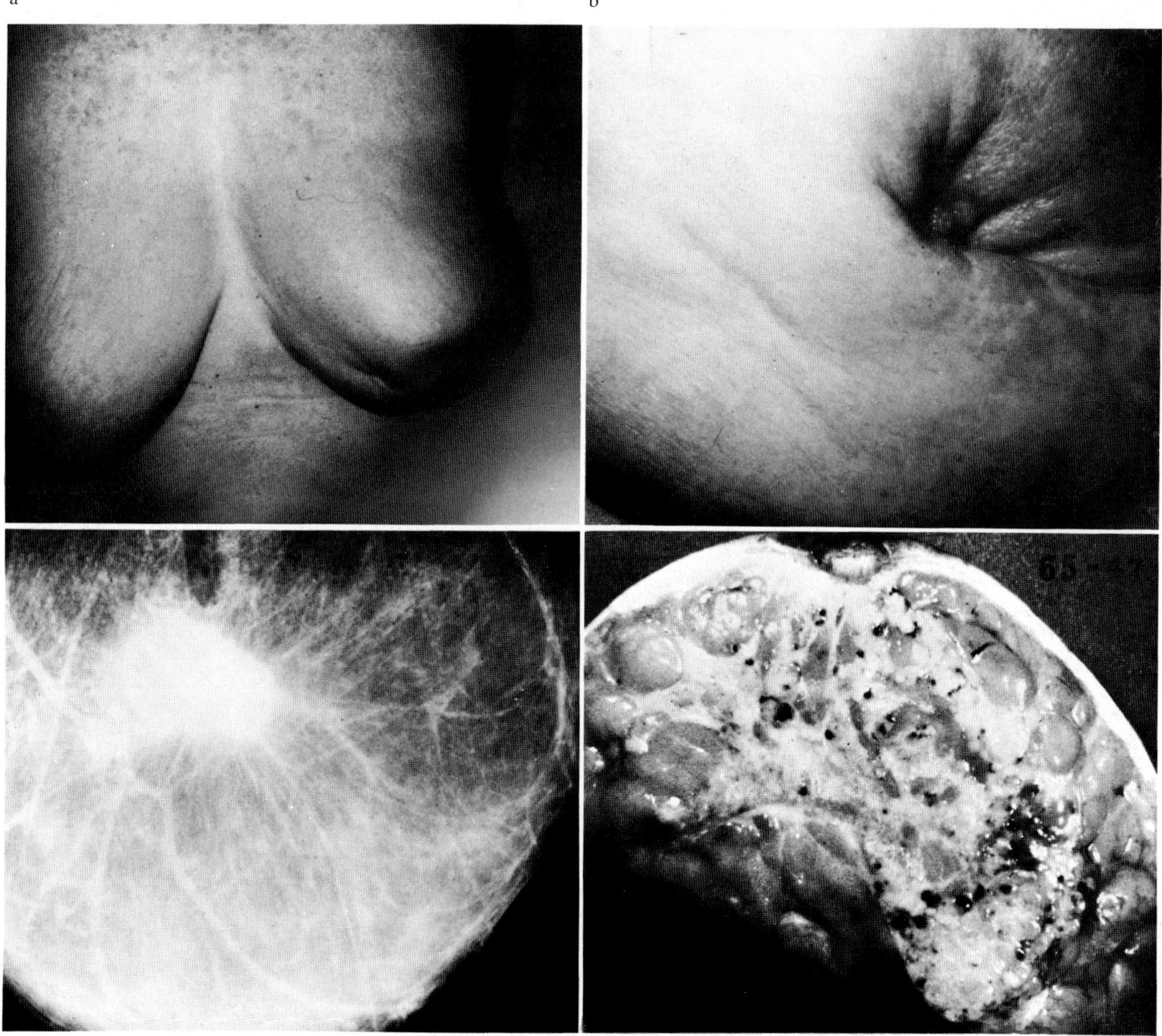

Fig. 16-4a–d. Breast cancer. (a) Normal breast; (b) retraction of the nipple as a result of loss of elasticity due to the development of a cancerous mass; (c) mammogram showing the normal lymphatic pattern obscured by a dense, absorbent mass; (d) gross section showing retraction of the nipple and infiltration of normal breast tissue (gray) by the tumoral growth (white). From Dr. Juillard

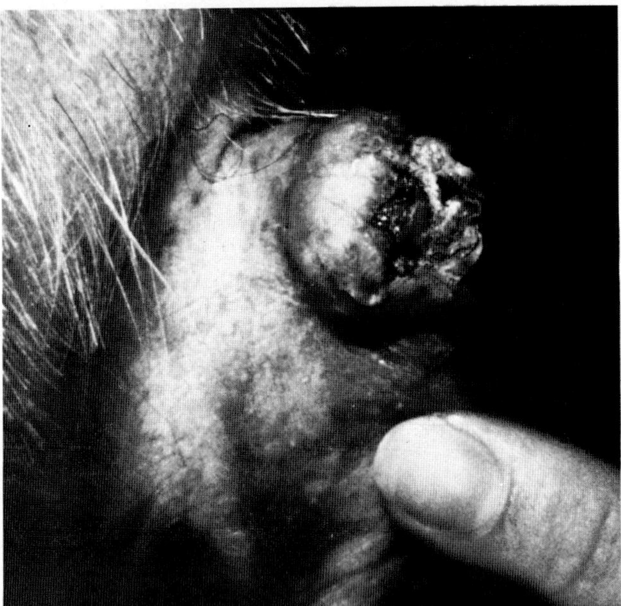

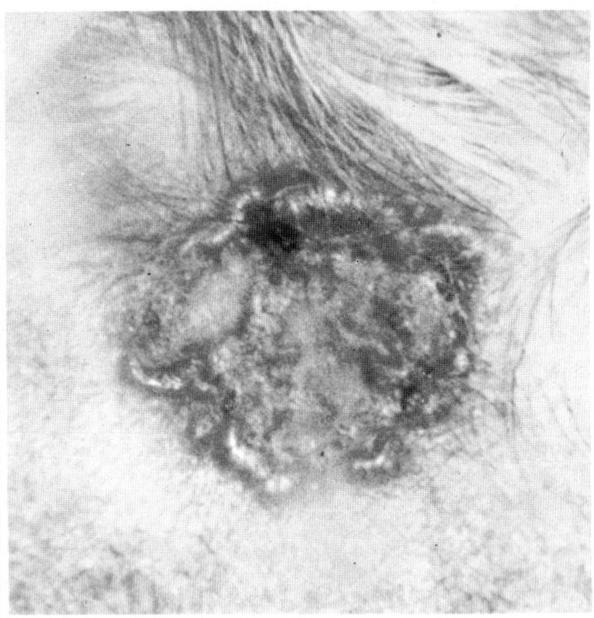

Fig. 16-5. Skin cancer. *Right,* squamous cell carcinoma, which produces large amounts of keratin and readily metastasizes; *left,* basocellular carcinoma, which is composed of cells resembling those of the basal layer of the skin and seldom metastasizes

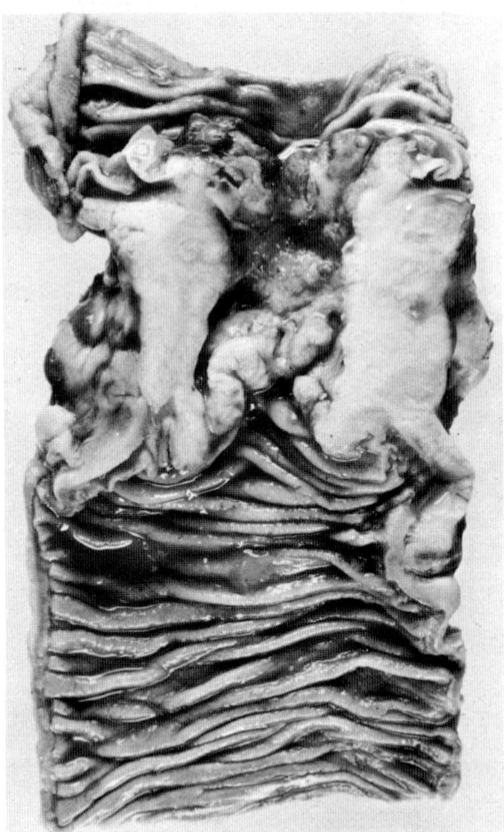

Fig. 16-6. Cancer of the colon. The cancerous mass forms a ring encircling the entire circumference of the intestine. In the center, meaty, budding masses emerge from the epithelial surface; at the periphery, the mucosa widens and all its layers are replaced by cancerous tissues

the cytoplasm, which is constant in normal cells, varies greatly in cancer cells as a result of variations in nuclear size and cytoplasmic volume. Often the cytoplasm of cancer cells is more basophilic than that of normal cells and greater amounts of RNA are found in cancer cells compared to normal. The normal constituents of the cytoplasm may vary a great deal in number, size, and shape. For example, mitochondria may be scarce or abundant; they may be small, large, or oddly shaped.

The appearance of the cytoplasm usually permits the pathologist to distinguish one type of cell from another. Distinct cytoplasmic features are the expression of cell differentiation. For example, the fibroblast elaborates collagen fibers; the epithelial cells of the gastrointestinal tract, mucus; the epithelium of the skin, keratin. Whereas some cancer cells differentiate to reproduce faithfully the structure of the mother tissue, others exhibit distortions of differentiation. All forms of distortions may be observed, including: disdifferentiation (*e.g.,* elaboration of products not normally found in the tissue from which the cancer is derived); hypodifferentiation or adifferentiation (*e.g.,* melanoma cells proliferating with little or no melanin production); hyperdifferentiation (*e.g.,* skin tumors producing excessive amounts of keratin).

Known modifications of the interaction of the cancer cell and its environment include invasion of surrounding tissues, distant metastasis, preying on the body's nitrogen sources, elaboration of toxic substances, and modification of antigenic properties.

In contrast to a normal cell, the cancer cell does not respect histological boundaries imposed by the regulation of cellular relationships in the host. Unlike benign tumors, the cancer cell does not permit the host to envelop the tumor by elaborating a fibrous capsule. On the contrary, the cancer cell aggressively attacks the surrounding tissue, sending prongs that invade its deepest furrow and slowly replace the normal histological structure with a cancerous mass. Cells may even become detached from the mother tumor, find their way in the lymphatics or bloodstream, seed distant tissues—such as lymph nodes, lungs, or bones—and grow into masses visible to the naked eye or with the microscope. Such distant proliferations are called metastases.

The biological significance of invasions and metastases will be discussed later. We will consider now only the clinical consequences. Invasion and metastasis may occur separately or in combination. They are the ultimate expression of clinical malignancy because they make the victim uncomfortable and cause death. Examples of gross manifestations of cancer are shown in Figs. 16-4 through 16-8 Fig. 16-9 illustrates the gross and microscopic appearance of skin cancer.

Now that a panoply of properties of the cancer cell has been described, the reader may wonder which of these properties signal malignancy: rapid division, disorder of differentiation, invasion, or metastasis. As we shall see later in greater detail, it is a fallacy to assume that cancerous cells divide fast. Cancer cells seldom divide as rapidly as those of some normal dividing tissue, such as the crypt cells of the intestine or the stem cells of the bone marrow. In fact, the rate of mitosis in malignant tumors is often slower than that in the homologous normal tissue.

To be sure, mitotic figures are often abundant in tumors, but they do not always indicate rapid cell proliferation. They may reflect an arrest in metaphase, as is seen after the administration of an antimitotic agent. If cancerous tissues do not grow fast, their

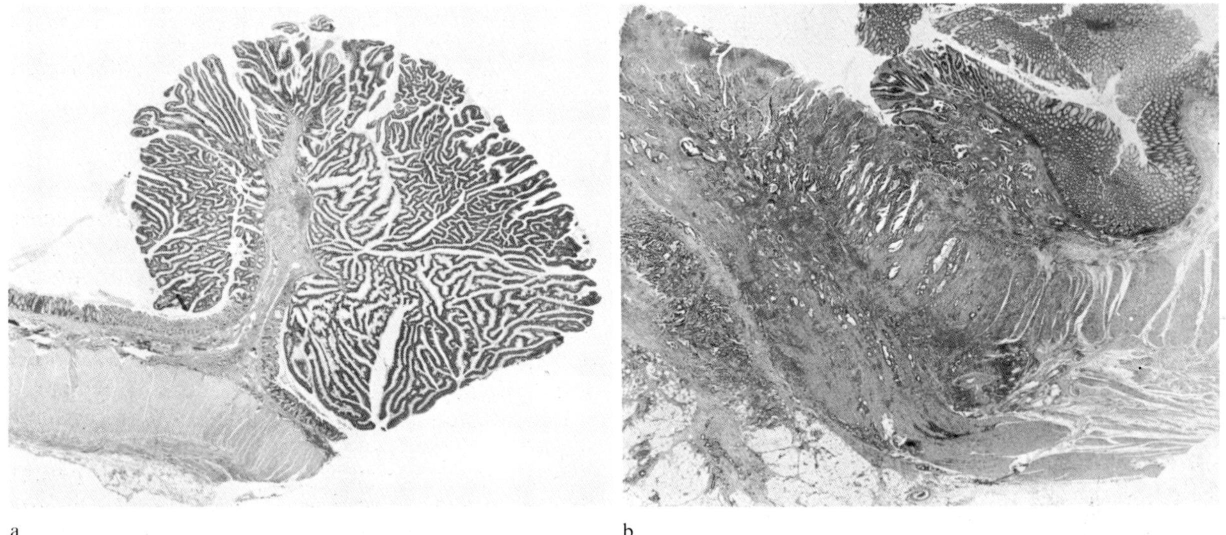

Fig. 16-7a, b. Polyp (a) showing expansion of the normal epithelium into a delicate arborization, yet normal histological features. Cancer of the colon (b); the normal epithelium *(extreme right)* becomes anaplastic and invades the submucosal tissues *(middle and left)*

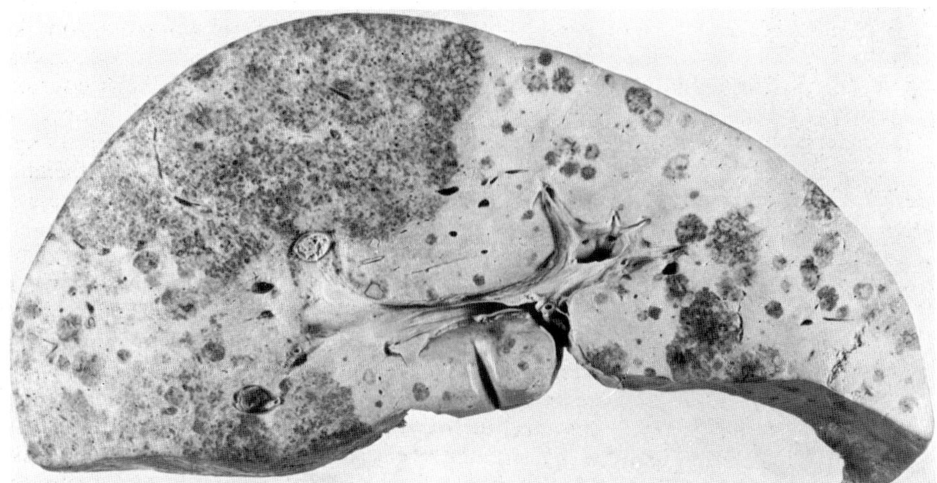

Fig. 16-8. Metastasis to liver from skin melanoma. Melanin-laden cells can be seen in the large *(left)* and small dark areas

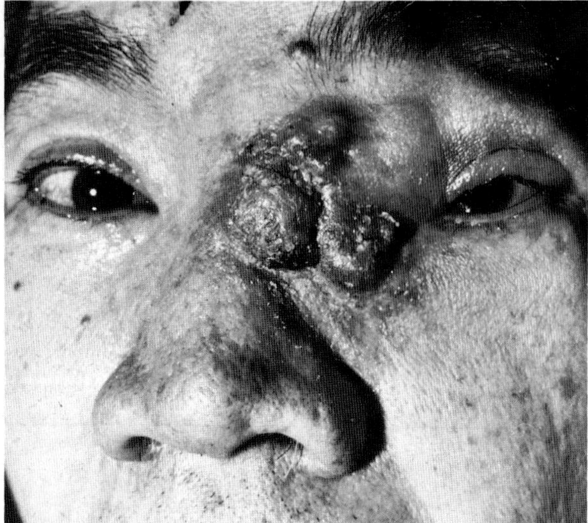
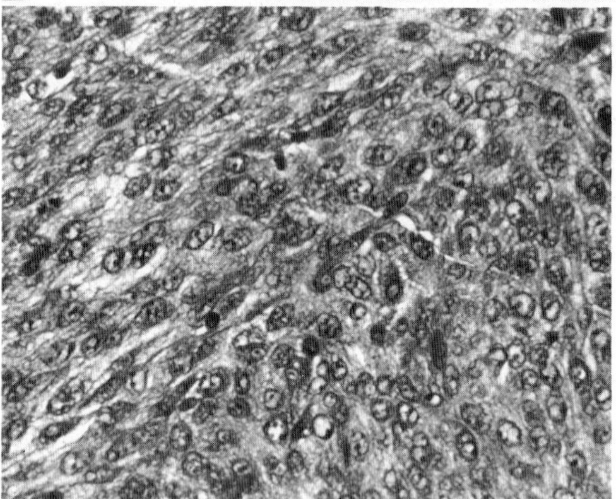

Fig. 16-9. Gross and microscopic views of basocellular carcinoma of the eyelid. Although the tumor is aggressively invasive, the histological appearance shows well-differentiated cells

growth is uninterrupted and not balanced by orderly elimination of differentiated cells. Such elimination, we have seen, is nothing but a form of ultimate differentiation, a natural form of cellular death. Therefore, the balance between life and death appears to be disrupted in cancer tissue, and this could be a manifestation of maldifferentiation. Needless to say, abnormal mitosis is not pathognomonic of cancer since abnormal mitosis occurs after various types of cellular injuries. Surely distortion of cellular differentiation is not the mark of malignancy. Some aggressively malignant tumors—for example, those of the thyroid and basal cell carcinoma of the skin—are well differentiated. Moreover, the immature stem cells that accumulate in the bone marrow of pernicious anemia patients cannot be considered cancer cells. Examples of the histological appearance of cancer are shown in Figs. 16-10 and 16-11.

Invasiveness is one of the most consistent properties of malignant tumors. Yet is it a prerogative of malignancy? Some stages in fetal development result from massive invasion and replacement of one type of cell by another.

Metastases are not unique to cancer. Macrophages migrate at a distance and may even proliferate. In embryonic development, cells can travel long distances and proliferate to colonize other tissue.

If none of the cytological features described is pathognomonic of cancer, how can one diagnose cancer cells at all? Cancer is diagnosed primarily through histological examinations. When it is diagnosed by examination of isolated cells, it is done so only by extrapolation of the knowledge acquired on studying the histological material. However, the profile of cellular and histological events permits cancer cells to be differentiated from those of normal tissue or benign tumors. This distinction will be better understood if we consider the evolution of cancer in its surrounding medium and in the body as a whole.

A malignant tumor develops in at least three successive stages: preinvasive, invasive, and systemic. We know little of what happens in the preinvasive stage. Do cancers start by the transformation of a single cell or a cluster of cells? Is there one starting point, or are the starting points multiple? Even observations of experimentally produced tumors have not permitted a conclusive answer to these questions, although the scientific world often operates on the assumptions that cancer originates from a group of cells and that cancer is often multicentric in origin.

Some information has been gathered about the preinvasive stage of cancer development by observing carcinomas *in situ,* or clusters of epithelial cells that are believed to be cancerous because they harbor nuclear and cytoplasmic alterations often observed in cancer tissues. Carcinomas *in situ* have been seen most frequently in the cervix, but they also occur in skin, stomach, breast and other tissues.

In an epithelial tumor, the invasive stage starts by disruption of the basal membrane by prongs of cells that penetrate the surrounding tissues in all directions, like the imprints a crab's legs leave in the sand. Soon the invading cells enter the lymphatic canal, and, through either direct extension within the lymphatic canal or embolization, the cells colonize the lymph nodes. Thus, the lymph nodes are the first relay of most primary tumors, and any physician who discovers a cancer anywhere in the body should automatically examine the adjacent lymph nodes by palpation or lymphography. Sometimes the invading cells fill the lymphatic channel so densely that they retrace the channels at the surface of the skin, reproducing the appearance of a multilegged crab (an analogy Hippocrates observed). Or the cells may invade the superficial tissue so rapidly that they infiltrate the dermis and replace it with a sheet of cancerous cells that compress the capillaries and cause anoxemia. The hardened, raised, irregular surface of the skin is also bluish as a result of anoxemia. The French refer to such forms of cancer as *cancer en cuirasse*.

When cancer cells enter the lumen of a vein, they are carried by the blood to distant organs. Favorite

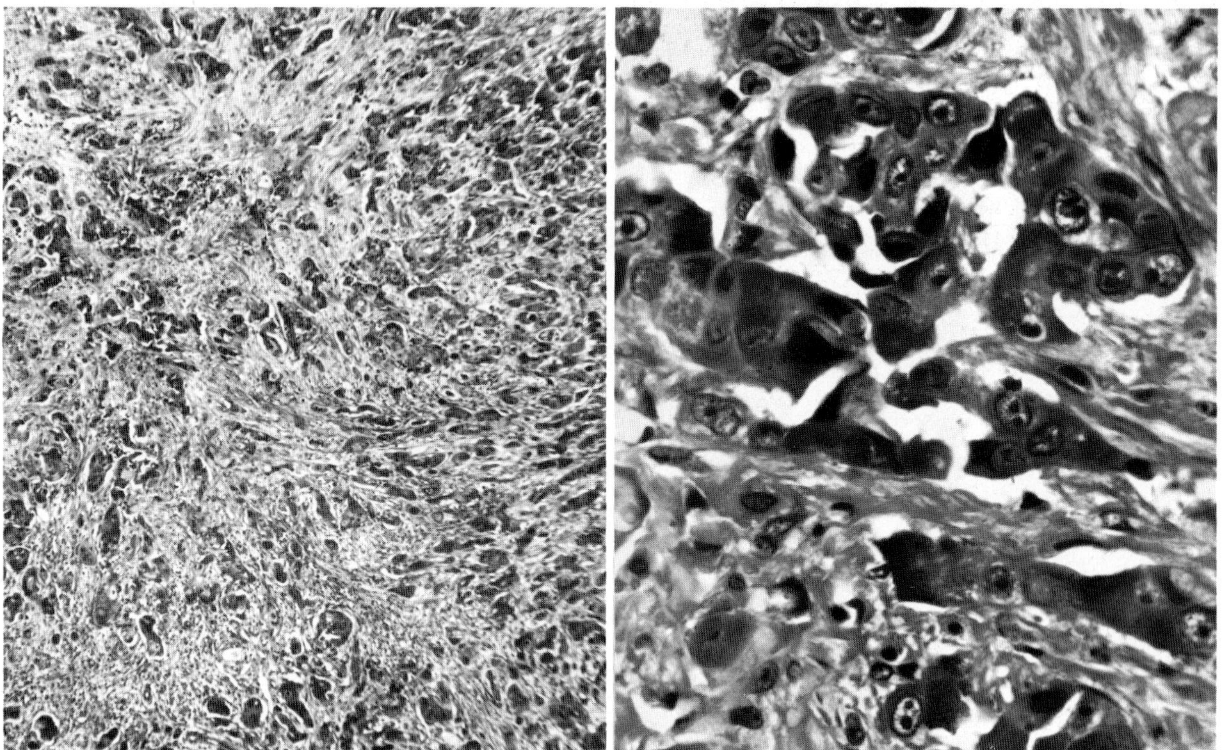

Fig. 16-10. Low- and high-power views of histological section of carcinoma of the breast showing destruction of normal architecture and cellular anaplasia

sites for metastasis are the liver (as a result of the invasion of the portal vein), the lungs, the bones, the brain, and the adrenals (as a result of invasion of the systemic circulation).

If it can be said that all cancers ultimately invade surrounding tissues, all cancers do not metastasize. A case in point is the basal cell carcinoma of the skin. However, a basal cell carcinoma originating in the mouth or any other mucosa readily metastasizes. There are no rigid correlations between the tendency to invade and metastasize. Whereas some cancers proliferate and kill their victims through invasion of the surrounding tissues, others remain small but metastasize early and extensively.

Why does cancer kill? The growth of even large-sized and multiple benign masses does not often kill its victim. The cause of death in cancer may result from local or systemic injuries, but it is usually complex. The local injuries include compression of vital organs (*e.g.*, brain or spinal cord), replacement of vital organs by cancer cells with loss of function, and occlusion of vital organs by tumor growth (cancers of the larynx, prostate, bladder, and esophagus). Occasionally, cancer outgrows its blood supply, and the mass becomes anoxemic and necrotic. The necrotic mass may then be a center for infection. If the cancer tissue grows to establish a connection between parenchyma (*e.g.*, the lung) and a hollow organ (*e.g.*, the esophagus) or between two hollow organs (*e.g.*, the trachea and the esophagus), and the tumor mass becomes necrotic with necrotic cells eliminated by lysis, artificial communications, or fistulas, are established. Often these fistulas may constitute a focus of infection resistant to antibiotic therapy.

Growth of the primary mass, invasion, and metastasis are not the only means by which cancer kills its victim. The cancer cells feed on the host for building blocks. A florid cancer functions as a nitrogen trap, depriving the host of necessary metabolites. As a result of this depletion of his resources, the victim may become so emaciated and weak that he is cachectic.

In addition to acting as a nitrogen trap, the cancer cells are believed by some to secrete toxic substances, polypeptic in nature, sometimes referred to as toxohormones. In some cases, as in cancer of the ovary, the cancer cells become detached from the primary tumor and seed the peritoneal cavity, eliciting a secretory reaction leading to massive ascites.

If the phenotypic manifestations of cancer cells' invasion, metastases and preying on the host resources are present in some normal cells (particularly embryonic cells) then all cells must contain the information needed to express the cancer phenotype in their genome. Such reasoning has brought Pierce and his collaborators [530] to raise an important question: is the cancer cell a more or less differentiated cell with limited potentiality whose gene expression is distorted and thereby expresses the cancer phenotype which includes invasion, metastasis, and dedifferentiation, or is the cancer cell a stem cell which after exposure to the carcinogen expresses in its phenotype the

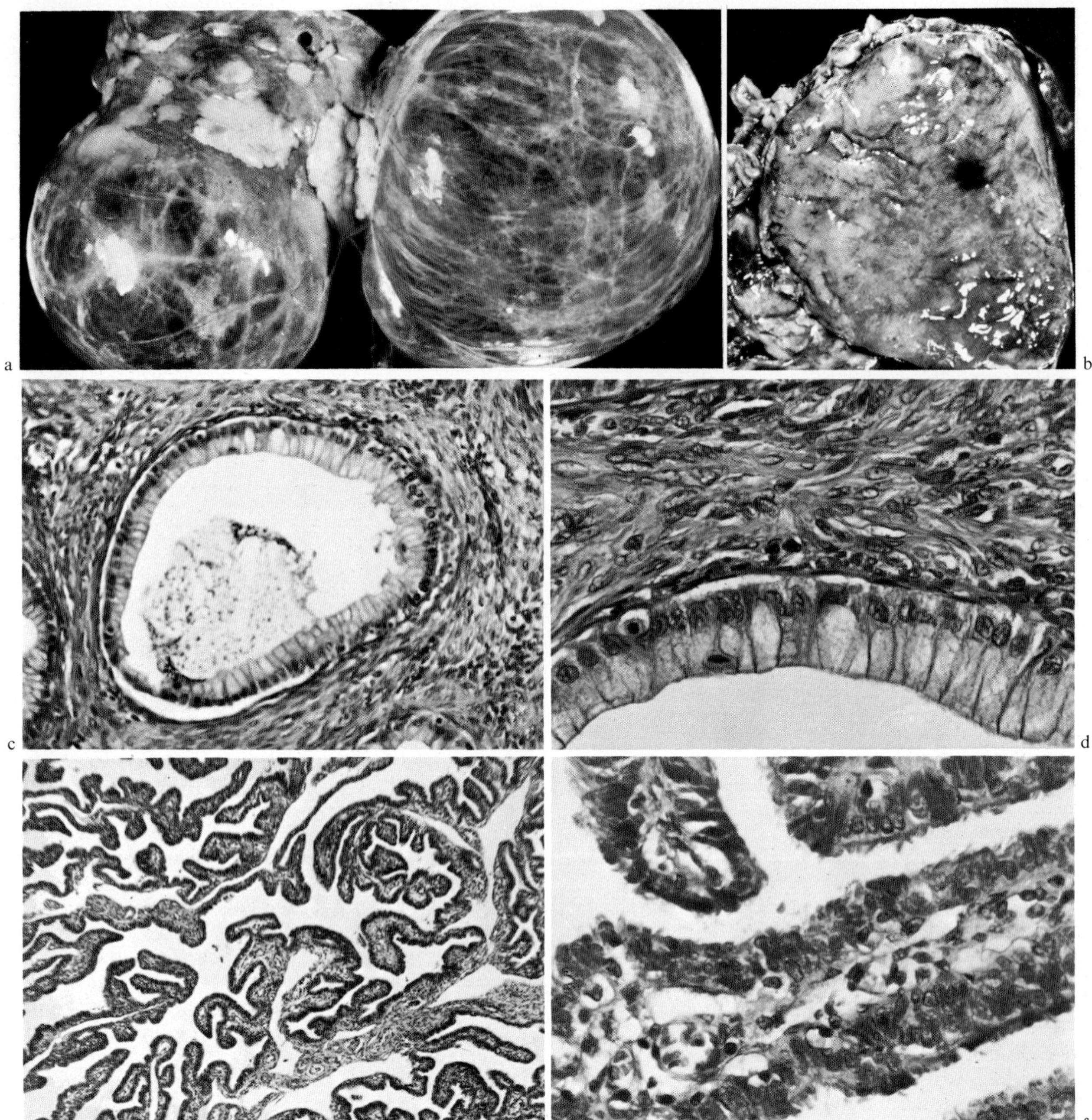

Fig. 16-11. (a) Ovarian cyst; (b) Cancer of the ovary. Notice the meaty appearance of the organ and the loss of normal histological structure. There is no capsule, and the cancer invades the organ's surface; (c-f) low- and high-power views of ovarian cysts upper left and right respectively and ovarian cancer. Lower left and right, showing the well differentiated appearance of the cells in the cyst and the anaplastic in the cancer

cancer characteristics, but remains still capable of differentiation into a normal cell?

Some ingenious experiments done with teratomas and squamous cells suggest that the latter alternative obtains at least for some cancer.

Induced or spontaneous teratomas derived from germ, gonial or early embryonic cells in mice provide a population of dividing cells with multipotentiality for differentiation. The cells can be transplanted and maintain their multipotentiality. As they grow they develop in a fashion similar to that of the embryonic cell by progressively directing their potential for differentiation. They are readily hybridizable and can be cloned to yield diploid cell cultures. Thus, the teratoma cell has properties intermediate between the multipotential embryonic cell and the multidifferentiated cancer cell and therefore, teratomas are a good model for the study of differentiation. Single embryonal carcinoma cells derived from teratomas were transplanted intraperitoneally in mice. Eleven percent of them yielded teratocarcinomas containing a dozen differentiated tissues. Clonal lines were developed from these tumors and each line yielded cellular elements representing the three germ layers and were therefore a teratocarcinoma. Thus, it was concluded that the teratocarcinoma cell is multipotential and differentiates in a broad spectrum of tissues.

When teratocarcinomas were converted to the ascitis [531], embroid bodies (resembling the benign desmoid cyst seen in the ovary) were formed. These findings suggested that the original cancer cell had differentiated into a benign tumor, possibly because of some favorable changes in the environment.

The conversion of cancer cells into benign cells was confirmed in another experiment in which Irish rat squamous cell carcinoma was used. In this tumor "squamous pearls" are surrounded by undifferentiated cells. Radioautographic studies suggested that the undifferentiated cells are converted into the squamous cells. When the pearls and the undifferentiated cells were dissected from the tumor with the use of a dissecting microscope and transplanted subcutaneously, the pearl did not yield cancer, but the poorly differentiated cells did. This led to the conclusion that the tumor starts with a population of stem cells, some of which mature in well-differentiated noncancerous cells.

Such an interpretation of the biology of the cancer cell led Pierce to propose an alternative to the traditional elimination therapy of cancer; namely, the stimulation of the normal process of differentiation in which the phenotypic properties of the cancer cells are excluded.

Such concepts have gained support from work in tissue culture. When Friend erythroleukemic cells are cultured in presence of dimethylsulfoxide (DMSO), their malignancy decreases and there is a marked enhancement of differentiation along the erythroid pathway [532]. Similar findings were made with neuroblasts and even fibroblasts.

Bendich *et al.* [533] showed that the addition of DMSO or dimethylformamide (DMF) to cells transformed by viruses and carcinogens brought them to grow in a much more regular fashion reminiscent of that of nontransformed cultures. When DMSO treated cells were injected to mice themselves treated with DMSO, no tumors appeared. Not only do these experiments indicate that tumor cells can differentiate into nonmalignant phenotypes, but they suggest that alterations of the cell membranes are in some way involved in the transforming process.

Cancer and Heredity

In Animals

The incidence of cancer is influenced by a variety of factors, such as heredity, chemical or physical carcinogens, and viruses. It is necessary to review the role of these factors to understand the biochemistry of cancer.

It would be impossible to review comprehensively the role of heredity in experimental tumors. However, some pertinent observations in animals and humans will be described. Slye [1] and Lynch [2] were among the first to study the influence of heredity in cancer. They showed that inbreeding of strains of mice prone to develop a given cancer markedly increased the incidence of that cancer. In contrast, the inbreeding of strains that were not prone to develop spontaneous cancer produced strains almost devoid of tumors. These early experiments led Slye to conclude that cancer is transmitted as a mendelian recessive character of low penetrance, while Lynch concluded that it is transmitted by a dominant gene. Both investigators agreed that cancer transmission is controlled by several genes.

These oversimplified conclusions were later strongly questioned on the basis of two major objections: first, the strains used in these early experiments were not genetically homogeneous, and second, the environmental conditions were not strictly controlled. Of course, at that time almost nothing was known of the role of environment in the genesis of cancer.

When pure strains of animals became available, it was further demonstrated that strains with a high incidence of a given cancer could be obtained by appropriate inbreeding. For example, strains referred to as CH_3 and DBA present a high incidence of mammary cancer. In contrast, those referred to as NH present a high percentage of spontaneous lung cancer in older mice.

The mechanism by which heredity influences the incidence of cancer is not clear. Does it act directly on the cellular potentialities to differentiate normally, or does it act on the internal environment of the individual by modifying, for example, its hormonal secretions or by increasing its susceptibility to carcinogens? Many investigators have designed and performed experiments with the hope of elucidating this important problem.

The evolution of our understanding of the genesis of breast cancer in mice illustrates the complexity of such investigations. As soon as Little demonstrated that a high incidence of carcinoma of the breast could be produced in pure strains of mice, it was observed independently in two different laboratories that the mother played a more important role than the father in transmitting the disease. In a remarkable series of experiments, Bittner [3] later demonstrated that he could reduce the incidence of carcinoma of the breast in a strain with a high spontaneous incidence simply by separating the mother from the newborn animals and by fostering the newborn animals with mothers obtained from a strain with a low incidence of breast carcinoma. This clearly demonstrated that the milk was responsible for the maternal influence observed by others to induce a high incidence of breast cancer. We shall see later that the milk factor is indeed a virus, and that various other factors—like hormones, nutrition, other maternal factors, and even male factors* of unknown origin—affect the incidence of breast cancer.

It was also demonstrated that the synergism of hereditary and environmental factors played a role in inducing many other experimental cancers, for example, leukemias and carcinomas of the adrenals.

Heredity not only influences the incidence of spontaneous cancers, but it also influences the susceptibility of the animals to experimental tumors such as those produced by carcinogens or induced by transplantation.

One may wonder how such a hereditary influence manifests itself in the human population, which is highly heterozygous and influenced by diverse environmental conditions. Strong [4, 5] has reproduced such situations experimentally and has obtained astounding results. Strong deliberately mixed three strains of mice. Each strain differed from the other considerably with regard to the incidence of developing spontaneous tumors. After mating the mice through several generations, he obtained a new homozygous strain with a rather low incidence of cancer (about 10%), but in which the histological variety of the tumor was much greater than in each of the original strains. Such tumors as breast and lung cancers were observed, as were lymphosarcomas and leukemias. Strong also investigated the influence of environmental factors; he injected methylcholanthrene, a potent carcinogen, in half of the animals and separated those mice that did not develop a local tumor from those that developed tumors at the injection site. He continued these injections through several generations and inbred those animals resistant to the development of local tumors. He finally obtained a strain of mice that did not develop tumors at the site of methylcholanthrene injection; however, among that group there was a high incidence of a great variety of tumors resembling the polymorphism of human cancer. What is even more astonishing is that this property was transmitted through the descendants even if the injection was interrupted.

Falconer and Bloom [6] have pursued an interesting problem concerning the relative contributions of chance genetic and environmental factors in induced lung tumor in mice. Their study led them to conclude that genetic factors caused important differences in the incidence of tumors in genetically heterogeneous strains. For example, in a so-called V_c strain, the genetic factors were responsible for 49% of the tumors. In contrast, in so-called LX strain, genetic factors were responsible for the incidence of 74% of the tumors. Chance and environment contributed 45% of the incidence in the V_c strain and only 25% in the LX strain.

All these experiments indicate that heredity plays a role in determining the incidence of tumors in animals. Furthermore, if some degree of ingenuity is introduced in programming the breeding, a pattern of cancer distribution reminiscent of the variety observed in man can be obtained. Whether the manipulation of the animal strain indeed reflects the distribution in the highly heterozygous human population remains to be established.

* If the ova of mice with a high incidence of cancer are implanted in the uterus of a mother with a low incidence of cancer, the incidence of spontaneous mammary cancer is reduced in the progeny.

In Humans

The descendants of cancerous parents have repeatedly been frightened by the possibility that cancer may be hereditary in humans. Except for a few rare cases involving rather exceptional types of cancer, the concept of hereditary cancer in humans rests on little concrete or convincing evidence. Among the arguments that are sometimes invoked in favor of hereditary influences in the incidences of cancer in humans are the existence of so-called cancer families and the accumulation of sometimes crude statistics. Warthin was the first in 1913 to identify families with high susceptibility to cancer. Ever since, all clinicians who have seen a large number of cancer patients have encountered cancer families. This appears to be an impressive argument supporting the hereditary transmission of cancer in humans. However, it is usually impossible to determine whether this increased incidence of cancer in a given family is due to hereditary factors or results from great similarities in the environment. The same dilemma arises when one attempts to interpret the occurrence of several cancers in the same patient.

In conclusion, except for a few specific tumors discussed below, there exists in humans no definite evidence that cancer is transmitted hereditarily because it has been impossible to trace the disease with strict criteria (such as histological diagnosis) for several generations, and at the same time, to eliminate the environmental factors that might lead to cancer. If there exists a hereditary predisposition to cancer in humans, most investigators agree that it consists of a general predisposition to all cancers. However, Gardner [7] and his associates disagree with this concept and, on the basis of their investigations, conclude that the hereditary predisposition concerns specific tumors.

The incidence of cancer in families of cancer patients has been investigated frequently [8–11]. Particular attention has been given to breast cancer, and on the basis of such studies, it has been concluded that the incidence of breast carcinoma is increased among the female relatives of patients affected by that kind of cancer. However, information on both controls and the cancerous patients is difficult to obtain because one must rely, with regard to the disease in the ancestry, either on the information given by the patient or on that given by death certificates. Both sources are often unreliable.

Murphy and Abbey [12] reviewed the literature on breast cancer in families and contributed a well-controlled study on a large number of individuals (over 2000). They concluded that there was no difference between the relatives of patients with breast cancer and controls with respect to the site and frequency of cancer. This contrasts with some studies of Jacobsen [13] on 200 cases of carcinoma in which he found a higher incidence of breast cancer in relatives of patients with breast carcinoma than among the general population, and some studies of Kemp [14] that led to the conclusion that relatives of patients with breast carcinoma have a nonspecific predisposition to cancer. Statistical analyses of Macklin [15] led to the conclusion that carcinoma of the breast is two to seven times more frequent in breast cancer relatives. Macklin also discovered that the incidence of carcinoma of the prostate is higher among relatives of patients with carcinoma of the breast. Similar observations have been made for carcinomas of the uterus and stomach and for leukemia.

Although some of the statistical studies on the distribution of carcinoma among relatives of cancer patients and in the general population may be criticized on various accounts, the studies in twins seem more reliable. There have been several reports of cancers occurring in identical twins at the same time and at the same site. In one study, 17 pairs of twins, of which 8 were identical, were observed. Carcinoma of the cervix was found in both members of one pair of identical twins simultaneously. When carcinoma of the cervix was found in nonidentical twins, only one of the twins was affected. A well-controlled study by Clemmesen [16] concerning 83 twins, of which 50 were monozygotic, suggested a slight increase (7%) of carcinomas among twins as compared with the general population.

Although it is difficult to accept beyond any shadow of a doubt that carcinomas of the breast or stomach are hereditarily controlled, it has been clearly demonstrated that precancerous lesions, such as those accompanying intestinal polyposis and xeroderma pigmentosum, and such tumors as retinoblastomas and neurofibromas, are under strict hereditary influence (see Table 16-1).

Familial polyposis is a rare disease (only 350 cases have been reported in the literature), and its incidence has been calculated as 1 in 30,000 individuals. The gene for polyposis is an autosomal dominant. Polyposis often leads to carcinoma of the colon and is therefore responsible for a hereditary form of that

Table 16-1. Hereditary cancer

Type	Mode of transmission Autosomal	Autosomal
Xeroderma pigmentosum	recessive	
Retinoblastoma	recessive	
Neurofibromatosis		dominant
Multiple polyposis		dominant
Polyendocrine adenomatosis		dominant
Hereditary multiple exostosis		dominant
Nevoid basal cell carcinoma		dominant
Medullary thyroid carcinoma		dominant

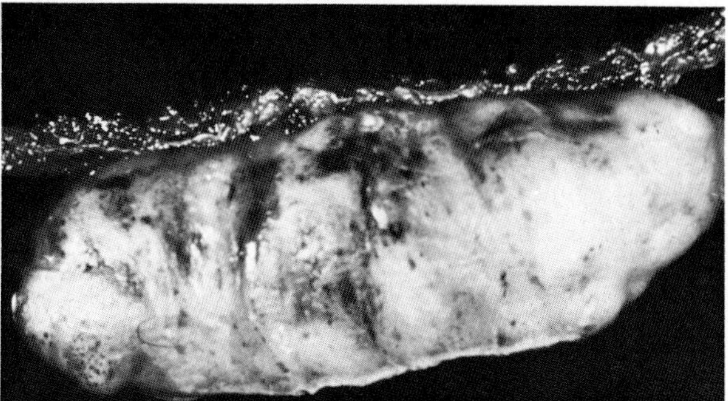

Fig. 16-12. Neurofibroma

carcinoma. A precancerous condition called xeroderma pigmentosum, characterized by dryness of the skin followed by pigmentation and ulceration, is known to be hereditary. It is transferred by a sex-linked gene (see chapter on radiation effects). Retinoblastoma, transmitted by a dominant gene, occurs at the rate of 5 in 100,000 and is usually fatal. Neurofibromatosis is transmitted by a dominant gene with a high degree of penetrance (see Fig. 16-12). For a review of cancer heredity in man see [534].

Chromosomes in Cancer

The chromosomal anomalies of the cancer cell suggest that cancer development may involve the genetic material of the afflicted somatic cells. However, the germ cells or other somatic cells of the cancer patient are generally morphologically normal.

In the normal cell, the shape of each chromosome and the total number of chromosomes are constant. The normal chromosome pattern is altered in many types of cancer cells. The alteration of the karyotypes involves changes in the number of chromosomes (heteroploidy) and changes in the shape of one or more chromosomes. Chromosomal changes have been observed in human or experimental tumors, in transplanted tumors, and in tissue cultures of malignant cells.

One of the most interesting observations on changes in chromosome structure was made by Nowell and Hungerford [17, 18] who described a consistent chromosome alteration in the immature granulocyte of patients with chronic myelogenous leukemia. In myelogenous leukemia, a chromosome belonging to group G (possibly chromosome 22) is shorter than its normal homolog; approximately half of the long arm of the chromosome is missing.

The abnormal chromosome has been called the Philadelphia chromosome, and the aberration is consistently found in the stem cell of the marrow and in the immature cell of the peripheral blood when these cells are grown under the influence of phytohemagglutinin. In fact, the abnormal chromosome also has been detected in preleukemic patients before the appearance of clinical symptoms [19]. The Philadelphia chromosome is absent in the mature granulocytes found in the peripheral blood of leukemic patients during periods of remission or after therapy. Even though treatment of chronic myelogenous leukemia induces a hematological remission in 80% of the patients, the Philadelphia chromosome of the immature cells is unaffected by therapy. The anomaly is certainly not congenital because the karyotype of the skin of patients with chronic myelogenous leukemia is normal. In view of the fact that Down's syndrome, or mongolism [20], is associated with trisomy of chromosome 22, it is interesting that the incidence of myeloid leukemia is 18 times greater in mongoloids than in the general population.

The mechanisms by which the chromosomal abnormality occurs are not clear, but a terminal deletion of chromosomal material is improbable because chromosomal material is seldom lost. Translocation of the lost pieces is more likely. Two possible types of mechanisms of translocation could account for the formation of a Philadelphia chromosome: reciprocal translocation (exchange of chromatin segments between two chromosomes) or interstitial deletion. Reciprocal exchange is unlikely because chromosome 22 would then be expected to combine occasionally with large pieces of chromatin, resulting from the break of another chromosome. Yet a chromosome 22 longer than normal has not been observed.

Two breaks in the same chromosome could lead to the deletion of part of the chromatin inside the chromosome, yielding an interstitial deletion followed by the adhesion of the terminal pieces to form a shorter chromosome. The small internal piece may be lost or may be translocated onto another chromosome; the translocation of the small piece cannot be detected because the piece is too small to be recognized when attached to another chromosome.

Whangpeng *et al.* have studied the genesis of the Philadelphia chromosome by the trypsin Giemsa banding technique and have shown in 5 patients that a single translocation occurs from the distal portion of the long arm of chromosome 22 at the 12 banding location to the end of the long arm of the chromosome [535].

On the basis of results obtained in a remarkable study in which the DNA content of individual chromosomes was measured by microspectrophotometry, Nowell and his associates were able to calculate the amount of DNA missing in the Philadelphia chromosome (0.02 pg of DNA, or 0.27% of the DNA content of the nucleus, 2×10^7 nucleotide pairs).

The link between the presence of the Philadelphia chromosome and the cancerous properties of the leukemic cells remains to be discovered, and the relationship between the chromosomal abnormality and the cancer can be interpreted only partially. An obvious but not necessarily correct interpretation of the presence of the Philadelphia chromosome in patients with chronic myelogenous leukemia is that the chromosomal alteration is responsible for a genetic deletion that leads to cancer; and it has been proposed that chronic myelogenous leukemia starts with the alteration of chromosome 22 of a single bone marrow stem cell.

Since the abnormal chromosome is found in all dividing cells of the bone marrow of patients with myelogenous leukemia, it would seem that in marrow only one type of stem cell later differentiates into the mature cells of the various lineages of hematopoietic cells. Inasmuch as neither the red nor the lymphoid cells of the marrow of patients with myelogenous leukemia become cancerous, it would also appear that the missing part of chromosome 22 is that part in which the information for differentiation into a granulopoietic cell is stored.

It does seem certain that chromosome 22 carries the genetic information responsible for the expression of alkaline phosphatase activity in the phenotype; the enzyme activity is decreased in chronic myelogenous leukemia, but is not altered in other forms of leukemia (myeloproliferative disorders) not associated with anomalies of chromosome 22. In contrast, in mongoloids alkaline phosphatase activity is increased.

Chromosomal changes have been observed in many other types of leukemia, but in contrast to what is found in chronic myelogenous leukemia, the chromosomal changes are not consistent.

Chromosomal changes have been observed in other types of cancers. Usually they are not as typical as in the Philadelphia chromosomes, and thus various but inconsistent structural changes in the chromosomes of cancer cells have been described. When an alteration is sufficiently consistent to permit a distinction between a normal cell and a cancer cell, the chromosomes thus altered are referred to as markers.

W.W. Nichols [21] has studied the chromosome pattern of the Schmidt-Ruppin strain of the Rous sarcoma. After transplantation, the original tumor and the tumor that develops after a few passages contain mostly normal chromosomal patterns, except for minor deviations in ploidy. But chromosomal breakage, translocation, and reunion occur when the cells that have undergone several passages are cultured.

Adding the virus to a culture of human leukocytes induces chromosome alteration after several divisions [22], an intriguing observation that has suggested to some that the oncogenic viruses, found in the biosphere and now assiduously cultivated in laboratories in a variety of animals, might manifest such nefarious effects in man if no rigid preventive measures are taken. Time will tell whether this assumption is right or wrong. But it should be kept in mind that the measles virus can induce chromosome breaks in human leukocytes without, as far as we know, affecting the incidence of leukemia. Other examples of chromosomal anomalies will be described as we discuss further the pathogenesis of cancer.

Since cancer, at least in part, is uncontrolled growth, it is not surprising that the number of mitoses is often greater in the tumor than in surrounding normal tissues. In addition to exhibiting an increased number of mitoses, cancer tissues also present a high proportion of abnormal mitoses. An abnormal mitosis may result from alterations: (1) of the duration of the mitotic cycles; (2) in spindle formation; and (3) in the number, length, and shape of the chromosomes.

The duration of the mitotic cycle is usually increased in the cancer cell, and prophase is affected primarily. The spindle may be completely absent or multipolar. In the first case, the newly formed chromosome cannot be separated and polyploidy occurs, whereas in the second case there is an irregular distribution of the number of chromosomes among the daughter cells.

Cancer cells are often heteroploid; in other words, their chromosomes make up a total number different from the usual diploid number observed in the somatic cell. The number of chromosomes in cancer cells has been found in great quantity in spontaneous and experimental tumors. Only a few examples will be presented here [23–26].

In counting the number of chromosomes in cancer cells obtained from preparations of adenocarcinomas of the cervix uteri, investigators observed that the average frequency peak for the number of chromosomes ranged between 42 and 76. As many as 346 chromosomes per cell have been found occasionally in adenocarcinomas of the intestine. In some tumors, the variations in the number yield polyploidy, whereas in others the changes lead to subploidy. For example, the number of chromosomes in human carcinomas of the colon may range from 10 to 45 with a peak between 25 and 30. In contrast, in liposarcoma, the tendency is toward polyploidy. The chromosome numbers range between 60 and 200 with two peaks—one between 65 and 75, and another between 145 and around 200. A similar situation occurs in the HeLa cell in which the number of chromosomes ranges from 40 to 200 with a peak between 80 and 90.

Heteroploidy seems to evolve in the following manner. A normal diploid cell becomes tetraploid because chromosome duplication is not followed by cell division. During subsequent division, either higher levels of polyploidy are achieved or the tetraploid cell divides and gives birth to cells with unequal numbers of chromosomes. Once chromosomal heterogeneity has been achieved, environmental conditions seem to determine which cell type has the best chance of survival.

Usually one type of heteroploid cell is found in the tumor in higher proportion than all other types of heteroploid cells. The predominant type of heteroploid cell is referred to as "stem line." In culture, the stem line tends to stabilize after several generations. For example, when mice mammary carcinoma is transplanted twice and the cells are cultured *in vitro*, the cells of the stem line contain 84 chromosomes. In contrast, if the same tumor is transplanted *in vivo* 186 times and then cultured *in vitro*, the cells of the stem line contain 73 chromosomes.

Occasionally, two stem lines may be present in the same tumor; a mouse tumor containing one stem line of 40 chromosomes and another of 80 chromosomes has been described. The properties of the stem line may change during the development of the cancer, and metastases may contain cells with chromosomal patterns different from those of the primary tumor.

An understanding of the relationship between chromosome observation and carcinogenesis is most likely to emanate from the study of a gamut of tumors that show different degrees of anaplasia but are all derived from the same tissues. Nowell has investigated the chromosomal alterations in a number of minimal deviation hepatomas. The results of these experiments will be described later, and at that time we will attempt to interpret the relationship between carcinogenesis and chromosome aberrations.

In conclusion, strains of mice in which the incidence of cancer is extremely high can be bred. However, there is no conclusive evidence that heredity plays a critical role in human carcinogenesis except in a few rare types of cancer, such as xeroderma pigmentosum, retinoblastoma, and familial polyposis.

With the possible exception of the Philadelphia chromosome in myelogenous leukemia, visible changes in the chromosomes do not constitute a primary event in carcinogenesis. Chromosome changes are more likely to result from a progressive loss of control of gene expression, including the loss of those regulatory factors that determine chromosome number and morphogenesis.

Hormones and Cancer

Because hormones affect growth and differentiation, it is not surprising that hormonal imbalances influence the incidence, location, and rate of cancer growth. Hormonal imbalances may be produced by injecting hormones, explanting or destroying the endocrine glands, or administering hormonal antagonists.

Breast Cancer

In mice, carcinoma of the breast occurs spontaneously only in females. We have seen that breast cancer development is influenced by heredity and maternal factors. That it is also influenced by female hormones was suggested by experiments which demonstrated that the incidence of carcinoma of the breast in mice could be reduced considerably by castration of the animal before puberty. In contrast, the implantation of ovaries in castrated animals increases the incidence of breast carcinoma as compared with its incidence in the castrate. Lacassagne [27–29] demonstrated that of the female hormones secreted by the ovaries, the estrogens primarily influenced the incidence of breast carcinoma. Indeed, the injection of estrogen to female or male castrated mice obtained from a strain predisposed to develop breast carcinoma considerably increased the incidence of cancer. This property of the estrogenic hormones was later shown to depend on their physiological effect rather than on their chemical structure, because compounds with different chemical structures but with similar physiological activities would all be active in increasing the incidence of breast carcinoma in mice.

Similar experiments in rats have shown that large amounts of estrogen induce breast carcinoma provided that spontaneous breast cancers occur occasionally in the strain used for the experiment. Furthermore, in rats, carcinomas of the breast have been produced by the simultaneous administration of estrogens and methylcholanthrene. (In contrast to 2-aminoacetylfluorene, which does induce breast carcinoma, methylcholanthrene alone does not induce carcinoma of the breast, at least in some strains of rats.)

The complexity of the hormonal interaction in mammary tumors is illustrated by studying the growth of mammary tumors produced with carcinogens. Breast cancer can be induced in rats by administering 5 mg of dimethylbenzanthracene (DMBA, see Section on carcinogenesis). Tumor growth is stimulated by the administration or artificial release of pituitary prolactin (which can be achieved by producing an electrolytic lesion in the median eminence of the hypothalamus). The stimulus prolactin provides for mammary cancer growth seems to depend, however, upon the presence of ovarian hormones, because in ovariectomized animals the tumors regress in spite of the high blood levels of prolactin.

From the preceding, it would seem that all endocrine imbalances that stimulate estrogen secretion have an effect similar to that of estrogen administration with respect to the incidence of breast carcinoma. If this is the case, it may be possible to explain the effect of adrenalectomy in C-3H mice. Adrenalectomy in these mice reduces the incidence of breast carcinoma to a rate similar to that observed after ovariectomy. Simultaneous adrenalectomy and ovariectomy lead to a greater reduction in the incidence of breast carcinoma than does simple castration. Furthermore, if ovariectomy is performed in mice at an early age (such as immediately after birth), the incidence of breast carcinoma is not considerably reduced. The adrenals are known to secrete estrogen, and if rabbits are ovariectomized at an early age, vicarious hypertrophy of the adrenals occurs, which is capable of maintaining the animals continuously under the influence of feminizing hormones.

The increased incidence of breast carcinoma in mice after the injection of hypophyseal hormones or by the implantation of the hypophysis in nonovariectomized animals probably results from the estrogenic stimulating effect of the hypophysis [30]. Indeed, if such procedures are applied to noncastrated males or castrated females, the incidence of breast carcinoma is not affected. Hypophysectomy reduces the incidence of breast carcinoma in mice even when they are deprived of the milk agent. Progesterone increases the incidence of breast carcinoma produced in rats by the administration of acetylaminofluorene. It has no such effect in mice.

Because they are simple to manipulate, rodents have been extensively used to study the pathogenesis and the histogenesis of cancer of the breast. The numerous experiments performed in the last 5 decades cannot be reviewed. The reader is referred to specialized articles [536, 537]. These studies leave no doubt that in rodents the genesis of cancer of the breast is influenced by a combination of hereditary, hormonal, viral and environmental factors. However, it is fair to raise the question as to whether the information assembled in the rodent is relevant to humans. Needless to point out that there are remarkable differences between the mouse and the human patient in the reproductive cycle. For example, the mouse has a nonfunctional corpus luteum. Moreover, in contrast to what is seen in women, the incidence of cancer of the breast in mice is less in virgins than in multiparous animals.

Cancer of the breast also occurs in dog and cat. It is, however, not likely that studies on these animals might shed new light on our understanding of cancer of the breast in humans.

Prolactin is also involved in development of experimental cancer of the breast in rodents. When prolactin blood levels of the host are decreased by any method such as hypophysectomy or the administration of antiserum, tumor growth is inhibited. In contrast, stimulation of prolactin secretion accelerates tumor growth.

Since estrogens were found to be unable to reactivate tumor growth after hypophysectomy, a direct stimulatory effect of estrogen on mammary tumor growth has been questioned and the suggestion has been made that the estrogens act indirectly through the hypophyseal stimulation of prolactin secretion. Previous evidence and recent studies by Leung *et al.* [538] leave, however, little doubt that the growth of mammary tumors induced in mice by the administration of the carcinogen 7,12-dimethyl-benz(a)anthracene is directly controlled by estrogens.

The role that prolactin plays in the pathogenesis of human breast cancer remains obscure. For review see [539].

According to Segaloff [540] the interaction of prolactin and estrogen is not the only hormonal factor influencing the growth of the cancerous mammary gland in rats. Ovariectomies followed by the administration of estrogens in the AXC rat suggest that in addition to estrogen the ovary produces another factor (not progesterone) which stimulates tumoral growth.

Inasmuch as prolactin and estrogen are mitogenic for the breast, it is not entirely surprising that they influence tumor growth. Whether either hormone is necessary for cancer initiation is, however, debatable. It seems more likely that the hormones stimulate the growth of a cell already transformed into a cancer cell. The interaction between prolactin and estrogen in breast cancer promotion remains to be clarified. Dao was recently able to induce breast cancers in organ culture *in vitro*. Such material might prove useful for the study of hormonal influences on tumor growth [541, 542]. In mammary adenocarcinoma of the Fisher rat, insulin seems to inhibit tumor growth.

In conclusion, the growth of mammary tumors in rodents is modulated by a number of hormonal factors which will be difficult to sort out unless a complete understanding of the molecular alterations that the hormone initiates is available. A step in that direction has been accomplished by studying the binding of hormones to the normal or cancerous mammary tissues grown *in vivo*.

Female rats treated with 7,12-dimethyl(a)anthracene develop breast cancers. When such treated animals are ovariectomized the growth of 80% of the tumor is arrested, but approximately 10% of the tumors continue to grow and one therefore distinguishes between ovarian dependent and ovarian independent tumors. One would reasonably anticipate that more binding sites for estrogen would be found in the dependent than the independent tumors. This is, however, not the case [543].

Similarly, Richards *et al.* [544] found no correlation between the susceptibility of a strain to develop mammary carcinomas and the binding capacity of the breast tissue for 17β-^{3}H estradiol.

Work in several laboratories and studies of large autopsy series seem to have established a relationship between the incidence of breast cancer and thyroid function. Autopsy series by Spencer [31] and Sommers [32] suggest that the incidence of breast carcinoma is higher among patients with goiters, usually adenomatous goiters. Thyroid atrophy has been proposed to lead to stimulation of the hypophysis, which secretes ovarian-stimulating hormones. As a result, the ovary is stimulated to secrete estrogens, which induce the breast tissue hyperplasia. Furth and his associates have described a hypophyseal tumor that produces TSH and also secretes ovarian-stimulating hormones such as LH and FSH.

It is difficult to reconcile the findings and the interpretation presented above with a recent observation of reduced incidence of mammary cancer in thyroidectomized rats fed methylcholanthrene.

Breast carcinoma continues to be common in women—each year in the United States 25 of every 100,000 women develop breast cancer. The likelihood that in humans the incidence and the development of breast carcinoma are influenced by hormones is suggested by a number of observations. Although common in women, breast cancer is extremely rare in men; the incidence of breast cancer is much lower in castrated than in normal women. Menopause and the development of breast cancer seem to be related. The incidence of cancer is greater after menopause. Women who have a late menopause are more susceptible to breast cancer than women with early menopause. Occasionally, when a cancer has been controlled in one breast, another may develop in the other breast, suggesting that a hormone factor influences the incidence of the tumor [10, 33–36].

Whether or not nursing influences the incidence of breast cancer in women remains to be established on solid grounds. Forced drying of the breast after pregnancy is often said to increase a woman's chances of developing breast cancer. Yet the number of women who do not nurse has increased in the last decades, and the incidence of breast cancer is unchanged. Similarly, estrogen administration after menopause to an increasing number of women has not affected the incidence of breast cancer. However, it has been reported that virgins and nulliparae are more prone to breast cancer than mothers of many children. The incidence of breast cancer is not significantly greater among pregnant women than among the general female population of the same age.

Cystic hyperplasia of the breast (Reclus' disease) seems to promote the development of breast cancer. The exact incidence of the cancer in organs affected by cystic hyperplasia is not known. The conflicting results published seem to derive from the authors' failure to distinguish between clinical and microscopic cystic hyperplasia. But it seems that at least 20% and possibly more of clinically obvious cystic hyperplasias are associated with cancer.

Therefore, it is significant that Goormachtig showed that chronic mastitis could be induced by injecting ovarian extracts in mice. Cystic hyperplasia can be induced in most rodents or primates by administering estrogen, but the animal disease differs from the human. Whereas in rodents the disease affects the entire breast, it is localized in women. As for primates, cystic and fibrotic changes develop without hyperplasia.

The relationship between breast carcinoma and cystic hyperplasia is of considerable practical importance. Cystic hyperplasia is often bilateral. Thus, when hyperplasia and cancer coexist, the surgeon must decide whether or not to excise the second breast, a difficult decision since it is impossible to determine in an individual case what the chances are for degeneration of the benign hyperplasia into malignancy.

The difficulties in identifying cystic hyperplasia as a precancerous state are not unique; recognition of a precancerous state is always difficult. Three methods are used in establishing a correlation between benign and malignant tumors: follow-up of a large number of patients for a long time; establishment of anatomical continuity between benign and malignant tumors on microscopic examination; experimental conversion of a benign into a malignant tumor.

Few so-called precancerous lesions of the breast satisfy all three criteria. The benign breast entities that are believed to have a higher incidence of malignancy include: virginal hypertrophy and excessive mammary development, residual lactation mastitis, aberrant mammary tissues, fibroadenoma (especially in pregnancy and at menopause), intraductal papilloma and chronic cystic mastitis.

The follow-up method indicates that patients with proliferative changes of the breasts present 7 times the expected incidence of cancer of breasts, while the expected incidence is doubled in patients with fibroadenoma. Follow-up studies do, however, not provide convincing evidence that either intraductal papilloma or the chronic cystic mastitis is precancerous.

Carcinoma of the Cervix

After unsuccessful attempts to produce carcinoma of the cervix in monkeys by administering estrogens, Gardner and his associates [37, 38] succeeded in inducing invasive and transplantable cervical cancers in mice. Cervical carcinomas are difficult to produce. The tumors develop only after administering high doses of estrogens for a long time to a strain susceptible to breast carcinoma. This procedure leads to the development of breast carcinoma, which is liable to be fatal before carcinoma of the cervix develops. Thus, the successful production of cervical carcinoma in those animals depends on the repeated elimination of the newly induced breast carcinoma.

In women, the incidence of carcinoma of the cervix is second to that of the breast. But although estrogens have been used to produce cervical cancer in animals, it seems that in the etiology of human cervical cancer, the influence of hormone factors is outweighed by the influence of environmental factors [39–42].

Epidemiological studies of cancer of the cervix have revealed that several socioeconomical elements influence the incidence of that cancer. Cancer of the cervix seems to be more common among the poor than among the well-to-do. It is rare among Jewish women and practically nonexistent among virgins (nuns). The incidence of cervical cancer has been claimed to be higher among prostitutes than among other women.

On the basis of some epidemiological observations, it has been proposed that the frequency of coitus might be a determining factor in the incidence of cancer of the cervix. Coitus could either cause repeated trauma or facilitate the introduction of carcinogenic substances into the uterus. In the latter case, one would have to further assume that the cervix is more responsive to the carcinogen than the vaginal mucosa. Because cancer of the cervix is said to be less common among women with circumcised partners, smegma has often been incriminated as the source of the carcinogen. Exact information on the relationship between the frequency of coitus and the incidence of cervical cancer seems difficult to obtain.

The role of pregnancy in the incidence of cervical cancer is not clear. Some claim that repeated pregnancies increase the incidence of cancer of the cervix because of the repeated trauma to the cervix, but others feel that the increased incidence is not linked to pregnancy *per se* but rather to a socioeconomic environment that also favors repeated pregnancies. The potential role of herpes virus in cancer of the cervix is discussed in the section cancer and virus.

Cancer of the Body of the Uterus

In the past, it was customary to state that cancer of the body of the uterus was rare. Indeed, this type of cancer occurs much less frequently than cancer of the cervix. But whereas the relative frequency of cancer of the cervix versus cancer of the body of the uterus used to be 1:5, the incidence of cancer of the uterus has increased so much in the last decades that this ratio is now 1:2. The reasons for these changes in incidence are not clear.

Cancer of the body of the uterus is difficult to produce experimentally [43, 45, 46, 47, 48]. An epithelial adenoma of the body develops spontaneously in the old female rabbit. The tumor is histologically well differentiated, yet it invades the surrounding tissues and metastasizes. The tumor has been claimed to develop spontaneously in rabbits that have given birth to several litters; it was proposed that the pregnancies were associated with a toxemia that damages the liver. As a result, the liver's ability to catabolize hormones is lost in part, and the increased blood level of hormones is thought to stimulate the development of uterine cancer by some unknown mechanism. The hypothesis is ingenious, but it surely requires further support [45].

Adenocarcinomas of the uterus have been produced in rats under the constant influence of estrus. This is achieved by implanting a newborn rat testicle into a newborn female. These results suggest a carcinogenic role of endogenously produced hormones.

From these experimental observations, one gains the impression that adenocarcinoma of the fundus is influenced by sustained high levels of estrogens and anovulation. Clinical histories of patients with carcinomas of the body of the uterus provide further support for these concepts. Carcinoma of the body develops more frequently among women who have a history of postmenopausal endometrial hyperplasia, a condition likely to result from the unchecked elaboration of estrogen. Novak has pointed out similarities among the clinical histories of patients with postmenopausal hyperplasia of the endometrium and those with adenocarcinoma of the uterus. Both groups frequently have a background of obesity, diabetes, and hypertension. Whether these similarities result from a common etiology or coincidence is not certain. However, several reports have appeared suggesting that a link exists between cancer of the endometrium and feminizing tumors of the ovaries, the incidence of cancer of the body being greater among patients with ovarian tumors. Furthermore, the incidence of cancer of the body seems to be higher among women who have received sustained estrogen therapy, while cancer of the body is practically nonexistent among castrated women.

Cutler *et al.* have reported a significant increase in the incidence of endometrial cancer in women treated with estrogens for gonadal dysgenesis [545].

Again the role of hormones in the development of cancer of the endometrium remains unclear. The development of cultures of endometrial epithelial cells in a defined medium will certainly help in elucidating this intriguing problem [546, 547].

Progestational therapy has resulted in objective remission in 12% of the patients with metastatic endometrial cancer. Patients with well-differentiated tumors respond better than those with undifferentiated carcinoma. Of course, remission is not permanent; often it lasts only a few months. Yet the literature contains reports of remissions that lasted up to 9 years.

Other Uterine Tumors

Leiomyoma, a benign tumor common in humans, occurs in the body of the uterus. A similar tumor can be produced easily in the guinea pig by estrogen administration. In contrast, mice and rats are resistant to uterine leiomyomas. In guinea pigs, the development of this tumor is induced by estrogen and inhibited by progesterone and testosterone administration. The relationship between guinea pig and human leiomyomas is not clear. In guinea pigs, the effect of the hormone is not restricted to the uterus but induces leiomyomas throughout the organism, particularly in the stomach and intestine.

The hormonal influence on the development of uterine leiomyomas is further suggested by the modification that the tumor undergoes when the bearer's hormonal balance is altered. A uterine leiomyoma may regress and become hyalinized and even calcified after menopause. It enlarges and proliferates during pregnancy.

Uterine polyps have been produced in rabbits by the continuous administration of estrogen. They appear during the estrogenic life of the animal and disappear at menopause. Deciduomas of the uterus, endometrial moles, and myxoid and several mesodermal tumors of the endometrial stroma have been produced by the concomitant action of trauma and estrogen injection. However, these tumors (leiomyomas, uterine polyps, deciduomas) all disappear as soon as hormone administration is curtailed [46–48].

Ovarian Tumors

Ovarian tumors have been produced experimentally in at least two ways: administration of X-irradiation and implantation of the organ in the spleen. Implantation experiments were done first by Li and Gardner [49] and by Biskind and Biskind [50, 51].

The ovary is implanted in the spleen of a castrated animal. All the hormones excreted by the ovary pass through the liver via the portal vein. In fact, the hormones never reach the general circulation because they are metabolized in the liver. (Adding thyroid powder to the diet of mice reduces the frequency of ovarian tumors in the intrasplenic graphs.) Consequently, the inhibitory effect on LSH and FSH secretion by the hypophysis is never manifested. Thus, the animal has a peculiar endocrinological situation—it possesses ovarian tissue that secretes large amounts of estrogen, but it remains continuously under the influence of the hypophyseal stimulus. This uninterrupted hypophyseal stimulus induces hyperplasia of the ovarian tissue first, and cancer later.

However, in addition to the hormone, other factors are involved in the induction of cancer, because if one attempts to produce ovarian cancer in a strain of rats with a low incidence of spontaneous tumors, the implanted ovary develops only benign tumors (luteomas or granulosa cell tumors, see Fig. 16-13). Metastatic and transplantable ovarian carcinomas (see Fig. 6-14) are obtained only after the concomitant administration of a carcinogen [52].

The administration of total body doses of X-irradiation or the local irradiation of both ovaries of mice induces ovarian tumors, probably by interfering with the ovariohypophyseal hormonal interrelation. Indeed, no tumor occurs if only one ovary is irradiated. Thus, the mechanism is probably analogous to the one that operates in the case of the intrasplenic graft.

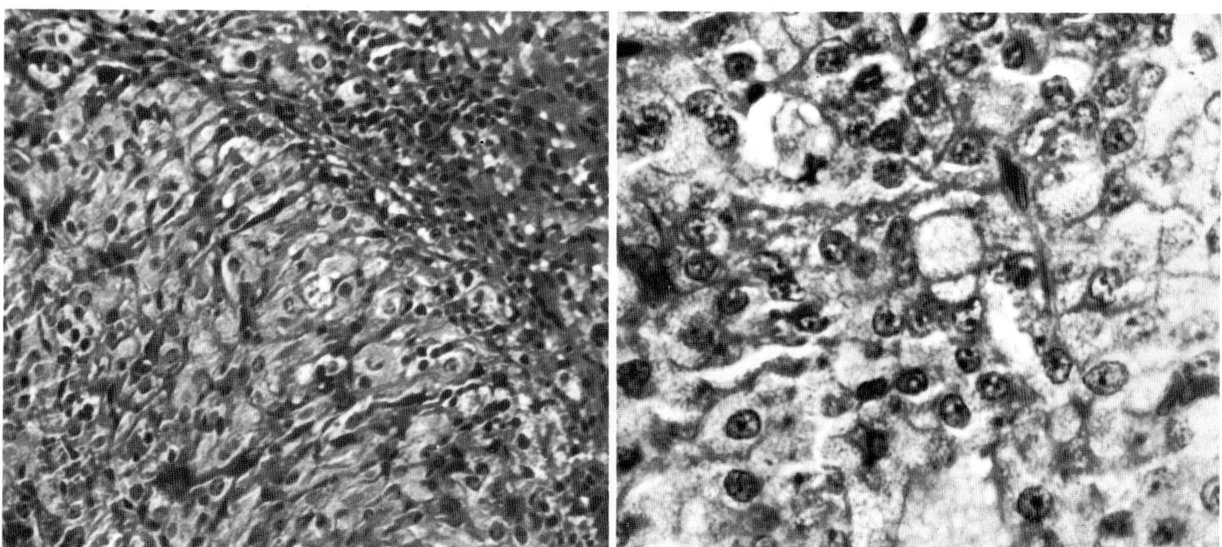

Fig. 16-13. Low- and high-power views of a luteoma produced by implantation of the ovary in a rat spleen

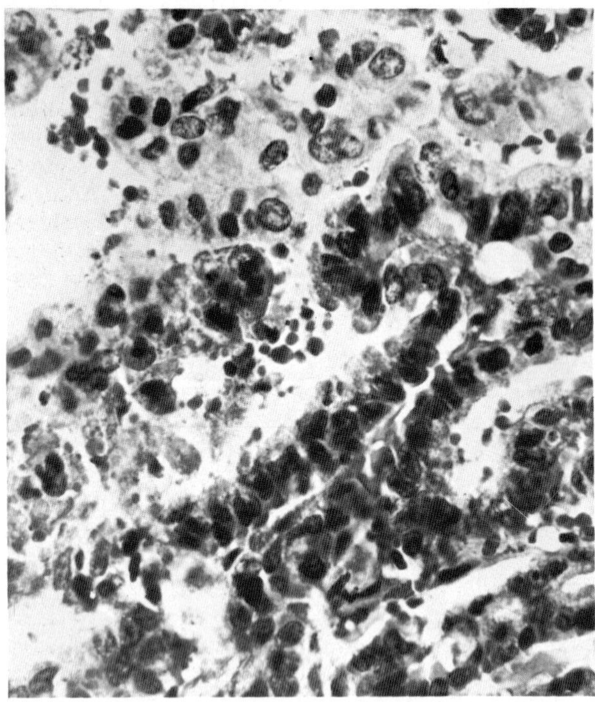

Fig. 16-14. Cancer of the ovary obtained after transplantation in spleen of rat whose vagina had been painted with methylcholanthrene weekly for 1 year

X-Irradiation interferes with the ovary's production of the normal quota of hormone, and there is less inhibition of the hypophyseal secretion of FSH and LSH. However, the responsiveness of the ovary to the gonadotropin, although disturbed by X-irradiation, is not completely abolished since the irradiated mouse may become pregnant and develop ovarian tumors after a few pregnancies. The appearance of ovarian tumors in irradiated animals is accelerated by methylcholanthrene administration or by parabiosis with castrated animals [44, 53–55]. In the latter case, the castrated animal contributes additional gonadotropins.

Cancer of the Adrenals

We have already mentioned that in castrated females a vicarious hypertrophy of the adrenal cortex develops soon after the operation. In mice, the hypertrophy evolves occasionally into a malignant tumor, which metastasizes and is transplantable. As a matter of fact, such tumors occur spontaneously in old female mice and may develop after feminization of castrated male mice. Although hypophysectomy, steroid injection, and the implantation of ovaries inhibit the development of these tumors, cortisone injection is without effect. Such results suggest that the adrenal tumor is under the influence of gonadotropins rather than ACTH.

In rats, ovariectomy leads only to a certain degree of adrenal hypertrophy. However, adrenocortical tumors have been produced in a special strain of rats by the administration of large amounts of estrogens. The transplantation of adrenals into the spleens of adrenalectomized rats leads to hypertrophy of the cortex, but no tumor develops.

Occasionally, pheochromocytomas have been observed in the adrenals of mice after castration or irradiation. These tumors are rare, and the mechanism of production is not clear. Pheochromocytomas occur spontaneously in the Wistar strain and can be induced by the administration of growth hormones in the Long-Evans strain of rats.

Cancer of the Hypophysis

Among experimental tumors, those of the hypophysis are of great interest because their study helped to elucidate some aspects of the physiology of the hypophysis and shed new light on the mechanism of carcinogenesis.

The hypophyseal tumors are interesting in at least two respects: (1) they secrete specific hypophyseal hormones, and (2) when transplanted, they go through various stages of dependency. Their survival at first depends on the hormonal environment in the host, but later the tumors may become autonomous [56–58].

The continuous administration of estrogens to mice leads to the formation of mammotropic tumors. The incidence of these tumors is modified by various factors: the strain of mice, the animal's sex, and the administration of androgens. Whereas mammotropic tumors develop readily in female C-57BL mice, only a few tumors develop in males. Furthermore, androgen administration inhibits the development of the tumors even in females. Extensive studies of C3H and CBA mice have failed to produce tumors of the hypophysis in those strains.

A thyrotropic tumor, different morphologically from the mammotropic tumor, can be produced in mice by ^{131}I administration or thyroidectomy. Thyrotropic tumors secrete large amounts of TSH, which can be detected by assaying the host's blood or by transplanting the tumor into hypophysectomized animals. Although TSH is the main hypophyseal hormone that is secreted, small amounts of gonadotropins are also found.

Total body doses or head irradiation leads to the development of adrenocorticotropic tumors of the hypophysis. These tumors are identified by: (1) their morphological characteristics, particularly the cells' staining properties (reaction with acid and basophilic reagent, the presence of PAS-positive material, and the reaction with aldehyde fuchsin); and (2) the nature of the hormone secreted, which occasionally may be detected by assaying the blood of the animal or by transplanting the tumor into a hypophysectomized host.

The animals in which adrenocorticotropic tumors have been transplanted present the following characteristics: (1) lipid depletion, enlarged cortical cells of the adrenals, leading to glandular hypertrophy; (2) atrophic lymphatic tissue, and (3) obesity.

Implantation of the adrenocorticotropic tumor leads to alteration in the host's adrenal. At first, nodules form in the adrenal cortex. These nodules contain tumors that are typical of the normal organ. In the next step, these nodules develop into dependent tumors, which may differ morphologically from their ancestors in the sense that they fail, for example, to react with the PAS reagent or the aldehyde fuchsin. The cells are thus completely agranular. It is interesting that these tumors continue to secrete large amounts of hormones—approximately ten times the normal values. Thus, the presence of the granules apparently is not related to the biosynthesis of the hormones, but rather to the hormone's storage mechanism.

Transplantation of the mammotropic tumor induces a proliferation of the ducts and the alveoli of the mammary glands; milk secretion is stimulated and the breast develops adenoid hyperplasia. Associated with this mammotropic effect is a marked somatotropic effect. The presence of these two different hormones in the same tissue raises an interesting question about the cellular origin of the two hormones: Are the mammotropic and somatotropic hormones secreted by a single cell or by two different cells?

When transplanted, most thyrotropic and mammotropic tumors are at first dependent—they grow successfully in hypophysectomized animals receiving estrogens or in thyroidectomized hosts. Some of these tumors metastasize, and even the transplanted metastases are dependent. However, after repeated transplantations, the tumors become autonomous and grow when transplanted even in normal hosts. All adrenocorticotropic tumors are autonomous from the beginning, even though their growth can be inhibited somewhat by the injection of adrenal secretions.

The passage from dependency to autonomy is progressive. In the first stages, the tumors are only relatively autonomous; they can still be influenced by the administration of antagonistic hormones (such as thyroid hormone in the thyrotropic tumor). In the last stages, the tumors become completely independent and are not influenced by hormone administration.

The molecular mechanism involved in the conversion of a hormone dependent into a hormone independent tumor is not known. Two sequences of molecular alterations have been contemplated: (1) a modification of the affinity of the receptor in the target organ for the hormone; (2) a modification of the genome. The first of these hypotheses is supported by work of Jensen and his associates [548, 549] who have shown that human mammary tumors, which are responsive to adrenalectomy, contain higher affinity and consequently more receptor sites for hormones than tumors which respond poorly to that procedure. Yet, we have seen that in animals a correlation between hormonal binding tumor incidence and growth does not always hold true. For further information on the role of receptors in cancer of the breast see [550].

The second hypothesis is in keeping with the hormone-gene theory. It postulates that the conversion of a hormone dependent into a hormone independent tumor results from a modulation of the mechanism regulating gene expression. Thus, normal response of the genome to hormonal stimulation would be lost in hormonal independent tumors. Although changes in RNA have often been described in cancer dependent on hormones for development, it remains to be established how these changes relate to hormonal carcinogenesis.

Tumors of the Prostate

Although common in man, prostate tumors are practically unknown in animals except dogs. In man, there are two types of prostatic tumors: benign hypertrophy and cancer of the prostate. Benign hypertrophy is a disease of old age. It occurs frequently after the sixth decade and consists of a benign hyperplasia of the periurethral glands. The tumoral process readily interferes with the evacuation of urine. Old dogs suffer from a similar disease, except that instead of being localized as in man, the disease involves all parts of the prostate.

Testosterone seems to be responsible for the development of the tumor in dogs. Testosterone injection stimulates the hyperplasia, whereas castration or estrogen administration prevents the development of the adenoma. Unfortunately, hormonal therapy seems to be of little help in man. Yet this does not preclude a hormonal origin of the disease. Indeed, prostatic adenomas have been claimed to be nonexistent in eunuchs and in patients suffering from pituitary infantilism.

In Britain and in the U.S., carcinoma of the prostate is responsible for at least 6% of the mortality among men. For some unknown reason, the disease is seldom encountered among Japanese and Chinese. Practically nothing is known of the etiology of carcinoma of the prostate. In fact, the disease is difficult to produce in animals experimentally. Prolonged administration of estrogens has led to squamous metaplasia of the prostatic epithelium in mice, and the development of spindle cell carcinomas has been described. But these tumors differ from the classic adenocarcinoma of the prostate observed in man. A tumor resembling the human adenocarcinoma in man has been produced by transplanting prostates in homologous hosts. However, cancer develops only if methylcholanthrene and testosterone are administered simultaneously.

The only clue as to the hormonal etiology of carcinoma of the prostate comes from the therapeutic effects of estrogens and castration. Huggins [59, 60] first made this important observation, one of the great contributions to cancer therapy. Estrogen administration retards, sometimes for a long time, the progress of cancer of the prostate even if metastases have developed. The patient's price for this lease on life at his advanced age is minimal: his breasts swell and he loses his libido. Castration seems to be even more efficacious than the administration of female hormones in controlling the progress of carcinoma of the prostate. Unfortunately, all patients do not respond to therapy, and the relief is seldom permanent. After a period of 6 months to several years, the tumor regains its original vigor and kills its victim.

Tumors of the Testicles

Interstitial cell tumors of the testicle rarely occur spontaneously in most experimental animals [61–64]. However, interstitial cell tumors are frequently observed in dogs, horses, and occasionally mice. The interstitial cell tumors observed in man are assumed to secrete androgen. They can be produced experimentally in mice by the administration of estrogens or a variety of compounds with estrogenic effects. In some experiments, the tumors were found to be transplantable, and metastases in the lymph nodes and lungs have been observed. The transplanted tumors can grow without estrogen administration; this autonomy depends upon the strain. Indeed, in some strains of mice estrogen administration must be continued to secure the survival of the transplant. The mechanism by which these tumors are produced is assumed to consist in the stimulation of the anterior lobe of the hypophysis under the influence of estrogens, which inhibit FSH secretion but stimulate ICSH secretion.

As would be expected, the administration of androgen or progesterone retards the development of the interstitial cell tumor. Thus, it is not surprising that interstitial cell tumors can be produced in castrated rats by implanting testicles in the spleen. However, such tumors do not metastasize and are not transplantable.

Teratomas of the testicles have been produced experimentally in roosters by administering zinc chloride during springtime. Similar tumors can be produced in other seasons if anterior hypophyseal hormone extracts are added to the zinc chloride. Partial resection of the testicles induces seminomas in birds. Partial destruction of the testicle by zinc chloride or partial resection of the organ is assumed to be responsible for stimulating the anterior lobe of the hypophysis.

Prolonged estrogen administration to cryptorchid mice of the BALB/C strain produces a high incidence of malignant Leydig cell tumors. The tumors develop even if the mice are hypophysectomized, which indicates that tumor development is not mediated through an indirect effect of estrogens on the hypothalamic hypophyseal systems.

When hypophysectomized cryptorchid mice are injected with diethylstilbestrol, 17-α-hydroxylase, 17-20 lyase, and 17-β-hydroxylase are reduced within 48 hours after the first injection. Three weeks after injection, the activity of these testicular enzymes drops to 10 or 15% of the control values. The hormone was not observed to affect other enzymes tested (glutamic oxalic transaminase, glucose-6-PO_4 dehydrogenase, lactate dehydrogenase, and isocitrate dehydrogenase). Estrogens added to the incubation mixture have no effect on the steroid enzyme. The steroid seems to interfere specifically with the biosynthesis of the enzyme involved in testosterone metabolism. The system provides a unique opportunity to follow the biochemical changes that take place in the formation of a malignant tumor [61].

Studies of the experimental production of testicular tumors have provided little information on their pathogenesis in human beings. Testicular tumors are rare in humans; they account for only 0.5% of malignant tumors in men. Four major histological types of testicular tumors are observed in men: seminomas, teratomas, Leydig cell tumors, and Sertoli cell tumors. Seminomas and teratomas account for more than 90% of testicular tumors; Leydig cell tumors, for 2 to 3%; and Sertoli cell tumors are very rare.

Most testicular tumors develop in men between the ages of 20 and 50. Undescended testes are ten times more susceptible to tumor development than normal testes. Whether the age incidence and the influence of cryptorchidism on the incidence of tumors indicate that the development of testicular tumors is hormonally influenced remains to be established. Many testicular tumors are associated with excessive hormone production, a point discussed elsewhere in this book.

Effect of Hormones on Cancer in Other Tissues

Hormones not only influence tumor production in the endocrine glands, but also affect the incidence of cancers of the kidney, bladder, lymphatic tissue, liver, skin, and subcutaneous tissue. Clear cell tumors of the kidney can be produced by estrogen administration in hamsters. But the incidence of tumors is reduced by the administration of other hormones, such as testosterone, progesterone, and deoxycorticosterone. The rate of development is accelerated by unilateral nephreotomy. The clear cell tumor has been transplanted in only one case as a dependent tumor. The acceleration of tumor growth by unilateral nephrectomy can be interpreted in two ways: either renal hypertrophy accelerates the development of the tumor, or a carcinogen is present in the urine and concentrated in larger amounts in a single kidney, rather than in both kidneys.

In mice, estrogens increase the incidence of lymphoma from 3 to 15 times. Castration enhances the effect of estrogen, but androgen administration reduces the incidence of spontaneous lymphoma in strains with a high incidence of leukemia and in mice exposed to X-irradiation. The administration of androgenic metabolic steroids is believed to induce hepatomas [551].

A retrospective study suggests that prenatal exposure to estrogens also leads to a number of benign conditions including transverse ridges (22%), abnormalities of the vaginal mucosa (56%) and adenosis (35%) [552].

Transplacental Cancer

Recent findings have generated new concern about the potential carcinogenicity of estrogen. A number of children born from mothers who received large doses of estrogen during pregnancy to prevent abortion developed clear cell adenocarcinomas of the vagina at an early age. Although this dramatic development is relatively infrequent even among children whose mothers received estrogens, the finding convincingly demonstrated that estrogen can be carcinogenic in humans. There is no explanation why only the vagina and not the breast or the ovary responded to the oncogenic stimulus.

Since these observations were made, a number of cancers, including brain tumors, have been produced experimentally by feeding carcinogens to pregnant rats [553, 554]. The mechanism by which large doses of estrogen cause cancer in humans is not known.

These problems assume particular significance because synthetic estrogens are, the world over, added to cattle feed. Therefore, it is fair to ask whether or not the inclusion of small amounts of estrogens in the diet might influence the incidence of cancer in the target organ in humans. At the present there is no straightforward answer to that question, but it would seem that the observation made of women who received iatrogenic doses of estrogen would tend to exclude the possibility. Indeed, the doses of female hormones ingested with meat are likely to be much lower than those administered iatrogenically [65, 66].

As for extending quantitative data obtained in mice to other species, it would be totally unrealistic at this point because of (1) the high susceptibility of the mice to cancer of the breast and (2) our lack of knowledge of the comparative biochemistry of estrogen in mice and men. Moreover, a great deal of epidemiological data have already been assembled in women who received prolonged administration of estrogen during and after menopause. These results do not suggest that iatrogenic amounts of estrogen are carcinogenic. If anything, they seem to delay the incidence of appearance of cancer of the breast. Inasmuch as these doses are much higher than what is likely to be absorbed by eating beef meat, the potential carcinogenicity of the hormones added to cattle feed seems to be academic. However, it is possible that beef would convert the hormone to an active proximate carcinogen which may be present in the meat we eat. Remote as it may be, the possibility may be worthwhile to explore, but this information cannot be obtained by administering estrogens to mice and will require instead that concentrated metabolic studies be made in cattle.

Some Biochemical Effects of Endocrine Cancer

Investigations during the last five decades have clearly established that the incidence, type, and growth of some cancers are influenced by hormones. Of course, some cancers produce excessive amounts of hormones that influence the host. This aspect of the relationship of cancer and hormones is discussed in another section of this chapter.

Hormones may either increase or reduce the incidence or the rate of growth of susceptible cancers. The susceptible cancer usually, but not necessarily, develops in a target organ. The hormone that normally stimulates the target organ also stimulates the cancer development, while the antagonistic hormone inhibits its development. Thus, tumors that are susceptible to the action of hormones respond in ways resembling the response of the normal tissues, and one can assume that the receptors and the regulators of the hormonal effect are intact in those cells. These dependent tumors become autonomous after several transplantations, and their growth and differentiation are no longer influenced by the hormonal environment of the host.

Although the study of the effects of hormones on cancer have revealed a new aspect of carcinogenesis, they have also raised such new problems as those concerning: (1) the mechanism of hormonal stimulation of tumor growth; (2) the nature of the molecular and cellular changes that take place when a tumor is converted from a dependent into an independent tumor; and (3) the importance of hormones in human cancer.

At least two major aspects of the mechanism of hormonal stimulation of tumor growth need to be considered: the mechanism by which the intracellular levels of activity of the stimulatory hormones are increased when spontaneous cancer of the target organ develops, and the mechanism by which the hormone stimulates cancer growth.

Despite many studies made in humans, there is little conclusive information on the hormonal levels in patients with cancer of the breast or prostate, for example. This aspect of the problem will be discussed below.

The levels of the stimulatory hormone might be increased in several ways: (1) increased production of the hormone by the source organ, (2) decreased inactivation or catabolism of the hormones by the specialized organs involved in these metabolic processes, or (3) increased responsiveness of the target organs. Although it is sometimes easy to determine what type of mechanism is operating in experimental tumors, little is known of what happens in spontaneous tumors.

Undoubtedly, comparative studies of hormone metabolism in normal and tumoral tissues should provide new clues as to the nature of this mechanism. Such studies have been undertaken in several laboratories; only a few examples will be discussed here. We have already mentioned the studies by Samuels' group on testicular tumors. Studies of steroid metabolism in normal and malignant lymphocytes have shown that 11-OH dehydrogenase, the enzyme that converts cortisol to cortisone, is active in normal and malignant lymphocytes. The dehydrogenase activity is reversible. When intact cells were incubated, it was found that the reductive reaction was prominent in the normal lymphocytes, while the oxidation was favored in the lymphoma cell. Unfortunately, these differences between lymphomas and normal cells disappeared when homogenates were prepared. Furthermore, the data are only suggestive because the results have not been subjected to rigid kinetic investigations or to statistical analysis. To attribute the metabolic changes to cancer would require comparing the malignant and the immature lymphocytes. The shift in the relative rates of conversion of cortisol to cortisone is more likely to be linked to cellular proliferation or immaturity than to carcinogenesis.

If more extensive studies were to support these differences between malignant and nonmalignant lymphocytes, the interpretation of the results proposed by Berliner and his associates [67] would become most attractive. These authors assume that a target cell controls its own fate (which may include proliferation, maturation, or death) by regulating the molecular concentration of the active hormone. Since in lymphocytes it is cortisol and not cortisone that limits growth and triggers maturation and death, the reduction of cortisone to cortisol should be prominent in the normal lymphocyte, whereas the reverse should occur in malignant lymphocytes. This theory is further supported by the studies of the effect of steroid hormones on the growth of fibroblasts in tissue culture.

Hormones with different molecular configurations have different inflammatory, gluconeogenic, and lymphocytolytic effectiveness *in vivo*. The effectiveness of the hormone *in vivo* correlates with the inhibitory effect of that hormone on fibroblast growth in tissue culture. The activities of the respective hormones vary both *in vivo* and *in vitro*, depending upon the structure of the molecule. It has been observed that the resistance of the fibroblasts to the effect of the hormone seems to depend upon their ability to catabolize it. Yet since fibroblasts may also develop resistance toward the biological effects of molecules that are not metabolized, resistance cannot always be the result of an increase in catabolic pathways. Other mechanisms, such as change in membrane permeability, must also come into play.

Sweat [68] has compared steroid metabolism in normal and malignant tissues of the female reproductive tract. On the basis of these studies, he was able to divide these tissues into two major classes: those that degrade and those that synthesize steroid hormones. The metabolic properties are related to the source of the tissue rather than to the passage from normal to cancerous tissue, although the rates of enzyme activity differ somewhat in normal and malignant tissues of the same origin. Normal endometrium and benign or malignant tumors derived from it have active catabolic pathways. Normal ovaries and functional, benign, or malignant tumors derived from them engage mainly in steroid synthesis. The key step is the 17-hydroxylation of progesterone. Tissues of endometrial origin are unable to perform this reaction; as a result, side chain cleavage and aromatization are impossible, and the steroid molecule is driven into the catabolic pathway. In contrast, ovarian tissues can perform 17-hydroxylation, which is then followed by side-chain cleavage and aromatization to yield androstenedione and finally estrogen. Although these findings may someday help us understand carcinogenesis, they are more directly related to the influence of the tumor on the host.

It is impossible to describe the role of hormones in converting a normal target cell into a cancer cell since the homones' mode of action and the intricacies of the first steps of carcinogenesis are not known. As we shall see, hormones probably play a role more likely to be stimulatory to that of a carcinogen.

Much effort has been devoted to testing metabolic products or synthetic derivatives of steroids for their carcinogenicity on other than target tissues, without much success. In spite of previous claims that steroids may be biologically converted into active carcinogens, it seems now well established that hormones are not carcinogenic *per se*, even at high and prolonged doses. There is usually a need for other factors—such as heredity, a cancer virus, or the administration of a carcinogen at a distance from the target site—to produce cancer with hormones. A typical example of this is the failure to induce ovarian cancer in rats by implanting the organ in the spleen, unless a carcinogen is also administered. For all these reasons, it seems more appropriate to consider hormones' effect on cancer development in light of the Berenblum theory of promoter and inducer.

The conversion of a dependent into an autonomous tumor seems to be a primary event in carcinogenesis. An accurate understanding of the nature of the factors that determine such a transformation would be valuable. One must keep in mind, however, that dependent cancers metastasize, invade, and kill. Consequently, carcinogenesis has already taken place when the tumor passes from a dependent to an autonomous state.

Therefore, the dependent tumor seems to lack many normal intracellular homeostatic mechanisms, and the passage from a dependent to an autonomous state appears to involve further derangements in the normal control mechanisms. To be sure, the passage from a dependent to an autonomous state is associated with: (1) histological changes (mainly in the direction of dedifferentiation), (2) alterations in the mosaic of enzyme activities, and (3) the appearance of chromosomal anomalies. These changes are several steps removed from the primary insult that triggers carcinogenesis. In fact, some cancers (for example, the so-called minimal deviation hepatomas, which will be discussed later) grow, metastasize, invade, and kill in the absence of such changes.

The relationship of cancer to hormones in humans is of considerable significance. Both men and women undergo drastic changes in their hormonal balance in a lifetime. Persistent distortion of the homeostatic balance in man might lead to cancer in the target organs. To contemplate the simplest example, one may wonder whether persistently high levels of androgens are responsible for the development of cancer of the prostate, or whether high levels of estrogen are responsible for the development of cancer of the breast or the endometrium. The correct answers to these questions presuppose knowledge of the molecular structure of the active hormone and its concentration in the target cell.

Studies of hormonal levels in blood, however, can provide clues as to the role that specific hormones might play in the development of a given cancer. Such studies must involve large population groups with different backgrounds, and the analysis must be repeated frequently. Modern methods of steroid analysis, especially the development of sensitive automated equipment, have made it possible to pursue such investigations with some hope of success.

The significance of these types of studies stems from two main observations related to the role of hormones in carcinogenesis: (1) the incidence of some cancer is related to the hormonal environment, and (2) a change in the hormonal balance can interfere with the growth of some tumors.

Obviously, interest in determining plasma and urine steroid levels is not new. It started soon after Beaston's observation [69, 70] that castration delays the progress of advanced breast cancer, and the work of Huggins [71–74], demonstrating that castration and estrogen administration delay the progress of cancer of the prostate. Analyses of plasma and urine steroids in cancer patients have been given a new impetus with the development of methods for steroid analysis (paper and gas chromatography, isotope techniques, automation).

In spite of the considerable interest in these types of studies, little convincing evidence has emerged. One of the earliest studies in this field was that of Dao and Huggins, who claim that one can determine whether a patient with breast cancer will respond to adrenalectomy by investigating two parameters: the titers of urinary estrogens measured by a biological method, and the histological features of the mammary tumor. The authors found that patients with well-differentiated tumors and high estrogen excretion responded best to adrenalectomy.

These results are in keeping with observations made on the effect of estrogens on experimental breast cancer. The empirical observations of Bulbrook, Hayward, and Ireenwood [75, 76] and Atkins [77] are somewhat more difficult to understand, yet these are some of the most publicized results, possibly because the investigators endeavored to develop a method that would be readily usable for determining whether a cancer patient should be subjected to such heroic therapy as hypophysectomy or adrenalectomy.

To determine whether a cancer patient should receive hormonal therapy is simple because either the patient responds or little harm is done. But a useless hypophysectomy or adrenalectomy can cause much unnecessary discomfort and pain. Therefore, a method for discriminating between responding and nonresponding patients is of the greatest value. The London group claims to have discovered such a method. These investigators measured urinary estrogens, gonadotropins, pregnanediol, 17-hydroxycorticosteroid, and the total and fractionated 11-deoxy-17-oxysteroids in patients with advanced breast cancer. The levels of two of the compounds studied varied consistently depending upon whether the patient was responding to the hypophysectomy or adrenalectomy. In the responding cases, the levels of the etiocholanolone were high and those of the 17-hydroxycorticosteroids were low. The reverse was found in unresponding cases.

On the basis of these observations, the authors were able to calculate a discriminant. When the value obtained for the discriminant is positive, the patient is responsive; when negative, the patient is unresponsive. Obviously, such important claims are not to be underestimated, and it is hoped that other institutions will try to develop similar or perhaps better methods of discrimination.

However, the results of Bulbrook and his associates have been criticized on various accounts. First, the correlation is much better with hypophysectomy than with adrenalectomy, and therefore the reliability of the test has been questioned. Further, one might question the significance of a test that compares the level of one 11-deoxy-17-ketosteroid with a population of 17-hydroxyketosteroids. Yet the important element in these studies is that they distinguish between responsive and unresponsive patients. Undoubtedly, more investigations are needed, and they should include more detailed studies of plasma and urinary steroid metabolites and investigations of the biotransformations of the hormones responsible for a specific pattern in blood and urine.

Dao [78] has applied the more sophisticated methods of gas-liquid chromatography to the study of urinary steroids of pre- and postmenopausal women. He compared the results obtained in normal patients with those found in patients with breast cancer and was unable to confirm Bulbrook's results, mainly because the use of gas liquid chromatography caused a marked elevation of the levels of 17-ketosteroids.

The Norwegian investigators Nissen-Meyer and Sanner [79] studied the urinary excretion of estrone, pregnanediol, and pregnanetriol in a series of breast cancers. Their studies provide evidence for the continuous secretion of female hormones at physiological levels up to 25 years after menopause. Immediately after the onset of menopause, the hormone levels decrease for a few years, then increase again and reach a new maximum between 10 and 15 years after the onset of menopause. The source of the hormones seems to be dual: the ovaries and the adrenal. The adrenal probably furnishes the major part of the hormone. The adrenal secretion of female hormones can be interrupted by the administration of a corticosteroid (prednisone); the ovarian secretion is blocked by irradiation of the ovaries. Although the administration of low doses of corticosteroids may interfere with the progress of metastasis, irradiation of the ovaries appears to have no effect on the progress of breast cancer in humans.

Results of hormonal studies of the blood or urinary distribution in patients suffering from cancer of the prostate are even more inconsistent than the reports on similar studies on patients with breast cancer. Gallagher [80] could find no substantial change in the androgen levels in patients with carcinoma of the prostate. But the possibility cannot be excluded that, even in the absence of quantitative differences, qualitative differences could be demonstrated if hormone levels were studied with modern methods of steroid analysis.

Stern and her associates [81] have claimed that the pattern of hormonal excretion in patients with cancer of the prostate and the breast differs from the pattern found in noncancerous individuals. Unfortunately, these investigators studied only a small number of patients, so a conclusive evaluation of the results is not possible.

Since human cancer can be influenced by hormone therapy, it is not surprising that the study of estrogen- or androgen-dependent breast cancer has been encouraged. Kim [82] has studied a rat mammary adenocarcinoma the growth of which can be influenced by a variety of hormonal treatments, including the administration of estrogens, progesterone, and a combination of progesterone and estrogen, and by adrenalectomy and ovariectomy. On the basis of these extensive investigations, Kim concluded that most of the hormonal effects were mediated through the pituitary and that the growth of a breast cancer is roughly related to the level of prolactin in the host's plasma. Kim claims that in addition to the effect of the steroids on the tumor, which is mediated through the hypophysis, there is a slight but significant direct effect. Tumor growth is inhibited by large doses of estrogen or small doses of androgen. Tumor growth is stimulated, especially in hypophysectomized animals, by the combined administration of estrogen and progesterone. As might have been anticipated, adrenalectomy is successful in controlling the growth of breast cancer in rats only if the function of the ovaries has been completely suppressed.

Japanese investigators have obtained an androgen-dependent mouse mammary tumor from a spontaneous mouse mammary tumor. The original tumor was hormone independent at the start. The tumor was transformed into an entirely androgen-dependent tumor by serial passage from male to male. The administration of estrogen to the castrated or noncastrated tumor-bearing males suppresses the growth and induces regression of the existing tumor. This is an unusual hormone dependency for a breast carcinoma, but it is reminiscent of the hormonal response of carcinoma of the prostate in man.

Carcinogens, Their Metabolism and Mode of Action

A great number of chemical substances with different structures produce cancer after local application, injection, or ingestion. Pure carcinogens have been extracted from natural substances (such as tar) and have been synthesized.

The first observation that the repeated local application of tar leads to cancer was made in 1775 by a clairvoyant clinician, Sir Percivall Pott [83], who described carcinoma of the scrotum in English chimney sweepers and suggested that the tumors were induced by the tar that accumulated in skin folds. Almost another 200 years passed before Yamagiwa and Itchikawa [84] demonstrated that tar is carcinogenic in animals. By painting the ears of rabbits with coal tar for months, these Japanese investigators produced metastasizing spindle cell carcinomas. This discovery stimulated investigators throughout the world to isolate pure substances responsible for the development of cancer. Tar was thus extracted with various solvents, and the extracts were distilled. These painstaking attempts to produce cancer with a pure substance were fruitless until Mayneord [85] remarked that the carcinogenic tar has three absorption bands: one at 4000 A, another at 4180 A, and another at 4400 A. Thus, by using spectral analysis as a criterion of fractionation, Sir Alexander Kennaway [86] finally succeeded in 1930 in producing cancers with the 1,2,5,6-dibenzanthracene. Since that historical discovery, numerous derivatives of anthracene, phenanthrene, and benzene pyrene have been demonstrated to be carcinogenic.

A large number of carcinogenic compounds ranging from minerals to steroids are now known. Classically, the most active chemical carcinogenic substances are divided into a number of groups: among them are the aromatic hydrocarbons, the derivatives of azobenzene, the derivatives of amino-4-stilbene, and aminofluorene.

The mode of action of a carcinogen varies with its molecular structure; for example, whereas polycyclic hydrocarbons induce cancer at the site of application, the administration of azo dyes and aminofluorene derivatives induces cancer at a distance.

Polycyclic Hydrocarbons

The polycyclic hydrocarbons with less than four conjugated benzene rings are not carcinogenic. Among those with four benzene rings, only benzene-3,4-phenanthrene is moderately carcinogenic, while benzo-1,2-anthracene and possibly chrysene are carcinogenic, but very mildly so. In contrast, 5 of the 15 five-ring conjugates of benzene are carcinogenic. Few of the polycyclic hydrocarbons with a higher number of benzene rings have been studied, but two of the various possible arrangements of a six-benzene ring polycyclic compound are carcinogenic.

1,2,5,6-Dibenzanthracene produces skin cancer but is even more effective in producing sarcoma when injected into connective tissue. Whereas the 1,2,7,8-dibenzanthracene is slightly active, the 1,2-benzanthracenes 1,2,3,4 and 1,2,6,7 are inactive.

A variety of substitutions may modify the carcinogenic properties of the naked conjugated rings. Among the substitutions, the addition of a methyl group plays a primordial role. In general, hydrogenation of the hydrocarbon leads to a reduction or a complete loss of the carcinogenic properties, while methylation activates the carcinogenic properties [85–88].

The addition of the methyl group to the polycyclic ring may influence its carcinogenicity in two ways: by the position of the methyl group on the ring and by the number of methyl groups added to the ring. Thus, methylation may generate carcinogenicity in a polycyclic ring that is normally noncarcinogenic, or it may enhance preexisting carcinogenicity. This is particularly true in the case of dimethyl derivatives versus monomethyl compounds. (There are exceptions, especially if the methyl group is substituted on one of the lateral benzene rings.) For example, anthracene and phenanthrene are noncarcinogenic, but the 1,10-dimethyl derivatives of phenanthrene are strongly carcinogenic. Similarly, although the benzo-1,2-anthracene is only a weak carcinogen, the 9-methyl derivative is moderately carcinogenic, and the 9,10-dimethyl is strongly carcinogenic.

The carcinogenicity of compounds made of 5-benzene rings is markedly increased when two hydrogens of one of the rings are substituted with methyl groups. Thus, 9,10-methyldibenzanthracene is one of the most potent carcinogens in mice. Sarcomas are produced with the injection of 0.4 gamma of that material. Methyl derivatives of anthracene are inactive.

The introduction of an intracyclic nitrogen to form acridines reduces the carcinogenic activity. Methyl derivatives of the acridines may or may not be carcinogenic, depending on the relative positions of the N-acridine and the methyl group. For example, whereas the 1,10-dimethyl derivative of benzo-5,6-acridine is noncarcinogenic, the 1,10, 2,10, and 3,10 derivatives of the benzo-7,8-acridines are carcinogenic. If a substitution involves the methyl group itself, the carcinogenic properties are usually reduced.

Among the carcinogenic derivatives of benzene pyrene, the 3,4-benzene pyrene, which is found in tar (800 mg/kg), occupies a prominent place. The compound was isolated from coal tar and prepared synthetically. It proved to be one of the most potent carcinogens available. The addition of an extra benzene group annihilates the carcinogenic properties. Some of the noncarcinogenic and carcinogenic polycyclic hydrocarbons are shown in Fig. 16-15.

Cholanthrene has four benzene rings and one pentene ring (see Fig. 16-16). Cholanthrene is only mildly carcinogenic, but the methyl derivative, 20-methylcholanthrene, is one of the most effective carcinogens and is frequently used in experimental carcinogenesis. This potent carcinogen can be synthesized from natural compounds, such as cholic acid and cholesterol.

This description of chemical carcinogens could be pursued almost indefinitely. Such an endeavor would be of interest, but the relationships between molecular structure and carcinogenicity may be more relevant.

Although it is now established that most carcinogens react with tissue constituents only after metabolic conversion, it was at first believed that the carcinogenic substance was directly responsible for the cellular changes that lead to cancer. This notion brought investigators to study the relationship between the carcinogen's electronic structure and its carcinogenicity. These early studies remain significant because if they did not permit direct identification of the mode of action of the carcinogen, they helped to recognize those portions of the molecule that were most likely to react with cellular macromolecules, including DNA and enzymes that might convert inactive into active metabolites.

I. UNSUBSTITUTED POLYCYCLIC HYDROCARBONS (NOT CARCINOGENIC)

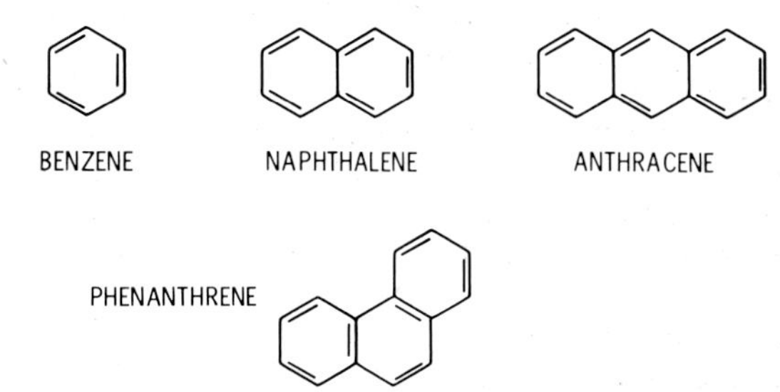

II. CARCINOGENS OF FOUR UNSUBSTITUTED CONJUGATED RINGS

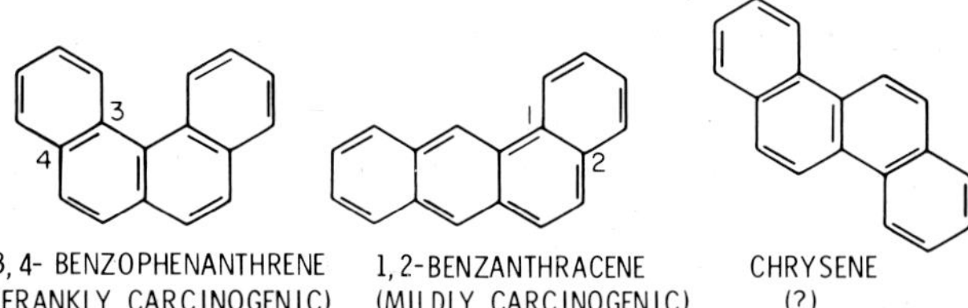

III. CARCINOGENS OF FIVE UNSUBSTITUTED CONJUGATED RINGS

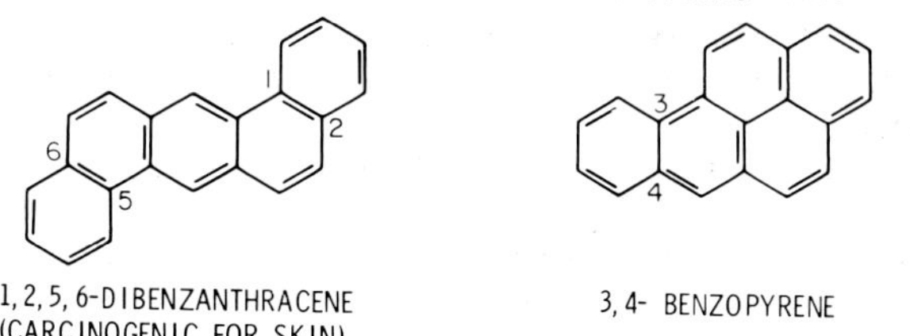

Fig. 16-15. Polycyclic hydrocarbons

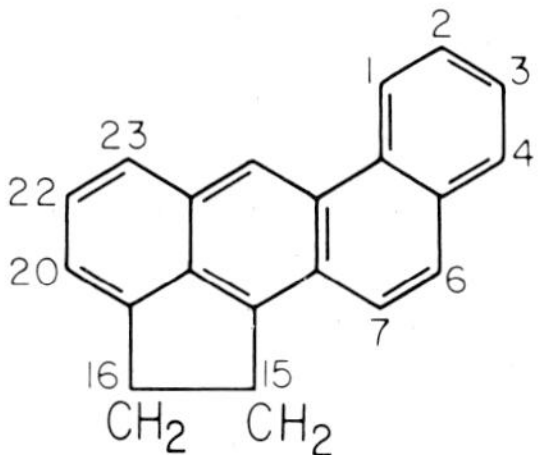

Fig. 16-16. Cholanthrene

Schmidt was the first (1938) to attempt to correlate the carcinogenic properties of aromatic hydrocarbons with their electronic structure. His hypothesis is of only historical value because it is based on an oversimplified concept of the electronic structure of the hydrocarbon.

Studies of the electronic structures of a variety of hydrocarbons led Pullman [90] to the following generalizations. First, the molecules of carcinogenic substances contain a region, called the "K region," that has a high electronic density (a region associated with a mesophenanthrenic type of bond and having a high index of mobile binding). Second, the carcinogen may or may not contain a second region ("L region") that is mesoanthracenic and characterized by a high free-valence index. And, third, a characteristic carcinogenic substance always contains a very active K region. Furthermore, if in addition to the K region an L region is present, the latter must be weak to insure carcinogenicity.

These assumptions imply that a carcinogenic substance combines with some vital biochemical component in the cell through the K region, while a combination at the L region interferes with binding through the K region. Therefore, if the L region is very active, the K region loses its capacity to react. That the presence of the K region is in someway linked to carcinogenicity has been verified in several laboratories through: (1) a quantitative theoretical verification, and (2) a chemical verification.

The first verification method consists of trying to define the K and L regions in a number of hydrocarbons using specific electronic indices. Then an attempt is made to find denominators common to all carcinogens on the basis of the quantitative results. These investigations led Pullman to the following general assumption: "the carcinogenic power of a polycyclic hydrocarbon is determined by an existence of a K region whose complex index, EOP+EPC minimum, is equal or inferior to 3.31 β. If the carcinogen also contains an L region, then the complex index EOP+EPC of the L region should be superior or equal to 5.66 β.* Thus, substances without a K region or with low K regions and a high L region are inactive. Many observations support this general concept. Indeed, a large number of compounds with an L region were found to be inactive as carcinogens. In contrast, dibenzanthracene 1,2 and 1,5 is active because the addition of lateral nuclei to the anthracenic molecule increases the reactivity of the K region and decreases that of the L region. Benzene-3,4-pyrene has a very active K region and no L region (see Fig. 16-17). (In fact, Pullman considered benzo-3,4-pyrene as a derivative of 1,2-benzanthracene in which the L regions had disappeared.)

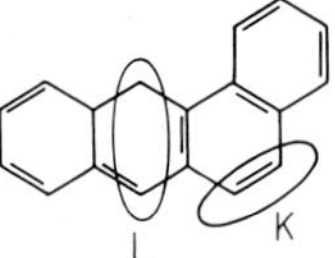

Fig. 16-17. The K and L regions of benzene-3,4-pyrene

Exceptions to this general rule are known. For example, the 3,4-benzophenanthrene and the dibenzophenanthrene 1-3, 1-4 both have K regions and no L region. However, neither compound is carcinogenic. Pullman thinks that in these two cases the departure from the general theory results from the fact that all his calculations were based on the assumption that the hydrocarbons' molecules are planar.

The notion that there exists a correlation between the electronic structure and the carcinogenic properties must be reconciled with the finding that the active carcinogen is often a metabolite of the former. The discrepancy between the Pullman theory and the new observation is not as formidable as it may seem at first, because the Pullman correlation may well express the capacity of cellular metabolism to transform the noncarcinogenic compound into a carcinogenic metabolite.

If the electronic calculations are correct, an investigator should be able to predict the chemical reactivity of the L and K regions. Furthermore, if the assumptions with respect to the correlation between the electronic structure and carcinogenicity are correct, it should be possible on the basis of such calculations to predict the carcinogenic activity of the substituted hydrocarbons. The Pullman theory is supported by the study of the carcinogenic properties of the methylated derivatives. Indeed, the addition of a methyl group to a carcinogen or a polycyclic hydrocarbon increases the reactivity for the K region and makes the region more electrophilic. These changes in the electric charge in the K region as calculated are paralleled by an increase in the carcinogenic properties of the methylated compound as compared to the naked conjugated ring. The methylation of position 9 of benzanthracene is most conspicuous in that respect.

Herndon has re-examined the K and L region hypothesis of Pullman and has provided further evidence in support of the correlation between electronic structure and carcinogenicity [555].

Various biological observations further support the Pullman theory of carcinogens' mode of action. These observations stem from the metabolic alteration of the carcinogen—namely, binding to protein and hydroxylation. In some cases, the carcinogens bind to protein in the area of the K regions.

It has been repeatedly observed that all carcinogenic substances are bound to proteins in tissue. However, some compounds that are not carcinogenic have been found to bind also. James and Elizabeth Miller first demonstrated the binding of carcinogens to liver proteins using amino azo dyes and later 2-acetylaminofluorene.

These studies have been extended by Heidelberger [91], who used labeled hydrocarbons and measured

* Translated from Pullman's *Cancérisation par les Substances Chimiques et Structure Moléculaire*. EOP=energy of orthopolarization; EPC=energy of parapolarization.

their binding to skin proteins at various times after a single application of the hydrocarbon. These authors found that in general there is a correlation between the amount of radioactive substance bound and its carcinogenicity, except for 1,2,3,4-benzanthracene, which is actively bound and is not carcinogenic. 2-6-Dimethylbenzanthracene (a very weak carcinogen) is also bound, but only slightly. The binding of 9-methylanthracene has been claimed also to occur extensively, but Heidelberger has shown that this is due to a high order of zero time binding.

Further investigations by Heidelberger demonstrated that the binding of active carcinogens to proteins is not due to absorption or to ionic or van der Waals bonds, but that true covalent bonds form between the carcinogen and the protein. By treating the protein with hydrazine, Heidelberger demonstrated that the binding occurred through the formation of a peptide bond. Furthermore, after treatment of the protein to which the labeled carcinogen is bound with pepsin, essentially no radioactivity is released. But if the peptides prepared by peptic digestion of the bound protein are further hydrolyzed with alkali, an acidic radioactive compound is obtained.

On the basis of the Pullman theory outlined previously, Heidelberger assumed that the acidic compound must be the 2-phenylphenanthrene-3,2′-dicarboxylic acid (PDA). The investigators tested the binding ability of PDA and found that it could not be bound to proteins. Tests with synthetic derivatives established that binding required an intact ring with an adequate K region.

These studies of Heidelberger and his group confirmed Pullman's predictions with respect to the binding site of the carcinogen with biochemical compounds. Yet they provide no evidence that the binding is part of the process of carcinogenesis.

Because of the role that metabolites might play in carcinogenesis, the elucidation of the metabolic conversion of the polycyclic hydrocarbons assumes special importance. Boyland has investigated the metabolism of phenanthrene, anthracene, and 1,2-benzanthracene. These studies were performed either by isolating the metabolites in urine or by incubating the hydrocarbon with microsomes in the presence of $NADH_2$. Such experiments reveal that two types of metabolites are formed: diols and mercaptopuric acids. Theoretically, the diols can be formed by two mechanisms—direct hydroxylation or intermediary formation of epoxides. Boyland believes that the biochemical conversion of the aromatic polycyclic hydrocarbons involves the intermediate formation of epoxide. Epoxides are highly reactive compounds that can be expected to react with water or glutathione to yield either dihydrodihydroxy derivatives or mercapturic acid precursors [7].

Enzymes were assumed to be involved in the metabolic perhydroxylation because the metabolite always contains a *trans* stereochemical configuration, whereas the perhydroxylation obtained by organic reactions has a *cis* configuration [87].

The first step in the metabolism of polycyclic hydrocarbons is carried out by the "mixed function oxidases" (see below). The product of the addition of molecular oxygen to the substrate may either be (a) reduced nonenzymatically and yield a phenol which will in turn form conjugates with glucuronic acid or sulfate, (b) be hydrated by an epoxide hydrase yielding the dihydrodiol, (c) react directly enzymatically with glutathione, or (d) bind with DNA, RNA or proteins [556] (Fig. 16-18).

Boyland has proposed that glutathione kinase or aryl glutathione transferase may be involved in the reaction of the epoxide with glutathione. The enzymic removal of glutamic and then of glycine residues yields the cysteine derivative, which by acetylation of its free amino group yields the mercapturic acid.

Inasmuch as the polycyclic hydrocarbon contains several double bonds that could react with oxygen to form epoxide, one might anticipate that various kinds of diols or mercapturic derivatives would be formed [90]. Boyland has shown that, indeed, a number of different metabolites are found in the urine after phenanthrene administration; and, judging from the relative amounts of metabolites formed, the epoxide's formation appears to proceed to extents that vary with the bond order. For example, in the 9:10 double bond, the bond order is 0.775, and it is 0.702 for the 3:4 bond. Substitutes of the 9:10 bond are more abundant *in vivo* (in urine) or *in vitro* (in microsomes). A similar correlation between bond order and metabolite formation has been observed for benzanthracene derivatives.

The reaction of the 5:6 bond of benzanthracene is of particular interest on two counts. First, it is reactive. Indeed, the 5:6 bond corresponds to the K region, which, according to previous beliefs, was not indispensable to metabolic conversion, except for binding to protein or nucleic acid. And second, the metabolite that results from the formation of an epoxide at the 5:6 double bond is a mercapturic acid, whereas diols are formed at the expense of the other double bonds. This selective reactivity of the 5:6 epoxide is explained by assuming that the 5:6 epoxide is a good substrate for the glutathione kinase.

Most of the epoxides that have been detected among the microsomal metabolites are "K region epoxides." It can, however, not be excluded that non K region epoxides are also formed and that the latter may play an important role in carcinogenicity. The complexity of the mode of binding of epoxides to DNA is illustrated by a study in which the product benzo(a)pyrene bound to cellular DNA was compared to the products of the reaction of benzo(a)pyrene, 4,5-oxide to DNA in aqueous ethanol solution. The products of the binding of benzo(a)pyrene *in vivo* were different from those formed when the oxide was bound *in vitro*. On the basis of these findings, Baird *et al.* suggest that the binding of polycyclic hydrocarbons to DNA may be more complex than the simple formation of K region epoxides [557].

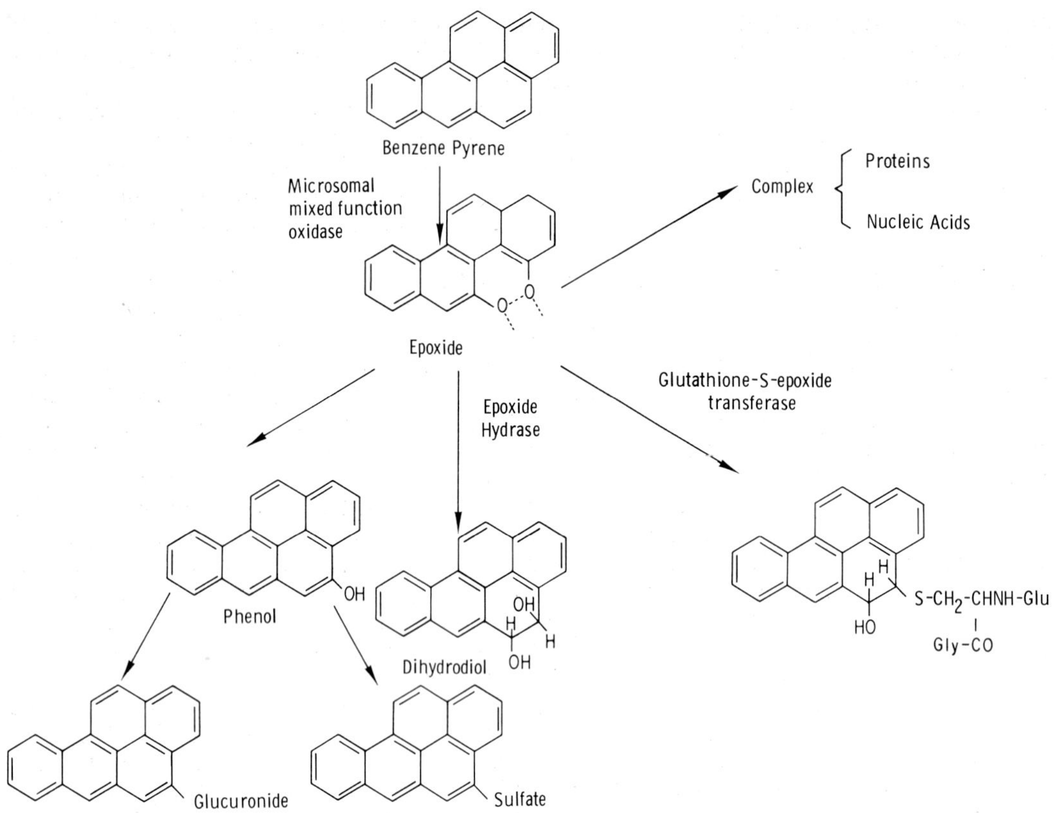

Fig. 16-18. Metabolism of K region epoxide

An important question that needs to be answered is whether the metabolites (diols and mercapturic derivatives) are products of detoxification or whether they are active carcinogens. Boyland believes that they are products of detoxification. As for the intermediate, the epoxide, it could alkylate nucleic acid (N_7 of guanine) or be rapidly converted to the inactive metabolite.

Although these assumptions were at first difficult to prove because when epoxides were isolated they were shown to be less carcinogenic than the parent compounds, it became clear that epoxides are formed *in vitro*, that they react with proteins and nucleic acids and that synthetic epoxides are more effective in inducing mutations in bacteria and in mammalian cells [558, 559].

The demonstration that epoxides are formed in microsomal preparations was made in several laboratories [19]. We will only briefly describe some experiments done by Heidelberger [560, 561] and his associates.

These investigators were able to demonstrate the formation of epoxides using labeled dibenzanthracene after inhibition of the epoxide hydrase which converts the highly reactive epoxide to the dihydrodiol.

It seems logical to link the binding of the carcinogen or its metabolite to macromolecules with the process of carcinogenesis. The binding of polycyclic hydrocarbon to proteins has already been described and if it cannot be excluded that such binding initiates the conversion of a normal into a cancer cell. Because binding to DNA is likely to initiate somatic mutation, it has been given a great deal more attention in the recent years. The binding of carcinogens to DNA will be discussed in more detail later.

One must distinguish between two modes of binding of the carcinogen to the nucleic acid, a weak form of binding involving the formation of complexes (charge transfer, van der Waals forces) and a strong type of binding involving the formation of covalent bonds. Boyland was the protagonist of the theory which proposed that the carcinogenic hydrocarbons are intercalated between the base pairs of the DNA molecules. In fact, Weil-Malherbe [92] in 1946 showed that free purine bases or their nucleosides facilitate the solubilization of hydrocarbons. De Santis and his associates [93] studied the molecular geometry of solutions containing a 1:1 solution of purine and pyrene molecules. They established that the purine and pyrene molecules were stacked on top of each other.

Boyland and Green [94] demonstrated the following for benzopyrene (carcinogenic) and pyrene (noncarcinogenic): (1) they were more soluble in DNA solution than in aqueous solution; (2) they lost their specific UV absorption band when dissolved in DNA; (3) the solubilization of the hydrocarbon was optimal when the ionic strength was low and when the DNA was present in a double-strand form; and (4) chloroform or cyclohexane readily removed the hydrocarbon that was complexed with the DNA. Boyland suggested that this interaction between the hydrocarbon and DNA results from the intercalation of the hydrocarbons between the base pairs. Of course, this is reminiscent of the properties of the amino acridines, which are known to intercalate between successive complementary pairs of purine-pyrimidine bases.

Brookes and Heidelberger [95], however, did not share Boyland's view. First, there is no correlation between the hydrocarbon's carcinogenicity and its ability to form complexes with DNA. Further, the reaction is not likely to be rigidly ordered, as it would have to be if intercalation occurred. Studies of the products obtained after degradation of DNA containing DMBA suggested covalent binding of the hydrocarbon to a DNA base, probably a purinic one.

Brookes and Lawley [96] also proposed an alternate mechanism to explain the binding of carcinogens to DNA *in vivo*; it involved covalent bonding, probably after conversion of the carcinogen to the epoxide. In further studies, these authors established a correlation between the carcinogenicity of a number of compounds and their ability to bind to DNA (but not to RNA or protein).

Harvey and Halonen [97] have shown that aromatic hydrocarbons bind to a variety of nucleosides (*e.g.*, uridine, thymidine, guanosine, and adenosine). But the mode of binding is not strictly correlated with the carcinogenic properties. Indeed, most hydrocarbons bind to the nucleosides whether they are potent or weak carcinogens.

Hennings and Boutwell studied the DNA inhibitory properties of a number of polycyclic hydrocarbons and could observe no relationship between carcinogenicity and inhibition of DNA synthesis [98].

The significance of each of these observations will be discussed after the mechanism of action of other carcinogens has been reviewed.

Gelboin [99] among others has demonstrated that the binding of [^{3}H]benzo[a]pyrene to DNA depends upon the catalytic activity associated with the microsomal fraction. The microsomes are believed to convert the hydrocarbons into an active metabolite of a composition still unknown (probably epoxides). The administration of polycyclic hydrocarbons enhances the microsomal enzyme activity. In fact, aryl hydrocarbon hydroxylase activity has been induced in tissue cultures with polycyclic hydrocarbons. Nevertheless, polycyclic hydrocarbons are not the only compounds to induce the activity of such an enzyme, and it is appropriate to discuss here some of the properties of the mixed-function oxidases [100]. The binding of carcinogens to DNA will be discussed further in the section devoted to carcinogenesis and DNA repair.

We constantly inhale or eat substances that are foreign to cellular metabolism by taking drugs, eating food (that contains contaminants), or simply breathing polluted air. Such substances are often poorly soluble, and when they enter the cell they are not readily eliminated and accumulate inside. If they are highly reactive, they may complex with metabolites or macromoleccules and cause cellular injury. The cell has devised a remarkable enzymic machinery to deal with those intruders by solubilizing and "detoxifying" them.

One group of such enzymes constitutes the mixed-function oxidases. The enzyme complex requires $NADPH_2$ and molecular oxygen for activity. These enzymes reduce one atom of oxygen while another atom is used in specific oxygenations or hydroxylations. In other words, the reaction occurs in a reductive step and an oxidative step. The sequence results in the binding of one atom of oxygen to the substrate. The reduction of the oxygen requires an electron source, which an electron transport chain provides. The attack of the complex on polycyclic hydrocarbons is believed to favor the formation of K-region epoxides, which then react with cellular macromolecules. In addition, a number of non-K-region diols and phenols are also formed, thus converting benzopyrene to a variety of diols and phenols and other hydroxylated products. Although only the action of the oxidases on benzopyrene will concern us here, it should not be forgotten that the same enzyme system acts on a number of drugs, including ethanol, hormones, and normal metabolites.

The multiple-enzyme system consists of a short electron transport chain, starting with $NADPH_2$, and ending with cytochrome p_{450}. The first and the last electron carriers are linked by $NADPH_2$ cytochrome c reductase and a cytochrome p_{450} reductase.

The administration of drugs or carcinogens induces the enzyme; induction is blocked by actinomycin and is associated with the incorporation of the appropriate precursors in heterogeneous nRNA and proteins, suggesting that the induction is at least partially regulated at the level of transcription [35, 36]. The level of induction that is achieved with a given carcinogen varies from animal to animal and from tissue to tissue and is controlled by simple mendelian genetics [562].

Histochemical methods have shown that the enzyme is present in almost all tissues examined.

The mixed-function oxidases have been partially solubilized from rat liver using increasing levels of sodium deoxycholate. The components of the mixed-function oxidases are under those conditions released from microsomes in three discrete steps. This partial solubilization of the components of the mixed-function oxidases is likely to shed new light on their mechanism of action [101, 566].

Although it is often assumed that drugs, insecticides and carcinogens are all oxidized by a single enzyme system, it cannot be excluded that at least classes of mixed function oxidases exist. Gurtoo *et al.* have shown that the mixed function oxidase which converts aflatoxin B_1 is different from that which reacts with benzenepyrene [563]. The heterogeneity of the mixed function oxidase system was further demonstrated by inducing the enzyme in rat liver with either phenobarbital or benzenepyrene. The enzyme induced by phenobarbital differed from that induced by benzenepyrene in that the metabolites of benzenepyrene produced with the former were different from those produced with the latter. Of particular significance is that the induction did not produce a benzenepyrene derivative that is mutagenic in bacteria. Moreover, phenobarbital did not induce the enzyme in the lung while carcinogens such as methylcholanthrene or dibenzanthracene did [564].

While phenobarbital can only induce the enzyme associated with the endoplasmic reticulum, the specific activity of enzymes located at the periphery of the nuclear membrane is increased 17 times after the intraperitoneal injection of methylcholanthrene [565].

The metabolic conversions of the carcinogen raise an important question as to whether the enzyme converts the foreign metabolite into a nontoxic compound or into an active carcinogen. The correlation between carcinogenesis and enzyme activity suggests the latter. Moreover, the administration of hydroxylase inhibitors—namely, benzoflavone—interferes with skin tumorigenesis by 7,12-dimethylbenz[a]anthracene and with the transformation of prostate fibroblasts by methylcholanthrene.

Thus, this complex enzyme machinery, which was developed for self-protection, fails to achieve its goals and elaborates the seed of the host's destruction. (Even more intriguing is the fact that the mixed-function oxidase system can be self-destructed by converting 2-allyl-2-isopropylacetamide into an epoxide, which binds with and ultimately destroys the cytochrome p_{450}. The decrease in cytochrome p_{450} which follows a single injection of the compound ultimately leads to experimental porphyria in rats and other species [102].) All investigators do not share these views; some believe that mixed-function oxidases may, at least in some cases, detoxify potential carcinogens.

The significance of the role of the mixed function oxidases is not only academic because aryl hydroxylases are induced by a number of compounds commonly used by some or even all of us. Cigarette smoking induces the formation of the hydroxylase in the lungs of mice [567]. Nicotine is likely to interfere with the aryl oxidase activity and reduces the metabolites of 3–4 benzenepyrene in the urine [568]. Indole-3-acetonitrite, indole-3-carbinol and 3,3′-diindolylmethane, compounds that naturally occur in cruciferous vegetables (brussels sprouts, cabbage and cauliflower), are inducers of the aryl oxidases [569].

Another example of the interaction between enzymes that metabolize carcinogens and environmental factors is the effects of the orgonophosphate insecticide, parathion, and its active metabolite, paraoxon, on the metabolism of benzenepyrene in rats. The administration of subacute doses of the active metabolites results in a decrease in the rate of biliary excretion of radioactive metabolites of benzene(a)pyrene 6 days after administration of the insecticide. In contrast, the level of intact benzene(a)pyrene in liver and other tissues is increased and the activity of the β hydroxylase in liver, small intestine and lung is inhibited. How the insecticide and the carcinogen interact to modulate the incidence of carcinogenesis in rats is not known [570].

It is now possible to present a general scheme for the metabolism of aromatic compounds. The conversion of aromatic compounds composed of one or more benzene rings to the corresponding phenols involves the formation of highly reactive arene oxides in which an aromatic double bond is converted to an epoxide. The fate of the epoxide is multiple: (1) it may isomerize spontaneously and yield the phenol; (2) it may be attacked by a microsomal enzyme "epoxide hydrase" which will convert it to the *trans*-dihydrodiols; (3) it may spontaneously react with nucleophiles including the thiol group of glutathione, protein and nucleic acids; (4) it may be complexed enzymatically to glutathione by an enzyme found in the cytosol, glutathione-S-epoxide transferase.

The epoxide hydrase has been partially purified from rat liver, but it is likely that more than one form of the enzyme exists. Similarly, at least two and possibly three different glutathione transferases have been found in rat liver.

The hepatic epoxide hydrase has been measured in neonatal and partially hepatectomized rats. It was found to be barely detectable in fetus one day old; it rose rapidly to adult values by 25 days of age. It was reduced after partial hepatectomy and falls to 68% of control values 48 hours after the operation. 1,1,1,-Trichloropropane oxide inhibits the enzyme [571].

The intermediate formation of K region epoxides has been convincingly established (using liver microsomal preparations in which the epoxide hydrase was inhibited) for naphthalene, phenanthrene, benzo(a)anthracene, dibenzo-(a,h)anthracene, pyrene, 4,5 benzo(a)pyrene, 7,12 dimethylbenzo(a)anthracene and other substituted benzo(a)anthracenes.

The significance of these findings resides in the fact that the K region epoxide might constitute the proximate carcinogen. Although initial experiments in which K region epoxides were administered *in vivo* showed that they were less active than the initial aromatic hydrocarbon, K region epoxides of benzo(a)anthracene, dibenzo(a,h)anthracene and 3 methylcholanthrene were shown to be more active in transforming cells *in vitro* than the parent hydrocarbon. An important consideration in the potential carcinogenicity of a given hydrocarbon is the steady state concentration of the arene oxides, which depends not only upon the rate at which they are formed, but also upon their proximity to critical macromolecules and their rate of conversion to phenol, dihydrodiols, etc. Therefore, the potential susceptibility of a given tissue to a specific aromatic hydrocarbon will be a function of the permeability of the cell to the compound and the interaction between the activities of the mixed function oxidase, the epoxide hydrase and the glutathione transferase. The situation will be further complicated in that covalent binding of the epoxide, for example to DNA, can at least in part be repaired [572].

Azo Derivatives

In 1934 Yoshida [103] produced hepatomas in mice, rats, and guinea pigs by the oral administration of aminoazotoluene in oil suspension. This first instance of parenchymal production cancer by ingestion of a carcinogen opened an entirely new field in chemical carcinogenesis. The carcinogenic properties of the ortho aminoazotoluene were not restricted to the liver; both subcutaneous administration and ingestion of the carcinogen induced a variety of tumors in a susceptible strain of mice. Among the tumors were subcutaneous sarcomas, pulmonary tumors, and hemoendothiomas.

Azobenzene is not carcinogenic; neither are the monobenzoic substitutes. However, the symmetrical 2-benzo substitutes, like α-α or (particularly in mice) β-β-azonaphthalene, are carcinogenic. In contrast, the asymmetrical α-β-azonaphthalene is noncarcinogenic. Amino-5-azobenzene is carcinogenic for rats. From it stem a number of derivatives that may or may not be carcinogenic, according to the type of substitution. Among the substitutions that need to be considered are alkylation of the rings and alkylation of the amino groups. The formulas of some of the carcinogenic and noncarcinogenic azo dyes are given in Fig. 16-19.

We will consider successively ring substitutions of aminobenzene, methylaminobenzene, and dimethylaminobenzene. Amino-4-azobenzene is generally more carcinogenic in mice than in rats. The substitution of methyls on the carbons of either ring may enhance the carcinogenicity. Such is the case for 3,2′-dimethylaminoazobenzene, which is very carcinogenic in mice and moderately carcinogenic in rats. However, methylation of the rings usually does not affect the carcinogenic properties of the compounds in rats, and it enhances carcinogenic properties only in mice. Furthermore, carcinogenic activity is increased only when the methylation involves the two rings of azobenzene. Thus, dimethyl 3,4′, 2,4′, 3,2′, and 2,3′ are all carcinogenic mice, whereas tetramethyl 2,5,2′,4′ [87] and pentamethyl 2′,3′,4′,5′,6′ are not carcinogenic. Furthermore, amination of the rings (*e.g.*, in position 4) does not affect the carcinogenic properties even when amination is combined with methylation of the same or of other rings.

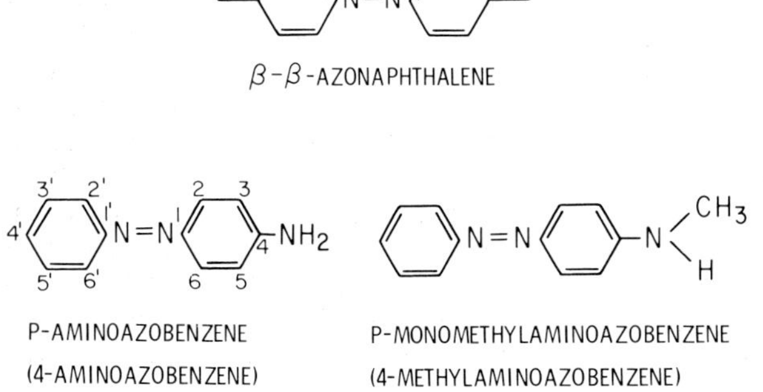

A few derivatives of monomethylaminoazobenzene have been investigated. Their behavior resembles that of homologous dimethylamino-4-azobenzene.

As for the dimethylamino-4-azobenzene, its carcinogenic properties vary according to the following general rule: hydroxylation of the ring annihilates the carcinogenic properties. The substitution of one halogen, particularly by fluorine,* enhances the carcinogenic properties considerably. Thus, fluoro 2,2′,3′ and 4′-dimethylamino-4-azobenzene are markedly carcinogenic. The chlorine derivatives (chloro 2′, chloro 3′, or chloro 4′, and dimethyl-4-aminoazobenzene) are only moderately carcinogenic. In contrast, methylation of the ring of 4-DAB may enhance the carcinogenic properties (as in methyl-3′-dimethylaminoazobenzene), or it may reduce or completely annihilate them. Thus, the methyl 2, methyl 3, and the methyl 4′ dimethylamino-4-azobenzene are less carcinogenic than 4-DAB.

A similar situation is observed with the nitroso derivatives where the 2′,3′ are carcinogenic, while the 4′ is not. Furthermore, although the substitution of more than one carbon by a chloro or a bromo derivative 2′,4′,6′ reduces the carcinogenic properties, the 2′,4′-difluorodimethylamino-4-azobenzene and the 2′,4′,6′-fluorodimethylamino-4-azobenzene present markedly increased carcinogenic properties. The methylation at two points of the same ring (2′,4′,2′,5′,3′,5′) annihilates the carcinogenic properties.

The substitution in the amino group also alters the carcinogenic properties. Thus, the dimethylaminoazotoluene is carcinogenic, as is the methylethylamino and methylaldehydamino. In contrast, when one of the methyl groups of 4-DAB is replaced by long alcohol chains, the carcinogenic properties are lost.

The position *para* of the amino group is not an absolute requirement for carcinogenicity. Indeed, the 6-amino-3,2′-dimethylazobenzene is carcinogenic in rats and mice. In contrast, the absence of the amino group eradicates the carcinogenic properties, except maybe for the hydroxy-4-dimethyl-3,2′-azobenzene. It seems that if the hydrogens of the amino groups are substituted by alkyl radicals, then the substitution of one of the hydrogens by a methyl group is required

AZOBENZENE

α-α -AZONAPHTHALENE

β-β -AZONAPHTHALENE

P-AMINOAZOBENZENE
(4-AMINOAZOBENZENE)

P-MONOMETHYLAMINOAZOBENZENE
(4-METHYLAMINOAZOBENZENE)

Fig. 16-19. Azo dyes

* The substitution of the hydrogen of various carbons of the ring by fluorine has been useful for investigating the site of the molecule that may be involved in the carcinogenic process. Indeed, if a fluoro-substituted molecule retains carcinogenic activity, then it is assumed that the positions involved are not immediately concerned with the carcinogenic process. It has even been suggested that such a procedure might be used to investigate other molecules.

for carcinogenic properties (thus, diethyl-4-aminoazobenzene is noncarcinogenic). But one of the methyl groups may be replaced by another alkyl radical, provided that it is not too large, or by an aldehyde, without abolishing the carcinogenic properties of the DAB derivative.

The metabolism of the azoic compounds has been studied extensively in rats. These compounds may be altered in various ways by demethylation, hydroxylation, reductive breakage of the azoic linkage, and protein binding.

Dimethyl-4-aminoazobenzene can easily be demethylated to mono-4-aminoazobenzene. This reaction is readily reversible. In contrast, the further demethylation of monomethyl-4-aminoazobenzene to 4-aminoazobenzene is irreversible. Demethylation was demonstrated both *in vivo* and *in vitro*. When 3′-methyl-4′-dimethylaminoazobenzene labeled in the N-methyl groups with ^{14}C is administered to rats, 70% of the ^{14}C is expired as $^{14}CO_2$. This indicates that a large portion of the methyl carbon is oxidized. In addition, part of the ^{14}C is recovered in protein-bound serine and in choline. The demethylation was reduced in the absence of folic acid and slightly increased in the presence of riboflavin. From these findings, it was concluded that the N-methylaminoazo dye underwent an oxidative demethylation in which the N-hydroxymethyl derivative is a possible intermediate. The products of the demethylation of N-monomethyl dyes are formaldehyde and the corresponding primary, aminoazo dye. The N-methyl groups of the dye are incorporated in the β-carbon of serine and in the methyl groups of choline.

Further studies in homogenate and cell fractions demonstrated that the enzymes that activate the demethylation of trimethyl-4-monomethylaminoazobenzene require oxygen, NADP, NAD, and hexose diphosphate for optimal activity. If glutathione is added to the reaction mixture, a highly polarized dye is formed that liberates the primary aminoazo dye upon acid treatment. Therefore, the N-hydroxymethyl derivative has been assumed to be a possible intermediate in the enzymatic demethylation of these dyes.

Rat liver homogenates fortified with diphosphopyridine nucleotide, nicotinamide, magnesium ions, hexose diphosphate demethylate, and hydroxylate-4-dimethylaminoazobenzene and yield 4′-hydroxy-4-dimethylaminoazobenzene. Hydroxylation of DAB occurs principally in the 4′ position. The intermediate formed in that reaction is unknown. Also unclear is the extent to which this reaction takes place *in vivo*.

Rat homogenates that contain glucose-6-phosphate, NAD, NADP, and nicotinamide catalyze a reductive cleavage of 4-dimethyl aminoazobenzene to yield a monophenylamine and N-paraphenylene diamine. Two enzyme systems are thus involved in the reductive cleavage: one that generates NADPH (a supernatant enzyme), and another that operates the cleavage (a microsomal enzyme). The cleavage of 4-DAB to inactive amines decreases when riboflavin is absent. Indeed, homogenates treated at 0 to 3° in a hypotonic medium with carbon dioxide lose the ability to cleave, but the ability to operate the reductive cleavage is restored if riboflavin is added to the medium. Thus, the protective action of riboflavin against liver tumors produced by 4-DAB in rats may result from riboflavin's effect on the cleavage of the carcinogen to inactive amines.

In 1938 Fisher suggested that carcinogens may act by combining with proteins. He thought that the combination might occur through the formation of S-S bridges. Studying the distribution of 3,4-benzene pyrene by fluorescence in mouse skin, Doniach, Mottram and Wagert [104] provided the first demonstration that carcinogens combine with proteins. These findings were conclusively extended by Miller and his associates [105–108] mainly to the azo dyes and later by Heidelberger and his associates [109–111] to the polycyclic hydrocarbons. Miller demonstrated that although the major share of the dye is metabolized in various ways (hydroxylation, demethylation, reductive cleavage of the azo linkage), a small percentage remains attached to the protein in the tissue. Thus, a polar dye can be released by hydrolysis of the protein-bound dye after feeding a rat with 4-DAB.

The significance of the binding of the aminoazo dye stems from the correlation that seems to exist between carcinogenicity and binding. The dyes are carcinogenic for the liver, and in that organ most of the binding occurs. When a species is not susceptible to cancer, little or no binding takes place. Thus, the livers of mouse and rat bind more dye than those of other rodents. The amount of dye that is bound correlates roughly with the carcinogenic activity of the azo dye. Although high carcinogenic activity correlates with protein binding of the dye, the ability to bind the protein of a compound with rather feeble or no carcinogenic properties does not correlate rigidly.

In fact, there are notorious discrepancies. For example, 3′-methyl-4-dimethylaminoazobenzene, 2-methyl-4-aminoazobenzene, and 3-methyl-4-monoethylaminoazobenzene all bind generously to liver proteins without having marked carcinogenic activities.

Binding would be meaningless if the dye were bound to all proteins indiscriminately. But this is not the case. Supernatant and microsomal proteins trap most of the bound dye.

3′Me-DAB has been found to bind principally to a cytosol protein which has been called H_25S and has been purified. The unconjugated protein, which has a sedimentation constant of 5 S and an electrophoretic mobility of the H_2 class, has been isolated. The molecular weight of the protein is 44,000 and its turnover 3.3 days [573].

The morphological changes that are associated with liver carcinogenesis have been investigated in several laboratories. We shall not present the results of these findings; suffice it to point out that the morphology of hepatomas varies considerably depending upon the type of animal, the type of carcinogen, and the time that elapsed between the application of the carcinogen and examination of the liver. Of course, one would assume that a correlation between carcinogenesis and histological changes can best be established at the early stages of hepatocarcinogenesis; therefore, many investigators have concentrated on these early changes.

Price [112, 113] and his collaborators showed an increase in basophilia 11 to 14 days after the administration of the dye, a finding in keeping with the higher RNA value measured at that time, particularly in the proliferating bile duct cells. Pyknosis and karyorrhexis were frequently observed, and bile duct proliferation was marked.

In general, the 3-methyl derivative of DAB has a greater tendency to induce bile proliferation and cirrhosis than 4-DAB. In contrast, 4-DAB alters more significantly than 4-fluoro-4-DAB the intracellular distribution of liver biochemical compounds. Price, Harman, Miller, and Miller [114] observed that the earliest microscopic alteration after the administration of an azo dye consisted in the development in the liver cells of hyaline bodies, which appear 7 days after feeding the azo dyes. These bodies first resemble sausages or horseshoes but later develop into hyaline, eosinophilic masses that surround the nucleus. These structures contrast sharply with the rest of the cytoplasm, which is finely granular.

There are two points of interest in the development of these hyaline masses. First, while they appear primarily in the peripheral lobules of the liver under the influence of 5-methyl-DAB, they develop primarily in the center of the lobule under the influence of 4′-fluoro-4-DAB. Secondly, correlated studies of the appearance of the hyaline structures and the amount of dye bound to proteins indicate that the development of the hyaline structures reaches a maximum when the proteins are bound maximally and the structures disappear when the latter decrease. The significance of that correlation is not clear.

Many investigators have studied the ultrastructural changes in the early stages of hepatocarcinogenesis. For a review, see the article by R.K. Murray and associates [115]. Up to now, no ultrastructural modification specific for carcinogenesis has been discovered. A number of alterations consistently are associated with hepatocarcinogenesis, but these changes also are observed when some noncarcinogenic toxins are administered. The alterations concern the presence of glycogen and the morphology of the endoplasmic reticulum. Glycogen is consistently decreased. There is disorganization of the rough endoplasmic reticulum with dissociation of ribosomes from the membrane and hyperplasia of the smooth endoplasmic reticulum. Other changes that have been described include alterations of the mitochondria (increase or decrease in the number of structural abnormalities), hyperplasia of the Golgi, and hyperplasia of the nucleolus.

The relevance of these changes to carcinogenesis is not convincing, and they probably reflect unspecific responses to the administration of a toxic agent. However, it cannot be excluded, as Murray and his associates pointed out, that yet undetected and more subtle changes take place after a carcinogen is administered—changes that might, for example, involve either the membrane or the chromosomes. We shall discuss the morphology of hepatomas further when we consider the biochemistry of the minimal deviation hepatoma.

Whereas the 2-methyl-DAB practically doubles the number of mitochondria per gram, the feeding of 3′-methyl-DAB leads to a reduction of about 40% of the original value. In contrast, the number of nuclei had doubled in those animals fed methyl-DAB and had dropped to 60% of the original number in animals fed 2-methyl-DAB. Examination of liver sections by the Chalkley method demonstrated that the parenchymal tissue had decreased considerably in the animals fed 3-methyl-DAB. Indeed, it fell to 55% of its original value, while it remained around 85, 90, or 91% for those animals fed 2-methyl-DAB. This reduction was obviously due to a reduction in the cytoplasmic fraction of the parenchymal cell because the area occupied by the nuclei remained constant. Therefore, it was concluded that the feeding of 3′-methyl-DAB led to a drop in mitochondria per cell.

Tissue fractionation studies performed on livers of animals fed 4-DAB, 4′-methyl-DAB, 4-DAB and 3′- and 4′-methyl-4-dimethyl-DAB had little effect on the composition of the liver. 3′-Methyl-4-DAB (a powerful carcinogen) and 4-dimethylaminoazobenzene (a moderate carcinogen) markedly altered the intracellular distribution of the cellular components. These changes consisted of: (1) an increase in the amount of proteins and DNA in the nuclear fraction; (2) a decrease in the protein and RNA associated with mitochondria and microsomal pellets; (3) a decrease in the amount of riboflavin associated with the microsomal pellet; and (4) an increase in the RNA associated with the supernatant and the nuclei. These changes were roughly proportional to the carcinogenicity of the compound. In addition, the liver of the hamster, which is unaffected by the aminoazo dye, shows no change in the intracellular distribution of its components. 2′,4-Methylaminoazobenzene produced an excessive increase in the mass of the mitochondria, which contained more proteins and riboflavin and less ribonucleic acid. Histological studies suggested that the alteration in the mitochondria resulted from an alteration in the parenchymal cells, whereas the alteration in the nuclei resulted from bile duct cell proliferation.

Fluorene Derivatives

Investigation of the toxicity of potential insecticides led to the discovery of one of the most interesting carcinogens—2-acetylaminofluorene (see Fig. 16-20). After ingestion or injection, this compound leads to the

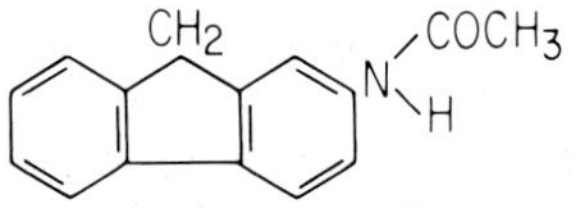

CH_2 / $COCH_3$ / N / H

Fig. 16-20. 2-Acetylaminofluorene

CH_2 / CH_3 / N / OH

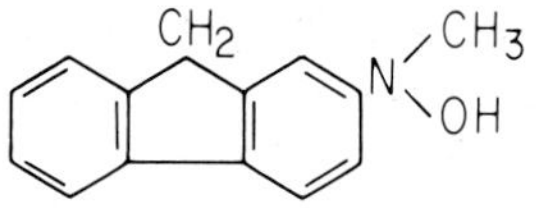

Fig. 16-21. N-Hydroxy-2-Acetylaminofluorene

development of tumors throughout the organism. The action of fluorene derivatives differs from that of the polycyclic hydrocarbons, which generally act only at the application site. It resembles that of the azo dyes inasmuch as it acts at a distance from the site of application, but it differs from the azo dyes in the great variety of tumors that it induces.

The basic skeleton of the group of carcinogenic compounds is fluorene, a compound that has been isolated from coal tar and consists of two benzene rings united by a methylene bridge. X-Ray crystallography has demonstrated that fluorene has a planar structure [87, 116]. (With regard to the structure and the mechanism of action of the carcinogens, which will be discussed in more detail later, it is worthwhile to remark that Pullman—from theoretical calculations—concluded that the 1 and the 4 positions of fluorene would be attacked first in the presence of reactants because they possess the higher electronic charge. In fact, the 2 position is first attacked by electrophilic substituents, then the other carbons are attacked in the following sequence: 7, 3, 1, and occasionally 5.)

The carcinogenic properties of numerous fluorene derivatives have been investigated. We need to consider separately those compounds substituted in position 2 and those substituted in another carbon of the ring. The substitution of the carbon 2 of fluorene includes amino and nitro derivatives. The 2-nitrofluorene is almost inactive, but the aminofluorene is a very active carcinogen. Thus, the presence of an amino group in position 2 seems to enhance the carcinogenic properties of the fluorene ring. If aminofluorene is further substituted by replacing one or two hydrogens of the amino group with acetyl radicals, carcinogenic compounds are produced. Similar substitutions by large alkyl or by aromatic groups, however, decrease or abolish the carcinogenic properties. The replacement of one or more of the hydrogen atoms of the methyl group of 2-methylaminofluorene by fluorine atoms does not abolish the carcinogenic properties. Miller and his associates [117–120] have observed that the introduction of 1-N-hydroxyl in the acetylaminofluorene (see Fig. 16-21) enhances the carcinogenicity of acetylaminofluorene considerably; therefore, the authors have proposed that the N-hydroxyl compound may be an active intermediate in the metabolism of acetylaminofluorene (see below).

Substitutions in the ring involve the carbons 7, 1, 3, 9, and 4. They consist of the addition of an acetamide, a halogen, a hydroxyl, and a sulfur group (among various other groups). Ring substitution may or may not be associated with the substitution of an acetamide in position 2. Thus, 1-acetylaminofluorene is moderately active; 4- and 9-acetylaminofluorene are inactive; 7-fluoro-2-acetylaminofluorene is very active; and 7-iodo and 7-chloro-2-acetylaminofluorene are either inactive or slightly active. In contrast, 3-iodo,2-acetylaminofluorene is markedly active in producing cancer of the ear, but only this type of tumor is produced. The introduction of a sulfur atom in position 9 of 3-acetylaminofluorene gives a moderately active compound. Finally, 7-hydroxy,2-acetylaminofluorene was found to be inactive.

Other fluorene derivatives that have been found to be slightly active or inactive include 9-hydroxy-2-acetylaminofluorene, 9-keto-2-acetylaminofluorene, 9-oxytriacetamide fluorene, 9-sulphoxytriacetamide fluorene, 2′-acetamide-9′-bifluorene, and 9-dimethyl-2-acetamide fluorene, among others.

The replacement of the methylene bridge by an atom of sulfur or oxygen decreases the carcinogenic activity of acetylaminofluorene.

Attempts were made to correlate the carcinogenic properties with such properties as ultraviolet absorption, molecular dimensions, oxidation-reduction potential, and condensation reaction of the compounds. Although most of these properties and the carcinogenic properties of the compound are not consistently related, it is worthwhile to consider the correlation postulated between the size of the molecule and its carcinogenic properties.

On the basis of what is known of the metabolism of the carcinogen—particularly its capacity to bind with protein, it seems quite possible that the size and orientation of the carcinogen may affect its carcinogenic properties. It is not surprising that attempts have been made to calculate the size of various carcinogenic and noncarcinogenic fluorene derivatives. Pauling [121] and Wheland [122] have shown that the N-dimethyl-2-fluorenylacetamide is 4 A thick, whereas the 2-fluorenylacetamide is only 2 A thick. Inasmuch as the dimethyl derivative is not carcinogenic, it was concluded that it may be too large to fit the size requirement for carcinogenic activity. With respect to size, it is interesting to note that the 7-iodo derivatives are not carcinogenic, although the 7-chloro and the 7-fluoro are. Fluorine does not increase the size of the molecule considerably, but bromine and iodine do. (The covalent diameters are hydrogen, 0.6 A; fluorene, 0.28 A; chlorine, 1.98 A; bromine, 2.28 A; and iodine, 2.68 A.)

Whether or not size is essential for the manifestation of fluorene's carcinogenicity is not certain. If it is essential for fluorene derivatives, it surely is not for polycyclic hydrocarbons. Change in size affects the molecules in various ways. It determines the geometrical specificity, solubility, and reactivity. By which mechanism size affects carcinogenicity is not known.

The carcinogenic properties of many of the fluorene derivatives can be modified considerably by a variety of factors [123] including the mode of administration of the carcinogen, the effect of diet, the hormonal environment, and the concomitant administration of other carcinogens. Oral administration is the most reliable means of testing the carcinogenic properties of fluorene derivatives.

Practically all strains of animals tested were found to respond to 2-AAF. Among the susceptible rodents are mice, rats, hamsters, and rabbits. Guinea pigs and cotton rats, in contrast, are resistant to the carcinogenic action of 2-AAF. Other species (fowl, cats, and dogs) were all found to be susceptible to the carcinogen. Among laboratory animals, rats seem to be the most responsive. Most frequently they develop cancer in the liver, the mammary gland, and the ear. Other tumors are occasionally found in the bladder, lungs, eyelids, skin, brain, thyroid, parathyroid, salivary glands, pancreas, gastrointestinal tract, kidney, uterus, renal pelvis, urinary tract, muscles, thymus, spleen, ovaries, and, finally, blood (leukemias). The site of appearance of the tumor depends on the strain of rats used for the experiment. For example, the Wistar rats develop urinary tract tumors or mammary gland cancers with predilection, whereas other strains are less prone to develop such tumors.

It was previously mentioned that the feeding of azo dyes is carcinogenic only under adequate dietary conditions. Of the dietary factors that influence the carcinogenic properties of azo dyes, riboflavin plays a prime role. In contrast, riboflavin or yeast extract has little effect on the carcinogenic properties of AAF. The effect of diet on the incidence of tumors after the administration of the fluorene derivatives has been studied extensively, and only one set of examples will be presented. Among the dietary effects that have been investigated, one must include the effect of a synthetic versus a regular diet and the importance of the protein, fat, and amino acid content of the diet. Synthetic diets have a deleterious effect on the animals fed 2-AAF because these animals are more sensitive to the toxic effects of the carcinogen. Low-protein diets have a dual effect on carcinogenesis by 2-AAF: they increase the latent period for the development of both mammary and duct tumors, and they increase the incidence of tumors produced.

One of the most interesting dietary effects is the role of tryptophan on the incidence of tumors produced by 2-AAF in rats. The tryptophan in these animals can be controlled by supplementing a tryptophan-free diet with known amounts of tryptophan. If small amounts of tryptophan (0.14%) are added to the diet, a triple effect can be observed: retarded growth, reduced life span, and decreased incidence and decreased latent period for the development of cancer of the liver. In contrast, if an amount of tryptophan 10 times as high (1.4%) is administered, the animals live from 1 to 3 months longer, they grow normally, and the incidence of liver tumors is decreased even though the latent period for the development of liver tumors is normal. Moreover, the incidence of cancer of the bladder increases up to 92 or even 100% in animals fed tryptophan and 2-AAF. (This synergic effect of a carcinogen and tryptophan is observed only with 2-AAF. Boyland tried without success to achieve similar results by administering benzidine and 2-naphthylamine.) However, the tryptophan *per se* is not necessary to produce carcinoma of the bladder by 2-AAF. The indoles or indolacetic acid (1% in the diet) combined with 2-AAF has a similar effect. The mechanism by which tryptophan produces this effect is not clear. Several hypotheses have been proposed, but none is supported by substantial evidence.

The effect of a high-fat diet on the carcinogenic properties of 2-AAF varies with the site of development of tumors produced. Although high-fat diets increase the incidence of mammary tumors in the female rat, low-fat diets increase the incidence of tumors of the eye originating in the harderian gland.

The effect of vitamins on 2-AAF carcinogenesis has been studied extensively. Vitamin B_{12}, ascorbic acid, and biotin have no effect on the carcinogenicity of 2-AAF. In contrast, the administration of 100 times the normal intake of pyridoxamine and riboflavin increases the incidence of the tumors in the ear duct. The effect of riboflavin has been studied most extensively. The normal levels of riboflavin do not seem to be maintained in rats fed 2-AAF, so the diet should contain at least 20 times as much riboflavin as normal to maintain standard levels of that coenzyme in the liver cells.

Several observations suggest that hormones may influence the incidence of tumors produced by 2-AAF. After 2-AAF administration, mammary tumors are common in females, but not in males. In contrast, liver tumors are more frequent in males. Castration has no effect on the incidence of liver tumors, but it reduces the incidence of mammary tumors considerably in females.

The effects of a variety of hormones and hormonal imbalances on the carcinogenic properties of 2-AAF have been investigated. They will not all be reviewed here, but suffice it to point out that the effects are varied, often contradictory, and often difficult to interpret. In spite of these difficulties, these studies have yielded many interesting observations, such as the fact that thyroidectomy or hypophysectomy interferes with the development of liver tumors either by completely abolishing the carcinogenic properties or by retarding the development of these tumors.

When 2-AAF and NN-dimethyl-2-azobenzene were fed simultaneously to rats, the incidence of tumors was greater than that for either carcinogen fed alone. In contrast, 2-AAF administered simultaneously with a weaker carcinogen did not affect the incidence of tumors. The incidence of liver cancer in animals injected with tannic acid can be practically doubled if 2-AAF is added to the diet. Indeed, the administration of tannic acid induces cirrhosis in 66% of cases, and 93% of the cirrhotic livers develop carcinomas if 2-AAF is added, in contrast to only 28% of carcinomas if 2-AAF is administered alone. The liver is not the only site where an irritant may act concomitantly with 2-AAF to produce tumors; the simultaneous administration of the carcinogen and irritants that produce local gastric ulcers leads to the development of carcinoma of the stomach. In contrast, the concomitant feeding of 3-methylcholanthrene, chrysene, dimethylbenzanthracene, 2-AAF, or 7-fluorol-2-fluorenylacetamide interfered with the carcinogenic properties of the fluorene compounds.

The metabolism of fluorene derivatives and the properties of the fluorene-induced tumors that are common to all other tumors will be discussed in another section of this chapter. But much effort was devoted to tracing the metabolism of aminofluorene derivatives in mammalian tissue by following the fate of 2-AAF or its derivatives in mammals by conventional chemical analysis of the compound or after the administration of radioactive carcinogens. These studies have led to the following general conclusions. After ingestion, the compound passes through the stomach without change and is absorbed in the intestine. From there, it is transferred through the ramification of the portal vein and reaches the liver, where it is metabolized. The chemical conversions in the liver include deacylation, acylation, hydroxylation, and combination to glucuronic acid or to a sulfate in a detoxification process. (Other metabolic transformations have been proposed, including methylation of the amino group, oxidation of the 9-methionine carbon to a ketone, and opening of the ring at the position 9 to yield derivatives of biphenylcarboxylic acid.)

The product of liver metabolism is excreted in the branches of the hepatic artery and from there carried in the general circulation and excreted in urine, or it is transferred from the hepatic cell to the bile ducts, concentrated in the gall bladder, and eliminated in the intestine. The metabolites that enter the intestine may be reabsorbed or excreted with the feces. The mechanism of absorption through the intestinal tract is not clear. It has been suggested that a carcinogen enters the liver through the mesenteric arteries because the right lobe is more prone to develop cancer than the left lobe, but this is not a consistent observation. (Partial hepatectomy interferes with the liver's capacity to metabolize aminofluorene derivatives; therefore, it is not surprising that neoplasms develop sooner in partially hepatectomized animals than in normal ones.)

Although the first insight into the metabolism of acetylaminofluorene was obtained by chemical techniques, only after ^{14}C-labeled aminofluorene was prepared [124, 125] was it possible to follow its metabolism with precision. Ray and Geiser prepared acetylaminofluorene labeled either in the acetyl group or in the ring. They observed that although acetyl-labeled compounds rapidly released their radioactivity in the form of respiratory CO_2, the radioactivity of the ring-labeled compounds remained intact. It was concluded that 2-AAF was deacylated to yield aminofluorene. Inasmuch as only small amounts of aminofluorene were found in urine, it was also suspected that other metabolites must be formed. The formation of hydroxylation products and of conjugated acetylaminofluorene derivatives with glucuronide or sulfate was demonstrated.

These observations, first made *in vivo*, were later extended by studies *in vitro*. Homogenates convert 2-AAF to 2-aminofluorene in the presence of oxygen. The reaction is enzymic in nature, but the enzymes involved have not been purified. Studies *in vitro*, however, have revealed some characteristics of the enzyme's specificity. The enzyme not only deacylates 2-acetylaminofluorene, but it acts also on N_2-naphthylacetamide, acetylacetamide-2-fluorol diacetamide and N-4-fluorolacetamide, and N-3-fluorenylacetamide and N-1-fluorenylacetamide. The deacylation of AAF is reversible because if 2-aminofluorene is used as a substrate in liver homogenate, 2-AAF can be rapidly recovered. Whether the same enzyme catalyzes the acetylation and the deacetylation is not known. There is some indication that acetyl CoA may be involved in the acetylation.

Bielschowsky [126] demonstrated that 2-AAF is hydroxylated in position 7 in rats, rabbits, and guinea pigs. Later, Weisburger and his associates [127, 128] found that hydroxylation products in positions 1, 3, 5, 7, and 8 were also present in the urine of rats given ^{14}C-labeled 2-AAF. Among the hydroxylated products, the 5 and 7 hydroxy were preponderant because positions 5 and 7 are most prone to be substituted chemically by electrophilic reagents when position 2 is already blocked.

The hydroxylation products are not excreted as such, but in the form of glucuronide mainly, or sulfate esters secondarily. N-7-hydroxy-2-fluorenylacetamide is the only compound excreted in the form of a sulfate conjugate. Thus, chromatographic analysis of the urine of animals injected with 2-AAF yields three groups of compounds: sulfuric acid conjugates, glucuronic acid conjugates, and the three fluorene derivatives.

Inasmuch as the deacetylated fluoreneamine undergoes oxidation, the free AAF derivatives found in urine also include 2-aminofluorenyl in addition to the acetylated AAF, the fluoreneamine, and the hydroxy derivatives. However, most of the hydroxy derivatives are transformed mainly by acetylation or by conjugation with glucuronide or sulfuric acid.

One may wonder which of these compounds is the active carcinogen. Miller and his associates have devoted much effort to this problem. They established that the N-hydroxy metabolites of 2-AAF exhibit greater carcinogenic properties than the parent compound. The difference is manifested in at least three ways: (1) the increased incidence of cancer at the site normally affected by the parent compound, (2) the development of tumors at sites not normally affected by the parent compound, and (3) the development of tumors in species (*e.g.*, guinea pig) usually not responsive to the carcinogenic effect of AAF.

Studies of the binding of different carcinogens further indicate that the N-hydroxy derivative is the active carcinogen. AAF binds to RNA and DNA;

in RNA, it is likely to be bound by the N-hydroxy intermediate, and the binding is likely to involve guanine bases. There is a good correlation between the amount of [^{14}C]AAF bound to protein and RNA and the carcinogenic properties. Thus, the N-hydroxy AAF is more efficiently bound than AAF, and the administration of methylcholanthrene, which interferes with carcinogenesis by both AAF and N-hydroxy AAF, reduces the amount of fluorene compound that is bound to proteins or RNA.

Acetylaminofluorene is not carcinogenic at the injection site, and N-hydroxy AAF is a poor local carcinogen. Tumors appear only after repeated injections of these carcinogens. For example, although no tumors appear after four injections, up to 80% of the rats develop cancer after sixteen injections. Thus, critical concentrations of the carcinogens must be reached repeatedly to produce tumors at the injection site. Miller's group has further investigated the carcinogenic properties of N-hydroxy AAF when it is slowly released at the injection site. This is achieved by combining the N-hydroxy AAF with various metals by chelation. The half-life of the chelate depends upon the nature of the metals. For example, ferric and cupric chelates have a half-life of 4 to 50 days at the injection site. In contrast, the half-life of magnesium chelate is only a few hours to 2 days. Chelates with short half-lives induce tumors at a distance from the injection site, but few tumors develop at the injection site. In contrast, the chelates with long half-lives induce fewer tumors at a distance, but are responsible for the development of appreciable numbers of sarcomas at the injection site [129].

The morphological events that follow the administration of N-2-fluorenylacetamide to rats are significant because they illustrate the complex relationship that links cellular hyperplasia and transformation into a cancer cell. All tissues that become cancerous after the administration of a carcinogen exhibit hyperplasia at some time after the agent is administered. In the liver, foci of young hepatocytes can be recognized microscopically and later grossly. The smallest foci are called areas; the largest, hyperplastic nodules. If the administration of the carcinogens is interrupted early enough (after 3 months' feeding), the evolution of the hyperplastic nodule into cancer can be prevented, and the hyperplastic nodules may disappear; yet after 1 more month of feeding cancer is inevitable.

Two mechanisms can be invoked to explain the relationship between carcinogenesis and hyperplasia. In the first, the triggering of hyperplasia and transformation are two separate events, but for reasons unknown, the triggering of transformation requires prolonged administration of the carcinogen. In the second, one single triggering event initiates both hyperplasia and transformation, and a sequence of specific molecular events links hyperplasia and carcinogenesis. A critical point of that sequence distinguishes a reversible from an irreversible state; to reach that critical point, a prolonged insult of the cell with the carcinogen is needed [130–132].

Aflatoxin and Cycasin

In 1960 English turkeys died in large numbers from a mysterious disease called turkey X disease. At autopsy, severe liver damage and in some cases cancer of the liver were found. A food contaminant was suspected. It was soon demonstrated that the disease resulted from a metabolite of a mold, *Aspergillus flavus*. The active compound isolated was named aflatoxin. Four different aflatoxins have been discovered: aflatoxins B_1 (see Fig. 16-22), B_2, G_1, and G_2. The aflatoxins differ by their chromatographic properties and fluorescence [130, 133–135].

Similarly, cancer of the liver in trout was quickly traced to the presence of an aflatoxin in their food. Aflatoxins are toxic for turkeys, ducks, chickens, cattle, sheep, pigs, rats, guinea pigs, dogs, cats, mice, rabbits, and monkeys, but there is no evidence that they cause cancer of the liver in humans.

The cycad nut, which grows in tropical and subtropical regions on a palmlike tree, is a source of food and medicine in Guam. The nut contains a toxin which, if not removed, causes a neurological disease. When untreated nuts were fed to rats, no neurological disease developed, but cancer appeared at various sites, including liver and kidney. Germ-free rats do not, however, develop cancer. It is now known that the toxic agent is cycasin. In the presence of a bacterial flora, cycasin (see Fig. 16-23) is converted to a methyl azyl C methanale which may be a proximal carcinogen.

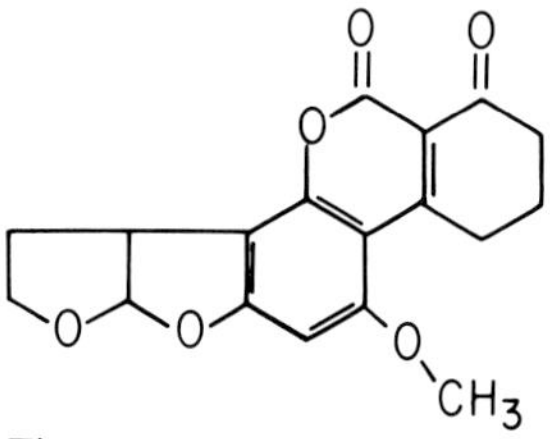

Fig. 16-22. Aflatoxin B_1

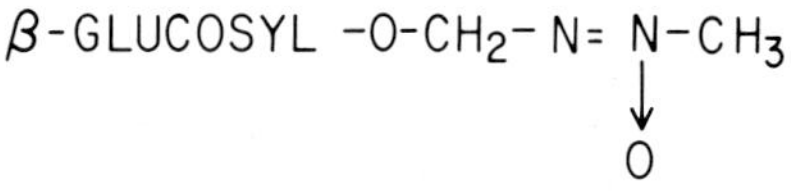

β-GLUCOSYL $-O-CH_2-N=N(\rightarrow O)-CH_3$

Fig. 16-23. Cycasin

Aniline Derivatives

It has been known for some time that the incidence of carcinomas of the bladder is unusually high among workers in the aniline, benzidine, and naphthylamine industries. At first, β-naphthylamine was thought to be the carcinogenetic agent responsible for the development of bladder carcinomas. However, Boyland and his group have established that the mechanism of carcinogenesis is much more complex. When 2-β-naphthylamine (see Fig. 16-24) is administered to the skin, the lungs, and the mouth, it is absorbed into the general

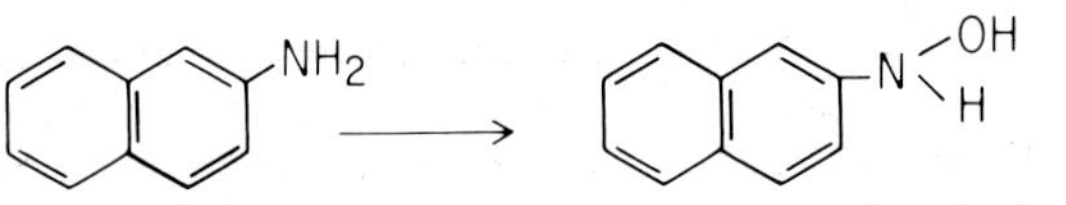

Fig. 16-24. 2-Naphthylamine and 2-naphthylhydroxylamine

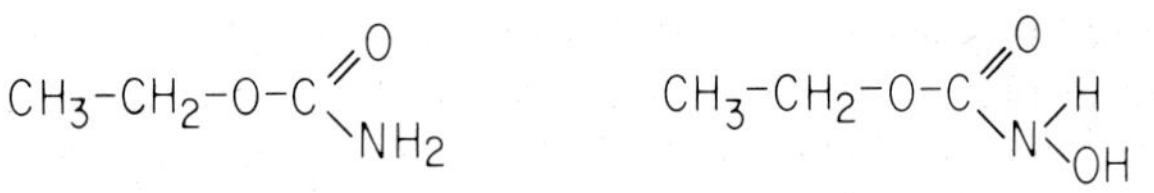

Fig. 16-25. Urethane and its N-hydroxy derivative

circulation and oxidized in the liver to yield a new compound that is very carcinogenic. Liver microsomes detoxify the carcinogen by conjugating it to either sulfate or glucuronide.

The conjugated carcinogen is excreted in the urine, but the β-glucuronidase—which is present in large amounts in acid urine—releases the glucuronic acid, and the active carcinogen acts on the cells of the bladder mucosa to induce cancer. The following arguments are used to support the theory: (1) β-naphthylamine is not carcinogenic after implantation in the bladder; (2) liver cells oxidize the 2-naphthylamine to aminonaphthol and conjugate the latter; (3) large amounts of glucuronides are found in the urine if glucuronidase is inhibited by 1,4-saccharolactone administered orally. However, the theory fails to explain why tumors are prone to occur in mice but not in rats, and why dogs are unable to convert 2-β-naphthylamine to sulfate or glucuronide derivatives. Dogs could resort to another mechanism of detoxification and, indeed, a 2-amino-1-naphthol mercapturic acid has been found in the urine of dogs.

Thus, Boyland's hypothesis postulates that β-naphthylamine is converted into a carcinogen, which is normally detoxified by the formation of a glucuronide that is split by the β-glucuronidase contained in the urine and then released in its active form. The molecular structure of the active carcinogen is not known, but it is believed to be 2-naphthylhydroxylamine.

All bladder carcinomas seen in the general population could result from similar mechanisms. Indeed, Boyland has found three natural metabolic compounds—3-hydroxyanthranilic acid, 2-amino-3-hydroxyacetophenone, and 3-hydroxykynurenic acid—that are chemically related to orthoaminophenol and appear during the normal metabolism of tryptophan. If these compounds are implanted in the bladders of mice (under adequate conditions), they lead to the formation of cancer in bladder. All these compounds are excreted in the conjugated form.

Urethane

Small doses of urethane (see Fig. 16-25) were administered to children for anesthetic purposes. The same compound is now used as an initiator of carcinogenesis of the lung, leukemias, and carcinomas of the skin. After urethane is adminstered, the metabolites N-hydroxyurethane and its N-acetyl derivatives and ethylmercapturic acid can be recovered in the urine of rat, rabbit, and man. Binding to nucleic acids and proteins has not been reported. Whether or not the N-hydroxy derivative is the actual carcinogen is not certain. In fact, N-hydroxyurethane was found to be less carcinogenic in mice than urethane itself. This may be due to the fact that the N-hydroxy form is rapidly reduced; it would seem, therefore, that the critical concentration of the carcinogen could be reached more safely by endogenous conversion of urethane to the N-hydroxy compound than by direct administration of the N-hydroxy compound.

Polymers

We stated at the beginning of this discussion that carcinogens were varied and numerous. We have discussed representative compounds among the group of classic carcinogens [136–140]. Several carcinogens, such as ethionine and dimethylnitrosamine, are also toxic to the liver. Their metabolism and modification have been discussed in another chapter.

To be comprehensive, this discussion on chemical carcinogenesis might be extended to metals, several alkylating agents, and so on. But the description of more carcinogens will add little to our understanding of the basic mechanisms of carcinogenesis. One should not, however, underestimate the importance of identifying potential carcinogens in the environment for the purpose of public health. Yet, before we conclude, we will consider one more group of carcinogens because the observations made on that group defy most existing theories of carcinogenesis.

The carcinogenic properties of plastics are most intriguing and cannot be neglected when the mechanism of action of carcinogens is interpreted. Practically all plastics investigated (including such unreactive compounds as polytetrafluoroethylene, or Teflon) lead to development of tumors after implantation. The form in which the plastic is presented is more important for its carcinogenic properties than its chemical structure. In the case of nylon, for example, tumors are easily produced by implantation of plain film. In contrast, nylon textiles have no carcinogenic properties, and the incidence of tumors after the implantation of perforated nylon plates is four times less than the incidence after implantation of plain film. Three theories have been proposed with respect to the mode of action of these plastics: direct chemical reaction, formation of free radicals, and biological interference with normal differentiation.

A small amount of the implanted plastic materials could be detached from the main implant and react as a carcinogen. But this theory is unappealing because most of the plastics used are markedly unreactive. Furthermore, the product of their breakdown would be water insoluble, so the tumor should develop at the site of implantation, but it occurs some distance from the implant. Using radioactive plastic, Oppenheimer and his coworkers demonstrated that the polymer was to some extent broken down and that the breakdown product could be recovered at some distance from the implantation site. These experiments also suggest that whatever the breakdown product may be, the monomeric form of the plastic probably is not responsible for tumor production because when monomers were used, they were not found to be carcinogenic, with the exception of vinyl chloride to be discussed later.

A different theory suggests that the friction of the plastic with the surrounding tissue induces the surface formation of free radicals, which migrate and produce tumors at some distance. The short life span of the free radicals and the numerous trapping agents present in biological specimens seem insurmountable obstacles to such a mechanism. Inasmuch as the mechanism of action of the plastic cannot be explained in molecular terms, other vague biologically interpretations have been proposed, such as local irritation, focal anoxemia, and interference with cellular differentiation. If irritation were responsible for tumor production by plastic sheets, it is difficult to conceive why intact plastic sheets are more efficient than the perforated sheets or the pulverized material. There is also no evidence that the implanted plastic sheets produce anoxemia, as some investigators have suggested. (Even if anoxemia is produced, it remains to be established that anoxemia is carcinogenic.)

At a loss for any rational explanation of the carcinogenic properties of plastics, Alexander and Horning [141] proposed a rather mysterious mechanism. Their hypothesis assumes that the connective tissue cell is fully aware of its role in the living, which is to fill some specific histological sectors with connective tissue fibers. The plain plastic sheet would then interfere with these connecting properties, and this interference is in some way signaled to the connective tissue cell, which responds by uncontrolled proliferation that ends in cancer.

A more plausible explanation, in our opinion, is that the plastic sheets are contaminated by active carcinogens that are slowly released into the surrounding tissues. When a critical concentration of carcinogens is reached repeatedly, normal cells are converted into cancer cells. Focal critical concentration can be reached only with intact film. If the film is perforated, or ground, the concentration of carcinogens is too low.

Mechanism of Chemical Carcinogenesis

Carcinogens clearly introduce in the cell a permanent change that is transmitted from cell to cell for many generations. Therefore, it seems inescapable that the carcinogen must alter the expression of the genome into the phenotype directly or indirectly. The major question that needs to be answered is whether the alteration of the expression of the genome results from a somatic mutation or from epigenetic alterations capable of exerting feedback influences on the expression of the genome.

Binding of carcinogens to DNA could result in a somatic mutation, and binding to proteins could cause deletion of proteins indispensable for regulating gene expression.

Whatever the mechanism of carcinogenesis may be, binding of the unaltered or the altered carcinogen to macromolecular constituents—nucleic acid, proteins, lipids, etc.—must be involved in carcinogenesis. On the basis of experimental data assembled in his and other laboratories, Miller has proposed a working hypothesis for the mode of action of the amino dyes and the aminofluorenes. When efforts were made to prepare N-hydroxy methylaminobenzene (MAB), the compound was found to be too unstable to isolate. To obviate this difficulty, Miller synthesized a compound that presumably would yield the N-hydroxy MAB *in vivo*. N-Benzoyloxy MAB, the benzoester of N-hydroxy MAB, was synthesized. Somewhat to Miller's surprise, this compound was a more active carcinogen than the N-hydroxy MAB. Benzoyloxy MAB produces carcinomas at the injection site and even kidney cancers in young rats. *In vitro*, N-benzoyloxy MAB reacts nonenzymatically at a neutral pH with DNA, RNA, guanosine, tryptophan, tyrosine, methionine, cystine, and a number of other nucleophiles. The molecular complex formed in such reactions is not always known. In methionine, it is speculated that a sulfonium derivative is formed, the 3-(methion-s-yl) MAB, which decomposes to yield the 3-methylmercapto MAB. The various metabolites of dimethylaminoazobenzene are given in Fig. 16-26, and the sequence of metabolic changes that occur *in vivo* is illustrated in Fig. 16-27.

Similarly, esters of N-hydroxy derivatives of fluorene are more carcinogenic than AAF and N-hydroxy AAF in the sense that the former produce carcinomas at the injection site. The N-acetoxy AAF has properties reminiscent of those of the N-benzoyloxy MAB and reacts with nucleophiles. With methionine, the ester yields the O-(methion-s-yl) AAF, which decomposes to yield O-methylmercapto-AAF. On the basis of the

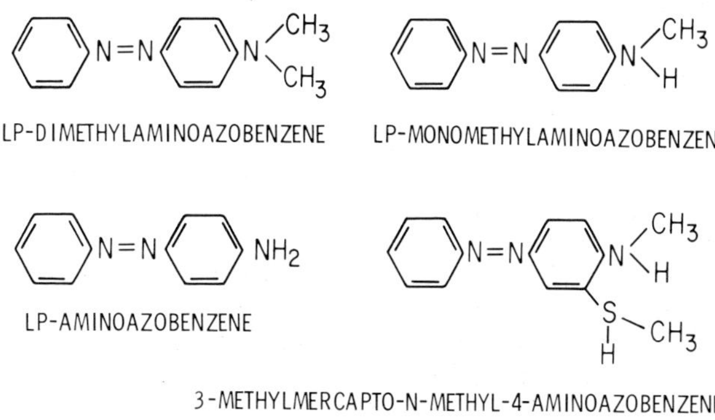

LP-DIMETHYLAMINOAZOBENZENE

LP-MONOMETHYLAMINOAZOBENZENE

LP-AMINOAZOBENZENE

3-METHYLMERCAPTO-N-METHYL-4-AMINOAZOBENZENE

Fig. 16-26. Metabolites of LP-dimethylaminoazobenzene

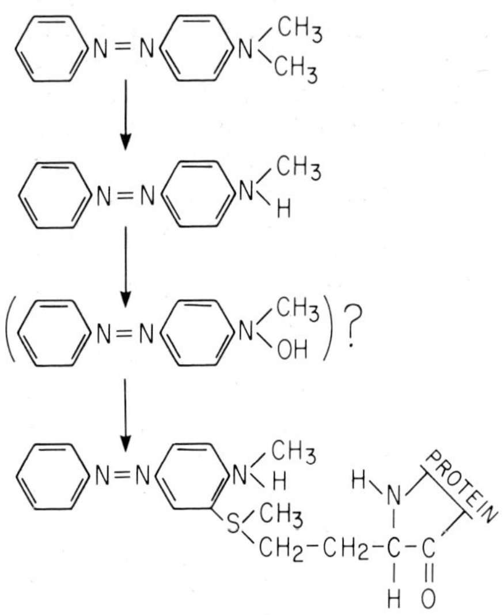

Fig. 16-27. Probable metabolic sequence of dimethylaminoazobenzene

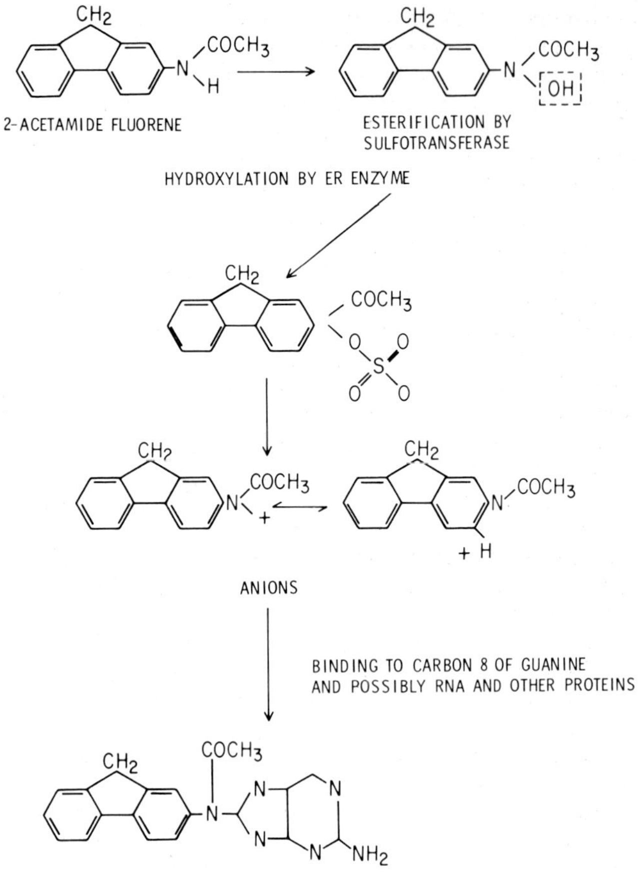

Fig. 16-28. Activation scheme of AAF. (After Miller and Miller [142])

findings made with both fluorene and MAB, Miller and his associates [142–145] have proposed a working hypothesis suggesting that the carcinogen is converted in a first step to an N-hydroxy derivative of the amine or the amide, which in turn is converted to a reactive ester that is capable of attacking nucleophiles such as DNA, RNA, and proteins. The binding then yields a cell with permanent losses of macromolecules regulating growth (see Fig. 16-28).

The development of inactive polycyclic hydrocarbons in active carcinogens has been explained in a similar fashion. For example, benzopyrene is converted to an active carcinogen. The conversion is catalyzed by the microsomal mixed hydroxylase system. In fact, liver microsome preparations can elaborate benzo(α)pyrene metabolites, which bind to DNA.

However, the exact molecular structure of the active carcinogen is unknown. In the polycyclic hydrocarbons, the K region epoxides have been suspected. Although it has been shown that K-region epoxides readily bind with purified preparations of macromolecules and transform hamster cells *in vitro*, isolation of DNA from mouse embryo cells cultured *in vitro* in the presence of [^{3}H]7-methylbenz[a]anthracene followed by DNA hydrolysis revealed that the hydrolysate contains hydrocarbon-deoxyribose nucleoside complexes different from those that are obtained by reacting DNA with K-region epoxides directly. Of course, these findings do not exclude the notion that K-region epoxides are the active carcinogens [146–149].

Conclusive evidence that the binding of carcinogens to nucleic acids is the cause of cancer has not yet been assembled. Even if binding of carcinogens to DNA causes cancer, the mechanism by which they do is likely to be complex because a number of factors could modulate the mode of binding: for example, the interaction of DNA with other macromolecules, the presence of competitors for binding sites, and the occurrence of DNA repair.

Although test tube experiments with purified macromolecular complexes have shown that 3,4-benzopyrene binding is lower when DNA histone preparations rather than deproteinized DNA are used, *in vivo* experiments indicate that mouse binding to satellite DNA (highly repetitive sequences that are part of heterochromatin) is of the same level as that of the rest of the chromatin [150–153].

Two-Stage Carcinogenesis

We have seen how the carcinogenic properties of some chemicals could be modulated in various ways. For example, the effect of a carcinogen can be activated by a hormone, or the concomitant administration of two carcinogens may result in the simple summation of the individual effects or in a multiplication of the effects, thus yielding combined carcinogenic properties greater than the sum of the carcinogenic power of the individual carcinogens. The administration of chloramphenicol or actinomycin can inhibit carcinogenic effects under some circumstances.

The significance of this modulation of chemical carcinogenesis, with respect to the pathogenesis of cancer in man, is obvious because substances that are in the environment at concentrations too low to be carcinogenic could become so with the proper stimulus. (The significance of the combination of carcinogenic effects is illustrated by a report indicating that the risk of developing cancer of the bladder is almost twice as great in smokers as in nonsmokers [154].) Unfortunately, the modulation of carcinogenic properties has proved difficult to measure. There is, however, one exception: experimental skin cancer.

Friedewald and Rous [155] were among the first to suggest that carcinogenesis in skin took place in two distinct stages. They based this conclusion on two sets of experiments. In one set, they painted rabbit ears with tar and found that tumors regressed if the applications were interrrupted. Later, when the applications were resumed, new tumors appeared at the sites of the old ones. These results suggested that the carcinogens had permanently damaged the cells in the painted area. In the second group of experiments, the application of the carcinogen, instead of being followed by the reapplication of another carcinogen, was followed by irritating the area in various ways. Even under those circumstances cancers developed. These results suggested that the carcinogens initiated some permanent damage in the cells that could promote carcinogenesis if an irritant was applied.

Extensive studies of two-stage carcinogenesis were then undertaken in Berenblum's [156] laboratory. The classic experiment consisted of a single application of methylcholanthrene, followed by repeated applications of croton oil. Such treatment yielded skin cancers. If the croton oil was applied before methylcholanthrene, no cancer developed. Croton oil alone is noncarcinogenic. A single dose of methylcholanthrene produces only a few tumors. Subsequent administration of croton oil increases the incidence of cancer and reduces the latent period for the appearance of cancer.

On the basis of these experiments, it was concluded that methylcholanthrene acts as an initiator, whereas croton oil acts as a promoter. It seemed logical to assume that the initiation induced a cellular injury that remained dormant until cellular proliferation took place. In such a case, one can anticipate that the incidence of tumors would depend upon the amount or number of applications of the initiator, and the rate of tumor production would depend upon the amount of promoter applied. Painstaking experiments of Berenblum and Shubik proved the assumption to be correct [157]. Other examples of two-stage carcinogenesis have been discovered. The systemic administration of urethane (initiator) followed by the topical application of croton oil (promoter) leads to the development of skin cancer at the application site.

Two-stage carcinogenesis is not restricted to the skin. It was already mentioned that in some strains of rats, cancers develop in ovaries implanted in the spleen only if a carcinogen is also administered. In some mice, leukemias can be produced with a single dose of X-irradiation (initiator) followed by the administration of urethane (promoter) [158].

The dissociation of the mechanism of carcinogenesis into two distinct steps has permitted investigators to determine whether the factors that modulate carcinogenesis act on the latent period or promotion. For example, the reduced incidence of tumors due to low caloric intake or the increased incidence of tumors caused by hormone administration appear to result from an influence on the promoter stage. Moreover, Van Duuren and his associates have isolated the active promoting factor in croton oil [159, 160]. The factor (12-O-tetradecanoyl-phorbol-13-acetate) is a fatty acid ester of a polyfunctional diterpin alcohol. The formula of phorbol is given in Fig. 16-29, and the formula of phorbol diester is given in Fig. 16-30. The structure of the active compound was determined by X-ray crystallography.

Although the compound is lipophilic-hydrophilic in nature, it would appear that the lipophilic-hydrophilic properties are not indispensable for tumor-promoting activity. The exact structural activity relationships have not been completely elucidated, but preliminary studies clearly suggest that the effect is highly specific. Studies with the radioactive phorbol ester also indicate that the compound may act somewhere on the cell membrane. As was the case with the crude croton oil, promotion with the phorbol ester is reversible. However, in contrast to croton oil, which exhibits no carcinogenic property, the phorbol ester is a weak carcinogen.

We know little of the molecular events associated with initiation or promotion. The general view is that initiation corresponds to a permanent molecular alteration of the cell, while promotion results in cell proliferation. Little is known of the permanent change that occurs during initiation, but it cannot be excluded that binding of the carcinogen to DNA or other macromolecules may be responsible for this change.

Although the initiation period is not associated with proliferation, it does require DNA synthesis. Paul [161] has shown that 9,10-dimethyl-1,2-benzanthracene

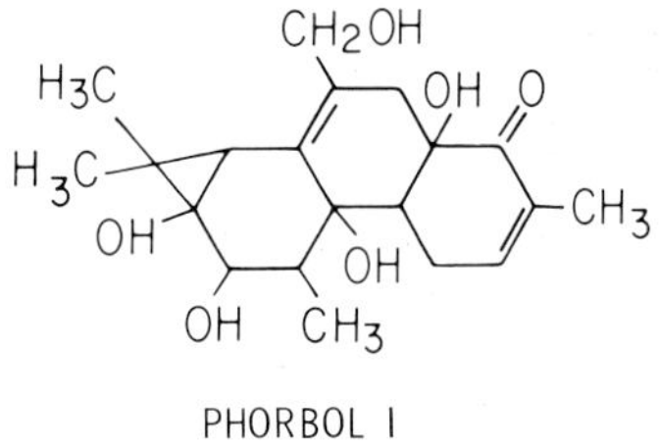

CH_2OH H_3C OH O H_3C CH_3 OH OH OH CH_3

PHORBOL I

Fig. 16-29. Phorbol I

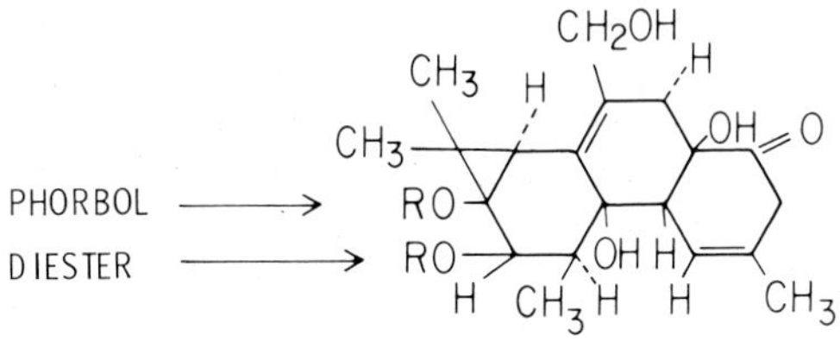

CH_2OH H CH_3 H CH_3 OH O PHORBOL → RO DIESTER → RO OH H H CH_3 H H CH_3

Fig. 16-30. Phorbol diester

(DMBA) induces DNA and RNA synthesis after a period of inhibiting such a macromolecular synthesis. In contrast, a weak carcinogen 1,2,3,4-dibenzanthracene (1,2,3,4-DBA) has no effect on DNA and little effect on RNA synthesis [100].

Antimetabolites that interfere with protein synthesis interfere with initiation, possibly by preventing the biosynthesis of the enzymes needed for proximate carcinogen formation.

Whatever the molecular mechanism involved in transformation by chemical carcinogens may be, it seems established (1) that transformation is inductive and not selective, (2) that transformation is independent of the toxicity of the carcinogen, (3) that transformation by chemical carcinogens is not likely to activate latent viruses, (4) that transformation *in vitro* is relevant to carcinogenesis *in vivo*.

Promotion with phorbol ester established that the promoter stimulates RNA, DNA, and protein synthesis. The events occur in sequence 18, 48, and 96 hours after application, respectively. The stimulation of DNA synthesis brought about by phorbol is not preceded by a period of inhibition of DNA synthesis as occurs with the initiator [162].

Tritium labeled phorbol-myristate-acetate was found to bind to cell membranes and to be localized in the portion of the membranes containing the potassium sodium ATPase. The addition of the phorbol esters to isolated cell membranes enhances the activity of both the ATPase and the 5′nucleotidase. One hour after treatment phorbol-myristate-acetate lowers the cyclic AMP levels in mouse skin and the reduction in cyclic AMP is maintained for 24 hours. Since theophylline inhibits the promoting effect it would appear that promotion is in some way linked to a decrease in cyclic AMP levels [574]. Phorbol-myristate-acetate induces a marked intracellular increase in the levels of cyclic GMP during the first minute after application. The cyclic GMP levels return to control levels after 3 minutes [575]. These studies clearly indicate that the primary site of action of the promoter is likely to be the cell membrane. It is, however, not clear what molecular alterations cause the enzyme changes and how the membrane events trigger other changes that follow the application of the promoter.

Phorbol esters 12-0-tetradecanoylphorbol-13-acetate, phorbol-12,13-didecanoate, and phorbol-12,13-benzoate were found to bind the microsomal and nucleolar membranes *in vitro*. The amount of phorbol ester that attaches to the membrane is modulated by the amounts of DNA added to the system [576].

Many laboratories have studied transformation *in vitro*. The first transformation with chemical carcinogens was achieved by Sachs [577], but the relevance of the transformation achieved *in vitro* to the *in vivo* situation needed to be established. This was mainly achieved in DiPaolo's and Heidelberger's laboratories.

DiPaolo's system consists of mixed hamster embryo cells plated on irradiated rat embryo feeder layers which are 6 to 24 hours after seeding and attachment treated with a carcinogen for periods ranging from half an hour to 7 hours. A number of morphological and biochemical criteria are used to evaluate transformation, but the most convincing is that the cell line derived from a transformed colony produces tumors when injected into the appropriate host [578]. Precautions were taken to exclude the possibility of viral contamination or activation. The transformed cells were tested for viral presence and reverse transcriptase was measured and shown to be absent.

In these experiments various doses of a given carcinogen and carcinogens of various potency *in vivo* were used. A linear relationship between the incidence of transformation and the dose of carcinogen was found. In addition, there was a good correlation between the potency of the carcinogen *in vivo* and its ability to transform *in vitro*.

Chemical Transformation in Vitro

Ever since methods have been available to culture cells *in vitro*, investigators have studied the effect of carcinogens on cells in culture. In 1953 Goldblatt and Cameron attempted to convert normal fibroblasts into cancer cells by depriving them of oxygen. Two years later, these investigators obtained some cultures that produced sarcomas after injection in intact animals. These experiments were not confirmed later, and the normal cells were probably converted into cancer cells spontaneously. Spontaneous transformations are known to occur with brain and liver cells [163] as well as with fibroblasts. The possibility of spontaneous transformation must, of course, be kept in mind in interpreting viral or chemically induced transformation in cell culture.

Further attempts involved the cultivation of fibroblasts in the presence of methylcholanthrene. The carcinogen was found to induce morphological changes in the cell; long and slender fibroblasts became plump, and the originally dispersed cells became compact and cohesive. Today cell cultures from various origins (liver, prostate, lung, mammary glands, brain) have been transformed with chemical carcinogens.

Various carcinogens have been used to achieve transformation *in vitro*, including polycyclic hydrocarbons, alkylating agents, and others. Transformation is accompanied by a number of alterations of the cellular, morphological, biochemical and functional properties, many of which were described when we considered viral transformation. These changes include changes in: membrane transport, membrane structure, adhesiveness to other cells and substratum, chromosomal number, growth characteristics, serum requirements, and morphological features. The relationship between any of these alterations and the transforming event is not known.

Heidelberger and his collaborators [164] transformed prostate cells with 3-methylcholanthrene; when the cells were injected in intact animals they produced sarcomas. The incidence of transformed cells was so high that it excluded the possibility of the carcinogen selectively facilitating the growth of preexisting malignant cells—a theory Prehn [166] proposed. The methylcholanthrene induces the development of the mixed-function oxidases in the culture cells, and benzoflavone inhibits transformation.

The chemically transformed clones are antigenic. This finding is in keeping with previous observations made on hydrocarbon-induced sarcomas in mice. Such sarcomas develop cell surface tumor-specific transplantation antigens that are individual and do not cross-react. Therefore, it is interesting that when pairs of transformed clones were picked from the same dishes, they were found not to be antigenically cross-reactive.

The study of chemical carcinogens *in vitro* may help to answer three important questions: (1) what is the relationship between chemical carcinogens and the oncogenic viruses; (2) is there any correlation between mutagenicity and carcinogenicity; (3) which of the biochemical changes that develop in the transformed cells are critical to the transformation process *in vitro* and carcinogenesis *in vivo*?

The oncogenetic theory proposes that chemicals and radiation produce cancer by activating a gene that may be of viral origin, but which invaded the genome maybe millions of years ago. If such is the case, one may expect that the cells transformed by chemical carcinogens will contain viral particles that should be infective for other cells. All available evidence seems to exclude this occurrence. However, the transformed cells could contain small amounts of the viral transcript that are not infective alone and cannot be detected with available methods.

If carcinogens cause the distortion of gene expression that is characteristic of cancer by altering the DNA, one may anticipate a close correlation between the carcinogen's ability to cause mutation and to cause cancer. Although the earlier studies done with bacteria did not suggest a correlation between carcinogenicity and mutagenicity, the extensive recent investigations, especially by DiPaolo's group [167] using mammalian cells, have established a correlation between mutagenicity and carcinogenicity whenever the metabolically activated forms of the carcinogens were used.

The relationship between mutagenicity and carcinogenicity is discussed below: maybe the most intriguing question raised by transformation, whether it be with viruses or chemicals, concerns the identification of the molecular events that are indispensable for the process. Clearly, the central event is a reprogramming of gene expression. We must discover what causes the reprogramming, and whether the pattern of reprogramming is random or nonrandom. Also, is there a single mechanism of transformation, or do a variety of molecular insults all ultimately result in a similar modification of cellular properties?

The alteration of gene expression could result from (1) direct alteration of the genome through a recent somatic cell mutation or a germ cell mutation, which would be transferred to the offspring and revealed later in life, or (2) through an ancestral germ mutation resulting in the inclusion of the oncogene in the genome.

Available evidence of chemical transformations does not exclude any of these possibilities, but the weight of existing evidence (*e.g.*, correlation between mutagenicity and carcinogenicity) seems to favor the somatic mutation. Although studies with chemical carcinogens strongly suggest that the alteration of gene expression is caused by direct damage to DNA, a modulation of DNA transcription induced by modification of the cell environment cannot be excluded. However, such a notion is difficult to reconcile with the fact that the properties of the transformed cell are transferred from one generation of cells to another, but the theory is compatible with the ubiquitous but varied alterations of the cell membranes that are associated with cancer.

The changes in the cell membrane may be the consequence or the cause of the alteration of gene expression. In transformed cells, it is not known which of these obtains.

However, the observation that N_6-2′-O-dibutyryl-3′,5′-cyclic adenosine monophosphate (DBcAMP) distorts normal morphology and leads to the transformation of fibroblasts is bound to stimulate further concern about the cell membrane's role in regulating cellular metabolism. Evidence that cyclic nucleotides also affect cellular proliferation came from observations indicating that increased levels of cAMP inhibited cell division, whereas inhibitors of enzymes generating cAMP stimulated replication. Cyclic GMP is suspected to influence cell division in phytohemagglutininstimulated lymphocytes, but its mode of action, or even the direction of its action, is not clear. The indications are that increased cGMP stimulates mitosis; therefore, the dynamic balance between the cellular concentration of cGMP and cAMP levels is believed to determine whether a cell divides or not.

cAMP-specific phosphodiesterases have been found to be activated when serum-free cultures of rat embryo cells are stimulated to divide, and the drop in the cAMP levels observed later in these growing cells is associated with the doubling of phosphodiesterase activity within an hour after serum stimulation. Ouabain and papavarine, which inhibit the phosphodiesterase, have been found to stimulate those systems that depend upon AMP for activity.

Another piece of evidence suggesting that the molecules of the cell membranes influence cellular proliferation comes from the observation that lymphocytes stimulated to proliferate increase their uptake of potassium. Inasmuch as this increase is inhibited by ouabain, the sodium potassium ATPase has been implicated. Moreover, calf serum, which stimulates cell growth in culture, has been found to influence ouabain binding sites.

The activites of K^+ and Na^+ ATPase and 5′-nucleotidase were found to be elevated in growing cells and reduced in the same cells when they were inhibited.

Chemical Carcinogenesis and DNA Repair

Many examples have been presented in which chemical carcinogens react directly or after metabolic conversion with many molecular constituents (nucleic acids, proteins, polysaccharides, molecules containing free SH groups, etc.). The relationship between covalent binding and the stepwise transformation of a normal cell into a cancerous cell, which exhibits survival advantages over all or most other cells in the environment, is not known. To be sure, binding to DNA molecules could be critical to transformation, but a clear link between DNA damage and oncogenesis has not been conclusively demonstrated. The study of the potential role of DNA binding in the carcinogenic process is complicated by the fact that repair of DNA to which carcinogens are bound has been demonstrated.

Thus, the single-strand breaks that are caused by the administration of acetylaminofluorene or benzopyrene progressively disappear, and unscheduled DNA synthesis occurs in cells in culture exposed to acetylaminofluorene or other carcinogens. The details of the enzymological steps involved in these repair processes are not known. Polynucleotide ligases have been found in various mammalian tissues and are likely to repair single-strand breaks. An enzyme has been purified from rat liver which knicks UV-irradiated DNA to which carcinogens are bound (acetylaminofluorene and bromoanthracene), thus permitting the distorted portion of the strand to be excised by $3' \rightarrow 5'$ exonucleases. The exonuclease and the DNA polymerase involved in excision repair in mammalian cells have not been identified.

If the purified enzymes responsible for DNA repair were available, they would help us understand the substrate specificity and kinetics of DNA repair, but such observations could provide only a somewhat distorted view of the happenings *in vivo*.

Although we know little of the molecular interaction of DNA with other macromolecules in the intact nucleus, in nonmetaphase nuclei some DNA molecules are transcribed while other are not. Therefore, a great deal if not most of the DNA's interact constantly with catalytic or structural proteins. It is thus fair to ask whether the nucleic acid-protein interaction restricts the accessibility of damaged DNA to the repair enzyme. If such restriction occurs, what portion of the DNA is most likely to be repaired, and what portion is not likely to be? In discussing the effect of X-irradiation on DNA synthesis, we concluded that only repressed DNA is not repaired. Whether a similar situation obtains for carcinogen-bound DNA remains to be seen.

Even the persistence of damage in DNA could be inconsequential to cell life, at least as long as such DNA is not transcribed or replicated. What happens if damaged DNA is transcribed or replicated is, at this point, purely speculative, but the consequences could include restoration of the integrity of the genome by mechanisms still unknown (*e.g.*, postreplicative repair), mutations, cellular death, and cancer.

Carcinogenesis and Mutations

There is little doubt that one of the major manifestations of cancer is a distortion of gene expression. Such distortions could be caused by various forms of molecular alteration, direct damage to DNA, inclusion of new DNA in the genome, as is the case with DNA or RNA tumor viruses, a permanent alteration of the types of DNA's that are derepressed.

A number of observations suggest that the primary event in carcinogenesis is a somatic mutation. For example, DNA is a major direct (*e.g.*, alkylating agents) and indirect (*e.g.*, epoxide, acetoxyacetylaminofluorene, etc.) target for carcinogen.

Patients with xeroderma pigmentosum in whom the DNA repair enzyme is missing are highly susceptible to cancer. Clearly, if carcinogens are mutagenic for mammalian cells *in vivo*, they should also be mutagenic *in vitro* and a simple test for detecting carcinogens could be devised. In the ideal experiment the incidence of mutation should be tested in mammals in the organ susceptible to develop tumors.

Maybe the most direct evidence that DNA is involved in transformation was obtained by Bendich who established that cells transformed in culture, by either carcinogens or viruses, were linked by intracellular bridges containing DNA. When nontumor cells were cultured together with tumor cells, the nontumor cells were transformed [533].

Not only must DNA be protected against damage, but it must also be protected from the introduction of foreign DNA within its molecules. The transcription of such foreign DNA would introduce new protein which not only would modify the phenotype, but could also be nefarious to the host.

In bacteria, specific endonucleases, called restriction endonucleases, protect against the introduction of foreign DNA by splitting it at specific sites. Such endonucleases fall into two major groups: one group, type I, consists of large enzymes composed of three subunits requiring ATP and S adenosyl methionine for activity; type II consists of small enzymes that function without these coenzymes. Also, both types require magnesium for activity. These enzymes cause double strand breaks apparently by recognizing a 6 base sequence on each strand. The sequence is unique in that it is symmetrical. If the double stranded 6 nucleotide sequence is divided into an upper ($5' \rightarrow 3'$) and lower ($3' \rightarrow 5'$) strand, and each strand split into two triads, the sequence of the triad at the $3'$ end of the upper strand is the mirror image of the triad at the $3'$ end of the lower strand. Similarly the triads at the two $5'$ ends are mirror images.

$5' \rightarrow 3'$
$\downarrow$
G—T—Py — Pu—A—C upper
strand
C—A—Pu — Py—T—G lower
$3' \uparrow \rightarrow 5'$

The DNA sequence is recognized by the type II restriction endonuclease prepared from *Hemophilus influenzae* (R enzyme). Notice that the central bases are not specified. That is because the enzyme specificity is not restricted by the type of base present in the center of the sequence. There is ambiguity of the bases in the center of the sequence [579].

Since such methods are not available, bacteria, mammalian cells in culture and host mediated assays have been used to test the mutagenicity of carcinogens. The first attempts to test the mutagenic properties of known carcinogens were disappointing mainly because bacteria are often devoid of the biochemical machinery necessary to convert inactive to active carcinogens, and it was only after exposure of the natural compound (*e.g.*, acetylaminofluorene) to microsomal enzymes that compounds were formed which were mutagenic for bacteria. In other cases the active product was extracted from urine after administration of the carcinogen [580]. Ames used histidine negative *Salmonella typhimurium* strains to test the mutagenicity of carcinogens. These bacteria are auxotrophs in which molecular changes of DNA in the histidine operon are well characterized. The operon that converts the 5 carbon chain of phosphoribosyl pyrophosphate to histidine exists on a single cluster. Ames *et al.* [581] tested 20 carcinogens in their system and found that 20 of the established carcinogens or proximate carcinogens were also mutagenic.

In other experiments *E. coli* mutants lacking polymerase I (pol AI) [708, 709] have been used to screen some carcinogens; namely, derivatives of nitrofuran. It was found that the nitrofuran derivatives were mutagenic for the *E. coli*, but not for the *S. typhimurium*. These results indicate that detection of potential carcinogens by bacterial mutation may require that several different bacterial systems be used.

The (pol A) strain isolated by Cairns from *E. coli* W 3110 (pol A+) was used to test the mutagenic properties of the greenhouse fungicide captan. The fungicide is mutagenic in bacteria, teratogenic in bird embryos and is an alkylating agent in mammals. One can hardly ask for more evidence leading to the suspicion that captan might be carcinogenic for humans.

The simple observation that carcinogens are mutagens is of considerable significance because it provides further evidence for the somatic mutation theory and it may help to identify the molecular damage caused by carcinogens. One may, however, wonder whether data collected on bacteria can be extrapolated to man. The uptake, metabolism and excretion of carcinogens in mammals vary considerably from that in bacteria and therefore, the correlation can only be qualitative. Moreover, the effect of a carcinogen *in vivo* may be altered by promoters, which may themselves not be mutagenic. There are, in fact, several carcinogens that were inactive as mutagens in bacteria, but are carcinogenic in humans and a few compounds that are mutagenic in bacteria are not carcinogenic in mammals because they are effectively detoxified. Therefore, studies of bacterial mutagenesis can only serve as a preliminary screening technique which must be followed by testing on mammalian cells and ultimately on mammals that behave as closely as possible to humans.

Because of these limitations of the bacterial system, other systems have been devised; namely, mammalian cells in culture and host-mediated assay. Those using cell cultures have used either cells obtained from individuals with known hereditary defects (galactosemia, etc.) or cells which have changed while in culture and have become drug resistant, have acquired new nutritional requirements or have changed in thermal sensitivity.

Auxotroph mutants are also often used. Most cells in culture can synthesize purines and pyrimidines, but as the line develops some cells lose their ability to synthesize bases, amino acids, etc. As a result of a spontaneous mutation, thanks to the advances made in tissue culture techniques such as single cell plating, clone isolation and the development of chemically defined media, it is possible to isolate the auxotrophic mutant and define its dependency. In absence of the needed nutrient, the dependent cells will not grow. If BUDR is added to the medium, the wild type, which continues to grow, picks up the BUDR. All cells whose DNA contains BUDR can readily be killed by exposure to near visible light (see Chapter 12). By transferring the surviving cells to media containing the defective nutrient, one can obtain the dependent cell lines. Auxotrophic mutants dependent on carbohydrate purine, pyrimidine, amino acids, etc. have been prepared.

When a population of 5×10^6 cells was examined for spontaneous mutation with the BUDR technique, no spontaneous mutants were observed, but a variety of auxotrophic mutants were found when the cells were treated with ethylmethanesulfonate, H-methyl-H^1-nitro-N-nitroguanidine, UV light, acridine mustard, N-nitrosodimethylamine, N-nitrosomethylurea and N-nitrosomethylurethane. These mutants are stable and have a diploid chromosome population [582].

In the host mediated assay an animal is injected with the mutagen or carcinogen and with a test organism such as the *S. typhimurium, Neurospora crassa, Saccharomyces cervisiae*. The test system is after an appropriate time removed from the host and mutations are scored. Using such an approach it has been established that certain types of mutations occur with certain types of carcinogens. For example, according to Malling and Chu polycyclic hydrocarbons induce predominantly base insertion and deletion, while alkyl carcinogen (dimethylnitrosamine) induces base pair substitutions [583].

Carcinogens in Humans

Undoubtedly, the combined efforts of organic chemists, biologists, and biochemists have dug deep tunnels into the unknown of cancer. Whether or not these inroads will lead to a cure of the disease is not certain. Yet one thing is clear: carcinogens exist in large numbers and in great varieties. Chemicals discretely but fatally pollute the water we drink, the food we eat, the air we breathe, and the smoke we inhale. Once these chemicals have been introduced into the body by mechanisms unknown and difficult to unravel—in part because of the multiplicity of factors that may affect carcinogenicity (hormones, age of other carcinogens, etc.)—these chemicals may, in a number of cases, convert one or more intact cells into cancer cells.

To deny that some of the carcinogens proved to be efficient in the laboratory are active in humans is unrealistic and dangerous. To be convinced, one needs only to review epidemiology and the geographic distribution of cancer [169–171]. In 1853 Paget vigorously attacked Sir Percivall Pott's interpretation of the pathogenesis of cancer of the scrotum in chimney sweepers and claimed that soot had nothing to do with cancer. Years later, Curling described a higher incidence of skin cancer among gardeners who used soot as a fertilizer. Workers who used to manipulate tar to build ships, roads, and shoes frequently presented warts that over the years developed into cancer. The warts sometimes appeared in unusual parts of the body, such as the ears of those carrying sacks full of coal, or the feet of those working barefoot. The weavers of Lancastershire, whose clothes were continuously splashed with lubricating oil, developed skin cancer at the site of maximum impregnation of their clothes. Paraffin workers develop carcinomas of the scrotum, forearm, and leg.

Perhaps the most dramatic illustration of the presence of carcinogens in the environment was observed among workers inhaling aniline vapors. In 1895 Rehn described several cases of cancer of the bladder among such workers. But before that, Granhomme had listed hematuria among the symptoms resulting from chronic aniline intoxication. This was less than 20 years after aniline dyes were first used in industry. Soon after Rehn's description, cancer of the bladder was observed among workers in many factories in Germany and Switzerland. Kennaway and his associates [172] in 1921 reported 5614 cases of cancer of the bladder and demonstrated that the incidence was four times greater among aniline workers than among farmers. The disease was practically unknown in the United States until the turn of the century. This may well reflect the fact that the aniline industry was introduced on the American continent only in 1893. That the repeated application of the crude material was related to the development of cancer could no longer be doubted once it became possible to produce cancer experimentally with the aid of the crude material and to extract pure carcinogens from most of the materials described above.

This brief outline by no means exhausts the large list of profession-related cancers due to chemical carcinogens, but it illustrates one of the most threatening socioeconomic problems of our times. The list is endless. Those working in coal mines frequently develop cancer of the nostrils. Asbestos workers develop mesotheliomas of the pleura. Workers exposed to benzol may develop leukemia. Those who work in arsenic smelters develop skin cancer.

Angiosarcoma of the liver is rare in man. Though it cannot be excluded that under some circumstances it can develop spontaneously, available evidence suggests that most cases are probably caused by the administration of chemical carcinogens. Vineyard workers in France and Germany, exposed to arsenical insecticide, have a high incidence of this tumor. A patient treated for psoriasis with sodium arsenite (Fowler's solution) developed a hemangioendotheliosarcoma.

In animals angiosarcomas can be produced by dimethylnitrosamine-1,1-dimethylhydrazine and diethylnitrosamine or by feeding the plant *Senecio longilobus,* which contains pyrrolizidine alkaloids. More recently angiosarcomas were seen among workers involved in the manufacture of polyvinyl chloride, the monomer of which vinyl chloride is believed to be the culprit.

In 1971 Violo *et al.* reported the development of cancers in animals exposed to vinyl chloride [584]. Vinyl chloride is a colorless gas, barely soluble in water, but slightly soluble in organic solvents such as ethanol. Polyvinyls contain 2 to 7% of vinyl chloride. Vinyl chloride has some narcotic property, but in large doses (500 parts per million), it's toxic to animals in which it produces pulmonary edema and hemorrhages, congestion of liver and kidney and interference with blood clotting. Higher doses (30,000 parts per million) will lead to degeneration of skeletal muscle and connective tissue with a histopathological picture similar to that seen in acroosteolysis of the hands [584–587].

Inasmuch as vinyl chloride is a rather unreactive compound, it is not believed to be the direct carcinogen and carcinogenesis is thought to be induced by a metabolite of the vinyl chloride, an epoxide, halo ethers or a free radical. For further information see [588].

Talc, a magnesium silicate, has been implicated in the high incidence of gastric carcinoma in Japan. Indeed, the Japanese consume a great deal of rice. The rice is coated with glucose and talc to produce a nutrient that is superior in appearance and taste. Talc is frequently contaminated with several types of fibrous silicates which are usually identified as asbestos.

The potential relationship between the development of benign hepatic adenoma and the use of contraceptives was suggested by Baum [589]. Since then the number of cases described have increased exponentially. Although the histology of the tumor varies, the lesions are always benign. The tumor may grow and undergo central necrosis, and occasionally may rupture and cause death. In other cases the tumor is associated with thrombosis of the main hepatic vein with congestion and hemorrhage (Budd-Chiari syndrome) [590].

When the relationship between the agent and cancer is obvious, as in the case of aniline and cancer of the bladder, prevention is easy, especially if it is a social rather than an individual responsibility. Sometimes even when the relationship between agent and cancer becomes convincing, all efforts to protect individuals fail. A case in point is the relationship between smoking and lung cancer. This type of cancer occurs almost exclusively among heavy cigarette smokers. Those that smoke pipes and cigars and do not inhale the smoke suffer few effects, if any. Today more people, and especially more young people, die of lung cancer in the civilized world than in all recorded medical history.

This is not the place to review the vast literature that has appeared on the relationship between smoking and cancer, and only a few salient observations will be mentioned. Although a correlation between smoking and cancer has frequently been observed by clinicians,* Doll and Hill [174, 175] were the first to establish this relationship on a solid statistical basis. Their study established a remarkable correlation between smoking histories and the incidence of lung cancer. These studies were criticized because they did not include an analysis of the role of other environmental factors, such as inhalation of polluted air, in the incidence of lung cancer. Of course, the participation of such environmental factors is difficult to eliminate, since practically the entire population of the Western world is exposed to high concentrations of soot, industrial fumes, and the products of automobile exhaust; and none of the existing studies on lung cancer has definitely excluded the participation of air pollution in eliciting lung cancer in man. Yet, statistical analyses of large populations in various industrial countries like England and the United States clearly indicate that the incidence of lung cancer is much higher among smokers than among nonsmokers, wherever they live. One can hardly underestimate the importance of a difference in incidence on the order of twenty on the side of smokers.

The painstaking double-blind histological studies of large populations of smokers and nonsmokers performed by Auerbach [176] strongly indicated that smoking alters the epithelium of the tracheobronchial tube. The lesions consist of basal cell hyperplasia with alteration of the normal epithelial cell into a more atypical cell, sometimes indistinguishable from cancerous cells. In fact, these atypical epithelial cells may even present signs of early invasion. Whether these lesions are precancerous remains to be seen. Yet similar lesions have been produced experimentally in smoking dogs, some of which ultimately developed cancer.

In 1967 it was estimated that 52,000 people, 42,000 men and 10,000 women, would die of lung cancer. There is enough suspicion about the relationship between smoking and lung cancer to warrant preventive measures. An example of lung cancer in a heavy smoker is shown in Fig. 16-31.

Because there is a great similarity between modes of consumption of marijuana and tobacco, it is important to determine whether or not the smoking of cannabis is carcinogenic.

The daily application of marijuana smoke condensates to the skin for 5 days in 10 albino Swiss and 10 black and white F_1 hybrid mice leads to ablation of the sebaceous glands, hyperkeratosis and acanthosis with focal enlargement, hyperchromasia of nuclei, and poor cellular polarity. Since complete ablation of sebaceous glands correlates with the carcinogenic properties of some compounds, the results suggest the possibility that marijuana condensates may be carcinogenic.

Compared to cigarette smokers, the amount of smoke inhaled by even heavy users of marijuana is very small. Therefore, unless marijuana contains high concentrations or an unusually effective carcinogen, it is unlikely that the incidence of cancer in humans by marijuana would be very high. Yet, the consequences of our lack of knowledge of the dangers of smoking cigarettes have been so tragic to the human race that it seems imperative to ascertain the carcinogenic potential of any drug likely to be used by a large number of consumers.

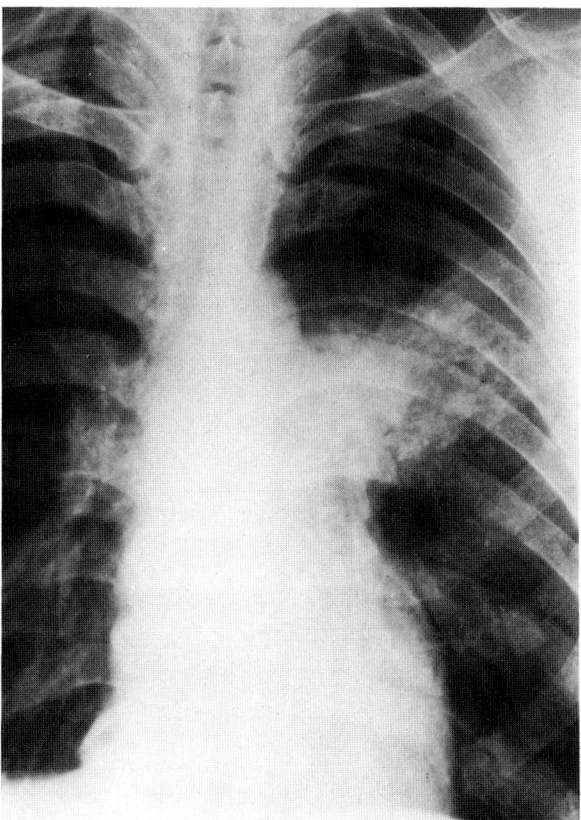

Fig. 16-31. Lung cancer in a heavy smoker

* John Hill, a physician who wrote operas, novels, and farces, seemed to have been the first to attract public attention to the carcinogenic properties of tobacco. He wrote a note entitled "Caution Against the Immoderate Use of Snuff," in which cancers of the nostrils were attributed to the abuse of snuff [173].

Our environment is likely to contain many unsuspected carcinogens. For example, aminoazotoluol, extracted from seemingly harmless buttercups, was used for coloring margarine, and was proven to be carcinogenic. Cosmetics, foods, and drinks are colored artificially; which coloring materials are carcinogenic? The carcinogenic properties of acetylaminofluorene were discovered by testing insecticides that were sprayed on cranberry bushes until the 1960s. Cyclamates are believed to be carcinogenic for the bladder. Carcinogenic polycyclic hydrocarbons have been detected in the smoke emanating from charcoal grills and have been found on the surface of broiled meats. The number of carcinogens in our environment is unknown, yet detecting them may be more beneficial to man's health than curing cancer, because once the cause is known, preventive measures can be taken.

The carcinogenic properties of nitrosamines are well established. Both nitrites and secondary amines can be found in the diet. Gastric juice is capable of stimulating the formation of nitrosamine by the combination of nitrites and the secondary amines; similarly enteric bacteria can form nitrosamine from nitrites and the secondary amines. At least one, nitrosamine dibutyl nitrosamine (NDB), is known to be carcinogenic for rodent bladder.

Whether a similar mechanism plays a role in carcinogenesis in the human gastrointestinal tract remains to be seen. Although the incidence of stomach cancer is reaching epidemic proportions in Japan, it is decreasing in the United States. A radiological view of a cancer of the stomach is shown in Fig. 16-32.

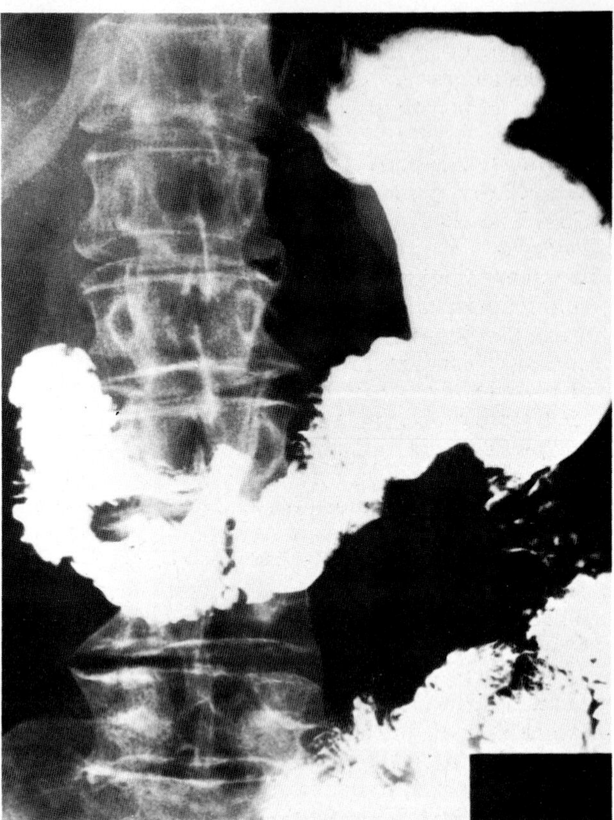

Fig. 16-32. Cancer of the stomach. Defective filling of the stomach with barium is due to the presence of a tumor in the antrum

The geographical distribution of cancer of the liver is somewhat unusual. Practically nonexistent in some countries like the United States, it is common in other parts of the world like Africa. In Mozambique the incidence of cancer of the liver is said to be 500 times that in the United States and 30 times that in Johannesburg. In Hong Kong, cancer of the liver is found in 30% of all autopsies. Carcinogens produced by fungi could be responsible for the high incidence of cancer of the liver in those areas. The carcinogenic properties of aflatoxin have already been discussed. In many of the countries where cancer of the liver prevails, aflatoxins have been found to contaminate the food. In addition, a number of other fungal toxins,often of quite different molecular structures, have been found to cause cancer not only of the liver, but also of the kidney and the stomach in experimental animals [177].

The list of drugs that are either proven or potential carcinogens increases every day. There is a serious question as to the propriety of their use in humans. An impressive number of antiseptics, antibiotics, analgesics, tranquilizers, and drug additives are known to be carcinogenic in animals or in humans when the humans are exposed to these compounds because of their professional activities.

Tars have been part of the therapeutic arsenal of dermatologists for generations. Chlorinated hydrocarbons, chloroform, and tetrachloroethylene have been used for many years as anesthetics; tetrachloroethylene has been used as an anthelmintic. Cancer of the liver has been reported in an individual using carbon tetrachloride as an extinguishing fluid. Whether chlorinated hydrocarbons are frequently involved in human carcinogenesis remains to be established.

Diethylene glycol, frequently used as a solvent for drugs, produces cancer of the bladder in rats. The carcinogen propylactone is used as an antiseptic to sterilize arterial grafts and serum for transfusion. Propionolactone produces fibrosarcoma when injected, carcinomas of the skin when painted, and carcinomas of the lung when introduced intratracheally in rats.

The β-propionolactone, which contains a four-membered strained ring, is highly reactive. It is an alkylating carcinogen. For example, it reacts with the sulfhydryl group of cysteine to yield S-2-carboxyethyl cysteine. Penicillin G is also a lactone group. Dickens' studies suggest that penicillin is a weak and slow-acting carcinogen which, after repeated injections, may produce carcinomas or fibrocarcinomas in rats. Some steroidal components and cardiac glycosides contain α- and β-unsaturated lactone rings. Although some of these glycosides have been known to be cytotoxic in tissue culture, evidence that they are carcinogenic is lacking.

Several petroleum products, such as mineral oil and petroleum waxes, may or may not contain carcinogenic hydrocarbons, depending upon their degree of refinement. A number of dyes (trypan blue, acid green, acridine, and creosote) used as antiseptics for local application or in gauze preparations for treating wounds are carcinogenic in animals. Acridine derivatives, such as acriflavine and quinoline, have been suspected to be carcinogenic, but no conclusive evidence has been provided.

Phenol acts as a promoter in skin cancer produced in mice with DMBA. Distillation of coal tar between 200° and 400° yields a population of compounds referred to as creosote. Creosol is a major component of creosote. Creosote produces skin cancer in mice, and reports have appeared of skin cancer with metastases developing in people working in the creosote industry. Tannins, long used in treating burns, induce hepatomas in rats. Reserpine, used in the treatment of hypertension, markedly accelerates the induction of hepatomas in animals.

Already in 400 B.C., Hippocrates recommended arsenical ointments for the treatment of skin ulcers. The use of arsenic was advocated in an incredible number of unrelated diseases: anemia, bronchial asthma, eczema, acne, epilepsy, and psychoneurosis. The efficacy of using organic arsenicals in therapy for syphilis and some parasitic diseases such as amebiasis and trypanosomiasis has been known for a long time. Arsenicals have been added to food to prevent parasitic disease in fish, poultry, and livestock. Inorganic arsenic, which has been generously prescribed in ointments and potions for centuries, is carcinogenic in man. Indeed, arsenical dust and fumes cause cancer of the skin and lungs in the smelter workers. The drinking water of Liechtenstein is polluted with arsenic and it is believed to have effected the increased incidence of cancer of the skin and viscera that afflicts the inhabitants of the small town. Increased incidence of skin cancer has been reported in patients with cirrhosis who are subjected to prolonged treatment with arsenic.

Both nickel and chrome, which are used in the preparation of nails and plates for bone surgery, are claimed by Heuper to be carcinogenic in man. Isoniazid, a drug that has helped eliminate tuberculosis, produces adenomas of the lung in mice. The intricacies of interpreting this finding will be reviewed later.

The discovery of the carcinogenicity of certain drugs raises the important and difficult problem of deciding whether a drug proved or suspected to be a carcinogen in animals or man should continue to be used in therapy. Moreover, should all drugs be tested for potential carcinogenicity, and, if so, what tests will be most revealing and will determine the decision of maintaining or withdrawing the drug from the market?

First, we must remind ourselves that the concept of carcinogenicity is a relative one. A given carcinogen is not carcinogenic for all animals, all species, all tissues in an animal, and at all times during a life span. Thus, the carcinogenic properties of a chemical vary considerably with age, strain, species, and type of cancer. Consequently, if a test for carcinogenesis is positive in one strain of animal, it cannot be concluded that it will be positive for all strains. Moreover, if one method of administration of the carcinogen is used, it cannot be concluded that introducing the drug by other methods will also cause cancer.

In contrast, if the results of the studies in animals are negative, the possibility that the drug could be carcinogenic in humans cannot be excluded. Therefore, the potential carcinogenicity of a given drug should be tested in a number of different species (rats, mice, hamsters, etc.), and testing should involve entire life spans of the animal (pregnancy, newborns, and adults). In all cases, the survey should include complete autopsies and examination of all lesions by a competent pathologist.

Two methods are available to determine whether a drug is carcinogenic in humans: the retrospective and the prospective approaches. Both methods obviously resort to statistical analysis of large amounts of information. In the retrospective approach, the incidence of cancer among patients who received the drug for a long time is investigated. But drug dosage and circumstances of use are difficult to survey accurately. We shall give an example of the difficulties involved when we discuss the carcinogenic role of therapeutic radiation.

In the prospective method, the survey is planned at the start, and follow-up studies of the patients and frequent examinations to detect cancer are planned. Such studies in humans are complicated by: (1) the long latent period between the time of administration of the carcinogen and the development of cancer; (2) the multiplicity and diversity of cancer that occurs in human beings; (3) the difficulty of obtaining a complete record of the intake of other drugs and of food additives—even if intake could be known, it is likely to vary considerably from one individual to the other; (4) the fact that carcinogenesis is complex and occurs in two phases—initiation and promotion; and (5) the difficulty in determining whether a drug acts as a promoter or an initiator. Despite these difficulties, careful epidemiological studies have occasionally linked the development of specific cancers (skin cancer and arsenic, lung cancer and cigarettes) to a specific carcinogen. In such cases, it is simple to propose the elimination of the carcinogen from the environment.

The case of isoniazid as described by Shubick is of particular interest. As mentioned before, isoniazid produces adenomas of the lungs in Swiss mice; but when investigators attempted to demonstrate isoniazid's carcinogenicity in other species, they were unsuccessful. Moreover, careful examination of the animals receiving isoniazid revealed that the drug, as it induced lung cancer, also reduced the incidence of some other cancer to which that strain of mice is prone (*e.g.*, breast cancer). In most cases, however, the decision to maintain or eliminate a potential carcinogen from the pharmacopeia rests on complex and sometimes conflicting data. In fact, Shubick's group reports that some fibroadenomas and breast cancer that had begun to appear receded after isoniazid was adminstered. In the face of these many, sometimes irreconcilable, facts, how is it possible to enounce wise rules for the use of drugs? Obviously, no drug should be used unless it is indispensable to the maintenance of the patient's physical and mental health, and only when needed should drugs be used for securing temporary comfort (elimination of pain).

Special consideration should be given to all drugs that are used for prolonged periods of time, such as hypotensive agents and anticoagulants. If the drug is carcinogenic in animals, physicians should attempt to replace it with a noncarcinogenic drug whenever possible. Carefully planned studies should be pursued in patients submitted to prolonged therapy with new drugs, keeping the possibility of cancer in mind.

If a drug is a proven carcinogen in humans, it should be eliminated from the market unless, of course, the condition of administration excludes the possibility of carcinogenesis, or the expected life span of the patient (because of age or disease) is much shorter than the latent period necessary for developing cancer.

Drugs that are not known to be carcinogens in humans or rats should not be considered safe until prospective studies in humans have established them to be. The chemical structure of the drug may serve as a guide for the detection of potential carcinogens.

Special precautions should be taken when the drug is to be administered to pregnant or lactating women or to newborns.

Several observations suggest that human cancers might frequently be caused by a combination of factors. For example, it would appear that the consumption of alcohol by itself does not increase the incidence of cancer of the mouth or the esophagus, but the combination of heavy drinking and smoking increases the risk of cancer considerably [591].

Viruses and Cancer Viruses

Introduction

Although viruses were not the first agents to be incriminated, the idea that cancer is propagated through infectious agents is not new. A number of clinical observations tended to implicate parasites in the pathogenesis of cancer. Fibiger [178] claimed to have identified and isolated a parasite, the *Congyglonema neoplastica,* that produced stomach cancer in the rats that had found a comfortable home in Copenhagen sugar factories. Whether the stomach tumors Fibiger observed were carcinomas or papillomas, or whether they were produced by the parasite or in part as a result of vitamin A deficiency, has long been debated.

Borrel [155] observed the frequent interaction between sarcoma of the liver and the presence of *Taenia crassicollis.*

A few investigators have devoted a large portion of their time in attempting to establish that bacteria cause cancer in animals and man. For example, Nebel claimed that some cancers were associated with the growth of a special kind of bacteria, the rather unusual life cycle of which ultimately yields active ultrafiltrates. Although other investigators identified tumor bacteria resembling those described by Nebel, they were never able to produce cancer experimentally with these bacteria.

Curtis and Bullock [180] produced liver cancer in a special strain of rats by infection with the taenia. Schistosomiasis on the southern coast of Asia has been repeatedly claimed to be associated with the development of cancer of the liver, and in Egypt, a relationship between the incidence of cancer of the bladder and schistosomiasis has frequently been claimed.

As with all new discoveries in the field of cancer, great hope was generated when viral tumors were found, but some confusion and even doubt arose. Early nebulous claims on the infectious nature of cancer had put future generations of investigators on their guard, and any new claim incriminating infectious agents in the pathogenesis of cancer was bound to be accepted with skepticism. For example, while Rous [181–183] claimed to have extracted a virus from an experimental cancer in the Plymouth Rock chick, Nakahara [160] was unable to confirm this finding. Soon some investigators became convinced that all cancers were due to viruses, while others claimed that the viral cancers were a rare occurrence unrelated to the pathogenesis of cancer in man (Murphy and Sturm).

Such confusion still prevailed in the early 1950s. To illustrate that state of mind, I would like to relate a brief encounter I had at Yale with Duran Reynal. In my naiveté, which only my youth could excuse, I asked the elegant and well-dressed gentleman if he thought that human cancers were caused by viruses. In a gesture worthy of a noble Spaniard, Reynal put his left hand on his chest and solemnly stated, "Yes, I feel it deep in my heart." Whether or not this was a humorous answer to a somewhat irresponsible question, I will never know. Yet today the answer and the question need to be reconsidered.

Sanarelli [185] had in 1848 established that infectious myxomatosis observed in domestic rabbits was a contagious disease and a virus was incriminated, but the tumor was not considered to be a cancer. The breakthrough came in 1910 [182] as the result of the remarkable observations made by Peyton Rous in a Plymouth Rock chick. This chick had a fusocellular sarcoma that could be transmitted with the aid of an ultrafiltrate. Rous' findings were confirmed within a year by the independent studies of Fujinami and Inamoto [186, 187].

There is at present no doubt that a number of animal cancers are caused by viruses, and viruses have already been incriminated in some known forms of human cancer, particularly leukemia and lymphoma.

Viruses

The world of viruses is unique, but at the same time, fundamental to the mechanisms of life, so that it would be unwise to consider cancer viruses separately from more general principles in the molecular and cellular biology of viruses.

The virus is essentially a complex of macromolecules capable of self-replication. The major macromolecular components are nucleic acids and proteins. Self-replication occurs with the aid of the biosynthetic machinery present in the living host cell. Thus, viruses are obligatory parasites. Viruses grow in bacteria, plants, and animals.

Jenner was the first to deal successfully with a viral disease without suspecting the nature of the agent. Later, Pasteur applied to the treatment of rabies the principles that he had learned from studying bacteria, in spite of the fact that the agent of rabies defied isolation and culture by classical microbiological methods.

Although Pasteur postulated that some diseases were caused by invisible agents, the proof of the existence of viral disease came only when tissue extracts filtered on Chamberland or Berkefeld filters were demonstrated to transfer the disease repeatedly. When a tissue extract is passed through such filters, the filtrate is usually free of cells and bacteria, yet when brain extracts of victims of rabies were used, the disease was found to be transmissible with such an extract free of cells and bacteria. Transmission is not caused by a toxin, because filtrates of brain of previously injected animals can be used to transmit the disease over and over again. Thus, the agent of rabies must replicate in the host.

But although many viral diseases were known to occur in humans and other mammals, early information of the structure and replication of viruses came from investigations of bacterial and plant viruses.

In 1898, Hankin [188] described a most intriguing observation in the *Annales de l'Institut Pasteur*. He had discovered that the water of the Ganges and the Yumma contained a heat-labile bactericidal agent especially efficient against the *Vibrio cholerae*. Although Hankin attributed the bactericidal effect to toxins elaborated by microorganisms, it was later suspected that the lysis of the Vibrio resulted from a bacteriophage in the water.

In 1915 Twart, for the first time, described transmissible bacteriolysis. Twart's observation was derived from a study of bacterial contamination of smallpox vaccine. He found that some of the bacterial colonies that were cultivated in a medium containing vaccine virus went through a lytic process. Furthermore, he could transfer indefinitely the lysing agent from one culture medium to another with the aid of a platinum wire.

In spite of these earlier findings, one can truly state that the history of bacteriophages started with Herelle, who discovered that the feces of patients convalescing from bacterial dysentery contained a factor bacteriolytic for bacilli of the coli of the typhic group. This observation was soon followed by the discovery of a large number of transmissible bacteriolytic agents. A controversy arose as to the nature of the agent. While Kobeshima claimed that the bacteriolytic effect resulted from a catalyst that stimulated a lytic enzyme present in bacteria, Bordet believed that the lytic factor was itself a lytic enzyme. Herelle had postulated at the start that the bacteriolytic factor was a virus. Bruynoghe [189] supported this view and proposed that different viruses existed for each type of bacteria. The marvel is that bacteriologists stubbornly pursued their investigation of bacterial viruses and thereby laid the foundations of modern molecular biology.

The general properties of bacteriophages and the influence that these studies had on the development of molecular genetics have already been described. Studies on plant viruses have also largely contributed to our knowledge of viral structure and chemistry. In 1892 Iwanowski demonstrated that the agents responsible for a disease observed in tobacco plants were ultrafiltrable. The infection of tobacco leaves proved later to be a marvelous means for obtaining large amounts of virus, which could then be studied for chemistry, infectiousness, and morphology.

Before we attempt to discuss the properties of viruses in greater detail, let us first consider the elementary molecular biology of viruses.

Introduction to the Molecular Biology of Viruses

We have seen that bacteriophages are composed of a nucleic acid core (DNA) and a protein coat. Only the nucleic acid enters the bacteria, where it dictates the biosynthesis of its own protein coat and the replication of its own DNA—all this by taking advantage of the host's enzymic equipment. Plant, insect, and animal viruses have molecular properties similar to those of the phage. In 1935 Stanley [190] isolated and crystallized the tobacco mosaic virus (TMV). This important discovery was followed by intensive studies of the chemical composition of the virus, which was found to have an RNA core and a protein coat. The two components can be dissociated from each other, and they can be recombined to generate an infective virus.

The first indication that the RNA of the virus was responsible for infectivity and self-duplication came from experiments of Markham and Smith. After ultracentrifugation of turnip mosaic virus, these English investigators were able to separate two different components, both containing proteins with identical immunological properties; yet only one of the components, the one that sedimented with the lower centrifugal forces, was infective. This heavy component contained RNA in addition to protein. These findings established that the nucleic acid is infective, but they did not prove that protein is uninvolved in infection. In fact, as late as 1955, many scientists believed that genetic information, in part, was stored in the amino acid sequence of proteins. Fraenkel-Conrat [191] in the United States and Schramm [192] in Germany observed that the separated protein was not infective, although the reconstituted viral RNA-protein complex was. Later, after painstaking efforts, Fraenkel-Conrat conclusively established that RNA alone was infective. His studies carefully excluded the possibility of contamination of RNA by intact virus. These studies finally established that in RNA viruses, RNA plays the role of DNA of the bacteriophages.

Properties of Viruses. With these introductory remarks, we can now examine some of the details of the properties of viruses. Viruses infect bacteria, plants, insects, and mammals. For unknown reasons, a large number of living organisms are free from viral infection.

The size of a virus varies from half the size of a small bacterium to the size of 5 to 10 hemoglobin molecules. Viruses are of various shapes—spheres, polygons, cubes, and others.

There is no immediate correlation between viral size, shape, and the host's susceptibility. As a result, an orderly classification of viruses is not easy. If the phylogenetic relationship between the different viruses were known, this information would naturally constitute the basis of the most logical classification. Since this is not possible, all classifications into groups and subgroups are bound to be arbitrary.

First of all, viruses are of two major types—RNA and DNA viruses. All plant viruses are RNA viruses, whereas all phages are DNA viruses; mammal and arthropod viruses may be either RNA or DNA viruses. The size of the nucleic acid component of the virus largely determines the size and complexity of the entire viral particle. For example, viruses containing a small DNA chain of 15,000 polynucleotides (mol wt 500,000) can code only for a total of 530 amino acid sequences in one single or several smaller polypeptide chains. Such viruses cannot contain more than a few proteins. In contrast, the DNA of T2 phage has a molecular weight of 130,000,000 and when introduced in the cell, it codes for large molecules of messenger RNA. With the aid of the bacterial ribosomes, the viral mRNA dictates the biosynthesis of a number of new enzymes: a new DNA polymerase, thymidylic acid synthetase and kinase, a dCTP deaminase, a DNA-glucosylating enzyme, and a deoxycytidylate hydroxymethylase. The DNA of the vaccinia virus has a molecular weight of 150×10^6. Such a template can dictate the biosynthesis of a number of proteins that participate in the structural buildup of the virus [193, 194].

Although the nucleic acid is responsible for viral infectivity and replication, the isolated nucleic acid molecules are very labile. Thus, an infectious nucleic acid core and a protective protein coat seem to be minimal requirements for effective virus action. Many small viruses have nothing more.

An elementary package of nucleic acid and protein is also found in more complex viruses, such as the myxoviruses. Yet these more complex viruses contain, in addition, structural or catalytic protein complexes that may or may not have been coded by the virus nucleic acid. Vaccinia virus contains enzymes that are foreign to the host cell. Myxoviruses contain specific proteins involved in the attachment to, and the penetration through, the membrane of the host cell. Finally, as they are expulsed from the host cell, some viruses are surrounded by an envelope derived from the cell membrane. Thus, viruses achieve various degrees of organization, but, again, no obvious phylogenic relationship links the simplest and the most complex viruses, and the complexity of the virus is not related to the nature of the host.

Obviously, structural studies of the simple viruses are of considerable significance for interpreting morphogenesis in general. Therefore, we shall pause for a moment to contemplate the marvels of the structural organization of the tobacco mosaic virus. A combination of chemical analysis, X-ray crystallography, and electron microscopy have enabled the reconstruction of the structure of the protein coat of the TMV, a small virus with a limited amount of nucleic acid yet a comparatively large amount of protein. The discrepancy between the amount of protein made and the amount of template available is compensated for by constructing a large polymer from a relatively small polypeptide. Each polypeptide chain carries three specific donors and three specific receptors. As a result, two polypeptides are bound to each other by three bonds, and a continuous network of polypeptides with helical symmetry is formed [195–199].

Within the polypeptide structure, no inherent property is capable of limiting the size of the helical shell. Restriction is achieved by the nucleic acid core. Furthermore, if the information contained in the nucleic acid is translated into a polypeptide sequence incorrectly, an abnormal capsid will be formed. Yet the abnormal shell will not be used to build a virus because the nucleic acid cannot fit inside the shell. Although the polypeptide units can be assembled without the nucleic acid, the empty shell is usually unstable. In contrast, the combination of the nucleic acid with the protein stabilizes the shell.

This strictly symmetrical helical structure of the shell, one in which every unit is surrounded by an identical environment, is an ideal state that can be achieved only when the rod-shaped virus has a perfectly straight axis.

Some viruses, like the myxoviruses, have a sinuous structure and take the shape of flexible rods. It is believed that their structure is helical also, but that in contrast to the rod-shaped viruses, there is no strong interaction between the successive turns of the helix in the flexible rods. Furthermore, in the flexible rods, each structural unit cannot be surrounded by an indentical environment; equivalence does not obtain, but a slight inflection may distort the size of the bond without changing the local bond pattern, thus permitting a quasi-equivalent relationship between the subunits of the protein.

All viruses are not rod-shaped; some have been shown by electron microscopy to be spherical. Crick and Watson proposed that spherical viruses were also made of small identical subunits. Regular bonding of identical units is achieved in three types of cubical symmetry: tetrahedral (12 sides), octahedral (24 units), and icosahedral (60 units or multiples of 60 units). Most spherical viruses are in reality icosahedral.

Among the icosahedral viruses, the turnip yellow mosaic virus has been investigated most extensively. Evidence for the icosahedral structure was obtained by three different methods of exploration: X-ray crystallography, electron microscopy, and chemical analysis. Chemical studies of the capsid established that it is made of subunits each with a molecular weight of 21,300.

X-Ray crystallography suggests that the capsomere has a 5:3:2 cubic symmetry, a finding compatible with the icosahedral structure.

A most important conceptual consequence of the elaboration of the structural models is that it brings the virus, a unit of living matter, closer to the more familiar realm of physical chemistry.

One can distinguish two steps in the elaboration of the protein coat: (1) the assembly of the amino acid sequence on the template, and (2) the self-assembly of the capsomeres to form the capsid. Self-assembly, like crystallization, obeys the laws of statistical mechanics, and the individual units fall together in an orderly fashion because this orderly arrangement is compatible with their lowest energy state. Yet, because of the presence of the nucleic acid, the self-assembly process differs from crystallization in at least two ways; the size of the capsid is self-limiting, and the ultimate product of the intermolecular arrangement, even in the simplest viruses, involves two molecules—a nucleic acid and a protein.

A true crystal is made of a single molecular type, and each molecule of the crystal is surrounded by exactly the same environment. We have already seen that in many types, if not in most viruses, rigid helical or icosahedral symmetry does not exist, and there is no equivalence of the environment surrounding the individual units; only quasi-equivalence is present. As Pirie [200] pointed out, such a state of quasi-equivalence is not unique to viruses—it exists in clarthrates, and it occurs when collagen is reconstituted from dispersed collagen fibers.

The self-assembly theory has been tested for a large number of viruses [201–204]. The best-known model is that of the TMV. Sometimes tobacco leaves become diseased and spotted. In 1892 the Russian botanist Ivanofskii found that the disease could be transferred with an ultrafiltrate of the juice of tobacco plants. Later the responsible virus was isolated.

As we have remarked, the virus is composed of a nucleic acid core and a protein coat. Under the electron microscope the assembled virus resembles a long cylinder 17 mμ in diameter and 300 mμ long.

The TMV protein has a molecular weight of 17,493 daltons and is composed of small monomers. The complete coat can be dissociated into its monomer under drastic conditions, such as low ionic strength and high pH. By following the reassociation of the monomers after producing progressively milder conditions of ionic strength and pH, investigators were able to follow the assembly of the entire protein coat.

The monomer is shaped like a piece of pie. When dispersed monomers are left to stand under the proper conditions for several hours, three of them join to form a trimer. In the trimer two of the pie-shaped proteins are placed side by side and support the third one. The trimers assemble to form discs composed of 34 monomers stacked in two layers, each composed of 17 monomers. The entire coat is constructed by the sequential piling up of discs [202] (see Fig. 16-33). Although it has been possible to self-assemble small viruses *in vitro,* this feat has not yet been achieved with more complex viruses. And although some viruses have been reconstituted by mixing complex intermediates, one may ask whether the self-assembly theory can be extended to viruses with more complex structures. Caspar and Klug [198] believe that their self-assembly theory can be extended to those viruses that, like the turnip crinkle virus or the papilloma virus, have two shells. Klug and his associates have proposed that there are in reality two concentric icosahedral shells, each put together by self-assembly of small units. It seems easy to make the step to larger isometric viruses by assuming that the complexity of their organization results from the repeated concentric deposition of icosahedral protein sheets, each sheet being put together by self-assembly. As for the viruses with lower symmetry, it can simply be assumed that the mechanism of assembling the units and the nature of the bonding are essentially the same as for isometric viruses, but in the viruses with lower symmetry, interactions with other components are responsible for a certain degree of distortion of the symmetry.

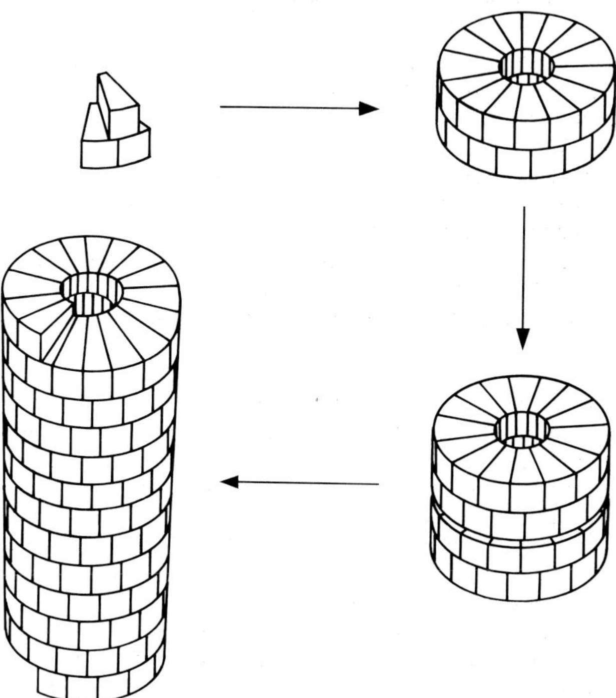

Fig. 16-33. Self-assembly of TMV viral coat protein

These concepts of virus morphogenesis undoubtedly harbor an important core of truth because the determinant step in morphogenesis is inescapably the formation of specific bonds between specific molecules. The bonding of a nucleic acid and a protein depends on the sequences of the two macromolecules and the nature of the environment. Genetic factors may intervene by determining the sequence of the protein or by indirectly modifying the environment—for example, by introducing other lipids, proteins, or enzymes. Furthermore, in complex morphogenesis, there is no need to assume that all the molecular elements that enter into the confection of a specific morphological structure are present all together and assemble at the same time. They could be elaborated in a rigid sequence, and the first formed could serve as a directional guide, a skeleton, or even a matrix for further elaboration. Kellenberger [205] has assembled evidence indicating that morphopoietic factors and morphopoietic genes are involved in elaborating phages with more complex morphologic features.

Viral Infection. We have already given an example of how a DNA phage enters the cell and takes over the controls of macromolecular synthesis to elaborate its own genome and capsid. Studies of the interrelationship between phage and bacteria most completely illustrate our knowledge in that field. In general, plant and animal viruses follow similar paths of infection and replication. First they become attached to cell membranes. They enter the cell, and the nucleic acid is disrobed. The naked nucleic acid directs its own replication and the biosynthesis of the proteins of the coat and possibly of other proteins. Finally, the nucleic acid and proteins are united in the process of maturation [206–213].

However, the individual steps of the general pattern of infection vary in many ways. In contrast to our detailed knowledge of the mode of attachment of certain phages, little is known of the ways by which animal viruses attach to the cell and release their nucleic acid inside it. One of the first observations in that field was made by Bachtold and his associates [214] with polio virus. The attachment of the virus to the monkey kidney cell was: (1) exponential, (2) sensitive to changes in salt concentration, and (3) relatively insensitive to temperature changes. It was concluded that the virus is attached to the membrane receptor mainly through an electrostatic process. Whether other factors are involved is not certain, but capsid sulfhydryl groups have been incriminated in binding virus to receptors. It seems that only the cells of susceptible animals can bind the capsid of the virus to the membrane receptor.

Infection of nonsusceptible species *in vitro* (tissue culture cells) or *in vivo* (intracerebral infection) with the naked RNA shows that when naked RNA is injected, intact virus can later be recovered from the host. These findings suggest that the susceptibility of the host cell depends on the presence, on its membrane, of specific receptors that bind electrostatically to specific donors in the capsid. In the case of polio virus, the attachment to the membrane is followed by alteration of the capsid, which modifies the antigenic properties of the protein and reduces its sensitivity to proteolytic enzymes. The activation of the capsid protein is temperature-sensitive and can be prevented by neutralizing antibodies. During this period of capsid alteration, the virus loses the infectivity and enters a so-called eclipse period.

Myxoviruses are bound to cell membrane receptors through the intermediate of the virus hemagglutinins.

Attachment of the virus to the cell membrane does not necessarily imply that the virus can enter the cell. For example, myxoviruses strongly adhere to the wall of red blood cells without ever entering them. Mandel [187] proposed a mechanism of penetration of polio virus involving a process akin to pinocytosis. Thus, after the nucleoprotein attaches to the membrane, it is soon engulfed into an invagination of the membrane which pinches off. Once the membrane-surrounded nucleoprotein is inside the cell, the membrane is shed and soon the virus is freed in the cytoplasm, going into the eclipse phase.

Electron microscopic studies with a number of viruses, including vaccinia, the adenovirus, and the influenza virus, have established the existence of an intimate contact between the cell membrane and the morphological particularities of the protein coat (spikes for influenza, tubules for vaccinia, and capsomeres for adenoviruses).

The viruses are believed to become engulfed in phagocytic vacuoles, and later, at least in the case of the adenovirus and the vaccinia, they become free in the cytoplasm. Although it would appear from these observations that viral phagocytosis is a fact, it remains to be established that phagocytosis is related to infectivity.

Types of Injuries Caused by Viruses

Viruses can inflict a wide range of injuries to the host. The virus may cuddle in the cell and keep silent; it may ravage the cell nucleus and its cytoplasm and kill the cell; it may surreptitiously infiltrate the genome of the host and in a slow but irreversible process turn it into a wild cancer cell. What a thrill the pathologist of the future will experience when he can describe in detail the molecular sequence for each type of injury. Yet the world of molecular biology, enchanting and elegant as it may be, is still too far from maturity to permit an accurate description of the pathological distortions.

We have already mentioned that the binding of the virus to receptors in the cell membrane partially determines the specific tropism for a given tissue and the susceptibility of a given species. McLaren and his associates [216] found that polio virus was not absorbed by nonsusceptible nonprimate cells, whereas the culture of susceptible cells absorbed virus at an exponential rate. Kunin [217] claims that the presence of sus-

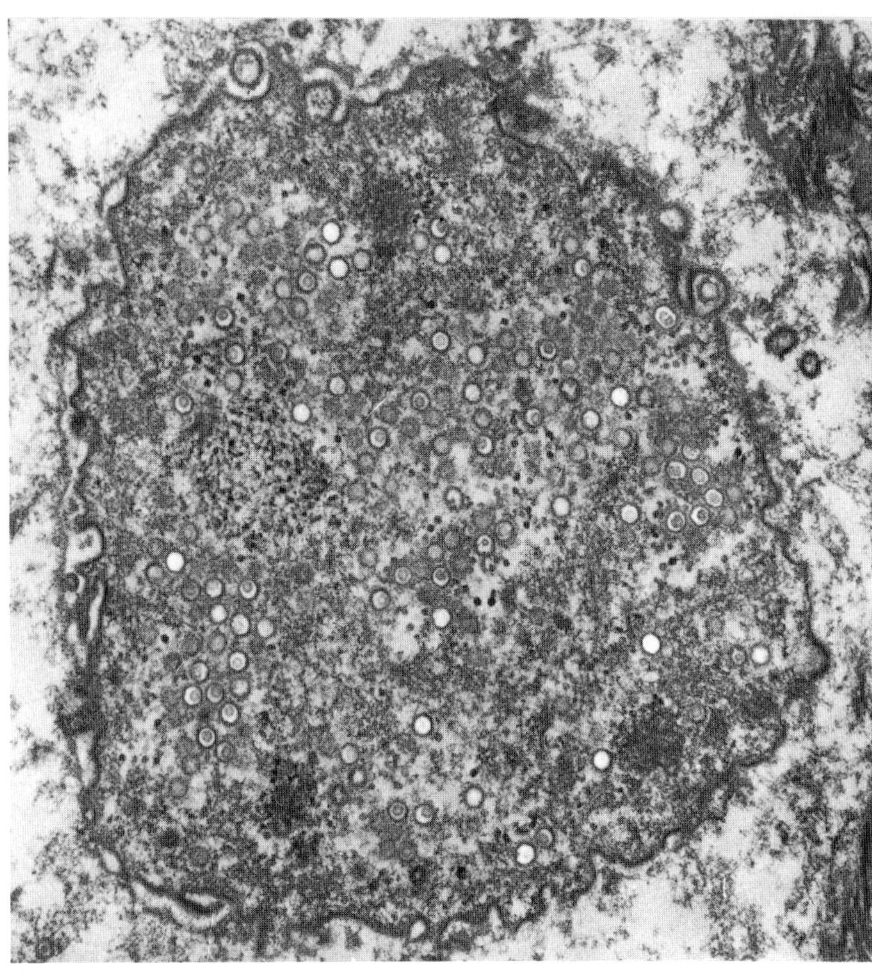

Fig. 16-34. Intranuclear herpes simplex virus particles in a vulvar epidermal lesion. (Zenker, glutaraldehyde and osmium fixation; uranyl acetate and lead citrate stain; ×30,000; provided by Miss Hart)

ceptible cells in a tissue can readily be estimated simply by testing the tissue for the existence of receptors. This is done by mixing a virus with tissue minces or homogenates and measuring the disappearance of the virus from the medium. For example, only tissue preparations obtained from male primates bind the virus. Furthermore, the binding ability decreases with age, a laboratory finding in good agreement with clinical observations. Little is known of the molecular reaction between the receptors and the surface of the cellular membrane and the acceptor on the viral coat.

The intensity of the cellular damage depends on the rate of virus multiplication, the site of multiplication, and the elaboration of viral toxins [218–220]. The following are general rules about the site of maturation: (1) DNA viruses mature in the nucleus, and (2) RNA viruses mature in the cytoplasm. There are exceptions; for example, the poxvirus (a DNA virus) matures in the cytoplasm. When viruses mature in the nucleus, numerous mature viral particles accumulate in the nucleoplasm. The accumulation of virus particles can readily be identified with the electron microscope. Sometimes, nonviral material crystallizes and accumulates in close proximity to the viral crystalline depositions. For example, the infection of tissue culture cells with adenovirus is followed by the intranuclear deposition of clusters of viral crystals, mixed with a crystalline protein of unknown origin which is not antigenically related to viral protein. We shall see later how these macromolecular deposits relate to the more classical inclusion bodies.

The intranuclear maturation of a virus leads to various types of nuclear injuries: (1) the formation of irregular lobules of nuclear membrane (almost a specific effect of adenovirus infection); (2) margination of chromatin (a frequent alteration after virus infection that is particularly striking after infection with K virus), and (3) alteration of the nucleolus. Examples of intranuclear viral infection are shown in Figs. 16-34 and 16-35.

As the infection progresses, nonspecific cytoplasmic alterations are detectable. Distant cytoplasmic vacuolization is an early event in cells infected by SV40. When virus proliferation is followed by rupture of the nuclear membrane, the virus particles, which matured in the nucleoplasm, may be spread into the cytoplasm. This is the case in cells infected by polyoma virus and SV40 virus.

Poxviruses mature in the cytoplasm; maturation is not restricted to small areas of cytoplasm but is diffuse, and areas of endoplasmic reticulum are replaced by a DNA-containing viroplasm, which is free of ribo-

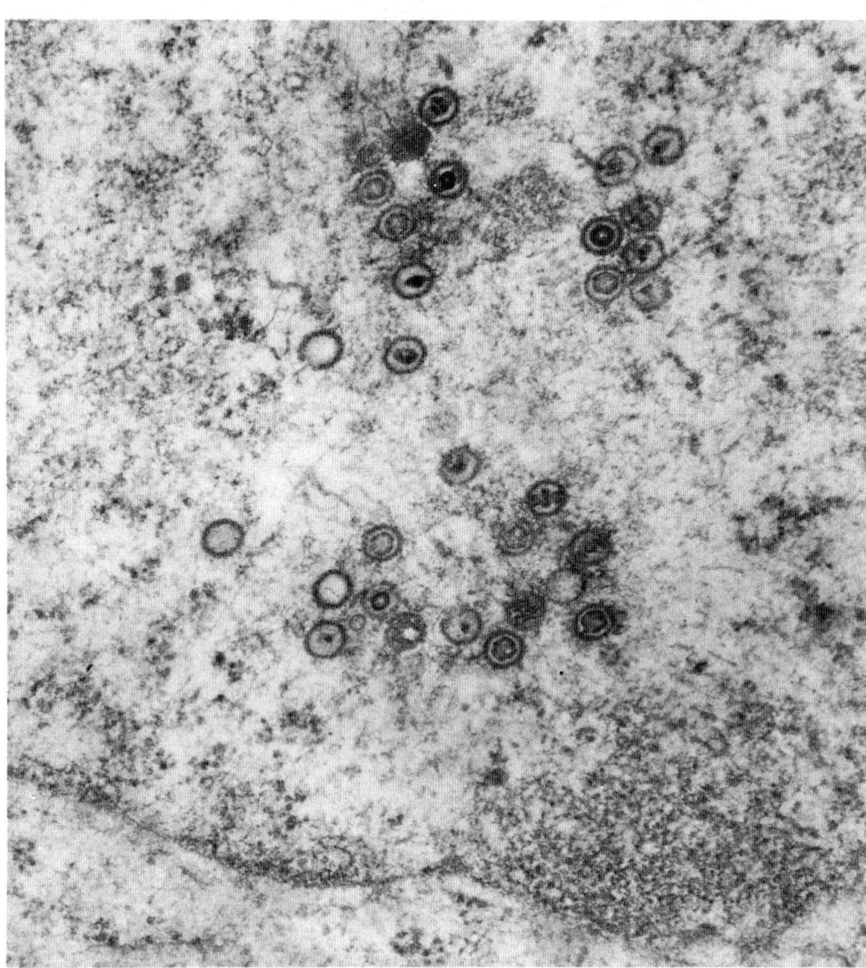

Fig. 16-35. Intranuclear cytomegalovirus isolated from lung of a patient with disseminated infection in WI-38 cell culture. (Osmium fixation; uranyl acetate and lead citrate stain; ×60,000; provided by Miss Hart)

somes. Sometimes the nucleic acid is mixed with protein, and a crescent-shaped virus matrix forms with a perinuclear distribution. These types of viral accumulations are readily recognizable under the microscope. Sometimes (*e.g.*, poliovirus infection) cellular death occurs so soon after infection that viral detection is difficult.

Most viruses that mature in the cytoplasm produce cytoplasmic injuries. Small RNA viruses seem to be particularly nefarious for the cytoplasm (vacuolization with virus particles). However, the injuries are not necessarily restricted to the cytoplasm. They may affect the nucleus also. Nonspecific nuclear alterations may develop at various times after infection depending upon the nature of the virus. Entovirus infection is associated with severe shrinking of the nucleus and marked chromatin margination.

The maturation of the influenza virus is of unique interest. The viral nucleic acid is likely to be synthesized in the nucleus. Of the proteins whose synthesis is dictated by the viral genome, some are synthesized in the nucleus, others in the cytoplasm. For example, the RMP antigen is of nuclear origin, whereas hemagglutinin is of cytoplasmic origin. The virus also contains lipids; some are preexisting cellular constituents, others are synthesized after infection (phosphatide). How these various components are assembled to form a mature virus is not certain, but the molecular assemblage of the influenza virus takes place on or near the surface membrane. The intracellular cycles of the parainfluenza, fowl plague, and the New Castle disease viruses probably resemble that of influenza virus.

Thus, the ultrastructural changes observed in a virus-infected cell are of two orders: changes specific for a group of viruses, and nonspecific cytocidal effects. The appearance of the specific changes is determined by the virus' maturation site, its morphology, and the accumulation of nonviral or incomplete viral material.

We have already discussed the different stages of macromolecular synthesis that ultimately yield the mature virus. We will now consider the relationship between the accumulation of mature viruses and the formation of inclusion bodies.

Even before the existence of viral diseases had been established, pathologists had described dense, round intracytoplasmic inclusion bodies. In fact, inclusion bodies were described for the first time in 1841 in a case of molluscum contagiosum. Although the presence of inclusion bodies in the cells of a biopsy or an autopsy specimen is pathognomonic for viral infection, viral infection cannot be excluded in the absence of inclusion bodies. Only 50% of viral infections are associated with the development of inclusion bodies. We shall describe a few of these inclusions as they are seen with the light microscope and then correlate the light microscopic with the ultrastructural changes.

Rabies is an infectious disease caused by a relatively large neurotropic virus. Man is usually infected as a result of being bitten by a rabid dog. Typical cytoplasmic inclusions, or Negri bodies, are found in a selected area of the central nervous system both in man and dog. These are sharply defined, round or oval acidophilic cytoplasmic inclusions. The size, number, and intracytoplasmic location of the bodies may vary considerably from one cell to another. Usually these inclusions are 5 to 10 μ, but sometimes Negri bodies only 1 μ in diameter or as large as 20 μ are seen. Negri bodies can be found anywhere in the nerve cell cytoplasm, including the dendrites. A cell may contain one or more Negri bodies. Negri bodies are found in greatest number in the pyramidal cells of the hypocampus, but they may also be found in the Purkinje cells of the cerebellum and in the cerebral cortex. Negri bodies may be difficult to find in patients who died soon after infection (48 hours), but they are usually prominent in older cases (9–10 days).

Thus, if the brain preparation is stained with eosin and the alkyline methylene blue of Unna, Negri bodies stand out as red corpuscles in the midst of the blue background.

Round, hyaline, eosinophilic masses are found in the skin cells of the victims of the benign skin infection molluscum contagiosum. In smallpox, the epithelial cells of the skin contain in their cytoplasm typical spherical eosinophilic bodies called Guarnieri's bodies. Similar cytoplasmic inclusion bodies are found in cowpox and vaccinia-infected skins. The cytoplasm of the liver cells of patients affected with yellow fever contains rounded areas of hyalin and eosinophilic material referred to as the Councilman bodies. Councilman-like bodies have been described in the hepatic cells of patients suffering from viral hepatitis.

Instead of being associated with typical cytoplasmic inclusion, some viral diseases are characterized by the development of typical nuclear inclusions. Examples are the nuclear inclusions found in zoster, varicella, and herpes simplex. In these diseases, the epidermal cells undergo a characteristic degenerative process. The cell cytoplasm swells and becomes intensely eosinophilic. As a result of the distention of the cell membrane, intracellular bridges are ruptured and the cells are separated from each other; the number of nuclei increases considerably, thus forming giant cells with four to eight nuclei. Typically, rounded eosinophilic inclusions are easily detectable within the nuclei of these balloon cells.

Intranuclear inclusions are found in a number of viral diseases. They may be a constant finding (as are the various types of inclusions found in the nuclei of alveolar cells in adenovirus pneumonia), or they may be seen only occasionally (as in cells infected with anterior poliomyelitis). Sometimes both nuclear and cytoplasmic inclusions are found in the same cell.

In measles giant cell pneumonia, multinucleated giant cells replace the normal alveolar lining. Usually these polykaryocytes contain numerous nuclear inclusions and an occasional cytoplasmic inclusion. Infrequently, nuclear inclusions are found in the hepatic cells of patients with yellow fever.

The cells lining the ducts of the salivary glands (mainly the parotid gland) of 10% of autopsied infants contain characteristic large nuclear inclusions (5–10 μ with a hyaline, eosinophilic center and a clear halo) and small PAS-positive cytoplasmic inclusions. In 10% of the infants whose salivary glands contain the cytomegalovirus, inclusions are found in the viscera (kidney and lung). In some cases, usually as a complication of some other systemic disease (leukemia, diabetes, pneumocystis carinii), the latent viral disease develops into an infection with pneumonia, jaundice, and leukoerythroblastic anemia.

The significance of inclusion bodies stems from their diagnostic value and their biological implication. If a child has been bitten by a rabid dog and the dog is captured alive within 10 days, its brain will contain Negri bodies, pathognomonic for rabies. In smallpox, cowpox, and vaccinia, the inclusion bodies are cytoplasmic. In herpes and varicella, they are intranuclear. Adams epidemic pneumonia, a giant cell pneumonia of viral origin, can be distinguished from measles giant cell pneumonia by the fact that nuclear inclusions are never found in the former.

Of considerable importance is the relationship between inclusion bodies and the virus. One could hardly expect that the early pathologists would have associated inclusion bodies with viral infection, since the virus is smaller than bacteria. Therefore, it is not surprising that Negri considered the cytoplasmic inclusions that he described to be parasites, and even today the exact origin of Negri and Councilman bodies remains obscure.

Electron microscopic studies of viral-infected structures coupled with histochemical examinations of the inclusion shed new light on the nature of at least some types of inclusion bodies. Maybe the most impressive illustration of the correlation between inclusion and virus growth is provided by observing viral infection in the polyhedroses, in which the virus consists of many-sided crystals. Polyhedroses are of two types: nuclear and cytoplasmic. We will consider the fate of the virus only in nuclear polyhedrosis.

In nuclear polyhedrosis, as the infection progresses [221], the nucleus becomes packed with viral crystals until it finally bursts and the virus spills into the cytoplasm. The virus particles are rods made of a central helical core of DNA surrounded by a protein capsid. Now that electron microscopy has permitted the inclusion bodies in nuclear polyhedrosis to be examined, the relationship between mature virus and inclusion bodies has become obvious. Similarly, it was established that the inclusion bodies found in the nucleus of cells infected with polyoma, papilloma, or SV40 virus were composed of mature virions.

It would be simple to state that viruses that mature in the nucleus yield nuclear inclusions and those maturing in the cytoplasm yield cytoplasmic inclusions. Unfortunately, the situation is much more complicated, and inclusion bodies are not always made of mature viruses. Other components, either alone or in association with mature viruses, may participate in inclusion body formation. Protein crystals of unknown origin accumulate in the nucleus in adenovirus infection. Cells of tissue infected with measle virus contain unidentified crystallike structures.

At the start of this section on inclusion, we remarked that inclusion bodies were not detectable with the light microscope in a large number of viral diseases. In many of these diseases, an "ultrastructural type of inclusion" has been detected. The composition of the ultrastructural inclusion varies considerably. They may consist of an accumulation of viral nucleic acid, viral protein coats, mature viruses, foreign protein, or a combination of these components.

In addition to inducing cellular death and cancer, viruses often lead to the appearance of giant cells, a phenomenon referred to as polykaryocytosis. Giant cells appear under pathological conditions, but they are also found in placenta and bone. These normal giant cells are susceptible to cancerization, and tumors may develop at their expense. However, giant cells may appear in any tumor, whatever its origin. Chronic infection processes, such as tuberculosis, syphilis, and mycosis, are associated with typical giant cell reactions. Sterile foreign bodies lead to the formation of giant cell-rich granulomas. Giant cells can theoretically arise in two ways: (1) repeated nuclear division, associated with cytoplasmic growth, but without cell division; and (2) coalescence of a number of individual cells.

Inasmuch as mitosis is rarely observed in giant cells, it was generally accepted that they formed by coalescense rather than by nuclear division. When the problem was reinvestigated using colchicine and tritium-labeled thymidine to block mitosis in metaphase, it seemed that cell division could also be involved in giant cell formation. Roizman [222] has investigated the histogenesis of multinucleated cells in virus infections. We have already seen that measles, herpes simplex, varicella, herpes zoster, and viral pneumonia may be associated with giant cell formation *in vivo*. In addition, a number of viruses lead to the formation of giant cells *in vitro*. Among them are mumps, measles, herpes simplex, varicella, herpes zoster, vaccinia, and adenovirus.

The administration of colchicine or X-irradiation has no effect on giant cell formation. Furthermore, the total number of nuclei does not increase during giant cell formation, and fusion of two cells or more can clearly be recognized with the light microscope as giant cells form *in vitro*.

Although mitosis may play a role in giant cell formation, the contribution of fusion of several cells is undeniable. Fusion could occur through phagocytosis of one cell by another. But this possibility seems to be excluded since macrophages are not found inside of the cytoplasm of other macrophages. Only intact cells can fuse; cells that take up trypan blue remain isolated.

If a polykaryocyte freshly induced by herpesvirus is treated with trypsin, it yields a number of individual cells equal to the total number of nuclei found in the giant cell. This finding suggests that polykaryocytes form as a result of the fusion of the membranes. Roizman proposes that the virus in some way alters the cell membrane of the infected cell. As a result, the membrane of the infected cell fuses with the membrane of an uninfected cell, and finally the fused membrane dissolves. Of course, the molecular alteration of the membrane is not known. Whether the mechanism of polykaryocyte formation in normal tumor and granulomatous tissue is the same as that observed *in vitro* in viral-infected cells remains to be established. Roizman remarks, however, that the formation of polykaryocytes in virus-infected cells is only an example of the alteration of the cell surface properties that viral infections are capable of inducing. Although it is not quite clear how these changes take place, it seems likely that new substances are elaborated in the infected cell and are then incorporated in the membrane to change its antigenic properties (agglutination), the rate of budding of microvilli, and possibly the normal charge distribution responsible for contact inhibition. Since little is known of the elaboration or the composition of cell membranes, the mechanism of these alterations can be only highly speculative. Whether changes in the structure of the cell membrane leading to alteration of the intracellular environment are indirectly responsible for changes in the rate of DNA synthesis or even cellular transformation remains to be established.

Antiviral Vaccination

The spectacular results Pasteur obtained in treating a young boy bitten by a rabid dog might have suggested that viral disease would be relatively simple to prevent. In fact, an efficient viral vaccine was extremely difficult to prepare. Among the most prominent sources of problems are the multiple antigenicity, the slow or poor propagation of the virus in nonhuman cells, and the possibility of contamination of the vaccine by an oncogenic virus.

Killed influenza vaccine can be extremely efficacious in protecting populations against the infection. However, the antigenic quality of the virus tends to change, and therefore, new antigenic forms of vaccine must constantly be prepared. Virologists have described over 50 different antigenic forms of rhinovirus. It is believed that there might be hundreds, if not thousands, of different antigenic forms of rhinoviruses. Such a widespread population of viruses makes it almost impossible to prepare an efficient and specific vaccine against the common cold.

The early discovery and the efficacy of smallpox vaccination stems from the fact that the same virus is responsible for the disease in cows and man. Jenner recognized that close relationship between human, bovine, and equine vaccine, but it was Ganner who, in Salzburg (1806), demonstrated that the human disease could be communicated to cows. When the human virus, which grows in cows, is reinoculated in man, it induces only a local infection. The virulence of the smallpox vaccine is attenuated during its passage from man to cow. The cow constitutes an excellent source of attenuated live virus that can be administered to the entire population.

Almost 200 years after Jenner's experiments, Pasteur attempted to prepare a second virus vaccine, the vaccine against rabies. He stumbled on a difficulty that would delay the preparation of the other vaccines for many years to come. The rabies virus could not be grown on ordinary culture media. To prepare his vaccine, Pasteur took fragments of dog brain and spinal chord and placed them in an oven to desiccate them. The vaccination process then consisted of injecting chord preparations of increasing virulence, the virulence being controlled by the degree of desiccation. Thus, the injection would start with dry tissue and end with fresh tissues. Of course, now viruses are grown on embryonated eggs and tissue culture. In many cases, enough virus can be produced to prepare efficient live or killed vaccine. For example, the Flury vaccine for rabies is now prepared by growing the virus on duck embryos, and this eliminates the danger of isoallergic encephalitis, which sometimes develops after injection of the nerve tissue preparation. In most cases, these newer methods have permitted the growth of enough virus to prepare adequate vaccine. The successful propagation of measles, mumps, and rubella viruses has permitted the preparation of either live or killed vaccines. In contrast, one of the difficulties encountered in preparing vaccine against rhinovirus is that this virus can be propagated only on human cells.

Obviously, primate tissues have frequently been used to prepare vaccines against viruses for which man is the principal host. Macacus kidney tissues are frequently contaminated by SV40, a virus oncogenic for hamster. Thus, SV40 contamination of live or killed vaccine must carefully be excluded when primate tissues are used. Yet in spite of all these difficulties, safe vaccines have been prepared against almost all known crippling viral diseases, except for some of the arboviruses and viral hepatitis. Yellow fever is the only disease caused by arboviruses that can be adequately prevented by a vaccine [223]. (Among the hundreds of viruses that propagate in insects, only a few are known to cause disease in man. Whether other diseases are caused by insect viruses remains to be established.)

Antiviral Chemotherapy

Although one may consider that medicine has been rather successful in preventing viral infections, little has been achieved in curing them. The problem of killing a virus without damaging the host seems almost insurmountable. To successfully challenge the cell survival, all that is required from the virus is that a polynucleotide template be introduced in the right place inside of the cell; once that is accomplished, viral and cell metabolism essentially use common pathways. Consequently, virus chemotherapy is not based on qualitative differences between the metabolism of the virus and that of the host, but on rather subtle quantitative differences. As a result, most antiviral agents are toxic to the host, and successful antiviral chemotherapy has been achieved only when active chemicals can be applied topically. The list of antiviral chemotherapeutic agents includes agents blocking protein or nucleic acid synthesis, "selective" inhibitors of virus multiplication and maturation, and inhibitors of virus release.

The halogenated pyrimidines can be applied topically. IUDR has proved to be highly effective in treating corneal infections due to herpes simplex. But even then the iodouridine interferes with reparative processes, especially in the stroma; furthermore, the antimetabolite may be incorporated into the DNA. Nevertheless, in topical therapy the efficacy of the drug in preventing catastrophic consequences outweighes the disadvantages of its use.

N′N′-Anhydrobis (β-hydroxyethyl) biguanide hydrochloride (ABOB) was claimed to selectively inhibit the multiplication of influenza virus without affecting the host. Convincing evidence of the efficacy of the drug is not available. N-Methylisatin 3-thiosemicarbazone blocks the maturation of the poxvirus. It has been used clinically to provide prophylaxis against nonimmunized individuals freshly exposed to infection. 1-Adamantanamine interferes with the penetration of myxoviruses in the host cells; the efficacy of the drug in clinical trials needs to be established.

If there is at the present little hope of developing efficacious chemotherapeutic agents, a better understanding of interaction between a virus and its biological environment may someday provide new means of therapy. When a bacteria, a plant, or an animal is infected by a virus, this infection interferes with the growth of another virus. Interference between the infection of one virus by another virus can take place through a number of mechanisms: (1) competition for site of absorption on the membrane or replication sites, (2) elaboration of viral products toxic for viruses, and (3) elaboration of host inhibitors. Sometimes the incorporation of one phage into the genome of the host builds up a resistance against infection by a related phage. When susceptible cells are placed in contact with UV-irradiated Newcastle disease virus, infection by nonirradiated viruses does not take place, possibly because the irradiated virus has blocked all cellular receptors. Antigens of adenovirus and the protein component of TMV interfere with the growth of each virus respectively [224].

One of the most intriguing forms of interference results from the elaboration of a cellular inhibitor different from antibodies. Isaacs has called this group of interfering substances "interferons."

One of the pioneering experiments in that field was performed by Isaacs and Lindenmann [225–227]. These investigators succeeded in extracting an acid-stable inhibitor of virus growth from chick embryo chorioallantoic membranes used to grow influenza virus. They established that the inhibitor was a polypeptide of cellular origin with antigenic properties different from those of the virus. The importance of interferon stems not only from its potential therapeutic value, but interferon production may determine the virulence of the virus and the establishment of persistent infections. Thus, it seems worthwhile to consider the properties, the mechanism of induction, and the mode of action of interferon. We will not consider interferon produced by nonviral compounds.

Little is known of the chemical properties of interferon molecules except that they are resistant to a wide pH range, and that their activity is lost after treatment with trypsin. It seems that a virus leads to the production of a wide range of molecular weights of interferon (18,000 to 100,000). Interferon is produced by the host cell independently of the genome of the virus. Thus, viral protein and interferon are not related immunologically. The specificity of interferon is not related to the infectant virus but to the species of the host cell. Although most interferons act on unrelated viruses, there is a strong cell species barrier to the action of interferon. Interferons derived from a given host may act alike on influenza, polyoma, and poxvirus grown in homologous host cells, but calf and chick interferons are not antiviral in heterologous cells [228–234].

The mechanism of production of interferons clearly involves the cell's machinery for protein synthesis. Host synthesis of DNA is not needed. In contrast, blockage of host messenger RNA synthesis with doses of actinomycin D that do not affect viral synthesis, or the administration of inhibitors of protein synthesis, interferes with the interferon formation by the host cell. In fact, the use of such inhibitors has permitted investigators to determine the time needed to elaborate interferon—1 to 2 hours after infection of chick embryo tissue and approximately 6 hours in tumor cells infected with Newcastle virus.

The mechanism by which interferon blocks viral replication is not clear. It seems certain that the polypeptide does not act directly. Little if any interferon binds to the infected cells [235]. But after interferon contacts the cell, the effect of interferon is considerably amplified, possibly through the biosynthesis of active antiviral agents. This is again suggested by experiments in which inhibitors of macromolecular synthesis were used. Whether the active agent is an RNA or a protein is not certain. In any event, the level of antiviral activity seems to be regulated by the rate of its induction by interferons and its rate of breakdown in the cell.

Interferons can induce the production of antiviral substances in noninfected cells. The effects of the active antiviral agents are manifested at the early stages of the virus' life cycle. Interferon blocks the formation of the double-stranded 16-S replicative RNA in cells infected with the encephalomyocarditis virus. Studies with cells infected with Mengo virus indicate that interferon not only blocks viral RNA synthesis, but it also abolishes the effect of the virus on cellular metabolism, particularly its inhibitory effect on the host mRNA synthesis.

Interferon has been shown to block the formation of RNA-dependent RNA polymerase in RNA virus infection and thymidine kinase in DNA virus infection. (Interferon blocks the biosynthesis of thymidine kinase of poxvirus infection when the virus is grown in chick embryo but not when it is grown in mouse embryo. Yet interferon blocks virus multiplication in mouse embryo.) The rearrangement of individual ribosomes to form, under the influence of viral mRNA, large viral polysomes for the purpose of fabricating viral protein is blocked by interferons with poxvirus, but not with Mengo virus.

The molecular mechanism of interferon induction is still unknown. It has been postulated that it involves derepression of at least two genes: one for interferon biosynthesis, the other for that of the antiviral protein. A hypothetical mechanism for repression and derepression based on Jacob and Monod's operon theory has been proposed. Thus, the interferon and the antiviral gene are both part of an operon. An I gene codes for a repressor, which combines with the O gene of the interferon operon and keeps the expression of that gene blocked. The inducer binds to the repressor and activates the interferon gene. Interferon is the inducer for the antiviral gene O. The repressor for the interferon gene is constitutively synthesized, but slowly, thus allowing time for enough interferon to accumulate before a critical concentration of interferon gene repressor will accumulate. It has been further proposed that interferon participates in the repression of its own operator gene. In this process monomeric interferon aggregates, and the aggregate binds to the "repressor," double locking the gene [236].

In conclusion, interferon acts at some early stage of viral replication; as a result, it abolishes the sequence of steps involved in the macromolecular synthesis of the virus. Yet the molecular nature of the first events that trigger the block in viral replication remains unknown.

As mentioned above, interferon can induce the formation of antiviral substances in uninfected cells. Other effects on uninfected cells—such as inhibition of nuclear oxidative phosphorylation, stimulation of glycolysis, block of DNA and RNA synthesis, and interference with mitosis—are still too controversial to be accepted without reservation.

Obviously, one important aspect of the studies of interferon is its relationship to virulence. An interesting molecular illustration of how interferon and virulence are related is provided by *in vitro* studies with viruses (such as picronavirus) that are known to block protein synthesis. As could be predicted from what we know of the mechanism of production of interferon and antiviral activity, picronavirus was found to prevent the development of interferon in infected cells and the development of antiviral activity in cells to which interferon was added.

The growth of picronavirus, however, was inhibited when cells were preincubated with interferon long enough that the interferon could induce the appearance of an active viricidal compound. Thus, the virulence of a virus may well depend upon its ability to prevent interferon formation by the host. Enders found that more interferon is produced in cells infected with an avirulent strain of measle virus than in cells infected with the virulent strain.

A successful attack on a living animal by a virus requires that after infection the virus reaches a target organ free of antiviral activity. How does interferon modify this situation in the infected animal? Let's consider poliovirus, an encephalomyelitis virus. After infection, poliovirus takes 24 hours to reach the target organ, yet interferon formation is stimulated within a few hours after infection, and injected exogenous interferon is known to reach distant organs (brain, kidney) within a few hours. Consequently, in the race between interferon and virus for the target organ, the smaller interferon molecule is bound to win, and target organ damage could conceivably be prevented if enough interferon were produced. Unless previous infection by the same virus has taken place, antibodies are not likely to play an important role in control during the early stages of viremia because large antibody molecules take too long to appear.

The circulating blood normally contains a background titer of interferon that may be increased during viremia. The source of the circulating interferon is not known. In fact, all the cells of the body could contribute to the pool of circulating interferon, either as a result of viral infection or because they have been stimulated to produce interferon by inducers other than viruses.

A number of agents other than viruses can induce interferon production,* among them mold products (statolon, cycloheximide, acetoxycycloheximide) or bacterial products such as *E. coli* or *B. abortus* endotoxin. Bacteria themselves can induce interferon formation. Whether the interferon produced by mold or bacterial products is the same as that induced by viruses is still debated. It seems that although the range of molecular weights of the interferon polypeptides is the same in all cases, the mechanism of production is different depending upon the nature of the inducer. A block in protein synthesis prevents interferon formation induced by viruses or bacteria, but it does not affect that produced by endotoxins. It has been proposed that inducers of interferon are polyanionic macromolecules, capable of combining with histone. As a result, DNA, which acts as a template for interferon biosynthesis, is derepressed. However, this theory does not explain the specific uncovering of the deoxypolynucleotide template for interferon and the difference between the mechanism of production of interferon induced by viruses and endotoxins.

When exogenous interferon is injected in mice, it disappears from the bloodstream very quickly (97% per hour). This contrasts with the stability of interferon produced in tissue culture. The mechanism of breakdown of circulatory interferon is not known. The relative rates of interferon formation and breakdown determine its concentration in the blood, and we have already seen that circulating interferon levels may determine the fate of the victim of a viral infection.

The therapeutic applications of interferon are meager up to date, principally because of the extreme difficulties that are encountered when investigators attempt to prepare and purify interferon in large quantities. One hope for the future resides in the fact that nontoxic agents can be used to stimulate the body to synthesize its own interferon. Time will tell whether such an approach is practical. The role of interferon in viral oncogenesis will be discussed below. Plants and bacteria develop interference with viral growth; whether this occurs through interferon elaboration, as in fish, birds, and mammals, is not known.

The inducers of interferon (the Newcastle disease virus) and polyinosinic-polycytidylic acid (PIC) inhibit the formation of B16 melanomas in CC7BL black mice, tumors in which viral particles have been seen. PIC is a better inducer of interferon that NDV and all available evidence from the author's laboratory suggests that the tumor inhibition is caused by a direct effect on the melanoma of interferon cells rather than by immunosuppression (the inhibition occurs in neonatally thymectomized and irradiated mice). A similar inhibition of growth of murine mammary adenocarcinoma was obtained with PIC.

Viral Toxins and Lysogeny

In addition to dictating their own replication, viruses elicit the formation of toxins that may play a considerable role in their cytocidal effect. One of the most fascinating discoveries of the 1950s and 1960s was that the diphtheria toxin is not produced by the *Corynebacterium diphtheriae* but by a toxigeniphage. Before we discuss this exciting subject, it will be necessary to devote a few paragraphs to another important concept in molecular biology—lysogeny.

The phage may either kill or live with the host; therefore, one speaks of virulent and temperate phages. When a virulent phage finds its way into a bacterium and proliferates, it kills the bacterium, which finally releases its host. This is the lytic cycle. When a temperate phage enters a bacterium, it establishes symbiosis with the bacterium in what is called the lysogenic cycle.

The notion of lysogeny was only recently accepted. Thus, in his concept of the relationship between bac-

---

* Recently a rather simple chemical, the diamine-2,7-bis-2-(diethylamino)-fluoren-9-one (Tilorone) has been found to increase the levels of circulating interferon in mice to which the compound is administered orally. Whether the increase results from *de novo* synthesis or from release of preexisting interferon is not established. The compound does not increase blood levels of interferon in man.

teria and infecting phage, Herelle maintained that infection always meant acute conflict between host and parasite, usually leading to the destruction of the host. Herelle refused to recognize the possibility of a peaceful coexistence securing symbiosis between phage and bacteria. It is now well established that some bacteria harbor invisible and silent viruses which, under special circumstances, are released without any contact with an infecting agent. Burnet's [237] experiments were critical in this area. He found that only a small fraction of phage-infected Salmonella contained the phage; yet when challenged to release the phage, all bacteria released it. The inescapable conclusion implied in such observations is that when a bacterium divides, at least one virus particle divides with it, and the replicate is transferred to the daughter bacteria.

André Lwoff [238] devoted much time to studying bacteriophage lysogeny and was among the first to regenerate the concept after it had fallen into disrepute for at least two decades. Lwoff established that one lysogenic bacterium contained one phage and yielded a replicate of the phage after one division. To call one virus particle a phage when it causes no damage was obviously a misnomer, and Lwoff proposed the term "prophage." It has since been established that prophage is the only genetic determinant of lysogeny. It is a deoxyribose polynucleotide. It becomes an integrated part of the bacterial chromosome in which it is located at a specific site. For example, at least 14 different prophages can live in symbiosis with *E. coli* K12. Crosses between nonlysogenic and lysogenic bacteria have demonstrated that all phages occupy specific sites on the chromosome.

If a prophage is silent, how do we know that it exists? This silent prophage can be converted into a virulent phage that goes into a lytic cycle. In fact, Burnet had already observed that a small fraction (0.1%) of lysogenic bacteria harbor prophages that become loose and enter lytic cycles. Later it was found that ultraviolet irradiation of a lysogenic phage disrupts the symbiotic relationship between bacterium and phage. After ultraviolet irradiation, the bacterium continues to grow for 45 minutes or so; but then the virus takes over, blocks bacterial metabolism, replicates, and kills the bacteria. As a result, each bacterium releases hundreds of phages [239].

The molecular biology of lysogeny has been investigated most intensively with the *E. coli* λ phage [240, 241]. The establishment of lysogeny requires that the λ genome be repressed and that its DNA be integrated in the *E. coli* genome. The λ phage genome, composed of double-stranded circular DNA, has been mapped out. Among other genes, it includes a group of regulatory genes (CIII, N, CI, CII, and q) and a group of genes (OP) involved in replication of λ DNA.

Lysis requires full transcription of the genome and production of new phage. In lysogeny, the genome has been inserted into the host's genome, and its transcription is blocked by a protein that binds to the CI regulatory gene, the so-called CI protein. Other phage-coded proteins are also needed to secure and maintain lysogeny, but their exact role is not clear. Neither is it clear whether the CI protein blocks RNA transcription by interfering with initiation, by preventing progress of transcription initiated at a proximal point, or by binding to RNA polymerase.

Relatively little is known about the mechanism of integration except that it is site-specific in the bacterial genome, and it requires the elaboration by the λ genome of a special protein, the int. protein.

When the λ phage enters the cell, it is believed to form circular DNA. A base sequence of 10 to 20 bases on the λ recognizes a specific base sequence on the DNA, either through base-to-base interaction or with the help of the int. protein. Once the two genomes are face to face, a site-specific recombination takes place which must involve: (1) nicking of the λ phage DNA, (2) nicking of the *E. coli* DNA, and (3) binding of each end of the λ phage (which is not broken into two pieces because it is circular) with the two fragments of the *E. coli* DNA.

Hopefully, this sketchy description of the molecular events of lysogeny illustrates the complexity of the interactions that involve the simplest host-parasite relationships. One can imagine the complexity of the events if phenomena similar to lysogeny involve viruses and mammalian cells, as may be the case with some oncogenes. Moreover, an accurate description of the molecular events in the "phage bacteria" system probably will bring us a new understanding of viral carcinogenesis.

Lysogeny plays an important role in the pathogenesis of viral infection. Some viral infections, such as herpetic infection, are silent for a long time. Furthermore, the asymptomatic host harbors an invisible virus. Yet a number of challenges, such as fever, sunburns, hormonal imbalance, and nervous excitation or stress, convert the latent into a full-blown symptomatic infection. In the latent herpesvirus, a sort of prophage is incorporated into epithelial or nerve cell DNA. What represses its expression into a cytocidal virus? What is the molecular mechanism of the derepressor? It is important to patient care that such questions be answered, and only the molecular biology of tomorrow can give such answers. The relationship between prophage and cancer viruses will become apparent later, but it is now time to return to the diphtheria toxin [242, 243].

Clinically, the bacteria that cause diphtheria do not cause injury by direct infection, but by spreading of the toxin that they elaborate. But this is not absolutely true because virulent diphtheria infections have been described in the absence of toxemia. Although not completely characterized, diphtheria toxin has been crystallized, and it is believed to be a polypeptide with a molecular weight of 72,000. We have described the cytocidal effects of the toxin; suffice it to remark here that although the toxin was thought to interfere with the electron transfer ability of cytochrome b, facts now suggest that the toxin might instead interfere with protein synthesis. The misinterpretation seems to have resulted from the nature of the experiment that was planned to test the effect of the toxin on the electron transport chain. Pappenheimer and Williams [244] observed that effective growth of the adult stage of the Cecropia silkworm, which was closely correlated with cytochrome biosynthesis, was inhibited by the toxin. In contrast, the toxin had no effect on the dormant pupal stage, which is devoid of cytochrome. These elegant but rather indirect observations led to the conclusion that diphtheria toxin blocks the cytochrome system. Yet it was later found that the toxin has no effect on ATP biosynthesis but interferes with the incorporation of amino acids into proteins. Pappenheimer's early findings probably can be explained by interference of the toxin with protein synthesis.

Until the 1950s, the toxin was believed to be elaborated by the virulent diphtheria bacterium, possibly when it lysed. In 1951 Freeman [245] found that a virulent bacteria (*Corynebacterium diphtheriae*) infected by a bacteriophage (b phage) became lysogenic and toxogenic. Groman and Eaton [246] went one step further by showing that the elimination of the prophage from the DNA complement of the bacterium was associated with the loss of toxigenicity.

Available evidence suggests that the toxin is elaborated after the prophage is converted into a virulent virus and appears concomitantly with viral replication. The amino acid sequence of the toxin is dictated by the genome of the phage, and the toxin is different from mature virus and capsid protein. However, some phages that cannot mature into complete viruses dictate toxin production. The antigenic properties of the toxin have nothing in common with the antigenic properties of the capsid. Iron needs to be present in the medium for the production of diphtheria toxin. The role of iron is not clear, but it has been linked to the release of the toxin by the bacteria.

A similar phage-host relationship has been invoked in the elaboration of some streptococcal and staphylococcal toxins. Scarlatinal strains of hemolytic streptococci induce an erythrogenic reaction that results from the release of a specific toxin. UV irradiation of lysogenic streptococci leads to the release of 10 to 20 more times of erythrogenic toxin.

Slow Virus Disease

There exists in humans and animals a number of diseases known or suspected to be caused by viruses which instead of being acute or causing cancer have an insidious onset. All the injuries caused by the infectious agent progress slowly until they cause death. In some cases the virus has been demonstrated, *e.g.*, measles in subacute sclerosing encephalitis, Papovirus (SV 40 and SC virus) in progressive multifocal leukoencephalopathy; in others it has not, *e.g.*, Kuru, Creutzfeldt-Jakob disease. The diseases are characterized by a long incubation period (1 month to 20 years) and the persistence of the virus throughout the entire duration of the disease.

Table 16-2. Slow virus diseases

Of known viral origin

Human subacute sclerosing encephalitis: measles
Progressive multifocal leukoencephalopathy: papovirus
Animal visna, viral encephalomyelitis of Islandic sheep: RNA virus with lipoprotein envelope
Zwoegerzichte (in Holland): same as visna
Mice lymphocytic choriomeningitis

Of unknown viral origin

Human
- Kuru encephalopathy, endemic to the Fore people in New Guinea
- Creutzfeldt-Jakob disease: rare presenile dementia

Animals
- Scrapies in sheep
- Transmissible mink encephalopathy

Human encephalopathies suspected to be caused by slow virus diseases

Multiple sclerosis
Guillain Barre syndrome
Amyotrophic lateral sclerosis
Parkinson's disease

When a known virus is the cause of the disease there is no obvious correlation between the morphology and the biochemistry or the mode of replication of the virus and the slow and progressive onset. The virus may be a DNA or an RNA virus with or without a lipid envelope. Antibodies to the virus are found in the blood of the victim. The virus can often be isolated and will produce damage when added to cells in culture.

When the virus is unknown, all that is solidly established is that the disease is transmissible from one animal to another with tissue extracts. Typical virions have not been isolated and specific antibodies have not been demonstrated. The slow virus usually affects the central nervous system. For a description of the clinical and morbid anatomic manifestation see [591–594].

It is possible that if the proper conditions of host virus relationships are induced, all viruses could lead to slow virus disease and therefore there is no unique feature that characterizes the slow virus.

The reasons why a given virus causes a slow virus disease are not clear. Certainly they must reside in a special host agent relationship which may vary in each case. For example, heredity is believed to play a role in Kuru, scrapies, Aleutian mink disease, and Creutzfeldt-Jakob disease.

The mode of inheritance of Kuru is not clear, but autosomal dominant inheritance is involved in Creutzfeldt-Jakob disease and autosomal recessive in scrapies. The fur of the Aleutian mink has a gun-gray color resembling that of the Aleutian fox. The mode of inheritance for the gene is autosomal recessive. Factors other than heredity are likely to be involved in determining the cause of the disease, although they are often unknown. For example, progressive multifocal encephalopathy usually occurs only in patients in an immunodeficiency state resulting from lymphoproliferative disorders or Hodgkin's disease. The exact participation of the immunodeficiency in the pathogenesis of the disease is, however, not clear.

Slow viruses may have some properties in common with the oncogenic viruses; for example, the visna virus, a RNA virus, contains reverse transcriptase and has caused transformation in murine cell culture. The significance of these similarities is not understood.

Viroids

A number of plant diseases (potato spindle tube disease, chrysanthemum stunt and citrus exocortis) are caused by what is the smallest known agent of infectious disease; namely, viroids. Viroids are composed of free RNA of low molecular weight, and virus particles are not present in the infected cells. It is not known if viroids also infect animal cells. The implication of the discovery of the viroids to pathology cannot as yet be predicted [595].

Viral Carcinogenesis

Viruses do not kill all mammalian cells; they can also live with them in symbiosis. Such symbiosis may leave the cell unchanged, or it may alter the host's flow of gene expression in such a fashion that the cell acquires a survival advantage over other cells in the organism. Thus, the cells proliferate actively, invade the surrounding tissue, metastasize, and are transplantable to other hosts. These so-called oncogenic viruses cause cancer to appear in fowl and mammals. (They also cause cancer in plants, but that process will not be discussed.) When such oncogenic viruses are introduced into cells cultivated *in vitro*, some morphological and biochemical changes take place in those cells, the sum of which is referred to as transformation. In the following pages we will briefly describe viral carcinogenesis in the intact animal, transformation, and the molecular mechanisms of viral carcinogenesis.

Experimental Viral Carcinogenesis

Avian Leukosis Viruses

Avian tumor viruses can be divided into two major groups: the avian leukosis virus and the Rous sarcoma virus. A family of closely related viruses (morphology, antigenicity) induce tumors in chicks, pheasants, ducks, quail, and turkeys. Various histological structures have been described, and classification varies with the investigator. However, it seems safe to state that fowl virus tumors can be grouped into a number of categories including lymphomatosis, leukemia, osteoporosis, endothelioma, and others.

Lymphomatosis consists of the proliferation of lymphoid cells in various visceral or neurological structures. Among the organs most frequently involved are the liver, the lungs, the spleen, and occasionally the nerves and the iris. Chicken leukemias, which have been observed by Furth [247] and by Ellerman and Bang [248], are of four types: lymphoid, myeloblastic, erythroblastic, and mixed. The leukemias can be transmitted by cells or by filtrates. Osteoporosis results from a proliferation of fibroblasts into the periosteum and endosteum, leading to an overgrowth of the bone; it may or may not be associated with lymphocytosis.

When the virus responsible for visceral lymphocytosis is passed from one animal to another, other types of tumors may develop—such as endotheliomas, hemangiomas, osteofibrosarcomas, and myxosarcomas. (The last can be retransmitted by cell filtrate.) These observations suggest that the same virus may, under appropriate conditions, lead to different tumors. However, the original tumor could contain a variety of viruses that might develop preferentially in different environments. Another possibility is that the original virus mutates. Burmester [249] has proposed a unifying theory to explain this variability in histological appearances. This author considers that the virus responsible for lymphomatosis is the wild type. After mutation and suitable transmission in an appropriate environment, the wild virus induces different types of tumors. Thus, the visceral lymphomatosis virus may, after several passages, be transformed into the virus responsible for: (1) the insults of osteoporosis, (2) hemangioendotheliomas, (3) sarcomas and fibrosarcomas, (4) erythroblastomas. The erythroblastosis virus may itself mutate into a virus that induces myxosarcomas, fibrosarcomas, myoblastomas, and osteochondral sarcomas.

This unified concept is not accepted by everyone. It has indeed been suggested that the visceral lymphomatosis virus and that responsible for osteoporosis are different for the following reasons: (1) there is no correlation between the incidence of the two diseases, and (2) while the lymphomatosis virus can be transmitted by contact, the osteoporosis virus cannot. Furthermore, it has been suggested that neurolymphomatosis is due to a virus different from that responsible for visceral lymphomatosis.

In spite of the confusion, an essential concept has emerged from all these studies on avian viruses—namely, that closely related viruses can induce different histological tumors. It is unlikely that the development of a given tumor type is fortuitous. It is much more likely that the histological type of the tumor is dictated by a close interrelationship between virus and host cell molecule. To be able to describe these molecular interrelations would constitute a great step forward in biology. Not only would such information shed new light on the mechanisms of carcinogenesis, but it would also give some clue as to the regulation of cellular differentiation. Unfortunately, too little is known at the present to permit a coherent interpretation of the viral host cell interrelation in terms of viral and cellular biochemistry.

Among the avian tumor viruses, the various strains of the Rous sarcoma virus occupy a special place. The various strains of the Rous sarcoma virus differ from the avian leukosis viruses in at least four ways. The avian leukosis viruses are ubiquitous in chickens, whereas the Rous sarcoma viruses occur rarely in nature. The leukosis viruses produce leukemia, but the Rous sarcoma viruses produce connective tissue tumors. Chickens can harbor the leukosis viruses for years without developing tumors, but the introduction of Rous sarcoma viruses appears to be followed by the rapid development of tumors or the viruses disappear. And, finally, the avian leukosis viruses do not damage tissue culture cells, whereas the Rous sarcoma viruses transform cultured fibroblasts into sarcoma cells. In contrast, all avian viruses contain RNA, and no crucial physical or chemical differences between the avian leukosis and Rous sarcoma viruses have been found. The physical and chemical properties of the Rous sarcoma viruses will be discussed in greater detail later [250–254]. Examples of tumors produced by Rous sarcoma viruses in chicken, rat, and monkey are shown in Fig. 16-36.

Shope Papilloma Virus

Shope demonstrated that the papillomatosis of cottontail rabbits of Kansas and Iowa was caused by a virus [255–259]. The evolution of the virus-induced disease varies depending upon the strain of rabbits used. In wild rabbits, the injection of the virus leads to hyperplasia of the epithelium with pigmented horny growth containing pseudokeratin. The papillomas develop in the ears and the thighs; usually they retrocede completely after a time. In contrast, in the domestic rabbit, the injection of the virus leads to papillomas that develop into metastasizing spinocellular carcinomas after 6 months. Many of these cancers can be transmitted by cellular transplantation but not with the aid of ultrafiltrates. Specific immunological reaction indicates, however, that the virus is present in the transplanted tumors. Thus, the tumors retain their antigenicity even after as many as 20 to 40 transplantations and even though the virus cannot be extracted from cancers produced in domestic rabbits.

Strangely enough, when fluorescent antibodies are applied to skin preparations containing the Shope papilloma, the antigen is found in the superficial undividing keratinizing cell layer, rather than in the dividing basal cells. Thus, whereas the virus is unmasked in the cells that are normally shed, it is masked in those cells where it affects cellular growth. Moreover, the masked virus is transferred from mother to daughter as these cells divide.

Carcinogens and hormones influence the development of the cancers induced by the Shope papilloma

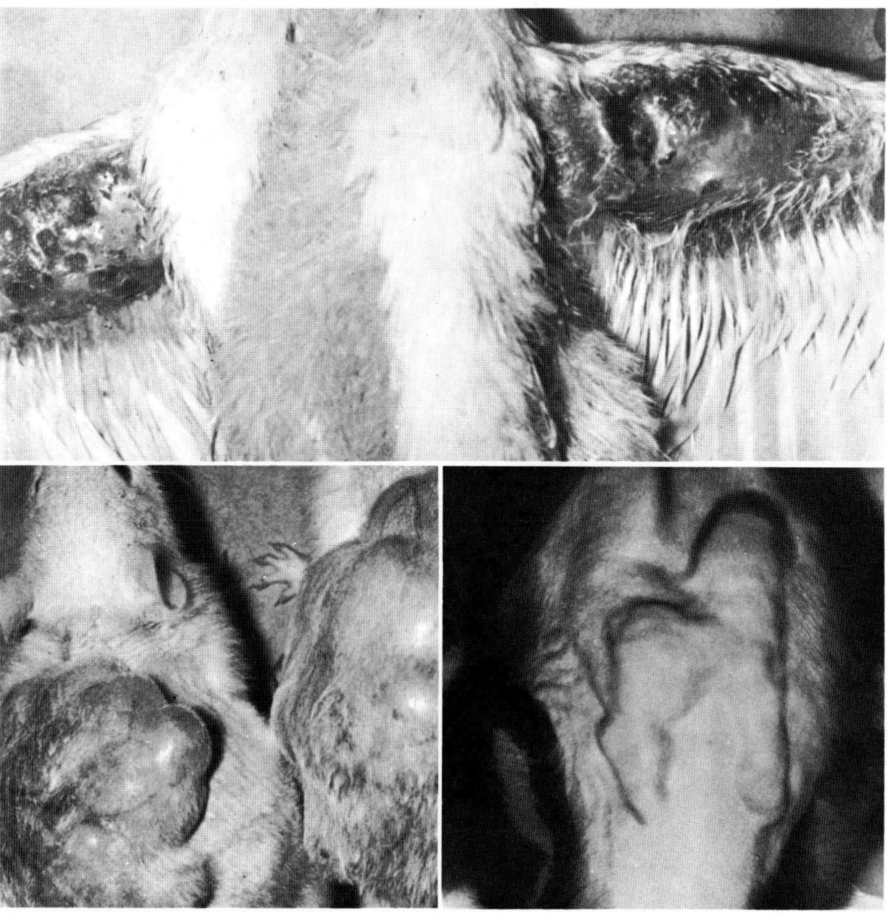

Fig. 16-36. Tumors produced in chicken, rat, and monkey by Rous sarcoma viruses (Van Lancker and McClure)

virus. If the virus is injected intravenously in animals whose skin has been painted with methylcholanthrene or 3,4-benzopyrene, papillomas develop that will undergo dramatic malignant transformation, even though it would have taken the carcinogen or the virus alone months to produce tumors.

Hypophysectomy prevents the development of tumors under the influence of the virus and induces the regression of those tumors induced by the virus.

Thus, the biology of Shope papilloma virus illustrates new aspects of the relationship between virus and tumor cell. The cellular alteration induced by the virus will vary with the host's genotype and environment. Wild rabbits develop benign tumors, but domestic rabbits develop cancer. The incidence and the degree of malignancy of the tumor are influenced by carcinogens and hormones.

A number of mammalian papillomas of the skin or the mucosa are caused by viruses. Such virus tumors have been observed in rats, rabbits, cats, and horses. In humans, warts, which have long been known to be contagious, are of viral origin. Ultrafiltrates transmit the tumor, and viral inclusions have been observed in histological specimens. (Human warts have been successfully transplanted to the conjunctiva of monkeys.) Viruses are also responsible for the development of connective tissue tumors (fibromas, myxomas, fibrosarcomas, and myxosarcomas) in rabbits, squirrels, and cats. A bladder tumor of dermal origin develops in cattle as the result of virus infection. Although the tumor is benign in Wisconsin cattle, it is not in mideastern cattle.

Bittner Virus

It was previously mentioned that three factors are required for the development of breast carcinoma in mice [260, 261]: natural hereditary susceptibility, estrogen administration, and the presence of virus. The virus is apparently present in all tissues but is transmitted from the mother to the progeny by the milk. This was demonstrated by cross-feeding experiments. By itself, the virus cannot induce cancer. Indeed, in some homozygous strains of mice that carry the virus, no more than 5% of the virgin females developed breast cancer, but 95% of the females who went through several pregnancies developed that tumor.

The oncogenic properties of the virus are restricted to mice and to the breast. The Bittner virus does not produce tumors in other animals or at other sites. However, all breast tumors are not produced by the Bittner virus. For example, the virus is not likely to be responsible for some experimental tumors produced in the NIHO Strong strain or for the spontaneous tumors appearing in some strains with a low incidence of breast tumors. Furthermore, when the virus is introduced into a strain of mice with a low incidence of breast cancer, it transforms that strain into a strain with a high incidence of breast cancer. This suggests a close interaction between virus and the mouse genotype [262–266].

Reports from Moore, Pollard, and Haagensen [267] have further complicated our understanding of the relationship between virus and host. The milk agent contains tumor-inducing (100–150 A) and tumor-inhibiting (40–50 A) particles. In addition to the particulate inhibitor, there is also a dialyzable inhibitor of low molecular weight.

Murine Leukemia Viruses

Gross found that ultrafiltrates of leukemic tissue obtained from AK or C58 mice (strains with a high incidence of leukemias) produce leukemia when injected into C-3H or C57 BL mice (strains that have a low incidence of leukemia) [268–270]. In addition, the progeny of the animals injected with the ultrafiltrate present a high incidence of leukemia. After 1 or 2 years, the new tumors can be transplanted to mice with a low incidence of leukemia, but they cannot be returned to the donor. It was later shown that the virus responsible for leukemia in mice is thermolabile and cannot be transmitted by the milk. Although no direct evidence is available, it is assumed that the virus is transferred through the germinal cells (vertical transmission) like that of chicken lymphomatosis.

Since Gross' original discovery, a number of murine viruses have been discovered. They differ in their size, host susceptibility, and the type of leukemia that they induce [271–273].

The Schwartz virus was first isolated from the brain of Swiss mice. On repeated cell-free passage, it produces lymphosarcomas in mice with hepatosplenomegaly more conspicuous than that observed in AK leukemia (Gross virus). The distribution of the virus in the host is puzzling; although present in lymphoid tissue, the virus cannot readily be recovered from that tissue. In contrast, the neural tissue of the inoculated mice is rich in virus.

Moloney has extracted a virus from a transplantable connective tissue neoplasm in mice. The virus produces lymphocytic neoplasms in almost all the inoculated mice. When injected in hamsters, it produces reticular cell sarcoma. Intravenous, intraperitoneal, intracerebral, and subcutaneous injections effectively transmit the disease. Horizontal transfer of the virus does not occur, but there are indications that the virus can be transferred through the milk or across extraembryonic membranes. A virus has been found in lymphoma induced by X-irradiation in C57 BL mice.

The Bregen-Moloney virus was derived from a plasma cell tumor of the ileocecal region of methylcholanthrene-treated C-3H mouse. It produces leukemia in BALB mice.

The Graffi virus was isolated from tumors of various strains of mice.* When injected, this virus causes bone

* The study on the Gross virus illustrates some of the difficulties involved in investigating tumor viruses. Indeed, many of the injected animals did not develop tumors when the ultrafiltrates of individual mice were used. Only when the ultrafiltrates were pooled were more reproducible results obtained.

marrow proliferation leading to myeloid leukemia, but never to the development of a tumor similar to the one from which the virus was extracted. The existence of the Graffi and the Schwartz viruses remains contested.

The Friend virus was obtained from Swiss mice injected with cell-free extract of Ehrlich carcinoma. This virus induces a systemic disease, a sort of panleukemia with erythroblastosis, lymphocytosis, and proliferation of the reticulum cells.

Although confusing, the pathology of the mouse leukemias is of considerable interest. In terms of the cells that dominate the leukemic picture, at least four types of murine leukemia can be distinguished: erythroleukemia, myeloid leukemia, lymphatic leukemia, and reticulum cell sarcoma. Except for the Friend and Rauscher viruses, which induce an erythroleukemic reaction starting in the spleen, most other mouse leukemia viruses can produce, depending upon the circumstances, any of the three other types of cellular proliferations just described.

Two factors determine the type of leukemia that develops: susceptibility and the presence of thymus. Newborn susceptible nonthymectomized mice develop a lymphatic leukemia that starts in the thymus. Mice from nonsusceptible strains, old, or thymectomized mice may develop myeloid leukemia or reticulum cell sarcoma.

The erythroleukemia starts in the spleen of the infected and from there extends to the liver and the bone marrow. Whether all proliferating cells participate in the neoplastic process is sometimes debated. Some investigators have claimed that only the proliferation of the reticulum cells of the spleen is neoplastic, and that the proliferation of the cells of the erythroblastic lineage is simply hyperplastic. Thus, this type of erythroleukemia might be a combination of erythrocytic polyerythema and leukemia.

The development of thymic lymphomas discussed in some detail in the section radiation carcinogenesis.

Four different phases have been described in the development of reticulum cell sarcomas: (1) proliferation of primitive reticulum cells in the spleen, (2) invasion of the splenic vein and the portal system, (3) reticulum cell proliferation in the liver, and (4) extension of the disease to the systemic circulation and the invasion of bone marrow with a myelofibrotic reaction. The latent period between viral inoculation or activation and the development of thymic lymphomas is so much shorter than the latent period between inoculation of either Graffi or Rich virus that mice with a high susceptibility to lymphomas are bound to die from thymic lymphoma before they develop myeloid leukemia.

The reticulum cell sarcoma develops in the lymph nodes. Its pathogenesis has been studied in the SJL/J mice. The first signs appear in the mesenteric nodes and consist of reticulum cell proliferation in the germinal centers. Reticulum cell proliferation spreads and soon obscures all normal lymphatic architecture. The proliferation is associated with cell lysis and phagocytosis by macrophages, plasma cell reaction, and scar formation. The histological picture is somewhat reminiscent of that seen in Hodgkin's disease in man. Whether Hodgkin's disease and the murine reticulum cell sarcoma are related remains to be established.

Polyoma Virus

During experiments on mouse leukemia, investigators observed that the ultrafiltrate obtained from leukemic tissues of the C-3H mice also led to the development of parotid tumors. Thus, this suggests that the development of parotid tumors is also due to a virus. Gross' [269] studies suggested that the leukemic and parotid viruses were two different viruses; the parotid virus was less thermolabile and could be separated from the leukemic virus by diluting the ultrafiltrate. Thus, diluted preparations did not induce leukemia, but only parotid tumors. Later, it became possible to separate the two viruses by ultracentrifugation.

Stewart and Eddy [273–278] isolated the virus responsible for parotid tumors by cultivating it on tissue culture cells of monkey kidney, chick embryo, and allantoic membrane cells. The administration of the virus to mice led to such a great variety of tumors that the responsible agent was called polyoma virus. The discovery of polyoma virus is so important in the history of carcinogenesis that it is worthwhile to elaborate on the technical evolution of that finding. The authors prepared cell-free extract mixes or homogenates of a good source of virus—for example, a parotid tumor. The virus was then propagated on monkey kidney or mouse embryo cultures, and the supernatant fluid was injected to other mice, who then developed a spectrum of tumors similar to that obtained by injecting the native leukemia cell-free extract. Furthermore, the new virus so obtained induced tumors not only in mice but also in rats, in the Syrian and Chinese hamsters, and in rabbits.

Practically all strains of mice tested are susceptible to the virus. The virus propagated on the mouse embryo culture is much more efficient in producing tumors than that cultured on the monkey kidney. Furthermore, in mice a variety of tumors have been described.

The most frequent of all tumors is a mixed tumor of the parotid, which may invade the surrounding tissue and lead to metastases. Although the parotid is a preponderant site for the development of such tumors, the submaxillary and the sublingual glands also participate in the carcinogenic process if enough virus is given. Renal sarcomas, thymomas, mammary carcinomas, hair follicle tumors, epidermoid carcinomas, osteosarcomas, mesotheliomas, hemangioblastomas, fibrosarcomas, carcinomas of the adrenal medulla, epidermoid carcinomas of the intestinal mucosa, visceral hemangiomas, squamous cell carcinomas of the stomach, sweat gland adenocarcinomas, and lung tumors have all been produced by this type of virus.

However, as pointed out previously, the incidence of a specific type of tumor varies considerably, and if, for example, the parotid is frequently involved (96%), gastric carcinoma rarely develops (1%). One observes in hamsters mainly sarcomas of the kidney, but occasionally other types of tumors have been recognized. A similar situation exists in the rat, in which the virus also induces mesenchymal sarcomas, particularly in the kidney. The virus also induces tumors in rabbits, but in contrast to mice and rat tumors, the rabbit tumors are nonmalignant (subcutaneous fibromas).

Morphological Characteristics of Tumor Viruses

The size of tumor viruses ranges from that of the larger viruses, like the smallpox virus, to that of some of the smallest known viruses, like the poliomyelitis virus. Thus, the virus responsible for rabbit myxomatosis has a diameter ranging between 220 and 260 mμ, whereas that of the polyoma virus is about 30 mμ. The Bittner virus, the viruses associated with mouse leukemia and chicken tumors, and the leukemia viruses all have sizes intermediate between one of these two extremes [279, 280].

Although the DNA viruses usually include medium-sized viruses, ranging from 40–120 mμ, and occasionally large ones of 120–150 mμ, RNA viruses are small or medium sized and do not include large viruses.

The morphology of tumor viruses does not differ from that of other viruses in any essential way. Tumor viruses include clarthroviruses, helical viruses, and the complex viruses. The first tumor virus that was examined in detail with the electron microscope was the adenovirus. The coat of the adenovirus forms an icosahedron with triangular faces that are covered with small projections of capsomeres. The capsomeres are polypeptides; their amino acid composition and sequence are not known, but it is believed that they are of two types, one made of six chemical subunits and another made of five chemical subunits. The SV40, the polyoma, the rabbit papilloma, and the human wart virus have symmetrical structures similar to that of the adenovirus. The capsids of the mouse leukemia virus, the mouse mammary tumor virus, the chicken leukemia virus, and the Rous sarcoma virus have a different type of symmetry, which is reminiscent of that of influenza, mumps, and Newcastle disease viruses. The capsid forms a helical structure surrounding the RNA core. The virus responsible for molluscum contagiosum and Shope fibroma has a complex structure similar to that of the poxvirus.

The intracellular site of multiplication of the virus has been studied with various methods, including the use of fluorescent antibodies, electron microscopy, and tissue fractionation. The DNA viruses develop in the nucleus, the helical RNA viruses develop either in the cytoplasm or in the cell membrane, and the complex viruses develop in the cytoplasm at the expense of a viroplasm similar to the one already described for poxviruses. In the cell, the virus particles may aggregate to yield intranuclear or intracytoplasmic inclusion bodies in which crystalline viral elements may sometimes be identified.

A number of ultrastructural alterations have been described in cells found in murine viral tumors. The origin and the role of these structures in viral oncology are not always certain. In some cases, however, these abnormal ultrastructures appear to result from combinations of virus and cytoplasmic structures. Bernard classified these structures in four different groups, referred to as A, B, C, and D.

Type A are donut-shaped structures formed by two concentric membranes, usually found near the Golgi apparatus and measuring 70–90 mμ.* The type A particle has been divided into three subgroups. A_1 (70 mμ) has an outer and an inner shell of approximately the same thickness. The outer shell is formed by budding of the cell's endoplasmic reticulum, and the inner shell seems to be elaborated *de novo*. A_2 has an outer shell thinner than the inner shell and a translucent center much larger than that of A_1. A_3 (85–90 mμ) is essentially the same as A_1 but has a larger diameter. The role of these particles in oncogenicity is still not clear. Type B particles are larger (105 mμ) and, in contrast to type A, they are mainly extracellular or found at the cell surface. B particles contain an eccentric nucleoprotein core surrounded by a lipoprotein membrane, which probably is of cellular origin.

The relationship between A and B types of particles is not clear, but A particles are believed to be progressively transformed into B. B particles are believed to be the agent responsible for mammary tumors. The B type has not been found in other mouse tumors; however, it has been detected in the milk of the mice with a low incidence of breast carcinoma. In contrast, the type A has been found in a dense cluster around the Golgi zone in a few other mouse tumors such as melanomas, sarcomas, plasmacytomas, and ascites tumors.

The type C virus, a larger particle with a larger nucleoprotein core, is found in cells obtained from involved areas (spleen, thymus, and lymph nodes) of leukemic AK mice. They are cytoplasmic viruses budding from the plasma membrane. Type D particles are found in polyoma and SV40 tumors. They are small intranuclear particles containing virus, surrounded by a thin membrane. Type D particles have been seen in a large number of nuclei in tumors produced by that virus. The dried virus measures 44 mμ, and the thin-section virus is 28–30 mμ.

---

* The dimensions of viruses observed under the electron microscope after fixation and embedding are considerably inferior to those of the native virus. This results partly from dehydration, partly from flattening of the virus during embedding, and partly from factors of an unknown nature.

Factors Modulating Viral Carcinogenesis in Vivo

Although one might have anticipated that the discovery of cancer viruses would have simplifed our understanding of carcinogenesis, it seems now more likely that it will complicate it further. At the present, no simple unifiying theory satisfactorily explains viral carcinogenesis. Some cancers in animals, are, in fact, caused by a wide range of viruses that are likely to act at different sites of the cell on different macromolecular systems. Therefore, the transformation of a normal cell into a cancer cell appears to be a stereotyped reaction to injury, several steps removed from the primary cellular insult. If this is true, it is important that we recognize it, because we have indications that the transformation is often irreversible. Furthermore, once transformation has occurred, the cancer cell uses metabolic pathways similar to those of the normal cell and, as a result, cancer cell proliferation cannot be blocked without also hurting normal cells. Consequently, our hope to control cancer resides not in studying the cancer cell, but in studying the precancerous state, and identifying the primary injury to the cell in each individual case.

If these paragraphs on viral carcinogenesis do not help to simplify our understanding of carcinogenesis, hopefully they illustrate the complexity of the problem, and emphasize the need for investigating those events that are closest to the primary molecular injury [281–283].

Any comprehensive theory on viral carcinogenesis must take the following observations into account: (1) the complex interrelationship between host and virus, (2) the effect of other helper viruses, (3) the role of carcinogens in viral carcinogenesis, and (4) the direct effect of the virus on the cell.

When mice are thymectomized 5 days after birth and then injected with the Gross leukemia virus, lymphoid tumors do not develop. However, some of these mice develop myeloid leukemia 12 months later. This clearly suggests that there is a scale of organ sensitivity to the viral transformation. Some tissues, in this case the lymphoid tissue, are more susceptible to transformation than others. Similarly, it has been shown that chickens surviving large doses of virus, without developing myeloblastosis, develop tumors of the kidney later. The tissue susceptibility to transformation is not necessarily linked to the organotropism of the virus. For example, we mentioned that some murine leukemia viruses are recovered in quantity from the brain rather than from lymphoid tissue.

A complex interrelationship between susceptibility to viruses and heredity is to be anticipated if one keeps in mind the number of factors that influence viral survival that are hereditarily controlled, such as structure of the cell membrane and immunological response to virus.

The role of heredity in breast cancer in mice has already been discussed. Similarly, leukemogenic viruses are limited in host range in various degrees. One possible restriction to host range may result from the mode of maturation of the virus. Electron microscopy suggests that the host cell membrane coats at least some virus particles, thereby conferring specific antigenicity to the virus, which as a result can be infective only to isoantigenic cells.

Several investigators have studied the susceptibility of chorioallantoic membranes of chicken to Rous sarcoma virus. Some have suggested that susceptibility to infection is controlled by a single pair of autosomal genes; some have assumed that the gene for susceptibility is dominant over the gene for resistance. However, this view is not accepted by all, and investigators have proposed that the gene for susceptibility manifests only a questionable degree of partial dominance. Whatever the details of the interaction between virus and host, it is clear from these experiments that the host's genome influences its susceptibility to the virus.

The complex interrelationship between viruses and host in viral carcinogenesis is further illustrated by the role of helper viruses in the Rous sarcoma virus (RSV). Studies of infections with various concentrations of RSV suggested that the relationship between host and tumor was somewhat peculiar when low concentrations of virus were used to induce tumors. These tumors would not yield mature viruses; however, when high concentrations of virus were used, mature RSV particles could be recovered from the homogenate of the tumor.

Burmester, Walter, and associates [284] also observed that animals injected with low concentrations of virus did not develop sarcoma after the expected latency, but developed leukemia later. Such a finding suggests that the RSV preparations are contaminated by the avian leukosis virus.

It was later established that high-titer strains of Rous sarcoma virus are unable to spawn infectious viral progeny unless a helper virus called the Rous associated virus (RAV) is also present. The helper virus is not necessary to effect transformation of fibroblasts into sarcoma cells by RSV, and after infection with RSV, the Rous sarcoma cell remains malignant through several divisions. Thus the RSV genome must be reproduced, yet the virus never matures in the infected cell. The maturation depends upon the presence of a helper virus. The helper virus apparently determines the biosynthesis of the capsid and, therefore, the antigenicity (see below).

Thus, the addition of RAV to cells infected with RSV activates the production of RSV. However, if cells are infected with RAV before RSV infection, the immunogenic reaction of the host interferes with RSV infectivity. Consequently, when chick allantoic membrane cells in culture are infected with enough RSV to infect single cells, only 10% of the cells are infected.

Two murine viruses capable of inducing sarcomas—the Harvey virus and the Moloney sarcoma virus—have been identified. These viruses appear to be defective like the RSV. Because defective viruses exist in birds and mice, it has been speculated that they might also exist in humans.

One needs to consider two aspects of the relationship between cancer viruses and carcinogens: (1) the presence of virus in chemically induced tumors, and (2) the effect of carcinogens on viral tumors [285].

Fowl, like most other animal species, are susceptible to the action of carcinogens, which may, for example, lead to the development of sarcomas when injected intramuscularly. Inasmuch as viruses transmit spontaneous tumors in fowl, it was quite natural for the investigators to look for a virus in the experimentally produced tumors. The problem is far from settled. The arguments in favor of the role of viruses in the development of fowl experimental cancers rest on two lines of information: the occasional transmission of chemically produced cancers by ultrafiltrates, and the development of antibodies to the transplanted tumors.

Carel was the first to claim that a tumor produced by tar in the Plymouth Rock chicken could be transmitted with an ultrafiltrate. Although Claude and Murphy [286] succeeded later in transplanting some of these chemically produced tumors by using intact cells, they could not reproduce Carel's findings. Many publications relating negative results followed the original paper of Carel. However, in 1950 Oberling and Guerin [287] extracted an active ultrafiltrate from a chemically produced tumor that had been transplanted repeatedly.

The effect of carcinogens on the virus tumors of breast cancer is much more complex. In general, the results in the literature can be summarized as follows. In contrast to hormones, which induce cancers only in strains that normally present a high incidence of tumors, carcinogens induce breast carcinoma in strains that normally have a low incidence of tumors. But carcinogens do not usually influence the incidence of breast cancer in strains containing the virus. (This should be correlated with the possible presence of viruses in tumors produced by carcinogens.) After several transplantations, a breast tumor produced by carcinogens in animals free of the Bittner virus could be transmitted by an ultrafiltrate. In this case, the carcinogen helped to reveal a virus in a tumor that did not seem to contain it, indicating that the virus was probably present at all times in a latent form.

Three interpretations can be invoked to explain the occasional presence of tumor viruses in tumors induced chemically: (1) contamination by known tumor viruses, (2) the spontaneous appearance of a yet unknown virus in an environment that has become favorable for its development, and (3) the presence of small amounts of a masked virus that is revealed only by repeated transplantation.

In conclusion, the relationship between carcinogens and tumor viruses is far from solved and deserves further investigation. A similar situation exists when it comes to evaluating the role of viruses in mouse lymphoma induced by X-irradiation (see Radiation Carcinogenesis).

Another aspect of the relationship between viruses and carcinogens resides in the effect of carcinogens on the development of the virus tumors. The most interesting effects have been observed in the Shope papilloma, in which carcinogen administration: (1) facilitates the transformation of the papilloma to cancer, (2) confines the site of carcinoma development to the area painted or injected with the carcinogen, (3) reduces the latent period for the occurrence of cancer, and (4) stimulates the growth, incidence, and malignancy of the tumor. Magee's findings may be relevant to the mechanism by which carcinogens affect viral oncogenesis. Magee claims that polycyclic aromatic carcinogens have an effect similar to that of actinomycin D on macromolecular synthesis in general, and on the biosynthesis of interferon in particular.

X-Irradiation modifies the capacity of cells to produce Rous sarcoma virus. In fact, the cell's radiosensitivity seems to be correlated with its ability to produce virus. The effect of X-irradiation on viral proliferation is manifested only if X-irradiation is administered before infection. If X-irradiation is administered 20 hours after infection, irradiation no longer affects viral proliferation.

The oncogenic properties of a tumor virus are not necessarily restricted to the species of the host from which it was isolated. The Fujimani virus of chickens can be transmitted to ducks, and both the Rous and Fujimani viruses can be transmitted to pheasants. In such cases, the ages of the donor and the recipient influence the adaptation of the virus. The chances of producing tumors are greater if the recipient is young.

The host's age is important in determining susceptibility to tumor viruses. Only extremely young animals are susceptible to the induction of tumors by some viruses, like the polyoma virus. Animals over 24 hours old become increasingly resistant to the induction of tumors by the polyoma virus. In others, the administration of the tumor virus leads to cell destruction, rather than to cell proliferation. Variations in the donor's age may also affect the oncogenic properties of the virus. Filtrates obtained from tumors of 3- to 10-month old chickens are active, while those obtained from 19- to 20-month old chickens are inactive.

When inoculated to a species foreign to the original host, the virus undergoes variation. It may induce new types of tumors in the foreign species or lead to unusual new lesions. For example, the Rous sarcoma virus, which classically leads to the development of lymphosarcomas in chickens, induces new lesions in ducks (a hemorrhagic disease and a variety of sarcomas in soft tissue or bones). Apparently, the more distantly the host is related to the chicken, the greater the variation in the virus.

From the morphological and biochemical description of the tumor virus, it clearly follows that they do not form classes that can be separated from other viruses on the basis of size, shape, chemical composition, or intracellular distribution. Furthermore, under appropriate conditions, many of the tumor viruses affect the organism or the cell as other viruses would. Thus, tumor viruses may be infectious and cytocidal.

Chicken lymphomatosis was a pure epizoic occurrence until purebred strains of chicken became available. Then the disease became infectious. Simple storage of Shope fibroma virus in glycerol is responsible for transforming the tumor virus into an agent capable of inducing lesions intermediate between tumor and inflammatory reactions. This new type of lesion is considered to be induced by a mutant strain of the virus.

In conclusion, both DNA and RNA viruses of various sizes, shapes, and biochemical compositions can cause various histological forms of cancer in a variety of animals.

Tumor viruses are clearly contagious, and transmission of disease follows epidemiological patterns common to all viruses. Diseases may be transmitted through: (1) direct contact (Rous sarcoma); (2) saliva, urine and feces (chicken lymphomatosis and polyoma virus); (3) insect transmission (mosquitoes in the infection of squirrels with Shope fibroma virus); (4) milk (Bittner virus and experimental murine leukemia); and (5) the mother or father—vertical transmission (AKR, C58 mice with a high incidence of spontaneous leukemia show a chromosomal pattern of transmission involving both parents).

The development of cancer is modulated by a number of factors including the immunological state, pedigree, and age of the host, the availability of helper virus, and exposure to chemical carcinogens and ionizing radiation.

Antigenic Properties of Viruses

Tumor viruses can be divided into two main groups with respect to their humoral antigenic properties. Some manifest clear-ut antigenic properties, like the polyoma virus and the Shope papilloma virus, and others exhibit little or no antigenic properties. The exact reasons for these differences are not clear. Sarah Stewart has suggested an explanation that seems logical, but it is not always in keeping with observations. She thinks that the origin of the protein component of the virus might be of considerable importance in determining its antigenic property.

In the Bittner virus, for example, the protein coat that surrounds the nucleic acid core is of cellular origin. It comes from cytoplasmic microvilli that surround the virus when it penetrates within the cells. The host cell cytoplasm leaves a protein coat around the core of viral nucleic acid. Thus, these proteins are not foreign to the host and they will not exhibit antigenic properties. In contrast, the Shope papilloma virus and the polyoma virus are found in the nucleus and are not encapsulated by a coat of cytoplasmic protein. Therefore, they are free to manifest antigenic properties. Consequently, it is not surprising that all rodents injected develop a high titer of antibodies.

Polyoma antibodies appear in the blood of all infected mice, even among those that do not develop tumors. Antibodies against the polyoma virus have appeared in monkeys kept close to infected mice, or in humans working with the virus. However, no polyoma antibody was ever found in ordinary hospital populations, regardless of whether the patients had cancer.

Studies using fluorescent antibodies prepared against mouse tissues infected with the various types of murine leukemia viruses have provided information on: (1) the intracellular localization of the virus, (2) the rate of appearance of antigen, and (3) the cross-immunity among leukemia viruses.

In the infected mouse, the antigen of the Friend virus first appears in the nucleus, but is later found in the cytoplasm of infected cells. Similarly, the antigen of the Rauscher virus appears in the nucleus but less consistently in the cytoplasm. The localization of the antigen in cultured cells seems to yield results different from those obtained in the intact animal. Although cytoplasmic staining with Friend fluorescent antibodies correlates with the degree of virus infections, no nuclear antibodies are found when Rauscher and Moloney fluorescent antibodies are used to stain infected culture cells or macrophages. But these studies confirmed previous electron microscopic studies that had established that the virus was found in close contact with the cell membrane. Cross-immunity has been known to take place between Friend and Rauscher viruses and between Rauscher and Moloney viruses, and it has even been claimed that Rauscher antigens were also found in human leukemia cells.

Cross-immunity among the various types of leukemia viruses is not surprising in view of the morphological and chemical similarities that exist among these viruses. Whether on the basis of these similarities, one should consider along with Gross that there is only a single murine leukemia virus, or whether one should along with Moloney consider the various mouse leukemia viruses as members of a single family is a debate it would be inappropriate to enter here.

A number of humoral antigens have also been identified in leukemic mice and tested for their cytotoxic effect against cells infected with one of the mouse leukemia viruses. At least four different humoral antigens have been described: FMR, G, TL, and E. (The reader should read specialized articles if he wishes to become more familiar with the techniques used in this type of study.)

The FMR antigen is cytotoxic for cells infected with Friend, Moloney, and Rauscher viruses. It is not antigenic for cells infected with the Gross virus. Lymphoid and leukemic cells of mice with a high incidence of spontaneous leukemia or lymphoid cells infected with the Gross virus yield an antigen G, which is cytotoxic for cells infected with the Gross virus and the Rich virus but not with the Friend, Moloney, or Rauscher viruses.

TL antigen is found in cells obtained from spontaneous or X-ray or chemically induced leukemia and in normal mouse thymus cells. Antigen E was found in the leukemic cells of C57 BL mice. The relationship between these tumor-specific antigens and the virus is not always clear. The role of viral antigens is discussed further in the chapter devoted to tumor immunology.

Biochemistry of Tumor Viruses

Although a large amount of biological information is available on tumor viruses, relatively little is known of their physicochemical properties. This results from the lack of appropriate antigen techniques, the similarities between virus and normal cell constituents, and the scarcity of the virus. To some extent, investigators have overcome part of the difficulties by harvesting the virus from the supernatant fluid obtained from tissue cultures, followed by further purifying the virus by chromatography on cellulose columns, by electrophoresis, or by fractionation in a cane sugar gradient [288–290].

Like most viruses, tumor viruses are composed of a core of nucleoproteins surrounded by a proteic membrane. Whereas the core is responsible for the reproductive and genetic properties of the virus, the coat confers the antigenic properties.

We will not discuss in detail all the biochemical properties of all tumor viruses. Instead, we shall briefly review two tumor viruses, a DNA virus (polyoma virus) and an RNA virus.

Polyoma virus is made of circular double-stranded DNA. However, purified polyoma virus DNA yields three different components upon centrifugation: a supercoiled circular duplex sedimenting at 20 S (mol wt 3×10^6, cytosine/guanine 49%), a nicked circular duplex sedimenting at 16 S, and linear host cell DNA strands. The 16-S fragment is thought to be a degradation product of the 20 S.* The supercoiled DNA duplex is supercoiled with 12 to 15 left-handed turns.

When the nucleic acid and the proteins of the polyoma virus are integrated to form the virion, each virion contains a core of supercoiled circular double-stranded DNA (3×10^6 daltons) surrounded by an icosahedral capsid containing a major capsid protein and 5 to 6 minor proteins.

The genome of the polyoma virus is composed of 5500 nucleotides and can code for 5–10 proteins.

About 12% of polyoma virus is DNA, the rest is protein. Polyoma proteins fall in three categories: 3 basic polypeptides, the capsid and 3 other polypeptides. The basic polypeptides are small, they have molecular weights ranging between 10,000 and 20,000 daltons. Available evidence suggests that these basic proteins are histones derived from the host. In addition, they are probably found inside of the virion in association with DNA. The capsid protein of polyoma DNA has a molecular weight of 46,000 to 50,000 daltons. Three other polypeptides are found in the complete virions: one has a molecular weight of 23,000 daltons, and two others have identical molecular weights of 35,000 daltons but slightly different electrophoretic mobility. For further information see [596–597].

A model for the inclusion of viral DNA in the DNA of the host genome has been proposed by Hill and Hillova [598]. The proviral DNA is single-stranded. The extended strand contains a sequence *hr* that codes for host range specificity and a sequence *tra* that codes for transformation. At each extremity of the proviral sequence there are inverted repetitive sequences which permit the formation of a single-stranded circle. Two enzymic steps are then put in gear: (1) the extended sequences are cut from the extremities; (2) the viral DNA is brought by a special enzyme in the replication fork of the host DNA where it is inserted and copied in a complementary strand.

The Rous sarcoma is the prototype of a group of viruses called the ribodeoxyviruses which consist of an envelope made of a lipid bilayer and external glycoprotein. The group includes the Rous sarcoma virus, the mouse mammary tumor virus and the visna virus. This group of viruses has a C type morphology and a core with no observable symmetry. The core contains RNA and a DNA polymerase.

The RNA of Rous sarcoma virus has been purified and some of the physicochemical properties have been investigated. The results suggest that the Rous sarcoma RNA moiety, like tobacco mosaic virus RNA, is made of a single-stranded RNA molecule.

RNA extracted from Rous sarcoma virus was found to have a rather high sedimentation constant (65 to 75 S). After treatment with heat or dimethyl sulfoxide, the sedimentation constant dropped to 35 S because of a change in conformation or more likely as a result of a drop in molecular weight. Since the mobility of the Rous sarcoma virus on the polyacrylamide gel electrophoresis increases after treatment with dimethyl sulfoxide, such treatment is believed to reduce the molecular weight of the viral RNA. Present hypotheses suggest that the RNA of the virion is composed of several aggregates, each of 3 to 4×10^6 daltons in molecular weight overlapping each other and forming hydrogen bonds between complementary sequences. The 35 S subunits are linear polynucleotides [599]. E lectrophoresis separates two kinds of subunits referred to as a and b. The a subunit is believed to carry the information needed to transfer a vision into a sarcoma cell.

In addition to the 70-S RNA, the RNA preparation obtained by extraction of Rous sarcoma virus yields 4-S, 7-S, 18-S, and 28-S fractions, and even small amounts of DNA. The significance and the role of these various RNA fractions or of the DNA remain to be established, but they are probably of cellular origin [292]. The DNA does not hybridize with viral RNA but anneals with cellular DNA. It is not believed to play any role in transformation.

There is surprisingly little difference between the known molecular properties of the various RNA tumor viruses. Sedimentation and chemical analysis indicate that the molecular weight of RNA per virus particle is 10^7 daltons per Rous sarcoma and the avian leukosis virus. The molecular weight of the RNA strand of the mouse leukemia virus has been estimated to be about the same as that of the Rous sarcoma virus. Inasmuch as the molecular weights of both are

* "Light" virus particles appear when cells are infected with large titers of polyoma virus. These are smaller circular duplexes that probably develop as a result of a deletion mutation. The light virus is also referred to as a defective virus [291].

known, it would appear that the RNA base composition is similar for both the avian and murine tumor RNA viruses. Studies on heat sensitivity and RNA resistance of purified Rauscher leukemia virus have indicated that the virus RNA is also single stranded.

All RNA tumor viruses contain 1% RNA, 2% carbohydrate, 20–30% lipids and 60–70% proteins. The protein population of RSV is complex and its description is made difficult because of the various nomenclatures used by different authors. The simplest nomenclature is that of Fleissner, who distinguishes two major groups of proteins: the glycoprotein and the structural protein. The two types of glycoproteins are referred to as m1 and m2. They contain galactose, fructose and glucosamine. m1 is a polymer with a molecular weight of 100,000, composed of subunits with molecular weights of 32,000. m2 is a monomer with a molecular weight of 70,000 daltons. The structural proteins are referred to as gsl (27,000 daltons), gs2 (19,000 daltons), gs3 (15,000 daltons), gs4 (12,000 daltons) and p5 (10,000 daltons). Except for the glycoproteins which form the spikes at the surface of the envelope and confer type (or subgroup antigenicity), the role of these proteins is not clear. The g proteins confer the group specific antigenicity and gs1, gs3, and p5 are believed to participate in the formation of the capsid.

The virus also contains reverse transcriptase which is not detectable except by its activity. The transcriptase is believed to be coded for by the viral genome. Other enzymes found in association with the virus, like ATPase, are probably from host origin.

Carbohydrate, lipid, and protein are arranged to form the viral C type structure. From the center to the periphery one can distinguish a spherical ribonucleoprotein nucleoid with a filamentous structure and which may possess some degree of helical conformation, a core membrane, a capsid shell made of subunits with a hexagonal structure, an outer envelope made of lipid, proteins, and phospholipids with a typical bilayer structure. The envelope is knobbed and the knobs or spikes are formed by glycoproteins. For further details on the biochemistry of RNA viruses see [600, 601].

Viral Replication

The replication pattern of DNA virus is necessarily different from that of RNA virus.

Studies of phages have provided adequate models of the replication of viral DNA and viral protein. Such models were described in the first part of this book.

Some still preliminary information suggests that there are some similarities between the mode of infection of animals and bacteria by DNA viruses. Once the virus has been absorbed at the cell surface and has penetrated inside the cell, the viral DNA is uncoated, and after a period of eclipse it serves as a template for its own replication.

Infection of rabbit kidney cells with pseudorabies virus is followed within a few hours by a block of cellular DNA synthesis. Because puromycin counteracts inhibition of DNA synthesis, viral DNA is believed to dictate the biosynthesis of a protein inhibitor of cellular DNA.

In HeLa cells infected with vaccinia, DNA synthesis starts between 1 and 1.5 hours after injection and reaches a peak approximately 2 hours later. The viral DNA is apparently synthesized in the cell cytoplasm in special cytoplasmic enclaves. Prior to the DNA synthesis, a new enzyme is made: thymidine kinase (the amino acid sequence of which is probably dictated by the virus nucleic acid). The rise of thymidine kinase occurs within half an hour after the infection. The activity of the enzyme per cell increases seven times between 12 and 60 hours after infection. The increased enzymic activity is likely to result from biosynthesis of a newly formed protein. Elaboration of new enzymes is blocked by antimetabolites that interfere with protein synthesis. The new enzyme has catalytic (Michaelis constant and temperature sensitivity) and antigenic properties different from the HeLa cell thymidine kinase. The viral DNA then dictates the biosynthesis of viral messenger RNA. The intracellular site of viral mRNA synthesis is not known. The viral mRNA uses the cell ribosome to dictate the biosynthesis of specific viral proteins.

As we shall see later, in transformed cells, DNA oncogenic viruses, in contrast to what follows traditional virus infection, do not go through the complete vegetative cycle and the viral DNA is incorporated into the genome.

As already pointed out, a crucial step in the multiplication of RNA viruses is RNA replication. The regular pathway for RNA replication is through RNA polymerase using DNA as a template. The fundamental assumption in molecular genetics is that the cell DNA sequence is unique. Thus, since the viral RNA sequence is also unique, cell DNA cannot be used to make virus RNA. Does the RNA virus make DNA prior to RNA replication? Is the viral RNA used as a template? Or does the host DNA in fact contain information for elaborating the viral DNA? We shall see that depending upon the circumstances, either of these mechanisms may obtain. The replication of viral RNA has been investigated with phage RNA.

Many RNA viruses—whether plant, bacterial, or animal viruses—are single stranded. This property raises an additional problem in replication. Is the single strand copied directly, or is it copied in a semiconservative fashion using a complementary chain as a template? The latter of these alternatives appears to prevail [293].

Thus, almost immediately after infection of the bacterial host, the newly introduced viral RNA becomes part of what has been described as a "replicative intermediate" with specific sedimentation properties and ribonuclease resistance. The exact composition of the replicative intermediate is still not known. But it is certain that it contains double-stranded RNA complexed with enzymes and possibly ribosomes. Thus, the formation of a complementary chain and double-stranded RNA appears to be intermediate between the parent virus and the newly formed virus single strands.

Virologists refer to single strands with a sequence identical to the infective virus as the "plus strand," while they call the complementary strand the "minus strand." Obviously, the synthesis of the plus strand is important for infectivity, and therefore the mechanism that favors plus over minus strand synthesis assumes particular significance.

The details of this mechanism are still unknown, but it is clear that in infected bacteria, radioactive precursors are incorporated much more rapidly in the plus than in the minus strand. Furthermore, although plus strands are readily displaced from the replicative complex, minus strands are not.

The enzyme machinery that is involved in the replication of RNA viruses is not completely known. Three different enzymes, all using RNA templates for RNA replication, have been prepared from *E. coli* infected with RNA phages: RNA polymerase, RNA synthetase, and RNA replicase.

RNA polymerase catalyzes the polymerization of complementary chains when exogenous or endogenous RNA is used as a primer. Thus, when phage plus strands are used, minus strands are formed predominantly. RNA synthetase uses single- or double-stranded minus strands as templates and catalyzes the formation of plus strands. The RNA replicase is more specific in its choice of template. It uses the virus RNA preferentially and catalyzes viral RNA replication in two successive steps: (1) minus strand formation; (2) plus strand formation.

In the case of RNA phage it has also been possible to identify in *"in vivo"* and *"in vitro"* systems the proteins that are specifically coded for by the phage nucleic acid. Three specific proteins are formed in some RNA phage-infected cells—the coat, the replicase, and the maturation protein [294]. In spite of the smallness of the genome, gene expression is strictly regulated in time and with respect to the relative amounts of proteins that are made. Thus, the replicase is made first, and when enough of it is available, its production is shut off. Little or no coat protein is made in the early stage of infection, but the amount of newly elaborated coat protein increases as the infection progresses, and ultimately the coat protein is the major new protein elaborated by the virus. Only small amounts of maturation proteins are synthesized at any time, but their production is constant during the cycle.

Each protein plays multiple and highly specific roles in regulating gene expression. The replicase makes viral RNA, but in addition, it prevents the access of viral messenger to ribosome. Only when the replicase levels have dropped is translation optimal. The maturation factor is needed for assembly of viral RNA and protein coat, but it is also believed to regulate translation of the parental virion (as opposed to the newly replicated virion). The coat protein maintains the structure of the nucleic acid, represses the expression of the viral genome, and exerts, by a yet unknown mechanism, a lytic effect on the host.

Much less is known about gene expression even in the simplest of animal viruses. The only thing that is certain is that the pattern varies from one type to another.

Let's first look at what happens when poliovirus infects cells in culture. The poliovirus belongs to the picornavirus class, the smallest among known animal RNA viruses (RNA molecular weight approximately 2.5×10^6; and the capsid proteins with molecular weights of 35, 28, and 24 6×10^3). After viral infection, a viral messenger is formed that has been isolated, but not proven infective. The messenger is translated in a single large "polyprotein," which is sequentially cleaved into smaller polypeptides. The cleavage enzyme has not been identified. Thus, in contrast to what happens in the RNA phage, all genes are expressed with equal frequency, and no other control mechanism for gene expression can exist except at the levels of initiation and termination. All animal viral RNA's are, however, not translated into a single polyprotein.

Other animal RNA viruses express themselves by different patterns of flow of information from viral RNA to viral protein. For example, the Newcastle virus and the mumps virus, which are double-stranded RNA viruses of the class of paramyxoviruses, are among the largest of the animal RNA viruses ($6 \times 7 \times 10^6$ daltons). They contain their own RNA polymerase. Only a portion of the virion RNA is transcribed. Thus, the viral messenger is translated in a number of proteins. The ratio of newly made viral proteins varies greatly. In some cases, post-transcriptional cleavage takes place for some of the polypeptides, but not for others. In other cases, no cleavage at all takes place. The mechanisms modulating transcription, translation, and cleavage are not known.

The influenza virus, a member of the myxovirus group, is composed of five distinct classes of double-stranded RNA's with molecular weights ranging from 10×10^5 to 2×10^5 daltons. The virion contains an RNA polymerase that transcribes the minus strands. The messengers have sizes identical to the segments of the virion RNA. The messengers are translated in a number of proteins, a few of which have been identified: the protein core (which is also responsible for the group-specific antigenicity), an inner membrane surrounding the ribonucleoprotein, and an outer envelope containing hemagglutinin and neuraminidase.

Several lines of investigation have indicated that DNA is necessary for the synthesis of at least some RNA viruses (mainly oncogenic viruses). Antimetabolites that block DNA synthesis (BUDR, IURD, mitomycin) interfere with the replication of RSV or RAV. However, once viral multiplication is underway, DNA synthesis is not necessary to maintain it. The need for DNA synthesis has also been claimed for the replication of influenza virus on the basis of studies with different inhibitors of macromolecular synthesis and hybridization experiments [295].

Temin [296–298] was the first to investigate the relationships between DNA synthesis and viral cancer. He proposed that DNA synthesis is necessary for the formation of RSV in the infected cell. At first, his evidence was indirect and was based on the inhibitory effects of actinomycin D and aminopterin. Actinomycin was found to block virus formation. Since actinomycin blocks DNA-dependent RNA synthesis, it was argued that DNA was indispensable for viral RNA synthesis. Temin later observed that aminopterin, which interferes with DNA synthesis, blocks virus formation. Temin's findings have been confirmed using BUDR, IUDR, mitomycin, and cytosine arabinoside. Although DNA synthesis is indispensable for initiation of viral production, it is not needed for viral proliferation.

The data are compatible with the following interpretation. The introduction of RSV RNA into the cell stimulates the formation of a DNA polymerase that uses RNA as a template. The new DNA is a provirus that is introduced in the host genome and can then dictate the biosynthesis of more viral RNA [299–306].

Temin's hypothesis found confirmation from: (1) the discovery of reverse transcription, (2) the demonstration of cytoplasmic DNA synthesis in viral infected cells, (3) the demonstration of a DNA complementary to viral RNA in the host genome, (4) the isolation from cells infected with RSV of infectious DNA containing the information for production of RSV and neoplastic transformation. In contrast, the Rous associated virus-O, another avian leukosis virus which contains DNA polymerase and the same group specific antigens as the RSV, does not contain the genome for transformation [602].

A somewhat similar situation obtains with the murine leukosis virus [603]. A single-strand DNA synthesized by using murine leukemia virus RNA extracted from AKR mice, a strain with high incidence of leukemia, contains 87% of the sequence present in 70-S viral RNA. In contrast, DNA of the NIH Swiss mouse, a strain which has low leukemic incidence, lacks some of the virus specific sequences found in the AKR mouse DNA. Thus, while the complete viral genome can be detected in the AKR mouse DNA, only fragments of the viral genome are found in the DNA of the NIH Swiss mice.

Only the transcriptase will be considered here.

Temin's group and the Baltimore group independently discovered that Rous sarcoma and mouse leukemia viruses contained an enzyme capable of transcribing RNA sequences into DNA sequences [307, 308]. The DNA that is transcribed in this manner hybridizes but is much smaller than the virion RNA (about one-tenth). The enzyme has been found in association with most tumor RNA viruses. There is, however, evidence that reverse transcription also occurs in at least some noncancerous cells. Therefore, reverse transcription could play a role in cellular differentiation by providing for amplification of the genome. We will return to the significance of reverse transcription when we discuss mechanisms of viral carcinogenesis.

In conclusion, both DNA and RNA viruses may replicate in the host, and one or more copies of the DNA virus and of the DNA transcript of the RNA virus may be incorporated in the host genome. As a result, the viral genome is partially or totally expressed in the host.

In the case of RSV, the genome contains the information for both multiplication and transformation. In the case of the RAV-O, the genome contains only the information for replication.

It may be appropriate to attempt to summarize what is known of the formation of viral RNA messenger RNA to contrast the formation of messenger in tumor viruses to that of other RNA viruses.

With RNA viruses one must distinguish between the genome RNA and the messenger RNA. The mechanism of transcription of the genome into the messenger falls into 4 classes: (1) in picornaviruses and arboviruses the genome is made of single-stranded RNA (25–30% of the virions). It contains poly A covalently attached to the 3′ terminus and includes the sequences necessary for initiation and termination of polypeptide synthesis. It can directly bind to ribosome and is translated as a monocistronic RNA. (2) The genomes of rhabdoviruses and paramyxoviruses are also made of single-stranded RNA (1–3% of the virion) closely associated with a capsid protein. The genome is not infectious and it is unable to act as messenger RNA. The virus contains an RNA polymerase which dictates for poly A and proper sequences for initiation and termination of the polypeptide chain and sites for ribosome binding. The mechanism by which poly A is attached to the RNA transcript of the genome is not known. (3) Influenza and diplornaviruses have an RNA genome which may be either single or double-stranded RNA. A virion-attached RNA polymerase transcribes the single-strand or one strand of the double-strand into a monocistronic messenger RNA. (4) In tumor viruses, the RNA genome is transcribed to DNA which is incorporated in the host genome and is in turn transcribed to RNA [597].

We will now describe the types of injuries that viruses may cause. Whatever the mode and the regulation of gene expression may be with either DNA or RNA oncogenic viruses, a number of biochemical changes are associated with viral oncogenesis. Some relate to the special mode of propagation of the virus, some to the passage of the cell from the normal steady state to that referred to as transformation.

For example, infection by polyoma or SV40 virus induces the following, among other biochemical alterations: (1) synthesis of host cell DNA, (2) synthesis of enzymes involved in nucleic acid biosynthesis, (3) synthesis of viral DNA, (4) transcription of viral DNA, (5) synthesis of surface antigen, and (6) alteration of the glycoprotein composition of the cell surface.

Polyoma and SV 40 viruses induce the synthesis of a number of enzymes, including thymidine kinase, DNA polymerase, dCMP deaminase, dTMP synthetase,

CDP reductase, CDR kinase, dTMP kinase, TDP kinase, and dehydrate folate reductase. The biosynthesis of these enzymes raises a number of questions. First, are the enzymes' are preexisting latent catalytic molecules activated or are new molecules elaborated? Second, what is the role of the viral genome in enzyme elaboration? Is the virus necessary for infection? Does the viral genome code for the elaboration of the proteins in question?

De novo protein synthesis takes place after viral infection, and the appearance of new enzymes requires transcription and is inhibited by actinomycin.

Although the virion is needed to elaborate new enzymes, it seems unlikely that the viral genome codes for all the proteins that appear after infection. Indeed, the genome sequence is too small to contain enough DNA molecules capable of coding for all the enzymes listed above. Therefore, it would appear that the virus activates the host genome either by further derepressing constitutive genes coding for the new proteins or by derepressing a gene normally repressed in the host. The protein elaborated by the derepressed gene could be of various kinds. It could be an enzyme similar to that already existing in the host, an enzyme with molecular properties different from that of the constitutive enzyme of the host, or a protein acting as an allosteric effector on the preexisting host enzyme. Although these questions are not answered in all cases, in some cases the enzyme that appears after viral infection has molecular properties different from those of the constitutive enzyme in the host.

A number of surface antigens appear in the transformed cells. They include two of viral origin—the T antigen and the transplantation antigen (TSTA), and one of host origin—the S antigen. Animals bearing virus-induced tumors develop new antibodies. If such immunofluorescent antibodies are prepared and placed in the presence of transformed cells, the existence of a specific viral antigen can be demonstrated. The viral antigens, referred to as the T antigens, are coded for by the viral genome. Thus, several identical T antigens are found in different host cells transformed by the same virus.

When animals are injected with cells transformed by either polyoma or SV40 virus, they develop antibodies that make them capable of rejecting further transplantation of viral transformed cells. These antibodies are directed toward a transplantation antigen, TSTA.

Immunofluorescent techniques have also demonstrated that a new surface antigen, the S antigen, appears in cells transformed with SV40 and polyoma virus.

Evidence suggests that whereas the T and TSTA antigens are viral coded (the same antigen appears in several types of cells of different species infected by the same virus), the S antigen is believed to be coded for by the host. Further evidence suggesting that T and TSTA antigens are of viral origin is provided by the observation of transformed cells, which revert to normal appearance and behavior after losing some chromosomes. When infected SV40 human cells were hybridized with mouse cells, reversion of the transformation process was concomitant with the loss of the human chromosome. Such observations have been interpreted to mean that the viral genome was associated with those chromosomes and, therefore, that the elaboration of the T and TSTA antigens was coded for by the virus.

Neoplastic transformation is associated with a number of alterations of the plasma membrane, including modification in the binding of substrates, increased refractivity, increased agglutinability by lectins, increased permeability, decreased ganglioside synthesis, increased phosphodiesterase activity, increased Na^+, K^+ ATPase activity, and decreased cyclic synthetase activity. In addition, cyclic AMP levels are decreased and there are transient changes in the concentrations of cyclic GMP inside the cell. Such observations raise three questions: (1) are the changes in the cell membrane that have been observed during transformation related to transformation or are they coincidental, (2) what molecular mechanisms are evoked to cause the changes, and (3) are all the changes caused by a single primary event after transformation?

To date, no answers to these questions are available. But for the purpose of focusing the discussion, let's concentrate on the changes in cyclic AMP and cyclic GMP that take place in transformation. Although the levels of cyclic AMP undoubtedly decrease during cell division and after transformation and transient changes in cyclic GMP develop during transformation, it is not clear how these changes come about. At least three mechanisms can be invoked in eliciting a decrease in either of the cyclic nucleotides: decreased permeability to precursors, increased catabolism, and decreased synthesis of the cyclic nucleotides. Each of these mechanisms can be caused by a variety of molecular changes. For example, an increase in catabolism or anabolism could result from *de novo* synthesis, or from allosteric activation or inhibition of the respective enzymes. The association of neoplastic transformation with decreased cyclic AMP synthetase and increased phosphodiesterase activities suggests that the changes in cyclic AMP are regulated by the balance between the anabolic and the catabolic enzymes.

In addition to the decrease in cyclic AMP that is observed after cell division or during transformation, changes in the cell permeability take place as well. Thus, the permeability of small molecules such as 2-deoxyglucose and α-aminobutyric acid increases after transformation. It is therefore pertinent to ask whether these changes cause the drop in cyclic AMP or whether they are the consequences of a reduction in cyclic AMP.

Transformation

Carcinogenicity is the property that distinguishes tumor viruses from other viruses; however, it is a property that tumor viruses share with a number of other carcinogenic agents. The cellular alteration most closely related to the carcinogenic properties of the virus is undoubtedly that of transformation.

Dulbecco has defined transformation as the process by which animal cells acquire inheritable properties different from those they had before infection [309–315].

A number of viruses cause transformations in cell cultures that are reminiscent of malignant alterations. They include Rous sarcoma virus, SV40, SE polyoma virus, and the virus of avian myeloblastosis. The phenomenon has been most extensively investigated with RSV and the polyoma virus.

Dulbecco has studied the transformation of cultured cells by the small papova viruses (SV40 and polyoma). Some cell lines are more readily transformable by a given virus than others. A line obtained from hamster, referred to as the BKH, is particularly suitable for transformation by polyoma virus, whereas another obtained from mouse, called the 3T3 line, is readily transformed by SV40. When either of these two cell lines is cultured in the presence of virus, colonies of transformed cells can easily be distinguished from normal colonies on morphological grounds. Thus, although the cells of normal colonies are regularly oriented with respect to each other, the cells of transformed colonies climb over each other forming irregular and somewhat chaotic cell clusters. The transformation is inheritable because when a transformed cell is changed to another medium, it yields a new transformed cluster. Since both normal and transformed cells were derived from the same class of cells (unexposed to virus), it seems logical to assume that the viral genome carries the information that leads to transformation. Derangement of the host's cell genome as a result of viral infection cannot be excluded.

Three groups of molecular changes are characteristic of transformation with DNA viruses: (1) the introduction of at least part of the viral genome into the host chromosomes; (2) the partial transcription of the viral genome; and (3) the phenotypic changes in the host.

The following observations suggest that the viral nucleic acids play a critical role in transformation: (1) nucleic acid deprived of its protein coat can still transform; (2) some mutations of the virus nucleic acid lead to loss of the transforming properties; and (3) the viral DNA persists in the transformed cell.

The third finding deserves further discussion. Does the viral DNA persist in extrachromosomal areas, or is it incorporated within the chromosome into infectious particles that can be isolated from transformed cells even after cell fusion? RNA-DNA and DNA-DNA hybridization studies have provided evidence that viral DNA is incorporated within the host DNA, but it is not known whether the inclusion is site specific or varies from one transformed cell to another. However, there is some evidence that multiple copies of the viral genome are present in most transformed cells. Moreover, studies of somatic hybrids suggest that these copies are found in several different chromosomes.

The discovery of methods that permit constitutive heterochromatin to be distinguished from euchromatin have raised the question as to whether transformation may be associated with alterations of the distribution of heterochromatin. Of course, heterochromatin forms zones of the chromosome in which the DNA is tightly condensed and not transcribed during interphase. The amount and distribution of the heterochromatin along the chromosome are believed to determine the cell's phenotype. Thus, if transformation is associated with distortion of gene expression, it is possible but not indispensable that the process will be associated with visible alterations of the constitutive heterochromatin. Studies from DiPaolo's laboratory with hamster cells transformed with chemical carcinogens suggest that although such alterations occur, in some cases they are not a *sine qua non* "condition" for transformation [316].

DNA viruses, like polyoma and SV40 viruses, code for a number of different proteins. In fact, the genome is believed to contain eight different genes. If complete transcription of the genome may be necessary for cell lysis,* is it for transformation? The use of temperature-sensitive mutants of polyoma virus has established that two viral gene functions are required for transformation. The names of the mutant—ts_a and ts_3—are used to refer to each function. The ts_a is needed to initiate transformation, and ts_3 is needed to maintain transformation and establish certain phenotypic properties of the transformed cell, such as changes in the cell surface properties. It is not known how ts_a or ts_3 determines the initiation and maintenance of transformation.

Studies with viral mutants demonstrate that incorporation of the viral genome into the viral DNA is indispensable for cell transformation, but they do not prove that transcription of the viral genome is needed. Hybridization experiments between purified viral DNA and labeled RNA obtained from transformed cells have established that the SV40 viral DNA is transcribed. The viral RNA is found in both the nucleus and on ribosomes. The nuclear component containing the viral RNA sediments at 45S. This was surprising because from the size of the SV40 virion (3×10^6 daltons) a messenger sedimenting at approximately 28S is expected. The fate of the SV40 45-S RNA has not been determined. It has also been established that cells transformed by adenovirus do not synthesize virions or virion structural proteins even though a large segment of the virus nucleic acid is transcribed. The fact that RNA's complementary to the viral nucleic acid are found attached to ribosomes suggests that the viral messenger is also translated during transformation.

---

* When a culture of mouse embryonic cells is exposed to a high titer of polyoma virus, a large number of the cells die. If the culture is maintained, it reaches a steady state; some cells die, others divide. Thus, an apparently homogeneous cellular population clearly reveals differences in the cellular susceptibility to the virus. The cause of this variation in susceptibility is not known.

However, the exact product of translation remains unknown.

The viral genome is believed to dictate the biosynthesis of only a few proteins. Among them are: (1) factors and enzymes that facilitate or are indispensable for DNA synthesis, (2) specific antigens, and (3) the coat protein of virus. It is not clear which of these expressions of the message contained in the genome is linked to transformation.

Because transformation does not usually take place until after several cell divisions, cell division was at first believed to be indispensable for transformation. However, transformation with RSV went on apparently unaffected when cell division in the host was blocked with vinblastine [317].

In conclusion, the viral DNA genome is incorporated at unknown sites of the chromosome. Incomplete transcription takes place, and translation is likely to yield products that initiate and maintain transformation.

The relationship between oncogenic RNA viruses and transformation is even more confusing. Is transcription of RNA into DNA critical for transformation, and if so, is the DNA complementary to the viral RNA transcribed? Furthermore, if the transcript is translated, what is the final product and how does the product affect transformation? We have mentioned that some RNA viruses contain an enzyme that synthesizes DNA duplexes using double-stranded RNA as a template. A search for the enzyme in a number of viruses indicates that it is always found in wild RNA oncogenic viruses and is absent in most typically infective viruses tested, except for a few in which its presence is uncertain [236].

In the test tube, the entire viral RNA can be transcribed into complementary DNA. Careful experiments of Baluda and Nayak [318] have established that viral RNA hybridizes increasingly with DNA of transformed cells. The inescapable conclusion in the face of such evidence is that information flows from viral RNA to complementary viral DNA to viral mRNA.

Reverse transcriptase has been isolated from Rous sarcoma virus. Like DNA polymerase it is a zinc containing enzyme [604]. The enzyme is composed of small (α; 60,000 daltons) and large (β; 100,000 daltons) subunits. The α subunits seem to possess all the catalytic properties of the enzymes. The purified enzyme is capable of exerting multiple catalytic activities: RNA directed DNA synthesis, DNA-DNA directed synthesis and selective degradation of the RNA bound to DNA-RNA hybrids (ribonuclease H activity). For further information on reverse transcriptase see [605, 607].

The nature of the messenger and its products remains unknown. But a number of observations, although not incompatible with the concept, raise serious questions as to the validity of this path of gene expression.

A mutant of RSV devoid of reverse transcriptase was found to transform cells as effectively as the wild virus. Therefore, one can ask whether all viral messenger is synthesized from viral RNA or from its complementary DNA. A number of explanations for the absence of RNA transcriptase enzymes, such as a peculiar liability of the protein that inactivates it when the viral extract is prepared for testing, can be invoked. Moreover, it cannot be excluded that the host cell's reverse transcriptase is used to transcribe viral RNA to DNA.

The ability to copy RNA into DNA is not restricted to reverse transcriptase. *E. coli* DNA polymerase I faithfully copies a variety of RNA templates.

Uninfected chickens have been shown to contain DNA that is complementary to RNA for several avian tumor viruses, but the amount of complementary DNA increases 3–10 times after infection [668].

The reverse transcriptase has indeed been found in a number of normal cells. Moreover, wild fowl that could not possibly have been contaminated by the laboratory virus have been shown to contain DNA sequences complementary to the viral RNA. The significance of that observation will become clear when we discuss the hypotheses on viral carcinogenesis.

Cancer and Viruses in Humans

Except for warts, there is no evidence that human tumors, benign or malignant, are caused by viruses. Yet although conclusive evidence is still lacking, there is a growing suspicion that viruses may play a role in the etiology of human cancer. This assumption is based on: (1) the observation that cancer virus occurs in many animal species, including primates, (2) the possibility of producing cancer in animals or transforming cells in culture with nucleic acids or viruses obtained from human tumors, and (3) the epidemiology of some human cancers and the identification of viruses in many human cancers.

Viruses cause cancer in amphibians [319], chickens, and mammals [320–323]. In view of the widespread occurrence of viral carcinogenesis in animals, it seems unlikely that human cancers are never produced by viruses. The identification of oncogenic viruses affecting humans is expectedly difficult. First, one must keep in mind that, in contrast to experimental animals, human populations are highly heterogeneous. As mentioned above, lymphomatosis in chickens became infectious only when purebred strains became available. There is thus *a priori* no essential difference between the epidemiology of chicken lymphomatosis and human leukemia. Human leukemia progresses in a heterozygous population, and it cannot be excluded that if homozygous human genetic material were available, leukemia would become infectious in humans as in chickens or rats [324]. Second, in humans, oncogenic or even nononcogenic viruses may work in combination with other carcinogens to produce cancer. The potential "cooperative" role that ordinary infectious viruses may play in human carcinogenesis by combining their effect with that of chemical carcinogens or X-irradiation has not yet been evaluated.

Several investigators have reported experiments in which ultrafiltrates prepared from such human tumors as those seen in Hodgkin's disease produced various carcinomas and sarcomas when inoculated into mice [325]. It remains to be established whether these human ultrafiltrates activate preexisting viruses or whether they truly induce these tumors. In one experiment, the nucleic acid preparation of human tumors or human lymphoma produced tumors in mice inoculated intraperitoneally. However, these results were inconsistent and have not been reproduced in other laboratories.

Viruses of human origin, such as the adenovirus, can produce transformation *in vitro*. Conversely, human cells have been infected and transformed by rodent oncogenic viruses modified in the laboratory [326]. Rous sarcomas have been transplanted from chick and rat to monkey [327, 328]. The significance of these findings is difficult to interpret. Although some claim to have produced by this means lymphoid tumors in the monkey that ultimately kill the animal, in our laboratory the transplantation of cell-free extracts of RSV obtained from chick or mouse to newborn monkey yielded gross tumoral masses that histologically were reminiscent of a proliferative inflammatory reaction rather than of a genuine lymphosarcoma. Moreover, all tumors regressed within 6 months after inoculation.

Perhaps the most compelling argument in favor of a viral etiology in some human cancers derives from epidemiological and electron microscopic observations. In fact, long before viruses had been discovered, the Academie des Sciences of Lyon awarded its prize to Bernard Peyrilhe, a French surgeon who proposed, on the basis of some epidemiological observations, that cancer is infectious. The familial incidence and the geographical distribution of leukemia, Hodgkin's disease, and Burkitt's sarcoma are often invoked as evidence of an infectious etiology. (A synopsis of the pathological findings in these diseases is presented at the end of this chapter.) Three observations support the hypothesis of the viral etiology of leukemia: the detection of clusters of cases, the coexistence of leukemia in children and their pets, and the high incidence of leukemia among children who have experienced repeated viral infections.

Clusters of cases have been reported in Texas and Illinois, and reports of coincidental hematological changes in children and their pets have led some to believe that domestic animals could serve as vectors for the virus. Viral particles have been found in sarcomas in cats, in leukemia in dogs, and in the milk of cows carrying lymphomas [329, 330]. Of course, if a viral etiology were established for leukemia, the relation of the virus to other pathogenic factors, such as X-irradiation, chromosome alteration, hormones, and chemicals, would need to be clarified.

The demonstration of reverse transcriptase activity in human leukemic cells has been offered as an argument for the viral origin of such cancers. However, the enzyme is found in normal lymphocytes as well.

More recently, Spiegelman and his associates [331] provided more compelling evidence of a molecular nature for the viral origin of human leukemias by: (1) demonstrating the presence of a viral RNA homologous to that of Rauscher leukemia in leukemic cells; (2) establishing that the transcriptase is associated with a particle with the density of the Rauscher leukemic virus; and (3) showing that the DNA of leukemic cells contains sequences that are homologous to DNA synthesized with the reserve transcriptase using Rauscher sarcoma RNA as a template.

Similar findings were made in human breast carcinoma in which evidence for a "temperate" cycle for the mouse mammary tumor virus was demonstrated. Spiegelman's studies prove that some of the molecular events described in the life cycle of the virus in rodents exist in humans, but they do not irrefutably establish that these events are in man associated with carcinogenesis, although one gains the feeling that the weight of the evidence favors a viral etiology of human leukemia and breast cancer.

Of particular interest is the epidemiology of Burkitt's lymphoma. Burkitt described a form of lymphoma that occurs in children and has a peculiar propensity to invade certain organs. Thus, in tropical Africa Burkitt's lymphoma is the most common tumor in children and is found in the kidney, adrenal and salivary glands, liver, testicles, and other sites. A special feature is the frequent involvement of the jaw.

Although Burkitt tumors have been described even outside Africa, the incidence of Burkitt's lymphoma seems to be high only in limited areas. The disease has not been described in the northern part of Africa, and only few cases have been reported in South Africa. Clusters of high frequency have been found in countries surrounding Lake Victoria, and geographical pathologists have concluded that a high-altitude barrier delineates the zone in which the disease is endemic.

Closer examination of the climate in which Burkitt's tumor prospers has suggested an influence of rainfall (mean minimum of 20 inches) and of temperatures (mean minimum of 60° F). Altitudes below 5000 feet, high rainfalls, and high temperatures are favorable breeding grounds for a variety of arthropods. These conditions are believed to favor the infection of some insects by a virus which, when transmitted to man, causes the disease. Thus, the distribution of Burkitt's tumor in Africa resembles that of sleeping sickness, and the similitudes between the epidemiologies of Burkitt's tumor and sleeping sickness lead to the conclusion that a mosquito must transmit the disease.

Investigators in several laboratories have found a herpes-like agent in Burkitt cells cultured *in vitro*. But the role of the herpes-like virus in the pathogenesis of the disease is far from clear. It is not known whether it is a passenger or the causative agent.

Apparently, two different types of herpesviruses exist. One causes lip lesions, and the other cervical lesions; the former has antigenic properties different from the latter. Thus, herpesvirus type I infects only above the waist, and herpesvirus type II causes infections below the waist. Type I is most likely transmitted by kissing, whereas type II is transmitted through sexual intercourse. Therefore, herpesvirus has been called the virus of love.

The herpesvirus is icosahedral, measuring 100–150 mμ in diameter. It is a DNA virus containing double-stranded DNA. Its capsid is composed of 162 cylindrical capsomeres, each made of 5 or 6 rodlike structural units.

Herpesvirus is a nuclear virus. In fact, contact of the virus with the cytoplasm destroys its activity. It is not known how the virus escapes passing through the cytoplasm during its release from the cells. Whether it is encapsulated in a vacuole for transport from nucleus to cell membrane or whether it travels through preconstructed tunnels has not been decided.

The virus genome dictates the biosynthesis of its own protein. However, it uses the cytoplasmic machinery of the host to elaborate the proteins. The viral protein is made within the cytoplasm and transported, again by some unknown mechanism, to the nucleus where it complexes with viral DNA.

The two major forms of infection by herpesvirus are the productive form and the so-called nonproductive form. In productive infections, fully infectious particles are made that ultimately kill the cells. In the nonproductive infections, no complete viral infectious particles are assembled, but the viral genome is undoubtedly present in some form within the nucleus because the cells that do not contain herpetic viral particles can, under appropriate conditions, produce infective virus.

Like most viruses, the herpesvirus alters the properties of the cell membrane through: (1) changing permeability, (2) promoting cell fusion, and (3) preventing contact inhibition. Little is known of the molecular changes that are responsible for these alterations of the cell membrane.

The primary infection to herpes occurs in childhood. Usually the victim is unaware of the infection because it does not differ from ordinary childhood infections.

Herpes simplex is a benign disease that leads to an epithelial inflammatory process on the lips or the cornea. Occasionally, it may affect the central nervous system, causing severe encephalitis. The skin lesions are called cold sores. Herpetic infections of the cornea result in keratitis, which was a serious condition before optical therapy with IUDR and BUDR.

When Epstein and his collaborators [332] succeeded in culturing Burkitt cells from a Burkitt's lymphoma biopsy, they observed a virus referred to as the Epstein-Barr virus. The virus found in Burkitt's tumors has been partially purified, and detailed electron microscopic studies revealed it to be a member of the herpes group. The capsid is made of 162 capsomeres, has a diameter of 900 A, and is coated with a distinctive layer of an amorphous substance (300 A thick).

Werner and Gertrude Henle [333] prepared an immunofluorescent antibody to the virus and demonstrated its presence in healthy people as well as in patients with Burkitt's tumors. The incidence of positive serum sample ranged from 80–90% in all persons tested. Since only a small number of individuals develop lymphoma, it must be concluded that if the EB (Epstein-Barr) virus is responsible for Burkitt's tumors, its transforming activity must in some way be aided by other factors.

The correlation between the presence of antibodies of the type II herpesvirus and cervical cancer is impressive. Among 35 women with cervical cancer, 81% had evidence of exposure to type II herpesvirus. In contrast, among 58 women without cancer, only 25% possessed antibodies to the virus. Such results have been reported by two laboratories, that of Nahmias and that of Melnick. Even more impressive are findings indicating that the antigens were present in the preinvasive and invasive stages in patients with cervical cancer. The antigen was restricted to the cancer and was not found in surrounding normal tissues of cancer patients nor in normal individuals. Thus, the appearance of the antigen is an early event preceding the transformation of a normal cell into a neoplastic one.

The association of herpesvirus with infectious mononucleosis is based on the fact that some patients who were devoid of herpes antigen before infection by infectious mononucleosis developed antigenicity after the infectious process. The relationship between infectious mononucleosis and leukemia is purely speculative and is based on the fact that occasionally an episode of infectious mononucleosis is followed, within a relatively short time after the infectious process, by the development of lymphomas in the victim. Similarly, the cytomegalic virus, a herpes relative, has been incriminated in Marek's disease, a lymphoproliferative disease observed in poultry. In fact, a vaccine against that virus has recently been obtained.

Relatives of the herpesvirus can cause lymphatic leukemia and reticulum cell sarcoma in monkeys. Finally, a herpesvirus is also believed to be responsible for Lucke's disease (kidney carcinoma) in frogs. The implications of these findings are enormous because they incriminate a virus that frequently infects humans as a major cause of cancer. Moreover, the herpesvirus is much more complex than the small DNA and RNA viruses. Therefore, our understanding of the mechanism by which herpesviruses cause cancer may prove a challenge because after all, even if one can establish a firm correlation between incidence of infection and the incidence of cancer, it will still be necessary to explain why only a relatively small number of infected humans develop that type of viral cancer.

The presence of C type virus-like particles has been demonstrated in hamster melanomas and in lymph node metastasis of human melanomas [608]. The fate of the virus in the pathogenesis of that cancer remains unknown.

The electron microscopic identification of viral particles in human laryngeal papillomas [341] and in liposarcomas [342] further supports the viral etiology of human cancer.

The incrimination of herpesvirus in human cancer has stimulated extensive research on the properties of the virus, its antigenicity, and its ability to transform cells *in vitro*. It is impossible to review recent findings here, and the reader is referred to some of the original papers [334–337]. For further information on the role of viruses in human cancer read [609, 610].

Hypothesis on the Mechanism of Viral Carcinogenesis

We have seen that most of the mammalian cancer viruses are RNA viruses (type C) and that available evidence suggests a flow of information from viral RNA→complementary viral DNA→messenger RNA. On the basis of these premises, two major theories of viral carcinogenesis have been proposed: the oncogenic gene theory of Todaro and Huebner, and the protovirus theory of Temin [338–340].

The oncogenic theory assumes that the original infection with the carcinogenic virus has occurred at some time during evolution, possibly at different times for each species. At that time, the viral RNA was transcribed in a complementary DNA that became part of the genome of every cell and was transferred vertically generation after generation. These "oncogenic genes" remain normally depressed, but environmental factors, such as radiation (UV and ionizing radiation) and chemical carcinogens, can under some circumstances that have not been clearly defined derepress the repressed "oncogene." The derepressed DNA is then transcribed, and the transcript is translated into a "transforming protein." The fact that C particles have been shown to appear spontaneously in normal mouse cell clones is in keeping with the theory. Moreover, hybridization experiments performed by Baluda and Nayak [318] showed that chickens that do not produce viruses nevertheless contain the viral genome. In fact, cultures from such cells can be induced to produce C particles with radiation or carcinogens.

The major advantage of the oncogenic theory is that it provides for a unifying pathogenic mechanism for all cancers. Whatever their clinical, morphological, and biochemical manifestations, all cancers are, according to this theory, manifestations of a single disease process. If true, such a concept would simplify our understanding of the pathogenesis of cancer, but it links carcinogenesis so closely with normal life processes that, at least for the present, it does not allow much hope for cure and prevention.

In conclusion, the oncogenic gene hypothesis proposes that, by a freak of evolution, mammalian and viral genomes have been forced to live in symbiosis. The mammalian cell has learned to control this intracellular "time bomb" by repressing it vigorously, but changes in the environment may trigger it.

Temin's protovirus theory postulates that the cell infected with the viral RNA transcribes the latter into complementary DNA. The theory does not require derepression of preexisting genes; it allows for different mechanisms for viral and chemical and radiation carcinogenesis and implies horizontal transmission of the virus.

Moreover, Temin believes that the gene responsible for the conversion of a normal cell into a cancer cell found in the RNA oncogenic virus arises from misevaluation of normal DNA. Thus, in Temin's scheme, normal DNA is altered to produce a viral genome which is transcribed into an RNA containing the viral RNA [602].

In conclusion, in animals viruses can cause cancer either spontaneously or experimentally. The same viruses transform cells *in vitro*. The oncogenic viruses exhibit no special properties except that they do not go through the complete vegetative cycle, and the genome of the virion is incorporated in the genome of the host directly with DNA viruses after transcription of RNA into DNA with RNA viruses. It is not known which portion of the viral genome needs to be expressed to cause cancer, but it is almost certain that that portion which is responsible for stimulating cellular proliferation is not indispensable for transformation. In humans, molecular, immunological, morphological, and epidemiological data have been assembled in support of a viral origin of at least some human cancers, in particular leukemia and breast cancer. Although most intriguing, the evidence is not conclusive.

Metabolic Pathways in the Cancer Cell

Introduction

Ever since the barrier between organic chemistry and biology was lifted, first with the synthesis of urea by Friedrich Wohler (1828) and later by solubilization from fresh yeast cells of the intracellular catalyst capable of digesting starch by Edward Buchner (1898), there has been a growing feeling among scientists that cancer would be understood through studying its chemistry.

The anarchic growth of cancer cells appears to constitute such an insult to orderly cellular proliferation and differentiation that drastic alterations from normal biochemical patterns were anticipated. Yet, even though cancer biochemistry has been studied worldwide by numerous investigators, a precise description of the primary molecular injury or injuries is not available.

In discussing cancer biochemistry, our purpose is not to be comprehensive. Even a careful distillation of the voluminous literature on cancer biochemistry could fill several volumes. Instead, our intention is to present illustrative examples of the two major lines of investigation in cancer biochemistry—the metabolism of the cancer cell and the effect of cancer on host metabolism.

When a normal cell has matured, it presents a typical morphology and performs a specific function. The code to this specificity is written into its molecular composition and interaction. The specificity of the smaller molecules and of some of the simpler macromolecules is dictated by the specificity of the enzymes that catalyze their biosynthesis. The specificity of the more complex macromolecules such as DNA, RNA, antibodies, and possibly membranes* is enshrined in a relatively stable structure, the DNA molecule, and is transferred through a relatively safe and somewhat complex machinery that involves template copying. When a cell divides, the specificity of its DNA, RNA, proteins, and membranes is transferred integrally to the daughter cells. As a result, the daughter cell has the same appearance and functions in the same way as the mother cell.

The cancer cell presents at least three abnormal behavior patterns, involving proliferation, differentiation, and its social relationship with neighboring cells. These changes in the biological patterns of cancer cells should have their counterparts in molecular composition. Since the intracellular presence of most of the smaller molecules is determined by the structure and concentration of the macromolecules, it would seem logical to assume that the primary distortion involves macromolecules—enzymes, membranes, or templates.

Detectable biochemical distortions can be quantitative or qualitative. Quantitative distortions may exist at two different levels. In the first, all molecules present in the normal cells are also found in the cancer cell, but at different concentrations. In the second, molecular components present in normal cells are deleted in the cancer cells. Changes in the concentration of a single molecule could have drastic consequences for the cell's economy. For example, the concentration of a rate-limiting enzyme could be altered as a result of the conversion of a normal cell into a cancer cell. The changes in the intracellular activity of the enzyme will, in turn, alter the concentration of the product of the reaction. If the availability of the product in some way regulates the rate of other biochemical pathways (by feedback inhibition, by acting as an activator of other enzymes, or by acting on the genome as an inducer or a repressor), an expansion of the original distortion in several other biochemical pathways can be expected. Or further, the biochemical alteration of the cancer cell could in an extreme situation lead to a complete deletion of a critical macromolecule, resulting in something akin to a localized and acquired error of metabolism.

Qualitative changes involving a substantial and detectable number of phenotypic molecules have never been described in cancer. No substance has been found exclusively in cancer cells. However, it is too early to exclude the possibility that qualitative changes exist in the cancer cell, even though they are difficult to detect for the reasons that follow.

* Cellular specificity is, however, not restricted to enzymes but is also manifested in the antigen-antibody reactions and in the membrane structures. Membranes have highly selective permeability properties, and the plasma membrane responds to neighboring cells in a unique fashion.

The mechanism determining specificity involves both replication of the template and amplification of the message. Thus, one molecule of DNA is transcribed to yield several molecules of messenger RNA whose code is translated to yield even more protein molecules, which may turn millions of molecules of substrate into product. Because the message is amplified, a single base alteration in DNA could lead to drastic quantitative changes and be itself undetectable with present methods of analysis. Any attempt to organize information on cancer metabolism is bound to reflect the author's prejudice. We hope to minimize the influence of preconceived views by first presenting an analytical, although sketchy, review of the pertinent observations on cancer metabolism and then evaluating the significance of the findings.

Glycolysis in Cancer

Glycolysis was the first biochemical pathway to be investigated successfully in tumors. Warburg may well be called the pioneer of cancer biochemistry. After developing manometric methods for the analysis of glycolysis under aerobic and anaerobic conditions in tissue slices, Warburg [343, 344] undertook to investigate the conversion of glucose to lactic acid in a number of normal tissues and tumors. He found that all cancer tissue had a definitely high sustained aerobic and anaerobic glycolysis. Thus, the Pasteur effect, the depression of glycolysis by oxygen, is relatively inefficient in tumors.* By implanting electrodes inside tumors, Voegtlin and his collaborators [345] also established that the administration of glucose to tumor-bearing animals was followed by a drop in pH of at least 0.5 units within the tumor.

Warburg himself and later Cori [346] and others extended the original finding made on tumor slices to *in vivo* situations. In such investigations, the arterial and the venous blood that went to or returned from a limb or a bird wing, which included a tumor transplanted or produced by other methods, was collected. The venous blood coming from tumors contained less glucose and more lactic acid than venous blood derived from normal tissue. The *in vivo* and *in vitro* observations led Warburg to propose: (1) that all cancer presented high rates of glycolysis; (2) that the high aerobic glycolysis resulted from a respiratory defect; and (3) that the transformation of a normal cell into a cancer cell resulted from the "morphological inferiority" of glycolytic energy over that of respiratory

* Nevertheless, the rate of glycolysis in tumors is so high that the absolute Pasteur effect may be more considerable than appears by expressing the ratio of lactic acid production in the presence and absence of oxygen. By shifting a tumor slice from anaerobic to aerobic environments, one can reduce the production of lactic acid considerably in the tumor slice and sometimes the absolute reduction is greater than the reduction observed in the corresponding normal tissue. However, if this Pasteur effect is expressed as a percent of the total production of lactic acid under anaerobic conditions, it is always lower in tumors than in normal tissue.

energy. We shall later examine the validity of the Warburg theory of carcinogenesis, but we shall first pursue this description of the studies on the performance of the bioenergetic pathways in the cancer cell.

Warburg's discovery of a single alteration in a critical bioenergetic pathway in cancer was bound to generate the hope that the cause and the cure of cancer were within reach. I remember hearing older oncologists speak with emotion of the thrills that seized the scientific world when the news of Warburg's discovery was announced. Unfortunately, this beam of light was soon clouded by confusing reports which sometimes became acrimonious polemics. Warburg was the first to show that some normal tissues have a high rate of anaerobic and aerobic glycolysis and low Pasteur effect. Such tissues include the retina, the renal medulla, the intestinal mucosa, the myeloid cells of bone marrow, the synovial membranes, and the tonsils. However, Warburg persisted in believing that a significant difference existed between the metabolism of glucose in normal and cancer tissue.

Warburg calculated the fermentation excess for a large number of normal and cancerous tissues,* and claimed that the values obtained for the fermentation excess were always negative in normal tissue and positive in tumors. Indeed, all normal tissues except the retina yield negative values for the fermentation excess. Although the values are positive for mouse tumors, several mouse tumors, such as spontaneous mouse tumors, sarcoma 37, or mouse myelomas, yielded negative values for fermentation excess, probably because these tumors have a high rate of respiration.

As new data were accumulated with the years, it became more and more obvious that high aerobic glycolysis and low Pasteur effect were not unique to tumors; therefore, these metabolic events could hardly be considered responsible for the cancer cell's abnormal behavior. Still, until the late 1960s, it seemed safe to state that although normal tissues and tumors overlapped considerably with respect to the pattern of glycolysis, all tumors examined had high anaerobic and aerobic rates of glycolysis.

Studies done by Weinhouse [347] may well have provided conclusive evidence that there is no causal relation between high glycolysis and carcinogenesis and the conversion from normal to cancerous behavior. In these experiments. Weinhouse used transplanted hepatomas with variable growth rates. As we shall see later, hepatomas can be produced that can be readily transplanted; some will grow faster than others. Those that have a relatively slow growth rate resemble the normal histological structure of the liver and are, therefore, referred to as "minimal deviation hepatomas." Those that grow fastest are more dedifferentiated.

The Novikoff hepatoma and the Morris 5123 hepatoma occupy extreme and opposite positions in this gamut of transplanted hepatomas. A Novikoff hepatoma is a rapidly growing tumor, and the 5123 is a slowly growing tumor. The rate of aerobic glycolysis is high in the Novikoff hepatoma; it is low in the Morris 5123, which resembles normal liver with respect to glycolysis.

The findings made in Aisenberg's and Weinhouse's laboratories clearly suggest that the shift from aerobic to a more "primitive" anaerobic pathway is not essential for the conversion from a normal to a cancerous behavior pattern.

The loss of enzyme regulation is not unique to tumors; it occurs in some inborn errors of metabolism and in benign tumors. Very few studies compare benign to malignant tumors. A study of the regulation of glycolysis in lipomas revealed that these benign tumors have lost their ability to regulate glycolysis by feedback inhibition of phosphofructokinase by citrate. Phosphofructokinase extracted from the tumor was less sensitive to inhibition by citrate than the enzyme extracted from normal tissues [611]. These results are believed to indicate that the loss of negative feedback control of regulatory enzymes is an early manifestation of neoplasia. The truth is that a lipoma seldom degenerates into a malignant tumor and therefore, the metabolic distortion described is peculiar to lipomas.

Whatever the relationship between anaerobic glycolysis and cancer, the molecular mechanism responsible for the metabolic distortion is of considerable interest and deserves further study. Such molecular studies could be significant because: (1) if a cancer cell at some time in its development becomes dependent on an anaerobic source of energy, it might be possible to devise methods for selectively depriving the cancer cell of that source of energy (and thereby killing it); and (2) changes in glycolysis may be an amplification of a more subtile primary injury, and more appropriate understanding of the molecular mechanism of the alteration would shed light on that primary injury.

Other Bioenergetic Pathways in Cancer

Glucose is a highly soluble organic compound, readily oxidizable and rich in chemical energy. It is therefore not entirely surprising that at some stage of evolution, it became a major source of food for a living organism.

As the multiplicity and the complexity of life evolved, the pathways for glucose became more and more numerous, and it may well be that the existing complexity of living forms could not have been achieved without alternative pathways for glucose oxidation. Whatever the significance of glucose metabolism may be in evolution, in living mammalian tissues glycolysis clearly does not constitute the sole metabolic pathway for glucose utilization.

Glucose may be reduced to sorbitol or dehydrogenated to gluconate; glucose reductase and NADPH

---

* In the Pasteur effect, one molecule of oxygen inhibits the formation of three molecules of lactic acids. The absolute Pasteur effect is measured by determing lactic acid in the presence and absence of oxygen. The fermentation excess is expressed by the difference between the number of molecules of lactic acid formed in the absence of oxygen and the number of moles of oxygen consumed.

are needed for the former reaction, and glucose dehydrogenase and atomic oxygen act in the latter. As we have seen previously, glucose-6-phosphate can enter the pentose pathway under the influence of glucose-6-phosphate dehydrogenase or the glucuronic pathway after conversion to the 6-phosphate gluconate. Of course, pyruvic acid derived from the oxidation of glucose may either be reduced to lactic acid or may enter the Kreb's cycle after decarboxylation. The Kreb's cycle pathway itself is closely linked to the generation of at least some amino acids and to fatty acid oxidation and synthesis. Thus, in mammalian tissues, glucose metabolism ramifies into a number of pathways that will generate coenzymes (NADPH), substrates (ribose and deoxyribose-5-phosphate), glucuronic acids, and amino acids that are indispensable building blocks for the biosynthesis of vital macromolecules.

Hatanaka [612] has investigated the transport of glucose, mannose, galactose, and glucosamine in chicken cells transformed with RSV and found that the transport of the sugars investigated was increased and that the increase coincided with the appearance of morphological changes. The permeability of the transformed cells to uridine, thymidine, leucine and phosphate was unchanged. Studies in which the uptake of nonmetabolizable sugar was investigated (2-deoxyglucose and 3,0-methylglucose) revealed that the increase in uptake resulted from changes in the carrier system, rather than changes in hexokinase activity. In fact, the hexokinase activity was approximately the same in normal and transformed cells. The relationship of the increase in sugar uptake to cell growth, cell transformation, or cellular metabolism (high aerobic glycolysis) is not known.

To determine whether cancer tissues were in fact deficient in certain oxidative enzymes, investigators measured oxygen uptake in tumor homogenates in the presence or absence of added substrates or enzymes. The experiments reported here were all done on normal or frankly malignant tissues. Experiments done on minimal deviation hepatomas, which turned out to be significant for interpreting the results, will be presented separately.

In view of the multiplicity of alternative pathways for glucose metabolism, it is not surprising that much research was devoted to studying the performance of bioenergetic pathways in tumors. This research started with a thorough investigation of the substrates and the enzymes of the glycolytic pathway. The studies on the Embden-Meyerhoff pathway were followed by similar studies on the Krebs cycle and the hexose monophosphate shunt. Furthermore, because of the interaction between glycolysis and respiration, much time was devoted to studying the pattern of respiration in cancer tissues.

Because adding hexose diphosphates to some tumor slices or extracts did not effectively stimulate lactic acid production, investigators proposed in 1937 that tumors might possess a nonphosphorylating pathway for glycolysis. This concept was abandoned when it was found that phosphorylated substrates did not readily enter cells. After a decade of laborious experimentation in some illustrious cancer laboratories, investigators established that glycolysis in cancer uses the same substrates, yields the same products, and involves the same enzymes as in normal tissue. Thus, LePage's work [348] clearly established that tumors contain all the enzymes needed for the classical Embden-Meyerhoff pathway, and that the energy derived from the glycolytic process is, in cancer as in normal tissues, collected in high-energy phosphate bonds. (In fact, Meyerhoff had concluded that glycolysis is in some way regulated by the interaction of hexokinase, which starts the pathway by phosphorylating glucose and ATPase, which breaks down ATP. Thus, according to Meyerhoff, when ATPase activity is low, the levels of intracellular organic phosphates are also low, and, as a result, glycolysis is inhibited by a lack of inorganic phosphate and inorganic phosphate acceptor.)

Once the individual steps of the Krebs cycle had been identified, workers in a number of laboratories—including those of Meister, Weinhouse, and Ochoa—examined tumor tissues for the individual enzymes involved in the cycle. The presence in a variety of tumors of condensing enzymes, aconitase, and the various dehydrogenases involved in the cycle, as well as lactic dehydrogenase, was soon established. When labeled intermediates became available, it was clearly demonstrated that tumor slices or homogenates were able to oxidize labeled glucose, lactate, pyruvate, and succinate.

Of course, it should be emphasized that, as was the case for the glycolytic enzymes, these studies involved the measurements of enzyme activities, rather than a direct determination of the number of enzyme molecules in the tumor. Therefore, tumors may contain enzymes with molecular properties different from those of the enzymes found in corresponding normal tissues.

Once it was established *in vitro* that all enzymes involved in converting pyruvic acid to CO_2 and oxaloacetate were present in the tumor tissue, it would have seemed unlikely that the cycle was not functioning *in vivo*. Yet it was imperative to study the performance of the cycle *in vivo* because the *in vitro* experiments did not exclude the possibility that marked differences in the performance of the cycle could take place in tumors *in situ*. These studies were started by Busch and Potter [349] and later pursued by Busch and his associate [350].

Although most normal tissues of fluoroacetate-treated animals accumulate fluorocitrate, Potter and Busch found that it is fluoroacetate that accumulates in tumors. Such a finding was interpreted to mean that tumors cannot convert acetate to citrate. Similarly, the injection of [^{14}C]acetate to tumor-bearing rats demonstrated that tumors were practically incapable of oxidizing this substrate, in contrast to normal tissues, which use the acetate through the Krebs cycle and convert it primarily to glutamate.

When labeled pyruvate was injected into tumor-bearing rats, it was found that the liver, kidney, intestine, brain, heart, muscle, and testis converted most of the pyruvic acid into amino acids synthesized through the Krebs cycle—alanine and aspartic and glutamic acids. In contrast, the tumor exhibited little or no transamination and converted over 50% of the pyruvic acid to lactic acid. Busch interpreted these results by proposing that the Krebs cycle, although active in the tumor tissue, played only a minor role in glucose oxidation. Additional studies using labeled glutamate and succinate established that *in vivo* the amino acids are converted to lactate through the Krebs cycle.

The findings made by Busch *in vivo* inescapably led to the conclusion that tumors have low oxidative properties, a conclusion that is diametrically opposed to that reached by those who studied the oxidative powers of tumors *in vitro*. Busch has attempted to explain the discrepancy between the capacity of tumors to oxidize acetate *in vitro* and their inability to do so *in vivo* by the presence of excess substrate and the high atmospheric oxygen tension prevalent in the *in vitro* experimental condition. *In vivo*, the combination of low substrate concentration, reduced intracellular pH, and low oxygen tension were thought to be responsible for the inability of the tumor tissue to convert fluoroacetate to fluorocitrate.

As a matter of fact, those investigators who have measured oxygen tension and pH in tumors have found these parameters to be lower in rapidly growing tumors than in normal tissues. In spite of the laudable attempts that were made to explain this discrepancy between the *in vivo* and *in vitro* oxidative powers of rapidly growing tumors, the findings made in Busch's laboratory continue to be disconcerting, because low oxidation could constitute an injury one step closer than glycolysis to that primary insult which converts a normal into a cancer cell. Whatever their relationship to high aerobic glycolysis might be, it is nevertheless unlikely that the changes in pH, oxygen tension, and *in vivo* ability to oxidize acetate constitute the primary insult in cancer. It appears more likely that these are changes that take place in the development of the tumor.

The pattern of the development of the research on fatty acid oxidation in tumors was similar to that already described for the oxidation of the Krebs cycle metabolites. The first studies in the field were done by adding substrates (fatty acids of various chain lengths) to minces or homogenates and later to mitochondria obtained from normal and cancerous tissue. The results suggested that the tumors' capacity to oxidize fatty acid was low compared to that of normal tissues. Thus, although the fatty acid would markedly stimulate oxygen uptake in preparations obtained from spleen, kidney, liver, or testis, it would have little effect on preparations obtained from tumors.

Weinhouse [351] compared the oxidation of labeled fatty acids by tumors to that observed with normal tissues. He found that although tumor tissues did not oxidize fatty acid as efficiently as normal tissues, they were perfectly capable of oxidizing the fatty acid.

The studies of fatty acid oxidation revealed that the specific activity of the CO_2 liberated in tumors was lower than that of CO_2 formed with normal tissues. This observation indicated that the tumors depend more than normal tissues the usage of endogenous fatty acids. (In contrast to the unesterified fatty acid, the methyl esthers of fatty acid made containing from 1 to 8 carbons were reported to stimulate oxygen uptake in tumors. On the basis of this finding, it was concluded that fatty acid oxidation, instead of being regular β in type, was probably of the ω type in tumors.)

Studies on fatty acid oxidation in hepatomas indicated that the oxidation pattern in hepatomas resembles that of the peripheral tissue rather than that of liver. After exhaustive studies of fatty acid oxidation in normal tissues and in tumors, Weinhouse was able to conclude that tumors could oxidize fatty acids and that although the values registered for tumors may be at the lower side of the normal, they fall well within the range of values obtained for normal tissues.

Furthermore, Aisenberg and Potter [352, 353] found that the inability of the Walker carcinoma and the Flexner-Jobling carcinoma to oxidize fatty acids did not entirely result from a deficiency in the enzymic machinery because the oxidative ability of the tumor could be largely increased by adding coenzyme A to the incubation mixture. Again, all the studies just described were performed on rapidly growing tumors, and the findings related to fatty acid oxidation were more likely to reflect the process of dedifferentiation, rather than being an indication of the primary event responsible for converting a normal to a cancerous cell.

Determinations of the enzymes' activities and measurements of the rate of conversions of the labeled substrate of the hexose monophosphate shunt suggest not only that the pathway exists in tumors, but also that it is at least as effective in tumors as in the corresponding normal tissue.

Before studies on the oxidative abilities of the Krebs cycle enzymes and on fatty acid oxidation appeared in literature, several laboratories investigated the metabolism of the enzymes in the electron transport chain. Studies of the intracellular content of the various components of the electron transport chain constituted a logical expansion of the Warburg theory of carcinogenesis. Although ingenious methods were used, most of these experiments were often inadequate in that they were disruptive and caused the loss of important amounts of catalysts. Thus, most of the experiments to be described did not measure accurately the enzyme content or actual intracellular level of activity.

Direct measurement of at least some of the components of the electron transport chain in a tumor tissue revealed that the concentrations of cytochrome oxidase and cytochrome c were relatively low in tumors, compared with such tissues as heart and kidney. The concentrations found in tumors were not lower than those found in spleen or lung. Moreover, Potter's studies suggested that the amount of various oxidative enzymes varied widely in normal tissue, and cancer tissues were grouped together at the low end of the normal range.

Potter's findings proved to be in agreement with studies of Slater, who compared oxygen consumption in tumor slices or suspension in the presence or absence of such substrates as succinate and paraphenylene diamine. Slater compared normal skin to squamous cell and basocellular carcinomas; normal kidney to sympaticoblastomas, hypernephromas, and adenocarcinomas; and normal rectal mucosa to metastatic carcinoma of the rectum. In normal tissues, the addition of succinate or paraphenylene diamine stimulated oxygen consumption 100% or more above the values obtained in the absence of substrate. The addition of the substrates to cancer tissue yielded small stimulatory effects or was slightly inhibitory.

Rosenthal and Drabkin [354] extended Slater's findings by studying a larger number of normal tissues and tumors. They concluded that whereas the normal tissues fell into two distinct categories—one in which the addition of substrate had a marked effect and another in which the addition of substrate to slices or suspension had little or no effect—adding substrate to any tumor preparation had practically no effect on the oxygen consumption.

Greenstein [355] added a new dimension to the studies of respiratory enzymes in tumors by adding cytochrome c to the incubation mixture containing acetone powder obtained from a number of normal and tumoral tissues. Such an approach provided Greenstein with what now may seem a crude procedure but which was at the time an imaginative method of measuring the relative concentration of cytochrome c and the activity of the cytochrome oxidase.

In his typical way, Greenstein studied an incredibly large number of normal and neoplastic tissues and found that tissues were of three types. In the first, the administration of cytochrome c to acetone powders elicited a slight oxygen response. This category included tissues with high oxidative metabolism such as heart, muscle, liver, kidney, and brain. Greenstein remarked that these tissues are rarely affected by neoplasia. In the second category of tissue, the oxygen response to the addition of cytochrome c was 5 to 60 times that observed in the first category; only tumors, usually highly malignant, were of this type. And the response in the third category of tissue was intermediate between the normal, with high oxidative metabolism, and that of the malignant tumors. It included a number of normal tissues as well as some benign and malignant tumors (with low degrees of malignancy or at early stages of their development).

Greenstein concluded that: (1) the ratio of cytochrome c concentration to cytochrome oxidase activity was great in those tissues with high oxidative properties; and (2) in general, tumors contained relatively low concentrations of cytochrome c. Except for the fact that he proposed that tumors ultimately converged toward a uniform type of metabolism, Greenstein carefully avoided expanding his metabolic findings into theories of carcinogenesis.

Although the content of certain respiratory catalysts may be low in certain tumors, tumors do not necessarily exhibit low respiration under normal stimuli. Furthermore, Chance and Castor [356, 357] have shown that intact ascites cells contain normal amounts of respiration catalysts, and Wu and Racker [358, 359] have found that intact mitochondria from ascites tumor cells respire actively. The oxidative phosphorylation levels of the ascites cell mitochondria are the same as in mitochondria obtained from normal cells.

While mitochondrial DNA of normal cells is made of double-stranded covalently closed circles, unicircular dimers of mtDNA have been found in neoplastic cells. The significance of this finding is not clear because first, it is not associated with known changes in informational content and secondly, because such unicircular dimers have also been found in normal human and beef thyroid and in benign tumors. Finally, many human and malignant tumors are devoid of the unicircular dimers [613].

Oxidative Phosphorylation in Tumors

Several investigators have studied oxidative phosphorylation in tumoral tissue and have reported somewhat conflicting results, depending upon the type of tumor and the substrates used. Potter and his associates were the first to study oxidative phosphorylation in tumor homogenates. Although the first preparations were made in water, later ones were made in isotonic KCl and in sucrose. Finally, when the technique became available, mitochondria were isolated by differential centrifugation.

Although these results may appear outdated and their validity questionable, the significance remains considerable and should not be ignored. The studies with homogenates revealed that tumors had a greater ability to break down ATP, and that potential ATP catabolism by far exceeds the tumors' ability to regenerate ATP by oxidative phosphorylation, and also that the ratio of potential breakdown to potential synthesis in tumors is greater than that in normal tissues.

Mitochondria of tumors could couple oxidation to phosphorylation as well as normal mitochondria. However, the total number of mitochondria in hepatomas was smaller than the total number of mitochondria in normal tissue. This finding is in keeping with some mitochondrial counts made by others. If these findings are still valid, they suggest that although the ability of the mitochondria to couple oxidation and phosphorylation is not changed in cancer, the total amount of ATP generated is lower in cancer tissue than in normal tissue for at least two reasons: an increased rate of breakdown and a smaller number of mitochondria. Although much evidence suggests that these findings cannot constitute the critical event in cancer, their occurrence at a later stage of cancer development could be responsible for the high rate of anaerobic glycolysis.

Williams-Ashman [360] studied oxidative phosphorylation in mitochondria of Jensen sarcoma and Walker 256 carcinosarcoma and demonstrated good oxidative phosphorylation ratios when succinate was used as a substrate. The P/O ratios were dependent on substrate conditions and were sensitive to dinitrophenol.

In contrast, Lindberg and his associates [361] studied ascites cell mitochondria and reported that the overall rate of respiration and phosphorylation expressed per milligram of nitrogen in the mitochondria was low. These findings were in conflict with those of Quastel and Bickis [362] and Emmelot and his associates [363], who demonstrated good P/O ratios in Ehrlich ascites cell mitochondria, Novikoff hepatomas, Walker 256 carcinosarcomas, and testicular and ovarian tumors. Furthermore, as Boyland showed previously, tumors destroy NAD rapidly, and consequently the levels of NAD in mitochondria and microsomes were found to be low. Good P/O ratios can be obtained with succinate as a substrate because in this situation NAD is not an intermediate in electron transfer.

Other tumors such as the mouse hepatoma and the Ehrlich ascites tumors show good oxidative phosphorylation ratios. Although as Aisenberg [353] pointed out, the high activities of ATPase and NADase could be responsible for the low levels of oxidative phosphorylation in some tumors, the possibility that changes in mitochondrial permeability take place as tumors develop has not been eliminated. In fact, when NAD and NADH ratios were measured in normal and tumoral tissues, the values for tumors fell within the range of those measured for normal tissue.

The failure of adequate phosphorylation may also be the result of a decreased number of mitochondria in tumors. The mitochondrial content of tumors has been investigated in a number of laboratories, usually by comparing hepatomas to normal and regenerating liver. The hepatomas were produced either with 4-dimethylaminoazobenzene or 2-acetylaminofluorene. The results from most laboratories seem to indicate that the number of mitochondria per cell decreases in the hepatoma during the preneoplastic period. The decrease in the number of mitochondria is accompanied by a decrease in the RNA nitrogen and enzymic content of the mitochondrial fraction. There has been no indication that the mitochondria of hepatomas are in any way different from the mitochondria of normal liver, although electron microscopists have described greater variations in the patterns of size in the mitochondria of tumors. Hogeboom and Schneider [364] have also claimed that ultracentrifugation of hepatoma mitochondria yields different distribution patterns of the fractions in the ultracentrifuge. A component in normal mitochondria seems to be absent in mitochondria obtained from tumors. To our knowledge, this intriguing observation has not been exploited in other laboratories.

Studies by Allard, who converted normal cells into cancerous ones, in rat hepatomas are in agreement with those obtained in mouse hepatomas. Allard further compared the mitochondrial population of normal liver to that of regenerating liver and showed that the total number of mitochondria decreased in regenerating liver. This finding suggests that the alteration and the number of mitochondria observed in hepatomas might be related to the rate of growth rather than to the primary insult which converts a normal into a cancer cell. Striebich, Shelton, and Schneider [365] described intriguing results with respect to the changes in the number of mitochondria after administering two different derivatives of 4-dimethylaminoazobenzene. These investigators administered 2-methyl and 3-dimethyl 4-dimethylaminoazobenzene to mice. The first of these two compounds is noncarcinogenic, but the second is highly carcinogenic.

The results obtained with the carcinogenic derivative were similar to those previously reported by these investigators with other carcinogens. However, the noncarcinogenic methyl derivative induced an increase in the number of mitochondria in liver, and the increase in the mitochondrial population was not associated with an increase in the total number of cells but was paralleled by increased succinoxidase activity. The levels of oxaloacetic oxidase, cytochrome c reductase, and total nitrogen did not increase in a parallel fashion with the increase in the number of mitochondria. On the basis of such findings, investigators concluded that the 2-methyl derivatives induced the formation of abnormal mitochondria.

The results of the studies of oxidative phosphorylation in tumors suggest that alterations may or may not occur, depending upon the type of tumor. Moreover, when phosphorylation is ineffective in tumors, it could be the result of several different primary injuries, such as activation of enzymes (ATPase, NADase), modification in mitochondrial permeability, or changes in the number of mitochondria. In any event, modifications in the level of oxidative phosphorylation can play only a peripheral role in cancer metabolism, because some tumors exhibit the typical biological behavior of cancer without presenting drastic changes in the pattern of oxidative phosphorylation. Aisenberg's [353] studies have shown that mitochondrial oxidation and the coupling of oxidation and phosphorylation are the same in the Morris hepatoma 5123 as in normal liver.

The relationship between glycolysis and respiration in tumors was reinvestigated in Weinhouse's [341] laboratory. These investigators used a new method of measuring oxidative phosphorylation; they used 2-deoxyglucose, which is readily phosphorylated in the presence of ATP but is not hydrolyzed or metabolized and will therefore accumulate in the medium. The amount of deoxyglucose-6-phosphate present in the medium is measured indirectly by determining the amount of deoxyglucose that participates in the glucose oxidase reactions. In these studies, the investigators found no significant difference between the oxygen uptake, in microatoms, and the 2-deoxyglucose conversion into deoxyglucose-6-phosphate, in micromoles (P/O ratio), in liver and hepatoma 5123. Furthermore, dinitrophenol uncoupled oxidative phosphorylation in the hepatoma in the same way as in the normal liver.

Results of studies on the aerobic glycolysis, oxygen uptake, and enzyme activities of the electron transport system in neoplastic and nonneoplastic ovarian tissue grafted into the spleen of C57 BL mice conflict with those reported for the minimal deviation hepatomas. Bruzzone transplanted ovaries in the spleen by the method of Lee and Gardner. Sixty days after transplantation, he measured oxygen uptake, aerobic lactic acid production, and the activities of reduced triphosphopyridine nucleotide oxidase, reduced triphosphopyridine nucleotide cytochrome c reductase, reduced triphosphopyridine nucleotide ferricyanide reductase, succinate cytochrome c reductase, and cytochrome oxidase. The results obtained on transplanted ovaries were compared with those obtained in normal ovaries.

At various stages of development of the transplant, the histological pattern of which resembles that of the normal ovary, the biochemical pattern differs considerably. Oxygen uptake decreases, aerobic glycolysis increases, and the activities of the five electron transport chain enzymes cited previously decrease. Mitochondrial counts were not made, so it is impossible to determine whether these changes in the activity of the enzymes of the electron transport chain result from a decrease in the number of mitochondria.

The decrease in aerobic lactic acid production observed by these investigators is intriguing. Indeed, the transplant is in a proliferating stage, and one cannot escape wondering what the source of chemical energy for proliferation might be.

Amino Acid Metabolism in Cancer

Roberts and his associate [366] studied the composition of the free amino acid pool in tumors, applying the two-dimensional paper chromatography techniques to their research in the field. They established that the pools of the various free amino acids were quite characteristic for a given tissue in a given strain of mice. In fact, some differences have been reported within a tissue—for example, when the white matter of the brain is compared with the gray matter. In contrast to normal tissue, different types of transplanted and spontaneous tumors all have a similar pattern of free amino acid distribution. Furthermore, according to Roberts, the free amino acid patterns remain constant in normal tissue (liver, kidney, muscle, and brain), in spite of severe inanition, dehydration, hypophysectomy, and thyroidectomy.

The amino acid patterns change after injury or hormonal imbalance. Examples of injuries or imbalances include: (1) a decrease in the amino acid concentration of the prostate of castrated males, restorable to normal by testosterone injection; (2) potassium deficiency (increase of lysine and arginine and decrease in glutamic and aspartic levels in kidney muscle); (3) myocardial infarct (decrease in the urine of alanine, glutamine, glutamic acid, aspartic acid, and glutathione); (4) insulin-produced hypoglycemia (large decrease in brain glutamic acid, isomolar increase in aspartic acid, and small decrease in aminoisobutyric acid); (5) fluoroacetate administration (decrease in glutamic and aspartic acids in brain); and (6) injection of lethal doses of ammonium acetate (increase of aspartic acid in liver and increase of glutamine in brain, testis, and muscle).

Although such patterns of amino acid distribution in various normal and injured tissues are difficult to interpret, they do constitute important reference points for studying the pattern of amino acid in tumors.

As already mentioned, most tumors that were studied (minimal deviation hepatomas were not included) have a similar amino acid pattern, a finding in keeping with the Greenstein generalization on tumor metabolism. Tumors contain relatively high levels of proline, alanine, and glycine, and low levels of aspartic acid, glutamine, and ethanolamine phosphate.

Tissues in general are practically impermeable to glutamic acid, yet glutamine passes the cell barrier readily. When glutamine is injected intraperitoneally to rats bearing the Yoshida sarcoma, the amino acid content of the ascitic fluid increases and the alanine, lysine, glutamine, threonine, serine, and glycine contents of the tumor decrease, possibly as a result of the displacement of the amino acids from the cell into the ascitic fluid. Control patterns of amino acid distribution reappear in fluid and tumors as the levels of glutamine fall in the peritoneal fluid. Inasmuch as glucose is a poor precursor of glutamic acid, it was proposed that glutamine may constitute an important precursor of glutamic acid in tumors. Deamination of glutamic acid converts it to α-ketoglutarate which serves as a substrate for the Krebs cycle. Two-dimensional paper chromatography of the amino acid patterns of tumors and of various tissues of tumor-bearing rats revealed: (1) low levels or absence of glutamine in the tumor, suggesting that the tumors are operating at marginal levels, and (2) no change in the tissues of the tumor-bearing rats until the terminal stage.

The levels of glutamine in the tissues of the host drop at the terminal stage. In humans with Hodgkin's disease or leukemia, low levels of plasma glutamine have been reported in association with increased levels of aspartic and glutamic acid and alanine. The low levels of glutamine in tumors were thought to result from special metabolic features of tumors, as in the following pattern: low level of synthesis of glutamine coupled with rapid uptake followed by almost instantaneous utilization of glutamine.

Some of the findings made *in vivo* found their counterpart in *in vitro* studies. The concentration of arginine in lymphoma cells was also found to be critical. When arginine is added to tumor cell lines, it causes interference with thymidine uptake and ultimately leads to cellular death [614].

The significance of such studies should not be underestimated because the studies could lead to successful methods of chemotherapy. The use of azaserine in cancer therapy is a case in point, although the efficiency of this antimetabolite is extremely limited, probably because of the rapid and extensive production of glutamine by normal tissues.

An interesting development in a similar vein was the discovery of the therapeutic effects of asparaginase. Guinea pigs are notoriously resistant to induced or transplanted tumors. Although this puzzling observation is still far from explained, a partial explanation is now available. In 1953 Kidd [367, 368] reported that guinea pig serum brought about the regression of transplanted lymphomas in mice, and Kidd thought that the interference with tumor growth resulted from immunological interactions. However, in 1961 Broome [369] showed that the effect of guinea pig serum resulted from its relatively high content of L-asparaginase. *E. coli* asparaginase was found to elicit the same effects as those of the guinea pig serum.

Results of therapeutic attempts in humans are still too preliminary to warrant objective evaluation of this mode of treatment. What seems certain is that the enzyme's toxicity to the host is minimal at levels capable of inducing temporary remission. Furthermore, the enzyme does not appear to pass the brain-blood barrier, and the pools of asparagine in nerve tissue are apparently separated from those that serve the rest of the body. Consequently, asparaginase seems to be unable to affect the growth of tumors of the central nervous system.

Amino acids are metabolites that are used or produced at crossroads of various metabolic pathways. For example, they may be deaminated and oxidized through the Krebs cycle or may serve as building blocks for gluconeogenesis or protein or nucleic acid synthesis. In spite of the multiplicity of routes for metabolism, the pattern of amino acid content in a given tissue appears to be constant under steady state conditions at a given stage in the development of that tissue, and it also seems to be relatively unalterable.

The inescapable conclusion is that one regulator controls, or several regulators operate simultaneously to control, intracellular amino acid levels. In cancer, the control mechanism is out of phase or it is nonexistent and amino acid levels are regulated by diffusion, penetration, and utilization in the cell.

The host can in some way restore normal amino acid patterns in tumors. Some strains of mice are susceptible and others are resistant to the transplantation of tumors. Two of such strains may differ from each other by a single histocompatibility gene. If a tumor with an aberrant amino acid pattern is transplanted in both types of mice, it grows and maintains its aberrant amino acid pattern in mice that are susceptible, while it regresses after a short growth period and the amino acid pattern reverts to normal in the resistant mice. Similar reversions to normal amino acid patterns have been reported for Yoshida sarcoma transplanted in resistant mice and for tumors regressing under the influence of antimetabolites. The amino acid pools in minimal deviation hepatomas are discussed below.

Amino Acid Incorporation in Tumor Proteins

Early studies on incorporation of labeled precursor into proteins were somewhat confusing. Sheman and Rittenberg concluded that [^{15}N]glycine was incorporated more slowly in tumors than in normal tissues. Similar reports originated from Griffin's [370] laboratory, who used [^{14}C]glycine but failed to separate proteins from nucleic acid. LePage [371] studied the incorporation of [^{14}C]glycine into protein and nucleic acid of liver, kidney, and Jobling sarcoma, carefully separating the proteins from the deoxyribonucleic and ribonucleic acids. He found that incorporation reached a peak soon after the isotope was injected and that the pattern of incorporation was similar in liver, hepatomas, and kidney. There were slight differences in the absolute incorporation; it was highest in liver and lowest in kidney.

Although there were some differences, depending upon the report, the studies of amino acid incorporation into proteins *in vivo* agree on one point: the incorporation of the labeled amino acid is not greater in tumor than in normal tissues. Yet all *in vitro* incorporation studies done with slices suggested that the rate of incorporation was greater in tumors than in normal tissues. It is believed now that *in vivo* the labeled amino acids are not readily available to the tumor because of poor peripheral circulation.

When the Ehrlich ascites cell carcinoma was made available in the United States, thanks to the efforts of Klein, LePage used this preparation for further studying [^{14}C]glycine incorporation into tumors. He compared the results in ascites cells with those obtained in cell suspensions of Gardner lymphosarcoma and mouse liver cell suspensions. Under these conditions, incorporation was much higher in the tumor than in the liver cells. LePage's incorporation studies included a comparison of the uptake of amino acid in the presence and absence of oxygen; no significant differences were observed in the tumor or in the liver.

Although the data LePage collected on tumors are reliable, his data on the liver cell suspension probably are not because the rate of incorporation in liver cell suspension differed from incorporation in liver *in vivo* or in liver slices. Therefore, like many of the early studies on precursor incorporation into proteins (especially those studies that attempted to evaluate the efficiency of the energy source), these first early studies of LePage lack adequate controls.

Zamecnik and coworkers [372] devoted much time to studying amino acid incorporation in tumors. Not only did he establish that hepatoma slices incorporate larger amounts of labeled amino acids into proteins than normal liver or even regenerating liver slices, but he proved also that tumor and normal tissues need a source of biochemical energy to synthesize proteins. Indeed, dinitrophenol interferes with amino acid incorporation in hepatoma slices.

Further studies by Farber and associates [373] established that the addition of glucose to incubation mixtures containing cell suspensions of Gardner lymphosarcoma stimulated [^{14}C]glycine incorporation in the presence or absence of oxygen. Krebs cycle substrates (pyruvate, citrate, malate, ketoglutarate, lactate) could not be substituted for glucose in stimulating amino acid incorporation. Similar results were reported by investigators who followed the incorporation of labeled methionine, phenylalanine, lysine, leucine, and valine in the Ehrlich ascites tumor.

Quastel [362] reexamined amino acid incorporation in tumors for the specific purpose of relating it to the source of energy available. The incorporation of amino acids into tissue proteins was measured under aerobic and anaerobic conditions, but always in the presence of glucose. Oxygen uptake, aerobic amino acid uptake, anaerobic glycolysis, and anaerobic amino acid uptake were measured in a number of proliferating tissues, including tumors (Ehrlich ascites carcinoma, Walker 256 carcinosarcoma, sarcoma 37), embryonic tissues, regenerating liver, and a variety of normal tissues, including some with a high rate of aerobic glycolysis, such as renal medulla and retina.

If the aerobic ATP generated is $6 \times QO_2$ and if one assumes that the P/O ratio is 3.0, then anaerobic ATP generated is Ql_a, if one assumes that one mole of lactate produced corresponds to one mole of ATP generated. Thus, on the basis of data that are relatively simple to collect, Quastel was able to compare the efficiency of ATP generated glycolytically with that generated aerobically.

In the presence of oxygen, the incorporation of amino acid per mole of ATP produced is the same whether glucose is present or not in the ascites cell tumors. Moreover, there is no difference in the rate of amino acid uptake in ascites tumors whether oxygen is present or not. Consequently, the ratio of aerobic to anaerobic efficiency for amino acid uptake is only slightly smaller than 1.0. In conclusion, tumors are indifferent to the source of ATP they use, whether generated through the Krebs cycle or through glycolysis.

Quastel's remarkable study compared the result obtained in tumors to those obtained in a number of normal tissues, and apparently all of them, even chick and rat embryos (rapidly growing tissues), the renal medulla, and the retina (tissues with high rates of aerobic glycolysis) have aerobic efficiency for amino acid incorporation greater than the anaerobic efficiency. To interpret these events, investigators suggested that normal tissues are unable to use extramitochondrial ATP for protein synthesis. These experiments on the relationship between the source of energy and the rate of incorporation of amino acids in tumors seemed to lead to the conclusion that tumors use anaerobic energy more efficiently than normal tissues for amino acid incorporation into proteins. (The major limitation of this type of study resides in the low absolute efficiency of amino acid usage for incorporation—only one amino acid molecule per 5500 molecules of ATP generated.)

Incorporation of Nucleic Acid Precursors in Tumors

In 1953 LePage [371] reported that there were few publications on the incorporation of precursors in nucleic acid *in vitro* compared to the wealth of information that had already been accumulated on amino acid incorporation into protein.

At that time, studies with nucleic acid precursors were tedious and laborious because it was often necessary to synthesize the needed precursor in one's own laboratory. Furthermore, since the intermediates for nucleic acid synthesis were not known, methods for their analysis were not available. Consequently, pool sizes were not known, and since much of the interpretation depended on the size of the pool, it is not surprising that the results were sometimes misleading.

Yet slow sifting of the data and accumulation of cross-check information obtained *in vivo* and *in vitro* not only permitted the step by step identification of the pathway or pathways for nucleotide and nucleic acid synthesis, but it also provided bridgeheads for major concepts in modern molecular biology.

Since we have already described several aspects of the research concerned with nucleotide biosynthesis, we shall restrict ourselves in this part of the book to describing a few experiments in which tumor tissues were used.

Several laboratories attacked the problem of nucleotide synthesis in tumors at about the same time. Abrams and Goldinger [374] studied the incorporation of purines and formate into the nucleic acid of rabbit bone marrow and concluded that hypoxanthine was a precursor of nucleic acid, adenine, and guanine. These conclusions proved to be essentially right, although it was later established that inosinic acid was the actual precursor of both AMP and GMP.

Studies in Buchanan's [375] and Greenberg's [376] laboratories in which labeled CO_2, formate, and glycine were used as precursors established that these smaller precursors were used to build the purine ring of hypoxanthine. LePage [371] extended this type of investigation to tumors. He followed the incorporation of [^{14}C]glycine in suspensions of liver, Ehrlich carcinoma, and Gardner lymphosarcoma cells. He separated the nucleic acid from the proteins, and although he did not separate DNA from RNA, he hydrolyzed the nucleic acid and separated adenine from guanine.

[^{14}C]Glycine was found to be much more effectively incorporated into guanine than adenine (the specific activity of the guanine was about five times that of adenine). In the carcinoma and the lymphosarcoma, the incorporation in liver cells was negligible in both adenine and guanine.

LePage added various bases, adenine and guanine, hypoxanthine, nucleosides (adenosine, guanosine, and uridine), and nucleotides (3-AMP, 5-AMP, 5-GMP, 5-CMP, 5-UMP, and 5-IMP) to the incubation mixture and studied the effects on [^{14}C]glycine incorporation into nucleic acids.

It was assumed that glycine incorporation would be reduced from the dilution of the pool of precursors by the added metabolite, which consequently would have to be used in a pathway for nucleic acid synthesis. Adenine and hypoxanthine markedly reduced the incorporation of [^{14}C]glycine into nucleic acid of both the carcinoma and the lymphosarcoma. Guanine had no effect on [^{14}C]glycine incorporation into the nucleic acid adenine and guanine of the carcinoma, but it reduced to one-third the incorporation of [^{14}C]glycine into the nucleic acid guanine of the lymphosarcoma. (The incorporation of glycine into the lymphosarcoma was one-tenth that in the carcinoma.)

Guanosine had no effect on the incorporation of glycine into nucleic acid adenine, but it diluted glycine incorporation into the guanine of carcinoma nucleic acids and reduced the incorporation of both adenine and guanine in nucleic acids of lymphosarcoma. Adenylic and inosinic acid reduced the incorporation into nucleic acid of guanine and adenine in both the carcinoma and the lymphosarcoma. Guanylic acid interfered only with the incorporation of glycine in the nucleic acid guanine in the carcinoma, but it interfered with the incorporation of glycine in both the guanine and adenine of the lymphosarcoma nucleic acid.

Although the interpretation of most of this data may appear simple in retrospect, an accurate interpretation was at the time difficult in the absence of separation of DNA from RNA and without an accurate evaluation of the intercellular pools. LePage wisely abstained from unwarranted speculation, yet some conclusions were inescapable. Tumors synthesize nucleic acid purines by two different pathways; one involves the condensation of small molecules to form the purine ring, and the other uses adenine directly. The difference in utilization of glycine for nucleic acid guanine synthesis (high in the carcinoma, low in the sarcoma) is still not readily explainable. The fact that nucleotides interfered with glycine incorporation suggested that they are on the pathway of nucleic acid synthesis.

At about that time, more sophisticated and reliable methods for tissue fractionation, nucleic acid analysis, and nucleoside separation were developed. In a remarkable paper that summarizes much of the knowledge of nucleic acid and protein synthesis up to that time, Tyner, Heidelberger, and LePage [377] describe the application of these various methods to the study of protein and nucleic acid synthesis in tumors. Truly, much of the data reported confirmed previous findings made in other laboratories. The paper constituted a comprehensive study of several parameters that led the authors to propose a scheme for the pathway of nucleic acid synthesis in tumors.

In these experiments, ^{32}P and [^{14}C]glycine were injected simultaneously to rats bearing Flexner-Jobling sarcomas. The nucleic acid and protein were extracted from nuclear, microsomal, mitochondrial, and supernatant fractions of the host's liver and the tumor. The authors confirmed a finding first made by Marshak [378] and later confirmed in several laboratories that nuclear RNA is labeled faster than cytoplasmic RNA.

An analysis of the incorporation of ^{32}P and [^{14}C]glycine led the authors to conclude that both glycine and ^{32}P were incorporated in some unknown precursors, thus suggesting the existence of a phosphorylated precursor. Therefore, an important facet of the study was that it confirmed *in vivo* previous findings made *in vitro* in Buchanan's laboratory with pigeon liver extract; namely, that the ribotide is an intermediate for deoxynucleotide synthesis.

Since adenine was also incorporated into nucleic acid, two pathways for nucleic acid synthesis—the *de novo* and salvage pathways—were proposed. Moreover, comparison of liver and tumor abilities to incorporate nucleic acid precursors revealed that the tumor used the same pathway as liver for RNA and DNA synthesis.

Similar studies were done in which ^{32}P incorporation in the DNA and RNA of various cell fractions of a transplanted mouse mammary carcinoma was carefully followed at various times after injecting the isotope. The studies led to the conclusion that both DNA and RNA were derived from a common precursor pool (a mixture of deoxyribose and ribose nucleotides was proposed), which was itself in rapid equilibrium with a common phosphorus donor (ATP was proposed). This conclusion thus hinted that ribose might be converted to deoxyribose at the nucleotide level.

Many of the studies on the incorporation of purines and pyrimidines or other nucleic acid precursors were done with the hope that they would reveal exploitable differences between cancer and normal tissue metabolism. Two important findings were made, which were related to purine and pyrimidine metabolism. Skipper and his associates found that cancer tissues use guanine much less efficiently than host normal tissues. Pretreatment of the host with a guanase inhibitor increased guanine utilization by the tumor. However, it has not been excluded that poor guanine utilization by tumors, compared to that of normal tissue, was not the result of greater availability of precursor through the circulatory system of normal tissues.

When ureosuccinic acid was administered to animals bearing transplanted human sarcomas, 7 hours after the precursor was injected the specific activity of the tumor nucleic acid (RNA and DNA) was higher than that of the host's spleen and liver nucleic acid. However, in contrast to some bacteria, which readily bypass *de novo* pathways, tumors do not preferentially use preformed precursors. It was important to establish this fact because tumor cells, like bacteria, grow in a relatively autonomous fashion.

When injected into rats, uracil labeled both DNA and RNA, but the specific activity of the RNA was much greater than that of DNA. In DNA, cytosine and thymidine were labeled equally well; in RNA, the specific activity of uracil was twice that of cytidine. Heidelberger [379] and his associates later established that uracil was used more effectively by tumors for DNA and RNA synthesis, probably as a result of a less efficient catabolic pathway for uracil breakdown.

Uracil utilization by liver was lower, and that of the intestinal mucosa higher, than that of the tumor. Except for these minor differences, there is to date no indication of any profound difference between metabolic pathways of tumors and those of normal tissue.

Studies of the incorporation of precursors into RNA did not differ in any essential way from those studies already described for the incorporation of precursor into DNA, except for the fact that attempts were made to study the specific activity of the various kinds of RNA. For example, rapidly labeled nuclear RNA and the various cytoplasmic RNA fractions obtained by differential centrifugation were subfractionated on sucrose gradient. The result of these experiments did not reveal any fundamental difference between the anabolic pathways for RNA synthesis in normal and cancer cells. Although there are some quantitative differences in the rate of incorporation of precursor in the various types of RNA, the pattern of precursor incorporation in tumors is essentially the same as that observed in growing tissue.

Even cells grown in tissue cultures that are derived from cancer cells do not have special metabolic pathways for purines or pyrimidines, which distinguishes them significantly from cells derived from normal tissue. In 1955, concluding a most laborious research program, Eagle reviewed his work in tissue culture of HeLa cells and fibroblasts. He established that adequate growth takes place in the presence of optimal concentrations of glucose, two antibiotics, dialyzed serum proteins, 13 amino acids, 8 vitamins, and 6 salts. The requirements were the same for the HeLa cells and the fibroblast.

Studies with such antimetabolites as aminopterin demonstrated that the mode of antimetabolite inhibition, judged by the accumulation of precursors, was the same in cancer tissues as in other growing tissue.

In conclusion, studies on the incorporation of labeled purine and pyrimidine precursors in tumors established that: (1) the pathways for nucleic acid biosynthesis are the same in tumors as in other proliferating tissues; (2) the antimetabolites that block metabolic pathways lead to the accumulation of the same precursors in tumors and other growing tissues; and (3) the relative rates of performance of the *de novo* and salvage pathways are essentially the same in tumor tissue and in other growing tissues.

These conclusions are of considerable importance with respect to the action of specific antimetabolites because they indicate that there are no qualitative, exploitable differences between cancer and normal cells. Differences should be of a quantitative order. Consequently, exploitable chemotherapy would require that tumors grow faster than the most rapidly growing normal tissue essential for survival.

Growth Rate of Tumors

The availability of tritium-labeled thymidine provided investigators with an opportunity for measuring the growth rate of tumors and comparing it with that of a number of normal tissues. Because tumors outgrow the boundaries of the tissues of origin and invade the surrounding tissues [338], it is usually believed that the rate of proliferation of tumor cells is greater than that of most normal tissues. Radioautographic studies with tritium-labeled thymidine combined with the administration of colchicine permitted investigators to measure the time that elapses between two mitoses in tumor cells.

The rate of cell division in most tumors is, in general, much slower than that of the most rapidly growing tissues, such as the bone marrow or the intestinal mucosa. Even leukemic cells do not divide as rapidly as the cells of the bone marrow. The mitotic rate in hepatomas is slower than that in regenerating liver. Studies of Baserga and Kisieleski [381], covering a large number of normal tissues and tumors, suggest that there is no correlation between the degree of malignancy and the growth rate.

In conclusion, although tumors usually grow at a rate equal to or somewhat faster than the rate of proliferation in the tissues of origin, the rate of cell division in tumors does not exceed that of the most rapidly growing tissues, some of which are vital for survival. This constitutes the major obstacle to efficient chemotherapy.

Studies of cell kinetics are of particular significance in therapy of human tumors. The data assembled on cell kinetics in leukemia may constitute a base line for studies on human solid tumors. A fundamental observation is that most chemotherapeutic agents, which are effective in leukemia, kill only those cells that are either undergoing DNA synthesis or mitosis. GO, G1 and G2 cells are not affected. When, however, a large proportion of the leukemic cells are killed, a number of the interphase cells are induced to divide and they do so in synchrony. The dividing cells then survive a second dose of the drug.

Cell kinetics of seven human tumors (lung, maxillary antrum, malignant melanoma, malignant schwannoma, colon cancer, and two breast cancers) have been studied by pulse labeling with ^{3}HTDR followed by repeated biopsies and radioautography. Three different techniques to measure the cell cycle were used [615, 616]: (1) a grain counting method, (2) the estimation of the percentage of labeled cells, (3) the total number of cells in mitosis per total number of cells counted. A computer model was devised to estimate the number of cells lost during the process of tumor proliferation. By using continuous intravenous injection of ^{3}HTDR, one can better identify the duration and distribution of intermitotic times as well as the size of the pool of nonproliferating cells during the period of infusion.

Results with four human tumors constantly perfused from 6 to 20 hours revealed that the percent of mitosis gradually increases with time to reach a peak only at 20 days (95%) after injection. This finding suggests that a large proportion of cells (approximately 30%) remains in interphase for as long as 20 days or more.

This is in contrast to normal epithelial cells in which 75% of the cells in interphase and 95% of the cells in mitosis were labeled on the 5th day.

It has been postulated that the low levels of incorporation of [^{3}H]TDR result from a defect in the conversion of [^{3}H]TDR to TMP through the catalytic action of thymidine kinase (salvage pathway). This assumption is, however, in conflict with studies by others who have not found any decrease in TDR kinase in tumors.

To explain the low level of incorporation of [^{3}H]TDR it was further assumed that the tumor contains excessive amounts of TTP which will have a dual effect: (1) a feedback inhibition of the kinase (and also of carbamyl aspartate synthetase) and (2) dilution of the pool of [^{3}H]TTP derived from [^{3}H]TDR. Other mechanisms of interference with labeling with [^{3}H]TDR may include a block in G2.

The administration of vincristine, cytosine arabinoside or methotrexate modifies cell kinetics considerably suggesting that these drugs bring the solid tumor cells that were arrested in G0 to divide more or less synchronously, thus making them available for further attack by antimetabolites of X-irradiation.

There is little doubt that our knowledge of cell kinetics in human tumors is scarce and certainly, except for some forms of leukemia, little has been learned of the modification of such kinetics by various chemical or physical therapeutic agents.

The fundamental strategy in cancer therapy is to hit every cell with the hope that all will be killed. Unfortunately almost always some escape. The reasons are numerous: (1) the state of the cell cycle; (2) changes in permeability of the cell to the drug; (3) the development in the tumor of alternative pathways which will neutralize the drug effects; (4) modification of the immunosuppressive state of the host; (5) modification of the host's ability to dispose of the drug; (6) ability of the cell to repair damage.

Thus, the changes in cell kinetics after drug administration result from a compilation of tumor and host alterations, variables which are difficult to measure.

It is, however, conceivable that the complexities and the multitude of the factors involved in modulating cell kinetics in tumors could be dumped in a black box and ignored, thus allowing the investigators to focus on the link between the drug administered and the observations made after injection of [^{3}H]TDR for the purpose of exploiting the changes in chemotherapy. Observations made on animal and human tumors suggest that cell kinetics vary considerably from tumor to tumor, and therefore it would appear that exploitable observations would require that the study be carried out on an individual basis. Even then there is no guarantee that what is seen in one biopsy will be representative of the whole of the tumor and its metastasis or that what is observed at one time may be representative of the response during the life span of the tumor.

DNA Content, Properties, and Metabolism in Cancer

Because two of the characteristics of cancer are persistent growth and alteration of the regular pattern of differentiation, much research has been devoted in the last 30 years to studying the concentrations, the biosynthesis, and the function of those macromolecules which in the second quarter of this century were suspected but are now known to be clearly involved in determining cellular specificity. Investigations with nucleic acids and proteins in cancer paralleled the development of macromolecular biology. And although the studies on cancer macromolecular biology might not have revealed any clue as to the pathogenesis of cancer, these studies have often wedged deeply into new fields of biochemistry and sometimes have provided information that later proved to be fundamental for the development of modern biochemistry.

Studies of the DNA content in cancer cells revealed that most, if not all, of the DNA was associated with the nuclear fraction and that the amount of DNA per cell was frankly increased in malignant tumors. This finding is not surprising since, in most advanced cancer, heteroploidy predominates. Thus, if the DNA content per unit weight or volume is increased in tumors, it must be as a result of polyteny, polyploidy, or of increased cellularity per unit volume. A number of laboratories, including those of Klein [382] and Kit [383], reported that the DNA content in cancer cell ascites lymphomas or carcinomas was approximately proportional to the chromosome number. Furthermore, the metabolic activity of these cells is related to the number of chromosomes. In tetraploid cells, it was twice that of diploid cells. Thus, the rate of respiration and glycolysis; the activities of succinoxidase, transaminase, and peptidase; and the content in nitrogen-free amino acids and histones were found to be, in the tetraploid cell, twice that of related diploid cells.

Metabolic activities vary considerably, however, when unrelated cells are compared. Thus, whereas the ratio of glycolysis to DNA is 30 in carcinoma cells, it is ten times greater in lymphoma cells. These findings suggest that even in cancer cells there is a quantitative relationship between DNA, RNA, protein content, and the number of chromosomes, provided, of course, that the cancer cell is compared with the related normal cell.

These reports contradict earlier reports on the studies of normal and cancer cells with the aid of ultraviolet microscopy, which revealed a significantly higher ratio of absorption of UV light at 260 mμ than at 280 mμ, suggesting that the ratio of the nucleic acids to protein was changed in the hepatoma or regenerating liver cell.

The diversity of the cell population of the biochemist's starting material may lead him astray. Using the Chalkley method, Stowell showed that hepatomas that develop in rats fed dimethylaminoazobenzene contain as few as 10% hepatoma cells and 60% connective and vascular tissues. Although cytophotometric methods do not provide rigid quantitative results, they allow the cell under investigation to be identified.

Mark and Ris [384] compared the DNA content of nuclei of identical size in normal liver, hepatomas, and cholangiomas using microspectrophotometric determination of the intensity of the Feulgen reaction. They concluded that the DNA content in nuclei of identical size was the same in all three tumors.

The constant relationship that links metabolic activity to chromosome number suggests that if one looks for the chemical differences in the genome that might be responsible for cancerization, he might have to resort to methods somewhat more sophisticated than those that consist of measuring the DNA or RNA content per cell. Thus, a number of laboratories have looked for physicochemical differences between the DNA of normal and cancerous tissues. Bendich [385] compared the physicochemical properties of DNA obtained from myeloid leukemic leukocytes with that of normal and lymphatic leukemic leukocytes. The patterns obtained by chromatography on ECTEOLA cellulose or of the sedimentation constant distribution curves varied with the source of the DNA. Furthermore, the effect of urea on the viscosity of myeloid leukemia DNA was different from its effect on normal leukocyte DNA. However, when Kit [383, 386] compared the chromatographic profiles of mouse spleen with transplanted lymphoma DNA, he found no differences. Similarly, no differences in the base composition of both types of DNA were detected.

It is not entirely surprising that the results of studies of DNA content and of the physicochemical properties of DNA in cancer tissues yielded negative and sometimes conflicting results. Such results surely do not exclude the possibility that alterations of the DNA molecules are, in fact, responsible for the shift from normal to cancerous behavior patterns. In such a case, the change in DNA that is responsible for cancerization could be quite small and difficult to detect with present methods of analysis. We may have to wait until DNA sequences can be determined completely. In evaluating the role of DNA in carcinogenesis, one cannot ignore the fact that at least some carcinogens are known to alter the DNA molecules.

Changes in the DNA molecules that are responsible for carcinogenesis must not necessarily involve the base sequence. Bacterial and mammalian DNA contain methyl groups that are enzymatically added to the base after they have been incorporated into the macromolecular system. Enzymes capable of catalyzing the methylation of mammalian DNA have been prepared from disrupted nuclei of rat liver, kidney, spleen, and brain. The activity of the enzyme is low in the Morris 5123 hepatoma and is undetectable in the Novikoff hepatoma. Although the biological function of methylation remains unknown, the presence of the methyl groups might be indispensable for reading the code correctly or for recognizing such enzymes as DNA polymerase.

As tumors grow, the cells must hypertrophy or divide. If cells proliferate and the DNA per chromosome and the number of chromosomes per cell are unchanged or increased, DNA must necessarily be synthesized as the tumors grow. Consequently, many laboratories have devoted much time to studying DNA synthesis in tumors. Three aspects of these studies of DNA synthesis in tumors must be distinguished: (1) the pathway used, (2) the rate of synthesis, and (3) the control of DNA synthesis in tumors.

One of the first studies using radioactive isotopes in biology consisted of following ^{32}P incorporation into DNA or growing sarcomas. When other nucleic acid precursors such as glycine, adenine, orotic acid, and thymidine became available, they were one by one used for studying their incorporation in the nucleic acids [387].

These experiments revealed that the pattern of incorporation of these precursors closely resembles that of growing tissues. Isotope dilution studies *in vivo* or *in vitro* using suspected intermediates indicated that the incorporation of the precursors into tumor nucleic acid, except in a few rare cases, followed the same pathways as in normal tissues.

The reported growth rates of tumors were sometimes misleading because of the choice of controls. Thus, LePage compared glycine incorporation into the soluble and acid-precipitable fractions of Ehrlich ascites carcinoma and Gardner lymphosarcoma with the incorporation of the same precursors into corresponding fractions of liver. Since the liver cells do not normally proliferate, it was easy to conclude that tumors grow faster than the normal tissues. But, of course, the most adequate control for liver tumors is regenerating rather than normal liver.

Although sketchy reports have appeared indicating that the nucleic acid precursors require energy for incorporation into the polynucleotide, the extensive and elegant studies of Quastel on the relative efficiencies of glycolytic and oxidative energies for protein biosynthesis have no counterpart in the field of nucleic acid biochemistry. There is evidence that ^{32}P incorporation in tumors is reduced in anaerobiosis. LePage's studies have shown that in the absence of oxygen, the incorporation of ^{14}C-labeled glycine and guanadine is reduced in mouse liver cells and in Ehrlich carcinoma cells, but incorporation in the Gardner lymphosarcoma is the same with or without oxygen. In contrast, [^{14}C]glycine incorporation in nucleic acid guanine is not affected by aerobiosis in liver carcinoma or lymphosarcoma cells.

Such data are difficult to interpret and they emphasize the need for more precise investigations of the relative efficiency of the two sources of ATP in nucleic acid biosynthesis.

RNA in Cancer

Most of the studies on RNA metabolism in tumors are concerned with the role of RNA in determining specificity and in controlling the rate of protein synthesis. These aspects of the study on RNA are discussed elsewhere.

In the late 1950s, several reports appeared in which RNA obtained from normal tissue was compared with that of tumors. One of the earliest reports emerged from a study of the carcinogenic effects of X-irradiation. A single dose of X-irradiation to the proper strain of mice is followed, after a latent period, by a high incidence of leukemia. Apparently, such a dose of irradiation also permanently changes the pattern of RNA distribution in the thymus and increases the RNA levels.

De Lamirande and coworkers [388] hydrolyzed RNA obtained from normal tissues and that obtained from tumors and claimed that the proportion of CMP is greater in tumor RNA. These findings did not agree with observations made by Kit, who hydrolyzed RNA obtained from normal and cancerous mouse tissues (spontaneous leukemia, transplanted lymphosarcomas, carcinomas, and medullosarcomas). Kit compared the base composition of RNA with that of DNA and concluded that although higher proportions of guanine and cytosine were consistently found in RNA, there was no convincing difference between tumors and normal tissue RNA.

Kit extended his investigation to the RNA composition of kidney and liver of newborn mice and again found no differences with adult tissues. Furthermore, analytic studies of microsomal and tRNA obtained from various origins, including normal tissues, revealed no difference in the composition of these types of RNA.

Busch and his associate [389] undertook a more sophisticated comparison of RNA of normal growing and tumoral tissue. Busch developed methods of isolating nucleoli which, to be sure, have their limitations; yet these methods have provided reliable information on the composition of the RNA that is firmly bound to that organelle. Busch's laboratory first investigated ^{32}P incorporation in nuclei of normal liver, regenerating liver, and Walker carcinoma and found that the RNA of the nuclei of the Walker tumor had a higher content of guanine and cytosine than the RNA of normal and regenerating liver.

The role of the nucleoli in carcinogenesis will be covered more extensively when we discuss metabolic controls and carcinogenesis.

An analysis of nucleotide composition and oligonucleotide frequencies (di- and trinucleotides) of rRNA extracted from lymphocytes of patients with acute myeloblastic leukemia, acute undifferentiated leukemia, myelocytic leukemia, lymphocytic leukemia, and lymphatic cell lines stimulated with phytohemagglutinin revealed no significant changes in the composition of the rRNA [617]. Whether such a finding will be substantiated in the future when more sophisticated techniques for the analysis of rRNA become available remains to be seen.

Schumm *et al.* [617–618] have described a system for the measurement of the release of nuclear RNA in the form of ribonucleoprotein. Nuclei whose RNA is prelabeled with orotic acid are incubated with dialyzed cytosol reinforced with a source of chemical energy. In this system the transport of RNA is twice as great when regenerating liver cytosol is used, compared to resting liver cytosol. In the cancer cell most of the RNA retained in the nucleus is released. The dialyzed plasma of tumor bearing rats or mice contains substances that stimulate messenger RNA release (80 to 300%) from isolated nuclei incubated with homologous cytosol.

These findings indicate (1) that the dialyzed cytosol contains macromolecules which generate the release of messenger RNA from nuclei to cytoplasm; (2) that there are quantitative differences in the ability of the normal regenerating liver and neoplastic cytosol to effectuate the release of intranuclear messenger RNA; (3) that the "regulatory" macromolecule is released in the plasma of tumor bearing animals.

Further studies of Cholon and Studzinski [619] suggest that neoplastic transformation is associated with some post-transcriptional alteration of messenger RNA which may involve processing and transport or stabilization of the processed RNA in the nucleus or the cytoplasm.

The aminonucleoside of puromycin interferes with the cell cycle of cultured fibroblasts by blocking it in G1 and G2. In contrast, the mitotic cycle of fibroblasts transformed with either SV40 or HeLa cells are affected by the aminonucleoside. The molecular nature of this difference in response to aminonucleoside remains unknown. What is certain is that the inhibitor blocks the appearance of messenger RNA (bound to poly A) in the normal cell, but has no such effect in the neoplastic cell. The coding properties of the excess messenger released in the neoplastic cells are not known, but it is suspected that the released RNA may contain the message for nonhistone proteins that are required to stimulate cell proliferation.

Metabolic Regulation and the Malignant State

Studies of the classical bioenergetic and biosynthetic pathways in cancer tissue reveal two major groups of alterations: one is related to alteration of metabolic regulation, the most typical example being the high anaerobic glycolysis, and the other is related to increased cellular proliferation, typified by increased DNA synthesis. Even those events associated with the second category of change are likely to result from distortions of the mechanism regulating the cell cycle.

During its life cycle, each cell of the mammalian body must adjust to modifications of the host (changes in nutrition, modification of the hormonal balance) and to cyclic modifications of the intracellular environment, such as proliferation and maturation. Biochemists have just begun to study the molecular aspects of regulation of cellular metabolism in quantitative terms.

Cellular metabolism is regulated essentially at three levels, regulation of: (1) the action of multiple-enzyme pathways, (2) gene expression, and (3) the permeability, movement, and social relationships of cell membranes. As mentioned above, the very nature of the cancer cells suggests that distortion of the regulatory mechanism is at the origin of the disease. However, at present there is no clear indication suggesting at which level the distortion takes place—genome, enzyme pathways, or cell membrane. Yet one can hope that a better understanding of the intricacies of regulation of cellular metabolism will open new avenues to our understanding of the pathogenesis of cancer.

We have no intention of reviewing all the work that has recently appeared in the field of metabolic regulations. We simply propose to illustrate the difficulties of the study by describing the complexity of a few of these regulatory events.

Control of Glycolysis

The major function of glucose is to provide the substrate for glycolysis in tissues. For that purpose, glucose needs to be available to all tissues in substantial amounts at all times. Reserves of glucose molecules are stored in a polymeric form of glycogen, which is readily available when needed. New glucose molecules can also be generated from amino acid through reversal of the Krebs cycle and the Embden-Meyerhoff pathway. Thus, the processes of glycolysis and gluconeogenesis function at the same time, and the organism must simultaneously dissimilate and assimilate glucose molecules.

Many biological molecules other than glucose can be diverted into biosynthetic or breakdown pathways, but usually the anabolic and catabolic pathways are entirely different. Glycolysis and gluconeogenesis are unique in that essentially the same pathway is used in one direction for glucose breakdown and in the other for the formation of new glucose molecules.

Although a large segment of the pathways for glucose metabolism are common to glycolysis and gluconeogenesis, a few steps are unique for glucose assimilation or dissimilation. Phosphofructokinase and pyruvic kinase are unique to glycolysis, whereas pyruvic carboxylase, phosphoenolpyruvic carboxykinase, and glucose phosphatase are unique to gluconeogenesis. Thus, the relative activities of the glycolytic versus the glucogenic enzymes determine whether different tissues or one tissue at different times may engage primarily in glucose anabolism or catabolism.

In the sequence of steps that dissimilate glucose to yield pyruvic acid, two steps are unique to glycolysis: the phosphorylation of fructose-6-phosphate to fructose diphosphate and the conversion of phosphoenolpyruvate to pyruvate. These are highly exergonic and relatively irreversible reactions. The first reaction is catalyzed by phosphofructokinase; the second by pyruvate kinase. Although both enzymes are indispensable for glycolysis, only one regulates the rate of glycolysis [390–394].

By methods that will be described later, biochemists have established that phosphofructokinase may be the rate-limiting enzyme in the glycolytic sequence. Consequently, the maximal catalytic capacity of this enzyme is a measure of the potential rate of glycolysis, and a comparison of the actual rate of glycolysis with the maximal catalytic capacity of the phosphofructokinase is a measure of the range of control of glycolysis.

Although metaphors are often a source of confusion, we shall unabashedly indulge in such a literary exercise to clarify the intricacies of the mechanism controlling glycolysis. Glycolysis can be compared to a long, wide channel with only one constriction close to the origin of the channel at the level of the phosphofructokinase reaction. The constriction restricts the overall flux from glucose to pyruvate. On the basis of measurements of the caliber of the constriction and the actual flux, it has become clear that a delicate mechanism capable of tightening and releasing the "sphincter" regulates the flux.

The phosphofructokinase reaction is now believed to be the site of a refined control mechanism regulating the rate of glycolysis. What evidence supports that idea? What molecular interactions are involved in the regulation? We shall try to answer these questions in the following paragraphs.

The most conclusive evidence supporting the regulation of glycolysis at the level of the phosphofructokinase reactions was obtained in crossover experiments. In biochemistry, crossover studies are studies in which intermediates of a pathway are measured during the transition between two steady states. (This, of course, is the technique that was used to identify the site of action of inhibitors on the electron transport chain.)

The usefulness of measuring metabolic intermediates for studying control mechanisms is clearly illustrated by the work of Lowry and associates. These investigators measured the glycolytic intermediates in tissues. However, these intermediates are found in such low concentrations that they are difficult to determine accurately. Lowry took advantage of the fact that all metabolites of the Embden-Meyerhoff pathway, or of the Krebs cycle for that matter, can serve as substrates in reactions that oxidize NADH or NADPH. Thus, the amount of a given substrate can be measured using sensitive enzyme techniques that involve simply spectrophotometric or, even better, fluorometric methods of determining the disappearance of the reduced pyrimidine nucleotide.

One major difficulty with this type of study is the rapid alteration of the concentration of the metabolite pools after anoxemia following death. In the brain, even a few seconds of anoxemia induces drastic changes in the concentration of glycolytic metabolites. Moreover, the conduction of heat in the tissues is so slow that it takes seconds to freeze tissues to a depth of 5 mm, even when the tissue are plunged in liquid air.

The flux of the glycolytic pathway can be altered several ways; it is decreased by oxygen and the addition or injection of fluoroacetate, and it is increased by anaerobiosis. When the flux is increased, all intermediates between fructose-6-diphosphate and lactate are increased, while the levels of glucose-6-phosphate and fructose-6-phosphate (F-6-P) decrease. Thus, a crossover is observed between F-6-P and fructose diphosphate (FDP), suggesting that either F-6-P becomes more readily available to the phosphofructokinase reaction or that the phosphofructokinase is activated.

In addition to the changes in the glycolytic intermediates that follow the installation of anaerobiosis, the levels of ATP decrease and those of AMP increase. Cory was the first to suggest that phosphofructokinase might play a role in the regulation of glycolysis. Aisenberg and Potter [352], who attempted to study the mechanism of the Pasteur effect by adding mitochondria to a reconstituted glycolytic system, concluded that the inhibition of glycolysis in aerobiosis resulted from the inactivation of phosphofructokinase by an intermediate of oxidative phosphorylation. Two years later, Lardy and Parks observed that ATP is a potent inhibitor of muscle phosphofructokinase, a finding which was soon confirmed using phosphofructokinase prepared from various sources. Later it was established that not only ATP but also citrate inhibited phosphofructokinase. A number of metabolites, including AMP, cyclic AMP, ADP, orthophosphate, and fructose-6-phosphate were found to antagonize the inhibitory effects of ATP and citrate.

The results of the crossover experiments and the discovery of the various effects emphasized the regulatory role of phosphofructokinase in glycolysis, and this was naturally followed by the investigation of the molecular mode of action of the effectors.

Kinetic studies of the interactions of various concentrations of ATP and F-6-P suggested that substrate and ATP each bind at different sites of the enzyme. Thus, there are at least two sites on the molecule, a catalytic site and an allosteric regulatory site. This interpretation of the effector's mode of action was further substantiated when the effects of other triphosphate nucleotides—GTP and ITP—on the phosphofructokinase reaction were investigated. Whereas low concentrations of GTP and ITP facilitate the phosphofructokinase reaction in the same way that ATP does, high concentrations of the alternate triphosphates are without effect on the phosphofructokinase reaction, indicating that ITP and GTP bind to the catalytic site but not to the regulatory site.

Further investigations of the mode of action of the various effector substances on phosphofructokinase led to the conclusion that all inhibitors act by reducing the K_m of F-6-P and, consequently, the F-6-P concentrations influence the effectiveness of the effectors. Since the regulatory efficiency of an effector decreases as the concentration of F-6-P increases, the substrate of the phosphofructokinase reaction is important in regulating the enzyme's activity. For example, in the transition from aerobiosis to anaerobiosis, the increase in the F-6-P concentration which ensues decreases the inhibitory effect of ATP.

It is not known whether in mammalian tissues the phosphofructokinase molecule is altered when passing from a less active to a more active form. Phosphorylation of the enzyme or reversible aggregation or disaggregation has been suggested to affect the transformation of a less active to a more active molecule.

Monsam has investigated the properties of phosphofructokinase in *Fasciola hepatica* and shown that the enzyme exists in two forms, active and subactive; the subactive enzyme sediments at 5.5 S, the active enzyme at 12.8 S. Activation by serotonin or cyclic AMP in the presence of ATP involves polymerization. A similar mechanism has been proposed but not convincingly established for the mammalian enzyme [395].

Pasteur Effect

Regulation at the level of the phosphofructokinase reaction has also been invoked to explain the Pasteur effect. In his studies on yeast fermentation, Pasteur discovered that oxygen depresses the fermentation of glucose. Ever since, biochemists have looked for a satisfactory explanation of the Pasteur effect. In anaerobiosis, glucose is oxidized to pyruvic acid, and lactic acid is formed. In aerobiosis, pyruvic acid is further oxidized through the Krebs cycle and, consequently, the Krebs cycle is much more efficient in producing ATP than the Embden-Meyerhoff pathway.

The theories on the mechanism of the Pasteur effect are of three types: (1) oxygen inactivation of the glycolytic enzymes, (2) accumulation of inhibitors of the glycolytic pathway, and (3) competition between aerobic and anaerobic processes for common intermediates or coenzymes.

Inhibition of the glycolytic process by oxygen has been demonstrated with redox dyes and with molecular oxygen *in vitro*. Oxygen is believed to reversibly oxidize the SH groups of the triphosphate dehydrogenase. However, there is no conclusive evidence establishing that such a reaction takes place *in vivo*.

The occurrence of the Pasteur effect has been explained on the basis of competition between aerobic and anaerobic processes for inorganic phosphate, ADP, or NAD.

In 1941 Lynen and Johnson and associates [396, 397] independently proposed that the Pasteur effect resulted from competition for inorganic phosphate and ADP. According to that theory, the lack of ADP and P_i that follows installation of aerobiosis is responsible for inhibiting the triose phosphate dehydrogenase reaction. This theory implies that the intracellular levels of ATP are much higher in aerobic respiration than in anaerobic glycolysis. Consequently, one would anticipate that reactions that required ATP would be accelerated in aerobiosis. In fact, glucose phosphorylation by hexokinase was found to be decreased under aerobic conditions.

To explain this inconsistency in the theory, investigators proposed that the ATP formed in aerobiosis is inaccessible to hexokinase because the ATP is concentrated in the mitochondria. Such an explanation is not very satisfactory because mitochondrial ATP can be used in a number of extramitochondrial ATP-requiring reactions, and there is no obvious reason for its ineffectiveness in the hexokinase reaction. Supporting the theory invoking competition for ATP was the fact that DNP, which uncouples oxidative phosphorylation and thus prevents the formation of ATP without interfering with respiration, is without effect on the rate of glycolysis.

NADH can be oxidized in numerous reactions, including the triose phosphate dehydrogenase reaction and respiration. Competition between glycolysis and respiration for the reduced pyrimidine was also invoked to explain the Pasteur effect. In such a case, uncouplers of oxidative phosphorylation should also depress glycolysis since they do not interfere with respiration.

The most plausible explanation for the Pasteur effect appears to be the one that proposes that in aerobiosis, substances which inhibit glycolysis accumulate. We have already stated that Aisenberg and Potter [352] concluded that the Pasteur effect resulted from the accumulation of an inhibitor formed during aerobic phosphorylation which acted at the site of the phosphofructokinase. These investigators used an ingenious system in which the Pasteur effect was reconstructed by adding liver mitochondria to brain or tumor glycolytic systems. These studies were criticized because it seemed unlikely that an effect identical to the Pasteur effect, as it occurs in living cells, could be produced in such a system. The mitochondria had been shown to inhibit glycolysis even under anaerobic conditions, and it was suspected that the effect of the mitochondria on the glycolytic system resulted from their ATPase content. Yet, it would now appear that a convenient way to interpret Potter's results is to assume that in aerobiosis the ATP accumulation results in the inhibition of phosphofructokinase. Whether or not enough cytoplasmic ATP is trapped to explain the decrease in hexokinase activity observed in aerobiosis is not known; however, such a possibility is unlikely since there is no interference with other ATP-requiring reactions.

A more likely explanation of the effect of aerobiosis on hexokinase is based on observations indicating that in aerobiosis, inhibitors also accumulate that block glucose transport or the hexokinase reaction. These experiments established that the depression of glycolysis by oxygen was not associated with the depletion of ADP or inorganic phosphate, but with an increase in fructose phosphate. Thus, aerobiosis leads to the inhibition of phosphofructokinase. This results in the accumulation of F-6-P and glucose-6-phosphate (G-6-P). G-6-P is known to inhibit the ascites cell hexokinase activity. However, it does not affect the activity of yeast hexokinase, and it has therefore been proposed that in yeast, G-6-P interferes with glucose transport.

However, if the G-6-P concentration increases, an increase in the pentose phosphate shunt should be expected as well. Yet this does not occur. No explanation for this is available at present.

Crabtree Effect

When high concentrations of glucose are added to ascites cells, cellular respiration decreases. This effect, which in some way is the reverse of the Pasteur effect, is called the Crabtree effect. But to refer to the Crabtree effect as if it were the reversal of the Pasteur effect is unfortunate because this implies that an identical mechanism is involved in both effects.

The availability of glucose would increase the levels of G-6-P and F-6-P provided that neither the hexokinase reaction nor glucose transport is rate limiting. High concentrations of fructose-6-phosphate would abolish the effectiveness of ATP inhibition on phosphofructokinase and thereby increase the glycolytic flux.

But how does glycolysis affect respiration? An increased rate of glycolysis is associated with rapid utilization of cytoplasmic ADP and P_i and increased levels ATP, which are bound to depress respiration.

Thus although the same biochemicals (ATP, ADP, and P_i) are responsible for the Crabtree and the Pasteur effects, the fundamental mechanism in eliciting these effects maybe different. In the Crabtree effect, the central event is an allosteric effect on phosphofructokinase.

Though this theory would explain why the Crabtree effect manifests itself even in the presence of iodoacetate, it does not satisfactorily explain why deoxyglucose can elicit a Crabtree effect and why the Crabtree effect is not relieved by the addition of pyruvate. These objections have been answered by assuming that deoxyglucose can generate the formation of NADPH; as for pyruvate, it is rapidly reduced to lactate in the presence of NADH. The mechanism of the Crabtree effect is discussed in the next section.

Hexokinase Regulation

Although the role of phosphofructokinase in controlling glycolysis is now well established, other steps in the glycolytic pathway could act as pacesetters. One of these steps is the hexokinase reaction. Glucose phosphorylation is a strong exergonic reaction that is virtually irreversible. It is located at the origin of the glycolytic pathway and could constitute an appropriate site for metabolic control. Still, all the evidence for the regulation of glycolysis at the level of the hexokinase reaction is of an indirect nature.

It has been proposed that in addition to its catalytic binding site for G-6-P, hexokinase contains an allosteric site for the binding of G-6-P molecules; the allosteric site is involved in regulating the enzyme activity. In addition, hexokinase is believed to have another binding site for orthophosphate molecules that modulate the inhibitory effect of G-6-P. Whether these regulatory mechanisms function *in vivo* is not certain.

Hexokinase phosphorylates glucose, and therefore competition between glycolysis and respiration for the substrates could explain the Crabtree effect. Chance and his associates have proposed that the addition of glucose to a suspension of ascites cells is followed by a rapid release of ADP, which results in a short increase of the rate of respiration. When all the ADP is converted into ATP, respiration slows down because of intramitochondrial ATP accumulation.

Another possibility that has been invoked to explain the Crabtree effect is that in some way the changes in pH that result from the lactic acid accumulation in cells inhibit the respiratory chain.

In ascites cells, the oxidation of fats appears to be primarily responsible for endogenous respiration. Therefore, it has been proposed that adding glucose to the ascites cells stimulates the hexose monophosphate shunt, which leads to the formation of extra NADPH. As a result, fatty acid synthesis is stimulated. Competition between the anabolism and catabolism of fatty acids is thought to be responsible for the decrease in the rate of respiration.

Cori and his associates [398] have devoted much effort to explain why the rate of glycolysis increases suddenly when the muscles contract anaerobically, and why glycolysis ceases as soon as the muscle relaxes. For that purpose, they stimulated electrically frog sartorii incubated in an anaerobic Ringer solution. These experiments clearly established that the conversion of glycogen to lactic acid provided the chemical energy needed for contraction. Glycogenolysis seems to be controlled at the level of the phosphorylase reaction, which catalyzes glycogen breakdown to yield glucose phosphate and P_i. Glycolysis appears to be controlled at the level of phosphofructokinase.

After stimulation, the activities of these two enzymes, phosphorylase and phosphofructokinase, increase simultaneously. However, measurements of intermediates in stimulated and relaxed muscle suggested that the changes were too small to explain the observed enzyme changes. Among the glycolytic intermediates, only the concentrations of lactate and glycerophosphate could be correlated with the rates of muscular activity. The levels of G-6-P, F-6-P, and fructose-1,6-diphosphate could not be correlated with the changes in enzyme activities. Thus, although these experiments have pointed toward phosphorylase and phosphofructokinase as the site of the control mechanism, they have not provided evidence of the mechanism that regulates their activity.

To reconcile the modern findings on the regulation of phosphofructokinase *in vitro* with the findings *in vivo*, Cori has invoked compartmentalization of the glycolytic enzyme, possibly in the muscle sarcoplasm.

The control of glycolysis has also been studied in the lens, which has an unusual source of chemical energy. In the lens, the aerobic phase of glucose plays only a minimal role in the production of ATP, which is generated primarily through glycolysis. The terminal metabolite of glycolysis is lactate, which can be eliminated only by diffusion, a slow process in the dense lenticular tissues. Thus, some mechanism must regulate glucose utilization so that enough ATP is generated without leading to deleterious changes in intracellular pH as a result of lactic acid accumulation. Again, the control sites seem to be located at the levels of the hexokinase and phosphofructokinase reactions. Thus, as ATP accumulates, it inhibits phosphofructokinase and fructose-6-phosphate accumulates. The ready reversibility of the isomerase reaction rapidly converts the F-6-P into G-6-P, which inhibits hexokinase and thereby limits the overall rate of glycolysis.

Hexokinase is also activated by citrate and other physiological anions. The mechanism by which hexokinase activity is altered by glucose 6-phosphate is not known. While in yeast hexokinase a slow conformation change in the monomer has been invoked [620], in brain hexokinase glucose 6-phosphate alters the conformation of the enzyme which leads to dimerization [621]. The dimerization is reversed by ATP and inorganic phosphate which antagonizes the effects of glucose 6-phosphate.

Gluconeogenesis

Already in 1929 the Coris had established that glucose was synthesized from pyruvic and lactic acids in mammalian organisms. Gluconeogenesis, or the synthesis of glucose or other hexose derivatives from molecules containing five carbon atoms or less, was from the start recognized to be of considerable physiological importance. One reason gluconeogenesis is such an important physiological phenomenon is that the functioning of the central nervous system depends on the maintenance of adequate concentrations of glucose in blood.

The importance of gluconeogenesis in overall metabolism is further emphasized by the appearance of the process during development. Although fetal dog liver slices are unable to convert alanine, glutamate, and CO_2 into glucose, chicken liver slices are capable of gluconeogenesis at a very early stage of development. The reason for this difference can probably be explained on the basis of glucose availability. The fetal dog receives glucose from the mother through the placenta; in contrast, in the chick embryo, the glucose reserves are depleted within 8 or 10 days after incubation, so the liver must provide new glucose molecules through gluconeogenesis. Gluconeogenesis is also indispensable for the maintenance of muscle glycogen levels. In mammals, gluconeogenesis occurs mainly in liver and kidney.

Under normal conditions of activity and nutrition, only small amounts of glucose are synthesized from smaller carbon units. However, gluconeogenesis can be activated considerably under some specific physiological and pathological conditions.

We have already discussed in Chapter IV some of the relationships between protein metabolism and gluconeogenesis. Amino acids are the major source of gluconeogenic precursors. The amino acids are released by muscle tissue and absorbed by the intestine. The amino acids are extracted by the liver. The major amino acid to flow from muscle to liver is alanine. The alanine is then converted to pyruvate by a transaminase [622]. Cori has shown that heavy work produces in muscle large amounts of lactic acid; this is transported to the liver, where 3-carbon compounds can be used for glucose synthesis. Fasting, not necessarily prolonged, leads to the breakdown of proteins in their constitutive amino acids and the release of glycerol from triglycerides. The amino acids can be used after deamination by reversal of the Krebs cycle and at least part of the glycolytic cycle for the biosynthesis of glucose molecules. Hormones from the adrenal medulla and cortex influence protein mobilization for gluconeogenesis. Protein gluconeogenesis is accelerated in diabetes, but is practically nonexistent in patients with Addison's disease.

For several decades it was believed that biosynthetic pathways occurred through the reversal of the catabolic pathways. In gluconeogenesis, it was assumed that the biosynthesis of glucose from smaller carbon units took place simply by reversal of the steps of the Krebs cycle and glycolysis. This assumption failed to recognize the thermodynamic incompatibilities of the reversible process.

Our modern understanding of the control of gluconeogenesis started when Sir Hanz Krebs showed investigators that three steps of the glycolytic pathway are strongly exergonic and virtually irreversible under physiological conditions. Those steps are: (1) the phosphorylation of glucose to glucose-6-phosphate by hexokinase, (2) the phosphorylation of fructose-6-phosphate to fructose-1,6-diphosphate by phosphofructokinase, and (3) the reaction catalyzed by pyruvic kinase. Once the thermodynamic limitations of the reversal of the glycolytic pathway were accepted, investigators started to look for new reactions that could reverse these three steps and thus were strongly endergonic in the direction of glucose synthesis.

Three enzymes are specific to the glucogenic process—pyruvic carboxylase, fructose diphosphatase, and glucose-6-phosphatase. Inasmuch as all other steps of gluconeogenesis are, in fact, reversals of glycolysis, it can be anticipated that: (1) a delicate control mechanism determines whether an intermediate is channeled in either the anabolic or catabolic pathway; and (2) the molecular control of gluconeogenesis is exerted at the level of one of the three enzymes specific for gluconeogenesis. However, in discussing the control of gluconeogenesis, we must distinguish between long-range changes in enzyme activity (such as those that take place in alloxan diabetes; for example, when the enzymes specific for glycolysis decrease while those specific for gluconeogenesis increase) and the acute changes in gluconeogenesis. The long-range change takes sometimes days or weeks, while the acute changes occur practically instantaneously. Whereas the long-range effects probably result from alterations in the concentration of enzyme molecules, the short-range alterations come about through the regulation of enzyme activity. Only the acute changes will be discussed here.

Properties of the Enzymes Involved in Gluconeogenesis

Before we describe the experiments that led to the conclusion that the site of control of gluconeogenesis is determined at the level of the phosphocarboxykinase reaction, it might be helpful to remind the reader of the molecular properties of pyruvic carboxylase, fructose diphosphatase, and glucose-6-phosphatase that make these enzymes good candidates for control sites. Studies on pyruvic carboxylase purified from chicken liver established that the enzyme contains a biotin-bound prosthetic group and requires acetyl CoA and magnesium for activity. The enzyme catalyzes a typical two-step, biotin-dependent carboxylation.

Two molecular properties of the enzyme are compatible with potential regulatory mechanisms: CoA activates pyruvic carboxylase and carboxylase is inhibited by ADP. Without CoA, pyruvic carboxylase disintegrates in the cold. Therefore, acetyl CoA has been assumed to strengthen the bonds between subunits of the enzyme. This activation of the carboxylase by CoA associated with the aggregation of subunits may be of considerable significance with respect to the control of gluconeogenesis.

The product of the carboxylase reaction is oxaloacetate. If the enzyme's activity is low, the level of oxaloacetate decreases. Inasmuch as oxaloacetate is indispensable for the oxidation of other intermediates in the Krebs cycle, the product of fatty acid oxidation, mainly acetyl CoA, cannot enter the Krebs cycle without oxaloacetate. Consequently, low carboxylase activity associated with low oxaloacetate concentrations leads to the accumulation of acetyl CoA, making CoA accessible for carboxylase activation. Increased activity of the carboxylase raises the rate of synthesis of oxaloacetate and activates the Krebs cycle, thus producing the intermediates for gluconeogenesis.

ADP inhibits pyruvic carboxylase and the inhibition is competitive with ATP. Nevertheless, the physiological significance of the effects of CoA and ADP on the carboxylase remains to be established.

A number of effectors are known to alter the activity of fructose diphosphatase. AMP noncompetitively inhibits the enzyme, and ATP converts it from an active to an inactive form. When purified enzyme is incubated with AMP, the protein binds reversibly three moles of AMP per mole of enzyme. The binding of AMP is believed to occur at allosteric sites because partial digestion of the enzyme with papain decreases the sensitivity of AMP inhibition without altering the enzyme's catalytic activity.

The diphosphatase exists in active and inactive forms. Fructose diphosphate and F-6-P partially inhibit while ATP induces the conversion of active diphosphatase to an inactive form. Again, the role of AMP and ATP on diphosphatase activity *in vivo* is not known, but while 5′-AMP and F-6-P inhibit fructose diphosphatase, the same substances activate phosphofructokinase.

If glucose-6-phosphatase and hexokinase functioned at the same time and at the same sites in the cell, no G-6-P would ever be available because it would be broken down as soon as it was formed. I have already mentioned that the hexokinase and the glucose-6-phosphatase are located at different sites in the cell, and it is thus possible, under conditions favoring glycolysis, that glucose-6-phosphate is not available to the glucose-6-phosphatase. In addition to the fact that the activity of glucose-6-phosphatase may be regulated by its association with the endoplasmic reticulum, some special molecular properties of the enzyme could also provide regulatory mechanisms for its activity. Glucose-6-phosphatase undoubtedly regulates the glucose level *in vivo*. In von Gierke's disease, which is characterized by absence or low level of glucose-6-phosphatase, there is hypoglycemia in addition to glycogen accumulation in liver and kidney.

Like crotonase, glucose-6-phosphate seems to be a multifunctional enzyme. It can catalyze: (1) the hydrolysis of pyrophosphate, (2) the phosphorylation of glucose to G-6-P in the presence of pyrophosphate, (3) the hydrolysis of G-6-P to glucose and P_i, and (4) the transphosphorylation of labeled glucose to the phosphate of an unlabeled G-6-P molecule yielding labeled G-6-P plus unlabeled glucose. Thus, the enzyme appears to combine with pyrophosphate, P_i, and sugar phosphate.

The interrelation of the various reactions catalyzed by glucose-6-phosphatase has been summarized in a scheme first described by Stetten and by Nordlie and Arion and summarized by Stadtman [393]. In this scheme, the hydrolysis of the pyrophosphate involves the binding of the enzyme with pyrophosphate. This step is followed by the release of one P_i molecule and the formation of a phosphoryl enzyme derivative, which is further hydrolyzed to release the enzyme and another molecule of P_i. Similarly, the hydrolysis of G-6-P first involves the binding of enzyme and sugar phosphate, followed by the release of the sugar and the formation of the phosphoryl enzyme derivative, which again is hydrolyzed to yield the enzyme and another molecule of P_i.

In this scheme, the formation of phosphoryl enzyme derivative is a common intermediate in the hydrolysis of pyrophosphate and G-6-P. It is believed that the pyrophosphate and glucose compete for the same catalytic site, and therefore the relative concentrations of pyrophosphate and glucose determine whether pyrophosphate or glucose phosphate is hydrolyzed. Whether such interpretations are relevant to the control of gluconeogenesis *in vivo* remains to be established.

Regulation of Gluconeogenesis

Several laboratories [399–401], including those of Lardy, Krebs, and Weber, have provided direct evidence for the *in vivo* control of gluconeogenesis. Some of the most interesting experiments on the control of gluconeogenesis were done in Lardy's [399] laboratory in Wisconsin. Lardy provided convincing evidence that the pyruvic carboxylase reaction constitutes the major site of control for gluconeogenesis and eliminated the possibility of a role for the malic enzyme in gluconeogenesis.

Maximal catalytic capacities of enzymes unique to gluconeogenesis are found in liver and kidney, yet small levels of enzyme activities may be found in non-gluconeogenic tissues such as brain, heart, and muscle. Three pathways can yield phosphoenolpyruvate from pyruvate: (1) the reaction of pyruvate plus ATP in the presence of pyruvate kinase, yielding ADP and phosphoenolpyruvate, (2) the reaction of pyruvate plus CO_2 in the presence of NADPH and malic enzyme to yield NADP and L-malate (malate will then, in the presence of malic dehydrogenase and NADH, yield oxaloacetate), and (3) the reaction of pyruvate plus CO_2 in the presence of ATP and pyruvic carboxylase to yield ATP plus P_i and oxaloacetate. The oxaloacetate is converted to phosphoenolpyruvate in the presence of GTP and phosphoenolpyruvate carboxykinase. GDP and CO_2 are byproducts of the reaction. The K_m values of pyruvic kinase for pyruvate largely exceed the probable concentration of the substrate in the cell.

Lardy and his associates studied the activity of phosphoenolpyruvic carboxykinase, pyruvic carboxylase, and the malic enzymes under a number of physiological or pathological conditions that are known to stimulate gluconeogenesis. Such conditions include fasting; lactate administration; injection of hormones, glucocorticoids, and glucagon; induction of diabetes (alloxan, mannoheptulose, pancreatectomy). The activity of the phosphoenolpyruvate carboxykinase is increased within 2 to 4 hours after installation of diabetes or the administration of hormones or lactate. Glucocorticoid administration has no effect on the pyruvic carboxylase, whereas the activity of the malic enzyme in livers of fasted and diabetic rats decreases. Such experiments convincingly establish that phosphoenolpyruvic carboxykinase modulates the rate of gluconeogenesis.

Lardy and his associates further provided direct evidence that the malic enzyme is not involved in gluconeogenesis. The levels of phosphoenolpyruvic carboxykinase and malic enzyme return to normal after a mixed diet is administered. However, if artificial diets are administered, the response of the activity of the malic enzyme varies considerably in the following ways: (1) the malic enzyme does not increase after the administration of a carbohydrate-free diet, (2) malic enzyme increases considerably with a diet rich in carbohydrates and devoid of fat, and (3) if corn oil is added to the high-carbohydrate diet, the malic enzyme activity drops.

Such findings led Lardy to suggest that the malic enzyme functions in some ways in relation to fats. Lardy visualized this role of the malic enzyme in fat synthesis in the following manner. The citrate produced in the Krebs cycle inside the mitochondria leaks out in the cytosol. In the presence of CoA and ATP and citrate cleavage, enzyme citrate yields two products: acetyl CoA and oxaloacetate. Acetyl CoA is used for fatty acid biosynthesis; oxaloacetate is either converted to phosphoenolpyruvate or reduced to malate in the presence of NADH and malate dehydrogenase. The malate in the presence of NADP and malic enzyme yields pyruvate, CO_2, and NADPH. Pyruvate returns to the Krebs cycle; the NADPH is used for fatty acid synthesis. The generation of NADPH by the malic enzyme in adipose tissue may be necessary for lipid synthesis since several investigators have established that the NADPH generated by glucose-6-phosphate and 6-phosphogluconate is not in keeping with the rate of lipid synthesis in adipose tissues.

In rat liver, pyruvic carboxylase is found in mitochondria. Yet, the phosphoenolpyruvate carboxykinase is found in the cytosol. Thus, two consecutive steps in gluconeogenesis are located in different compartments of the cell. This situation is further complicated by the fact that the oxaloacetate generated inside the mitochondria does not diffuse into the cytosol. The oxaloacetate that is formed inside the mitochondria under the influence of pyruvic carboxylase does not accumulate but either reacts with acetyl CoA or is transformed into malate by reduction or aspartate by transamination.

Elegant experiments in Lardy's laboratory have clarified this puzzling situation. The investigators added radioactive bicarbonate to isolated mitochondria and found that labeled malate, citrate, α-ketoglutarate, and fumarate, but not oxaloacetate, appear in the cytosol. Furthermore, when ammonia or glutamine was added to the incubation mixture, substantial amounts of radioactive aspartate also appeared in the cytosol. It was established that the intermediates that appear in the cytosol retained the radioactive bicarbonate. Consequently, they could not be derived from the oxaloacetate that is generated through the Krebs cycle, so they had to be formed by carboxylation of pyruvic acid through the pyruvic carboxylase reaction.

The oxaloacetate formed in the pyruvic carboxylase reaction and which contains the labeled CO_2 yields by reduction a molecule of labeled malate which can then generate labeled intermediates of the Krebs cycle. Since the mitochondrial membrane is permeable to these intermediates, they leak out into the cytosol. There the malate by reduction and the amino acid by transamination regenerate oxaloacetate, which in the presence of GTP and pyruvic carboxykinase yields phosphoenolpyruvate. In keeping with this concept is the existence of two different glutamate oxaloacetate transaminases—one in mitochondria and one in the cytosol. Furthermore, the activities of the glutamic transaminases are enhanced in conditions that favor gluconeogenesis, such as hydrocortisone administration, fasting, and alloxan diabetes. The situation in the rat is somewhat unique. Indeed, in several other animals, pyruvic carboxylase is found in the cytosol, and the complex mechanism of transfer from mitochondria to cytosol need not be invoked.

From this scheme, one can visualize a number of molecular events that could influence the pyruvic carboxylase and the pyruvic carboxykinase reactions. A high ATP/ADP ratio would favor carboxylation. In fact, if a phosphate acceptor system is added to the mitochondria, the amount of fixed CO_2 is moderately reduced, suggesting that extramitochondrial processes requiring ATP, such as the hexokinase reaction, compete effectively with the intramitochondrial pyruvic carboxylase for mitochondrial ATP. Inasmuch as the oxaloacetate produced in the mitochondria in the pyruvic carboxylase reaction needs to be reduced to malate before it can pass the mitochondrial barrier, a high NADH/NAD ratio inside of the mitochondria would seem to favor gluconeogenesis.

Pyrimidine nucleotides in mitochondria are in a relatively reduced state only when a phosphate acceptor is lacking and, consequently, when the ATP/ADP ratio is high.

Also, the levels of free fatty acids may regulate the rate of gluconeogenesis in liver and kidney. Evidence suggests that the effect of free fatty acids is not restricted to the activation of pyruvic carboxylase by acetyl CoA but also manifests itself at several other metabolic sites. In 1963 Wheeland and his associates had shown that fatty acyl CoA thioester inhibited citrate synthetase and explained ketogenesis on that basis. Lardy suggested that the inhibition of citrate synthetase also forces oxaloacetate into the reductive pathway and leads to the formation of malate and aspartic acid, which are used for gluconeogenesis.

Williamson and associates [402] established that when fatty acids were added to isolated perfused rat livers, fatty acids stimulated gluconeogenesis from 3-carbon precursors. The enhanced gluconeogenesis observed after glucagon administration was interpreted to result from its lipolytic effect. Indeed, glucagon stimulates the formation of cyclic AMP by adenylic cyclase, and cyclic AMP activates the mobilization of free fatty acids and glycerol from triglyceride in liver and adipose tissue. In liver, the free fatty acids are either reesterified to yield triglyceride or oxidized to yield acetyl CoA, acetoacetate, and β-hydroxybutyrate. The increased level of acetyl CoA not only seems to activate pyruvic carboxylase, but it also inhibits pyruvic decarboxylation and the biosynthesis of malonyl CoA and citrate (through inhibiting citrate synthetase). Thus, it would seem that most of the pyruvate would be forced into the oxaloacetate pathway, and the oxaloacetate would have to be reduced to malate since it cannot be used for citrate biosynthesis. In addition, Weber's work suggests that free fatty acids inhibit the activity of the enzymes unique to glycolysis. Thus, the availability of free fatty acids seems to act as a three-way switch, which, once turned on, inhibits the conversion of oxaloacetate to citrate, enhances the conversion of pyruvate to oxaloacetate, and reduces the glycolytic flux. As a result, the effect of the fatty acid tilts the metabolic balance in the direction of gluconeogenesis.

Glucose administration to fasted rats depresses the activity of pyruvic carboxykinase. If glucose and puromycin are administered simultaneously, the depressive effect of glucose is abolished, suggesting that protein synthesis is needed for glucose to express its effect on enzyme activity.

Let's return to the original question that we raised at the beginning of this chapter. What is the mechanism for the increase in activity in the acute state? We will give special consideration to the effect of adrenocortical hormones on gluconeogenesis. Although it cannot entirely be excluded that the adrenocortical hormones stimulate the formation of RNA and thereby the formation of new proteins and possibly new enzyme molecules, this event is unlikely since Lardy has shown that hydrocortisone stimulates gluconeogenesis in normal and adrenalectomized rats, even though enzyme induction was prevented by actinomycin. In considering this hormonal effect, one must keep in mind, however, that adrenocortical hormones can stimulate, within an hour or two after administration, the biosynthesis of tryptophan pyrrolase, and tyrosine transaminase.

Studies of gluconeogenesis in isolated hepatocytes might help to further clarify the kinetics of gluconeogenesis [623]. Assays of concentrations of different gluconeogenic substrates were studied with preparations of liver cells. The rate of gluconeogenesis was found to vary with the concentration of the substrate. Low concentrations of glyceraldehyde (1.5 mM) stimulated gluconeogenesis. Concentrations above 1.5 mM inhibited gluconeogenesis. In contrast, dihydroxyacetone is maximally converted at concentrations of 1.5 mM, but continues to be converted albeit at a slower rate at high concentrations. D-fructose was converted at a constant rate up to concentrations of 11.3 mM. Alanine, the major amino acid source of gluconeogenesis, was converted slowly; pyruvate was converted at a rate intermediate between that of the amino acid and the trioses. cAMP stimulated gluconeogenesis from dihydroxyacetone (30%), but had relatively little effect when lactate and pyruvate were used as substrates.

The findings of the usage of the various substrates in isolated hepatic cells are at present difficult to relate to the regulation of gluconeogenesis *in vivo* because the concentrations of the substrates *in vivo* are not known and the isolated hepatocyte might not respond identically to liver cells *in situ*. For example, although the isolated hepatocyte seems to respond to glucagon, the response is inconsistent.

Control of Glycogen Metabolism

Two enzymes are believed to play a key role in glycogen metabolism—phosphorylase and glycogen synthetase, or UDP-glycogen glycosyl transferase. The mechanism controlling the activity of these two enzymes is so complex that, as Larner pointed out, it is sometimes reminiscent of the mechanism controlling blood coagulation. Phosphorylase exists in two major forms: phosphorylase B and phosphorylase A. Phosphorylase B is the less active form and is absolutely dependent upon the presence of 5′-AMP for activity. Under some conditions, 5′-AMP activates phosphorylase A, but it is not indispensable for the activity of the A form of the enzyme. We shall consider here three major aspects of the regulation of phosphorylase activity: (1) the regulation of the activity of phosphorylase B; (2) the regulation of the conversion of phosphorylase B to phosphorylase A; and (3) some pathological implications of the phosphorylase activity control.

The effectors of phosphorylase B can be classified as activators, modulators, and inhibitors. 5′-AMP activates the enzyme by reducing the K_m for the formation of the complex between enzyme and substrates (P_i and glycogen). The effect of 5′-AMP can be modulated positively or negatively. ATP and glucose-6-phosphate act antagonistically toward the effect of AMP, while glucose-1-phosphate acts synergetically with AMP. Consequently, as the precursors of glycolysis (glucose, etc.) increase, the activity of phosphorylase B decreases. In contrast, the precursor of glycogen (glucose-1-phosphate) reduces the rate at which glycogen is broken down.

GTP, 6-phosphogluconate, NADH, malate, UDP-glucose, and phosphoenolpyruvate inhibit the activities of phosphorylase A and B. When the products of the hexose monophosphate shunt, the glucuronic pathway, or the gluconeogenic pathway accumulate, glycogen breakdown is inhibited.

We have already discussed in some detail the molecular changes that take place when phosphorylase B is converted to phosphorylase A, the independent form of phosphorylase. Phosphorylase B can be converted into phosphorylase A in three ways. One is an enzyme mechanism involving a specific kinase, ATP, and magnesium; the second involves a protein of an unknown nature and calcium; and the third involves partial hydrolysis with trypsin.

The activity of the kinase system can be modified in a number of ways. There are several activators, the most efficient of which is 3′,5′-cyclic AMP, generated under the influence of epinephrine and glucagon. The activity of the kinase system also seems to be stimulated by glycogen and heparin. These activations of the kinase result from the conversion of an inactive into an active form. At least in liver, there is at present no indication that this conversion involves dimerization of monomers. The most likely mechanism is that conformational changes occur in the protein molecules.

The second mechanism of activation involves calcium and an unknown protein sometimes referred to as KAF (kinase-activating factor). The protein has not been identified, and little is known about its mechanism of action. There are at least three possibilities concerning the protein's mode of action: it could act as an enzyme and exhibit catalytic properties, it could provide a structural support for all the factors involved in converting phosphorylase B into phosphorylase A; or it could act like a coenzyme and combine stoichiometrically with the kinase. The difference between these types of mechanism is of considerable importance because epinephrine stimulates the first of these three mechanisms by stimulating the generation of 3′,5′-cyclic AMP. In contrast, electrical stimulation of the frog sartorius muscles probably stimulates the conversion of phosphorylase B into phosphorylase A by the effect of calcium and the unknown protein.

The elucidation of the mechanisms controlling glycogen breakdown has provided an explanation for the pathogenesis of some symptoms in anoxemia and glycogen storage disease. In anoxemia, the rate of glycogenolysis in the heart is high, and this occurs in the absence of a conversion of phosphorylase B to phosphorylase A. The special situation can be explained by the difference in the ratio of AMP (which obviously increases after anoxemia) over ATP (which decreases). The decreasing ATP levels are associated with decreases in G-6-P concentration and increases in P_i, all changes in the steady state which influence the rate of glycogenolysis.

Again, AMP activates phosphorylase B while ATP is an inhibitor. In von Gierke's disease, glycogen accumulates in the liver as a result of the block of glycogenolysis.

Studies in a number of rat tissues (liver, kidney, skeletal muscle, heart, and brain) regarding the relative activities of glycogen synthesis and glycogen breakdown have revealed that the capacity for breakdown exceeds that for synthesis in all tissues. Yet under some conditions, glycogen is actively synthesized in liver, skeletal muscle, and heart (and to a much lesser degree in kidney and brain where glycogen metabolism is usually low). Although there is no good explanation for these tendencies of various tissues to favor breakdown, it indicates that a delicate mechanism controlling the relative rates of breakdown and synthesis must exist.

We have seen that the activation of glycogenolysis involves a central event, the conversion of an inactive to an active phosphorylase. The inactive phosphorylase requires the presence of activators to express its catalytic properties. The activator is not necessary for the active phosphorylase. The mechanism of conversion of the inactive to the active form is a complex one which may vary depending upon the stimulatory effect.

The mechanism controlling the expression of the catalytic activity of glycogen synthetase is reminiscent of that which controls the expression of phosphorylase activity. Thus, like phosphorylase, glycogen synthetase exists in two forms, one relatively inactive (I) and another relatively active (D). The D form of glycogen synthetase is a phosphorylated form of the I form, and it is dependent upon the presence of glucose-6-phosphate for activity. The I form can be converted to the D form by three mechanisms similar to those described for the conversion of phosphorylase B to phosphorylase A: (1) the phosphorylation of I to D in the presence of ATP, magnesium, 3′,5′-cyclic AMP, and a specific kinase; (2) the combined effect of calcium and an unknown protein; and (3) partial hydrolysis with trypsin.

Carboxylic acids that are intermediates (e.g., citrate) in glycolysis or the Krebs cycle stimulate the I form of glycogen synthetase. The stimulation occurs even in absence of glucose-6-phosphate. Such stimulation is believed to coordinate the deposition of glycogen in tissues with the levels of activity of glycolysis and that of the Krebs cycle [624].

Glucose-6-phosphate increases the velocity of the D form of the enzyme and, as a result, causes a decrease in the apparent K_m for UDP-glucose. The activator acts at an allosteric site, possibly by inducing conformational changes in the enzyme molecule. Glucose-6-phosphate is known to protect the enzyme activity against the inhibitory effect of parachloromercuric benzoate.

In von Gierke's disease, the amount of glycogen that accumulates in the liver does not exceed three or four times that amount found in normal liver. This finding has long been interpreted by assuming that a negative feedback control existed between the amount of glycogen present in the hepatic cell and the rate of synthesis of the biopolymer. This effect of glycogen is believed to result from inhibition of the conversion of the I into the D form of the glycogen synthetase.

Although both the kinases involved in activating phosphorylase B and glycogen synthetase are stimulated by cyclic AMP, it is not likely that the phosphorylase kinase and the synthetase kinase are identical. Larner purified phosphorylase kinase and showed that the ratio of activity of phosphorylase to that of synthetase could be increased 100-fold.

Regulation of Cholesterol Metabolism

Like glucose, cholesterol in the body has two sources: exogenous, through intestinal absorption, and endogenous, through synthesis in the body. The details of the steps involved in the biosynthesis of cholesterol and many aspects of the regulation of cholesterol metabolism were discussed in the chapter on arteriosclerosis. Only the most salient points will be reviewed here.

Practically every tissue of the body is capable of synthesizing cholesterol. Maximum synthesis occurs in liver; next in line are the cells of the intestinal wall. Minimum levels of synthesis are observed in muscle.

To understand the regulation of cholesterol metabolism, consider various stages: the intestinal, the bloodstream, and the liver stages. The intestinal phase can be divided into two periods: the luminal phase, during which the ingested cholesterol is, in the presence of bile, incorporated into micelles and absorbed in the intestine, and the intracellular phase. The cells of the wall of the intestine participate in cholesterol metabolism in at least two ways: they synthesize new cholesterol molecules from acetate, and they incorporate cholesterol of exogenous and endogenous origin into chylomicrons. Chylomicrons are excreted in the lymph, transported in the bloodstream, and cleared by the liver. The liver participates in cholesterol metabolism in various ways: (1) as mentioned above, it is the major site of *de novo* synthesis of cholesterol; (2) it possesses an enzyme machinery that degrades cholesterol into bile acids; (3) it excretes cholesterol into the biliary system; and (4) it exchanges the cholesterol from exogenous or endogenous origin with extrahepatic pools.

How are the relative rates of absorption, excretion, synthesis, and degradation of cholesterol regulated to achieve homeostasis? Obviously, a delicate feedback loop must connect these various paths of cholesterol metabolism. The most obvious connections have already been identified, but many of the details of the interactions remain to be clarified. Cholesterol and bile acids play key roles in regulating cholesterol metabolism.

An important feedback loop is that which links cholesterol absorption and cholesterol synthesis. The biosynthesis of cholesterol in liver is reduced in cholesterol-fed animals. Cholesterol inhibits its own biosynthesis by interfering with the reduction of β-hydroxy-β-methylglutaryl CoA. However, the feedback inhibition of cholesterol synthesis appears to occur only in liver and not in the intestinal mucosa.

The mechanism regulating the activity of the hepatic β-hydroxy-β-methylglutaryl CoA reductase is intriguing. It seems not to involve allosteric sites on the enzyme; thus, neither cholesterol nor bile acids inhibit the enzyme (although bile contains a β-lipoprotein that irreversibly inactivates HMG-CoA), and the depression in activity is believed to result from depressing a cyclic rise in the reductase without affecting the cyclic decline. The rise is due to enzyme synthesis; therefore, cholesterol must suppress HMG-CoA synthesis. This mode of interference with enzyme activity by modulation of gene expression is lost in hepatomas [403].

All factors that influence cholesterol absorption indirectly affect cholesterol synthesis. Among those factors are the bile acids, which facilitate cholesterol micelle and chylomicron formation. Although it has also been claimed that bile acids inhibit cholesterol biosynthesis in the intestine, such a direct effect has never been convincingly established. What seems certain is that increased concentrations of bile acids in the intestinal lumen inhibit intestinal cholesterol formation, whereas decreased concentrations accentuate it [404].

Coenzymes and Metabolic Regulation

One or several metabolic pathways may also be regulated by adjusting the levels of coenzyme available. We discussed many examples of such regulation in the section on vitamin deficiency. To illustrate the intricacies of such a form of regulation, we shall briefly describe postulated mechanisms regulating nicotinic acid metabolism and, consequently, NAD and NADH formation in various organisms.

The levels of nicotinic acid in a given tissue or in the blood depend on: (1) the balance of the biosynthetic and catabolic pathways, and (2) the usage of nicotinic acid as a precursor of NAD and NADP.

Little is known of the exact site of control of NAD metabolism in organisms, but one can, on the basis of the known pathways, predict the site of action of the control mechanisms. In microorganisms, the immediate preferred precursor of NAD and NADP seems to be nicotinamide, or nicotinic acid (nicotinic acid can be used only if the organism contains the appropriate deaminase). When the vitamin is absent from the growth medium, nicotinic acid is synthesized from tryptophan. When for some reason the tryptophan pathway cannot function, such as in some microorganisms under anaerobic conditions, a more extensive *de novo* pathway takes over, and niacin is synthesized from aspartic acid and glycerol. Niacin is known to inhibit through a negative feedback loop the incorporation of aspartic acid in quinolinic acid in some microorganisms. (There is no evidence that plants can synthesize NAD from tryptophan. In plants the most likely pathway for NAD biosynthesis is through aspartic glycerol condensation with quinolinic acid.)

In animal cells, the aspartic glycerol pathway contributes little or nothing to NAD biosynthesis. The tryptophan pathway exists in liver and kidney exclusively, but it seems to operate only when neither nicotinic acid or nicotinamide is present in the diet. The macromolecular interaction responsible for briniging the tryptophan biosynthetic pathway into gear is not clear. It has been proposed that niacin or nicotinic acid might exert feedback inhibition on the rate-limiting enzymes catalyzing one of the early steps in the sequence of tryptophan conversion to quinolinic acid.

When the vitamin is absent from the diet, many animals can initiate a *de novo* pathway by relieving the inhibition of the existing enzyme or stimulating the synthesis of a new enzyme, and thereby minimizing the risk of deprivation of an essential coenzyme.

Yet in the course of evolution most of the animal cells except those of liver and kidney have lost the ability to synthesize nicotinic acid from tryptophan. All animal cells have lost the *de novo* pathway starting with the aspartic glycerol pathway.

Metabolic Regulation in Cancer Cells

As we shall see in more detail later, gene expression is distorted in the cancer cell in a fashion that provides these cells with survival advantages over the host. Among the manifestations of the distortions of gene expression are anomalies in metabolic regulation; the high aerobic glycolysis is a classical example (albeit its mechanism is not understood). Many other forms of loss of metabolic regulations involving other metabolic pathways have been described. At present generalizations relating distortion of metabolic regulation and the special properties of the cancer cells cannot be made. We must content ourselves to list a few examples here. Others will be described in other sections of this chapter.

In fact, in many cases cancer cell lines have been used to study metabolic regulation and it is not known if the findings are different from what obtains in normal cells.

Sterol biosynthesis is feedback regulated by cholesterol. The rate limiting step in biosynthesis of sterols is the conversion of 3-hydroxy-3-methylglutaryl coenzyme A to mevalonic acid. The enzyme catalyzing the reaction is the HMG-CoA reductase. The loss of feedback inhibition is believed to be characteristic of neoplasia. Kirsten and Watson demonstrated that HMG-CoA activity in a cell line derived from the minimal deviation hepatoma 7288C was responsive to changes in the serum lipoprotein composition. The reductase activity was 4 times lower in cells maintained in a medium poor in lipoproteins than in cells cultured with high levels of lipoproteins. The increase induced by the presence of lipoproteins is not affected by actinomycin, but it is inhibited by cycloheximide, suggesting that the activity of the HMG-CoA is regulated by modulating its biosynthesis at the posttranscriptional level [625].

Similarly, purine biosynthesis is inhibited when cells are incubated with purines probably by either feedback inhibition of the amidophosphoribosyltransferase or 5-phosphoribosyl-1-pyrophosphate synthetase, which are both feedback inhibited by purine nucleotides in cell free systems. Moreover, the added purine, which in the conversion to nucleotides through the salvage pathway utilizes PRPP, and the levels of PRPP may be rate limiting for the *de novo* pathway.

Bagnara *et al.* [627] have attempted to identify which among these three regulatory mechanisms of purine biosynthesis obtains in intact cells, namely, Ehrlich ascitis cells. The level of amidophosphoribosyltransferase is unchanged, but the level of PRPP is decreased as a result of its utilization in the salvage pathway and an inhibition of its synthesis. Again, it is not certain that what obtains for the cancer cells is also true for normal cells.

In the discussion on purine pyrimidine metabolism we have seen that the activities of glutamine-dependent carbamyl phosphate synthetase and orotidine decarboxylase are regulated by product and substrate. Thus, UTP allosterically feedback inhibits and PRPP activates the enzyme activity. Orotidine decarboxylase is inhibited by CMP and UMP. Although both enzymes are under regulatory control, it is not known which of the two regulates the rate of pyrimidine synthesis.

Hoogenraad and Lee [626] have shown that uridine interferes with pyrimidine synthesis in hepatoma cells in culture. The removal of uridine from the medium restores normal levels of pyrimidine synthesis after a period of approximately 8 hours. Restoration is impaired by actinomycin and cycloheximide. Measurement of the activities of enzymes involved in pyrimidine synthesis indicates that orotate phosphoribosyltransferase is the rate limiting enzyme in the biosynthesis of pyrimidine nucleotides. These studies suggest that at least in hepatoma cells the regulation of pyrimidine nucleotide synthesis is affected by the final product UMP, but that the effect of the product is not allosteric, but manifests itself directly at the level of transcription of the rate limiting enzyme. Whether these findings can be extended to normal tissues remains to be established.

Green and Martin have shown that hepatoma cells in continuous culture have an increased rate of *de novo* pathway for purine biosynthesis because the PRPP synthetase has lost its sensitivity to the feedback inhibition by purine or pyrimidine nucleotides [628].

When liver slices are incubated with oxygen for a short period, the rate of glycolysis is markedly increased when the slices are switched to an anaerobic milieu. Such a rate of increase does not occur in tumor, but neither does it in embryonic tissue. This suggests that the alteration of the rate of glycolysis by preincubation of oxygen is linked to the rate of growth. A study of the stimulation of glycolysis by preincubation with oxygen in transplantable hepatomas with various degrees of growth did not support this hypothesis [629].

Regulation of Gene Expression and Differentiation

In the preceding paragraphs, we described changes in enzyme activity which resulted from the modification of properties inherent in the enzyme molecule. They consist of modification of the enzyme's affinity for its substrate as a result of changes in substrate concentration, the presence of competitive or allosteric inhibitors, alteration by effectors, or catalytic modification of the enzyme molecule itself.

Such changes in enzyme activity usually provide rapid but not sustained adaptation to the environment. Sustained adaptation often requires the elaboration of new enzyme molecules and, enzymes being proteins, the machinery involved in gene expression must be put in gear to secure the biosynthesis of new enzyme molecules. Thus, bacteria respond to changes in the environment by expressing or repressing genes involved in the biosynthesis of specific enzyme. The mechanisms regulating the masking and unmasking of genes are at the center of metabolic regulation, not only in bacteria and viruses, but also in eukaryotes. But in eukaryotes the situation is much more complex because the fertilized ovum does not simply give rise to cells identical to the mother cell. In contrast, as the fetus develops and throughout life, most cells of the eukaryotes have specialized functions reflected by unique morphologies and molecular composition [405–407].

Enzymes play a key role in determining cellular specificity. Consequently, any theory of gene expression in eukaryotes must account for the fact that in each cell the gene potential far exceeds the expression of the genome in the phenotype, and that throughout development and differentiation, the pattern of gene expression is modified by repressing or unmasking genes, which are or are not expressed in the embryo. The progress made in molecular biology during the last two decades has established the fundamentals of gene expression.

Information stored in DNA molecules is transcribed into RNA molecules, which in the presence of ribosomes, tRNA, and the appropriate enzymes, can serve as templates for the elaboration of the polypeptide chain.

The mechanism regulating each step of protein synthesis can modulate gene expression; unfortunately, little is known of such regulatory mechanisms, especially in the mammalian cell.

In the biosynthesis of DNA, RNA, and protein, determination of the specificity of the product not only resides with the substrate-enzyme reaction, but also involves specific templates. Therefore, the regulation of such macromolecular synthesis involves two aspects: the initiation and termination of the reading of the template, and the regulation of the amount of macromolecular product.

The regulation of total RNA and protein produced is modified by nutritional conditions, hormonal shifts, and a number of other endocellular and exocellular factors, many of which have been discussed in other chapters of this book.

In theory, gene expression could be regulated at each step of protein synthesis. Gene expression is modified by direct alteration of the DNA only in rare situations either as a result of loss of DNA (as in erythrocytes) or possibly because of the elaboration of increased amounts of certain DNA molecules. Quantitative modifications of the oocyte DNA content have been reported just before gastrulation. Qualitative changes in the composition of the DNA molecules are not known to occur during gene expression. Theoretically, they could include base modification, methylation, or glucosylation.

Regulation at the level of transcription has been clearly established in bacteria in enzyme induction. In bacteria, individual genes are arranged to form operons, which contain operator, structural, and regulator genes. Unmasking the operator gene unleashes the transcription of several structural genes. Proteins called repressors bind to specific DNA sequences and control the expression of the genetic information stored in the DNA by preventing RNA transcription. For example, in *E. coli*, the lactose operator gene is a specific DNA sequence that reacts with a specific repressor protein (lactose repressor). The usage of lactose by bacteria requires that two enzymes be made—a permease and a β-galactosidase. The system is not induced by lactose itself, but galactose and especially isopropyl-β-thiogalactoside function as inducers.

During induction, the inducer binds with the regulator gene. "Anti-inducers," or corepressors, are substances that favor repression. The repressors of the λ phage proteins and of the lac operon have been purified, and many of their properties have been investigated. The lac operon repressor was shown to bind at the operator site of the gene. Conclusive evidence that it inhibits transcription has not been provided (see also Chapter 2, Determination of Cellular Specificity).

Although it is safe to predict that the molecular events of repression and derepression as we known them in bacteria must play a key role in gene expression, in most cases we have little information of the details of the mechanism that triggers or stops gene expression in bacterial cells, let alone in mammalian cells. Development and differentiation in mammalian tissues are much more complex events than adaptation in bacteria. These processes result in the functional and structural specialization of a group of cells and therefore must involve switching off or switching on of a large number of individual genes or gene complexes.

An understanding of gene expression is fundamental to the understanding of the molecular distortion responsible for the conversion of a normal into a cancer cell. Distortion of gene expression is the hallmark of the cancer cell. It is manifested morphologically, metabolically and functionally. We have already described some of the morphological changes that take place; the metabolic changes include loss of metabolic regulation, a switch from adult to fetal enzyme, changes in isoenzyme patterns.

Studies of cell differentiation during embryonic life and adult life are varied and numerous. We have already described such events in the red blood cell, the gastrointestinal tract, and other sites. Winick and McCrory have reviewed phases of cell differentiation in the kidney [408]. Mainly to provide a factual framework for further discussion, we shall briefly review the studies of Wessels [409] and Rutter and his collaborators [410–413] on phases of differentiation in pancreatic cells.

The pancreas is a double organ composed of exocrine and endocrine glands. The major proteins secreted by the exocrine pancreas are hydrolases, which attack polypeptides, polynucleotides, polysaccharides, and lipids. The key proteins elaborated by the endocrine pancreas are two polypeptide hormones: glucagon and insulin.

On the ninth day of gestation in the mouse, and on the eleventh day in the rat, a group of cells of the upper portion of the intestine proliferate and form a bulge at the surface of the epithelium. Later, the connection between the evagination and the intestine narrows, and only a duct (the future pancreatic duct) links the evagination to the intestinal wall. The endodermic tissue of the evagination then penetrates the surrounding mesodermic tissue, and the endodermic cells are modified in three ways: active proliferation, arrangement into primitive acini and islets, and differentiation of zymogen granules and β-granules.

A study of the appearance of enzymes, polypeptide hormones, and ultrastructural changes can now be superimposed upon the light microscopic description of pancreatic morphogenesis. This was made possible by the development of microassays for the enzymes and immunofluorescent techniques for the hormone determinations. Wessells and Rutter found that the activities of the hydrolases develop in three identifiable stages: a period of slow rise, a period of rapid rise, and a leveling off of the enzyme activity.

All hydrolases, chymotrypsin, carboxypeptidase A and B, ribonuclease, and lipase A and B follow the same pattern of development, which yields an S-shaped curve when the concentration of the enzyme molecule is expressed in a function of the embryo's age. However, the curves obtained for each enzyme cannot be superimposed because some enzymes appear faster* (*e.g.*, chymotrypsin) and others slower (*e.g.*, lipase); the significance of the dephasing between the curves is not clear. Although this finding suggests that the regulation of gene expression for these enzymes is not coordinate, coordination of unmasking of the structural genes could occur with the rate of elaboration of each enzyme regulated separately.

In any event, it is significant that the endoplasmic reticulum and the Golgi apparatus, which are, of course, implicated in the development of zymogen granules, become readily apparent precisely at a time in between the period of slow and rapid growth. The pattern of insulin and glucagon development is similar to that of the hydrolase.

Further embryological experimentation has permitted four stages in the development of the organ to be distinguished: a predifferentiated stage, a protodifferentiated stage, a differentiated stage, and a modulated adult level.

The notion of a protodifferentiated stage is based on the result of organ culture experiments. If intestinal cells are obtained from that portion of the intestine in which pancreas will develop and are cultured *in vitro*, they will develop into pancreatic cells, provided that the tissue is obtained not earlier than 18 hours before the pancreatic bud becomes visible and that both the endodermic and mesodermic components are present at the same time. This experiment established that the endodermic cell reaches a definite point at which development into a pancreatic cell is irrevocably predetermined and that the mesoderm is involved in pancreas formation. The mesoderm seems to elaborate substances capable of stimulating the proliferation of the cells in the pancreatic bud. Thus, the critical events in pancreatic development appear to occur when the genetic potential of an endodermic cell is determined to be expressed in such a manner that pancreatic morphology and function evolve. Such an event can be defined as a cytodifferentiating event, and it obviously precedes the elaboration of proteins specific for structure and function.

Whatever mechanism may be put into gear later to modulate the cytodifferentiating event, that event must be triggered at the level of the DNA or the mRNA, either by the elaboration of new genes or by the unmasking of unexpressed genes.

As mentioned, the genome is a constant of the cell and it is only rarely changed during differentiation. Consequently, the cytodifferentiating event must involve either new transcription or activation of preexisting messenger.

Because actinomycin administration, in most cases tested, interferes with the appearance of the proteins normally triggered by the cytodifferentiating event, transcription of new messenger is believed to be involved. Some competitive hybridization studies of RNA formed during enzyme induction or other forms of gene expression have revealed the appearance of new types of RNA. But the results of studies of enzyme induction in intact animals are difficult to interpret because too many potential variables escape control by the investigators.

Therefore, attempts have been made to investigate enzyme induction in cells in culture. Inasmuch as satisfactory cultures of liver cells were not available when these studies were begun, cell lines derived from rat minimal deviation hepatomas were used. Although these cells resemble normal liver cells morphologically, they are heteroploid and lack some of the proteins found in normal liver (*e.g.*, tryptophan pyrrolase).

The finding made on the hepatoma cells probably reflects the *in vivo* situation because the pattern of enzyme induction *in vitro* often resembles that observed *in vivo*.

Rather than attempting to discuss all forms of enzyme induction here, we will confine our discussion to that of tyrosine aminotransferase. (Enzyme induction is not restricted to bacteria or animal cells. Environmentally determined modifications of enzyme activities have been observed in plants, and in some cases [*e.g.*, hydrolase increase], the enzyme changes were shown to result from *de novo* synthesis [414].)

When the synthetic corticosteroid dexamethasone is added to HTC cells grown in the midlogarithmic stage, the activity of tyrosine aminotransferase increases within less than an hour. The activity of the enzyme rises sharply between 1 and 10 hours after the hormone is added to the culture medium, later levels off, and stays high as long as the steroid is present in the medium. If the steroid is removed, the activity of the enzyme drops rapidly.

The increase in activity could result from activation of latent enzyme, interference with enzyme degradation, or *de novo* synthesis of new enzyme molecules. Studies in which HTC cells were incubated during induction with labeled amino acid revealed increased incorporation in the anti-TAT-immune precipitate.

Such findings indicate that the appearance of new enzyme activity is associated with new protein synthesis. According to Thompkins and his associates, all the new activity that develops after induction can

---

* Similar findings were made in regenerating pancreas (see chapter on regeneration).

be accounted for by *de novo* synthesis. Attempts to demonstrate levels of enzyme degradation have failed.

The hormone does not stimulate cell division, increase overall RNA protein synthesis, or modify the kinetics of the cell cycle. Alteration in the HTC stickiness has, however, been observed in steroid-treated cells. The relationship of the membrane alteration and enzyme induction is not clear. Therefore, the hormone's effect seems to be rather specific for the enzyme induction.

When HTC cells that have been induced by the steroids are incubated in the presence of an inhibitor of translation (*e.g.*, cycloheximide or puromycin) and the inducer and inhibitor are removed from the culture several hours later, there is an immediate increase in TAT activity without the usual lag period. If the induced cells are incubated in the presence of actinomycin and cycloheximide, no new enzyme synthesis occurs when inhibitors and inducers are removed. These results have been interpreted to mean that during the lag period the inducer stimulates the production of a specific mRNA, which accumulates in the cells and can be translated once the inhibitors of translation are removed.

Although 3′,5′-cyclic AMP is known to mediate many hormonal actions, there is no evidence that cyclic AMP is involved in steroid induction of aminotransferase, at least *in vitro*.

Although transcriptional control of TAT synthesis has clearly been demonstrated, new insight suggesting posttranscriptional control in the mechanism regulating protein synthesis has been provided by the superinduction of TAT. When induced cells are incubated with amounts of actinomycin that block 90% of RNA synthesis, TAT activity increases dramatically. Although some believe that this increase in activity results from interference by actinomycin with enzyme degradation, there seems to be enough evidence to indicate that in most cases the increased enzyme activity during superinduction results from *de novo* synthesis. The finding thus suggests that post-transcriptional control of protein synthesis exists.

To explain post-transcriptional regulation, investigators have postulated the existence of cytoplasmic repressors. The repressor is believed to be a protein coded for by a regulatory gene. The repressor protein combines with the mRNA and regulates both its translation and degradation. When large doses of actinomycin are added to an induced cell, a pool of inactive mRNA is activated by removing the repressor. The active messenger is translated and believed to be resistant to degradation.

The interrelationship between TAT induction and the cell cycle are of interest. The cycle can be divided into noninducible and inducible phases (mitosis, last one-third of G1 and G2). The turning off of gene transcription during the cell cycle is not steroid sensitive, but it is believed that during that period neither the TAT nor the repressor message is made as a result of nonspecific blocking of all gene transcription. Thus, only the preexisting TAT message continues to be translated. The translation is much more effective because under those circumstances the repressor is not present and, as pointed out above, only the combination messenger and repressor is susceptible to degradation.

The addition of 5% bovine serum to chemically defined culture medium enhances TAT synthesis even in the presence of actinomycin. It has been suggested that the effect of serum is to stimulate the aggregation of ribosomes into polysomes. Insulin and glycogen both stimulate TAT synthesis. The mechanism of action of insulin is not clear; it does not involve glucose or amino acid uptake. One possibility is that insulin stimulates polysome formation. Nothing is known of the mode of action of glycogen.

Tomkins' group has recently been able to induce tyrosine aminotransferase activity in cell-free extracts of cultured hepatoma cells; this system has great promise for furthering our understanding of gene expression in mammalian cells.

Most of the findings on the transaminase induction in hepatoma cells were confirmed by Gerschenson using hepatic cells in a chemically defined medium [630].

Thompson established a cell line called the HTC cell. The line was derived from a hepatoma HTC cell which, as we shall see later, responds to some, but not all regulatory stimuli, especially hormonal stimuli. For example, glucocorticosteroids, insulin, glucagon and catecholamines can all induce tyrosine aminotransferase activity in liver. The induction is preceded by the activation of adenylcyclase, formation of cyclic AMP and phosphorylation of protein kinase. Tyrosine aminotransferase is only induced by glucocorticosteroids and insulin in HTC cells.

When an inducible hepatoma cell is hybridized with a noninducible diploid liver cell, the hybrid is never able to respond to the glucocorticoid by synthesizing TAT. Thus, when the HTC cell is complexed with the hepatic cell, the hepatoma cell appears to acquire the ability to repress its TAT synthesis. Although the result of such experiments can readily be explained by the existence of a cytoplasmic repressor, some other regulatory mechanism of gene expression could develop in the hepatoma cells under the influence of the normal liver cells.

The hepatoma cell appears to contain 10^5 cytoplasmic receptors for glucocorticoids. The receptors are believed to be proteins with properties similar to those described for receptors of other hormones in other target tissues (*e.g.*, estrogen receptors in the uterus, progesterone receptors in the oviduct, and dehydrotestosterone receptors in the prostate). Thus, the protein aggregates at low ionic strength, and this aggregate at high-salt concentration has a sedimentation coefficient of 4 S.*

---

* See Gordon Thompkins' paper in Advances in Cell Biology, Vol. 2, Chapter 6, p. 299, Specific Enzyme Production in Eukaryotic Cells [652]. A chapter on enzyme synthesis and degradation in mammalian systems, editor M.C. Rechcijl, by Thomas D. Cellehrter, Regulatory Mechanism of Enzyme Synthesis, Enzyme Induction, p. 165–199, [653].

The identification of the regulatory defect in the sequence of events which followed the administration of the hormone is of obvious interest. Chromatography on DEAE cellulose shows that the HTC cell is defective in one major cyclic AMP stimulated protein kinase, probably because of the absence in HTC cells of the cyclic AMP binding fraction. It is possible, but not proven, that this defect and others in protein kinase activity are responsible for the lack of response of the HTC cell to hormone stimulation.

Although there seems to be no doubt that in mammalian tissue, at least in certain cases, gene expression or the cytodifferentiating event requires new transcription, the mechanism of gene unmasking remains unknown.

In mammalian cells, as in bacteria, the "repressor" is at the center of the problem. What are the repressors in mammalian cells? The requirements for mammalian repressor are as follows. The substance must be specific for the DNA sequence of one gene or more. It must be released from DNA by an agent that derepresses the gene. It must be available and recombine with DNA when the "derepressants" are gone. DNA complexed with the repressor should not be able to serve as a template in the RNA polymerase reaction.

Although studies with hepatoma cell lines have proven most useful for improving the understanding of gene expression in mammalian cells and it is likely that the findings made with hepatoma cells will largely be substantiated by studies with isolated hepatocytes, a great number of investigators have attempted to prepare clean suspensions of hepatocytes. The results of these studies are often difficult to evaluate because either cell lines were prepared and they yielded spontaneous transformation and, in the case of primary cultures, adequate controls for hepatocyte function and conclusive elimination of other cellular contaminants were missing. However, acceptable primary cultures seem to be available in several laboratories. For a presentation of the technique and the results see [631].

It is not possible to review here all these studies, but for the purpose of illustrating the general approach we shall briefly summarize some of the studies now underway in Dr. Potter's laboratory [632].

The group used the collagenase perfusion technique to prepare liver cell suspension. The hepatocytes were separated from contaminating cells. The investigators were aware of the properties of the freshly isolated cells and found that they were incapable of retaining small molecules, such as amino acids and inorganic ions. Moreover, the fresh cells also lose mitochondrial enzymes and lactic dehydrogenase and as a result one may expect that their production in ATP may be reduced. We have seen in the chapter on necrosis that the role that low levels of ATP play in alteration of cell function is difficult to evaluate, but it cannot be argued that if one is to study hepatocyte function, it is best to use a cellular population which generates normal levels of ATP.

In normal liver the preparation of liver cells that divide is less than 0.1%. Therefore, dividing liver cells are not appropriate for studies of liver cell functions during the steady state. Keeping these restrictions in mind Potter's group chose to let the prepared hepatocytes recover and eliminated cells unable to attach. They selected a number of criteria to determine whether they were dealing with hepatocytes: the presence of adult rather than fetal isozymes, their ability to synthesize arginine from ornithine, their ability to perform gluconeogenesis, their morphological identity with the normal hepatocyte and the absence of cellular division. The preparation contained the adult type of pyruvate kinase and aldolase, was rich in glucokinase and presented the morphology of hepatic cells. Tyrosine aminotransferase and orotidine decarboxylase were inducible. The availability of intact liver cells will undoubtedly help the study of differentiation and of transformation of a normal to a malignant cell.

Because histones are synthesized at the same time as DNA, forming nucleoprotein complexes with DNA, and interfere with the template activity of DNA in RNA polymerase reactions, they are often believed to constitute a population of mammalian repressors. Although histones are likely to play a secondary role in repression of the mammalian genome, the lack of specificity from species to species and their relatively small number seem to exclude the possibility of specific recognition of DNA sequences.

We have already mentioned that in addition to DNA and histones, the chromosome also contains nonbasic protein and RNA. The complex of chromosomal DNA, RNA, and histones is called chromatin. Dahmus and Bonner [415] have isolated chromatin from various sources. This method has provided the authors with a new tool for dissecting the transcription event. Indeed, the DNA of the chromatin isolated from cells of higher organisms is partially repressed.

When the template ability (for RNA polymerase) of purified DNA is compared with that of DNA in chromatin, the incorporation of the triphosphate nucleotides into the RNA (on a weight basis) is with chromatin DNA only one-fifth of the incorporation when purified DNA is used. This type of result suggests that at least four-fifths of the DNA associated with chromatin is derepressed, provided, of course, that the *in vitro* experiment depicts the *in vivo* reality.

Hybridization experiments indicating that the RNA synthesized *in vitro* resembles or is identical to the RNA synthesized *in vivo* suggest that the *in vitro* indeed reflects the *in vivo* situation.

Bonner and his associates further investigated which of the components of chromatin were responsible for restricting template activity. The template activity increases as histones are removed. When all histones have been eliminated, the template activity of the chromatin DNA equals that of purified DNA.

Huang and Bonner [416] have isolated a special chromosomal RNA, which is made of small molecules (40 nucleotides long) that hybridize readily with 5% DNA. The hybridization process is species specific, indicating that the base sequence of the chromosomal RNA is complementary to species-specific sequences in DNA.

All components of chromatin (DNA, nucleoproteins, and RNA) are separated from each other in 2 M sodium chloride. After solubilization in 2 M sodium chloride, chromatin with template activities similar to the original preparation can be reconstituted simply by dialysis. Hybridization studies using the RNA produced with reconstituted chromatin strongly suggest that the product of the RNA polymerase reaction resembles or is identical to that obtained when fresh chromatin is used.

Such a finding indicates that after dissociation, the histones find, during reconstitution, their exact same place on the DNA. In contrast, when chromosomal RNA was digested with RNase, sequence-specific reconstitution of the chromatin did not take place. Consequently, the chromosomal RNA appears to seek out the DNA sequences that are repressed by histones.

These data clearly suggest that histones restrict [417] chromatin transcription, and they are in keeping with the fact that cytochemical studies of dividing cells ranging from frogs to beef kidney show that condensed chromatin (which is not transcribed) contains less nonhistone proteins than regions of extended chromatin (which are transcribed). Yet, they do not exclude the possibility that other nuclear proteins play a key and possibly a principal role in determining gene expression.

The role of nonhistone chromosomal proteins needs to be elucidated, but they are very likely to play an important function in regulation of gene expression [633]. Although like histones they are synthesized in the cytoplasm, their concentration in chromatin varies with the level of transcription. The non-histone proteins are more abundant in chromatin obtained from cells in which protein and nucleic acid anabolism is highest. Moreover, while the types of histones are limited, the non-histone chromosomal proteins are much more heterogeneous. Of course, these findings do not prove that non-histone chromosomal proteins are involved in gene expression, but they are compatible with such a notion.

The process of cell division results from a well-orchestrated reorganization of gene expression and therefore, the study of the fate of non-histones in continuously dividing cells or in cells stimulated to divide may help us understand their role in regulation of gene expression.

Cell division can be induced in regenerating liver, lymphocytes or salivary gland cells by partial hepatectomies, phytohemagglutinin or injection of isoproterenol, respectively (Chapter 15). The cells that are in G1 pass into an S phase and a mitotic phase. DNA is synthesized during the S phase and the synthesis of histones is tightly coupled to that of DNA. In contrast, in all those cases the development of DNA synthesis is preceded by the *de novo* synthesis of nonhistone chromosomal proteins and such synthesis continues through the cell cycle. Moreover, all the nonhistone proteins are not synthesized at once, but specific ones are elaborated in a rigid sequence which parallels that of the cell cycle.

The messenger for the non-histone protein is stored in the cytoplasm, thus the administration of actinomycin D even before the induction of the proliferative process does not interfere with the biosynthesis of the acidic proteins.

Chromatin can be dissociated into its main components—DNA, histones and nonhistone proteins. The elementary components can then be mixed again to reconstitute the original chromatin. When chromatin is isolated from continuously dividing HeLa cells, it is observed that the template capacity is decreased during the mitotic phase compared to the S phase. In such experiments it was found that histones are more effectively bound to DNA during mitosis than during the S phase. It is believed that nonhistone proteins regulate the binding of histones during the S phase and mitosis and thereby influence the transcription of the DNA. Thus, if one attempts to reconstitute chromatin using DNA histones and S chromatin, the binding of the histone to the DNA is weaker than if one attempts to reconstitute chromatin with DNA, histones and M proteins.

Thus, present views propose that histones act as unspecific repressors of the DNA molecules. Whenever the pattern of gene expression is modified, histones are displaced by acidic proteins. Such a mechanism implies that the acidic proteins recognize specific DNA sequences from which they displace the histone permitting the transcription of the freed DNA. It is not known if, in fact, the variability of the nonhistone proteins is great enough to provide for a multitude of different modes of gene expression. Although as we have seen, different nonchromosomal proteins appear at different stages of the deployment of steps involved in the cell cycle and that each tissue has a unique and reproducible pattern of nonchromosomal proteins, there is overlap from one tissue to another.

The mechanism by which nonhistone chromosomal proteins displace histone also remains unknown. Phosphorylation of nonchromosomal proteins has been incriminated. Phosphorylation would increase the negative charge on the nonhistone chromosomal proteins and thereby tighten their binding to histone which supposedly would then be released from DNA.

Phosphorylation of nuclear proteins is known to occur and it appears that 90% of the phosphorus taken up by nuclear proteins involves the serine residue of nonhistone chromosomal proteins.

Clearly the discovery of some of the properties of nonhistone chromosomal proteins has brought about new working hypotheses on the mode of gene expression in mammalian cells, but much remains to be learned about the exact molecular interaction between DNA, histone, and nonhistone chromosomal proteins before a detailed and accurate description of mammalian gene expression can be available.

As may be anticipated, RNA transcribed directly from DNA will be different from RNA transcribed from chromatin. Only a portion of the DNA sequences are translated in the latter. Competitive hybridization studies have shown that RNAs synthesized from chromatin of different tissue clearly reveal differences in the RNA sequences. Various methods have been designed to dissociate chromatin into its major basic components. The methods are rather drastic and degradation of histone and nonhistone proteins has been reported [634]. Nevertheless, it was shown by Gilmour and his associates [635] that when dissociated chromatin is reconstituted (DNA, histone and acid protein), the RNA synthesized is similar to that directly synthesized on normal chromatin. In contrast, no hybridizable RNA was synthesized when DNA was combined with histones alone. Hybridization studies of the RNA synthesized with DNA and acid protein of various origins suggest tissue specificity of the type of RNA synthesized. Similar conclusions were reached in studies in which the immunospecificity of the nonhistone protein DNA complexes were studied.

Kleinsmith [636] has proposed a tentative mechanism for such displacement. The hypothesis is based on the fact that acidic nuclear proteins are phosphorylated, probably at a greater rate than histones, by a protein kinase under the control of cyclic AMP. Moreover, histones stimulate phosphorylation. Thus, the negatively charged acid proteins may interact with positively charged histones and displace them from the DNA after conversion of condensed to extended chromatin.

Gilmour [635] has proposed that the acidic proteins bind to special sequences of the DNA, called "address site," and that as a result of such binding supercoiled DNA is unwound and made accessible to RNA polymerase. The fact that histone increases the level of phosphorylation of the acidic protein may facilitate the combination of the latter with histones. Other hypotheses propose that the acidic protein binds specifically to DNA sequences or may activate RNA polymerase.

Studies done in Bonner's laboratory have led to an attractive model for the interaction of histones and acidic proteins [637].

Regenerating and partially hepatectomized livers have frequently been used to study derepression. Of course, little is known about the chromosome of rat liver except that it contains DNA, protein and RNA. The DNA can be divided into three major categories: (1) single copies with a sequence made of about 800 base pairs; (2) satellite or centromeric DNA made of 200 base pairs repeated one million times, but which are never copied; and (3) redundant DNA which is composed of under 50 base pairs and is interspersed between the single copies. The proteins fall into two major categories: histones and nonhistone proteins. DNA covered by histones is never transcribed. Chromosomal RNA is a small RNA made of a 4 or nucleotide sequences and rich in dihydropyrimidines. The changes that are known to take place before DNA synthesis occurs in regenerating liver include (1) an increase in template activity for RNA polymerase which is associated with a decrease of all known histones, probably as a result of an attack on the histones by neutral protease (nothing is known of the mechanism that tells the protease which kind of histone should be digested); (2) an increase in one of the specific acidic proteins; and (3) an increase in chromosomal RNA. Obviously any interpretation of the sequence of events that lead to derepression of the genome is, at this point, incomplete. One can, as Bonner did, reason by analogy with what is known from derepression with hormones and arrive to some acceptable working hypothesis for derepression in regenerating liver. Bonner has proposed that an effector molecule of unknown nature binds to an effector binding protease to form a complex which recognizes a sensor gene specifically and is capable of derepressing the sensor gene. The sensor gene is then copied into a high molecular weight RNA including some chromosomal RNA. The chromosomal RNA complexes to repetitive segments of the histone covered gene and permits the removal of the histone. The sensor gene is either copied into chromosomal RNA or in some cases, into RNA which is later translated into nonhistone chromosomal proteins [637].

Clearly in spite of the multiple efforts to design models for the molecular structure of chromatin [639], none at this point are definitely established.

The significance of such research is illustrated by the different responses to injuries depending upon the conformation of chromatin.

Silverman and Mirsky [638] have compared the availability of chromatin in intact nuclei and included a preparation of deoxyribonucleoproteins with respect to their ability to serve as templates on both DNA polymerase and DNA dependent RNA polymerase. They found that only a very small fraction of the DNA is accessible to these enzymes in intact nuclei, while DNA in extracted chromatin is somewhat more accessible to the enzyme. When chromatin is irradiated *in vitro*, it is more sensitive to UV radiation than free DNA. Moreover, twice as many thymine dimers are formed in heterochromatin than in euchromatin [640]. When fibroblasts are grown in presence of BUDR, 20% of the thymine residues are replaced by the analogue. When the altered DNA is transcribed, the transcript contains more GMP and less AMP than a transcript derived from a normal DNA template. The incidence of transcriptional errors is increased when chromatin is used as a template. Baserga and his colleagues [641] compared changes introduced into DNA and chromatin by circular dichroism and temperature denaturation and found that the changes introduced by the analogue were greater in chromatin than in DNA. The investigators interpreted the result to mean that the introduction of BUDR in the DNA causes alterations of the interaction between DNA and chromosomal proteins.

The distortion in gene expression that manifests itself in various ways in cancer cells, for example switching to different types of isozymes, appearance of fetal antigens and formation of hormones that are usually not made by the corresponding normal tissue, must in some way be associated with a corresponding alteration in the genome. Histones are not primarily altered in cancer, but nonhistone proteins, with immunological properties different from that of the normal, have been detected.

Stein *et al.* [642] studied chromosomal proteins in poorly differentiated hepatomas and found that the total amount of histones in liver and hepatoma was the same, but that the quantity of nonhistone chromosomal protein is increased in the tumors compared to normal liver. Arnold *et al.* [643] have described differences in the electrophoretic pattern of rapidly growing hepatomas compared to minimal deviation hepatomas. Similar results were reported in studies comparing mouse breast carcinomas with normal mice breast [644].

Whatever the restrictive mechanism, it has been shown that the restriction of chromatin transcription compared to that of native DNA results from the decrease in the number of available initiation sites for RNA polymerase on chromatin.

The study of the products of chromatin transcription is likely to help our understanding of gene expression in mammalian cells; therefore, some of the recent developments in that field are of considerable interest.

Transcription of rat liver chromatin with homologous enzymes, mainly an RNA polymerase form B, obtained from liver has yielded RNA's with molecular weights ranging between 18 and 45 S. Although the size of this RNA transcript is closer to that which is found *in vivo*, it is still smaller than that of the heterogeneous high molecular weight RNA [418] (see Chapter 1).

There is no evidence that the transcript of chromatin can be translated, but the product of transcription of duck reticulocyte chromatin was shown to be globin mRNA. This was achieved by experiments [419] in which the product was hybridized with DNA synthesized with messengers obtained in a cell-free system through the reverse RNA polymerase reaction. Chromatin prepared from liver is incapable of globin RNA synthesis, which is in keeping with the restriction imposed on chromatin by differentiation.

The possibility that special chromosomal RNA might regulate gene expression was investigated using a completely different approach. A somewhat unexpected finding was at the origin of these observations. It had been anticipated that since the cells of mammalian tissues contain much more DNA than do bacteria, the chances of reassociation of specific DNA sequences after separating the two strands would be small with mammalian DNA. Yet, reassociation was more effective with mouse than with bacterial DNA. To explain this finding, Britten assumed that in mammalian DNA some sequences are frequently repeated.

Britten and Kohne [420] measured the time necessary for reassociation of a DNA sequence and thereby determined the incidence of repeated sequences. To study DNA reassociation, an investigator passes the DNA through a column of hydroxyapatite, which separates single- from souble-stranded DNA under the conditions of the experiment. The DNA solution is kept at 60° (only 25° below that which dissociates DNA). As a result, the double-stranded DNA sticks to the column while most of the single-stranded DNA passes through.

If DNA sequences are not repeated, the time necessary to secure reassociation of complementary strands will be strictly proportionate to the DNA concentration. If some of the DNA sequences are frequently repeated, the concentration of that portion of the DNA will be greater than that of other DNA, and the repeated portion of the DNA will reassociate faster than the remaining DNA. Thus, by measuring reassociation in function of time, one can determine the incidence of repeated sequences. The incidence of repeated sequences was found to be low in virus and bacteria and increased in more highly evolved organisms. By coupling this finding with existing knowledge of molecular biology, Britten and Davidson proposed a new theory for gene regulation of higher cells [421]. Britten and Davidson remarked that even though changes in the state of differentiation in higher animals are triggered by a single event (hormone, substrate, etc.), the changes require coordinated activation of a large number of genes which, at least in some cases, are known not to be contiguous (*e.g.*, the genes for polypeptide chains of hemoglobin).

Therefore, these investigators postulate that the single event that triggers a change in differentiation activates one or more of the so-called batteries of genes. A battery of genes is activated with a sequence-specific RNA called "activator RNA." Special genes, or "integrator genes," code for the sequence of the activator RNA. These integrator genes are believed to be linked together and are part of sets of genes. All the gene sets can be activated by a single event.

Each set of genes is composed of a number of "producer genes" that, according to the definition of Britten and Davidson, code for messenger, ribosomal, and transfer RNA. In addition, Britten and Davidson have postulated the existence of two more types of genes—receptor genes and sensor genes. The receptor gene is linked to the producer gene, and it regulates the transcription of the producer gene. Transcription takes place only when the DNA of the receptor gene forms a base-specific complex with activator RNA.

Sensor genes are linked to integrator genes. They bind to the "inducer" (the triggering event in the change of the state of differentiation). Binding between inducer and integrator is specific and is determined by the sensor gene's base sequence. For the model to work, that is to say, before the coordinated biosynthesis of a large number of proteins can be triggered, some genes—either the regulator or the integrator genes—must be redundant [422]. The model also calls for regulation of gene expression through gene-specific RNA, rather than through histones.

Even if they are at the present purely hypothetical, such models are most useful to planning further experiments. Davidson and Britten [421], pursuing these studies using the DNA-RNA hybridization techniques, have provided data suggesting (1) that structural genes constitute nonrepetitive sequences, represented once or possibly twice in a haploid chromosome; (2) that the structural gene sequences are usually longer (800–1200 nucleotides) than the repetitive sequences; (3) and that structural genes are orderly interdispersed with repetitive genes, approximately 300 nucleotides long.

Although these findings do not as yet form an unshakable basis for a plausible theory of regulation of gene expression in mammalian cells, it is fair to ask how they relate to existing concepts. The mature mammalian cell is characteristically made of a mosaic of specific structural, transport, messenger, and catalytic proteins. Structure and function depend upon the orderly interaction between macromolecules, the catalytic products and the nutrients provided by the environment. The key to this specificity lies with the DNA. The DNA is the same in all cells and therefore, the expression in the phenotype of any protein made at any time by any other cell of the organism is potentially feasible provided that the gene which is silent in that cell is brought to express itself. In reality only a small proportion of the genes present in every cell is expressed, and such expression is selective in that only the genes needed for the elaboration of the protein mosaic of that cell are expressed. Moreover, panoplies of genes are expressed in a given cell. For example, it is useless for a cell to make lactic dehydrogenase without a glycolytic pathway. The expression of one enzyme of the *de novo* purine biosynthetic pathway is of little significance if those other steps involved in the biosynthesis are not expressed. To account for such coordination Britten has proposed that groups of genes are expressed: such groups are called "batteries," and the specificity of the repetitive sequences, which we now know are intercalated between chains of structural genes, determines the site of action of specific "activation" which brings the "battery" to be transcribed into messenger RNA.

The concept of gene "batteries" regulated by the intercalation of repetitive sequences does not answer all questions raised by gene expression in mammalian cells, but it provides a base for further thinking and planning new experiments. A corollary of this hypothesis is that the specific mode of expression in each cell is determined by the interaction of repetitive and nonrepetitive sequences and thus, while damage to structural genes would lead to deletion, nonsense or mis-sense mutation, damage to repetitive sequences, would result in distortion of gene expression. Consequently, cancer could result from alteration of one or more repetitive sequences which result in a phenotype with survival advantages over that of other cells.

For further details on the model, the reader is referred to the original paper. Suffice it to point out that although much evidence is still needed to support the model, it constitutes a serious attempt to resolve the complexity of the events in gene expression in mammals and has the advantage of taking into account the existence of both redundant DNA sequences and chromosomal RNA.

Moreover, Tomkins has expanded the existing theories on gene expression in higher organisms, primarily on the basis of studies of the effect of steroids on the activity of tyrosine aminotransferase in mammalian cells in culture. (Enzyme induction is not restricted to bacteria or animal cells. Environmentally determined modifications of enzyme activities have been observed in plants, and in some cases [*e.g.*, hydrolase increase], it was established that the enzyme changes result from *de novo* synthesis [414].) During enzyme induction, the structural gene is transcribed and the messenger is translated to form the enzyme. At the same time, a regulatory gene is transcribed whose messenger codes for the production of a protein which can specifically bind to the messenger coded for by the structural gene. Complexing of structural messenger and regulatory proteins is believed to lead to the degradation of the messenger. When enough of the regulatory protein is formed, all structural messenger is inactivated as it is produced, and a noninducing state is reached.

The noninducing state can be reverted to the inducing state under the influence of the inducer, which by an unknown mechanism inactivates the regulatory protein and frees the structural messenger so that it can be translated again. This is a form of post-transcription regulation which precedes the translational stage.

Of course, post-transcriptional control of gene expression does not exclude the possibility of the existence of transcriptional control. Tomkins and associates have suggested that whereas transcriptional control is most important in the sequential gene activation of development, post-transcriptional control is likely to be more important during enzyme induction [423].

When we described some of the properties of mRNA, we pointed out that although bacterial messengers seem to have short life spans, the functional half-life of mammalian mRNA is much longer. Echinoderm eggs elaborate mRNA, which is transferred to the cytoplasm but not translated, even though other messenger is selectively translated. Long template life span and the presence of nontranslated messenger in cytoplasm led some to believe that the control of the biosynthesis of some protein must be post-transcriptional.

This has to be the case for hemoglobin biosynthesis in the erythrocyte since in the enucleated reticulocyte, transcription is excluded. In fact, some evidence suggests that heme regulates the biosynthesis of globin by acting at some step of translation. Similarly, insulin stimulates protein synthesis in muscle ribosome in the absence of new mRNA synthesis. While the retina develops, glutamic synthetase appears in the presence of actinomycin. (Glutamic synthetase develops in the retina in two phases: an early actinomycin-sensitive phase and a later actinomycin-independent phase.) All these facts and many others suggest that certainly post-transcriptional or even translational control sites for protein synthesis must exist. Yet the exact mechanism of these controls remains obscure.

tRNA molecules are believed to regulate protein synthesis at the level of translation of the messenger. A shift in the relative concentrations of the tRNA's has been described when gene expression takes place in bacteria (phage infection, sporulation), in plant cells (differentiation of the wheat seedling), and in animal cells (virus-infected and developing chick erythrocyte).

Investigators at the National Institutes of Health have reported an increase in 4S RNA coinciding with an increase of tRNA in the oviduct of chick embryos stimulated to differentiate under the influence of estrogen. Whether this increase in tRNA results from activation of new DNA sequence, increased rate of transcription, or decreased rates of breakdown has not been decided. The multiple control sites of differentiation have been reviewed by Wright, who studied the differentiation of social amoeba [422].

Because of its complexity, the mammalian genome is much more difficult to dissect than the bacterial. Consequently, functional units of DNA have not been identified in the mammalian chromosome. In fact, rarely has it been possible to assign a specific function to a specific chromosome. However, two techniques are likely to help advance our knowledge of the function of the components of the mammalian genome: nuclear transplantation and cell hybridization experiments [425].

A group of investigators in Paris discovered that when two different types of mammalian cells were cultured simultaneously, a new cell type appeared in the cultured medium with properties belonging to both original types. Ways were soon discovered to increase the proportion of hybridized cells by designing media on which they would grow selectively. For example, by placing aminopterin in the incubation medium, one prevents thymidylic acid formation through the *de novo* pathway; consequently, any cell lacking thymidine kinase does not survive. Similarly, the addition of BUDR to the incubation medium interferes with the biosynthesis of thymidylic acid in cells that depend on thymidine kinase through the salvage pathways for thymidine biosynthesis. Thus, if a group of cells depending primarily on the *de novo* pathway and a group of cells depending primarily on the salvage pathway are cultured in such a medium, the selection will be in favor of the hybrids, which will have the thymidine kinase in their enzyme arsenal.

Green and his collaborator [426] discovered that when attempts are made to hybridize cells obtained from human culture with mouse culture cells, only a small number of human chromosomes participate in the hybridization. Thus, the hybrid cell has most of the mouse characteristics and only a few of the human characteristics. The hybrids produced between human diploid fibroblasts in an established line of mouse cells maintain the entire chromosome complement of the mouse, but during cultivation the hybrid progressively loses human chromosomes. The method is of considerable importance because it permits chromosomal assignments of human genes. In fact, by such methods a single human chromosome can be introduced into a mouse cell and make a mouse cell that is thymidine kinase independent. However, after repeated transplant of these thymidine kinase-independent cells, the human chromosome disappears, but the thymidine independence persists. The human chromosome carrying the thymidine kinase is a submetacentric member of groupe E. That the human characteristic persists in the mouse even when the human chromosome has disappeared indicates that either the human DNA was translocated to mouse chromosome or the human chromosome introduced in the mouse cells carries with it a derepressor for the thymidine kinase, a derepressor that is lacking in the mouse genome.

Although these techniques have as yet not yielded new surprises in molecular genetics, they have already provided some interesting information. For example, it was known that the lactic dehydrogenase of rat has an amino acid composition and molecular properties different from the lactic dehydrogenase of mouse. When rat cells are hybridized with mouse cells, the hybrid cells synthesize both types of lactic dehydrogenase as well as a new form of the enzyme that is composed of subunits derived from both mouse and rat parent cells.

The technique is pregnant with promises. Consider the findings relating to the identification of the human regulatory gene for inducible tyrosine aminotransferase in rat human hybrid cell [424]. The enzyme can be induced in rat human cell hybrid, but induction is consistently inhibited when the X chromosome survives in the hybrid, even though the same amount of corticoid receptors is present on both inducible and noninducible cells. On the basis of these experiments and others, investigators have concluded that the repressor for the induction of TAT is located on the X chromosome.

Gene reactivation has also been demonstrated in the dormant nucleus of the chicken erythrocyte when such cells were hybridized with human cells that synthesize DNA and RNA. There seems to be no doubt that the cytoplasm influences gene expression. This has been clearly demonstrated by nuclear transplantation experiments. It is possible to select embryonic nuclei with various types of dominant metabolic activities—such as DNA, mRNA, rRNA, or tRNA synthesis. In the Xenopus embryo, no nRNA synthesis can be detected during the first 10 divisions after fertilization. Later, at the midblastula stage, the cell synthesizes a large RNA molecule population, which is believed not to include rRNA and is unlikely to include mRNA. Toward the end of the blastula stage, mRNA synthesis is first detected. This is followed a few hours later, during gastrula formation, by the synthesis of rRNA. For further details see [645].

When eggs that have reached a specific metabolic stage are transplanted into enucleated eggs, they adopt the pattern of RNA synthesis that existed in the host at the time of enucleation. For example, studies of the regulation of DNA synthesis in enucleated cells in which are transplanted nuclei that normally do not synthesize DNA have shown that the initiation of DNA synthesis depends not so much on the availability of precursor and DNA polymerase as upon some type of expansion of the nucleus with an extension of the chromosomes. According to Gordon, these changes make the chromosomes accessible to activation by cytoplasmic substances. Although the molecular structure of the activiating substances is not known, these experiments leave no doubt that gene expression (in this instance, DNA synthesis) is, in part, determined by cytoplasmic factors.

Gene Expression and Regulation of Cell Divison

If contraction by muscle cells, chemical conversion in liver cells, and absorption and secretion by intestinal and kidney cells are astonishing events that are difficult to comprehend, the fact that such specialized cells are capable of cell division is not less amazing. During division, the cell must not only secure integral replication of the genome potential, but it must also make sure that only those genetic functions expressed before cell division are also those expressed in the daughter cells after division.

Methods for studying mitosis have included light microscopy, electron microscopy, radioautography, and biochemical analysis.

Light and electron microscopy have permitted biologists to observe chromosome deployment during the various phases of mitosis and to study the formation of the spindle and nuclear membrane (these events have already been described).

Radioautographic studies have aimed primarily at studying DNA and protein synthesis during the cell cycle. In fact, on the basis of such studies various stages of the cell cycle were described.

The first radioautographies were done with ^{32}P- and ^{14}C-labeled precursors, but this technique reached new levels of precision when it was discovered that a tritium-labeled precursor provided better resolution than ^{14}C-labeled precursors.

In any event, on the basis of studies of the kinetics of cell division in *Vicia faba*, investigators divided the generation cycle into four successive stages: postmitotic interphase (G1), DNA synthesis (S), premitotic interphase (G2), and mitosis (M). In molecular terms, one can distinguish three major nuclear events during cell division: duplication of the chromosomal material, formation of the contractile protein—which distributes the chromosomes between daughter cells, and reconstitution of two new nuclear membranes.

Chromosome duplication involves duplication of DNA. The properties and mechanism of synthesis of DNA and nucleoproteins have been discussed in Chapter 2, Determination of Cellular Specificity. Here we shall be concerned only with what is known of the regulation and the coordination of DNA and protein synthesis during chromosome replication. These events are assumed to result from the sequential activation of several genes. We shall focus our discussion on the replication of mammalian chromosomes, and events in bacteria will be referred to only as they are relevant to the mammalian cell cycle. This should not be interpreted to mean that studies in bacteria are not fundamental to interpreting events in mammalian cells, and we refer the reader to the reviews of Lark [427] and Maale and Kjelgaard [428] for further details on studies in bacteria.

The biochemistry of cell division in mammalian cells has been investigated with synchronized cell systems *in vitro* or *in vivo*. Mammalian cells growing logarithmically in culture can be brought to synthesize DNA and enter mitosis in synchrony. For that purpose, it suffices to add to the culture medium antimetabolites that interfere with the usage of deoxyribonucleotides for DNA synthesis or agents such as colchicine or vinblastine, which block mitosis in metaphase.

The generation time of the HeLa cell, 24 hours, is divided into a period of 6 hours for G1, 1 hour for DNA and chromatin synthesis, 2 hours for G2 and mitosis, and 15 to 16 hours for interphase. Mueller and his associates [429] have exploited this technique of cell synchrony with success for studying the biochemistry of mitosis. As mentioned above, the G1 period lasts in HeLa cells for 16 hours, and some time during G1 the decision is made for the cell to enter the next period of DNA synthesis and mitosis. This decision is likely to involve gene activation, and one may thus anticipate that it will require synthesis of new RNA and new proteins. By using transcription inhibitors, investigators have been able to demonstrate that RNA is necessary for passage from the G1 to the S stage. Whether the RNA synthesized is mRNA is not known. Some enzyme activities, including that of thymidine kinase, are known to increase at the end of G1 and during the S period. Inhibitors of protein synthesis prevent this increase in activity. Whether new templates for thymidine kinase are made in HeLa cells during G1 is not certain.

It was established in a number of laboratories including those of Taylor [430], Painter [431], and Rusch [432] that even though most cells in culture go through the metabolic steps of cell division in synchrony, DNA synthesis occurs in an asynchronous fashion in each cell. Thus, DNA synthesis does not start at the same time in all chromosomes, and within a chromosome some portions of the DNA are replicated faster than others. The findings made in synchronized HeLa cells have their counterpart in Physarum, as Rusch and his associates showed [432].

Thus, at the chromosomal level one may distinguish two kinds of DNA with respect to replication kinetics: an early and a late replicating fraction. Using bromodeoxyuridine for DNA, investigators further suggested that cell growth and survival depend more on the replication of the early DNA than on that of the late DNA. In fact, DNA replicating late seems to be associated with heterochromatin, a portion of the chromatin believed to be repressed in the mature cell.

DNA synthesis can be interrupted by inhibiting RNA synthesis during the early phases of the S period. Inhibition of RNA synthesis during the second half of the S phase interferes little with DNA synthesis. These findings suggest that the establishment of the S period depends upon the elaboration of new RNA molecules during the early stages of the S period. Once these molecules have been made, further interference with DNA synthesis does not occur. Although not proven, it is assumed that the new RNA molecules are templates for the biosynthesis of proteins indispensable for DNA synthesis. That active protein synthesis takes place during the S period has been established by radioautographic methods and the use of inhibitors of protein synthesis. Prescott [433] found heavy incorporation of amino acid into proteins concomitantly with DNA synthesis in S in Euplotes; Baserga [434] found this in mammalian cells. DNA synthesis in these systems is sensitive to puromycin, cycloheximide, and other antibiotics.

Experiments in *Physarum polycephalum*, a large multinucleated slime mold in which all nuclei enter the generation cycle in synchrony, have shown that continuous protein synthesis is needed during the S period, and that the DNA made in the early stages is necessary for the biosynthesis of protein indispensable for elaborating that DNA which is made in the later stages of the S period.

Although protein synthesis is indispensable for DNA synthesis, little is known of which proteins are involved. In reviewing DNA synthesis in regenerating tissues, we have seen that it is unlikely that DNA synthesis is regulated by the activity of the enzymes involved in the last steps of DNA synthesis. Histones are synthesized concomitantly with DNA. If the cell is to make sure that selective parts of its genome are repressed, it would seem that histones must be made at the same time as DNA is made, but it would not necessarily follow that a feedback loop must link histone synthesis to DNA synthesis in such a fashion that interference with histone synthesis would ultimately interfere with DNA synthesis. Interference with DNA synthesis, however, blocks histone synthesis in mammalian cells. Such findings differ from those made on slime molds in which the block of DNA synthesis does not prevent histone synthesis but leads to an increase in the amount of histones (three times the normal level).

Histones have been shown to be synthesized in the cytoplasm, and a cell-free system composed of microsomes and cytosol performs the reaction *in vitro*. Histone synthesis is blocked if microsomes are obtained from HeLa cells in which DNA synthesis is interrupted, but it is fully active when microsomes are obtained from cells in which the block of DNA synthesis has been lifted. But if RNA synthesis is blocked after DNA synthesis has resumed, the microsomes prepared from such cells remain incapable of synthesizing DNA. As Mueller pointed out, this suggests that the coupling between DNA and histone synthesis is mediated through RNA. An 8-S RNA made during the S period is believed to be the messenger for the histone synthesis.

In regenerating pancreas a lysine rich histone fraction decreases in concentration per cell (in comparison to the total histone content) prior to DNA synthesis and is restored to normal concentration after DNA synthesis. The same histone fraction is absent from the polyacrylamide gel preparation in embryonic pancreas, but appears 3 to 5 weeks after birth.

Further investigation of the relationship of the lysine rich histone content and the rates of DNA synthesis in other tissues revealed an inverse relationship between these events. Thus, the histone is absent in duodenum, spleen or lymph nodes, is high in liver, breast and pancreas.

The very lysine rich histone is phosphorylated prior to DNA synthesis as shown in regenerating pancreas and liver. In Morris hepatomas, with various degrees of growth, the level of phosphorylation of the F1 histone increases with the degree of malignancy. Ord and Stocken [654] have shown that the F1 and F3 lysine rich fractions isolated by a special procedure contain adenosyl diphosphate ribose.

In contrast to other histones, F1 and F3 histones are readily removed from DNA with low salt concentration, are more readily phosphorylated and are labile. Although their function is not known, it has been proposed that they are involved in cross-linking of DNA strands and that their removal is indispensable prior to DNA synthesis.

The F1 fraction has been further subdivided into two separate groups of lysine rich histones; one called F1 which is ADP ribosylated, the other referred to as P1 which is phosphorylated. F1 is suspected to dissociate a repressor from the genome opening it for phenotypic expression.

During the early stages of the development of sea urchin embryos, the number of nuclei increases considerably (20 times), without a net change in the total mass. Gross and his collaborators [435] have investigated the phenomenon biochemically. They have shown that during this period of cleavage, 40 to 60% of the protein synthesized accumulates in the nucleus. Among these newly synthesized proteins, 40% are acid soluble. When embryos are treated with actinomycin, the accumulation of the new protein in the nuclei is 20 to 40% less than that in the control. The synthesis of the acid-soluble protein is inhibited more severely than that of others. However, a large amount of the protein continues to be synthesized. Exponential synthesis of DNA during that period of rapid replication is a part of nuclear replication. The cell cycle is 28 to 32 minutes at 23° C and is characterized by almost uninterrupted DNA synthesis followed by mitosis. Thus, at this stage of development of the sea urchin, there is no G1 or G2; consequently, it would seem that if new proteins are made, it may just be for S and M. Cultured sea urchin embryos are synchronous with respect to S and M for the first three cycles.

Evidence suggests that nuclear proteins are synthesized in the cytoplasm and accumulate in the nucleus after a brief delay. At the 128-cell stage, about half of the protein synthesized by the embryo appears to be molecules that find their way into nuclear structures. Since the newly made proteins that accumulate in the nucleus seem to be rich in lysine and poor in tryptophan, they are believed to be histones or histonelike proteins.

Synthesis of histonelike proteins is, in part, linked to the production of new RNA templates. Available experiments do not allow us to decide whether the new RNA's are messengers for the lysine-rich, tryptophan-poor protein, or are indirectly responsible for activating messenger synthesized during embryogenesis. Since nuclear proteins, specifically those associated with chromosomes, continue to be synthesized in the presence of actinomycin, some of the new RNA could serve as template for a different class of proteins, perhaps regulating histone synthesis.

Mueller and his associates have discovered a cytoplasmic factor found in the cytosol, which is thermolabile, sensitive to proteolytic enzymes, and indispensable for DNA synthesis in lysates of HeLa cells.

Nonhistone nucleoproteins are also synthesized during the S period. However, there is no rigid coupling between their synthesis and that of DNA. Their role is even less understood than that of histones (see chapter on determination of specificity and regeneration).

Sometimes in the late S or early G2 phase, the cell decides to deploy its chromosomes and distribute them equally between two portions of the cytoplasm. A critical event during that period is spindle formation. What is known of the biogenesis and biochemistry of the spindle has been briefly reviewed in the chapter on cellular specificity.

Investigators have proposed that prophase is brought about by an increase in the intracellular concentration of sodium, which takes place when threshold values of the surface volume ratio are reached. If this is the case, it may be anticipated that the membrane potential level will have a significant regulatory influence on metabolic preparation for mitosis [436]. Some have even postulated that the autonomous division of the malignant cell could result from a stable abnormality in the electro-osmotic balance of the cell.

That polyribosomes disaggregate during metaphase has been established by sucrose gradient analysis and electron microscopy. The polyribosome breakdown is associated with a sudden and transient decrease in protein synthesis. Therefore, during metaphase, a mechanism regulating protein synthesis not in existence during the rest of mitosis is put to work. The absence of RNA synthesis during metaphase does not explain the rapid breakdown of polyribosomes, because it has been estimated that in the HeLa cells, messenger half-life is 3 to 4 hours, whereas metaphase lasts only 15 minutes. The mechanism by which polyribosomes are broken down has not been established [437].

Little is known of what determines the entrance in G2. The elaboration of new RNA during late S or early G2 is suggested from experiments in which dactinomycin was used. Moreover, the existence of a puromycin-sensitive step in G2 has been established.

If RNA synthesis is blocked in such a way that the block can be lifted by removing the inhibitor, then the cells are again capable of entering mitosis. Surprisingly, a block of DNA synthesis with a deoxyriboside antimetabolite also blocks the development of G2 and mitosis. It would appear from studies in which radioautography was combined with the use of inhibitors of RNA synthesis that cells whose RNA synthesis had been blocked in late S were unable to synthesize the last 3% of their DNA contingent. The results with DNA and RNA inhibitors were interpreted to mean that a DNA indispensable for mitosis is synthesized during the late stages of DNA synthesis.

Experiments in *Physarum polycephalum* done in Rusch's laboratory indicate that the plasmodium, which normally enters a G2 period after DNA synthesis, can be induced to enter mitosis as soon as the S period is completed, indicating that G2 is not an indispensable portion of the generation cycle, at least in Physarum.

G2 is likely to be a period during which substances needed in the cytoplasm are accumulated. RNA and protein synthesis do not appear to be needed during mitosis and, thus, all components needed for migration of the centriole and assemblage of the spindle are elaborated during interphase or the S period. Migration of centriole and spindle assembly are inhibited by colchicine.

Important steps in DNA synthesis and mitosis seem to require new RNA and new protein synthesis as if they were the products of new gene expression. Thus, DNA synthesis and mitosis seem to result from the orderly and sequential unmasking of genes. It is not known if the mechanism that triggers DNA synthesis needs to unmask more than one gene. The decision to enter cell division must be made some time during interphase. Must the cell make more decisions after that first, or does it simply implement the decision by transferring the order from gene to gene until DNA synthesis and mitosis are complete? What keeps the cell from dividing during interphase? These questions are relevant to the regulation of cell division and, as such, to the pathogenesis of cancer. Yet none can be answered at this time.

Available data suggest that only one decision needs to be made, and that thereafter each step of the cell cycle is inexorably put into gear unless interrupted artificially. Thus, during G1 new RNA and new proteins indispensable for DNA synthesis are made. It is also likely that, at about the same time, proteins are made that will serve as building blocks for the elaboration of the mitotic apparatus. DNA synthesis enters its successive phases and, as Rusch's work on Physarum suggests, the DNA synthesized in the early phase is indispensable for that DNA made in the late phase of the S period. Moreover, Mueller's work indicates that the DNA made at the end of the S phase (3% of the total DNA synthesized) is indispensable for mitosis. When mitosis occurs, apparently all the messengers and proteins necessary for the process have already been assembled. Thus, each step of the sequence is in some way dependent upon the previous one, and it would seem that simply triggering the process would be sufficient to deploy the full sequence.

In fact, the cell might store in its nucleus mRNA molecules that would be used as soon as the cycle has been triggered, thus reducing to a minimum the number of genes that need to be unmasked during DNA synthesis and mitosis.

Experiments done in bacteria are of interest to the mechanism triggering DNA synthesis. In bacteria, the triggering of DNA synthesis is coordinated with cell mass, and DNA synthesis has been demonstrated to start at a fixed point on the chromosome. This initiation depends on the elaboration of a new protein (σ protein), which is believed to bind tightly to segments of the DNA at the beginning of replication.* It has been assumed that initiation requires the cooperation of a large number of the σ-protein molecules. In this fashion, initiation could simply be regulated by the overall rate of protein synthesis. Thus, whenever the cellular mass reaches a critical point, DNA synthesis would be initiated.

Reversion of Gene Expression in the Cancer Cell

Distortion in gene expression is a fancy word for distortion of differentiation. But in the beginning of this chapter we pointed out that the processes of transformation and malignancy can, in some cases, be reversed.

We have already discussed the Pierce hypothesis of the malignant stem cell and will not elaborate further on it [646]. We shall give a few examples which support Pierce's view which proposes that attack on the cancer cell should include attempts to convert a poorly differentiated tumorigenic cell into a well-differentiated nontumorigenic cell.

Under some circumstances malignant cells grown in culture can be brought to differentiate. For example, the neuroblastoma NBE cells grow rapidly. They are poorly differentiated and produce tumors when injected subcutaneously to male mice. These cells will undergo spontaneous differentiation when exposed to 4-(3-butoxy-4-methoxybenzyl)-2-imidazolidone, an inhibitor of adenosine 3′5-monophosphate diesterase. The differentiation is associated with a reduction of the rate of growth, restoration of neuronal morphology and reappearance of enzymes (tyrosine hydroxylase, choline acetyl transferase, acetyl cholinesterase) that are absent in the malignant form and elevation of intracellular levels of cyclic AMP [647]. The process is irreversible and associated with inhibition of cell division. The differentiated cells have lost their ability to produce tumors when injected in intact animals.

Bondy *et al.* [648] also determined the amounts of RNA containing polyadenylic acid in the cytoplasm of the undifferentiated and the differentiated cells and found that although differentiation is associated with a reduction of total cytoplasmic RNA, the rate of synthesis of poly (A) containing RNA is relatively increased. Since poly (A) is bound to messenger RNA, these findings would suggest that the differentiation process is associated with a relative increase in the formation of messenger RNA. Moreover, an increase in RNA synthesis takes place during regression of mammary tumors after castration or reduction of secretion of the mammotrophic hormone [649].

Mouse leukemia cells can be induced to differentiate *in vitro* into macrophages by a factor, thermolabile and nondialyzable, found in ascitic fluid of mice bearing Yoshida tumors [650]. The Friend leukemic virus blocks erythropoietic maturation in the proerythroblast. Treatment of infected cells with dimethyl sulfoxide (DMSO) allows at least some cells to differentiate. The process of differentiation is manifested by the formation of mRNA for globin, the formation of hemoglobin, the appearance of δ-aminolevulinic acid in the cell and of a specific erythrocyte membrane antigen with loss of tumorigenicity [651].

The Cell Membrane and the Malignant State

More than any other cell structure except the nucleus, the cell membrane makes the cell unique. To look upon the cell membrane as an inert envelope is to underestimate its function grossly. Many important decisions in the cell's life are made at the level of the cell membrane. In addition to preventing the exclusion of some basic constituents of the cell, the membrane determines the transport of components from the environment into the intracellular space and, *vice versa,* from the intracellular space into the environment. Enzymes and sources of energy within or close to the membrane determine active and passive transport. Many of the cell's social relationships are selected by the membrane, which may displace the cell by active movements on interphases or may establish contact with certain types of cells and repell others.

Because the membrane is at the confines of cell life, the cell has established feedback mechanisms between membrane and genome that regulate cell division and possibly other aspects of gene expression. In view of the importance of the cell membrane in cellular economy, it seems safe to predict that the elucidation in molecular terms of the structure and function of the cell membrane will have as much impact on cellular biology as the elucidation of the structure of DNA

---

* A protein that binds in cluster to DNA has been isolated, even under conditions of large DNA excess. It has been prepared from T4 phage. The protein has a negative charge at pH 7, and bacteriophage mutant, which lacks the protein, is believed to be blocked at an early stage of genetic recombination. Moreover, DNA replication is markedly slowed down in these mutants. DNA synthesis is not indispensable for recombination of T4 in T-infected cells; thus, the protein is assumed to act on genes that regulate both events.

and the transfer of specificity from the genome to the finished protein. Therefore, much work has been devoted in recent years to the cell membrane, and several models for its structure have been proposed.

Function of the Plasma Membrane

Transport

The plasma membrane is a specialized cell structure that modulates the interaction between the cell interior and the surrounding environment and communicates with other cells. The cell membrane influences the composition of the cell by serving as a barrier and by regulating transport.

The cell membrane prevents the extrusion of cellular constituents in the medium and penetration of some of the chemicals that are undesirable or unnecessary for the cell's economy. But of more significance to cellular metabolism is the selective permeability of the membrane, permitting transport from the inside of the cell into the environment and *vice versa*. A great variety of molecules can be transported from the environment into the intracellular space through the cell membranes. They range from simple ones—such as water, ions, sugar, and amino acids—to extremely complex macromolecules—such as lipids (chylomicrons) and even other cells (as in phagocytosis).

The four major mechanisms of transport are: (1) free diffusion, depending primarily on the solubility properties of the compound to be transported; (2) passage through pores, a process essentially limited by the size and possibly the charge of the compound; (3) engulfment in expansions of the cell membrane (pinocytosis and phagocytosis); and (4) carrier-mediated transport.

The carrier concept assumes that the membrane contains segments of special molecular composition and configuration involved in transporting specific molecules. Carrier-mediated modes of transport are of three types: facilitated diffusion, exchange diffusion, and active transport. The types of molecules that are transported and the mode of transport vary with the cell. Many examples (such as water, ion, sugar, and amino acid transport) have been given in other chapters.

Transport is far from unidirectional. Secretion and excretion products are transported from the inside of the cell into the environment. Again, the cell may secrete molecules as simple as HCl or secrete complex enzymes or even entire organelles, such as the zymogen granules. Secretion and intracellular transport are modulated by hormones—aldosterone for sodium, insulin for glucose, etc. Some of these hormones attach to the cell membrane to exert their function. Therefore, the membrane must have included in its structure some specialized segments that function as receptors for the attachment of the hormones (see Chapter 8).

Two cellular properties govern the relationship of one cell with another: movement and the ability to establish or reject contact with another cell. Cellular movement and communication are properties of the cell membranes. They play key roles in embryogenesis, morphogenesis, inflammation, wound healing, and cancer (invasion and metastasis).

The ultimate in transport cells may be the intestinal cells, which can absorb all components from small ions to gammaglobulin. At their luminal end, epithelial cells of the intestine have a special differentiation of their membranes. Long, slender, fingerlike projections develop on the luminal border of the cell. These structures are called microvilli, and the assemblage of microvilli constitutes the brush border. The brush border is permeable to lipid-soluble and small water-soluble compounds, but many important nutrients—electrolytes, sugar, amino acids and special vitamins, gammaglobulin, and triglycerides—are brought into the cell by active transport. In most cases, specialized membrane structures are likely to be involved in the transport mechanism. In fact, in sugar transport, specific carrier systems have been identified.

Gammaglobulins are absorbed by pinocytosis. This process provides a number of animals (pigs, cows, horses), which at birth are devoid of antibodies, with immune protection. A single feeding with colostrom brings the gammaglobulin level of the blood to that of the adult.

In view of these varied absorbent functions of the intestinal cell, it is not surprising that a number of enzymes have been found in the brush border. Some are hydrolases found in granules similar to those found in the pancreas, while others are hydrolases believed to be directly associated with the membrane structure. They include potassium-dependent phosphatases, aminopeptidase, phosphatidase, phosphohydrolase, ATPase, etc.

Available evidence suggests that enzymes found in the plasma membrane are not distributed at random, but are part of functional units. Maybe the most dramatic example of such an arrangement was provided by the studies of Crane [438] on the intestinal brush border. By controlled homogenization of intestinal scraping followed by differential centrifugation, Crane isolated the brush border of the intestine. Enzymic studies demonstrated the presence of a number of hydrolases in the brush border. The following enzymes are predominantly or exclusively associated with the brush border: maltase, lactase, invertase, isomaltase, trehalase, alkaline phosphatase, and leucylaminopeptidase. In addition, significant activity of an alkaline and a neutral ATPase as well as acid phosphatase were found in association with the brush border.

A number of biochemical experiments, including enzyme identification in cell membrane fractions, suggested that disaccharides are hydrolyzed in the superficial portion of the cell membrane. Thus, phlorizin and the absence of sodium do not stop disaccharidase action, but they do prevent monosaccharide accumulation, indicating that in the intestine the transport of at least some sugars is sodium dependent. On the basis of such findings, Crane proposed a model in which the membrane could be divided into two compartments referred to as the digestive surface and the diffusion barrier. The digestive surface, the most superficial, contains hydrolases and is permeable to glucose, fructose, sodium, etc. The diffusion barrier is located at the internal aspect of the digestive surface. Fructose diffuses freely, independent of sodium, but glucose transport requires a mobile carrier system, which is rependent on sodium penetration.

Not much is known about the carrier system, but it is believed to be made of a specific protein with specific binding sites for sugar and sodium. According to Crane, the mobile carrier can equilibrate sugar concentration across the brush border membrane, but the accumulation of sugar against the concentration gradient is believed to depend on the constant operation of the energy-dependent sodium pump.

Of the components needed for sugar transport that we have mentioned, sodium potassium ATPase has been identified in the cell membrane, and the sodium pump has been isolated as a discrete entity from the cell membrane. Thus, it is tempting to imagine a function or unit in which disaccharidases, a mobile carrier, and the sodium pump form intimate molecular complexes permitting sodium and glucose transport through the membrane of the brush border. But not all elements of this scheme are proven, and some are in question. On the basis of histochemical data, some investigators have argued that the disaccharidases are not an integral part of the cell surface but are located in organelles inside the cell. Others have claimed that the disaccharidases are simply absorbed at the cell surface. (The substrate of the sodium-dependent sugar carrier process includes glucose, galactose, 3-methylglucose, and xylose; that of the sodium-independent process includes fructose, 2-deoxyglucose, mannose, and sorbitol. Nilsson and Ronist [439] have shown that an erythrocyte membrane devoid of cytoplasmic contaminants contains glycerol triose phosphate dehydrogenase, phosphoglyceride kinase, and adenylate kinase.) As Crane pointed out, it is interesting that in the inherited malabsorption diseases, no brush border can be detected by electron microscopy.

Two forms of disaccharide intolerance have been described: sucrose and lactose intolerance. Sucrose intolerance is always associated with isomaltase intolerance and is found only in children. Lactose intolerance has been found in children and adults. The respective disaccharidases of the brush border are almost completely absent in both forms. These diseases are now believed to result from a failure of differentiation, including that of specific enzymes of the outer coat of the membrane.

Movement

To move, individual cells must either swim or crawl. Two types of crawling movements have been described; one has been primarily studied with amoeba, the other with fibroblasts.

Although not universally accepted, Goldacre's model [440] will be presented here. Amoeba move by expanding pseudopods. After the cell has established a point of contact with a solid surface, that portion of the cell referred to as the tail contracts. The contraction projects a stream of cytoplasm in the opposite direction, distending a portion of the membrane into a pseudopod, which contacts the solid surface. The molecular structure of the "motor" that generates the movements is not known. A number of hypotheses are available: (1) the tail contains contractible protein; (2) the peripheral cytoplasm is reversibly converted from sol to gel; (3) the elaboration of the new membrane provides the motive force. Although available evidence does not permit us to determine which of these mechanisms is responsible for cellular movement, the third mechanism appears to be unlikely, since a rapid turnover of the constituents of the amoeba membrane has not been demonstrated.

It has long been known that fibroblasts and many other mammalian cells are capable of movement. Some of the details of the movement were revealed only when interference and surface contact microscopy became available.

Abercrombie and Ambrose [441, 442] investigated the movement of fibroblasts. The moving fibroblast adheres to the solid surface and forms a "ruffled edge." The waving movement of the periphery of the cytoplasm, which is responsible for the development of the ruffled edge, secures displacement along the solid surface. The faster the cells move, the more rapidly their membranes develop the undulations that intermittently contact the solid surface. Again, the locomotive force is believed to be a contractible protein, forming short filaments inside of, and parallel to, the membrane. ATP is, of course, the source of chemical energy.

Although the molecular interactions involved in generating movement in the metazoan cells are likely to be complex and are surely far from elucidated, the following facts seem to have been established: (1) several types of filaments exist in various cultured cells—microtubes (see elsewhere) and 10-nm and 6-nm filaments; (2) the intracellular changes in the distribution of the filaments coordinate well with the deployment of cell movement; (3) actomyosinlike proteins are present in metazoan structure although their exact role in cell movement and distribution among the microfibrils is not clear [443].

The direction of the cell movement can be determined by three different mechanisms: contact guidance, chemotactism, and contact inhibition. In contact guidance, the solid substrate to which the cell must adhere for motion also determines the path of the cell because it is made of fibers (collagen) or grooves. Without such contact guidance, the movement of the cells is random, and that is exactly what happens on smooth glass surfaces.

The role that chemotactism plays in the movement of inflammatory cells has already been discussed. Clear-cut evidence for positive or negative chemotactism of other types of mammalian cells has never been convincingly established.

Contact Inhibition

When we discussed wound healing, we described how in a circular piece of excised amphibian skin, the cells at the free edge start to move toward the center of the wound until they meet the cells that migrated from the opposite direction, then they stop. For the purpose of investigating the inhibition of locomotion by contact with other cells, Abercrombie [444] studied the movement of fibroblasts by placing two explants in suspension in culture medium on a glass coverslip. The cells of each explant move at random as they proliferate, forming the ruffled edges that we have already described. The cells that move away from their respective explant toward the other explant come in contact in between the two. As the cells make intimate contact at some point of their membrane, the ruffled edges disappear and the cells stop moving. Abercrombie calls this impairment of cell movement as a result of contact "contact inhibition."

The mechanism of contact inhibition is not known. There is no obvious reason why cells should stop moving after they have established contact. Why couldn't they move together? A number of hypotheses have been proposed to explain contact inhibition. They include increased adhesiveness between cells and between cells and substrate. If adhesiveness is the mechanism, the molecules that hold the cells together and to the substrate remain to be identified. Later we will discuss adhesion further.

The notion that interference with contact making results from immobilization of the cell has been challenged. Films of cell movements in confluent monolayers have suggested that the inhibition results instead from a lack of tendency of the cells to crawl over each other or to overlap. Therefore, investigators have proposed that the phenomenon of contact inhibition be referred to as "contact inhibition of overlapping" [445].

Contact inhibition is not a random but a rather specific event. Every cell will not stop the locomotion of any other cell; for example, contact inhibition does not take place between fibroblasts and leukocytes or even between fibroblasts obtained from normal connective tissue and those obtained from sarcoma.

Obviously, directed cell migration coupled with specific contact inhibition could go far in explaining embryogenesis and histogenesis of tissues. The special cellular mosaic that composes a tissue may at least in part result from the regulation of cell movement and contact inhibition. Of course, little is known of the factors that influence these cellular properties. In embryogenesis large segments of the cell population are destroyed after migration and proliferation into a specific area, which suggests that other mechanisms in addition to cell movements are involved in the selection of the cell population that constitutes an organ.

On the basis of what we have just mentioned on cell movement and its arrest by contact inhibition, these events clearly are bound to play determinant roles in the biology of the organism. Therefore, detailed understanding of the molecular interaction involved in these events would be helpful in interpreting histogenesis and possibly carcinogenesis. These events are complex first because they occur at a level of magnitude that far exceeds even the most complex macromolecular interaction. Moreover, they are likely to involve multiple interactions between a large number of molecules of sizes ranging from that of small ions to that of large lipoproteins.

The problem can be examined by two different approaches—a rather theoretical one in which the interacting cells are considered to be charged masses in motion in a conductive fluid, and a direct one in which membrane components are taken apart and molecular complexes responsible for movement and contact inhibition are identified. Neither of these approaches has as yet yielded decisive information.

Adhesion

Weiss has reviewed the physical aspects of contact phenomena [446]. Two opposing forces determine cell contacts: a repression force that is electrostatic and develops because any particle suspended in an electrolyte solution is surrounded by double layers of ions, and an attraction force due primarily to van der Waal's forces. Physicists have derived appropriate equations for these forces, and the interested reader is referred to specialized reviews.

To reproduce these formulas here would serve no purpose because most of the variables entered cannot at this point be measured accurately in biological systems. Suffice it to point out that the repulsion forces decrease exponentially with the distance, whereas the attraction forces decrease inversely with the distance between particles. The resultant energy expressed in function of distance yields a sharp peak, the summit of which measures the potential barrier. On each side of this potential barrier are attractive troughs—one at short range and the other at long range. Thus, two cells can make contact in two ways: they find themselves within distances that are shorter than those at which the potential barrier develops, or the potential barrier is reduced.

The potential barrier can be reduced by increasing the attractive forces (little can be done about that) or by decreasing the repulsion forces. The latter can be achieved by altering the ionic milieu, reducing the dielectric constant of the medium, reducing the radius of curvature of approaching cell processes, and reducing surface potentials of approaching cells. The significance of all these parameters in determining cell contact remains unknown.

As Weiss pointed out, conventional physical treatment of the potential barrier in terms of particles simply submitted to brownian movement does not reflect the biological reality. The reality is a crawling cell in which the energy of movement may be great enough to bypass the potential barrier. When the potential energy has been overcome, adhesion between cells becomes possible. The forces that secure adhesion are not known. They could involve chemical (electrostatic) covalents of hydrogen bonds or van der Waal's forces. They may be direct from membrane to membrane, or indirect, involving protein or ions in the medium. The physical components involved in biological adhesion have been reviewed by Baier and his associates [447].

Some examples of adhesion between macromolecules (fibrin) and platelets are discussed in the chapter on blood coagulation. Whether these events can serve as models for cell adhesion remains to be seen.

Some observations made on mammalian cells have given some lead as to the mode of binding involved in cell adhesion. First, electron microscopy reveals that the points of contact are small relative to the cell size. Second, a protein must be involved in adhesion, since proteolytic enzymes facilitate separation. Third, exposure of the cell surface to neuraminidase also facilitates cell detachment, suggesting that sialic acid might be involved in cell adhesion.

Calcium's role in contacts of adult cells remains to be established. Calcium seems to affect the attachment of embryonic cells, and thus embryonic cells are readily separated by treatment with EDTA. Studies from Gasic's laboratory indicate that at least in sponge cells, reaggregation is impaired if disulfide bond formation is blocked.

In this discussion we have not considered the specificity of the attachment, yet Moscona and Moscona showed that when embryonic cells are dissociated and then allowed to reaggregate, they do so by sorting out according to cell type. After the cells have segregated, groups of cells are distributed in the aggregate according to patterns similar to those found in the embryo [448]. The selectivity of cell aggregation may be the consequence of qualitative specificity of the molecules involved in cellular adhesion (*e.g.*, special configuration of surface proteins as Weiss proposed [449], or selectivity may result from quantitative differences in strength of adhesion as Steinberg [450] proposed.

What mechanism obtains in the completed organ has not been settled. Evidence for the existence of special adhesive substances has been assembled in Moscona's laboratory. Cell products were isolated that specifically enhanced reassociation of dissociated sponge or chick embryo cells [451].

A compound apparently present in the cytosol of the cells of the living embryonic neural retina promotes histogenic aggregations of these cells. The compound is specific for retinal cells and will not aggregate liver, heart, or kidney cells. Little is known of the molecular structure of the compound.

Investigators have proposed that glycosyl transferase is involved in holding the cells together. If this were the case, the affinity between cells would depend on the molecular structure of the enzyme and that of the acceptor molecules on the membrane surface.

Two observations (modification of agglutination properties and analysis of glycolipid structures) emerging from the study of surface glycoproteins in cancer and normal cells have indicated that a surface alteration—a glycoprotein isolated from wheat agglutinates cells transformed by tumor viruses—takes place in the development of malignancy, but this does not affect normal cells.

However, normal cells are also agglutinated if they are treated with papain, indicating that a kind of superficial protein is lost during transformation. Similarly, leukemic or transformed cells are agglutinated by concanavalin A, a compound unable to agglutinate normal cells unless they are first treated with proteolytic enzymes. (Concavanalin A specifically binds to the α-methylglucopyranoside of the D-mannose or D-glucose configuration.)

Changes in the glycolipid composition of the cell surface have been demonstrated in a number of laboratories after viral transformation of cells. We shall consider only changes in ganglioside composition as an example.

We have seen that gangliosides are made of a ceramide moiety on which a polysaccharide side chain, as was the case for glycoproteins, is elaborated in a stepwise fashion by the successive actions of specific transferases. In transformed cells, the activity of these specific transferases appears to be decreased or lost altogether. For example, a decrease in UDP-N-acetylgalactosamine hematoside-N-acetylgalactosamine transferase has been observed in SV40 and polyoma transformed viruses.

In both cases, appropriate alterations in the glycolipid structure of the membrane are associated with the enzyme defect. Whether these changes are linked with malignancy is not certain. They could indeed be several steps removed from it and simply reflect changes in cell physiology accompanying transformation.

Because cellular aggregation is not thermodynamically reversible, the investigation of the molecular events involved in cellular adhesions is complicated further. One can never be certain that all the bonds that make the cells adhere to each other are broken after pulling the cells apart. Regular reactions as we know them are usually thermodynamically reversible. Thus, if molecule A is reacted with molecule B to yield complex C, and the conditions are right, C can be split to restore the exact molecules A and B. However, evidence does not suggest that when cell α and cell β are made to adhere to each other, they can be again separated to restore the cell α and the cell β integrally.

This notion can best be grasped by considering a metaphor. If a carpenter glues together a piece of redwood and white pine and tries to separate the two pieces by shearing after the glue has dried, pieces of the redwood adhere to the white pine and *vice versa*. The two boards will be even harder to separate if the joints were dovetailed. The same is true of an attempt to separate two adhering cells. After separation, each of the cells retains some fragments of the other. The irreversibility of adhesion is best illustrated by experiments in which cells are shaken off their glass support. The cohesion of the glass molecules is such that no glass remains attached to the cell, but cell fragments remain attached to the glass and leave what have been referred to as "tracks" or "footprints."

The tracks contain mucopolysaccharides, proteins, and even RNA. What effects a cellular fragment may have on its separated neighbor are not known, but fragments that include RNA and possibly DNA may affect the future of the segregated cell. That such cellular interactions are possible is suggested by electron microscopic observation. Cytoplasmic continuity between macrophages and lymphocytes in the lymph nodes and between the cells of peritoneal exudates of mice have been demonstrated by electron microscopy. Bridges containing DNA have been observed between tumor cells and peritoneal exudate cells of rats and mice [452].

Cellular Communication

These considerations brings us to examine the concept of cellular communication. For a long time, it was assumed that all cells were autonomous. Thus, each cell was believed to occupy a specific geographical position in the tissue mosaic and be metabolically independent. Regulation of genome expression or rate of activity of bioenergetic pathways would thus be the privilege of each cell. This belief collapsed when two simple but elegant experiments were performed in Loewenstein's laboratory [453]. In one experiment, an electric current was discharged in one cell and it propagated to other cells. In another, macromolecules were injected in one cell, and they were transferred to other cells.

It was later established that the presence of calcium in the medium is indispensable for intracellular communication. Moreover, the increasing of the intracellular concentration of calcium to levels similar to those found in the extracellular fluids abolished intracellular communication. The cell membrane is believed to contain binding sites for calcium, and when all binding sites are occupied by calcium ions, the cell membrane is impermeable. When cells are in contact, the calcium attached to the binding site at the points of contact is in the presence of all intracellular media with low concentrations of calcium. Consequently, the calcium at the points of contact is released from its binding sites, making the junction permeable for intercellular communication. Although it is suspected that growth factors are transferred from cell to cell, it is not known what type of information passes through these intercellular communication paths.

Electron microscopists have described three major types of physical contacts between cells: desmosomes, tight junctions, and gap junctions.

Most of the epithelial cells—namely, those sheets of cells that form the skin and cover the surface of the gastrointestinal and respiratory tracts—are hooked together, not by a continuous glue molding the surface like the cement of a brick wall, but by joints that are specifically located at the membrane surface. These areas of physical contact between two cells have been known for a long time and are called desmosomes. Desmosomes were long considered to be sites of focal thickening of each membrane, but electron microscopy has revealed that this is not so. Thus, at the desmosomes two normal bilayer membranes are separated by a normal intermembrane space, which is filled with an electron-dense material probably proteic in nature. For unknown reasons, a similar electron-dense condensation is found at the internal aspects of the membrane at a point exactly opposite the membrane junction. The role of desmosomes is believed to be purely mechanical—they hold cells together.

Some cell contacts, the tight junctions, involve the complete fusion of the two cellular membranes. Under the electron microscope, the surfaces of the two cells are closely apposed at the site of the tight junction, and the classical appearance of the two electron-dense lines of the bilayered membrane has disappeared, as has the intercellular space. There are only three electron-dense lines, suggesting that the external layers of the bilayered cellular membranes have fused together.

The function of the tight junctions has been derived from their anatomical location. They are indeed preponderant whenever a clear separation between two cell types or between a cell layer and the intracellular fluid is indispensable. For example, after intravenous administration, many substances never reach the brain, although they may reach all other tissues. The tight junction is believed to be the anatomical counterpart of the physiological barrier (the blood-brain barrier, see section on reaction to injury in the nervous system, Chapter 10). Thus, those cells that line the blood vessels of the brain are held together by tight junctions; in contrast, such junctions are not seen in cells that line blood vessels anywhere else in the body.

The third type of junction, the gap junction, forms channels between two cell membranes, penetrating intercellular spaces and connecting the cytoplasm of each cell. The gap junctions are probably critical to communication from cell to cell. Their precise role is not known. However, the incidence of gap junctions varies with the developmental level of tissues. Thus, gap junctions are present in the blastula of some fish, but they disappear at later stages of embryogenesis. They are also believed to channel the electrical communications between cells. These conclusions emerge from experiments with the electric organ of the electric eel. Rather than being adjacent to each other, the motor neurons that control that organ are linked together by gap junctions, which suggests that the junctions serve to secure synchronization of the electric discharge [454].

Regulation of Cellular Metabolism

Little is known of the cell membrane's role in regulating gene expression and the rate of cellular proliferation. The influence of the cell membrane on cell proliferation and differentiation will become more obvious when we discuss the modification of the membrane in cancer cells. Both in the embryo and in tissue culture, cell proliferation is slowed down or stopped when cells make contact.

Continued synthesis of chondroitin sulfate in cartilaginous cells is dependent on cell apposition, and the interaction between cells stabilizes the cell surface and allows continued chondroitin sulfate synthesis. These findings suggest that a feedback loop exists between the cell membranes and the genome.

The mechanism of pinocytosis has been investigated in *Amoeba chaos* fed paramecia. The inducer of pinocytosis leads to a structural change and an electrical change in membrane resistance. The electron-transparent core of the lamella of the unit membrane is at least twice as thick in areas of the membranes involved in phagocytosis than in others, and the electrical resistance of the membrane is reduced 50-fold in these areas. These morphological and electrical changes have been associated with the formation of typical tunnels and vacuoles that appear during pinocytosis. The formation of the pinocytic vacuoles depends on the concentration of external calcium. If the calcium in the medium is increased, the changes associated with pinocytosis are rapidly reversed.

With this information in mind, it is now easier to visualize how events occurring at the level of the cell membrane may influence cellular metabolism. We shall mention only three examples: regulation of genome expression, protein synthesis, and respiration.

We have seen that the sodium pump requires ATP for activity. The ATP can be provided by aerobic or anaerobic bioenergetic pathways. Abolition of the aerobic pathways reduces the effectiveness of active transport mechanisms. In turn, active transport can influence the rate of respiration. Indeed, the cell membrane contains an ATPase that seems to be involved in sodium pumping by converting ATP to ADP. The ATP is provided from the intracellular bioenergetic pathways in which the mitochondria play the major role. The level of respiration in the mitochondria is itself regulated by the levels of ADP. The higher the levels of ADP, the higher the stimulation to respiration. Consequently, one may anticipate that when the sodium pump is activated, the levels of ADP will increase inside the cell, and the level of respiration will be affected. Such interrelationships between ion transport and cellular respiration have been demonstrated in brain and in kidney [455].

The transfer of amino acids from amino acyl tRNA to a polypeptide chain during protein synthesis requires optimal concentrations of potassium. Potassium depletion produces a block in the late stage of protein synthesis. When potassium levels are low, the cell continues to synthesize RNA but not protein. How the variation in potassium concentration regulates protein synthesis during development or during the steady state is not known, but potassium's effect on protein synthesis provides a new potential link between cell membrane and regulation of intercellular metabolism [456].

In regenerating liver, the potassium-sodium-activated ATPase system is increased, reaching a maximum of increase 3 to 6 days after partial hepatectomy. The increase does not exceed 57% of the total of the activity in the normal. At the same time, the passive influx of rubidium 88, which indirectly measures the influx of potassium, was decreased between 1 and 6 days after operation. The increase in cation transport associated with a decrease in the passive cationic influx is believed to be responsible for the increased potassium and decreased sodium levels observed in the regenerating liver cell.

At the beginning of this section on the cell membrane, we stated that we would not describe the properties of the bacterial cell membrane in detail. Nevertheless, we will briefly mention the relationship between permeases, cell membrane, and gene expression. In bacteria, the rate-limiting step in the utilization of lactose is the activity of an α-galactoside permease, which is induced by the substrate. At low concentrations of inducers, the amount of newly synthesized enzyme hydrolyzing galactose β-galactosidase parallels that of new permease. One of the products of galactose breakdown is glucose. Glucose is known to inhibit many permeases.

Although the evidence is not conclusive, it is believed that the permease is directly inhibited by ATP, the terminal product of glucose utilization, rather than by glucose. Admittedly, this constitutes an oversimplification of a rather complex chain of metabolic interactions. But in this complex chain, the permease is the first enzyme and ATP is the last product, and it has been suggested that ATP is an allosteric inhibitor of the permease. This example taken from observations in bacteria and yeast illustrates the complex feedback loop that links cell membranes, genome, and bioenergetic pathway [457].

In his Nobel prize lecture, Luria [458] briefly but lucidly described the role and function of the protein antibiotic, colicine. Some bacteria produce proteins that kill susceptible strains of coliform bacteria by blocking macromolecular biosynthesis (nucleic acids and proteins). A single colicine molecule appears to be able to find its proper receptor on the bacterial surface and kill it. Although the inhibition of nucleic acid and protein synthesis is simultaneous with the arrival of colicine at the membrane, the metabolic blocks do not take place when the *E. coli* are grown in strict anaerobiosis. Therefore, investigators have concluded that colicine interferes with macromolecular synthesis indirectly by blocking oxidative phosphorylation. Later experiments revealed that the effect of the antibiotic was not directly on oxidative phosphorylation but probably resulted from an alteration of the permeability of the cell membrane. Thus, colicine-treated cells leaked out glucose-6-phosphate, fructose-1,6-diphosphate, dihydroxyacetone phosphate, and 3-phosphoglycerates. Moreover, a block in the conversion of pyruvate to acetate was also detected. Luria therefore proposes that an earlier effect of the colicine is to induce a reversible alteration of the cytoplasmic membrane. The alteration of the membrane becomes evident only in the presence of oxygen. Changes in membrane permeability result in reduction of ATP levels and, consequently, in reduction of all ATP-dependent processes. If colicine affects the configuration of the cell membrane, then the experiment illustrates the possibility of amplification of a small interference with the membrane into a complete block of macromolecular synthesis.

Molecular Composition of the Cell Membrane

Plasma membranes are made primarily of proteins and lipids. The proportion of proteins to lipids varies considerably, depending upon the method used for isolating and extracting the various components and the source of the membranes. We shall first concentrate on the chemical composition of the membranes of erythrocyte ghosts, although some have questioned whether erythrocyte ghosts are representative of cell membranes in other tissues.

The erythrocyte membrane contains three kinds of lipids—neutral, polar, and complex. Thirty per cent of the lipids contained in the erythrocyte ghosts are extracted with chloroform. The major portion (between 76 and 90%) of the neutral lipids of the erythrocyte ghosts is cholesterol. The remaining lipids are cholesterol esters, mono-, di-, and triglycerides, and fatty acids. Polar solvents extract approximately 60% of the lipids in the erythrocyte ghosts. Lecithin and sphingomyelin are among the polar lipids found in the highest proportion (respectively, 30% and 15% of the lipid phosphorus), followed by phosphatidylethanolamine and phosphatidylserine (14% and 11% of the lipid phosphorus, respectively). The remaining polar lipids are made of plasmalogens, monophosphoinositides, and phosphatidic acid.

Plasmalogens are acetal phospholipids or phosphoglyceracetals. They are thus phosphoglycerides containing a monovinyl ester and a mono fatty acyl group. Ethanolamine plasmalogen is a typical example. Thus, the plasmalogens constitute a group of phosphoglycerides in which the α position of the glycerol is involved in a vinyl ester linkage with a long-chain aliphatic aldehyde, while the β position forms an ester linkage with a fatty acid. Mammalian tissues contain ethanolamine, choline, and serine plasmalogens. Ethanolamine plasmalogen is usually the most abundant. (The diphosphatidylglycerol, cardiolipin, has been found in mitochondria.)

Little is known of the biosynthesis or the breakdown of plasmalogens. However, enzymes that catalyze the hydrolysis of the vinyl ester linkage of plasmalogen have been found in mammals. The enzyme that attacks the ethanolamine plasmalogen yields a lysophosphatidylethanolamine and a fatty aldehyde. A similar but different enzyme has been found to act on the choline plasmalogen. The erythrocyte ghost contains approximately 4% of choline plasmalogen and ethanolamine plasmalogen each, and less than 1% of serine plasmalogen (in percent of the total lipid phosphorus). The role of the plasmalogens in the cell membrane is unknown.

Although most lipids in the plasma membranes have structural roles, some of the lipids may contribute actively to membrane function. We have already mentioned the rapid modification of the turnover of some phospholipids in the sodium-potassium exchange and during phagocytosis. Membrane lipids are also believed to be involved in the effect of hormones such as insulin and TSH. At least in the endoplasmic reticulum, the activity of some enzymes is modified by the presence of lipids.

At first, studies of the protein component of the cell membrane were plagued by the fact that protein is not very soluble, so drastic methods of extractions were necessary. Therefore, it is difficult to be sure of what portion of protein has been lost and what portion is absorbed during the preparation. Consequently, it has proven almost impossible to establish the relevance of the protein extracted to the structure and the function of the membrane. In view of this, it is also not surprising that the reported ratio of lipids to proteins varies considerably from one laboratory to another. Because so little is established or understood about the protein composition of the cell membrane, even a comprehensive review of the available literature would not permit us to make a definite generalization about the participation of proteins in the structure and the function of cell membranes. Consequently, we will briefly review a few examples of the work done on the protein composition of the cell membrane, primarily to illustrate the difficulties involved in studying these problems.

Several investigators have attempted to study the protein composition of erythrocyte ghosts. Erythrocyte ghosts are particularly convenient for this type of study because the mature erythrocyte contains no cellular organelles, and thus after hemolysis the plasma membrane provides most if not all of the membrane structure of the ghost.

Neville [459] has isolated a pure protein from erythrocyte ghosts; but the most systematic studies were done in Bakerman's laboratory on human erythrocyte ghosts. Bakerman [460] and his associates isolated cell membrane preparations that were subjected to repeated washings until the levels of RNA content were minimized. Whether low levels of RNA are a criterion of purity of the cell membrane preparation remains to be seen, because it has been claimed that RNA is found in the cell membrane. Bakerman's membrane preparation is composed of 44% protein, 35% lipids, and 10% carbohydrates. The membrane preparation was virtually free of ATPase activity. Because of the relatively high and somewhat surprising carbohydrate content, Bakerman chose to refer to the membrane component as a lipoglycoprotein. Bakerman emphasized the similarities between the properties of the rat liver and the human erythrocyte plasma membrane with respect to overall solubility; relative proportions of lipids, carbohydrates, and proteins; and the relative proportions of polar and nonpolar amino acid side chains in the protein's moiety.

A systematic study of the solubility properties of the membrane component showed that high pH (pH 13) facilitates solubilization in anionic detergent. The soluble compound was then chromatographed on polyacrylamide gel; the details of these experiments cannot be described here, but the data suggested that the membrane was depolymerized to large aggregates by pH elevation and further depolymerized to two different subunits in the presence of detergents. The final product of depolymerization had a molecular weight of 40,000 and a lipid-protein ratio similar to that in the original membrane, sedimented in a single peak in the analytical centrifuge, and its amino acid composition was the same from one preparation to another. On the basis of the lipid and amino acid content, investigators calculated that the molecular weight of the protein segment must be of the order of 22,000. Bakerman has referred to the 40,000 molecular weight unit as the erythrocyte structural unit and to the protein moiety as the erythrocyte structural protein. He compared the molecular weight of the erythrocyte structural protein with that of the mitochondrial structural protein isolated in Green's laboratory and pointed out the similarity in molecular weight (22,500 for the mitochondrial structural protein). The amino acid composition of the mitochondrial structural protein is different from that of the erythrocyte structural protein. In conclusion, Bakerman's studies suggest that the erythrocyte cell membrane contains a repeated lipoprotein structural unit with a molecular weight of 40,000. A similar repeating unit was found in cell membranes in human liver, suggesting that the repeating unit is the same in both organs. Whether or not these repeating units are species specific remains to be seen.

Zwaal and Van Deenen [461] have prepared proteins from erythrocyte ghosts after solubilization by methods somewhat different from those used by Bakerman. The erythrocyte membranes of humans, rabbits, pigs, oxen, and sheep were solubilized by N-butanol fractionation of the ghost suspension. In the human erythrocyte, this method had yielded only small amounts of soluble materials in Bakerman's hands. The reasons for the differences in solubility are not explained. After solubilization in N-butanol, the pattern of protein distribution on polyacrylamide gel varied considerably from one species to another.

A combination of immunological studies and specific hydrolytic procedures has permitted investigators to establish the relative positions of glycolipids and glycoproteins on the membrane surface.

Treatment of cells with papain or pronase removes 15% of the dry weight of the cell without affecting its viability. As a result of such manipulation, 74% of the cell's sialic acid is lost. Similarly, treating the cell with neuraminidase removes 80% of the sialic acid. These findings indicate that the sialoglycoproteins are located at the cell surface. In contrast, glycolipids are located more centrally then the glycoproteins. For example, erythrocytes are not agglutinated by antibodies of ceramide tetrahexoside unless they have previously been treated with papain.

Meritorious as all these studies are, it is still difficult to determine the protein content and composition of the cell membrane. Because of differences in methods used, various laboratories have isolated different kinds of protein. The isolated proteins differ in their solubility and chemical properties, but probably also in their function. Three major categories of proteins can thus be distinguished: (1) those that participate in elaborating a lipoproteic structural unit (*e.g.*, the protein Bakerman isolated in the erythrocyte and the liver cell membrane); (2) those responsible for cell recognition; and (3) the catalytic proteins, which are more or less closely associated with the membrane and are involved in such membrane functions as transport and secretion.

However, as Marchesi [462, 463] pointed out, these studies also clearly established that membrane proteins are glycoproteins unusually rich in carbohydrates (up to 60%) that carry the antigenic group for the ABO and MN blood groups and serve as receptors for agglutinins. In addition, sialic acid is a preponderant component of the carbohydrate population, which indicates that this charged carbohydrate is responsible for the negative surface charge of the erythrocyte.

Marchesi and his collaborators used a simplified method of extracting erythrocyte membranes—namely, the treatment of erythrocyte ghosts with lithium diiodosalicylate (LIS); all proteins are solubilized, and can be separated by gel electrophoresis. Among a number of minor components, one protein, glycophorin, constitutes the major glycoprotein component of erythrocyte membranes. (Spectrin is another protein found in large amounts in erythrocyte membranes. It represents approximately 40% of the total membrane protein and appears to be extrinsic to the lipid hydrophobic region.)

Glycophorin is made of 131 amino acid residues to which 16 oligosaccharides are attached and can be divided into three essential portions: the N-terminal half to which most of the sugars are attached, the C-terminal, which contains a cluster of charged amino acids, and the middle portion. The sugars form small oligosaccharide chains (*e.g.*, tetrasaccharides) which may, for example, contain N-acetylgalactosamine, galactose, and sialic acid, but longer chains, made of 8 to 12 monosaccharides are also found. The carboxy-terminal end contains charged amino acid, the middle portion of the molecule is hydrophobic.

What is peculiar to the glycophorin molecule is the clear dissociation of the hydrophobic and the charged residues. This arrangement provides for a liposoluble central strand held by two water-soluble ends, and, as we shall see, a new model for membrane structure has been proposed on the basis of the intramolecular distribution of charges in glycophorin.

To represent the erythrocyte membrane as a lipid layer into which a single protein, glycophorin, is dissolved would be inappropriate because the erythrocyte ghost contains several minor components with unknown functions and a number of specific enzymes. We shall return to this matter when we consider membrane models.

The study of the constituent proteins of membranes obtained from sources other than the erythrocyte ghosts has been reviewed [464, 465] and will not be outlined in detail here. Suffice it to state that: (1) often tissues composed of various cell types were used; (2) little effort was made to quantitate the yield of plasma membranes obtained, so the isolated preparation is not necessarily representative of the whole; (3) few investigators have checked their preparation with appropriate morphological (electron microscopy) and biochemical (enzyme activities) markers. Even when markers were used, available techniques were limited. To prepare membranes from intact tissue, an investigator must homogenize cells, separate the cell components by differential centrifugation, and further concentrate the membrane preparation by separation on continuous or discontinuous gradients—for example, sucrose, dextrans, or ficolls.

When preparations obtained in this fashion are examined under the electron microscope, they appear as small vesicles that are believed to be fragments of plasma membranes that have curled up. Unfortunately, fragments of the endoplasmic reticulum or of the Golgi apparatus after homogenization yield similar vesicles; therefore, unless some special method is used to eliminate, or special criteria are used to assess, contamination of the plasma membrane preparation, one cannot be certain of what one is working with. Histochemists have established that some enzymes (for example, the 3-diphosphoglycerate phosphatase in erythrocyte membranes or sialidase in the liver cell membranes) are primarily, if not exclusively, associated with the plasma membrane.

Even histochemistry has its limitations. The demonstration of an enzyme in one cell fraction by histochemical techniques may provide conclusive evidence for the presence of the enzyme in that fraction; however, it does not necessarily exclude the presence of latent enzyme, inaccessible to the substrate, in other fractions. Some form of the enzyme activity that is used as a marker for the plasma membrane almost certainly will also be found in other cell fractions, particularly the endoplasmic reticulum where they are synthesized. Thus, unless one has also available, in addition to the plasma membrane marker, a good marker for the endoplasmic reticulum (*e.g.*, glucose-6-phosphatase in liver), it may be impossible to evaluate the level of endoplasmic reticulum contamination of the plasma membrane.

Few attempts have been made to separate the plasma membranes from other cell membranes on the basis of their charge. This is assuming that clear-cut differences in charge will be found by electrophoretic methods. Among the most promising methods of preparing plasma membranes is that devised by Warren and his associates, who found that the cell membranes of cells in culture could be toughened by adding compounds containing heavy metals, such as zinc chloride or fluorescein mercuric acetate. These compounds are believed to attach to the available SH group of the surface membrane. After such a procedure, the cell contents can be expelled from their surface envelope by gentle homogenization in hypotonic media, and density centrifugation permits further purification of the membrane preparation.

Similar procedures have been developed for cells obtained from intact animals. A solution of zinc chloride is injected, the tissue is homogenized, and the plasma membranes are separated from other cellular components by the two-phase system described above. Although the fixation method probably provides membrane components that are pure and in greater yield, it is not certain how representative they are of the intact intracellular membrane because the effects of the heavy metal on membrane structure and function are not known. Many catalytic proteins have been found in association with cell membrane preparations and, of course, with mitochondrial and endoplasmic reticulum fractions. Definite proof that the enzyme is part of the cell membrane is seldom available unless typical histochemical studies have been pursued.

Whether an enzyme is genuine to the plasma membrane is often difficult to demonstrate. Glucose-6-phosphate activity is usually used as a marker for contaminating endoplasmic reticulum, but it has been claimed that glucose phosphatase is also present in the plasma membrane. Only when an enzyme is unique to the plasma membrane can one feel secure that it is genuine to that structure.

The enzymes associated with cell membranes can be classified in three functional groups: (1) those involved in transport, (2) those involved in secretion, and (3) those that affect the source of energy. We have already discussed the sodium-potassium-sensitive ATPase, the diglyceride kinase, and the role of the phosphatidic acid cycle in cell membrane function in the salt gland. When the cell secretes salt, phosphatidylinositol is reduced to a diglyceride, which in the presence of ATP is converted to phosphatidic acid. The reaction is reversible as soon as the cell stops secreting salt; the phosphatidic acid is reconverted to phosphatidylic inositol.

Enzymes necessary for this cycle—diglyceride kinase and phosphatidic acid phosphatase—have been found in the erythrocyte membranes by Hokin and Hokin. In bacteria, permeases with a high degree of stereospecificity toward transported substrates have been found. Examples are the β-galactoside permease and the α-metaglucoside permease.

The enzymes associated with the plasma membrane have seldom been extensively purified and isolated. They have been identified only by their catalytical properties.

Relationships between protein and lipid in the cell membrane may not be only for structural arrangement. A number of enzymes have been shown to be activated by lipids. For example, phospholipase C is activated by phosphatidylcholine and lysophosphatidylproline.

A number of phosphohydrolases of the plasma membrane of the liver are activated by the presence of lipid or inactivated by lipid removal. Such findings were made for ATPase of sarcoplasmic reticulum and glucose-6-phosphatase of the liver endoplasmic reticulum.

Molecular Organization of the Cell Membrane

Unless the cell membrane is made of a coded macromolecule similar to DNA, the multiplicity of its function would bring one to anticipate a rather complex structure. That DNA can be a macromolecule of relatively uncomplicated composition storing a triplet code is understandable because the function of DNA is relatively simple. It binds to a few enzymes, including DNA or RNA polymerase, and makes two different kinds of templates—its own complimentary DNA chain and an RNA chain.

In contrast, the function of the cell membrane is varied. In fact, in addition to highly specialized functions, such as transport, many of the major cellular functions are represented in the membrane. It would seem that only the plasticity and the diversity of protein molecules could provide the membrane with such far-reaching potentials. Yet so little is known of the protein structure of the cell membrane that it is surprising that so many attempts have been made to build membrane models and, even more astonishing, that some of the oldest models are likely to depict large segments of the membrane structure.

When we discussed the pathology of the nerve cells, we also described the structure of myelin and pointed out how the study of the myelin sheaths combined with physicochemical investigation of membrane permeability, electron microscopic examinations of cell membranes of various sources, and X-ray diffraction studies of some membranes led somewhat unexpectedly to the concept of the unit membrane. Today the two major hypotheses for the membrane structure are the unit membrane and subunit structure [466–468]. We will examine them only briefly because a conclusive description of membrane structure will come about only when the molecular composition and the intermolecular reactions in the cell membrane are clearly understood. Although physicochemical, electron microscopic, and X-ray diffraction studies might provide a wealth of information to buttress one hypothesis or another, only laborious chemical breakdown of the cell membrane into its components will provide the definite answer.

Already in 1925 Gorter and Grendel [469] proposed that cell membranes were made of lipid bilayers, but Danielli [470, 471] developed the concept into what has become the classic model of membrane structure. Danielli proposed that the membrane is composed of a continuous bimolecular lipid layer in which the molecules are rigidly arranged. The hydrophobic bonds face inward, while the hydrophilic groups face outward. Consequently, polar groups are found at both sides of the membrane, and the lipid layers are believed to be covered with a continuous protein layer at their inner and outer sides, the protein being attached to the polar groups of the lipid. Obviously, only phospholipids can play such a role in the bimolecular lipid layer.

The proportion of proteins to lipids satisfies the requirement of the model, and, as we have seen, the model is in keeping with the three-layered appearance of the membrane in electron micrographs. If the chemical analyses are not absolutely convincing, they are not in conflict with Danielli's model.

Nevertheless, in recent years many objections have been raised against Danielli's model. Perhaps the most important concerns its rigidity and its inadequacy in explaining the functions of the cell membrane. Studies with X-ray crystallography, infrared spectroscopy, nuclear magnetic resonance, and *in vitro* reconstructed models seem to indicate that the lipid layer, rather than being a typical bilayer, has a thickness less than twice the length of the phospholipid molecule. The fatty acid chains of the membrane interior are now believed to be in a disordered state approaching that of a liquid hydrocarbon. As Stoeckenius and Engelman pointed out [472], the functional consequences of this liquidlike hydrocarbon region have not been explored. Neither is there much knowledge of the lipid-protein interaction in the membrane.

As it is described in Danielli's model, the membrane cannot provide for the variety of multimolecular interactions necessary for some of the membrane functions described previously. The subunit theory proposes that the cell membrane is composed of self-assembled structural or functional subunits or both. In the cell membrane, the concept is purely hypothetical since such subunits have not been identified morphologically.

The difficulty that surrounds the demonstration of subunits in a given membrane is illustrated by what we have already said about the mitochondria, in which two types of subunits have been identified. The first is a morphological subunit, often referred to as the inner membrane particle or the elementary particle, and it constitutes a repeating unit of the membrane that has been isolated and demonstrated to contain mitochondrial ATPase. The ATPase can be separated and rebound to the membrane. Whether the combination of the singular enzyme with the membrane qualifies as a subunit is debatable.

The second type of subunit that has been described in mitochondria is a functional one known as the respiratory chain. Green claims to have separated four lipids associated with some of the proteins of the respiratory chain which, after separation, reassociate to form a functional subunit having the properties of the respiratory chain.

These findings have been challenged because some believe that the components separated are not pure lipids and proteins but also contain membrane fragments. If, indeed, the individual lipids and proteins of the respiratory chain remain attached to some membrane fragments, one may anticipate that these membrane fragments would spontaneously reaggregate without constituting a genuine subunit. Functional subunits are not found only in mitochondria. We have already discussed the possibility of the existence of functional units in the intestinal brush border.

Several investigators have reviewed the merits and disadvantages of the lipid bilayer and the subunit theory, but we cannot enter this controversy here; the reader is referred to specialized papers. We will simply describe the position taken by Stoeckenius and Engelman [472]. After exhaustively reviewing the subject, these investigators concluded that the membrane is likely to be made of a continuous lipid bilayer that would provide the passive permeability required for cell survival. However, this bilayer is different from the traditional one. Instead of having a rigid arrangement of the bimolecular layers, the lipids form a disordered central hydrocarbon region. Proteins are believed to be located predominantly at the surface of the lipid layer to which they are connected by both hydrophobic and ionic bonds. Thus, the general permeability and the barrier property of the cell membrane are contributed by the lipid bilayer, whereas the selective permeability and function are contributed by special arrangement and conformation of the protein. Whether the specific properties of the membrane require that either lipid and protein or proteins alone are arranged in a special mosaic to form a special subunit is not settled.

This theory of cell membrane structure reconciles some of the basic concepts of a unit membrane with the various functions of the membrane. Thus, all membranes would have a fundamental suprastructure, a bilayer of lipids coated with protein arranged in a disorderly fashion and detectable by electron microscopy. In addition, a much more diversified infrastructure is made of a combination of lipids and protein molecules. The infrastructure varies considerably from one side of the membrane to another, from one type of cell membrane to another, and within the cell from one type of organelle membrane to another.

This concept of a membrane composed of a fluid lipid bilayer [473] containing floating proteins has been expanded into a more precise model thanks to the discovery of some special properties of cytochrome b_5 and glycophorin. The tripartite amphipatic (a central hydrophobic core and two hydrophilic ends) structure of glycophorin has already been described. Similarly, cytochrome b_5, a hemoprotein found in microsomal membranes, the polypeptide chain of which is composed of 100 amino acid residues, has its heme group protruding at the surface of the membrane (it can be clipped off with proteolytic enzymes). The amino acid sequence of the rest of the molecule indicates that it is highly hydrophobic, making the molecule well suited to mix with lipids. In fact, when cytochrome b_5 is separated from the membrane, lipids and then protein and lipids are again mixed together; the cytochrome instantaneously attaches to the membrane.

Rhodopsin is also believed to span the lipid bilayer of the retinal disk membrane. In addition, when the retina is exposed to light, calcium enters the membrane. This is believed to occur at the rhodopsin sites which form transmembrane channels similar to those formed by gramicidin [655, 656].

On the basis of these findings, a new model for the relation between proteins and lipids in the membrane has been proposed in which the protein is believed to stretch from one end of the lipid layer to the other. Thus, the middle hydrophobic portion of glycophorin sinks into the lipid pool while its edges emerge from the pool. The inside end is loaded with the carbohydrate and the outside end with charged amino acids. This new concept is sometimes referred to as the iceberg model, comparing the protein with an iceberg swimming in a pool of lipids. The new model is entirely compatible with available electron microscopic pictures of membranes obtained by freeze etching, with the physicochemical status of lipids in the membrane, and with membrane function.

In the freeze etching technique, membrane preparations are frozen in liquid nitrogen, cleaved under a vacuum, and the cleaved surfaces are sprayed with vaporized platinum and carbon. The vapors solidify and form a replica that can then be examined under the electron microscope.

Experiments with labeled ferritin, which attaches exclusively to the exterior membrane, have established that the cleaved surfaces never contain ferritin. This finding strongly suggests that the cleaved surface represents not the exterior but the internal surface obtained after fracture of the lipid bilayer. Studies with the erythrocyte membrane have shown that 10–20% of the total membrane is represented by globular particles 75 A in diameter and proteic in nature, which span the membrane width and penetrate both the inner and outer surfaces. This confirms the prediction of Bretscher, who was the first to propose that the major glycoproteic component of the cell membrane spans the lipid bilayer and carries much of the carbohydrate and most of the sialic acid of the cell surface [474].

Among the properties that the composition of the lipid bilayer can be expected to modulate, one must include the physicochemical state of the membrane and the permeability of membranes to polar groups. Although the details of all the molecular interactions are far from known, the tightness with which two lipid molecules interact is reflected by the melting point of the molecular complex. Thus, the heating of lipid preparations brings about a switch from a state of "crystalline gel" to that of a liquid crystal." The increment of temperature needed for the passage of one state to another is called the transition temperature. By measuring transition temperatures of pure compounds and comparing them with those of bacterial or cell membrane preparations, one can determine whether the sample is in the crystal gel or the liquid crystal form. The existence of the latter form is, of course, of great significance because the liquid crystal state facilitates the passage of organic molecules that can dissolve in the membrane.

At least three factors help to determine whether the membrane or a portion of the membrane exists in one form or another: (1) the presence of cholesterol, (2) the length of the fatty acid chain, and (3) the degree of saturation of these chains. At least in bacterial membranes, some portions of the membrane are in the crystalline gel configuration while others appear in the liquid crystal structure. *E. coli* react to the lowering of growth temperature by increasing the level of unsaturated fatty acids in their membrane lipids. The physiological implications of these differences are not always clear. Variations in the physicochemical appearance of the membrane have been observed in poikilodermic animals. Fish are known to adjust the fatty acid composition of their lipids to suit the water temperature.

Studies of mammalian cell membranes suggest that they all exist in the liquid crystal state, sometimes for different reasons.

The concept of a lipid fluid membrane in which proteins are dissolved is compatible with membrane function. For example, consider the carrier mechanism. The membrane, primarily composed of a phospholipid bilayer, is impermeable to substances from the exterior, and a carrier is responsible for transferring substances from the outside to the inside or *vice versa*. A carrier has been postulated to function by diffusing substances through the membrane and by operating as a revolving door.

The antibiotic valinomycin makes the membrane permeable to potassium ions but not to sodium ions. In other words, it modifies the membrane permeability in a selective fashion carrying a specific ion. Valinomycin is believed to achieve these roles by combining with the phospholipid layer membrane, then grabbing the potassium ion in the environment and diffusing it through the membrane. Once the potassium ion has reached the opposite side of the membrane, it is dissociated from the complex and released. This can be achieved because valinomycin is a nonpolar, fat-soluble polypeptide that can easily mix with the lipid bilayer of the membrane.

A floating protein could more readily revolve in the lipid fluid and act as a revolving door to carry compounds from the outside to the inside of cells, or *vice versa*. The model is also compatible with the notion of transport through channels. Thus, it has been proposed, for example, that some substances penetrate the membrane through channels that are lined with four constitutive membrane proteins that span the distance between the periphery and the inside of the cell.

If valinomycin is the prototype ion carrier in biological membranes, gramicidin A a pentadecapeptide, facilitates ion transport through channels or pores. Although the details of the tertiary structure of gramicidin A are not known, the pentadecapeptide is believed to be twisted by formation of hydrogen bonds into a β pleated helix. Two helical molecules of gramicidin A form head to head dimers which are embedded in the lipid bilayer where they form channels which act as a pore. For further information on molecular models for membrane carriers and pores see [667].

Immobilization of the lipid bilayer by cooling the cell in cultures at 32° C inhibits adenylcyclase, indicating that a close interaction between membrane lipids and proteins exists.

Biosynthesis of the Cell Membrane

Since so little is known of the chemical composition of the cell membrane, one can hardly anticipate that the mechanism of cell membrane biosynthesis could be known, except of course for the elaboration of the building blocks—fatty acids for lipid, and amino acids for protein synthesis. Even less is known about the metabolism of plasma membranes than about that of the endoplasmic reticulum. A new plasma membrane must be elaborated after cell division, and the new membrane differentiates, thus developing specialized functional and morphological properties. Moreover, even in the steady states there is some protein turnover, and the rate of turnover varies from one protein to another. For further detail, see Siekevitz's article [475].

The dynamic properties of the cell membrane can be better understood if one keeps in mind some of the performance of the cell membrane during the life span of some cells. At the onset of life the sperm cell, by mechanisms still unknown, pierces the membrane of the egg. This penetration makes a hole which must be repaired by fusion of the remaining membranes. Every time a cell divides, the single membrane that surrounds the two cytoplasms and nuclei must in some way invaginate until it meets the membrane at the opposite site, and fuse with it to allow the separation of the two cells. In the process of pinocytosis, the membrane sends out evaginations which engulf the material to be pinocytized; but to secure the inclusion of the pinocytic vacuole, portions of the evaginated pockets must fuse. A similar, but reverse process occurs in exocytosis; thus membrane fusion is a frequent and sometimes a vital part of cell life. During embryogenesis, myeloblasts fuse to form muscle microfibrils. Some primitive cells fuse to form osteoclasts and after conception, cells are fused to form the syncitial trophoblast.

We have concentrated this discussion on cell membranes on the plasma membrane. However, it should be kept in mind that at least 8 different types of membranes are found in the eukaryotic cell and even more are found in plants. These membranes outline special compartments in which metabolic constituents are present in different concentrations. Thus, they generate gradients of concentrations between the different compartments and the extracellular environment. The maintenance of these gradients is essential for the maintenance of life. To maintain the integrity of the cellular environment and the intracellular compartments, the cellular membranes must remain uninterrupted at all times (except for discontinuities compatible with selective permeability) and must, during cell division, maintain spatial and functional continuity.

The biosynthesis of cell membrane involves the elaboration of its building blocks, lipids, proteins, etc. The building blocks must be transported to the site of assembly and be assembled with the macromolecular structure of the membrane.

When new membranes are synthesized, the existing membranes could be destroyed and be replaced by a new and enlarged membrane system. Such a mechanism would undoubtedly interrupt membrane continuity. Membranes could also be formed by expanding pre-existing membranes simply by including new molecular components.

Evidence assembled in Palade's laboratory on differentiating hepatocytes and after induction of the endoplasmic reticulum with drugs, which is still too preliminary to be described in detail here, suggest that the latter mode of membrane biosynthesis obtains, at least under those conditions.

One may also ask whether all the individual molecules that constitute a membrane are introduced in the membrane multimolecular structure at the same or at different rates. Again, studies on differentiating hepatocytes or induction of endoplasmic reticulum after phenobarbital suggest that the expansion of the membrane is a multistep event. For example, after induction with phenobarbital the reductase levels in the membrane increase before that of cytochrome p_{450}. In contrast, the levels of cytochrome b_5 which are not involved in the mixed function oxidase activity do not change. There is further evidence that the biosynthesis of the membrane proteins involves a set of polyribosomes different from those used in the biosynthesis of proteins made for other intracellular functions or for export. Glucose-6-phosphatase, which is low before birth, increases after birth. Within a given cell it is randomly distributed within the endoplasmic reticulum. Such dispersion of the enzyme implies that either the enzyme is inserted in the membrane at random, or that after being introduced in special areas, it diffuses throughout the membrane. Studies in *Clamidonomas* support the findings made in hepatocytes.

In conclusion, available evidence suggests that during cell differentiation and induction and cell division, the new membranes are formed by expansion of preexisting membranes. In the case of cell division, once enough membranes are made, two processes take place: (1) thickening of the membranes to be associated with each individual cell and (2) fusion of the separate membranes to reconstitute the continuity of the compartments in each cell.

Furthermore, the cell periphery is composed of that portion of the cell including the cell membrane and ectoplasmic structures which contain microtubules and actin-like microfilaments. According to modern concepts, the cell periphery is composed of a collection of molecular domains. Ninety percent of the matrix is formed of a lipid bilayer containing fatty acids, cholesterol, phospholipids, etc. The lipids are in a dynamic state and can either rapidly rotate and be displaced laterally or can travel more slowly across the membrane in what is referred to as a flip-flop motion.

The fluidity or the viscosity of the membrane varies depending upon the cell type and depends upon the lipid composition of the membrane. High concentrations of long chain fatty acids decrease the viscosity, while the presence of high concentrations of sterols and unsaturated fatty acids increases the intrinsic viscosity.

The relationships between proteins and the lipid bilayer are of three types: (1) The protein may be deposited at the internal or external aspect of the bilayer without penetrating it. This is the case for the spectrin, actin and tubulin molecules found at the internal aspect of the membrane. These tubular or fibrous proteins may, however, be anchored to proteins that penetrate the membrane. (2) Proteins may be partially buried into the lipid layer with one end protruding at the exterior or the interior. (3) Proteins may be amphipatic and span the width of the membrane with small segments extending beyond the inner or outer aspect of the membrane (*e.g.*, glycophorin, rhodopsin, cytochrome b). Glycolipids are usually found inside of the lipid bilayer.

When new membranes are formed it is through a multistep macromolecular synthesis expanding preexisting membranes.

The membrane receives signals from the outside and forwards signals that are emitted from the periphery of the cell to the inside. Among the components that issue signals are either virus coded proteins (*e.g.*, new protease) that appear at the surface of the transformed cells or the binding of hormones on specific receptors. The signals received by the cell surface are transmitted inside the cell either by activating surface enzymes, such as adenylate cyclase and the Na^+-K^+ adenosine triphosphatase, or by modulating the internal structures (microtubules and actin filaments) or the cell periphery.

Cancer and Cell Membranes

In previous sections of this chapter we have described various alterations of the cell membrane in cancer cells; they include reduced adherence, changes in electrical conduction, loss of contact inhibition of movement, appearance of virus transplantation antigens. In this section we will briefly review some of these changes and others such as alteration in membrane agglutinability caused by lectins and the alteration in surface glycolipids and glycoproteins [651–661].

While normal cells do not grow beyond the monolayer, transformed cells grow over each other to form multiple layers.

Transformed cells have little or no serum requirement for growth. This is believed to result from the presence of inhibitors which are elaborated in normal, but absent in transformed cells, or from the presence in serum of factors necessary to the growth of normal cells, but not for that of cancer cells. Among the growth factors are insulin, nonsuppressible insulin-like activity (somatomedin), the sulfation factor and the multiplication stimulating activity (MSA). The growth stimulating properties of insulin, somatomedin and sulfation factors have been described in Chapter 8. MSA is a small protein (10,000 molecular weight) with the properties of both somatomedin and the sulfation factor. It can substitute for serum in inducing incorporation of thymidine in chick embryo cells.

Treatment of cells in culture with a number of substances that modify the surface membranes, such as hyaluronidase and digitonin, are as effective at stimulating DNA synthesis as a fresh change in serum. Neuraminidase stimulates cell division and mitosis in chick embryo.

Mild and short treatment of cells in culture with protease (trypsin, papain, chymotrypsin or pronase) releases the cells from density inhibition of growth (which refers to the inability of normal cells to grow beyond the monolayer low density).

Moreover, as we have seen already, protease causes nonagglutinable cells to agglutinate. Thus, proteases do confer to normal cells at least some of the properties of transformed cells. However, the cells do not maintain these properties. After one or two rounds of cell division the cells recover their density dependent inhibition of growth and their agglutinability. Protein inhibitors inhibit the growth of transformed 3T3 cells or of tumor cell cultures *in vitro*.

A number of laboratories have shown that viral transformed cells, but not normal fibroblasts, hydrolyze fibrin. Only DNA and RNA transforming viruses, but not cytolytic viruses, induce the fibrinolysis. The fibrinolytic activity of tumors involves two proteases; one is plasminogen which is present in all vertebrate sera and an arginine specific protease (38,000 daltons) found in small amounts in transformed cells which hydrolyzes a single peptide bond in plasminogen. It has been suggested by Reich and his coworkers that transformed cells have receptors for plasmin that are not found in normal cell cultures and that the binding of plasmin and fibrinolysis are responsible for the changes in morphology and mobility observed in the transformed cells. In fact, the role of the fibrinolytic system in transformation remains to be clarified [662].

Further evidence that release of growth control is associated with changes in cell membranes is provided by experiments in which cells are treated with a 2 M urea. Such treatment induces agglutinability and abolishes density dependent inhibition of growth. Removal of urea restores the cells to normal. Restoration was prevented by inhibition of protein synthesis (*e.g.*, cycloheximide) suggesting that *de novo* synthesis of membrane proteins is needed for the restoration.

Lectins are plant or vertebrate proteins that react with the cell surface. At least 10 have been described and characterized; they include: concanavalin (Con A) which was isolated from jack beans and crystallized (molecular weight of 100,000 to 120,000); soya bean agglutinin, a tetrameric glycoprotein with a molecular weight of 100,000; wheat germ agglutinin, a dimeric protein with a molecular weight of 35,000; phytohemagglutinin, a protein extracted from the red kidney bean, with a molecular weight of 29,000 to 30,000. The main interest in these proteins resides in their ability to agglutinate cells and in general, it can be said that transformed cells are more readily agglutinated than normal cells.

One can distinguish two steps in the agglutination process: the binding of the agglutinin to the cell and the attachment of cell to cell. The binding of the agglutinin to the cell surface is not unlike that of IgG to lymphocytes. IgG attaches to accessible receptors on the cell surface, the attachment is followed by the "capping" or clustering of the receptors at one point of the surface of the membrane and endophagocytosis of the antigen antibody complex. The clustering is believed to be a passive process involving the cross-linking of bivalent or polyvalent antibody.

The binding of lectins to the cell surface occurs through a similar mechanism, attachment to accessible receptors, clustering of the receptors and cross-linking of the polymeric agglutinins. Data indicating the need for ATP during the binding process are controversial.

The clustering of the receptors is intriguing. It agrees with the "fluid dynamic theory of the cell membrane," if, in fact, the membrane is immobilized by treatment with glutaraldehyde which will cross-link proteins; binding of agglutinin does not take place. There is evidence that clustering requires an intact microtubular system; colchicine and vinblastine inhibit agglutination of fibroblasts and polymorphonuclears. A role of microfilaments in clustering is suspected, but not established.

Nothing is known of the molecular mechanism by which lectins bind cells together. Two mechanisms have been proposed: the formation of covalent cross-links between lectin, and the clustering of hydrophobic sites in the fluid membrane which facilitates adherence between cells through hydrophobic bonds.

One can distinguish several classes of cells with respect to their binding properties to lectin. Some cells cannot bind lectins because the receptor is either absent or buried. Buried receptors can be brought to the surface by treatment in some cases with glycosidase, in others with protease. The exteriorization of receptors by proteases does not necessarily imply that the receptor is entirely coated with proteins. In fact, the splitting of only a few peptide bonds seems to be necessary to uncover the receptor, indicating that only a few critical sites need to be uncovered. Some normal cells can bind agglutinin, but the binding is not followed by agglutination. There is no satisfactory explanation for this special property.

Some cells bind the agglutinin and agglutinate. This includes cells transformed by either viruses or carcinogens. Thus, in most cases transformation induces changes in the surface membrane which leads to altered agglutinability.

The property to agglutinate in presence of lectins is, however, not restricted to transformed cells. Embryonic cells agglutinate, but in most cases they lose this property when they differentiate. Lectins may agglutinate normal cells, but then the agglutinability of the normal cell is usually weaker than that of the corresponding transformed cell. There are exceptions however, lentil agglutinin agglutinates hepatic more effectively than hepatoma cells.

The reasons for the reactivity of transformed cells with agglutinin is not known. Increased electronegativity or membrane flexibility, emergence of buried receptors either through the action of peptidase or glycosidase, *de novo* synthesis of receptors under the influence of the virus or the chemical carcinogens have all been proposed with little convincing evidence.

Some segments of the membrane may be more rigid than others. They usually contain rigid molecules such as cholesterol. There seems to be a relationship between membrane fluidity and membrane function. Inbar and Sacks have found that differentiated cells release a protein which induces undifferentiated leukemic myeloblasts to differentiate. However, all leukemic cells do not differentiate. The cells that differentiate form caps or clusters at the cell surface with fluorescent-tagged concanavalin A, while the cells that do not differentiate have no tendency to do so. Thus, the receptors are more mobile in the cells that differentiate than in those that do not differentiate. It was further observed that the receptor sites are more mobile in normal lymphoid than in lymphoma cells. (This finding contradicts previous observations made on normal and transformed fibroblasts.)

Changes in the distribution of ATPase activity on the surface of the cell membrane have been observed during the preneoplastic phase in hepatocytes of rats fed N,N′-dimethylaminoazobenzene [669].

Large portions of the cellular carbohydrate polymers (except hyaluronic acid and glycogen), whether they are located at the cell surface, found between cells like the ground substance, or are part of the circulating glycoproteins, are covalently bound to lipids or proteins.

Two types of binding prevail, N-glycosidic and O glycosidic linkages. The N-glycosidic linkage occurs more frequently than the O-glycosidic. The N-glycosidic linkage involves an asparagine residue of the protein and a N-acetylhexosamine residue of the reducing end of the polysaccharide. The O-glycosidic linkage occurs between the hydroxyl of either a serine, threonine or hydroxyproline residue of the protein and the terminal reducing sugar of the polysaccharide.

Biosynthesis of the polysaccharide side chains takes place by the sequential addition of sugar moieties to a growing polysaccharide chain. The unchanged sugar moiety is not a good substrate for the building of the polysaccharide chain. The effective precursor is a UDP derivative of the sugar in question. The transfer of the sugar from the UDP derivative to the growing polysaccharide chain is catalyzed by glycosyl transferase. Such transferases are highly specific for both donor and receptor sugar and consequently the structure of a specific polysaccharide side chain is determined by the sequential catalytic action of specific transferases.

Two cell structures are involved in the biosynthesis of glycoproteins; the endoplasmic reticulum and the Golgi. Clearly, the protein moiety for glycoproteins as for other proteins is synthesized on a polysomal scaffold. Intracellular proteins (*e.g.*, ferritin) are synthesized on free polysomes, while proteins for export (*e.g.*, serum glycoprotein) are synthesized on polysomes attached to membranes (rough endoplasmic reticulum).

It has been proposed, but not convincingly established, that hexosamine is bound to the protein while the protein is still attached to ribosomes. What is certain is that glycosylation is pursued as the glycoprotein is removed from and moves along the channels of the smooth endoplasmic reticulum. The Golgi apparatus appears to be the major center of glycosylation; the protein which has been partially glycosylated in the channels of the smooth endoplasmic reticulum is transferred to the Golgi where radioautographic studies have demonstrated that extensive glycosylation takes place. It now appears that both excreted and endogenous glycoproteins are glycosylated in the Golgi. In fact, transferases catalyzing the transfer of a N-acetyl glucosamine, galactose, and N-acetylneuraminic acid have been found in association with the Golgi. These transferases act in sequence when an appropriate acceptor is present.

A comprehensive discussion of the properties of glycoproteins will not be presented here. Suffice to point out (1) that they constitute a broad population of proteins, some of which are secreted (mucoproteins), while others are found in plasma and others exist in the form of insoluble collagen or surface antigens; (2) that their polysaccharide moiety includes D-glucose, D-galactose, D-mannose, D-xylose, N-acetyl-D-glucosamine, N-acetyl-D-galactosamine and L-fucose; (3) that the carbohydrate content may vary considerably (from 1 to 80%).

Glycoprotein alterations in transformed cells have not been as extensively investigated as those of glycolipids. But it appears that a lack of sialyl transferase leads to incomplete synthesis of glycoproteins deficient in terminal sialic acid. In some carcinomas, increased amounts of fucose have been found in the membrane glycoproteins. Moreover, there is a deletion of A and B blood group antigenicity in premalignant lesions and malignant tumors.

In normal cells glycolipids are believed to be involved in cellular recognition and growth regulation through surface receptors. Therefore, it is not surprising that a great number of studies were devoted to the analysis of the glycolipids of the surface of cancer cells.

Rapport demonstrated that homogenates of human tumors are more effective in eliciting an immune response against lipid antigens than normal tissues. Lactosylceramide was shown to be the haptene of the lipid antigen. In cell lines transformed by polyoma virus, the levels of glycolipids per mg of protein were reduced by half. The reduction was associated with a switch in the relative proportion of glycolipids. The levels of the hematoside were reduced 4 times, while that of lactosylceramide is increased 10 times and a decrease in the activity of the enzyme that catalyzes the addition of N-acetylgalactosamine to hematoside was observed. In general, it appears that tumor glycolipids have incomplete carbohydrate chains. However, there are no exceptions; for example, there are no changes in glycolipids in some human hepatomas.

As we have seen previously (Chapter 3), the cell surface contains a number of gangliosides which differ from each other by the length of the carbohydrate chain.

It is generally accepted that most cellular glycosphyngolipids are found in the plasma membrane.

Brody and Fishman have further investigated the changes in gangliosides observed after transformation with polyoma or SV40 virus and spontaneously transformed cells. They found (1) that different analogs of sialic acid were present in the transformed cells, N-acetylneuraminic acid and N-glycosylneuramic acid; (2) different fatty acids in the ceramide moiety; (3) the absence of gangliosides with carbohydrate chains longer than that found in GM_3; and (4) a decrease in the activity of the hematoside N-acetylgalactosaminyl transferase.

What is the relationship between the virus transformation and the change in hematoside, N-acetylgalactosamyltransferase activity? The existence of specific activators in normal cells or of specific inhibitors in virus transformed cells has been excluded. However, when normal and transformed cells were cultured together, the enzyme activity was depressed in the normal cell suggesting that the virus transformed cell secretes a regulatory substance possibly a repressor. The possibility that the viral genome is inserted in a portion of the host genome critical to the expression or regulation of the enzyme activity can, however, not be ignored.

Conclusion

In the last decennium a great deal of progress has been made in the study of function and molecular structure of cellular membranes, yet, we are still far from understanding how structure and function are integrated. But it has been possible to describe plausible models for membrane structure which are not incompatible with membrane function.

A number of functional and molecular changes have been discovered in membrancs of neoplastic cells and some have, in fact, proposed that the primary site of injury in carcinogenesis occurs at the level of the cell membrane. Although such a mechanism of transformation cannot be excluded, it seems more likely that the membrane changes are secondary to alterations of the genome. Still, the changes in membrane function and structure raise a number of puzzling questions. First, how does the integration of the viral genome into the cell genome lead to membrane alterations? Second, why do changes in membrane function lead to uncontrolled growth, increased DNA synthesis and alterations of gene expression which provide the cancer cell with survival advantages over the cell of the host. We have seen that in the case of cell growth the second messengers cyclic AMP and cyclic GMP might be involved.

However, much remains to be learned before meaningful generalizations of the role of cell membranes in neoplasia can be enounced.

Whatever their significance, functional and molecular changes in the cell surface of transformed cells have been observed. The changes include: (1) enhanced transport of various nutrients including sugars and amino acids. This alteration is probably responsible for an increase in the concentration of cell nutrients with accelerated growth. (2) Loss of contact inhibition of cell movement and growth. Thus, while normal cells do not grow beyond the monolayer stage, transformed cells grow over each other to form multilayers. (3) Loss of cell communication as shown by electron microscopy and charge transfers. The lack of normal communication between cells makes the tumor cell metabolically more autonomous than normal cells. (4) Presence of tumor specific antigens. (5) Decreased surface adhesiveness which may or may not be related to the ability of tumor cells to metastasize. (6) Agglutination by lectins.

These changes in function must in some way be correlated with molecular alterations of the cell membrane after transformation. The changes include (1) alteration in the relative proportions of sugars to sialic acid residues in the membrane; (2) an increase in the negative charge at the surface; (3) alteration in glycolipids (incomplete synthesis and absence of synthetic enzymes); (4) changes in glycoproteins. To date it is impossible to correlate the molecular with the functional changes.

Metabolic Regulation in Minimal Deviation Hepatomas

Although our review of the various mechanisms regulating enzyme activities, membrane selectivity, gene expression, and cellular proliferation is far from complete, it illustrates the complexity of the interaction involved in maintaining the steady state and adapting to shifts in the steady state.

Inadequate as such an exercise may be, it is worthwhile to distill from what we have discussed some elementary concepts on metabolic regulation because such concepts may help us understand the nature of cancer. Three kinds of elementary functional units can be distinguished in the cell: units of determination of specificity, units of catalytic activity, and units of selectivity.

The basic components of the units of determination of specificity are

$$\text{DNA} \rightarrow \text{mRNA} \rightarrow \text{proteins},$$

rRNA
tRNA
ER

The elementary components of the unit of catalytic activity are

$$\text{E (coenzyme)} + \text{S} \rightarrow \text{P}$$

(where S is the substrate and P the product), and E is the enzyme.

The elementary components of the units of selectivity (membranes) are only partially known; they include structural lipoproteins and carriers. The three kinds of units are not regulated independently, and the functions of one influence those of the other. Thus, the catalytic activities are modified by changes in enzyme concentration resulting from *de novo* synthesis.

Feedback loops connect some membrane functions with DNA synthesis in such a fashion that cell contact inhibits DNA synthesis.

Gene expression is regulated by modification of translation or transcription. The latter includes mutation of the DNA molecule and alterations of the template. Template alteration yields ineffective or effective templates. When effective, the polypeptide translated on the message may have a normal amino acid sequence or it may be in an abnormal product. An alteration of the template may also modify its sensitivity to breakdown mechanisms and thereby increase or decrease its life span.

Modification of gene expression at the transcriptional level may also result from shifts in the patterns of transcription because of interaction of DNA with repressors or derepressors or from acceleration or deceleration of transcription as a result of specific activation or deceleration of RNA polymerase.

Translational regulation of gene expression includes modification of: (1) the binding of mRNA to ribosomes; (2) the interaction between ribosomes, messenger, and membranes of the endoplasmic reticulum; and (3) the rate of translation as a result of modification in the availability of substrates (*e.g.*, amino acids) or anticodons (tRNA).

Regulation of catalytic function in the absence of *de novo* enzyme synthesis depends upon: (1) the accessibility of enzyme to substrate and *vice versa*; (2) the modifications of enzyme activity by the availability of coenzymes or metals, hydrogen, and other molecules that participate in the molecular composition and react with the enzyme or modify the conformation of its active center through allosteric effectors or inhibitors.

How selective exchange between cell and surrounding milieu is regulated at the level of the cell membrane is not known in detail. Hormones often modify the membrane's permeability to specific molecules. The relevance of knowledge of metabolic regulation to the cancer problem will become clear if we contemplate the biological behavior of the cancer cell. Some manifestations of the cancer cell are maldifferentiation, metastasis, invasion, and uninterrupted growth.

In human and experimental cancers—whether produced by carcinogens, hormones, or viruses—there are grades of malignancy, and thus tumors in the same species and same tissues may be more or less malignant according to their invasiveness. Sometimes during the patient's lifetime a tumor evolves from a state of low to high malignancy.

Thus, cervical tumors may grow slowly and have a low tendency to invade and metastasize; others may be poorly differentiated, aggressively invasive, and rapidly growing. When tumors produced by hormones are repeatedly transplanted in animals, a tumor that first depended on the presence of the hormone for growth later grows autonomously. Thus, the distortion of metabolic regulation or gene expression is not the same in all cancers, and it may not be the same in all the cells that compose a given tumor. To understand the mechanism of conversion from low to high malignancy, one should distinguish the events as they occur at the cellular and the tissue levels.

At the cellular level, the disregulation can be amplified in parallel or in series. Thus, an initial distortion (*e.g.*, a defect in gene expression) could cascade into more and more complex disregulation (*e.g.*, loss of feedback inhibition→accumulation of substrate→inhibition of some pathways and acceleration of others, etc.). Also, distortions similar to the initial one could occur repeatedly, bringing about new and unpredictable metabolic distortion. At the tissue level, the passage from low- to high-level malignancy is likely to result from the amplification of the original distortion in only a few cells that grow at the expense of the others.

Whatever the mechanism of conversion of low to high malignancy may be at the cellular level, there must exist a "minimal distortion" or a "minimal deviation" (see below), which is transmitted irreversibly and is the signature of cancer. A molecular description of these minimal deviations would yield clues as to the cause of cancer, hence the importance of studying minimal deviation hepatomas.

Minimal Deviation Hepatomas

By feeding different carcinogens, each with different carcinogenic potencies, to rats, Morris was able to produce a great variety of liver tumors. These tumors are called hepatomas because they are believed to orginate from the hepatic cell. All the experimental liver tumors were transplantable and metastasized. The tumors differed from each other by their growth rate and their degree of differentiation. Thus, the full spectrum of experimental hepatomas in rats ranges from rapidly growing and poorly differentiated tumors to slowly growing and well differentiated tumors. There is, in fact, a 25-fold difference between the growth rates of the fastest and slowest growing hepatomas.

The name "minimal deviation hepatoma" was coined by Van Potter to refer to the slow-growing and well-differentiated tumors. These tumors resembled normal liver so closely that they were sometimes difficult to distinguish from the normal tissue, and special methods of identification had to be devised. (Rose bengal is actively taken up by hepatic cells. The more differentiated the tumor, the more pink it is after intravenous injection of rose bengal. In contrast, poorly differentiated tumors appear as white nodules in a pink liver.)

Reuber [476] performed an exhaustive morphological study of transplanted hepatomas of both the type produced by Morris and of a similar gamut of tumors produced by Firminger in a special strain of rats fed N-1-fluorenyldiacetamide (2-diacetylaminofluorene). According to Reuber, most minimally deviated hepatomas obtained by Morris do not fall in the highly differentiated category but in the well-differentiated category.

When highly differentiated hepatomas were transplanted to another host, the transplant could hardly be distinguished from normal liver. Although the tumor cells were somewhat larger than normal hepatic cells or cells of well-differentiated carcinomas, microscopically and ultrastructurally the tumor cells were organized as in normal liver. Differences between normal liver and a tumor are more obvious with the less differentiated hepatoma. The more dedifferentiated types grow as gray-white nodular masses.

Histologically, the cells proliferate in a disorderly fashion with chordlike structures. The cells are irregular with large vesicular nuclei and frequent mitoses. Ultramicroscopic examination reveals the absence of microbodies, irregularity, a paucity of mitochondria, and small amounts of endoplasmic reticulum. The cells contain no bile, serum, or glycogen. The normal architecture of the liver is distorted. Although the cells proliferate in a chordlike fashion, the proliferation is disorganized and cohesion between cells is lacking. Connective tissue and Kupffer cells are sparse.

When morphological appearance was correlated with biological behavior, two major groups of observations were made. First, there is a close correlation between the success of transplantation, the growth rate, the incidence of metastases, and the degree of differentiation. Second, a given tumor tends to differentiate further after successive transplantations. Thus, highly differentiated carcinomas are difficult to transplant and grow slowly. They do not metastasize or kill the host. In contrast, undifferentiated carcinomas are easy to transplant, and they kill the animal by metastasis or cachexia within 14 or 20 weeks after transplantation. The growth rate and the incidence of metastases increase similarly. If highly differentiated tumors contain some well but not highly differentiated cells, after several generations the highly differentiated tumors turn into well-differentiated tumors.

The biological behavior of well-differentiated carcinomas is intermediate between that of highly differentiated and poorly differentiated or undifferentiated carcinomas. The well-differentiated tumors are difficult to transplant in the first generation, but transplantation becomes easier after two or three generations.

After the second generation, the speed at which the tumor kills the host is accelerated. Although the growth rate increases somewhat with successive transplantations, there is no histological change in the well-differentiated tumors until about the 15th or 20th transplantation. The tumor may then become undifferentiated or poorly differentiated.

The relationship between transformation of the solid transplanted nodule into an ascitic form and the degree of differentiation of the original tumor is remarkable. When a solid tumor is passed asceptically through a tissue press, and the tissue gruel (which contains intact cells) so obtained is injected into the intraperitoneal cavity, some of the cells proliferate into a special kind of tumor formed by a large number of rapidly growing individual cells rather than by nodular masses. Such tumors are called ascitic cell tumors. The ability of a hepatoma to be converted into the ascitic form depends on the degree of differentiation of the original tumor. Poorly differentiated tumors are converted in three cases out of four, although only one out of eight well-differentiated tumors acquires the ascitic form. Even then, the well-differentiated carcinoma grows into a form intermediate between the nodular and the classical ascitic tumor.

The incidence of metastasis is also related to the degree of the differentiation of the original tumor. Well-differentiated carcinomas take between 2.5 and 3 times as long to develop and kill the animal as do poorly differentiated carcinomas. The volume of tumor material appearing in the ascitic form was much smaller (sometimes 10 times less) with well-differentiated than with poorly differentiated tumors. With well-differentiated tumors there was usually little ascitic fluid, but enormous numbers of tumor nodules were in the peritoneal cavity.

The significance of these histological and biological studies resides in the fact that they have provided the investigator with a wide gamut of tumors all derived from the same organ and the same type of cell, the hepatic cell. The gamut spreads from highly differentiated and poorly transplantable to poorly differentiated and readily transplantable tumors. The easier the tumor is to transplant, the more effectively it is converted into an ascitic form. The tissue of origin, the liver, provides an excellent control because it can be studied when all cells are at interphase (normal liver) or when a large number of the cells are dividing (regenerating liver). Moreover, we probably know more about the biochemistry of rat liver than about any other organ. It is therefore not surprising that many of the leading laboratories in cancer research have studied the biochemistry of the minimal deviation hepatomas. Thus, most of the biochemical generalizations that emerged between 1930 and 1960 to explain the cause of cancer were reexamined in minimal deviation hepatomas.

Before we describe the biochemical changes, we should state that this range of differentiation in malignancy is not unique to hepatomas. Tumors with various degrees of differentiation can be produced experimentally or observed in human patients. As pointed out above, sometimes at the early stages of its development while the tumor is still highly differentiated, an important, irreversible change takes place. The change is transmitted from cell to cell, and it converts the normal cell into a cell with the characteristics of cancer—proliferation, invasion, metastasis, etc.

Glycolysis in Minimal Deviation Hepatomas

Studies of the biochemistry of minimal deviation hepatomas aim at identifying the primary lesion. It could have been predicted on the basis of the behavior of normal tissues and the existence of well-differentiated cancer in humans that two of the classical generalizations of cancer could not relate to the primary cause of cancer, but must have been a consequence of the progress of the injury.

A drastic shift in the cell's enzyme mosaic from normal to a so-called malignant pattern (*e.g.*, decrease in activity of tissue-specific enzymes, low cytochrome levels) is not a necessary concomitant of the malignant state, because the enzyme mosaic of minimal deviation hepatomas is essentially the same as that of normal liver. Only discrete changes in the enzyme composition of the minimal deviation hepatomas have been observed.

Inasmuch as tissues may exhibit high aerobic glycolytic rates without becoming cancerous, it seemed unlikely that high aerobic glycolysis could be linked with the primary injury in cancer. The facts that glycolysis is normal or even low in minimal deviation hepatomas and glycine uptake into protein in the absence of aerobiosis is impossible in slices of minimal deviation hepatomas strongly indicate that high aerobic glycolysis is not indispensable for a cell to be cancerous. This conclusion, which Weinhouse reached long ago, has now been accepted by most cancer investigators and the arguments brought against it by Warburg [344] are not convincing.

Warburg's major argument rests on the work of Woods, Burk, and Hunter [477], who established a correlation between glycolysis and the velocity of growth. Stilbestrol is known to depress glycolytic activity in normal liver. Burk and his associates further established that the ability of stilbestrol to depress glycolysis decreases as tumors grow more rapidly. The mechanism by which stilbestrol interferes with glycolysis is not known. It has been suggested that it might interfere by activating mitochondrial ATPase, thus generating more ADP.

When the velocity of growth is expressed in function of fermentation, an almost linear curve is obtained. The investigators extrapolate the curve to zero and thus claim that the correlation holds with minimal deviation hepatoma. However, there is no direct evidence that such a mathematical extrapolation reflects biological reality, but even if it did, the correlation between high glycolysis and rapid growth does not establish a relationship of cause to effect. Consequently, we shall adopt the view that the high rate of glycolysis, important as it may be in the description of cancer metabolism, is part of the progressive lesion rather than the primary cause of cancer.

In fact, the curve of Burk, Woods, and Hunter is not rigidly linear. The rate of increase in the anaerobic glycolysis is slowed in intermediate hepatomas and then rises rapidly as one uses more and more dedifferentiated hepatomas. Moreover, differences between minimal deviation hepatomas and normal liver are small and at the limit of significance.

As we have already mentioned, Morris [478] has shown that certain minimal deviation hepatomas have paradoxically low rates of glucose utilization and lactic acid production. Studies from Weinhouse's laboratory established that the low level of glucose utilization in these tumors resulted from low levels of hexokinase activity. The low level of hexokinase activity could further be correlated with preferential oxidation of fatty acids and low levels of ketone body production, as well as with slow growth. In contrast, rapidly growing tumors have high hexokinase activity, oxidize little or no fatty acid, and produce no ketone bodies.

As we have remarked before, Weinhouse and his collaborators [347] demonstrated the existence of a special glucokinase in liver. The enzyme is unique in that it requires insulin for activity, is induced by glucose, and has a low affinity for glucose. Thus, it will catalyze the conversion of its substrate only if the concentrations of glucose in the medium are relatively high. Weinhouse studied the activity of this enzyme in a number of tumors and found that it was low or nonexistent in most tumors. There seemed to be no correlation between hexokinase activity and the glucokinase in the tumors. Thus, some tumors with high hexokinase activity may be completely deprived of glucokinase. Usually the more differentiated the tumor, the lower the glucokinase activity, except in the tumor 9098, which is well differentiated, contains both glucokinase and hexokinase, but is unresponsive to glucose in the diet with respect to induction of glucokinase. These findings brought Weinhouse to conclude that no retention or deletion pattern appears in the conversion of a normal to a cancerous cell.

Although allosteric inhibition of enzyme pathways has been best investigated with bacterial enzymes, their existence has been clearly demonstrated in mammalian systems. Many of the studies on allosteric inhibition in mammalian tissues were concerned with purine and pyrimidine metabolism. In all cases except one, the feedback loop that functioned in the normal also existed in the neoplasm. However, Bresnick [479] reported that inhibition of thymidine kinase by CTP was abolished in Novikoff hepatomas. The most remarkable example of loss of feedback inhibition was described by Siperstein, Fagan, and Morris [480] with respect to cholesterol biosynthesis. Cholesterol interferes with its own biosynthesis by inhibiting the activity of hydroxymethylglutaryl CoA reductase. This allosteric inhibition of the enzyme is abolished in 5123 and human hepatomas.

Weber [481] studied the enzymes involved in glycolysis and gluconeogenesis in the hepatomas and observed that they could be classified in three groups according to their activity and depending on the growth rate. The enzymes that play a key role in glycolysis increase with growth; the enzymes that are rate determining in gluconeogenesis from 3-carbon precursors decrease with growth; and those enzymes that are involved in the reversible steps of glycolysis are unaffected by growth. Such a finding would seem to suggest that the regulation of gene expression is disturbed during carcinogenesis.

Amino Acid Pools in Minimal Deviation Hepatomas

When minimal deviation hepatomas became available (see below) a reinvestigation of the amino acid pools in those tumors became necessary.

Thus, in their studies of the amino acid pools in hepatoma, Roberts and Simonson [664] found that the amino acid pool of the hepatoma resembled that of other neoplasms more than that of liver. A reinvestigation of the amino acid pools in minimal deviation hepatomas was carried out by Moyer and Pitot [665].

Amino acid pool sizes depend upon: the permeability of the cell membrane to the amino acid, the rate of transport through the membrane, the metabolic conversion to precursors of glycolysis, gluconeogenesis and other pathways, and the rate of incorporation in proteins. Therefore, interpretation of pool changes is difficult without a comprehensive analysis of all the metabolic components involved in the regulation of amino acid pools. The evaluation of the data is further complicated by the fact that the amino acid pool is divided into two compartments.

In minimal deviation hepatoma, although the paterns of the amino acid pool in the hepatomas 7300 and 9618A are similar in liver and hepatomas, there is, however, a tendency toward low values in the hepatoma except for high lysine in 9618A hepatoma. The decay of carboxyl-labeled [^{14}C]leucine is the same in 7800 hepatoma and normal liver, but it is slowed down in the 9618A.

Enzyme Induction in Minimal Deviation Hepatomas

Among the most intriguing findings made on minimal deviation hepatomas are the studies on enzyme induction in hepatomas. The bulk of that work was done in the laboratories of Potter, Pitot, and Weinhouse.

Fiala and Fiala [482] were the first to show that acute administration or chronic feeding of the carcinogen trimethyldiaminobenzene impaired the liver's ability to respond to tryptophan administration by elaborating tryptophan pyrrolase. Auerbach and Waisman [483] were unable to induce the formation of tryptophan pyrrolase by administering tryptophan in hepatomas. Similar results were later obtained using ethionine-produced carcinomas, Dunning hepatomas, etc.

Pitot and associates investigated some of the biochemical properties of the hepatoma 5123 [484–487]. After first demonstrating that the number of diploid chromosomes (42) of this type of tumor was normal,* Pitot pursued his studies by measuring the activity of a large number of enzymes in the hepatoma and then comparing it to the distribution of enzymes in more rapidly growing tumors. The enzyme mosaic of the hepatoma 5123 resembled that of liver. While marked deviation from the enzyme patterns of liver could be observed in rapidly growing hepatomas, chromosome and enzyme patterns remained stable even after several transplantations.

On the basis of these preliminary investigations, Pitot and his collaborators concluded that the hepatoma 5123 constituted an ideal material for investigating the conversion of a normal into a malignant hepatic cell. The tumor is indeed devoid of some of the most dramatic changes usually seen in tumors, changes (high anaerobic glycolysis and rapid growth) that probably reflect the development of cancer rather than being related to its primary cause. For these reasons, the discovery that in most cases the response of multiple-enzyme systems to physiological changes (diet, shift in hormone administration or substrate injection) differed in the tumor and in the host—even

* Nowell and Morris [488] studied the chromosome pattern of a large number of transferable hepatomas produced chemically; they found nine that had the normal number of 42 chromosomes, but only two of them, 9618A and 9633, had what they considered a completely normal karyotype. An important finding was that chromosome patterns changed from one transplantation generation to the next. For example, tumors 9618B and 9611B, which were diploid in generation two, became anaploid (43 and 44 chromosomes) in generation three. After a long-range follow-up of the chromosome pattern of minimal deviation hepatomas, Nowell and Morris concluded in 1969 that only tumor 9618A and 9633 had normal karyotypes.

though the enzyme pattern of the minimal deviation hepatoma is identical to that of liver—is of considerable significance.

Knox and his collaborators [489] had demonstrated that tryptophan administration induces the formation of tryptophan pyrrolase in normal liver. In contrast, tryptophan administration to animals carrying transplanted hepatomas 5123 had no effect on the level of the enzyme in the transplant. Yet, the enzyme increased markedly in the liver even if the liver was somewhat cirrhotic. Similarly, the induction of tryptophan pyrrolase with cortisone was prevented in the hepatoma. Induction of tryptophan pyrrolase was found to be altered in a number of other minimal deviation hepatomas, except the Reuber hepatoma H35, in which tryptophan pyrrolase was induced with the substrate and cortisone in the intact animal. However, if the animal had been adrenalectomized, the hepatoma did not respond to the administration of tryptophan and cortisone.

Pitot further extended his studies to the induction of threonine dehydrase in the Morris 700 hepatoma and demonstrated that the enzyme could not be induced by substrate or hormones. However, both tumor and host liver had marked increases in threonine dehydrase after a high-protein diet was administered.

Tyrosine glutaryl transaminase is induced by corticoids. The enzyme is found in liver and in the hepatoma 5123. Cortisone administration increases the level of tyrosine glutaryl transaminase in liver markedly, but has little effect on the enzyme in the tumor. Hepatoma 5123 is characterized by a high level of tyrosine glutaryl transaminase when the tumor is transplanted in an intact host. When the tumor is transplanted in an adrenalectomized rat, the tumor has levels of enzyme activity that approach those of the liver of the normal host. When cortisone is given to these animals, the transaminase levels increase in both tumor and liver.

These pioneering experiments demonstrated that minimal deviation hepatomas differ from normal liver in their ability to respond to stimulus. As Van Potter pointed out, this was the first observed biochemical difference between the minimal deviation hepatoma and normal liver.

Potter and Ono [490] used glycogen formation and glucose-6-phosphate dehydrogenase activity as indicators of the ability of minimal deviation hepatomas to respond to physiological stimuli; although normal liver responds to fasting followed by glucose administration with increases in glycogen synthesis and the activity of glucose-6-phosphate dehydrogenase, the Morris 5123 hepatoma does not. Similar studies were carried out with other types of minimal deviation hepatomas, and investigators observed that the response to the physiological stimuli varied markedly, an observation that led Potter to state that no two of the minimal deviation hepatomas were identical and that probably hundreds of enzyme patterns are compatible with the malignant state.

Watanabe, Potter, and Morris [491] have shown that although methylcholanthrene was able to induce hydroxylase activity in Morris hepatoma, the level of activity induced was always lower than in the host liver. Of considerable interest is that these investigators compared induction in hepatomas to that in fetal rat liver and found that induction was low in fetal liver as well. Thus, it would appear that the induced levels of the enzyme depend on the age of the liver.

These findings raise an important question. Is the great variety of enzyme patterns found in hepatomas linked directly to carcinogenesis, or does this variety reflect some modification in the cyclic activities of the enzymes coupled with subtle changes in response to stimuli that are related more to growth than to carcinogenesis? Potter has reviewed this concept [492].

Kishi and coworkers [493] demonstrated that although the glycogen content of transplantable rat hepatoma was low, it did not vary with fasting and feeding as it would in the normal liver. The response of minimal deviation hepatomas to cortisone administration varies depending upon the type of hepatoma, although the response is low in all of them. Thus, the Morris hepatoma 5123 deposits small amounts of glycogen after cortisone administration, whereas the 7800 and the 3924 hepatomas do not.

Lueders and collaborators [494] studied glucuronyl transferase activity in transplantable rat hepatomas (Morris 7787, 7316A, and 7794A, and Reuber H35 and HI39) and learned that the activity of the enzyme is higher in those hepatomas than in normal liver. This finding shows that hepatomas are not devoid of all drug-metabolizing enzymes as some believe.

Hopefully, some of the studies started on a variety of hepatomas will be pursued on tumors of other organs with a similar spectrum of differentiation. Knox and his collaborators have obtained a line of rat mammary tumors transplantable by chemical application or radiation at the site of origin. Like the hepatomas, the transplantable tumors range from highly differentiated to poorly differentiated tumors. All that is known about them is that growth rates are proportional to the glutaminase content per cell or per gram.

It would be pointless to describe more examples of the responses of hepatomas to dietary and hormonal enzyme induction. They all lead to the same conclusion. Metabolic regulation is altered in virtually every tumor examined. The metabolic alteration precedes the morphological changes, the alteration in chromosome patterns, or even the drastic alteration in enzyme mosaic. No generalization emerges except that the pattern of alteration of regulatory metabolism is unique for each cell.

Isozymes in Cancer

If one manifestation of cancer is a distortion of the expression of the genotype into normal phenotypical patterns, then one may anticipate that distortions in the enzyme pattern will also occur and take various forms. Thus, an enzyme in a normal cell of the tissue of origin may disappear, and enzymes not found in the normal cell of origin may appear in a cancer cell. In florid cancers the former usually prevails; for example, glucose-6-phosphate activity is lost in advanced hepatomas, or peptidase activity is lost in advanced stomach cancer.

Chapter 1 contains many examples of enzymes that catalyze the same reaction but exhibit different molecular properties. The difference in molecular properties can be evaluated by determining kinetic, electrophoretic, chromatographic, isoelectric focusing, or immunological properties of the enzyme. Let's illustrate this concept by one more example: Pitot and Inoue [495] studied the serine dehydrase in rat livers and showed that the enzyme exists in at least two isozymic forms that can be separated by polyacrylamide gel electrophoresis. The significance of the separation is borne out by the fact that the levels of activity of the two forms of the enzyme are modulated differently. Tryptophan administration yields equal levels of the two enzymes; glucagon elicits the formation of one form, and cortisone that of the other form.

In the normal cell, the isozyme pattern is transmitted from cell to cell and maintained as long as the steady state persists. If under the influence of various stimulators, the cell switches from one functional state to another, the isozyme pattern may change also but always predictably. In the cancer cell, the isozyme pattern is often altered.

One of the main purposes of studying isozyme patterns in cancer was to determine whether the pattern of alteration was random or programmed. If the switch is random, one can anticipate a myriad of changes. In contrast, if the switch is programmed, one can expect a consistent pattern of isozymic alterations [496].

Weinhouse and his collaborators [497–499] were among the first to study the distribution of isozymes of carbohydrate metabolism (glucose ATP phosphotransferases, aldolases, pyruvate kinases, and glycogen phosphorylases) in minimal deviation hepatomas exhibiting various degrees of differentiation and growth. Each of these catalytic properties is represented by various molecular forms in the liver, one of which is typical for fetal liver and usually does not appear until several days or several weeks after birth. In well-differentiated hepatomas, the isozyme pattern is identical to the one in adult liver. In contrast, in poorly differentiated hepatomas, the isozyme pattern in liver is usually the type that predominates in the embryo.

Isozyme patterns have been studied in a number of transplanted hepatomas. When isozyme patterns could be correlated with the rates of growth and departure from differentiation, investigators found that the pattern tended to switch from the adult to the fetal type. For example, the liver contains two isozymic forms of glutaminase. One form is prevalent, is also found in the kidney, and does not require phosphorus for activation. The other is found in liver only and functions at low concentration. The kidney type of phosphorus-independent isozyme is present in fetal liver; it disappears in adult liver but is found again in some hepatomas.

Lawson *et al.* measured the two isozymes of carbamyl phosphate in rat liver and in a variety of hepatomas with slow and rapid growth and differentiation. Carbamyl phosphate synthetase I, a mitochondrial enzyme restricted to liver and involved in the urea cycle, was high in slow growing hepatomas and low in rapidly growing hepatomas. Carbamyl phosphate synthetase II, an enzyme found in the cytosol of most tissues and probably primarily involved in purine biosynthesis, was found in liver and all hepatomas, but changes in activity did not correlate with rates of growth [666].

The study of enzyme induction and isozyme distribution in minimal deviation hepatomas has revealed a paradox. The cancer cell loses the ability to respond to the inducer of some enzymes, and at the same time the enzymes that were present in the fetal liver reappear.

The absence of induction of an enzyme in hepatomas may result from gene deletion or from interference with gene expression. The findings of Pitot and Morris [485], which showed that under special conditions tyrosine transaminase can be induced in well-differentiated hepatomas (9618A), indicate that at least in this special case, interference with enzyme induction does not result from gene deletion, but from alterations of the mechanism of gene expression.

The mechanism regulating the appearance of enzymes in adult liver that are absent in fetal liver is not clear, but it is likely to result from derepression after fetal life of genomes repressed in the fetus, and it may resemble what happens when fetal liver cells are cultured *in vitro*. When rat fetal liver is cultured *in vitro,* tyrosine aminotransferase activity develops in ways quite similar to its development *in vivo*. The development of activity is not affected by humoral factors in fetal or adult rats. Hydrocortisone and glucagon enhance the development of activity but cannot initiate it. Actinomycin blocks the appearance of the tyrosine aminotransferase.

Alterations in the cellular protein mosaic are not unique to hepatomas. They are found in most, if not all cancers. The alterations found in leukemia will be an example.

Leukemia cells, like other cancer cells, are characterized by a distortion of gene expression associated with survival advantages over the host. As a result the pattern of protein synthesis in leukemic lymphocytes is often abnormal. Depending upon the type of leukemia, the cell may be defective in enzyme receptors or other functional proteins. For example, some leukemic cells are defective in cytidine deaminase and as a result are sensitive to cytosine arabinoside. Unfortunately the drug induces the enzyme to reappear. Others lack 5′-nucleotidase. Sensitivity to glucocorticoids depends upon the presence of appropriate receptors and in some cases they are missing. Granulocytes include at least two factors with respective molecular weights of 35,000 and 1330 daltons which stimulate colony formation in spleen. The factors are present in normal serum, but often are absent in the serum of leukemic patients.

In other forms of leukemia some of the factors involved in inflammation are lost. A peptide that activates connective tissue has been found in many cells including leukocytes and platelets. The protein induces messenger RNA and protein synthesis in the fibroblast. The latter responds by increasing glucose utilization and produces excessive amounts of lactic acid and hyaluronic acid. The activation of fibroblasts by the protein is mediated through cyclic AMP. The protein has a molecular weight of 15,318 daltons and is made of 142 amino acids. Its amino acid sequence is known. The factor is suspected to play a role in the proliferation of connective tissue in inflammation and in the desmoplasmic reaction in cancer.

Invasion, Metastasis, and Host Reactions

Many of the biochemical changes in the cell membrane that develop during the conversion of a normal into a cancer cell were described in the discussion of viral and chemical transformations. The significance of these changes with respect to cell function is difficult to evaluate because too little is known of the chemical properties of the cell membrane. Certainly, one of the most dreadful consequences of the alteration of the cell membrane in cancer is the disregard of the cancer cell for its neighbor cells. In this section we will discuss some of the alterations of the cell membranes that may be relevant to development of invasion and metastases.

Cancer would not be the dreadful disease that it is if it were simply an acceleration of local growth. What kills the patient is invasion and preying on the host's resources in the process of cachexia. To illustrate the importance of invasion in the pathogenesis of cancer, consider the case of a young man who developed a malignant melanoma. All his life he had a mole that had never bothered him on his left thigh. The mole was deep black, oval, 2 cm long, 1 cm wide, and elevated with an irregular surface. In the army, he wounded the mole while jumping from a truck.

Within a matter of weeks, the wounded area was bluish and the surrounding dermis had become infiltrated with newly formed, pigmented cells. Lymph nodes appeared in his groin. When the nodes were removed, they were found to contain black material. A chest X-ray revealed numerous dense, round masses distributed to both lungs. A few months later, the patient died. At autopsy, masses containing black pigment were found in the lungs, liver, and even the brain. It was not the local growth of the tumor that had killed the patient, but its dissemination. Cancer cells disseminate in two ways—through directly invading the surrounding tissue and by seeding distant tissues. The seeding of normal tissue away from the primary site of the tumor is called metastasis.

Invasion

In contrast to benign tumors, which are usually surrounded by a connective tissue capsule, cancers, except cancer *in situ,* are invasive. In a basal cell carcinoma of the skin, the proliferative cells resemble the germinal cells of the epithelium, but they do not remain in the epithelial layer. On the contrary, the cancer develops prongs that penetrate the basal membranes and enter the connective tissue and even the vascular wall. Walling of the cancer by a connective tissue does not occur. A number of interactions between cancer cells and host surrounding tissue modulate cancer invasiveness.

In addition to the changes in membrane properties that are likely to be fundamental to invasion, the development of the tumor favors invasion in at least two ways—pressure and elaboration of substances toxic to the host. That the pressure of the growing mass may facilitate invasion by disrupting basement membranes and compressing vessels and cells seems obvious. Yet it does not explain the development of prongs of cancer cells into healthy tissue.

Hamperl [500] believes that the cancer cells push aside normal structures and use existing gaps for expansion. However, pressure cannot be a sufficient cause for invasion since benign tumors may grow into large masses that compress the surrounding tissues without actually invading it.

Histological examination of cancer tissue reveals the existence of discrete or even massive signs of cellular necrosis and fiber degeneration at the periphery of the cancerous mass. Cells lose their tinctorial properties, their nuclei are pyknotic, or the chromatin is fragmented. Collagen fibers swell and disintegrate, muscle fibers are degraded, and remnants of nondigested, tapered-off muscle fibers are found among the cancer cells.

Although cancer invasion undoubtedly is associated with the necrosis of the surrounding tissue, the mechanism by which this degradation takes place is still debated. Whereas Hamperl believes that pressure plays a key role, others, like Sylvén [501] emphasize a more aggressive participation of the cancer cell in invasion. Cancer cells could favor the degradation of the surrounding tissues in at least three ways: by elaborating cytotoxic substances, by elaborating hydrolytic enzymes, and by generating an environment favorable to hydrolysis.

In 1905 Battelli and Stern [502] discovered that a water extract of beef spleen inhibited catalase. Later, chloroform extracts of cancer were also found to inhibit catalase, a finding in keeping with the low catalase activities that were detected in liver of tumor-bearing animals. The catalase inhibitor was believed to be a toxic principle elaborated by cancer cells and was called toxohormone.

Toxohormone has been partially purified; it is believed to be a peptide. The amino acid composition reported by Yunoki and Griffin [503] shows that toxohormone contains 16 different amino acids and is especially rich in aspartic acid (10%), glutamic acid (11%), and leucine (14%). The polypeptide has a minimum molecular weight of 4200 to 6400. The amino terminal is believed to be arginine. At the earliest stages of preparation, toxohormone is found in association with neutral lipid, but there is no indication that the lipid is needed for activity.

Toxohormone's role is not clear. In addition to depressing catalase activity in liver and kidney, the injection of the toxin leads to anemia with reduced plasma iron; enlargement of the liver, kidney, and spleen; and involution of the thymus. Whether toxohormone exerts a cytotoxic effect on the cells of the surrounding tissue is not known. However, toxohormone's identifying characteristic is its effect on catalase activity. The inhibition occurs in liver and kidney and is somewhat proportional to the size of the tumor. The inhibitory effect is observed with almost all rapidly growing transplantable tumors, and it is reversible, as indicated by experiments in Greenstein's laboratory [504] in which the tumor was transplanted in rat tails and later clipped off.

Of course, the critical question is whether toxohormone is specific for cancer. More recent investigations have suggested that toxohormonelike substances are found in all autolyzed tissue, and that the appearance of toxohormone in rapidly growing tumors results from autolysis rather than from neoplasia per se [505].

Sylvén has claimed that cytotoxic polypeptides with amino acid compositions different from that of toxohormone are elaborated by cancer cells. These are believed to be small polypeptides containing only eight different amino acids. Although the amino acid composition and sequence of the compound are not known, Sylvén believes that an amino acid grouping including Tyr-Cys-Tyr-Cys constitutes the center of a mitotic poison that acts by blocking vital biosynthetic pathways before mitosis.

Vague as they are, these assumptions deserve to be reckoned with because even if the development of cytotoxic agents is a consequence of necrosis rather than neoplasia, it cannot be excluded that clarification of their molecular structure and mode of action may open new avenues in chemotherapy.

Although no true collagenases or elastases have been found in tumors or in surrounding interstitial fluid, the interstitial fluid surrounding tumors is especially rich in hydrolases, particularly those that catalyze the hydrolysis of the carbamide bond (amino peptidase, dipeptidase, amino acyl naphthylamidase, cathepsin). Increases in hyaluronidase have been described in Rous sarcomas in chickens. The presence of these hydrolases in the interstitial fluid surrounding the cancer raises two questions: what role do these hydrolases play in killing and scavenging the surrounding tissue during cancerous invasion, and where do they come from? There are no satisfactory answers for either of these questions.

Some have claimed that the enzymes are elaborated inside the tumor cells and leak out as a result of alteration of the permeability of the plasma membrane. Leaking of enzymes (*e.g.*, lactic dehydrogenase) has in fact been observed in cultures of cancer cells. Yet it is not excluded that some of the hydrolases that accumulate around the tumor are the products of healthy host cells, such as inflammatory cells, or are released in the interstitial fluid as a consequence of necrosis of cancer cells, inflammatory cells, or both.

The increased hyaluronidase activity has, at least in some cases, been linked with the presence of contaminating bacteria. The cancer may sometimes contribute to the destruction of the surrounding cells by releasing its metabolite in the intercellular fluid (lactic acid and chelating agents such as small polypeptides that may trap vital ions). Again, these events are not likely to be indispensable to invasion since high glycolytic rates are not observed in all invading tumors. The host tissue may react in various ways with the invading cancer. It may develop edema, provide a stromal network—a vascular bed on which the tumor thrives, or elicit inflammatory and reticuloendothelial reactions. Edema fluid sometimes surrounds the cancerous mass; its causes and its role in the dissemination of the cancer cell are not known.

Much has been written about the cancer connective tissue framework or stroma, but almost nothing is known of the role of the stroma in dissemination. Tumors vary greatly with respect to the histology of their connective tissue framework. Some have little; others, like the scirrhous carcinoma of the breast and stomach, have a dense connective tissue framework. The stroma of a transplanted tumor is entirely derived from fibroblasts of the host, but the distribution and the density of the collagen fibers are determined by the tumor. Although not much concrete evidence for or against the participation of the stroma in tumor dissemination *in vivo* is available, the stroma could influence tumor dissemination in at least three ways: by providing tracts for cell migration, by creating barriers toward cellular progression, and by facilitating or interfering with the flow of nutrients and the elimination of catabolites.

Metastasis

At first approximation, one is tempted to consider metastasis as a special form of invasion in which clusters of cells penetrate the vascular tissue and form emboli that ultimately settle in distant organs to grow. However, one or more features of the cancer cell must determine whether an invasive cancer metastasizes because some cancers grow for a long time, invading the surrounding tissues extensively before they metastasize, whereas others metastasize at an early stage of their development.

Nothing is known about the molecular changes that make cancer cells detach themselves into clusters to metastasize at a distance. In fact, surprisingly little work has been done on the factors that trap cancer cells in lymph nodes, viscera, muscle, connective tissue, and bone marrow. It is not clear why the colonized tissue tolerates or even encourages the growth of the intruder. Cancer cells migrate through available natural paths, free tissue space, blood and lymph vessels, and occasionally natural canals.

Lymphatic invasion, the most common type, results in the formation of metastases in the lymph nodes adjacent to the tumor. Theoretically, the tumoral cells may travel from the tumor to the lymph nodes through growth in the lymphatic channel or by embolization in the lymphatic stream and filtration in the lymph node. When lymphatic infiltration is marked, the lymphatic pattern may be mapped out in relief in the shape of an arborization surrounding the tumor mass.

After lymphatic dissemination, dissemination through the blood vessels is the most frequent. One or a cluster of cells becomes detached, penetrates the lumen of veins and arteries, is transported in the blood flow, and ultimately settles in some organ to grow at the expense of the existing tissue.

The journey of the metastatic cell from tumor to a distant locus is not without challenge. The cells must become detached, travel in connective tissue, traverse basal membranes and endothelial walls, survive the attack of antagonistic substances in the blood flow, in some circumstances traverse organs without settling there, and finally grow some distance from the original tumor. Moreover, all tissues are not equal with respect to their ability to host metastases. Some (heart, spleen, uterus) are rarely the site of metastasis; others (lung, liver, lymph nodes) are common sites of metastasis.

Although it was believed at first that metastases reach a lymph node by directly permeating the lymphatics draining the area of the tumor, we know now that most if not all lymph node metastases occur as a result of embolization. Special anatomical and mechanical events explain why some lymph nodes are sometimes skipped and why retrograde metastases occur. Little is known of the interaction between lymph node and cancer cell, except that cells are trapped in the nodes and proliferate in spite of a mild reticuloendothelial reaction. The proliferation is often so extensive that on microscopic examination the normal architecture of the lymph node may be entirely replaced by chords, plaques, and masses of cancer cells.

In many experimental cancers in animals and in spontaneous cancers in humans, cancer cells are found in the blood if it is carefully examined. Tissue culture and transplantation studies have proven that at least some of the circulating cancer cells are viable. According to Fisher and Fisher [506, 507], in animal experiments the incidence of metastasis can be correlated with the amount of cells injected in the blood. The significance of the presence of cancer cells in the human blood is not clear, primarily because it is impossible to determine in humans what chances the circulatory cells have of producing carcinoma. No convenient correlation between the incidence of metastasis and the presence of cancer cells in blood has been established.

Once the cancer cells have reached the lumen of the blood vessels, a triple fate awaits them: they die, they are trapped in thrombi, or they traverse the blood vessel wall to infiltrate the intercellular tissue. Although no strict quantitative evaluation is available, it is believed that most of the cancer cells that reach the blood flow die. This does not imply that humoral factors kill cancer cells; Fisher claims categorically that there is no evidence for the existence of such humoral factors.

Many of the cancer cells that reach the bloodstream adhere to the endothelial wall. This adhesion is a paradox because the adhesiveness of the cancer cell is believed to be reduced. Nevertheless, adhesion to the endothelial wall may involve factors related to blood coagulation. Indeed, cancer cells are rich in a thromboplastinlike substance, and heparin or plasmin injections reduce the incidence of metastasis in experimental animals.

The fate of the cancer cells trapped in thrombi made of fibrin and platelets is not certain, but many of these cells may be viable and may find their way through the vascular wall, becoming the seed of metastasis in the extracellular space. Some of the cells that adhere to the endothelial wall manage to pass through it, reach the intercellular space, and become the source of new metastases. The molecular properties of the cancer cell that make it able to traverse the vascular wall are not known, but it seems that at least part of these special molecular properties, if not all of them, must be associated with the cancer cell membrane.

Inasmuch as metastases colonize some tissues in preference to others, the role of the soil in determining the implantation of metastasis is inescapable. The question is not so much whether the soil plays a role in trapping and favoring the proliferation of cancer cells, but whether this role is simply anatomical and mechanical or involves a genuine metabolic environment fertile for the growth of metastases. The truth probably lies between these two extremes, and the incidence of metastases may be determined in part by the anatomy of the organ and in part by its biochemistry.

Still, little is known of the factors that determine the incidence of metastasis in a given organ. Many of the original observations on the biology of metastasis were made in cancer patients and these observations continue to be of considerable significance in the management of cancer patients. Such observations did not answer some fundamental questions concerning the incidence and the fate of metastasis, and most of our understanding of the mechanisms of metastasis comes from experimental studies. In fact, few laboratories have endeavored to study this phenomenon. The Fishers and Zeidman are among those who devoted much of their effort to the problem.

Fisher and Fisher demonstrated the existence of dormant cells. These investigators injected 50 cells in the portal veins of two groups of rats. One group was first inspected 13 weeks after inoculation of the tumor cells and then reinspected weekly by laparotomy; the other was not inspected at all until the 20th week. At the 20th week, the incidence of metastasis was high in the first group and nonexistent in the second. Therefore, Fisher and Fisher concluded that the repeated trauma to the liver due to examination stimulates mitosis, which makes the dormant cells proliferate.

Other studies made in the Fishers' laboratory indicated that liver trauma (chloroform or carbon tetrachloride administration, cirrhosis) increased the incidence of metastasis. The mechanism by which trauma influences metastasis has not been discovered, but anoxemia has been eliminated as an important determinant factor. The possibility that the increased incidence of metastasis results from an increased trapping of injected cells has been eliminated in experiments in which labeled cells were injected intraportally. This finding suggested that liver trauma affects the incidence of metastasis more by modifying the metabolic environment than by mechanically influencing the organ or by affecting hepatic cell relationships.

By developing relatively accurate methods of measuring both the number of cells injected in the blood on lymphatic circulation of experimental animals and the number of cells that settle in a given organ at a given site, Fisher and Fisher were able to measure the incidence of takes of injected cells after local irradiation or inflammation. The findings suggested that neither irradiation nor inflammation affected the dissemination of tumor cells.

However, these findings contrast with results obtained when labeled Walker tumor cells were injected intravenously or via the aorta in normal rats and in rats whose hind limbs had been submitted to surgical or mechanical trauma. Trauma increased the number of injected cells that nestled in the limb. Moreover, adequate heparinization, which reduced the number of cells settling in the untraumatized limb, did not affect the traumatized limb.

The Fishers' experiments suggest that the incidence of metastasis is not affected by the host's plasma calcium levels. Zeidman [508] devised a method in which a suspension of cancer cells is injected into a lymphatic. This technique provided a pattern of metastasis distribution resembling that observed in man. Thus, cancer spread from the popliteal to the pelvic node resembling the chainlike pattern of lymphatic spread sometimes seen in human cancer.

Such experiments further revealed that tumor cell emboli in afferent lymphatics are arrested in the subcapsular tissue of one or more nodules of the corresponding node. The cells do not immediately spread from one node to another, but such a transfer takes place after about three weeks. Although the metastasis readily grows in the lymphatic node, it does not develop a lymphatic system of its own. Consequently, when a dye is injected in the lymphatic system, it does not reach the metastasis.

These methods for following the pathogenesis of metastasis have helped to clarify the mechanism of development of a long debated clinical sign and an anatomical phenomenon referred to as Troisier's sign and Virchow's node, respectively.

In man, abdominal cancer often metastasizes to the lymph node of the mediastinum and the supraclavicular region. Troisier described a lymph node in the supraclavicular region as a sign of abdominal cancer. Such metastases could develop in various ways, including detachment from a metastasis to the lung and retrograde embolization through the thoracic duct (blockage of the thoracic duct would be responsible for retrograde lymphatic flow and embolization).

Zeidman's experiments [509] suggest that none of these interpretations needs to be invoked because cancer cell emboli may be carried directly from the thoracic duct through efferent lymphatic channels to mediastinal intercostal and supraclavicular nodes. Of course, such results imply that the thoracic duct, as believed previously, empties not only into the veins of the base of the neck, but that part of the lymph flowing in the duct is carried through afferent lym-

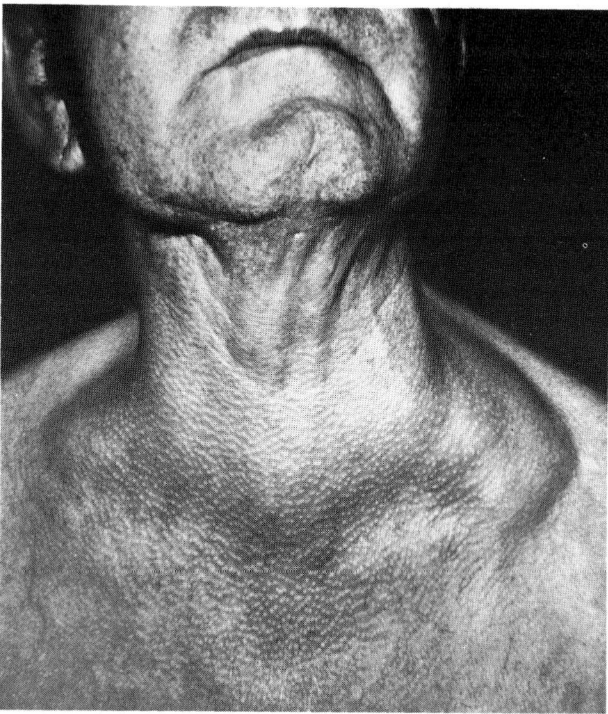

Fig. 16-37. Lymphatic invasion of the scapular nodes in a patient with lung cancer

phatics to adjacent nodes and returned from the nodes to the duct through efferent lymphatics. In this transfer, the cancer cells are filtered out and remain in the node.

Although retrograde progression of the metastasis need not be invoked to explain the Virchow nodes, observations in humans suggest that retrograde progress of metastasis does occur. Zeidman has shown that tumor cells injected directly into the pelvic lymphatic system pass backward through circuitous collateral lymphatics, which empty into afferent lymphatics of the popliteal node.

The arrest of the emboli is necessary for metastatic formation; it is facilitated by cortisone, which increases the incidence of metastasis, and decreased by anticoagulants. Although a necessary condition for metastasis, arrest of the tumor cell embolus is not a sufficient condition for metastasis.

Thus, Greene has shown that disseminated malignant cells are present in many organs early after transplantation of a malignant tumor. Yet these trapped cell clusters do not succeed in producing metastasis unless the primary tumor is removed. Madden and Karpas [510] compared the ability of tissues to arrest tumoral cells in their capillary bed with their ability to develop metastasis. Their studies show that tissues vary greatly in their ability to arrest tumoral cells, but there is no correlation between the proportion of cells arrested in a tissue and ability to develop metastasis. Such findings indicate that specific tissue factors or special tissular metabolic conditions favor the settling of metastasis.

The role of the lymph node in the development of metastasis is of particular significance, because if the lymph node filters cancer cells that will multiply in it and generate a new center from which more embolic clusters can be released to seed other nodes, it should be removed. On the contrary, if the node exerts a noxious effect, immunological or other, on the tumor cells that are arrested in its sinuses, it should be left in place. Most surgeons agree that node removal, especially in cancer of the breast, colon, head, and neck, significantly improves the patient's chances of survival. Still, some surgeons have recommended that negative nodes not be excised in breast cancer. (The difficulty with such recommendations rests on the fact that it is impossible to determine whether a lymph node is negative on the basis of gross examination.)

In cancer of the stomach and lung, Madden claims that the lymph node acts as a barrier to dissemination. The concept of a barrier to dissemination rests on some observations made on the phagocytic properties of the lymph node reticuloendothelial cells toward charcoal particles, lymphocytes, and other substances.

Tumor cells may not be subject to trapping by lymph nodes in the same fashion as foreign particles and normal cells. Fisher and Fisher have shown that although irradiation and inflammation modify the uptake of injected erythrocytes in lymph nodes, they are without effect on the number of tumor cells that are trapped in the lymph nodes. Moreover, several laboratories have established, with a number of different techniques, that cancer cells may traverse lymph

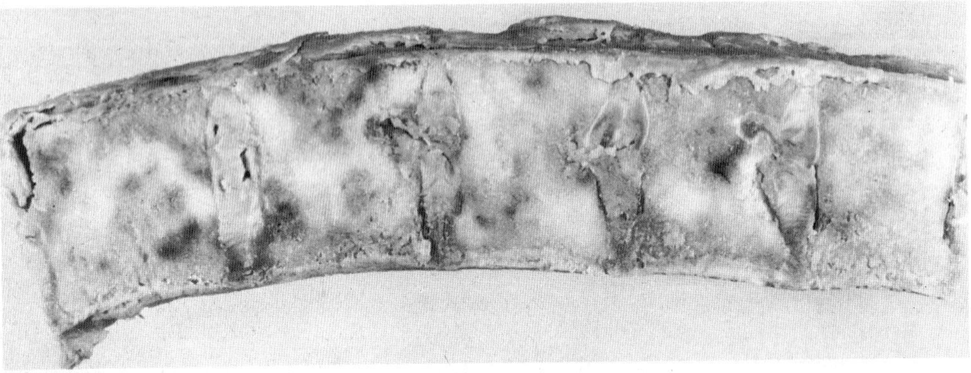

Fig. 16-38. Several vertebrae invaded by osteoblastic metastasis of breast cancer

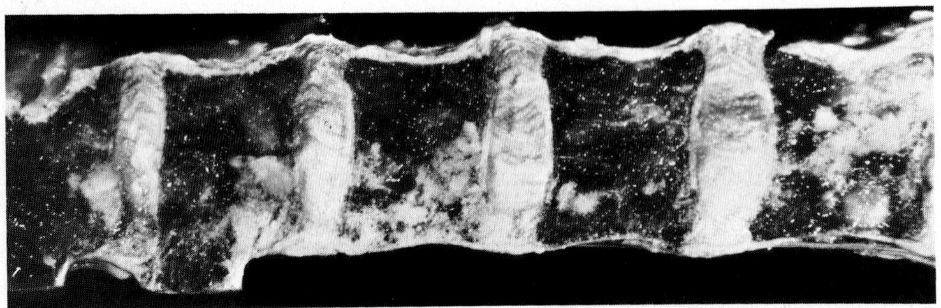

Fig. 16-39. Metastasis in vertebrae; normal bone tissue is replaced by whitish, meaty cancerous tissue

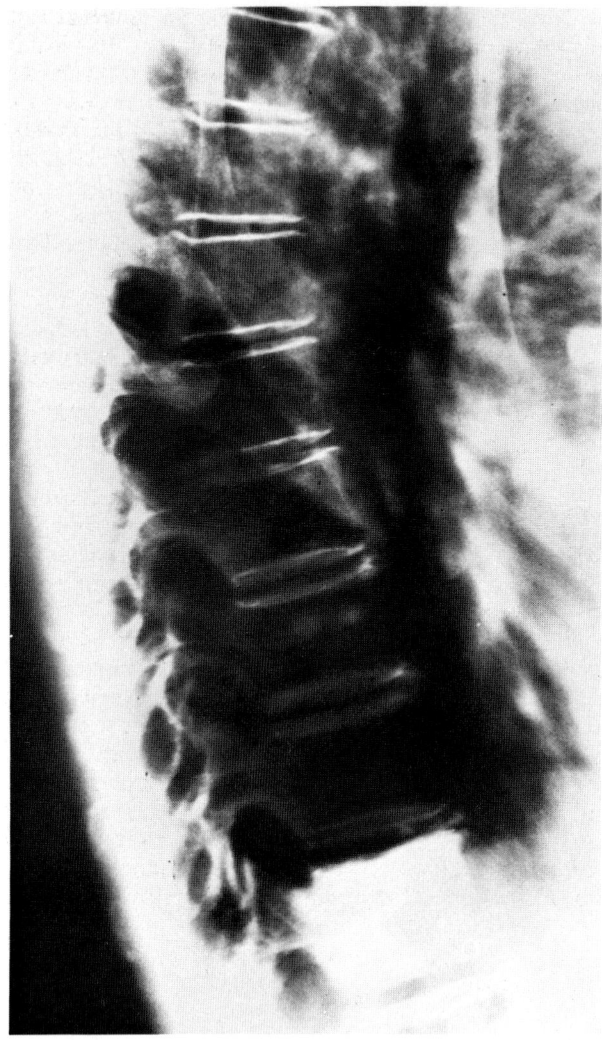

Fig. 16-40. Osteoblastic metastasis of cancer of the prostate in vertebrae; notice the dense ivory bone

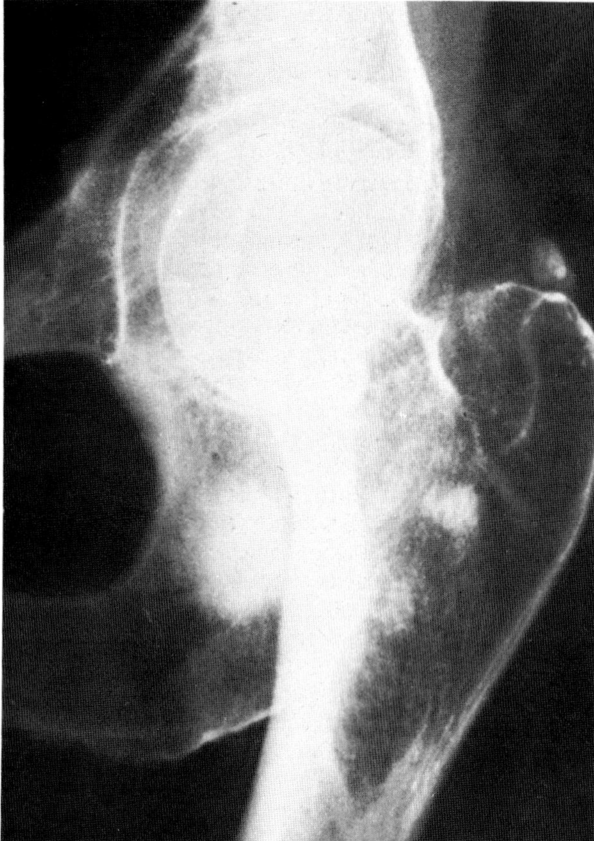

Fig. 16-41. Osteolytic metastasis showing an area of radiolucency in the trochanter

nodes. In fact, studies made in Madden's laboratory suggest that even the presence of tumors in the node does not prevent sieving of injected tumor cells. Therefore, widespread vascular dissemination could occur in the absence of positive nodes. Moreover, the presence of a positive node cannot be considered as an indication that the nodes have successfully filtered all the cancer cells. Examples of lymphatic invasion and bone metastases are shown in Figs. 16-37, 16-38, 16-39, 16-40, and 16-41.

Membrane Alteration in Invasion and Metastasis

Although cancer invasion has been known since classical Greek times, the concept of metastasis was accepted and developed much later into what we understand it to be today. Metastases presumably develop from a single or a group of cells that have become detached from the main tumor mass to seed some distant organs. This interpretation of the formation of metastasis is now so obvious that it is surprising that Virchow refused to accept it and proposed that metastasis resulted from the combination of body juices with existing fibroblasts. Hunter also thought that the development of metastasis was unrelated to the primary tumor.

Whatever may cause invasion and metastasis, these phenomena must involve the cell membrane; therefore, much research on the properties and the structure of the cancer cell membrane is under way. Light microscopists, of course, knew for a long time of changes in the cancer cell membrane. Cancer cells are often separated from their neighbors and thus loose the size and shape usually imposed on them by contact with other cells. Connections normally seen between cells (tonofibrils) often disappear in cancer. Phagocytic properties usually not exhibited by the normal counterpart appear in the cancer cell.

Three properties emerge from all attempts to distill the most prominent features of cancer from a multitude of biological, biochemical, and morphological alterations associated with the malignant state: (1) the cancer cell divides in an uninterrupted fashion; (2) it progressively surrenders the control of its metabolism; and (3) it is readily detached and invades and metastasizes.

Whether changes in the plasma membrane constitute the primary injury of cancer, as Wallach proposed [511, 512], and whether this primary injury is amplified through distortion of the feedback loop leading to secondary injuries in the genome* or in the intermediary metabolism** is far from settled. The hypotheses are intriguing and further emphasize the need for detailed knowledge of the molecular configuration and interaction at the level of the cell membrane.

Physiological, physicochemical, and biochemical methods have been used to study membrane alteration in cancer cells. The physiological studies include investigations of contact inhibition, phagocytosis, cell permeability, and ion transfer from one cell to another. The physicochemical studies include investigations of the cell's adhesiveness and electronegativity. The biochemical studies include biochemical analysis of cell constituents.

Since we know so little about the structure of the normal cell's plasma membrane, meaningful generalizations on the alteration of the cancer cell membrane are not likely to be available. In fact, much of the data accumulated on the cancer cell membrane are not readily interpretable because (1) adequate control cells were not used or were not available; (2) the cell population studied included necrotic cells; (3) the results are not consistent but vary considerably, sometimes in opposite directions, depending upon the type of tumor used; or (4) the changes observed are not really linked to carcinogenesis *per se* but to uninterrupted proliferation.

At least two changes in the cell membrane are related to invasion: the loss of adhesiveness and a change in intercellular communication.

Coman made the major contribution to the study of cell adhesion in cancer. The bend assumed by special needles was calibrated using a known force (weights). The needles were then used to separate cells in a delicate micromanipulation. The bend of the calibrated needles measured the force needed to separate cells. The force required to separate cells of human lip and cervical cancers was only 15 to 25% of that needed to separate cells of the epithelium of the lip or cervix.

Calcium probably influences adhesiveness; indeed, hepatoma cells dissociate readily after perfusion with EDTA. In contrast, cells of normal livers remain attached to each other. In general, cancer cells are also readily separated by passing some tumors through a syringe. However, cellular adhesiveness is not always decreased in the cancer cell. Halpern and associates studied cultures (grown in an agitated medium) of cell lines derived from malignant and normal cells and found that adhesiveness was greater in cancer cells [513].

Although electron microscopists have described various types of morphological contacts between cells (zona occluteus, loose junctions, gross cytoplasmic continuity, and desmosomes), electric currents or macromolecules were not thought to pass from cell to cell. Nevertheless, Loewenstein showed that such communications occur [453].

It is therefore remarkable that the intracellular electrical techniques used in Loewenstein's laboratory also clearly revealed that cancer cells had lost the cell-to-cell communication that in normal cells permits the free diffusion of cellular substances. In fact, when cancer cells are transplanted into normal liver, the communication between the normal liver cells, which are found near the cancer cells, is abolished.

The interruption of cell communication clearly is not linked directly to cellular proliferation, since normal communication persists in regenerating liver cells and healing eroded skin, tissues in which the rate of cell proliferation is greater than that in many tumors. Thus, in the normal cell communication is the rule and is compatible with prolonged interphase or mitosis. In the cancerous tissue cell, communication is abolished during both interphase and mitosis.

Whether the loss of cell communication is in some way linked with the disregulation that leads to uninterrupted mitosis or metastasis is not clear. The absence of cell communication is not inevitably associated with uninterrupted mitosis because macrophages and lymphocytes, which wander as individual cells, seldom divide [514]. However, cancer cells do not always separate. Cone has reported the formation of cytoplasmic bridges (cytopons) between cancer cells as a result of the merging of pseudopods from adjacent cells and incomplete separation of dividing daughter cells. Cone believes that these bridges transmit signals from cell to cell, and that initiation of mitosis in one cell triggers a wave of mitosis in neighboring cells.

Ambrose has compared the movement of the fibroblast on a glass surface with that of an earthworm. The peristaltic wave generated at the moving edge flows from the edge toward the nucleus, making the membrane undulate and securing intermittent contact between membrane surface and glass support.

Using a phase-contrast microscope, Ambrose compared the movements of cancer cells and normal cells. The phase-contrast microscope contains a 60-degree glass prism that reflects all light. Thus, when the investigator looks through the ocular, no light passes through and only a dark field is seen. When a specimen is examined with a phase-contrast microscope, the angle of reflection is distorted and light becomes visible wherever the cell contacts the glass surface.

On the basis of such observations, it appears that it is not the malignant cell's mode of locomotion that is responsible for invasion and metastasis, but its inability to stop the movement by contact inhibition. Thus, whereas fibroblast's movements are stopped by contact inhibition, cancer cell movements are not inhibited by contact with fibroblasts. The loss of contact inhibition appears early after neoplastic conversion by oncogenic viruses. Surprisingly, tumor cells that are not inhibited by homologous

---

* Distortion in the programing of transcription.

** *E.g.*, anomaly of mitochondrial membrane results in modification of permeability for NAD and ADP, and as a result leads to disregulation in glycolysis.

tumor cells can be inhibited occasionally by normal cells or by different tumor cells. These observations suggest that contact inhibition is extremely specific.

Contact inhibition is believed to result from a two-way signal: reception from the neighboring cell and transmission from the original cell to the neighboring cell. It would appear that a cancer cell can receive the message from cells that have an intact signal system (reception and transmission), but it cannot transmit the signal to other cells.

Experiments from several laboratories suggest that contact inhibition, as observed *in vitro*, is not unrelated to the behavior of the tumor *in vivo*. For example, Pollack and Teebor [515] have prepared hamster cell lines with various degrees of contact inhibition *in vitro*. Contact inhibition *in vitro* is inversely related to the capacity to initiate tumor growth *in vivo*. Thus, contact-inhibited sublines were less able than densely growing sublines to initiate tumor growth. However, there is no correlation between the morphology and tumor patterns and the degree of contact inhibition *in vitro*.

Movement and contact inhibition are not the appanage of the cancer cell. Although most blood cells are simply carried passively by blood flow, macrophages are capable of active locomotion. Leukocytes that can invade normal tissues are not contact inhibited by fibroblasts *in vitro*. We have seen how Abercrombie devised methods of measuring contact inhibition in fibroblasts by putting two fibroblast explants suspended in serum on a glass support. When fibroblasts were replaced by carcinoma cells in one of the explants, movement was not inhibited when the carcinoma cells touched the fibroblasts. Similarly, cells transformed with the Bryant strain of Rous sarcoma virus show clear-cut homologous contact inhibition but not heterologous inhibition for fibroblasts, even if the fibroblasts are of embryonic origin. However, depending upon the source of the transformed cell, the degree of heterologous inhibition seems to vary widely, ranging from almost nothing to complete inhibition.

A number of investigators have compared the electrophoretic mobilities of isolated cancer cells and normal cells. Both types of cells are suspended in a container filled with buffer through which a mild current travels. The mobility of the cells is a measure of the total charge. It has been claimed that cancer cells are more electronegative than their normal counterparts. Thus, the mobility of cells obtained from rat hepatomas produced with aminoazotoluene (butter yellow) and of those obtained from kidney tumors produced with stilbestrol was compared with the mobility of normal liver and renal cortical cells. Tumor cells always have a higher mobility than their homolog. The increase in mobility could be reduced by neuraminidase, and therefore is believed to result from the carboxylic groups of sialic acid. In fact, in human erythrocytes, 90% of the surface charge per unit area can be removed by treatment with neuraminidase.

Ambrose has devised a means to distinguish between charges contributed by the carboxyl group of sialic acid and the phosphate group of phospholipids. The sialic acid groups can be removed by neuraminidase, but the phosphate groups have a great affinity for calcium. By successive treatment with neuraminidase and calcium, it has been possible to show that the charge varies with the type of tumor investigated. So whereas in some leukemias the charge is entirely due to sialic acid, in other types of tumors (such as Ehrlich's carcinoma) phospholipids also participate. Ambrose then attempted to determine whether shifts in the proportion of the phospholipid relative to the sialic acid charges determined the alteration of the overall charge in the tumor cells. For that purpose he used transformed fibroblasts.

He observed that hamster fibroblasts transformed with polyoma virus have much higher mobility and much greater variation in mobility than the normal fibroblast. Treatment with calcium, which covers the phospholipid charges, did not abolish the difference in mobilities between normal and cancer cells. However, when the fibroblasts were treated with neuraminidase, all differences between normal and cancer cells disappeared, suggesting that the sialic acid content is responsible for the differences in electrophoretic properties of normal and cancer cells.

This finding correlates with a histochemical observation made in Gasic's laboratory [516] that demonstrated that after transformation with polyoma virus, embryonic hamster cells develop a mucopolysaccharide coat that disappears after treatment with neuraminidase. Ambrose has further shown that the fibroblast is covered by a sialopeptide, which can be removed by combined treatment with neuraminidase and trypsin. The peptide portion of the sialoprotein has an amino acid composition reminiscent of that of collagen; whether these sialopeptides play a role in tumor antigenicity remains to be seen.

The relevance of the changes in the cell charge to the primary injury in cancer remains to be established and, in fact, is doubtful. Studies on a variety of tumors suggest that there is a close correlation between the charge changes and the tumor's growth rate. Moreover, the electrophoretic charge of regenerating liver cells is 40% greater than that of normal cells.

Weiss and Sinks [517] have studied the electrophoretic mobility of human peripheral lymphocytes and circulating malignant cells obtained from patients with acute and chronic leukemia. They also compared cultures of normal lymphoblasts with those of lymphoblasts derived from Burkitt's tumors. No consistent differences between the electrophoretic mobilities of the isolated cells were found. However, treatment with ribonuclease modified the electrophoretic mobility of these cells so that they could be categorized in two groups. Exposure to the enzyme reduced the mobility of normal lymphoblasts and peripheral lymphocytes but had no effect on the mobility of cultured Burkitt cells or circulating leukemia cells. These findings illustrate the great differences in the patterns of total RNA synthesis among the various types of cells investigated.

In conclusion, the increase in negative surface charge of the neoplastic cell appears to result from increased surface sialic acid. However, there is no indication that this charge might constitute the primary injury in cancer, but evidence suggests that the change in surface charge might correlate with the growth rate.

Tumor Host Relationships

Tumors affect the host in many ways: (1) by the simple presence of their mass, or through invasion or metastasis; (2) by elaborating antigens; (3) by elaborating normal or abnormal products that appear in blood and urine and may distort the host's physiological balance; and (4) by selectively consuming cellular metabolites [518].

The effect of metastasis on the host has already been discussed, and the immunological properties of tumors will be reviewed separately.

Ectopic Hormones

We have already discussed the pathogenesis of (1) primary aldosteronism associated with cancer of the adrenals, (2) hypertension associated with pheochromocytoma, (3) hypoglycemia in tumors of the pancreas, (4) hyperparathyroidism in tumors of the parotid, and (5) secretion of gonadotropins in tumors of the testes and the placenta. In all these cases, the hormone is a normal product of the tissue from which the tumor originates, and the humoral disturbance is the consequence of cellular hyperplasia and overproduction.

The identification of nonmalignant tumors leading to the production of substances with hormonal activity is of importance for the pathogenesis, diagnosis, and therapy of such tumors. The hormonal disturbances that have been observed in association with the proliferation of nonendocrine tumors include: Cushing's syndrome (ACTH or ACTH-like hormones), diabetes insipidus (ADH), diabetes or increased glucose tolerance test (unknown factor), hypoglycemia, hypercalcemia, TSH secretion without hyperthyroidism, and gonadotropin elaboration [519–521].

The association of Cushing's syndrome with nonendocrine cancer was first described by Brown in 1928 [522]. Since then, the syndrome has been observed in many types of tumors including oat cell carcinomas of the bronchi, carcinomas of the pancreas, thyroid, parathyroid, prostate, ovary, colon, and mammary glands, thymus tumors, sympatheticoblastomas, pheochromocytomas, and carcinoid tumors (see Fig. 16-42).

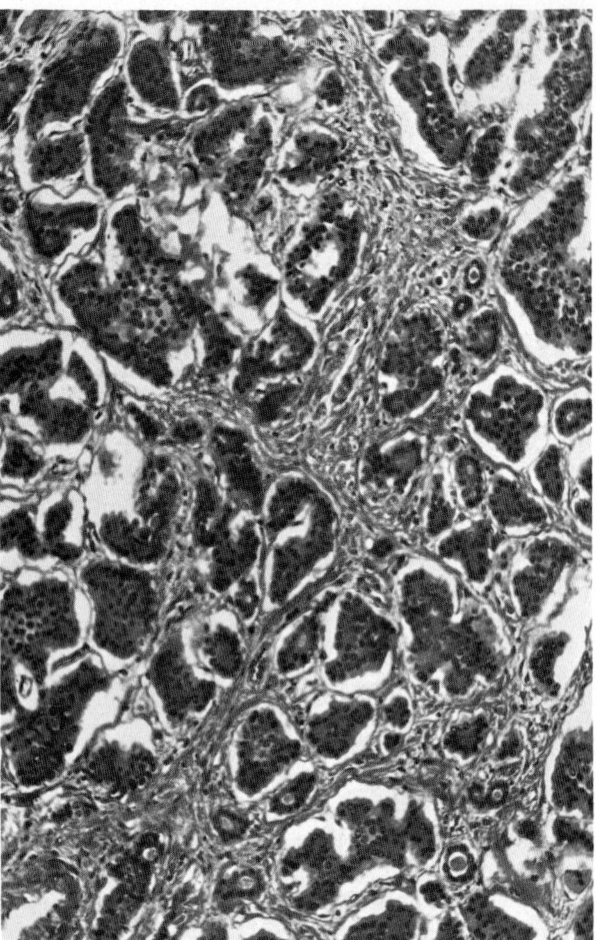

Fig. 16-42. Carcinoid tumor of small intestine

The substance that is produced has been shown to be either ACTH or an ACTH-like compound. The hormone induces hypertrophy of the adrenal cortex and is responsible for the development of the cushinoid syndrome. The cushinoid syndrome observed in these cancer patients differs from what is observed in the classical Cushing's syndrome. In cancer patients the moon-shaped face and the lipodystrophy of the trunk or the thighs are exceptional, but the electrolyte imbalances—especially hypocalcemia and alkalosis—are typical. The reasons for these differences in the clinical manifestations are not known. An obvious interpretation is that the hormone elaborated by tumors is different from that secreted by the hypophysis [523].

Undifferentiated lung carcinomas (oat cell carcinomas) have also been observed to produce antidiuretic hormone with hyponatremia, hypo-osmolality of the serum, and increased sodium secretion in hyperconcentrated urine. Hypocalcemic factors have been described in nonparathyroid tumors of rats and humans. Although these factors are different from those of the traditional parathyroid tumors, their exact composition has not been established. Hypersecretion of chorionic gonadotropin has been observed in liver tumors, breast cancers, and malignant melanomas as well as in bronchial carcinoma.

Some bronchial carcinomas have been found to be associated with the hypersecretion of thyrotropic hormones. In most cases, the increased TSH levels in the serum and in the tumor are not associated with hyperthyroidism.

Abnormal glucose tolerance tests have been observed in almost 40% of patients with advanced cancer. Up to 10% of cancer patients reportedly have frank diabetes. The mechanism producing diabetes and hyperglycemia is not known.

Hypoglycemia is observed in association with large peritoneal spindle cell carcinomas and advanced liver cancer. In liver cancer, hypoglycemia is believed to result from sequestration of large amounts of glycogen in the tumors.

Growth factors of unknown origin are sometimes produced by tumors. In leukemia, the liver and kidney are sometimes enlarged even though they are not infiltrated with leukemic cells. Such changes result from enlargement of the individual hepatic and kidney cells.

The appearance of unscheduled hormonal activities in cancer cells is disconcerting, but not totally unexpected. A mechanism frequently invoked to explain such an occurrence is derepression in the tumor of genes repressed in the normal cells. Therefore, the appearance of new hormones in these cells would simply reflect the general distortion of gene expression that takes place in cancer.

When the source of the ectopic hormonal secretion can be traced, extirpation of the tumor may be expected to eliminate the symptoms resulting from hormonal hypersecretion.

Cancer and the Host's Nutrition

If it does not by itself constitute an absolute diagnostic criterion, weight loss is often a sign of the existence of cancer.

Sometimes even a small tumor is responsible for the progressive wasting away of the host. The patient loses his fat reserve, and he also uses muscles and other tissue proteins to feed insatiable and wasteful cancer cells.

The severe emaciation and weakness that accompany the development of cancer is called cachexia, a word derived from the Greek $\kappa\alpha\kappa o\varsigma$ (bad), which literally means a bad state of affairs.

Cachexia occurs in many diseases. In fact, most severe chronic or acute infections lead to cachexia. Balzac, Zola, and many other novelists have given moving, if not always accurate, descriptions of the "consumption" of their characters with tuberculosis. We have already described the cachexia associated with the loss of function of the hypophysis.

Cancer patients often show a negative nitrogen and phosphorus balance, and although force feeding may induce a temporary weight gain, the gain is usually transient. Such observations lead clinicians and investigators to conclude that normal tissues yield their components to the cancer cell.

Since most of the cellular components are constantly replaced through cell renewal or discrete molecular turnover, it is not necessary for the cancer cell to kill cells to deplete the host. The cancer cell needs only to be more efficient than host cells in uptake of nutrients.

Among the biochemicals that are lost to the cancer cell, proteins are most critical. The cancer cell has an advantage over the host cell because the former can function as a "nitrogen trap."

Experimental proof of the existence of the nitrogen trap was obtained principally in the laboratories of Mider [524, 525] and LePage [526, 527]. The concept of the nitrogen trap rests on three basic findings: (1) tumors continue to grow in animals fed a protein-free diet; (2) the nitrogen used to build up tumor protein is derived mostly from the carcass of the animal; (3) once incorporated in the tumor cells, the nitrogen is not released to the host even under conditions of fasting.

Miscellaneous Alterations in Cancer Patients

Anemia

Cancer is often associated with anemia. The pathogenesis of some of the anemias is easy to explain because anemia results from repeated hemorrhage or interference with absorption of vitamin B_{12}, trapping and overuse of folic acid, or massive invasion of bone marrow by cancer cells. Nevertheless, in some cases none of these pathogenic mechanisms can be invoked, yet red cells die and anemia develops. In those cases, structural or molecular alterations of the red cells cannot be demonstrated, and the anemia is believed to result from the presence of hemolytic factors in the cancer patient's blood. Zucker believes that in some cancer patients the anemia may result from unresponsiveness of the bone marrow to erythropoietin [670].

Degeneration

Peripheral neuritis and even degeneration of the cerebellum have been described in patients with severe leukemia. Although in most cases the symptoms can be explained by direct leukemic infiltration or hemorrhages, sometimes the pathogenesis is unclear.

Uric Acid Accumulation

Serum and urine uric acid levels are often increased in patients with acute leukemia. In those cases, the pools of uric acid are most frequently normal or borderline, but they may occasionally be increased. The pathogenesis of hyperuricemia in cancer patients is likely to involve increased *de novo* biosynthesis of nucleic acid followed by excessive breakdown.

Angiogenesis in Tumors

When cells are cultured in semisolid agar, they grow to form a little sphere that regularly expands in three dimensions. In the beginning all cells are alive because diffusion permits the usage of nutrients and elimination of catabolites. In a second stage, the cells at the center of the mass die, but the peripheral cells continue to divide, further expanding the size of the sphere. In a third stage, growth comes to a standstill, not because the cells stop dividing, but because an equilibrium is reached between the cells that die in the center of the mass and the cells that proliferate at the periphery [528, 529].

Similarly, when Green implanted tumors in the anterior chamber of the eye, the cells proliferated, but proliferation was again limited by diffusion.

In contrast, if the cells were implanted close to the iris and became vascularized, these cells grew at a pace 100 times that of the unvascularized mass. Pathologists have known for a long time that the development of an adequate vasculature is essential to growth of solid tumors. In fact, whenever a tumor grows so fast that the proliferation of the tumor cells exceeds that of the endothelial cells, the tumor cells die once they have exceeded the limit of diffusion. Vascularization of tumors can result only from capillary proliferation. The vasculature of the tumor is unique in that tumors usually do not contain veins and arteries, but a rich network of capillaries bound only by an endothelial epithelium. This form of capillary proliferation is not unique to tumors, it occurs in granulation tissue. The mechanism that triggers endothelial cell proliferation is unknown [671].

Chalkley and Warren proposed that capillary proliferation was induced by a humoral factor in the tumor cells. The experiments of Greenblatt and Shubik have provided evidence in support of this view. These investigators implanted ear chambers in the cheek pouch of hamsters. They placed tumor cells in the mass and observed capillary proliferation in the surrounding tissue. In some of these experiments, the tumor cells were separated from the surrounding environment by Millipore filters. This excluded the possibility of cell migration. The results clearly indicated that the tumors elaborated a substance that stimulates endothelial growth, and they also established that the humoral factor influences the pattern of capillary growth, and that this pattern depends on the type of tumors used for transplantation.

The molecular structure of the "angiogenic" factor remains to be established with certainty. Folkman and his associates claim that the factor is present in both cytoplasm and nucleus. They have partially purified the factor from the nucleus and, surprisingly, found it to be part of chromatin; they believe it to be a nonhistone protein bound to RNA. The factor is unusually painstaking to purify because rigid asepsia is required throughout.

Cancer Immunity

Introduction

At least three generations of cancer researchers and clinicians have dreamed of preventing cancer by immunization or curbing it by exploiting the immune responses. Although the antigenicity of tumors was already suspected in 1910, conclusive evidence for tumor antigenicity has only been available in the last two decennia. Whether the majority of human tumors are able to mount an effective immune response is still in doubt. If, indeed, the properties of the tumors are to be readily exploitable for prevention, diagnosis, or therapy, not only must the tumor be antigenic, but it must also trigger an immune reaction against the antigen which destroys the cancer cell and which cannot be overcome either by clonal mutation or by the elaboration of substances that interfere with the immune response.

Two clinical observations, among many others, suggest that the growth of human cancers is, at least under some circumstances, controlled by immunological responses, spontaneous regression and the high incidence of cancers among patients with immunodeficient diseases. I never had the good fortune to see one spontaneous recovery among the thousands of cancer patients that I have had the opportunity to observe from onset to outcome; however there is documented evidence that some cancers regress without intervention. This finding has for long been at the source of the hope that some day a more effective form of therapy will become available. It is now believed that spontaneous regression is caused by an immunological response to the tumor and hence, attempts are made to enhance the immunological response against those cancers that do not regress spontaneously. The relatively higher incidence of cancer among patients afflicted with either immunodeficient or autoimmune disease has led clinicians to believe that cancer is controlled immunologically. Similarly, most immunosuppressive agents, such as X-ray or purine and pyrimidine analogues, bring about an increase in cancer incidence. It can, however, not be excluded that the association between these conditions simply results from the fact that all these are caused by increased susceptibility to mutation [672–676].

For the purpose of illustrating the immunological aspects of cancer we shall return to our original example, the melanoma. Melanomas represent 15% of the spontaneously regressing cancers. Because often no primary can be found even in cases of widely metastasizing melanomas, it is believed, but difficult to prove, that in such cases the primary regressed. Melanoma cells can be found in the circulation which seem to have undergone cellular deterioration as a result of the immune response mounted against them. Pathologists are accustomed to seeing tumors that are generously infiltrated with lymphocytes and plasmocytes and naturally they came to suspect that such infiltration results from the immune response of the host. Melanomas are characteristically infiltrated with lymphoid cells. There even exists a benign lesion in which central necrosis of the proliferating melanocytes is typically observed (halo nevus, leukoderma acquisitum centrifugum). Similar lesions are sometimes seen in malignant melanomas.

Using a battery of tests various groups of investigators have demonstrated changes in humoral and cell mediated immunity in patients with melanoma [677–679]. Humoral antibodies directed against melanoma cells have been detected by indirect fluorescence and cellular cytolysis via complement–antigen-antibody complexes. The antibodies are directed toward a specific melanoma antigen similar to those found in viral tumors in animals and toward an antigen unique to the host, similar to those found in tumors produced with the aid of chemical carcinogens (see below). When the antibodies are tested against autologous cells, humoral antibodies against melanoma are found in 100% of the patients. When they are tested against cells of other patients with melanoma, 68% contain the antibodies. Only 20% of normal individuals have antimelanoma antibodies.

It is generally assumed that the immunological defense against cancer is primarily of the cellular rather than the humoral type. If extracts of melanoma are inoculated in the same fashion as tuberculin, patients respond to autologous melanomas, but not to benign pigmented tumors or normal skin. Such a finding clearly suggests that the organism mounts a cellular immune reaction to the malignant tumor, a conclusion confirmed in experiments using lymphocyte stimulation and macrophage inhibition tests.

It is fair to ask why most victims of established melanomas die a tragic death within a short time. The answer is not known, but either the immune response is ineffective from the start or at some point the tumor finds it within its power to tilt the balance in its own favor either by specifically neutralizing the immune response or by unspecifically generating an immune deficiency state. For these reasons the evaluation of the immune deficiency status is considered to be of prognostic significance in patients with melanoma. This is achieved by determing the response to tuberculin and to 2,4-dinitrotrochlorobenzene. While the first test measures sensitivity to old, the second measures sensitivity to recent antigenic exposure.

A defect in the immune response of cancer patients is not restricted to melanoma. A state of anergy has long been known to occur in patients with Hodgkin's disease and leukemias. Such an observation is not surprising since the malignant transformation involves immunocompetent cells. Evidence of defective immune response in human patients afflicted with other types of cancer is less conclusive. Morton and his associates have studied 52 patients with various types of cancers including carcinoma, melanoma and sarcoma. They studied the *in vitro* response of the patients' lymphocytes to blastogenesis and to the *in vivo* response to 2,4-dinitrochlorobenzene stimulation and the recall reaction to microbial antigens [680]. Impairment in skin test reaction and blastogenesis were seen in most cases. The patients with carcinoma had mostly impairment of skin test while the patients with melanoma had more marked impairment of lymphocyte function and less impairment in skin test. Depressed levels of rosette formation have been observed in patients with carcinoma of the lung [681]. Patients with transitional carcinoma of the urinary tract have been found to have a serum factor that induces lymphocyte mediated antitumor toxicity.

The existence of anergy in cancer patients and that of immunological protective mechanisms in other cases have encouraged the development of immunotherapy of cancer. One means of stimulating the immune response of the T cells is to administer a vigorously immunological agent such as BCG (bacilli de Calmette-Guerin), the agent responsible for tuberculosis. The success of such therapy is at present difficult to evaluate, although objective temporary remissions have been recorded. The therapy is not without hazards. Granulomatous hepatitis and mycobacterial pneumonia have been reported in patients treated by such means [682–686].

Various modes of administration of BCG have been used in humans. BCG has been administered orally and injected systemically or within the lesion. BCG seems to be most effective when administered within the tumor, as is the case, for example, for skin melanoma. When the tumor is not accessible paralesional administration is attempted. For example, in patients with lung cancer, BCG is administered either in the form of aerosols or injected into the pleura. Systemic administration is usually reserved for patients with disseminated cancers like myelogenous leukemia.

More recently the use of killed *C. parvum* injected systemically or inside the tumor or injection of the antihelmintic drug levamisole has been used as adjuvant for the purpose of stimulating the immune response.

Other forms of immunotherapy of tumors include the stimulation of host lymphoid cells *in vitro* with transfer factor and immune RNA obtained from cured patients. The stimulated lymphocytes can then be reintroduced in the host and hopefully will interfere with tumor growth.

A number of investigators have found that irradiation of the field of implantation of syngeneic tissues enhanced the growth of the transplant. Similarly, Kaplan and Murphy found that sublethal irradiation of transplanted syngeneic mammary tumors facilitated the formation of lung metastasis. The studies of Vaage *et al.* [687] suggest that these "abscopal" effects of radiation result from immunosuppression. While radiation interfered with tumor growth of implanted sarcoma in mice, extensive field radiation facilitated the growth of tumors in unirradiated parts of the animals.

Whatever the role of the immune system may be in controlling the growth of human cancers, the findings of the last decennium present the oncotherapist with a crucial dilemma. Except for surgery all anticancer agents (ionizing radiation and antimetabolites) are immunosuppressant. The fact is that in most cases the oncotherapist has little choice since these agents are the only ones proven effective against some advanced cancers at this time.

Tumor antigens have been found in a number of human cancers: Burkitt's lymphoma, neuroblastoma, melanoma, osteogenic sarcoma, liposarcoma, leukemia, retinoblastoma, hepatoma, Wilms' tumors, kidney hypernephroma, squamous and basal cell carcinoma of the skin, and carcinoma of the colon, lung, pancreas, bladder, stomach, esophagus, breast, thyroid and parathyroid. The antigens have not always been identified. In the case of Burkitt's lymphoma, the antigen of one patient is recognized by that of other patients with Burkitt's lymphoma on observation, suggesting that the tumor may be of viral origin. In colon carcinoma and hepatoma and possibly pancreatic carcinoma, specific fetal antigens appear at the surface of the cancer cell during oncogenesis.

Animal Experiments

If the observation made in man inspired studies on the immunological response in animals, the animal studies clarified our understanding of the immunological response to cancer in man, and it is therefore appropriate to briefly review modern knowledge of cancer immunity. Although a great deal had been written around 1920 about cancer immunity, it was at the time difficult to distinguish whether the immunity mounted against cancer was aimed at a unique antigen or at histocompatibility antigens. The earliest experiments performed for the purpose of demonstrating an immunological response to cancer were not conclusive and were ignored. Thus, in 1943 Gross demonstrated that mice could be immunized against tumors obtained from syngeneic animals. Prehn and his co-workers, fourteen years later, showed that the capacity to reject the tumor was not linked to that of rejecting skin grafts from the donor bearing the tumor, thus indicating that the antigens mounting the immunological response against the tumor were not histocompatibility, but tumor specific antigens. This finding was confirmed by an elegant and simple experiment of Klein in which a tumor was produced by injection of benzene pyrene in a mouse leg. The florid mass was amputated and transplanted to another animal for preservation. Then the three-legged bearer of the original tumor was immunized repeatedly with irradiated cells obtained from the tumor. When transplantation of the original tumor was performed there was no take. Since these were autologous tumors that were transplanted, the experiment left no doubt that the antigens were tumor specific. Further studies in a large number of laboratories using chemically induced tumors clearly established that although specific antigens existed, the antigens were different for each tumor.

Different results were obtained when tumors of viral origin, such as those caused by the polyoma virus, were studied for their antigenic properties. Such tumors, even when produced in animals of different strains, possess various specific antigens. Thus one can immunize a rat against the virus with mouse tumor cells. Some tumors, such as the mouse mammary tumor, were later found to contain two types of antigens: a specific one characteristic of chemically produced tumors and a common one characteristic of virus produced tumors.

Since we have already discussed some of the antigenic properties of viral cancers we shall focus our attention on chemically produced cancers.

Studies of the antigenic properties of experimental tumors produced by chemical carcinogens have revealed three types of changes: (1) appearance of new antigens, (2) disappearance of normal surface antigens, (3) reappearance of antigens which exist in the fetus, but not in the adult.

The new antigens of those tumors produced by chemical or physical carcinogens are not the same for all such cancers. In fact, these types of cancers characteristically vary considerably in their antigenic properties. Moreover, carcinogens which produce strongly antigenic tumors, for example, methylcholanthrene sarcoma, at one site may yield nonantigenic tumors at others, for example, mammary tumors induced by methylcholanthrene. Even a more intriguing finding is that the antigens of each chemically or physically induced tumor are different. In fact, when the antigenicity of four different hepatoma nodules produced in the same rat was determined, each nodule proved to have different antigens.

Immunofluorescence and tissue fractionation studies (see below) have established that the tumor specific antigens are located on the cell membrane. Antigens that cross react with other tissues or fetal rat serum, but not normally present in the tissue of origin have, however, been found in the cell sap or other cell constituents in some DAB induced tumors. Some of the new antigens that appear in DAB tumors are detected at the time when maximum binding to protein occurs. Antibodies prepared against protein bound acetylaminofluorene complexes react with antigens of microsomes and cytosol of AAF induced hepatomas. In some cases it has been possible to isolate tumor specific antigens from concentrated membrane fractions. The yield of recovered antigens compared to the amount found on the surface of the complete cell is, however, low (10–15%). The antigen can be solubilized from membrane fragments, chromatographed, and separated by centrifugation or electrophoresis on polyacrylamide gel. Antigens with molecular weights of 55,000 and 75,000 to 150,000 daltons have been isolated from amino azo dye (rat) and dimethylnitrosamine (guinea pig) induced hepatomas, respectively. Very little is known of the chemistry of tumor antigens, but available evidence suggests that they are protein-carbohydrate-lipid complexes and that each moiety is involved in antigenic determination.

Weilu demonstrated in 1952 that organ specific antigens were lost in the course of development of rat hepatomas. Later antigenic loss was demonstrated to occur in a number of chemically produced tumors; namely, DAB induced hepatoma in rat, dimethylnitrosamine induced hepatoma in guinea pigs, amino azo toluene induced hepatoma in rats, 2 AAF induced hepatoma in rats. Similarly, deletion of kidney specific antigens has been observed in kidney tumors induced by diethylstilbestrol or in transplanted tumors originally induced by X-irradiation. Although the molecular structure of the missing antigens has not been identified, the lost antigens can be grouped in three categories: intracellular antigen, normally found in the microsome or the cytosol, carcinogen binding proteins and cell surface proteins.

Normal mouse antigens are lost in methylcholanthrene induced sarcoma and normal epidermal antigen in the methylcholanthrene induced squamous cell carcinoma. It is possible that the loss of intracellular antigen reflects the distortion of the normal enzyme mosaic that takes place in cancer cells. The loss of surface antigens is of particular significance. It includes loss of H_2 antigen in mouse hepatoma, lymphoma and polyoma tumors as well as HL-A antigens in human lymphoma and liver specific antigen at the cell surface of DBA induced hepatomas. Such losses may reflect the cell surface alterations observed in cancer cells by either morphological or biochemical methods. The relationship between antigen loss and tumorigenesis is not known, but it raises several questions. Could, for example, the loss include (a) proteins or other substances regulating cell growth, such as chalones; or (b) substances controlling cellular interactions and normally preventing invasion of surrounding tissues? The fact that the antigenic loss is most marked at the periphery of the tumor may be an indication that the loss of antigens and invasion are related. There seems to exist an inverse relationship between the amount of H_2 antigen present on the surface and the immunogenicity of the tumor, the more H_2 antigen present the less immunogenicity and vice versa. Such a finding would suggest that H_2 antigens are replaced by neoantigens in the process of cancerization. Direct evidence for such a possibility is not available and it cannot be excluded that molecular rearrangements during cell transformation are responsible for the loss of some and appearance of other antigens.

Hepatomas produced with α amino azotoluene, diethylnitrosamine or N-2 fluorenylacetamide synthesize "α fetoprotein" a substance found in fetal but not adult serum [688–690]. These antigens are present in the cytosol of the liver cell and therefore must differ from the tumor specific antigens which are located on the cell surface. Moreover, this type of fetal antigen does not contribute to tumor regulation by immunization. In the case of SV-40 induced tumors, embryonic antigens have, however, been found at the surface of the cell by cross reaction between SV-40 tumors and fetal cells and by reacting tumor cells with multiparous rat serum. Similarly, methylcholanthrene induced tumors may have embryonic antigens associated with the cell membranes.

Becker *et al.*, using a radioimmune inhibition assay, were able to demonstrate the appearance of α_1-fetoprotein after the administration of minimal doses of N-2-fluorenylacetamide [691]. Further studies indicate that the synthesis of α_1-fetoprotein and cell proliferation are coupled [692]. An oncofetal complex believed to be specific for pancreas has also been described in humans [693].

In conclusion, it appears that experimental chemical carcinogenesis is associated with the derepression of genes that code for a large gamut of embryonic antigens, some of which are not, while others are associated with cell membranes. Whether or not all cell membrane tumor antigens are embryonic antigens is not known.

In human, like in animal tumors, the distortion of gene expression associated with cancer results in the reappearance in the tumor of antigenic molecules which are normally present in the fetus. Two human fetal antigens associated with human tumors stand out: the carcinoembryonic antigen and the α fetoprotein. When sera of patients with cancer of the colon are absorbed on normal colon tissue and then injected to rabbit, the rabbit develops antibodies specifically directed against the tumor antigen. The antigen was found to be present in all cancer of endodermic origin and in fetal intestine, liver and pancreas [694–701].

CEA is a heat stable, water soluble sialoglycoprotein with β electrophoretic mobility. It is located in the membrane of the epithelial cells. When the purified antigen is chromatographed on DEAE-cellulose columns, several antigenetically active components (at least 8) are resolved [695].

The appearance of fetal enzymes and fetal antigens raises intriguing questions independently of the mode of gene activation. First, is fetal gene reactivation always associated with cancer? Second, is fetal gene activation indispensable for providing the cancer cell with the survival advantages it exhibits or is it simply a coincidental manifestation of distortion of gene expression not directly related to the fundamental properties of the cancer cell? The first question can be answered negatively without hesitation. Cases at point are the appearance of fetal hemoglobin in cases of severe anemia or the development the carcinoembryonic antigens in diseases other than cancer.

The levels of CEA vary with the clinical stage of the cancer. The more advanced the disease the more CEA is found in the serum. Therefore the CEA assay is a better indicator of widespread disease than of early carcinoma. It is not very useful as a screening test; first, because many patients with early cancer of the colon have normal levels of CEA. Secondly, because high levels of CEA have been found in patients with other colonic disease such as ulcerative colitis, Crohn's disease, multiple polyposis, etc. In fact, high levels of CEA have been found in a substantial percentage of patients with other cancers such as hepatomas, carcinomas of pancreas, breast, lung, cervix, endometrium, ovary, testis, prostate, kidney, and bladder, neuroblastoma, leukemia, and lymphoma.

The second question remains unanswered in spite of extensive research. If the answer is positive, fetal antigens can be expected to be found in all cancers. Whether such occurrence will then be exploitable for diagnosis or therapy remains to be seen. The fetal genome, because it contains paternal genes, has by necessity a phenotype different from that of the mother. Some of the proteins expressed in the phenotype are antigenic and therefore are bound to affect the maternal immune system. The response of the maternal immune system varies in different species. It includes tolerance, enhancement, antibody formation and lymphocytic sensitization. The interaction between the fetal and maternal immune systems is not completely understood.

The existence of tumor antigens raises a number of questions. Are they capable of mounting an immune response and if so, of what type: humoral or cellular? Is the immune response of a magnitude sufficient to prevent tumor growth at least under some circumstances? Can the immune response be enhanced to secure regression of a florid tumor [702–704]?

Evidence of an immune response to animal and human tumors has been obtained through both *in vivo* and *in vitro* experiments. With rare exceptions the immunological response to the presence of the tumor is believed to be elicited through cellular (sensitized lymphocytes) rather than humoral (circulating cytotoxic antibodies*) immunity; in spite of the fact that both cellular and humoral responses are elicited. Burnet [702] and Thomas [704] have gone so far as to propose that the very purpose of the development of cellular immunity during evolution is to check tumor growth (see section on immunosurveillance). In contrast, the effect of humoral antibodies on tumor dynamics is confusing. Not only have they often been found ineffective in inhibiting tumor growth *in vivo*, but under some circumstances they have been claimed to enhance the rate of growth. Such a phenomenon is referred to as "immunological enhancement" [686]. Moreover, as we shall see later, such antibodies are likely to interfere with cytotoxic effects of sensitized lymphocytes.

We have already described some of the *in vivo* observations which indicate that at least some human or animal tumors are capable of mounting an effective immune response against the tumor cell. If such were the case for all cancers, the cancer cell would be a curiosity, uncovered only through the laborious histological examination of autopsy material. The fact is that most cancers grow apparently unchallenged. There seem to be two obvious reasons for unchallenged growth of tumors: the absence of antigenicity or a depressed immunological status of the host. It is not certain that all tumors are antigenic. There seems, however, to be little doubt that suppression of the immune response by thymectomy, X-irradiation, antimetabolites and antilymphocyte sera enhances tumor growth and tumor incidence at least in some cases. In that context it must be kept in mind that some chemical carcinogens are also immunosuppressant and therefore, their role in carcinogenesis may not only include, for example, their action as mutagens or modulators of cell membranes, but also their function as immunosuppressants. A more puzzling observation is that the size of the tumor mass may influence the immunological response. If mice bearing 10 to 30 day old sarcomas are challenged with a second transplant, the latter is rejected only in those mice carrying the smaller tumors (10 days old). Similarly, it has been shown that although sensitized lymphocytes appear early after tumor transplantation, the cellular immune response decreases as the tumor grows.

In vitro studies of the immune response to tumor growth have provided partial explanations for this paradoxical relationship between tumor growth and the immune response. Before we enter this discussion it will be helpful, however, to describe the colony inhibition test tersely. The discovery of that test is indeed an important landmark in our understanding of tumor immunology because it provided a sensitive assay for measuring the response of tumor cells to humoral or cellular immunity. When a dilute suspension of tumor cells is spread on a Petri dish, the cells are widely dispersed. As the cells proliferate each one becomes the parent of a distinct small colony which can easily be seen and counted. If one kills a proportion of the plated cells, the number of colonies is directly related to the number of cells that survive. Therefore, the number of colonies that appear, for example, after exposure of the plated cell to sensitized lymphocytes or humoral antibodies, is an indirect measure of the cytotoxic effect.* The colony inhibition test clearly indicated that sensitized lymphocytes are cytotoxic for a number of animal and human tumors, but it also revealed that the serum of tumor bearing hosts contains circulating factors that interfere with cell mediated immunity. Whatever

* Some experimental lymphomas are, however, believed to be kept in check by humoral cytotoxic antibodies.

* Of course it remains to be proven that the total cytotoxic effect results from antigen antibody reactions.

other factors may be involved it seems established that specific circulating antibodies participate in the "blocking role." Thus if one plates cells obtained from a DBA induced hepatoma in rats, the serum of those rats blocks only colony inhibition of those cells and has no effect on other types of hepatomas. The blocking antibodies are likely to be 7S antibodies of the IgG type. Antibodies of the IgM type are believed to be devoid of blocking properties.

Blocking antibodies are believed to interfere with cell mediated immunity by combining with lymphocyte surface antigens forming antigen antibody complexes. As a result the surface antigens which serve as detectors of the cancer cells are dimmed and the lymphocyte is unable to identify its target.

Coggin *et al.* have explored why the immune response elicited SV40 hamster sarcoma does not lead to the destruction of the tumor. They found that shortly after the appearance of the tumor, antibodies inhibitory to the growth of the tumor cells appear, but the antibodies are not cytotoxic and moreover, they probably reduce the tumor antigenicity. Later cell mediated immunity against the tumor develops, but is ineffective in preventing tumor growth and formation of metastasis. Circulating antigens released by the growing tumor are believed to bind to circulating lymphocytes and prevent their attack on the intact neoplastic cell [705].

In humans the unresponsiveness of cancer to the immune reaction against it has been correlated with the appearance of a circulating immunosuppressive component [706].

It is often assumed that the only mechanism interfering with the cancer growth involves specific immunological reactions such as the formation of blocking antibodies. But it cannot be excluded that some cells adapt to the hostile immune environment by altered gene expression which, when it appears in the phenotype, allows the cell to escape the immune attack. Hyman has studied and provided some evidence for such a mechanism [707].

This brief introduction to some of the immunological properties of tumors allows us to discuss the concept of "immunosurveillance," the role of immunity in the steady state of human tumors and the hopes for tumor prevention or cure by immunological approaches.

Immunosurveillance

The term immunosurveillance was coined by Burnet [702]. The concept postulates that the initial clone of cancer cells mounts an immune reaction which ultimately disposes of the clone or prevents its growth. This simple and appealing interpretation of the regulation of cancer cells fails, however, to take into account many other factors regulating the process and ignores the paradoxical interaction between tumor cells and the immune response.

Among the clinical evidence used to support immunosurveillance one must include (1) the increased incidence of cancer with old age and immunosuppression, (2) the fact that only a fraction of the population exposed to carcinogens develops cancer, and (3) the existence of a latent period between the time of application of the carcinogen and the development of the tumor.

There is evidence to suggest that in man maximal immunological capacity is reached between the ages of 5 and 30 and decreases some time during or after the third decade. Most cancers develop after the fourth decade. This apparent correlation between the decrease in immunological capacity and the increase in the incidence of cancer is often taken as an argument in favor of immunosurveillance against cancer. Such an assumption, intellectually appealing as it may be, is difficult to prove. Moreover, mechanisms of tumor surveillance, other than immunological ones, could control tumor growth. For example, there is little doubt that the hormonal status of the host modulates the incidence of cancer of the prostate and breast in man and animals (see cancer and hormones).

Cancers are not rare in young people. Melanoma, Hodgkin's disease, acute leukemia, Wilms' tumors, neuroblastoma, Burkitt's tumor, etc. occur between the ages of 5 and 25 frequently. In such cases it has been argued that the transformation into and cloning of the tumor cells might have taken place soon after birth, thus escaping tumor immunosurveillance. Why then did the tumor not grow rapidly during the earliest age and why should it proliferate during an age with maximum immunological capacity? To be sure in some, but by no means all young patients with cancer, both the humoral and the cellular immune responses are depressed; it is, however, not certain whether this is the cause or the effect of cancer.

The fact that all smokers do not develop cancer of the lung is intriguing and could be attributed to the individual immune response. Yet, so many unknown and uncontrollable factors are involved in determining the incidence of cancer of the lung in a human population (smoking habits, the presence of other carcinogens or cocarcinogens in the environment, the capacity to eliminate carcinogens, the ability to repair molecular damage) that to assume that control is exclusively by immunosurveillance risks being a gross oversimplification.

We have seen that individuals exposed to carcinogenic chemicals (*e.g.*, β-naphthylamine) develop cancer at the site of accumulation (*e.g.*, bladder) years after exposure. Similarly, patients X-irradiated for curable diseases may develop cancer at the site of irradiation 10 to 20 years after exposure. The latent period for cancer is often explained by assuming that the original cancer cells are maintained under control through "immunosurveillance." To appreciate the plausibility of such an assumption, it must again be placed into the context of what is known about the mechanisms of chemical carcinogenesis. One can conceive of two extreme means of inducing cancer with chemical or physical agents: single or repeated exposures to the carcinogen. Clearly the length of the latent period is impossible to estimate in the case of repeated exposures. Therefore, for the sake of simplicity let's consider the instance of a single application of a carcinogen in a single cell. If the carcinogen enters the cell, it may be metabolized, rendered ineffective, or it may be converted into an active carcinogen which binds to a macromolecular complex essential to cellular integrity. If the damage to the cell is not repaired, cell function may be altered and as a result the cell may either die or survive and become susceptible to mutations. Some mutations may lead to metaplasia with little survival advantages, others to transformation with the survival advantages of the cancer cell. Transformation may not always take place in the first generation, but it may occur after repeated cell division and therefore, the manifestation of a florid cancer may take a long time after the initial exposure for detection. Consequently the latent period may not be caused by immunosurveillance, but by the dynamics of cancer development. Moreover, it cannot be excluded that even after transformation some yet unknown factor can reverse the cellular status and bring it back under the operation of normal metabolic controls.

Prehn [703] has reviewed the role of immunosurveillance in experimental cancer and points out that the issue is no longer whether or not immunity plays a role in the biology of cancer, but how important that role may be.

We have already mentioned that to secure immunosurveillance the tumor must be antigenic, stimulate the immune response and the host must be immunologically competent. Prehn reviews the antigenicity of neoplasms of animal origin and remarks that tumors arising by the spontaneous transformation of mouse cell in tissue culture have little or no antigenicity and that most spontaneous tumors have low or no antigenicity. Moreover, even some experimental tumors, for example, lung adenomas induced by urethane and rat mammary carcinomas induced by 2-acetylaminofluorene, are seldom antigenic.

The proponents of immunosurveillance could argue that the very lack of antigenicity of tumors supports the concept because only nonantigenic tumors could grow by selection of a clone of cells which escape surveillance. Such immunoselection cannot, however, account for the lack of antigenicity of cells spontaneously transformed in culture.

If immunosurveillance is real, the immune response should operate primarily against small, incipient neoplasms because it is well known that large numbers of tumor cells overwhelm the immune system. It is therefore intriguing that a small neoplasm may often grow without stimulating the host immune reaction to a size so large that it can no longer be controlled by the immune reaction.

In conclusion, experimental and human cancers elicdit both a T cell (cellular immunity) and a B cell (humoral immunity) response.

The cancer cell antigen can react directly with B-lymphocytes, T-lymphocytes and macrophages. The B-lymphocytes produce soluble antibody that may attach to the cancer cell. They may act alone or in cooperation with T-lymphocytes that elaborate a helper factor. The T-lymphocytes sensitized by the cancer cell antigen elaborate factors that immobilize macrophages and stimulate it to process antigen which is fed to more T-lymphocytes; these are then also sensitized. After proliferation the T-lymphocytes become cytotoxic for the cancer cell. The possibility that macrophages can directly be activated by the tumor antigen and attack the tumor cells has not been excluded.

In spite of this multicellular response, tumor growth is not arrested because of either mutations in the cancer cells, formation of blocking antibodies or release of tumor antigens which complex with T-lymphocytes and thereby prevent their attack on tumor cells.

General Conclusions

Cancer results from the proliferation of a population of cells that have acquired survival advantages over other cells and replace them through invasion or metastasis. The survival advantages derive from a reprogramming of gene expression, and these advantages are transferred from one generation of cells to the next.

The central questions in cancer are: what causes the distortion, and what pattern of distortion is essential to carcinogenesis? Because the alteration is transmitted from one generation of cells to the next, it seems that at least some stage of carcinogenesis must involve a permanent alteration of the genome (somatic mutation*). Although a permanent alteration brought about by environmental changes that cause injury outside of the genome—for example, at the cell membrane—cannot be excluded, the mode of action of known carcinogens strongly suggests a direct insult to the genome. Viruses, chemical carcinogens, ionizing radiation, and UV light all alter DNA: the DNA viruses by direct incorporation of the genome into the DNA, the RNA viruses by transcription of the RNA into DNA complementary strands that are incorporated in the genome; the carcinogens by binding to DNA, UV radiation by causing the formation of thymine dimers; X-irradiation by causing strand breaks, cross-links, and base alteration.

* However, it cannot be excluded that recent mutations in the germ cell under the influence of environmental factors are transmitted to the offspring where they are responsible for the appearance of a "neo-oncogene," which is normally repressed and becomes derepressed under the influence of carcinogens later in life. The difference between such a concept and the classical oncogene hypothesis is that the acquisition of the oncogene is not ancestral but recent. Therefore, one would not expect the "neo-oncogene" to be present in the entire mammalian population, and one can predict that the incidence of cancer would be greater in some families.

If we can accept that the distortion of gene expression observed in cancer is caused by primary alteration of the genome, we must also ask whether the alteration of the genome is the same for all cancers? One oncogenic hypothesis (that of the oncogene) proposes that the mutation is ancestral and is revealed by derepression, and that other known carcinogens (radiation and chemicals) act as derepressors.

It has also been proposed that the mutation is acquired in the somatic cells as a result of incorporation of the viral genome or alterations of DNA by chemicals or radiation. The discovery of DNA repair has introduced a new parameter in our understanding of chemical and radiation carcinogenesis. If the only function of repair with respect to carcinogenesis is to prevent cancer, those factors that restrict repair (availability of the enzyme, susceptibility of the substrate, etc.) must be critical to carcinogenesis. Also, repair itself could cause the DNA alteration through mispairing of bases.

Whatever the role of DNA repair may be, a comprehensive understanding of chemical and radiation carcinogenesis will require that the specifics of DNA repair be known.

In the oncogene hypothesis, the virus plays a critical role in carcinogenesis in the cooperation between virus and carcinogens, but one could also conceive of a model of carcinogenesis in which the chemical or radiation plays the principal role. For example, these agents cause breaks in the DNA strands, and this might facilitate viral integration.

In our discussion of cancer, we have presented each hypothesis on carcinogenesis separately, as if only one pathogenic mechanism exists. However, there is no reason to assume that all cancers are produced in the same way. Moreover, the versatility of pathogenic mechanisms for other diseases makes it difficult to resist the temptation of favoring a pluralistic theory for the triggering of carcinogenesis.

Assuming that the primary injury in cancer is in DNA, and assuming that it proves impossible to correct the primary injury, the distortion of gene expression that follows could be interrupted or reversed, and, therefore, cancer could be cured or prevented. Consequently, an accurate understanding of the sequence of macromolecular alterations that occur in carcinogenesis is important. The morphology and the enzyme mosaic of florid cancer seem to vary infinitely, suggesting that a distortion in gene expression is random. However, some cancers resemble closely the tissues from which they develop, and experimentally it has been possible to produce hepatomas with morphological features almost identical to those of normal liver (minimal deviation hepatomas). This suggests that when it occurs, randomization of gene expression is a late consequence of carcinogenesis rather than an early event.

The study of the biochemistry of minimal deviation hepatomas has yielded some clues as to the early events in carcinogenesis, including the development of isozymes, interference with enzyme induction, and development of new antigens. Enzymes often are not induced in the fetus. The hepatomas switch from one pattern of isozymes typical for the differentiated cells to that found in the fetal cell, and the antigenic properties result from the appearance in the adult of proteins that were present in the fetus. Thus, at some stage of the conversion of the normal cell into a cancer cell, the pattern of gene expression is switched from that which had evolved in the adult to that which exists in the fetal cell. Whether this switch constitutes the minimal deviation in gene expression associated with carcinogenesis is not certain. Neither is it known whether it results from earlier reversible changes—for example, changes in the structure of the cell membrane.

References

1. Slye, M.: The inheritance behavior of cancer as a simple Mendelian recessive. Studies in the nature and inheritability of spontaneous cancer in mice. J. Cancer Res. **10**, 15–49 (1926)
2. Lynch, C.J.: Studies on relation between tumor susceptibility and heredity; influence of heredity upon incidence of lung tumors in mice. J. exp. Med. **54**, 747–760 (1931)
3. Bittner, J.J.: The breeding behavior and tumor incidence of inbred Albino strain of mice. Amer. J. Cancer **25**, 113–121 (1935)
4. Strong, L.C.: Genetic analysis of induction of tumors by methylcholanthrene; absence of the sex influence when a large dose of the carcinogen is administered. Arch. Path. **36**, 58–63 (1943)
5. Strong, L.C.: Genetic analysis of induction of tumors by methylcholanthrene; induced and spontaneous adenocarcinomas of stomach in mice. J. nat. Cancer Inst. **5**, 339–362 (1945)
6. Falconer, D.S., Bloom, J.L.: A genetic study of induced lung-tumours in mice. Brit. J. Cancer **16**, 665–685 (1962)
7. Gardner, E.J., Stephens, F.E.: Cancer of the lower digestive tract in one family group. Amer. J. hum. Genet. **2**, 41–48 (1950)
8. Papadrianos, E., Haagensen, C.D., Cooley, E.: Cancer of the breast as a familial disease. Ann. Surg. **165**, 10–19 (1967)
9. Lynch, H.T., Krush, A.J., Larsen, A.L.: Heredity and multiple primary malignant neoplasms: six cancer families. Amer. J. med. Sci. **254**, 322–329 (1967)
10. Lynch, H.T., Shaw, M.W., Magnuson, C.W., Larsen, A.L., Krush, A.J.: Hereditary factors in cancer. Study of two large midwestern kindreds. Arch. intern Med. **117**, 206–212 (1966)
11. Krush, A.J., Lynch, H.T., Magnuson, C.: Attitudes toward cancer in a "cancer family": implications for cancer detection. Amer. J. med. Sci. **249**, 432–438 (1965)
12. Murphy, D.P., Abbey, H.: Cancer in families. Cambridge, Massachusetts: Cancer Commonwealth Fund 1959
13. Jacobsen, O.: Heredity in breast cancer. A genetic and clinical study of 200 probands [thesis; transl. by Robert Fraser]. Forlag, Copenhagen 1946
14. Kemp, T.: Heredity in human cancer. Brit. J. Cancer **2**, 144–149 (1948)
15. Macklin, M.T.: Comparison of the number of breast-cancer deaths observed in relatives of breast-cancer patients, and the number expected on the basis of morality rates. J. nat. Cancer Inst. **22**, 927–951 (1959)
16. Clemmesen, J.: Statistical studies in the aetiology of malignant neoplasms, vol. 1. Copenhagen: Munksgaard 1965
17. Nowell, P.C., Hungerford, D.A.: The etiology of leukemia: Some comments on current studies. Semin. Hemat. **3**, 114–121 (1966)
18. Nowell, P.C., Hungerford, D.A.: Chromosome changes in human leukemia and a tentative assessment of their significance. Ann. N.Y. Acad. Sci. **113**, 654–662 (1964)
19. Nowell, P.C.: Prognostic value of marrow chromosome studies in human "preleukemia." Arch. Path. **80**, 205–208 (1965)
20. Wegelius, R., Väänänen, I., Koskela, S.L.: Down's syndrome and transient leukaemia-like disease in a newborn. Acta paediat. scand. **56**, 301–306 (1967)
21. Nichols, W.W.: Relationships of viruses, chromosomes, and carcinogenesis, Hereditas (Lund) **50**, 53–80 (1963)
22. Nichols, W.W., Levan, A., Coriell, L.L., Goldner, H., Ahlstroem, C.G.: Chromosome abnormalities *in vitro* in human leukocytes associated with Schmidt-Ruppin Rous sarcoma virus. Science **146**, 248–250 (1964)
23. Miles, C.P., O'Neill, F.: Chromosomes of some heterotransplanted human tumors. II. H.Ep. #1, H.Ep. #3, and H.Ep. #5. J. nat. Cancer Inst. **35**, 435–458 (1965)

24. Makino, S., Sasaki, M.S., Tonomura, A.: Cytological studies of tumors. XL. Chromosome studies in fifty-two human tumors. J. nat. Cancer Inst. **32**, 741–777 (1964)
25. Koller, P.C.: Chromosome behavior in tumors: readjustments to Boveri's theory. In: Cell physiology of neoplasia. 14th Annu. Symp., Fund. Cancer Res., p. 9–48. Austin, Texas: University of Texas Press (1960)
26. Bicknell, J.M.: Chromosome studies of human brain tumors. Neurology (Minneap.) **17**, 485–490 (1967)
27. Lacassagne, A.: Apparition de cancers de la mamelle chez la souris mâle, soumise à des injections de folliculine. C.R. Acad. Sci. (Paris) **195**, 630–632 (1932)
28. Lacassagne, A.: Modifications progressives de l'utérus de la souris sous l'action prolongée de l'oestrone. C.R. Soc. Biol. (Paris) **120**, 1156–1158 (1935)
29. Lacassagne, A.: Les rapports entre les hormones sexuelles et la formation du cancer. Ergeb. Vit.- u. Horm.-Forsch. **2**, 259–296 (1939)
30. Loeb, L., Kirtz, M.M.: The effects of transplants of anterior lobes of the hypophysis on the growth of the mammary gland and on development of mammary gland carcinoma in various strains of mice. Amer. J. Cancer **36**, 56–82 (1939)
31. Spencer, J.G.C.: The influence of the thyroid in malignant disease. Brit. J. Cancer **8**, 393–411 (1954)
32. Sommers, S.C.: Endocrine abnormalities in women with breast cancer. Lab. Invest. **4**, 160–174 (1955)
33. Taylor, H.C., Jr.: Evidence for endocrine factor in etiology of mammary tumors. Amer. J. Cancer **27**, 525–541 (1936)
34. Olch, I.Y.: Menopausal age in women with cancer of the breast. Amer. J. Cancer **30**, 563–566 (1937)
35. Geschickter, C.F.: Diseases of the breast. Philadelphia: J.B. Lippincott Co. 1943
36. Oliver, C.P.: Genetic factors in breast cancer. In: 5th National Cancer Conference Proc., p. 133–142. Philadelphia: J.B. Lippincott Co. 1964
37. Gardner, W.U., Smith, G.M., Allen, E., Strong, L.C.: Cancer of mammary glands induced in male mice receiving estrogenic hormone. Arch. Path. **21**, 265–272 (1936)
38. Gardner, W.U.: Testicular tumors in mice of several strains receiving triphenylethylene. Cancer Res. **3**, 92–99 (1943)
39. Lombard, H.L., Potter, E.A.: Epidemiological aspects of cancer of the cervix. II. Hereditary and environmental factors. Cancer (Philad.) **3**, 960–968 (1950)
40. Pratt-Thomas, H.R., Dennis, E.J., Williamson, H.O., Brown, R.R.: Research on the relation of smegma to cervical cancer. In: 4th Nat. Cancer Conf. Proc., p. 337–341. Philadelphia: J.B. Lippincott Co. 1961
41. Rothman, A., Rapoport, L.P., Davidsohn, I.: Carcinoma of the cervix in Jewish women. Amer. J. Obstet. Gynec. **62**, 160–162 (1951)
42. Weiner, I., Burke, L., Goldberger, M.A.: Carcinoma of the cervix in Jewish women. Amer. J. Obstet. Gynec. **61**, 418–422 (1951)
43. Lipschütz, A.: Hyperplasie expérimentale de l'endomètre avec prolifération atypique de l'épithèle utérin après des interventions ovariennes. Gynéc. et Obstét. **36**, 408–426 (1937)
44. Schmidt, I.G.: Influence of normal ovary on formation of typical irradiation tissues in X-rayed ovary. Anat. Rec. **71**, 406–412 (1938)
45. Ayre, J.E., Bauld, W.A.G.: Thiamine deficiency and high estrogen findings in uterine cancer and in menorrhagia. Science **103**, 441–445 (1946)
46. McKay, D.G.: A review of the status of endometrial cancer. Cancer Res. **25**, 1182–1187 (1965)
47. Hertz, R.: Hormonal relationships of the endometrium in animals. Cancer Res. **25**, 1188–1189 (1965)
48. Kelley, R.M., Baker, W.H.: The role of progesterone in human endometrial cancer. Cancer Res. **25**, 1190–1192 (1965)
49. Li, M.H., Gardner, W.U.: Granulosa cell tumors in intrapancreatic ovarian grafts in castrated mice. Science **106**, 270 (1947)
50. Biskind, G.R., Biskind, M.S.: Atrophy of ovaries transplanted to the spleen in unilaterally castrated rats; proliferative changes following subsequent removal of intact ovary. Science **108**, 137–138 (1948)
51. Biskind, G.R., Biskind, M.S.: Experimental ovarian tumors in rats. Amer. J. clin. Path. **19**, 501–521 (1949)
52. Van Lancker, J., Maisin, J.: Le sort des greffes intraspleniques d'ovaires et de testicules. Unio Internat. Contra Cancrum Acta **7**, 354-359 (1951)
53. Furth, J., Butterworth, J.S.: Neoplastic diseases occurring among mice subjected to general irradiation with X-rays; ovarian tumors and associated lesions. Amer. J. Cancer **28**, 66–95 (1936)
54. Furth, J., Boon, M.C.: Induction of ovarian tumors in mice by X-rays. Cancer Res. **7**, 241–245 (1947)
55. Furth, J.: Relation of pregnancies to induction of ovarian tumors by X-rays. Proc. Soc. exp. Biol. (N.Y.) **71**, 274–277 (1949)
56. Furth, J.: Discussion of problems related to hormonal factors in initiating and maintaining tumor growth. Cancer Res. **17**, 454–463 (1957)
57. Furth, J., Kim, U., Clifton, K.H.: On evolution of the neoplastic state; progression from dependence to autonomy. Nat. Cancer Inst. Monogr. **2**, 149–177 (1960)
58. Clifton, K.H.: Problems in experimental tumorigenesis of the pituitary gland, gonads, adrenal cortices, and mammary glands: a review. Cancer Res. **19**, 2–22 (1959)
59. Huggins, C.: Control of cancers of man by endocrinologic methods. Cancer Res. **17**, 467–472 (1957)
60. Huggins, C.: Endocrine-induced regression of cancers. Science **156**, 1050–1054 (1967)
61. Huseby, R.A., Dominguez, O.V., Samuels, L.T.: Function of normal and abnormal testicular interstitial cells in the mouse. Recent Prog. Hormone Res. **17**, 1–51 (1961)
62. Uchikawa, T., Huseby, R.A., Zain-ul-Abedin, M., Samuels, L.T.: Changes in testicular DNA produced in BALB/c mice by diethylstilbestrol. J. nat. Cancer Inst. **45**, 525–533 (1970)
63. Kiyoshi, K., Huseby, R.A., Baldi, A., Samuels, L.T.: Effects of diethylstilbestrol on hybridizability of mouse testicular RNA. Cancer Res. **33**, 1247–1252 (1973)
64. Samuels, L.T., Matsumoto, K., Samuels, B.K.: Localization of enzymes involved in testosterone biosynthesis by the mouse testis. Endocrinology **94**, 55–60 (1974)
65. Folkman, J.: Transplacental carcinogenesis by stilbestrol. New Engl. J. Med. **285**, 404–405 (1971)
66. Greenwald, P., Barlow, J.J., Nasca, P.C., Burnett, W.S.: Vaginal cancer after maternal treatment with synthetic estrogens. New Engl. J. Med. **285**, 390–392 (1971)
67. Sweat, M.L., Berliner, D.L., Bryson, M.J., Nabors, C., Jr., Haskell, J., Holmstrom, E.G.: The synthesis and metabolism of progesterone in the human and bovine ovary. Biochim. biophys. Acta (Amst.) **40**, 289–296 (1960)
68. Sweat, M.L.: Metabolism of steroid hormones in human proliferative endometrium and myometrium. Fed. Proc. **24**, 384 (1965) (Intersociety Sessions, Abstracts)
69. Beatson, G.T.: On the treatment of inoperable cases of carcinoma of the mamma; suggestions for a new method of treatment, with illustrative cases. Lancet **1896II**, 104–107, 162–165
70. Beatson, G.T.: The treatment of inoperable carcinoma of the female mamma. Glasgow med. J. **76**, 81–87 (1911)
71. Huggins, C.: The adrenal component in mammary cancer. Int. Union Against Cancer **10**, 67–69 (1954)
72. Huggins, C.: Endocrine methods of treatment of cancer of the breast. J. nat. Cancer Inst. **15**, 1–25 (1954)
73. Huggins, C., Bergenstal, D.M.: Inhibition of human mammary and prostatic cancers by adrenalectomy. Cancer Res. **12**, 134–141 (1952)
74. Huggins, C.A.: Two principles in endocrine therapy of cancers: hormone-deprival and hormone-interference. Cancer Res. **25**, 1163–1167 (1965)
75. Bulbrook, R.D., Greenwood, F.C., Hayward, J.L.: Selection of breast-cancer patients for adrenalectomy or hypophysectomy by determination of urinary 17-hydroxycorticosteroids and aeticholanolone. Lancet **1960I**, 1154–1157
76. Hayward, J.L., Bulbrook, R.D., Greenwood, F.C.: Hormone assays and prognosis in breast cancer. Mem. Soc. Endocrinol. **10**, 144–149 (1961)
77. Atkins, H.: A preoperative assessment of response to the operations of adrenalectomy and hypohphysectomy. Unio Internat. Contra Cancrum Acta **18**, 885–889 (1962)
78. Dao, T.L.: Studies on mechanism of carcinogenesis in the mammary gland. Progr. exp. Tumor Res. (Basel) **11**, 235–261 (1969)
79. Nissen-Meyer, R., Sanner, T.: The excretion of oestrone, pregnanediol and pregnanetriol in breast-cancer patients. I. Excretion after spontaneous menopause. Acta endocr. (Kbh.) **44**, 325–333 (1963)
80. Gallagher, T.F.: Summary of informal discussion on steroid hormone concentrations and tumor responses. Cancer Res. **25**, 1140–1145 (1965)
81. Stern, E., Hopkins, C.E., Weiner, J.M., Marmorston, J.: Hormone excretion patterns in breast and prostate cancer are abnormal. Science **145**, 716–719 (1964)
82. Kim, U.: Pituitary function and hormonal therapy of experimental breast cancer. Cancer Res. **25**, 1146–1161 (1965)
83. Pott, P.: The chirurgical works of Percivall Pott, F.R.S., and Surgeon to St. Bartholemew's Hospital, Hawes, W. Clarke, and R. Collins, London 1775
84. Yamagiwa, K., Ichikawa, K.: Experimental study of the pathogenesis of carcinoma. J. Cancer Res. **3**, 1–21 (1918)
85. Mayneord, W.V., Roe, E.: Fluorescence spectrum of 1:2-benzpyrene. Biochem. J. **30**, 707–708 (1936)
86. Kennaway, E.L., Hieger, I.: Carcinogenic substances and their fluorescence spectra. Brit. med. J. **1930I**, 1044–1046
87. Pullman, A., Pullman, B.: Cancérisation par les Substances Chimiques et Structure Moléculaire. Paris: Masson 1955
88. Pullman, B., Pullman, A.: Quantum biochemistry. New York: Interscience Publishers 1963
89. Boyland, E.: Some aspects of the mechanism of carcinogenesis. In: International Symposium on the Electronic Aspects of Biochemistry (Pullman, B., ed.), p. 155–165. New York: Academic Press 1964
90. Pullman, A.: The description of molecules by the method of molecular orbitals. In: Molecular biophysics (Pullman, B., and Weissbluth, M., eds.), p. 81–115. New York: Academic Press 1965
91. Heidelberger, C.: The relation of protein binding to hydrocarbon carcinogenesis. In: Ciba Symposium on Carcinogenesis: Mechanisms of Action (Wolstenholme, G., and O'Connor, M., eds.), p. 179–196, London: I. & A. Churchill, Ltd. 1959
92. Weil-Malherbe, H.: The solubilization of polycylic aromatic hydrocarbons by purines. Biochem. J. **40**, 351–363 (1946)
93. De Dantis, F., Giglio, E., Liquori, A.M., Ripamonti, A.: Crystallography: Molecular geometry of a 1:1 crystalline complex between 1,3,

7,9-tetramethyluric acid and pyrene. Nature (Lond.) **191**, 900–901 (1961)

94. Boyland, E., Green, B.: The interaction of polycyclic hydrocarbons and nucleic acids. Brit. J. Cancer **16**, 507–517 (1962)
95. Brookes, P., Heidelberger, C.: Isolation and degradation of DNA from cells treated with tritium-labeled 7, 12-dimethylbenz(a)anthracene: studies on nature of binding of this carcinogen to DNA. Cancer Res. **29**, 157–165 (1969)
96. Brookes, P., Lawley, P.D.: Evidence for the binding of polynuclear aromatic hydrocyrbons to the nucleic acids of mouse skin: relation between carcinogenic power of hydrocarbons and their binding to deoxyribonucleic acid. Nature (Lond.) **202**, 781–784 (1964)
97. Harvey, R.G., Halonen, M.: Interaction between carcinogenic hydrocarbons and nucleosides. Cancer Res. **28**, 2183–2186 (1968)
98. Hennings, H., Boutwell, R.K.: The inhibition of DNA synthesis by initiators of mouse skin tumorigenesis. Cancer Res. **29**, 510–514 (1969).
99. Gelboin, H.V., Kinoshita, N., Wiebel, F.J.: Microsomal hydroxylases: induction and role in polycyclic hydrocarbon carcinogenesis and toxicity. Fed. Proc. **31**, 1298–1309 (1972)
100. Gielen, J.E., Nebert, D.W.: Microsomal hydroxylase induction in liver cell culture by phenobarbital, polycyclic hydrocarbons, and p,p′-DDT. Science **172**, 167–169 (1971)
101. Lu, A.Y.H., Levin, W., West, S.B., Jacobson, M., Ryan, D., Kuntzman, R., Conney, A.H.: Liver microsomal enzyme system that hydroxylates drugs, other foreign compounds and endogenous substrates. VI. Different substrate specificities of the cytochrome P-450 fractions from control and phenobarbital-treated rats. J. biol. Chem. **248**, 456–460 (1973)
102. Sweeney, G.D., Rothwell, J.D.: Spectroscopic evidence of interaction between 2-allyl-2-isopropylacetamide and cytochrome P-450 of rat liver microsomes. Biochem. biophys. Res. Commun. **55**, 798–804 (1973)
103. Yoshida, T.: Development of experimental hepatoma by the use of Q-aminoazotoluene with particular reference to gradual changes in the liver up to the time of development of carcinoma. Jap. path. Soc. Trans. **24**, 523–530 (1934)
104. Doniach, I., Mottram, J.C.: On the effect of light upon the incidence of tumours in painted mice. Amer. J. Cancer **39**, 234–240 (1940)
105. Miller, E.C.: Studies on the formation of protein-bound derivatives of 3,4-benzpyrene in the epidermal fraction of mouse skin. Cancer Res. **11**, 100–108 (1951)
106. Miller, E.C., Miller, J.A.: Symposium on immunogenetics and carcinogenesis; *in vivo* combinations between carcinogens and tissue constituents and their possible role in carcinogenesis. Cancer Res. **12**, 547–556 (1952)
107. Miller, J.A., Miller, E.C., Finger, G.C.: On the enhancement of the carcinogenicity of 4-dimethylaminoazobenzene by fluorosubstitution. Cancer Res. **13**, 93–97 (1953)
108. Miller, E.C., Miller, J.A.: Biochemistry of carcinogenesis. Annu. Rev. Biochem. **28**, 291–320 (1959)
109. Heidelberger, C., Weiss, S.M.: The distribution of radioactivity in mice following administration of 3,4-benzpyrene-5-C^{14} and 1,2,5,6-dibenzanthracene-9,10-C^{14}. Cancer Res. **11**, 885–891 (1951)
110. Heidelberger, C., Rieke, H.S.: The synthesis of 3,4-benzpyrene-5-C^{14} and of 2-acetylaminofluorene-9-C^{14}. Cancer Res. **11**, 640–643 (1951)
111. Heidelberger, C.: Studies on the mechanism of hydrocarbon carcinogenesis. Unio Internat. Contra Cancrum Acta **15**, 107–113 (1959)
112. Price, J.M., Miller, E.C., Miller, J.A., Weber, G.M.: Studies on the intracellular composition of livers from rats fed various aminoazo dyes; 4-aminoazobenzene, 4-dimethylaminoazobenzene, 4′-methyl-, and 3′-methyl-4-dimethylaminoazobenzene. Cancer Res. **9**, 398–402 (1949)
113. Price, J.M., Miller, E.C., Miller, J.A., Weber, G.M.: Studies on the intracellular composition of livers from rats fed various aminoazo dyes. II. 3′-methyl-2′-methyl- and 2-methyl-4-dimethylamino-azobenzene, 3′-methyl-4-monomethylaminoazobenzene and 4′-fluoro-4-dimethylaminoazobenzene. Cancer Res. **10**, 18–27 (1950)
114. Price, J.M., Harman, J.W., Miller, E.C., Miller, J.A.: Progressive microscopic alterations in the livers of rats fed the hepatic carcinogens 3′-methyl-4-dimethylaminoazobenzene and 4′-fluoro-4-dimethylaminoazobenzene. Cancer Res. **12**, 192–200 (1952)
115. Murray, R.K., Khairallah, L., Ragland, W., Pitot, H.C.: The biochemical morphology and morphogenesis of hepatomas. Int. Rev. exp. Path. **6**, 229–283 (1968)
116. Burns, D.M., Iball, J.: Molecular structure of fluorene. Nature (Lond.) **173**, 635 (1954)
117. Miller, E.C., Miller, J.A., Sandin, R.B., Brown, R.K.: The carcinogenic activities of certain analogues of 2-acetylaminofluorene in the rat. Cancer Res. **9**, 504–509 (1949)
118. Miller, J.A., Cramer, J.W., Miller, E.C.: The N- and ring-hydroxylation of 2-acetylaminofluorene during carcinogenesis in the rat. Cancer Res. **20**, 950–962 (1960)
119. Miller, E.C., Miller, J.A., Hartmann, H.A.: N-Hydroxy-2-acetylaminofluorene: A metabolite of 2-acetylaminofluorene with increased carcinogenic activity in the rat. Cancer Res. **21**, 815–824 (1961)
120. Miller, E.C., Miller, J.A., Enomoto, M.: The comparative carcinogenicities of 2-acetylaminofluorene and its N-hydroxy metabolite in mice, hamsters, and guinea pigs. Cancer Res. **24**, 2018–2032 (1964)
121. Pauling, L.: The nature of the chemical bond and the structure of molecules and crystals, 2nd ed. Ithaca, New York: Cornell Univ. Press 1948
122. Wheland, G.W.: The theory of resonance and its application to organic chemistry. New York: Wiley 1944
123. Weisburger, E.K., Weisburger, J.H.: Chemistry, carcinogenicity, and metabolism of 2-fluorenamine and related compounds. Advanc. Cancer Res. **5**, 331–431 (1958)
124. Ray, F.E., Geiser, C.R.: 2-Acetylamino-9-C^{14}-fluorene. Science **109**, 200 (1949)
125. Ray, F.E., Geiser, C.R.: Synthesis of 2-acetylaminofluorene-9-C^{14} and 2-acetylaminofluorene-ω-C^{14}. Cancer Res. **10**, 616–619 (1950)
126. Bielschowsky, F.: A metabolite of 2-acetamidofluorene. Biochem. J. **39**, 287–289 (1945)
127. Weisburger, J.H., Weisburger, E.K., Morris, H.P.: Urinary metabolites of carcinogen N-2-fluorenylacetamide. J. nat. Cancer Inst. **17**, 345–361 (1956)
128. Weisburger, J.H., Weisburger, E.K., Morris, H.P., Sober, H.: Chromatographic separation of some metabolites of carcinogen N-2-fluorenylacetamide. J. nat. Cancer Inst. **17**, 363–374 (1956)
129. Poirier, M.M., Miller, J.A., Miller, E.C.: The carcinogenic activities of N-hydroxy-2-acetylaminofluorene and its metal chelates as a function of retention at the injection site. Cancer Res. **25**, 527–533 (1965)
130. Teebor, G.W., Becker, F.F.: Regression and persistence of hyperplastic hepatic nodules induced by N-2-fluorenylacetamide and their relationship to hepatocarcinogenesis. Cancer Res. **31**, 1–3 (1971)
131. Epstein, S., Ito, N., Merkow, L., Farber, E.: Cellular analysis of liver carcinogenesis: the induction of large hyperplastic nodules in the liver with 2-fluorenylacetamide or ethionine and some aspects of their morphology and glycogen metabolism. Cancer Res. **27**, 1702–1711 (1967)
132. Reuber, M.D.: Development of preneoplastic and neoplastic lesions of the liver in male rats given 0.025 percent N-2-fluorenyldiacetamide. J. nat. Cancer Inst. **34**, 697–723 (1965)
133. Newberne, P.M., Butler, W.H.: Acute and chronic effects of aflatoxin on the liver of domestic and laboratory animals: A review. Cancer Res. **29**, 236–250 (1969)
134. Butler, W.H., Greenblatt, M., Lijinsky, W.: Carcinogenesis in rats by aflatoxins B_1, G_1, and B_2. Cancer Res. **29**, 2206–2211 (1969)
135. Epstein, S.M., Bartus, B., Farber, E.: Renal epithelial neoplasms induced in male Wistar rats by oral aflatoxin B_1. Cancer Res. **29**, 1045–1050 (1969)
136. Klein, G., Sjogren, H.O., Klein, E.: Demonstration of host resistance against sarcomas induced by implantation of cellophane films in isologous (syngeneic) recipients. Cancer Res. **23**, 84–92 (1963)
137. Oppenheimer, E.T., Willhite, M., Stout, A.P., Danishefsky, I., Fishman, M.M.: A comparative study of the effects of imbedding cellophane and polystyrene films in rats. Cancer Res. **24**, 379–387 (1964)
138. Zajdela, F.: Production de sarcomes sous-cutanés chez le rat au moyen de membranes cellulosiques de porosité connue. Bull. Cancer **53**, 401–408 (1966)
139. Hueper, W.C.: Cancer induction by polyurethane and polysilicone plastics. J. nat. Cancer Inst. **33**, 1005–1027 (1964)
140. Brand, K.G.: Induction of neoplasms by plastic implants. Bull. Path. **9**, 209 (1968)
141. Alexander, P., Horning, E.S.: Observations on the Oppenheimer method of inducing tumours by subcutaneous implantation of plastic films. In: Ciba Foundation Symposium on Carcinogenesis, Mechanisms of Action (Wolstenholme, G., and O'Connor, M., eds.), p. 12–25. 1959 London: J. & A. Churchill, Ltd.
142. Miller, J.A., Miller, E.C.: The metabolic activation of carcinogenic aromatic amines and amides. In: Progress in experimental tumor research (Homburger, F., ed.), vol. 11, p. 273–301. Int. Symp. on Carcinogenesis and Carcinogen Testing. Basel: S. Karger 1969
143. Scribner, J.D., Miller, J.A., Miller, E.C.: Nucleophilic substitution on carcinogenic N-acetoxy-n-arylacetamides. Cancer Res. **30**, 1570–1579 (1970)
144. Miller, J.A.: Carcinogenesis by chemicals: An overview—G.H.A. Clowes Memorial Lecture. Cancer Res. **30**, 559–576 (1970)
145. DeBaun, J.R., Miller, E.C., Miller, J.A.: N-hydroxy-2-acetylaminofluorene sulfotransferase: Its probable role in carcinogenesis and in protein-(methion-S-yl) binding in rat liver. Cancer Res. **30**, 577–595 (1970)
146. Baird, W.M., Dipple, A., Grover, P.L., Sims, P., Brookes, P.: Studies on the formation of hydrocarbon-deoxyribonucleoside products by the binding of derivatives of 7-methylbenz[a]anthracene to DNA in aqueous solution and in mouse embryo cells in culture. Cancer Res. **33**, 2386–2392 (1973)
147. Wang, I.Y., Rasmussen, R.E., Crocker, T.T.: Isolation and characterization of an active DNA-binding metabolite of benzo(a)pyrene from hamster liver microsomal incubation systems. Biochem. biophys. Res. Commun. **49**, 1142–1149 (1972)
148. Ames, B.N., Sims, P., Grover, P.L.: Epoxides of carcinogenic polycylic hydrocarbons are frameshift mutagens. Science **176**, 47–49 (1972)
149. Huberman, E., Kuroki, T., Marquardt, H., Selkirk, J.K., Heidelberger, C., Grover, P.L., Sims, P.: Transformation of hamster embryo cells by epoxides and other derivatives of polycyclic hydrocarbons. Cancer Res. **32**, 1391–1396 (1972)
150. Lesko, S.A., Jr., Smith, A., Ts'o, P.D.P., Umans R.S.: Interaction of nucleic acids. IV. The physical binding of 3,4-benzpyrene to nucleosides, nucleotides, nucleic acids, and nucleoprotein. Biochemistry **7**, 434–447 (1968)

151. Zeiger, R.S., Salomon, R., Kinoshita, N., Peacock, A.C.: The binding of 9,10-dimethyl-1,2-benzanthracene to mouse epidermal satellite DNA *in vivo*. Cancer Res. **32**, 643–647 (1972)
152. Toft, D.O., Spelsberg, T.C.: A distinction between 3-methylcholanthrene and estrogen binding in the uterus. Cancer Res. **32**, 2743–2746 (1972)
153. Singer, S., Litwack, G.: Identity of corticosteroid binder I with the macromolecule binding 3-methylcholanthrene in liver cytosol *in vivo*. Cancer Res. **31**, 1364–1368 (1971)
154. Cole, P., Monson, R.R., Haning, H., Friedell, G.H.: Smoking and cancer of the lower urinary tract. New Engl. J. Med. **284**, 129–134 (1971)
155. Friedewald, W.F., Rous, P.: The pathogenesis of deferred cancer; a study of the after-effects of methylcholanthrene upon rabbit skin. J. exp. Med. **91**, 459–484 (1950)
156. Berenblum, I.: The two-stage mechanism of carcinogenesis as an analytical tool. In: Cellular control mechanisms and cancer (Emmelot, P., and Mühlbock, O., eds.), p. 259–267. Amsterdam: Elsevier 1964
157. Berenblum, I., Shubik, P.: Role of croton oil applications, associated with single painting of a carcinogen, in tumour induction of the mouse's skin. Brit. J. Cancer **1**, 379–382 (1947)
158. Berenblum, I.: The possible role of a "transmissable factor" in leukemia induction by radiation plus urethan. In: Viruses, nucleic acids, and cancer. Proc. 17th Annu. Symp. Fund. Cancer Res., p. 529–543. Baltimore: Williams & Wilkins 1963
159. Van Duuren, B.L.: Tumor-promoting agents in two-stage carcinogenesis. Progr. exp. Tumor Res. **11**, 31–68 (1969)
160. Sivak, A., Van Duuren, B.L.: RNA synthesis induction in cell culture by a tumor promoter. Cancer Res. **30**, 1203–1205 (1970)
161. Paul, D.: Effects of carcinogenic, noncarcinogenic, and cocarcinogenic agents on the biosynthesis of nucleic acids in mouse skin. Cancer Res. **29**, 1218–1225 (1969)
162. Baird, W.M., Sedgwick, J.A., Boutwell, R.K.: Effect of phorbol and four diesters of phorbol on the incorporation of tritiated precursors into DNA, RNA, and protein in mouse epidermis. Cancer Res. **31**, 1434–1439 (1971)
163. Ambrose, E.J., Easty, D.M., Wylie, J.A.H.: The cancer cell *in vitro*. London: Butterworths 1967
164. Heidelberger, C.: Current trends in chemical carcinogenesis. Fed. Proc. **32**, 2154–2161 (1973)
165. Weinhouse, S.: Metabolism and isozyme alterations in experimental hepatomas. Fed. Proc. **32**, 2162–2167 (1973)
166. Prehn, R.T.: A clonal selection theory of chemical carcinogenesis. J. nat. Cancer Inst. **32**, 1–17 (1964)
167. DiPaolo, J.A., Donovan, P.J., Nelson, R.L.: Quantitative studies of *in vitro* transformation by chemical carcinogens. J. nat. Cancer Inst. **42**, 867–874 (1969)
168. Huberman, E., Donovan, P.J., DiPaolo, J.A.: Mutation and transformation of cultured mammalian cells by N-acetoxy-N 2-fluorenylacetamide. J. nat. Cancer Inst. **48**, 837–840 (1972)
169. Shimkin, M.B., Triolo, V.A.: History of chemical carcinogenesis: some prospective remarks. Progr. exp. Tumor Res. **11**, 1–20 (1969)
170. MacMahon, B.: Epidemiologic methods in cancer research. Yale J. Biol. Med. **37**, 508–522 (1965)
171. Truhaut, Rene (ed.): Potential carcinogenic hazards from drugs; evaluation of risks. Proc. Symp. U.I.C.C. Commission on Cancer Control. Berlin-Heidelberg-NewYork: Springer 1967
172. Henry, S.A., Kennaway, N.M., Kennaway, E.L.: The incidence of cancer of the bladder and prostate in certain occupations. J. Hyg. **31**, 125–137 (1931)
173. Redmond, D.E., Jr.: Tobacco and cancer: the first clinical report, 1761. New Engl. J. Med. **282**, 18–23 (1970)
174. Doll, R., Hill, A.B.: A study of the aetiology of carcinoma of the lung. Brit. med. J. **1952II**, 1271–1286
175. Doll, R., Hill, A.B.: Lung cancer and other causes of death in relation to smoking. A second report on the mortality of British doctors. Brit. med. J. **1956II**, 1071–1081
176. Auerbach, O.: The role of smoking in the development of lung cancer. In: Fifth National Cancer Conference Proceedings, p. 497–501. Philadelphia: J.B. Lippincott 1964
177. Enomoto, M., Saito, M.: Carcinogens produced by fungi. Annu. Rev. Microbiol. **26**, 279–312 (1972)
178. Fibiger, J.: The nematode [Spiroptera Sp. n.] and its capacity to develop papillomatous and carcinomatous tumors in the ventricle of the rat. Hosp.-Tid. (Kbh.) 5.R., **6**, 417, 469, 473, discuss. 441–448 (1913)
179. Borrel, A.: Parasitisme et tumeurs, Ann. Inst. Pasteur **24**, 778–788 (1910)
180. Bullock, F.D., Curtis, M.R.: Spontaneous tumors of the rat. J. Cancer Res. **14**, 1–115 (1930)
181. Rous, P.: An experimental comparison of transplanted tumor and a transplanted normal tissue capable of growth. J. exp. Med. **12**, 344–366 (1910)
182. Rous, P.: A transmissible avian neoplasm (sarcoma of the common fowl). J. exp. Med. **12**, 696–706 (1910)
183. Rous, P.: Transmission of a malignant new growth by means of a cell-free filtrate. J. Amer. med. Ass. **56**, 198 (1911)
184. Nakahara, W.: Survival of the cells of a chicken sarcoma through the process of desiccation or glycerination. Gann. **20**, 13–21 (1926)
185. Sanarelli, G.: Das myxomatogene virus: Beitrag zum Studium der Krankheitserreger außerhalb des Sichtbaren. [Vorlaufige Mitt.] Zbl. Bakt. **23**, 865–873 (1898)
186. Fujinami, A., Inamoto, K.: Über eine transplantable Hühnergeschwulst (II. Mitt.). Gann **5**, 13–15 (1914)
187. Fujinami, A., Inamoto, K.: Über Geschwülste bei japanischen Haushühnern, insbesonders über einen transplantablen Tumor. Z. Krebsforsch. **14**, 94–119 (1914)
188. Hankin, E.H.: La propagation de la peste. Ann. Inst. Pasteur **12**, 705–762 (1898)
189. Bruynoghe, R.: Manuel de bacteriologie. Louvain, Belgium: Librairie Universitaire 1949
190. Stanley, W.M., Valens, E.G.: Viruses and the nature of life. New York: E.P. Dutton 1961
191. Fraenkel-Conrat, H.: Infectious ribonucleic acid. Surv. Biol. Progr. **4**, 59–92 (1962)
192. Schramm, G., Engler, R.: The latent period after infection with tobacco mosaic virus and virus nucleic acid. Nature (Lond.) **181**, 916–917 (1958)
193. Sinsheimer, R.L.: Replication of the nucleic acids of the bacterial viruses. In: Viruses. Nucleic acids, and cancer. Proc. 17th Annu. Symp. Fund. Cancer Res., p. 246–251. Baltimore: Williams & Wilkins 1963
194. Kay, D.: A comparative study of the structures of a variety of bacteriophage particles with some observations on the mechanism of nucleic acid injection. In: Viruses, nucleic acids, and cancer. Proc. 17th Annu. Symp. Fund. Cancer Res., p. 7–26. Baltimore: Williams & Wilkins 1963
195. Caspar, D.L.D., Klug, A.: Structure and assembly of regular virus particles. In: Viruses, nucleic acids, and cancer. Proc. 17th Annu. Symp. Fund. Cancer Res., p. 27–39. Baltimore: Williams & Wilkins 1963
196. Horne, R.W.: Electron microscope studies on the structure and symmetry of virus particles. In: Viruses, nucleic acids, and cancer. Proc. 17th Annu. Symp. Fund. Cancer Res., p. 40–62. Baltimore: Williams & Wilkins 1963
197. Mayor, H.D.: Icosahedral viruses—a geometric approach to their maturation. In: Viruses, nucleic acids, and cancer. Proc. 17th Annu. Symp. Fund. Cancer Res., p. 63–67. Baltimore: Williams & Wilkins 1963
198. Caspar, D.L.D., Klug, A.: Physical principles in the construction of regular viruses. Symp. quant. Biol. **27**, 1–24 (1962)
199. Wildy, P., Watson, D.H.: Electron microscopic studies on the architecture of animal viruses. Symp. quant. Biol. **27**, 25–47 (1962)
200. Pirie, N.W.: Biological organization of viruses. In: Principles of biomolecular organization (Wolstenholme, G.E.W., and O'Connor, M., eds.). Proc. Ciba Symp., p. 136–157. London: J & A. Churchill Ltd. 1966
201. Klug, A., Durham, A.C.H.: The disk of TMV protein and its relation to the helical and other modes of aggregation. Symp. quant. Biol. **36**, 449–460 (1971)
202. Fraenkel-Conrat, H.: Reconstitution of viruses. Annu. Rev. Microbiol. **24**, 463–478 (1970)
203. Klug, A.: Assembly of tobacco mosaic virus. Fed. Proc. **31**, 30–42 (1972)
204. Eiserling, F.A., Dickson, R.C.: Assembly of viruses, Annu. Rev. Biochem. **41**, 467–502 (1972)
205. Kellenberger, E.: Control mechanisms in bacteriophage morphopoiesis. In: Principles of biomolecular organization (Wolstenholme, G.E.W. and O'Connor, M., eds.). Ciba Symp., p. 192–228. Boston: Little, Brown & Co. 1966
206. Yarmolinsky, M.B.: Influence of phages on the synthesis of host enzymes of bacteria. In: Viruses, nucleic acids, and cancer. Proc. 17th Annu. Symp. Fund. Cancer Res., p. 151–172. Baltimore: Williams & Wilkins 1963
207. Zinder, N.D.: The functions of the RNA of bacteriophage f2. In: Viruses, nucleic acids, and cancer. Proc. 17th Annu. Symp. Fund. Cancer Res., p. 173–179. Baltimore: Williams & Wilkins 1963
208. Roizman, B.: The programming of herpes virus multiplication in mammalian cells. In: Viruses, nucleic acids, and cancer. Proc. 17th Annu. Symp. Fund. Cancer Res., p. 205–223. Baltimore: Williams & Wilkins 1963
209. Kit, S.: Early changes following virus infection: thymidine kinase induction in cells infected with vaccinia and herpes simplex viruses. In: Viruses, nucleic acids, and cancer. Proc. 17th Annu. Symp. Fund. Cancer Res., p. 296. Baltimore: Williams & Wilkins 1963
210. Franklin, R.M., Baltimore, D.: Changes in RNA and protein synthesis in mammalian cells infected with a virulent virus. In: Viruses, nucleic acids, and cancer. Proc. 17th Annu. Symp. Fund. Cancer Res., p. 310–326. Baltimore: Williams & Wilkins 1963
211. Darnell, J.E., Jr.: Early events in poliovirus infection. Symp. quant. Biol. **27**, 149–158 (1962)
212. Attardi, G., Smith, J.: Virus specific protein and a ribonucleic acid associated with ribosomes in poliovirus infected HeLa cells. Symp. quant. Biol. **27**, 271–292 (1962)
213. Kerr, I.M., Martin, E.M., Hamilton, M.G., Work, T.S.: The initiation of virus protein synthesis in Krebs ascites tumor cells infected with EMC virus. Symp. quant. Biol. **27**, 259–269 (1962)
214. Bachtold, J.G., Bubel, H.C., Gebhardt, L.P.: The primary interaction of poliomyelitis virus with host cells of tissue culture origin. Virology **4**, 582–589 (1957)
215. Mandel, B.: Studies on the interactions of poliomyelitis virus, antibody, and host cells in a tissue culture system. Virology **6**, 424–447 (1958)

216. McLaren, L.C., Holland, J.J., Syverton, J.T.: The mammalian cell-virus relationship. I. Attachment of poliovirus to cultivated cells of primate and non-primate origin. J. exp. Med. **109**, 475–485 (1959)
217. Kunin, C.M.: Virus-tissue union and the pathogenesis of enterovirus infections. J. Immunol. **88**, 556–569 (1962)
218. Chanock, R.M., Johnson, K.M.: Infectious disease: respiratory viruses. Annu. Rev. Med. **12**, 1–18 (1961)
219. Godman, G.C.: The cytopathology of enteroviral infection. Int. Rev. exp. Path. **5**, 67–110 (1966)
220. Kunin, C.M.: Cellular susceptibility to enteroviruses. Bact. Rev. **28**, 382–390 (1964)
221. Smith, K.M.: The arthropod viruses. In: Viruses, nucleic acids, and cancer. Proc. 17th Annu. Symp. Fund. Cancer Res., p. 72–84. Baltimore: Williams & Wilkins 1963
222. Roizman, B.: Polykaryocytosis. Symp. quant. Biol. **27**, 327–342 (1962)
223. Hilleman, M.R.: Immunologic, chemotherapeutic and interferon approaches to control of viral disease. Amer. J. Med. **38**, 751–766 (1965)
224. Baluda, M.A.: Loss of viral receptors in homologous interference by ultraviolet-irradiated Newcastle disease virus. Virology **7**, 315–327 (1959)
225. Lindenmann, J., Burke, D.C., Isaacs, A.: Studies on the production, mode of action and properties of interferon. Brit. J. exp. Path. **38**, 551–562 (1957)
226. Isaacs, A.: Production and action of interferon. Symp. quant. Biol. **27**, 343–349 (1962)
227. Isaacs, A., Lindenmann, J.: Virus interference. I. The interferon. Proc. roy. Soc. B **147**, 258–267 (1957)
228. Wagner, R.R.: The interferons: cellular inhibitors of viral infection. Annu. Rev. Microbiol. **17**, 285–296 (1963)
229. Baron, S., Levy, H.B.: Interferon. Annu. Rev. Microbiol. **20**, 291–318 (1966)
230. Wagner, R.R., Smith, J.J.: The interferons: Some unsolved problems of action and biosynthesis. In: 1st Int. Conf. Vaccines Against Viral and Rickettsial Diseases of Man, p. 616. Washington, D.C.: Pan Amer. Health Org. 1967
231. Merigan, T.C.: Various molecular species of interferon induced by viral and nonviral agents. Bact. Rev. **31**, 138–144 (1967)
232. Lockart, R.Z., Jr.: Recent progress in research on interferons. Progr. med. Virol. **9**, 451–475 (1967)
233. Merigan, T.C., Jr.: Interferon and interferon inducers: the clinical outlook. Hosp. Prac. **4**, 42–49 (1969)
234. Merigan, T.C.: Interferons of mice and men. New Engl. J. Med. **276**, 913–920 (1967)
235. Friedman, R.M.: Interferon binding: the first step in establishment of antiviral activity. Science **156**, 1760–1761 (1967)
236. Kleinschmidt, W.J.: Biochemistry of interferon and its inducers. Annu. Rev. Biochem. **41**, 517–542 (1972)
237. Burnet, F.M.: The bacteriophages. Biol. Rev. **9**, 332–350 (1934)
238. Lwoff, A.: Interaction among virus, cell, and organism. Science **152**, 1216–1220 (1966)
239. Jacob, F., Wollman, E.L.: Genetic aspects of lysogeny. In: The Chemical basis of heredity (McElroy, W.D., and Glass, B., eds.), p. 468–500. Baltimore: John Hopkins Press 1957
240. Echols, H.: Lysogeny: viral repression and site-specific recombination. Annu. Rev. Biochem. **40**, 827–854 (1971)
241. Borek, E., Ryan, A.: Lysogenic induction. Prog. Nucleic Acids Res. Mol. Biol. **13**, 249–300 (1973)
242. Zabriskie, J.B.: Viral-induced bacterial toxins. Annu. Rev. Med. **17**, 337–350 (1966)
243. Signer, E.R.: Lysogeny: the integration problem. Annu. Rev. Microbiol. **22**, 451–488 (1968)
244. Pappenheimer, A.M., Jr., Williams, C.M.: The effects of diphtheria toxin on the Cecropia silkworm. J. gen. Physiol. **35**, 727–740 (1951)
245. Freeman, V.J.: Studies on the virulence of bacteriophage-infected strains of *Corynebacterium diphtheriae*. J. Bact. **61**, 675–688 (1951)
246. Groman, N.B., Eaton, M.: Genetic factors in *Corynebacterium diphtheriae* conversion. J. Bact. **70**, 637–640 (1955)
247. Furth, J.: Lymphomatosis, myelomatosis, and endothelioma of chickens caused by a filterable agent. I. Transmission experiments. J. exp. Med. **58**, 253–275 (1933)
248. Ellermann, V., Bang, O.: Experimentelle Leukämie bei Hühnern. Zbl. Bakt. **46**, 595–609 (1908)
249. Burmester, B.R.: The vertical and horizontal transmission of avian visceral lymphomatosis. Symp. quant. Biol. **27**, 471–477 (1962)
250. Rubin, H.A.: Virus in chick embryos which induces resistance *in vitro* to infection with Rous sarcoma virus. Proc. nat. Acad. Sci. (Wash.) **46**, 1105–1119 (1960)
251. Burmester, B.R., Waters, N.F.: The role of the infected egg in the transmission of visceral lymphomatosis. Poultry Sci. **34**, 1415–1429 (1955)
252. Harris, R.J.C.: Biological and structural properties of Rous sarcoma viruses. In: Viruses, nucleic acids, and cancer. Proc. 17th Annu. Symp. Fund. Cancer Res., p. 331–343. Baltimore: Williams & Wilkins 1963
253. Beard, J.W., Bonar, R.A., Heine U., de The, G., Beard, D.: Studies on the biological, biochemical, and biophysical properties of avian tumor viruses. In: Viruses, nucleic acids and cancer. Proc. 17th Annu. Symp. Fund. Cancer Res., p. 344–373. Baltimore: Williams & Wilkins 1963
254. Rubin, H., Temin, H.M.: Infection with the Rous sarcoma virus *in vitro*. Fed. Proc. **17**, 994–1003 (1958)
255. Shope, R.E.: Infectious papillomatosis of rabbits. J. exp. Med. **58**, 607–624 (1933)
256. Greene, H.S.N.: The induction of the Shope papilloma in homologous transplants of embryonic rat skin. Cancer Res. **13**, 681–683 (1953)
257. Israeli, E., Sachs, L.: Cell-virus interactions with the Shope fibroma virus on cultures of rabbit and rat cells. Virology **23**, 473–485 (1964)
258. Evans, C.A., Rashad, A.L.: Virus content of Shope papillomas of Cottontail rabbits. Cancer Res. **27**, 1011–1015 (1967)
259. Kreider, J.W., Breedis, C., Curran, J.S.: Interactions of Shope papilloma virus and rabbit skin cells *in vitro*. I. Immunofluorescent localization of virus inocula. J. nat. Cancer Inst. **38**, 921–931 (1967)
260. Bittner, J.J.: Some possible effects of nursing on the mammary gland tumor incidence in mice. Science **84**, 162 (1936)
261. Bittner, J.J.: Possible relationship of the estrogenic hormones, genetic susceptibility, and milk influence in the production of mammary cancer in mice. Cancer Res. **2**, 710–721 (1942)
262. Hairstone, M.A., Sheffield, J.B., Moore, D.H.: Study of β particles in the mammary tumors of different mouse strains. J. nat. Cancer Inst. **33**, 825–836 (1964)
263. Pitelka, D.R., Bern, H.A., Nandi, S., DeOme, K.B.: On the significance of virus-like particles in the mammary tissue of C3Hf mice. J. nat. Cancer Inst. **33**, 867–885 (1964)
264. Lyons, M.J., Moore, D.H.: Isolation of the mouse mammary tumor virus: Chemical and morphological studies. J. Cancer Inst. **35**, 549–565 (1965)
265. Bentvelzen, P., Daams, J.H., Hageman, P., Calafat, J.: Genetic transmission of viruses that incite mammary tumor in mice. Proc. nat. Acad. Sci. (Wash.) **67**, 377–384 (1970)
266. Moore, D.H., Lyons, M.J.: Studies of replication and properties of the Bittner virus. In: Viruses, nucleic acids, and cancer. Proc. 17th Annu. Symp. Fund. Cancer Res., p. 224–242. Baltimore: Williams & Wilkins 1963
267. Moore, D.H., Pollard, E.C., Haagensen, C.D.: Further correlations of physical and biological properties of mouse mammary tumor agent. Fed. Proc. **21**, 942–946 (1962)
268. Gross, L.: "Spontaneous" leukemia developing in C3H mice following inoculation, in infancy, with AK-leukemic extracts or AK-embryos. Proc. Soc. exp. Biol. (N.Y.) **76**, 27–32 (1951)
269. Gross, L.: A filterable agent, recovered from AK leukemic extracts, causing salivary gland carcinomas in C3H mice. Proc. Soc. exp. Biol. Med. **83**, 414–421 (1953)
270. Gross, L.: Properties of a virus isolated from leukemic mice, inducing various forms of leukemia and lymphomas in mice and rats. In: Viruses, nucleic acids and cancer. Proc. 17th Annu. Symp. Fund. Cancer Res., p. 403–426. Baltimore: Williams & Wilkins 1963
271. Moloney, J.B.: The rodent leukemias: virus-induced murine leukemias. Annu. Rev. Med. **15**, 383–392 (1964)
272. O'Connor, T.E.: Murine-leukemia viruses—a review. In: Viruses inducing cancer (Burdette, W.J., ed.), p. 3–12. Salt Lake City, Utah: Univ. of Utah Press 1966
273. Rich, M.A., Siegler, R.: Virus leukemia in the mouse. Annu. Rev. Microbiol. **21**, 529–572 (1967)
274. Stewart, S.E., Eddy, B.E., Borgese, N.G.: Neoplasms in mice inoculated with a tumor agent carried in tissue culture. J. nat. Cancer Inst. **20**, 1223–1243 (1958)
275. Eddy, B.E., Stewart, S.E.: Physical properties and hemagglutinating and cytopathogenic effects of the SE polyoma virus. Canad. Cancer Conf. **3**, 307–324 (1959)
276. Eddy, B.E., Stewart, S.E., Berkeley, W.: Cytopathogenicity in tissue cultures by a tumor virus from mice. Proc. Soc. exp. Biol. (N.Y.) **98**, 848–851 (1958)
277. Eddy, B.E., Stewart, S.E., Stanton, M.F., Marcotte, J.M.: Induction of tumors in rats by tissue-culture preparations of SE polyoma virus. J. nat. Cancer Inst. **22**, 161–171 (1959)
278. Eddy, B.E., Stewart, S.E., Young, R., Mider, G.B.: Neoplasms in hamsters induced by mouse tumor agent passed in tissue culture. J. nat. Cancer Inst. **20**, 747–761 (1958)
279. Dmochowski, L.: Viruses and tumors in the light of electron microscope studies: a review. Cancer Res. **20**, 977–1015 (1960)
280. Dmochowski, L.: The electron microscopic view of virus-host relationship in neoplasia. Prog. exp. Tumor Res. **3**, 35–147 (1963)
281. Habel, K.: Tumor viruses. Yale J. Biol. Med. **37**, 473–486 (1965)
282. Green, M.: Oncogenic viruses. Annu. Rev. Biochem. **39**, 701–756 (1970)
283. Rich, M.A., Siegler, R.: Virus leukemia in the mouse. Annu. Rev. Microbiol. **21**, 529–572 (1967)
284. Burmester, B.R., Gross, M.A., Walter, W.G., Fontes, A.K.: Pathogenicity of a viral strain (RPL12) causing avian visceral lymphomatosis and related neoplasms. II. Host-virus interrelations affecting response. J. nat. Cancer Inst. **22**, 103–127 (1959)
285. Roe, F.J.C., Rowson, K.E.K.: The induction of cancer by combinations of viruses and other agents. Int. Rev. exp. Path. **6**, 181–227 (1968)
286. Claude, A., Murphy, J.B.: Transmissible tumors of the fowl. Physiol. Rev. **13**, 246–275 (1933)

287. Oberling, C., Guerin, M.: L'existence d'un ultra-chondriome dans les cellules normales et tumorales. C.R. Acad. Sci. (Paris) **231**, 1260–1262 (1950)
288. Green, M.: Chemistry and structure of animal virus particles. Amer. J. Med. **38**, 651–668 (1965)
289. Tamm, I., Eggers, H.J.: Biochemistry of virus reproduction. Amer. J. Med. **38**, 678–698 (1965)
290. Summers, D.F.: Biochemistry of animal virus replication. New Engl. J. Med. **276**, 1016–1023 (1967)
291. Rapp, F.: Defective DNA animal viruses. Annu. Rev. Microbiol. **23**, 293–316 (1969)
292. Eckhart, W.: Oncogenic viruses. Annu. Rev. Biochem. **41**, 503–516 (1972)
293. Weissmann, C., Ochoa, S.: Replication of phage DNA. Progr. Nucleic Acid Res. **6**, 353–399 (1967)
294. Sugiyama, T., Korant, B.D., Lonberg-Holm, K.K.: RNA virus gene expression and its control. Annu. Rev. Microbiol. **26**, 467–502 (1972)
295. Bader, J.P.: The requirement for DNA synthesis in the growth of Rous sarcoma and Rous-associated viruses. Virology **26**, 253–261 (1965)
296. Temin, H.M.: The participation of DNA in Rous sarcoma virus production. Virology **23**, 486–494 (1964)
297. Temin, H.M.: The mechanism of carcinogenesis by avian sarcoma viruses. I. Cell multiplication and differentiation. J. nat. Cancer Inst. **35**, 679–693 (1965)
298. Temin, H.M.: Nature of the provirus of Rous sarcoma. Nat. Cancer Inst. Monogr. 17, Int. Conf. on Avian Tumor Viruses, p. 557–570 (1964)
299. Bader, J.P., Bader, A.V.: Evidence for a DNA replicative genome for RNA-containing tumor viruses. Proc. nat. Acad. Sci. (Wash.) **67**, 843–850 (1970)
300. Scolnick, E.M., Aaronson, S.A., Todaro, G.J.: DNA synthesis by RNA containing tumor viruses. Proc. nat. Acad. Sci. (Wash.) **67**, 1034–1041 (1970)
301. Spiegelman, S., Burny, A., Das, M.R., Keydar, J., Schlom, J., Travnicek, M., Watson, K.: DNA-directed DNA polymerase activity in oncogenic RNA viruses. Nature (Lond.) **227**, 1029–1031 (1970)
302. Duesberg, P., Helm, K.V.D., Canaani, E.: Properties of a soluble DNA polymerase isolated from Rous sarcoma virus. Proc. nat. Acad. Sci. (Wash.) **68**, 747–751 (1971)
303. McDonnell, J.P., Garapin, A.C., Levinson, W.E., Quintrell, N., Fanshier, L., Bishop, J.M.: DNA polymerases of Rous sarcoma virus: delineation of two reactions with actinomycin. Nature (Lond.) **228**, 433–435 (1970)
304. Riman, J., Beaudreau, G.S.: Viral DNA-dependent DNA polymerase and the properties of thymidine labelled material in virions of an oncogenic RNA virus. Nature (Lond.) **228**, 427–430 (1970)
305. Rokutanda, M., Rokutanda, H., Green, M., Fujinaga, K., Ray, R.K., Gurgo, C.: Formation of viral RNA-DNA hybrid molecules by the DNA polymerase of sarcoma-leukaemia viruses. Nature (Lond.) **227**, 1026–1028 (1970)
306. Spiegelman, B., Burny, A., Das, M.R., Keydar, J., Schlom, J., Travnicek, M., Watson, K.: Synthetic DNA-RNA hybrids and RNA-RNA duplexes as templates for the polymerases of the oncogenic RNA viruses. Nature (Lond.) **228**, 430–432 (1970)
307. Temin, H.M., Mizutani, S.: RNA-dependent DNA polymerase in virions of Rous sarcoma virus. Nature (Lond.) **226**, 1211–1213 (1970)
308. Gerwin, B.I., Todaro, G.J., Zeve, V., Scolnick, E.M., Aaronson, S.A.: Separation of RNA-dependent DNA polymerase activity from the murine leukaemia virion. Nature (Lond.) **228**, 435–438 (1970)
309. Dulbecco, R.: The induction of cancer by viruses. Sci. Amer. **216**, 28–37 (1967)
310. Dulbecco, R.: Transformation of cells *in vitro* by DNA-containing viruses, carcinogenesis. J. Amer. med. Ass. **109**, 721–726 (1964)
311. Temin, H.M.: Malignant transformation of cells by viruses. Perspect. Biol. Med. **14**, 11–26 (1970)
312. Dulbecco, R.: Cell transformation by the small DNA-containing viruses. Harvey Lect. Series **63**, 33–46 (1967–68)
313. Green, M.: Effect of oncogenic DNA viruses on regulatory mechanisms of cells. Fed. Proc. **29**, 1265–1275 (1970)
314. Rubin, H.: The behavior of cells before and after virus-induced malignant transformation. Harvey Lect. Series 117–143 (1965–66)
315. Black, P.H.: The oncogenic DNA viruses: A review of *in vitro* transformation studies. Annu. Rev. Microbiol. **22**, 391–426 (1968)
316. DiPaolo, J.A., Popescu, N.C.: Distribution of chromosome constitutive heterochromatin of Syrian hamster cells transformed by chemical carcinogens. Cancer Res. **33**, 3259–3265 (1973)
317. Bader, J.P.: Virus-induced transformation without cell division. Science **180**, 1069–1071 (1973)
318. Baluda, M.A., Nayak, D.P.: DNA complementary to viral RNA in leukemic cells induced by avian myeloblastosis virus. Proc. nat. Acad. Sci. (Wash.) **66**, 329–336 (1970)
319. Lunger, P.D.: The isolation and morphology of the Lucke-Frog kidney tumor virus. Virology **24**, 138–145 (1964)
320. Olson, C., Pamukcu, A.M., Brobst, D.F.: Papilloma-like virus from bovine urinary bladder tumors. Cancer Res. **25**, 840–849 (1965)
321. Dutcher, R.M., Larkin, E.P., Marshak, R.R.: Virus-like particles in cow's milk from a herd with a high incidence of lymphosarcoma. J. nat. Cancer Inst. **33**, 1055–1064 (1964)
322. Hardy, W.D., Geering, G., Old, L.J., De Harven, E., Brody, R.S., McDonough, S.: Feline leukemia virus: occurrence of viral antigen in the tissues of cats with lymphosarcoma and other diseases. Science **166**, 1019–1021 (1969)
323. Schneider, R.: The natural history of malignant lymphoma and sarcoma in cats and their associations with cancer in man and dog. J. Amer. vet. med. Ass. **157**, 1753–1758 (1970)
324. Yokoro, K., Ito, T., Imamura, N., Kawase, A., Yamasaki, T.: Synergistic action of radiation and virus in induction of leukemia in rats. Cancer Res. **29**, 1973–1976 (1969)
325. Hays, E.F.: Transmission of mouse leukaemia with purified nucleic acid preparations. Nature (Lond.) **192**, 230–232 (1961)
326. Fischinger, P.J., O'Connor, T.E.: Productive infection and morphologic alteration of human cells by a modified sarcoma virus. J. nat. Cancer Inst. **44**, 429–438 (1970)
327. Munroe, J.S., Southam, C.M.: Oncogenicity of two strains of chicken sarcoma virus for rats. Nat. Cancer Inst. J. **32**, 591–607 (1964)
328. McClure, H.M., Van Lancker, J.: Unpublished results
329. Newell, G.R., Harris, W.W., Borman, K.O., Boone, C.W., Anderson, N.G.: Evaluation of "virus-like" particles in the plasmas of 255 patients with leukemia and related diseases. New Engl. J. Med. **278**, 1185–1191 (1968)
330. Porter, G.H., Dalton, A.J., Moloney, J.B., Mitchell, E.Z.: Association of electron-dense particles with human acute leukemia. J. nat. Cancer Inst. **33**, 547–556 (1964)
331. Hehlmann, R., Baxt, W., Kufe, D., Spiegelman, S.: Molecular evidence for a viral etiology of human leukemias, lymphomas and sarcomas. Amer. J. clin. Path. **60**, 65–79 (1973)
332. Epstein, M.A., Achong, B.G.: Fine structural organization of human lymphoblasts of a tissue culture strain (EBI) from Burkitt's lymphoma. J. nat. Cancer Inst. **34**, 241–253 (1965)
333. Henle, G., Henle, W.: Studies on cell lines derived from Burkitt's lymphoma. Trans. N.Y. Acad. Sci. **29**, 71–79 (1966–67)
334. Rabson, A.S.: Herpesviruses and cancer, introduction. Fed. Proc. **31**, 1625–1668 (1972)
335. Allen, D.W., Cole, P.: Viruses and human cancer. New Engl. J. Med. **286**, 70–82 (1972)
336. Henle, G., Henle, W.: EB virus in the etiology of infectious mononucleosis. Hosp. Pract. **5**, 33–41 (1970)
337. Klein, G.: Herpesviruses and oncogenesis. Proc. nat. Acad. Sci. (Wash.) **69**, 1056–1064 (1972)
338. Todaro, G.J., Huebner, R.J.: N.A.S. Symposium: new evidence as the basis for increased efforts in cancer research. Proc. nat. Acad. Sci. (Wash.) **69**, 1009–1015 (1972)
339. Temin, H.M.: The RNA tumor viruses—background and foreground. Proc. nat. Acad. Sci. (Wash.) **69**, 1016–1020 (1972)
340. Temin, H.M.: Mechanism of cell transformation by RNA tumor viruses. Annu. Rev. Microbiol. **25**, 609–648 (1971)
341. Dmochowski, L., Grey, C.E., Sykes, J.A., Dreyer, D.A., Langford, P., Jesse, R.H., Jr., MacComb, W.S., Ballantyne, A.J.: A study of submicroscopic structure and of virus particles in cells of human laryngeal papillomas. Tex. Rep. Biol. Med. **22**, 454–491 (1964)
342. Morton, D.L., Hall, W.T., Malmgren, R.A.: Human liposarcomas: tissue cultures containing foci of transformed cells with viral particles. Science **165**, 813–815 (1969)
343. Warburg, O.: The metabolism of tumours. English Translation, Frank Dickens, London, Constable (1930)
344. Warburg, O.: The prime cause and prevention of cancer. Lect. at Meeting of Nobel Laureates, June 30, 1966, K. Triltsch, Würzburg, Germany 1967
345. Voegtlin, C., Kahler, H., Fitch, R.H., II: The estimation of the hydrogen-ion concentration of tissues in living animals by means of the capillary glass electrode. U.S. nat. Inst. Hlth Bull. **164**, 15–27 (1935)
346. Cori, C.F., Cori, G.T.: The carbohydrate metabolism of tumors. II. Changes in the sugar, lactic acid and CO_2-combining power of blood passing through a tumor. J. biol. Chem. **65**, 397–405 (1925)
347. Weinhouse, S.: Glycolysis, respiration, and enzyme deletions in slow-growing hepatic tumors. In: U.S.-Japan Joint Conf. on Biological and Biochemical Evaluation of Malignancy in Experimental Hepatomas, Kyoto, 1965, Gann Monograph 1, 99–115. Tokyo: Jap. Cancer Assoc. 1966
348. LePage, G.A.: A comparison of tumor and normal tissues with respect to factors affecting the rate of anaerobic glycolysis. Cancer Res. **10**, 77–88 (1950)
349. Busch, H., Potter, V.: Studies on tissue metabolism by means of *in vivo* metabolic blocking techniques; metabolism of acetate-1-C^{14} in malonate-treated rats. Cancer Res. **13**, 168–173 (1953)
350. Busch, H., Baltrush, H.A.: Rates of metabolism of acetate-1-C^{14} in tissues *in vivo*. Cancer Res. **14**, 448–455 (1954)
351. Weinhouse, S.: Oxidative metabolism of neoplastic tissues. Advanc. Cancer Res. **3**, 269–325 (1955)
352. Aisenberg, A.C., Potter, V.R.: Studies on the Pasteur effect. II. Specific mechanisms. J. biol. Chem. **224**, 1115–1127 (1957)
353. Aisenberg, A.C.: The glycolysis and respiration of tumors. New York: Academic Press 1961
354. Rosenthal, O., Drabkin, D.L.: The oxidative response of normal and

neoplastic tissues to succinate and to ρ-phenylenediamine. Cancer Res. **4**, 487–494 (1944)
355. Greenstein, J.P.: Biochemistry of cancer, 2nd ed. New York: Academic Press 1944
356. Chance, B., Castor, L.N.: Some patterns of the respiratory pigments of ascites tumors of mice. Science **116**, 200–202 (1952)
357. Chance, B.: A digital computer representation of chemical and spectroscopic studies on chemical control of ascites tumor cell metabolism. In: Amino acids, proteins, and cancer biochemistry (Edsall, J.T., ed.), p. 191–212. New York: Academic Press 1960
358. Wu, R., Racker, E.: Regulatory mechanisms in carbohydrate metabolism. IV. Pasteur effect and Crabtree effect in ascites tumor cells. J. biol. Chem. **234**, 1036–1041 (1959)
359. Racker, E., Wu, R., Alpers, J.B.: Carbohydrate metabolism in ascites tumor and HeLa cells. In: Amino acids, proteins, and cancer biochemistry (Edsall, J., ed.), p. 175–189. New York: Academic Press 1960
360. Williams-Ashman, H.G.: Studies on the Ehrlich ascites tumor; oxidation of hexose phosphates. Cancer Res. **13**, 721–725 (1953)
361. Lindberg, O., Ljunggren, M., Ernster, L., Révész, L.: Isolation and some enzymic properties of Ehrlich ascites tumor mitochondria. Exp. Cell Res. **4**, 243–245 (1953)
362. Quastel, J.H., Bickis, I.J.: Metabolism of normal tissues and neoplasms *in vitro*. Nature (Lond.) **183**, 281–286 (1959)
363. Emmelot, P., Bos, C.J., Brombacher, P.J.: Fatty acid oxidation in normal and neoplastic tissues. Enzymatic activities and optical densities of mitochondrial suspensions prepared from normal and neoplastic tissues of the mouse. Brit. J. Cancer **10**, 188–201 (1956)
364. Hogeboom, G.H., Schneider, W.C.: Intracellular distribution of enzymes. VIII. The distribution of diphosphopyridine nucleotide-cytochrome C reductase in normal mouse liver and mouse hepatoma. J. nat. Cancer Inst. **10**, 983–987 (1950)
365. Striebich, M.J., Shelton, E., Schneider, W.C.: Quantitative morphological studies on the livers and liver homogenates of rats fed 2-methyl- or 3-methyl-4-dimethylaminoazobenzene. Cancer Res. **13**, 279–284 (1953)
366. Roberts, E., Simonsen, D.G.: Free amino acids and related substances in normal and neoplastic tissues. In: Amino acids, proteins, and cancer biochemistry (Edsall, J., ed.), p. 121–145. New York: Academic Press 1960
367. Kidd, J.G.: Regression of transplanted lymphomas induced *in vivo*, by means of normal guinea pig serum. I. Course of transplanted cancers of various kinds in mice and rats given guinea pig serum, horse serum or rabbit serum. J. exp. Med. **98**, 565–582 (1953)
368. Kidd, J.G.: Regression of transplanted lymphomas induced *in vivo*, by means of normal guinea pig serum. II. Studies on the nature of active serum constituent. Histological mechanism of regression. Tests for effects of guinea pig serum on lymphoma cells in vitro: discussion. J. exp. Med. **98**, 583–606 (1953)
369. Broome, J.D.: Evidence that the L-asparaginase activity of guinea pig serum is responsible for its antilymphoma effects. Nature (Lond.) **191**, 1114–1115 (1961)
370. Griffin, A.C., Bloom, S., Cunningham, L., Teresi, J.D., Luck, J.M.: The uptake of labeled glycine by normal and cancerous tissues in the rat. Cancer (Philad.) **3**, 316–320 (1950)
371. LePage, G.A.: *In vitro* incorporation of glycine-2-C^{14} into purines and proteins. Cancer Res. **13**, 178–185 (1953)
372. Zamecnik, P.C., Loftfield, R.B., Stephenson, M.L., Steele, J.M.: Studies on the carbohydrate and protein metabolism of the rat hepatoma. Cancer Res. **11**, 592–602 (1951)
373. Farber, E., Kit, S., Greenberg, D.M.: Tracer studies on the metabolism of the Gardner lymphosarcoma. I. The uptake of radioactive glycine into tumor protein. Cancer Res. **11**, 490–494 (1951)
374. Abrams, R., Goldinger, J.M.: Formation of nucleic acid purines from hypoxanthine and formate in bone marrow slices. Arch. Biochem. Biophys. **35**, 243–248 (1952)
375. Hartman, S.C., Buchanan, J.M.: Nucleic acids, purines, pyrimidines (nucleotide synthesis). Annu. Rev. Biochem. **28**, 365–410 (1959)
376. Greenberg, D.M.: Amino acid metabolism. Annu. Rev. Biochem. **33**, 633–666 (1964)
377. Tyner, E.P., Heidelberger, C., LePage, G.A.: Intracellular distribution of radioactivity in nucleic acid nucleotides and proteins following simultaneous administration of P^{32} and glycerine-2-C^{14}. Cancer Res. **13**, 186–203 (1953)
378. Marshak, A.: Evidence for a nuclear precursor of ribo- and desoxyribonucleic acid. J. cell. comp. Physiol. **32**, 381–406 (1948)
379. Heidelberger, C.: Chemical carcinogenesis, chemotherapy: cancer's continuing core challenges, G.H.A. Clowes Mem. Lect. Cancer Res. **30**, 1549–1569 (1970)
380. Post, J., Hoffman, J.: Cell renewal patterns. New Engl. J. Med. **279**, 248–258 (1968)
381. Baserga, R., Kisieleski, W.E.: Comparative study of the kinetics of cellular proliferation of normal and tumorous tissues with the use of tritiated thymidine. I. Dilution of the label and migration of labeled cells. J. nat. Cancer Inst. **28**, 331–339 (1962)
382. Klein, G.: Comparative studies of mouse tumors with respect to their capacity for growth as "ascites tumors" and their average nucleic acid content per cell. Exp. Cell Res. **2**, 518–573 (1951)
383. Kit, S.: The nucleic acids of normal tissues and tumors. In: Amino acids, proteins, and cancer biochemistry (Edsall, J.T., ed.), p. 147–174. J.P. Greenstein Memorial Symp. New York: Academic Press 1960
384. Mark, D.D., Ris, H.: A comparison of deoxyribonucleic acid content in certain nuclei of normal liver and liver tumors. Proc. Soc. exp. Biol. (N.Y.) **71**, 727–729 (1949)
385. Di Mayorca, G., Rosenkranz, H.S., Polli, E.E., Korngold, G.C., Bendich, A.: A chromatographic study of the deoxyribonucleic acids from normal and leukemic human tissues. J. nat. Cancer Inst. **24**, 1309–1318 (1960)
386. Kit, S., Griffin, A.C.: Cellular metabolism and cancer: a review. Cancer Res. **18**, 621–656 (1958)
387. Carter, C.E.: Paper chromatography of purine and pyrimidine derivatives of yeast ribonucleic acid. J. Amer. chem. Soc. **72**, 1466–1471 (1950)
388. De Lamirande, G., Allard, C., Cantero, A.: Ribonucleic acid composition in cytoplasmic fractions isolated from rat liver cells. J. biophys. biochem. Cytol. **6**, 291–292 (1959)
389. Muramatsu, M., Busch, H.: Studies on nucleolar RNA of the Walker 256 carcinosarcoma and the liver of the rat. Cancer Res. **24**, 1028–1034 (1964)
390. Scrutton, M.C., Utter, M.F.: The regulation of glycolysis and gluconeogenesis in animal tissues. Annu. Rev. Biochem. **37**, 249–302 (1968)
391. Koshland, D.E., Jr., Neet, K.E.: The catalytic and regulatory properties of enzymes. Annu. Rev. Biochem. **37**, 359–410 (1968)
392. Cleland, W.W.: The statistical analysis of enzyme kinetic data. Advanc. Enzymol. **29**, 1–32 (1967)
393. Stadtman, E.R.: Allosteric regulation of enzyme activity. Advanc. Enzymol. **28**, 41–154 (1966)
394. Holzer, H.: Regulation of enzymes by enzyme-catalyzed chemical modification. Advanc. Enzymol. **32**, 297–326 (1969)
395. Mansour, T.E.: Kinetic and physical properties of phosphofructokinase. Advanc. Enzyme Rgul. **8**, 37–52 (1970)
396. Lynen, F., Hartmann, G., Netter, K.F., Schuegraf, A.: Phosphate turnover and Pasteur effect. In: Ciba Foundation Symp. on the Regulation of Cell Metabolism (Wolstenholme, G.E.W., and O'Connor, C.M., eds.), p. 256–276. London: J. & A. Churchill 1959
397. Johnson, M.J.: The role of aerobic phosphorylation in the Pasteur effect. Science **94**, 200–202 (1941)
398. Cori, C.F.: Problems of cellular biochemistry. In: Currents in biochemical research (Green, D.E., ed.), p. 198–214. New York: Interscience Publishers 1956
399. Lardy, H.A.: Gluconeogenesis: pathways and hormonal regulation. Harvey Lect. Series **60**, 261–278 (1964–65)
400. Weber, G., Lea, M.A., Convery, H.J.H., Stamm, N.B.: Regulation of gluconeogenesis and glycolysis: studies of mechanisms controlling enzyme activity. Advanc. Enzyme Regul. **5**, 257–300 (1967)
401. Herrera, M.G., Kamm, D., Ruderman, N., Cahill, G.F., Jr.: Nonhormonal factors in the control of gluconeogenesis. Advanc. Enzyme Regul. **4**, 225–235 (1966)
402. Williamson, J.R.: Effects of fatty acids, glucagon and anti-insulin serum on the control of gluconeogenesis and ketogenesis in rat liver. Advanc. Enzyme Regul. **5**, 229–255 (1967)
403. Rodwell, V.W., McNamara, D.J., Shapiro, D.J.: Regulation of hepatic 3-hydroxy-3-methylglutaryl-coenzyme A reductase. Advanc. Enzymol. **38**, 373–412 (1973)
404. Krebs, H.A.: The regulation of the release of ketone bodies by the liver. Advanc. Enzyme Regul. **4**, 339–353 (1966)
405. Gross, P.R.: Biochemistry of differentiation. Annu. Rev. Biochem. **37**, 631–660 (1968)
406. Epstein, W., Beckwith, J.R.: Regulation of gene expression. Annu. Rev. Biochem. **37**, 411–436 (1968)
407. Kornberg, A., Spudich, J.A., Nelson, D.L., Deutscher, M.P.: Origin of proteins in sporulation. Annu. Rev. Biochem. **37**, 51–78 (1968)
408. Winick, M., McCrory, W.W.: Renal differentiation: a model for the study of development. Birth Defects, Original Article Series IV, 1–14 (1968)
409. Wessells, N.K.: DNA synthesis, mitosis and differentiation in pancreatic acinar cells *in vitro*. J. Cell Biol. **20**, 415–433 (1964)
410. Rutter, W.J.: Ontogeny of specific proteins during pancreatic development. Science **150**, 383 (1965)
411. Rutter, W.J., Wessells, N.K., Grobstein, C.: Control of specific synthesis in the developing pancreas. Nat. Cancer Inst. Monogr. **13**, 51–65 (1964)
412. Rutter, W.J., Clark, W.R., Kemp, J.D., Bradshaw, W.S., Sanders, T.G., Ball, W.D.: Multiphasic regulation in cytodifferentiation. In: Epithelial-mesenchymal interactions (Fleischmajer, R., and Billingham, R., eds.), p. 114–131. Baltimore: Williams & Wilkins 1968
413. Wessells, N.K., Rutter, W.J.: Phases in cell differentiation. Sci. Amer. **220**, 36–44 (1969)
414. Filner, P., Wray, J.L., Varner, J.E.: Enzyme induction in higher plants. Science **165**, 358–367 (1969)
415. Dahmus, M.E., Bonner, J.: Nucleoproteins in regulation of gene function. Fed. Proc. **29**, 1255–1260 (1970)
416. Huang, R.C.C., Bonner, J.: Histone-bound RNA, a component of native nucleohistone. Proc. nat. Acad. Sci. (Wash.) **54**, 960–967 (1965)

417. Zirkin, B.R.: A cytochemical study of the non-histone protein content of condensed and extended chromatin. Exp. Cell Res. **78**, 394–398 (1973)
418. Maryanka, D., Gould, H.: Transcription of rat-liver chromatin with homologous enzyme. Proc. nat. Acad. Sci. (Wash.) **70**, 1161–1165 (1973)
419. Axel, R., Cedar, H., Felsenfeld, G.: Synthesis of globin ribonucleic acid from duck-reticulocyte chromatin *in vitro*. Proc. nat. Acad. Sci. (Wash.) **70**, 2029–2032 (1973)
420. Britten, R.J., Kohne, D.E.: Nucleotide sequence repetition in DNA. Annu. Report of the Director of the Department of Terrestrial Magnetism, Carnegie Institution, p. 78–125 (1965–66)
421. Britten, R.J., Davidson, E.H.: Gene regulation for higher cells: a theory. Science **165**, 349–357 (1969)
422. Wright, B.E.: Multiple causes and controls in differentiation. Science **153**, 830–837 (1966)
423. Tomkins, G.M., Gelehrter, T.D., Granner, D., Martin, D., Jr., Samuels, H.H., Thompson, E.B.: Control of specific gene expression in higher organisms. Science **166**, 1474–1486 (1969)
424. Croce, C.M., Litwack, G., Koprowski, H.: Human regulatory gene for inducible tyrosine aminotransferase in rat-human hybrids. Proc. nat. Acad. Sci. (Wash.) **70**, 1268–1272 (1973)
425. Gurdon, J.B.: Transplanted nuclei and cell differentiation. Sci. Amer. **219**, 24–35 (1968)
426. Weiss, M.C., Green, H.: Human-mouse hybrid cell lines containing partial complements of human chromosomes and functioning human genes. Proc. nat. Acad. Sci. (Wash.) **58**, 1104–1111 (1967)
427. Lark, K.G.: Initiation and control of DNA synthesis. Annu. Rev. Biochem. **38**, 569–604 (1969)
428. Maale, O., Kjelgaard, N.O.: Control of macromolecular synthesis; A study of DNA, RNA, and protein synthesis in bacteria. New York: Benjamin 1966
429. Mueller, G.C.: Biochemical events in the animal cell cycle. Fed. Proc. **28**, 1780–1789 (1969)
430. Taylor, J.H.: Asynchronous duplication of chromosomes in cultured cells of Chinese hamster. J. biophys. biochem. Cytol. **7**, 455–464 (1960)
431. Painter, R.B.: Asynchronous replication of HeLa S3 chromosomal deoxyribonucleic acid. J. biophys. biochem. Cytol. **11**, 485–488 (1961)
432. Rusch, H.P.: Some biochemical events in the growth cycles of *Physarum polycephalum*. Fed. Proc. **28**, 1761–1770 (1969)
433. Prescott, D.M.: Symposium: synthetic processes in the cell nucleus. II. Nucleic acid and protein metabolism in the macronuclei of two ciliated protozoa. J. Histochem. Cytochem. **10**, 145–153 (1962)
434. Baserga, R.: A radioautographic study of the uptake of [^{14}C]-leucine by tumor cells in deoxyribonucleic acid synthesis. Biochim. biophys. Acta (Amst.) **61**, 445–450 (1962)
435. Kedes, L.H., Gross, P.R., Cognetti, G., Hunter, A.L.: Synthesis of nuclear and chromosomal proteins on light polyribosomes during cleavage in the sea urchin embryo. J. molec. Biol. **45**, 337–351 (1967)
436. Cone, C.D., Jr.: Electroosmotic interactions accompanying mitosis initiation in sarcoma cells *in vitro*. Trans. N.Y. Acad. Sci. **31**, 404–427 (1969)
437. Yatvin, M.B.: Polysome morphology: Evidence for endocrine control during chick embryogenesis. Science **151**, 1001–1003 (1966)
438. Crane, R.K.: Structural and functional organization of an epithelial cell brush border. Int. Soc. Cell Biol. Symp. **5**, 71–102 (1966)
439. Nilsson, O., Ronist, G.: Enzyme activities and ultrastructure of a membrane fraction from human erythrocytes. Biochim. biophys. Acta **183**, 1–9 (1969)
440. Goldacre, R.J.: On the mechanism and control of ameboid movement. In: Primitive motile systems in cell biology (Allen, R.D., and Kamiya, N., eds.), p. 237–255. New York: Academic Press 1964
441. Abercrombie, M., Ambrose, E.J.: Interference microscope studies of cell contacts in tissue culture. Exp. Cell Res. **15**, 332–345 (1958)
442. Abercrombie, M., Ambrose, E.J.: The surface properties of cancer cells: a review. Cancer Res. **22**, 525–548 (1962)
443. Porter, K.R.: Microtubules in intracellular locomotion. In: Locomotion of tissue cells. Ciba Foundation Symp. #14 (New Series), p. 149–169. Amsterdam: Assoc. Scientific Publishers 1973
444. Abercrombie, M.: An *in vitro* model of the mechanism of invasion. In: Mechanisms of invasion in cancer (Denoix, P.F., ed.), p. 140–144. Berlin-Heidelberg-New York: Springer 1967
445. Steinberg, M.S.: Cell movement in confluent monolayers: a re-evaluation of the causes of "contact inhibition." In: Locomotion of tissue cells. Ciba Foundation Symposium #14, p. 333–341. Assoc. New York: Scientific Publishers 1973
446. Weiss, L.: The cell periphery, metastasis, and other contact phenomena. Amsterdam: North-Holland Publishing Co. 1967
447. Baier, R.E., Shafrin, E.G., Zisman, W.A.: Adhesion: mechanisms that assist or impede it. Science **162**, 1360–1368 (1968)
448. Moscona, A., Moscona, H.: The dissociation and aggregation of cells from organ rudiments of the early chick embryo. J. Anat. (Lond.) **86**, 287–301 (1952)
449. Weiss, P.: The biological foundations of wound repair. Harvey Lect. Series **55**, 13–42 (1959–60)
450. Steinberg, M.S.: The problem of adhesive selectivity in cellular interactions. In: Cellular membranes in development (Locke, M., ed.), p. 321–366. New York: Academic Press 1964
451. Lilien, J.E., Moscona, A.A.: Cell aggregation: its enhancement by a supernatant from cultures of homologous cells. Science **157**, 70–72 (1967)
452. Lindholm, L., Britton, S.: Possible presence of DNA in intercellular bridges. Exp. Cell Res. **48**, 660–665 (1967)
453. Loewenstein, W.R.: Intercellular communication. Sci. Amer. **222**, 78–86 (1970)
454. Pappas, G.D.: Junctions between cells. Hosp. Prac. **8**, 39–46 (1973)
455. Whittam, R.: The interdependence of metabolism and active transport. In: The cellular functions of membrane transport (Hoffman, J.F., ed.), p. 139–154. Englewood Cliffs, New Jersey: Prentice-Hall 1964
456. Lubin, M.: Cell potassium and the regulation of protein synthesis. In: The cellular functions of membrane transport (Hoffman, J.F., ed.), p. 193–211. Englewood Cliffs, New Jersey: Prentice-Hall 1964
457. Kepes, A.: The place of permeases in cellular organization. In: The cellular functions of membrane transport (Hoffman, J.F., ed.), p. 155–169. Englewood Cliffs, New Jersey: Prentice-Hall 1964
458. Luria, S.E.: Phage, colicins, and macroregulatory phenomena. Science **168**, 1166–1170 (1970)
459. Neville, D.M., Jr.: Fractionation of cell membrane protein by disc electrophoresis. Biochim. biophys. Acta (Amst.) **133**, 168–170 (1967)
460. Bakerman, S., Wasemiller, G.: Studies on structural units of human erythrocyte membrane. I. Separation, isolation and partial characterization. Biochemistry **6**, 1100–1113 (1967)
461. Zwaal, R.F.A., Van Deenen, L.L.M.: Protein patterns of red cell membranes from different mammalian species. Biochim. biophys. Acta **163**, 44–49 (1968)
462. Marchesi, V.T.: The structure and orientation of a membrane protein. Hosp. Pract. **8**, 76–84 (1973)
463. Marchesi, V.T., Jackson, R.L., Segrest, J.P., Kahane, I.: Molecular features of the major glycoprotein of the human erythrocyte membrane. Fed. Proc. **32**, 1833–1837 (1973)
464. Oseroff, A.R., Robbins, P.W., Burger, M.M.: The cell surface membrane: biochemical aspects and biophysical probes. Annu. Rev. Biochem. **42**, 647–682 (1973)
465. DePierre, J.W., Karnovsky, M.L.: Plasma membranes of mammalian cells: a review of methods for their characterization and isolation. J. Cell Biol. **56**, 275–303 (1973)
466. Robertson, J.D.: The unit membrane and the Danielli-Davson model. In: Intracellular transport (Warren, K.B., ed.). Symp. Int. Soc. Cell Biol., vol. 5, p. 1–31. New York: Academic Press 1966
467. Korn, E.D.: Structure of biological membranes. Science **153**, 1491–1498 (1966)
468. Korn, E.D.: Cell membranes: structure and synthesis. Annu. Rev. Biochem. **38**, 263–288 (1969)
469. Gorter, E., Grendel, F.: On bimolecular layers of lipoids on the chromocytes of the blood. J. exp. Med. **41**, 439–443 (1925)
470. Danielli, J.F., Davson, H.: A contribution to the theory of permeability of thin films. J. cell comp. Physiol. **5**, 495–508 (1935)
471. Danielli, J.F., Harvey, E.N.: The tension at the surface of mackerel egg oil, with remarks on the nature of the cell surface. J. cell comp. Physiol. **5**, 483–494 (1935)
472. Stoeckenius, A., Engelman, D.M.: Current models for the structure of biological membranes. J. Cell Biol. **42**, 613–646 (1969)
473. Singer, S.J., Nicolson, G.L.: The fluid mosaic model of the structure of cell membranes. Science **175**, 720–731 (1972)
474. Bretscher, M.S.: Membrane structure: some general principles. Science **181**, 622–629 (1973)
475. Siekevitz, P.: Biological membranes: the dynamics of their organization. Annu. Rev. Physiol. **25**, 15–40 (1963)
476. Reuber, M.D.: Histopathology of transplantable hepatic carcinomas induced by chemical carcinogens in rats. In: U.S.-Japan Joint Conf. on Biological and Biochemical Evaluation of Malignancy in Experimental Hepatomas, Kyoto, 1965, Gann Monograph 1, 43–54. Tokyo: Jap. Cancer Assoc. 1966
477. Woods, M., Burk, D., Hunter, J.: Factors affecting anaerobic glycolysis in mouse and rat liver and in Morris rat hepatomas. J. nat. Cancer Inst. **41**, 267–286 (1968)
478. Morris, H.P.: Studies on the development, biochemistry, and biology of experimental hepatomas. Advanc. Cancer Res. **9**, 227–302 (1965)
479. Bresnick, E.: Feedback inhibition of aspartate transcarbamylase in liver and in hepatoma. Cancer Res. **22**, 1246–1251 (1962)
480. Siperstein, M.D., Fagan, V.M., Morris, H.P.: Further studies on the deletion of the cholesterol feedback system in hepatomas. Cancer Res. **26**, 7–11 (1966)
481. Weber, G.: The molecular correlation concept: studies on the metabolic pattern of hepatomas. In: U.S.-Japan Joint Conf. on Biological and Biochemical Evaluation of Malignancy in Experimental Hepatomas, Kyoto, 1965, Gann Monograph 1, 151–178. Tokyo: Jap. Cancer Assoc. 1966
482. Fiala, S., Fiala, A.E.: Prevention of adaptive formation of tryptophan peroxidase by a carcinogenic azo dye. Nature (Lond.) **183**, 1532–1533 (1959)
483. Auerbach, V.H., Waisman, H.A.: Amino acid metabolism of Novikoff hepatoma. Cancer Res. **18**, 543–547 (1958)
484. Pitot, H.C., Potter, V.R., Morris, H.P.: Metabolic adaptations in rat hepatomas. I. The effect of dietary protein on some inducible enzymes in liver and hepatoma 5123. Cancer Res. **21**, 1001–1008 (1961)

485. Pitot, H.C., Morris, H.P.: Metabolic adaptations in rat hepatomas. II. Tryptophan pyrrolase and tyrosine α-ketoglutarate transaminase. Cancer Res. **21**, 1009–1014 (1961)
486. Pitot, H.C.: Some biochemical essentials of malignancy. Cancer Res. **23**, 1474–1482 (1963)
487. Pitot, H.C., Heidelberger, C.: Metabolic regulatory circuits and carcinogenesis. Cancer Res. **23**, 1694–1700 (1963)
488. Nowell, P.C., Morris, H.P.: Chromosomes of "minimal deviation" hepatomas: a further report on diploid tumors. Cancer Res. **29**, 969–970 (1969)
489. Knox, W.E., Auerbach, V.H., Lin, E.C.C.: Enzymatic and metabolic adaptations in animals. Physiol. Rev. **36**, 164–254 (1956)
490. Potter, V.R., Ono, T.: Enzyme patterns in rat liver and Morris hepatoma 5123 during metabolic transitions. Symp. quant. Biol. **26**, 355–362 (1961)
491. Watanabe, M., Potter, V.R., Morris, H.P.: Benzpyrene hydroxylase activity and its induction by methylcholanthrene in Morris hepatomas, in host livers, in adult livers, and in rat liver during development. Cancer Res. **30**, 263–273 (1970)
492. Potter, V.R.: Recent trends in cancer biochemistry: the importance of studies on fetal tissue. Canad. Cancer Res. Conf. Proc. **8**, 9–30 (1969)
493. Kishi, S., Fujiwara, T., Nakahara, W.: Comparison of chemical composition between hepatoma and normal liver tissues. V. Glycogen, glucose and lactic acid. Gann **31**, 556–567 (1937)
494. Lueders, K.K., Dyer, H.M., Thompson, E.B., Kuff, E.L.: Glucuronyltransferase activity in transplantable rat hepatomas. Cancer Res. **30**, 274–279 (1970)
495. Inoue, H., Pitot, H.C.: Regulation of the synthesis of serine dehydratase isozymes. Advanc. Enzyme Regul. **8**, 289–296 (1970)
496. Weber, G.: Ordered and specific pattern of gene expression in neoplasia. Advanc. Enzyme Regul. **11**, 79–102 (1973)
497. Weinhouse, S., Shatton, J.B., Criss, W.E., Farina, F.A., Morris, H.P.: Isozymes in relation to differentiation in transplantable rat hepatomas. In: Isozymes and enzyme regulation in cancer (Weinhouse, S., and Ono, T., eds.), Gann Monograph on Cancer Res. 13, 1–17. Tokyo: Jap. Cancer Assoc. 1972
498. Weinhouse, S.: Glycolysis, respiration, and enzyme deletions in slow-growing hepatic tumors. Gann Monograph on Cancer Res. 1, 99–115. Tokyo: Jap. Cancer Assoc. 1966
499. Weinhouse, S.: Metabolism and isozyme alterations in experimental hepatomas. Fed. Proc. **32**, 2162–2167 (1973)
500. Hamperl, H.: Early invasive growth as seen in uterine cancer and the role of the basal membrane. In: Mechanisms of invasion in cancer (Denoix, P.F., ed.), p. 17–25. Berlin-Heidelberg-New York: Springer 1967
501. Sylvén, B.: Biochemical factors accompanying growth and invasion. In: Endogenous factors influencing host-tumor balance (Wissler, R.W., Dao, T.L., and Wood, S., Jr., eds.), p. 267–276. Chicago: Chicago University Press 1967
502. Battelli, F., Stern, L.: Recherches sur l'anticatalase dans les tissues animaux. J. Physiol. Path. gén. **7**, 919–934 (1905)
503. Yunoki, K., Griffin, A.C.: Composition and properties of a highly purified toxohormone preparation. Cancer Res. **21,** 537–544 (1961)
504. Greenstein, J.P., Jenrette, W.V., White, J.: The liver catalase activity of tumor-bearing rats and the effect of extirpation of the tumors. J. nat. Cancer Inst. **2**, 283–291 (1941–42)
505. Olivares, J., Callao, V., Montoya, E.: Toxohormone from normal tissues. Science **157**, 327–328 (1967)
506. Fisher, E.R., Fisher, B.: Host-tumor relationship in the development and growth of hepatic metastases. In: Endogenous factors influencing host-tumor balance (Wissler, R.W., Dao, T.L., and Wood, S., Jr., eds.), p. 149–166. Chicago: Chicago University Press 1967
507. Fisher, B., Fisher, E.R.: Biologic aspects of cancer-cell spread. In: Fifth National Cancer Conference Proceedings, p. 105–122. Philadelphia: J.B. Lippincott 1964
508. Zeidman, I.: Fate of circulating tumor cells. 3. Comparison of metastatic growth produced by tumor cell emboli in veins and lymphatics. Cancer Res. **25**, 324–327 (1965)
509. Zeidman, I.: Experimental studies on the spread of cancer in the lymphatic system. III. Tumor emboli in thoracic duct. The pathogenesis of Virchow's node. Cancer Res. **15**, 719–721 (1955)
510. Madden, R.E., Karpas, C.M.: Arrest of circulating tumor cells versus metastases formation. Arch. Surg. **94**, 307–312 (1967)
511. Wallach, D.F.H.: Cellular membranes and tumor behavior: a new hypothesis. Proc. nat. Acad. Sci. (Wash.) **61**, 868–874 (1968)
512. Wallach, D.F.H.: Generalized membrane defects in cancer. New Engl. J.Med. **280**, 761–767 (1969)
513. Halpern, B., Pejsachowicz, B., Febvre, J.L., Barski, G.: Differences in patterns of aggregation of malignant and non-malignant mammalian cells. Nature (Lond.) **209**, 157–159 (1966)
514. Loewenstein, W.R., Kanno, Y.: Intercellular communication and tissue growth. I. Cancerous growth. J. Cell Biol. **33**, 225–234 (1967)
515. Pollack, R.E., Teebor, G.W.: Relationship of contact inhibition to tumor transplantability, morphology, and growth rate. Cancer Res. **29**, 1770–1772 (1969)
516. Gasic, G., Baydak, T.: Adhesiveness of mucopolysaccharides to the surfaces of tumor cells and vascular endothelium. In: Biological interactions in normal and neoplastic growth (Brennan, M.J., and Simpson, W.L., eds.), p. 709–719. Boston: Little, Brown, and Co. 1962
517. Weiss, L., Sinks, L.F.: The electrokinetic surfaces of human cells of lymphoid origin and their ribonuclease susceptibility. Cancer Res. **30**, 90–94 (1970)
518. Wissler, R.W., Dao, T.L., Wood, S., Jr.: Endogenous factors influencing host-tumor balance. Chicago: Chicago University Press 1967
519. Kase, N., Cohn, G.L.: Clinical implications of extragonadal estrogen production. New Engl. J. Med. **276**, 28–31 (1967)
520. Faiman, C., Colwell, J.A., Ryan, R.J., Hershman, J.M., Shields, T.W.: Gonadotropin secretion from a bronchogenic carcinoma; demonstration by radioimmunoassay. New Engl. J. Med. **277**, 1395–1399 (1967)
521. Fusco, F.D., Rosen, S.W.: Gonadotropin-producing anaplastic large-cell carcinomas of the lung. New Engl. J. Med. **275**, 507–516 (1966)
522. Brown, W.H.: A case of pluriglandular syndrome. Lancet **1928 II**, 1022–1023
523. Steel, K., Baerg, R.D., Adams, D.O.: Cushing's syndrome in association with a carcinoid tumor of the lung. J. clin. Endocr. **27**, 1285–1289 (1967)
524. Mider, G.B.: Some aspects of nitrogen and energy metabolism in cancerous subjects: a review. Cancer Res. **11**, 821–829 (1951)
525. Mider, G.B., Tesluk, H., Morton, J.J.: Effects of Walker carcinoma 256 on food intake, body weight and nitrogen metabolism of growing rats. Unio Internat. Contra Cancrum Acta **6**, 409–420 (1948)
526. LePage, G.A., Potter, V.R., Busch, H., Heidelberger, C., Hurlbert, R.B.: Growth of carcinoma implants in fed and fasted rats. Cancer Res. **12**, 153–157 (1952)
527. Henderson, J.F., LePage, G.A.: Utilization of host purines by transplanted tumors. Cancer Res. **19**, 67–71 (1959)
528. Folkman, J.: Tumor angiogenesis: therapeutic implications. New Engl. J. Med. **285**, 1182–1186 (1971)
529. Folkman, J.: Anti-angiogenesis: New concept for therapy of solid tumors. Ann. Surg. **175**, 409–416 (1972)
530. Pierce, G.B.: Cellular heterogeneity of cancers. In: Chemical carcinogenesis (Ts'o, P.O.P. and DiPaolo, J.A., eds.), part B, p. 463–481. New York: Marcel Dekker, Inc. 1974
531. Pierce, G.B., Dixon, F.J., Jr.: Testicular teratomas. I. II. Cancer (Phila.) **12**, 573–589 (1959)
532. Friend, C., Scher, W., Holland, J.G., Sato, T.: Hemoglobin synthesis in murine virus-induced cells *in vitro*: stimulation of erythroid differentiation by dimethylsulfoxide. Proc. nat. Acad. Sci. (Wash.) **68**, 372 (1971)
533. Bendich, A., Borenfreund, E., Higgins, P.J., Sternberg, S.S., Stonehill, E.H.: Experimental approaches to problems in carcinogenesis. In: Chemical Carcinogenesis (Ts'o, P.O.P., and Di Paolo, J.A., eds.), part B, p. 515–530. New York: Marcel Dekker, Inc. 1974
534. Lynch, H.T.: Hereditary factors in carcinoma. In: Recent results in cancer research (Rentchnick, Geneve), vol. 12. Berlin-Heidelberg-New York: Springer 1967
535. Whang-Peng, J., Lee, E.C., Knutsen, T.A.: Genesis of the pH^1 chromosome. J. nat. Cancer Inst. **52**, 1035–1036 (1974)
536. Nandi, S., McGrath, C.M.: Mammary neoplasia in mice. In: Advances in cancer research (Klein, G., Weinhouse, S., and Haddow, A., eds.), vol. 17, p. 353–404. New York and London: Academic Press 1973
537. Hamilton, J.M.: Comparative aspects of mammary tumors. In: Advances in cancer research (Klein, G., Weinhouse, S., and Haddow, A., eds.), vol. 19, p. 1–38. New York and London: Academic Press 1974
538. Leung, B.S., Sasaki, G.H., Leung, J.S.: Estrogen-prolactin dependency in 7,12-dimethylbenz(a)-anthracene-induced tumors. Cancer Res. **35**, 621–627 (1975)
539. Smithline, F., Sherman, L., Kolodny, H.D.: Prolactin and breast carcinoma. New Engl. J. Med. **292**, 784–792 (1975)
540. Segaloff, A.: The role of the ovary in estrogen production of mammary cancer in the rat. Cancer Res. **34**, 2708–2710 (1974)
541. MacMahon, B., Cole, P., Brown, J.: Etiology of human breast cancer: a review. J. nat. Cancer Inst. **50**, 21–42 (1973)
542. Dao, T.L.: Nature of hormonal influence in carcinogenesis: studies *in vivo* and *in vitro*, in Chemical Carcinogenesis (Ts'o, P.O.P., and DiPaolo, J.A., eds.), part B, p. 503–514. New York: Marcel Dekker, Inc. 1974
543. Boylan, E.S., Wittliff, J.L.: Specific estrogen binding in rat mammary tumors induced by 7,12-dimethylbenz(a)anthracene. Cancer Res. **35**, 506–511 (1975)
544. Richards, J.E., Shyamala, G., Nandi, S.: Estrogen receptor in normal and neoplastic mouse mammary tissues. Cancer Res. **34**, 2764–2772 (1974)
545. Cutler, B.S., Forbes, A.P., Ingersoll, F.M., Scully, R.E.: Endometrial carcinoma after stilbestrol therapy in gonadal dysgenesis. New Engl. J. Med. **287**, 628–631 (1972)
546. Gerschenson, L.E., Berliner, J., Yang, J.J.: Diethylstilbesterol and progesterone regulation of cultured rabbit endometrial cell growth. Cancer Res. **34**, 2873–2880 (1974)
547. Sonnenschein, C., Weiller, S., Farookhi, R., Soto, A.M.: Characterization of an estrogen-sensitive cell line established from normal rat endometrium. Cancer Res. **34**, 3147–3154 (1974)

548. Jensen, E.V.: Estrogen binding and clinical response of breast cancer. In: Cancer medicine (Holland, J.F., Frei, E., III, eds.), p. 900–907. Philadelphia: Lea & Febiger 1973
549. Jensen, E.V.: Some newer endocrine aspects of breast cancer. New Engl. J. Med. **291**, 1252–1254 (1974)
550. Hähnel, R., Vivian, A.B.: Biochemical and clinical experience with the estimation of estrogen receptors in human breast carcinoma. In: Estrogen receptors in human breast cancer (McGuire, W.L., Carbone, P.P., and Vollmer, E.P., eds.), p. 205–245. New York: Raven Press 1975
551. Farrell, G.C., Joshua, D.E., Uren, R.F., Baird, P.J., Perkins, K.W., Kronenberg, H.: Androgen-induced hepatoma. Lancet **1975I**, 430–432
552. Herbst, A.L., Poskanzer, D.C., Robboy, S.J., Freidlander, L., Scully, R.E.: Prenatal exposure to stilbestrol. New Engl. J. Med. **292**, 334–339 (1975)
553. Ivanokovic, J.: Intrauterine induction of cancer by the experimental application of chemical substances (Grundman, G.E., ed.), vol. 44, p. 16–20. Berlin-Heidelberg-New York: Springer 1972
554. Lanier, A.P., Noller, K.L., Decker, D.G., Elveback, L.R., Kurland, L.T.: Cancer and stilbestrol. A follow-up of 1,719 persons exposed to estrogens in utero and born 1943–1959. Mayo Clin. Proc. **48**, 793–799 (1973)
555. Herndon, W.C.: Theory of carcinogenic activity of aromatic hydrocarbons. Trans. N.Y. Acad. Sci. **36**, 200–217 (1974)
556. Sims, P., Grover, P.L.: Epoxides in polycyclic aromatic hydrocarbon metabolism and carcinogenesis. In: Advances in cancer research (Klein, G., Weinhouse, S., and Haddow, A., eds.), vol. 20, p. 165–274. New York-San Francisco-London: Academic Press 1974
557. Baird, W.M., Harvey, R.G., Brookes, P.: Comparison of the cellular DNA-bound products of benzo(a)pyrene with the products formed by the reaction of benzo(a)pyrene-4,5-oxide with DNA. Cancer Res. **35**, 54–57 (1975)
558. Ts'o, P.O.P., Caspary, W.J., Cohen, B.I., Leavitt, J.C., Lesko, S.A., Jr., Lorentzen, R.J., Schechtman, L.M.: Basic mechanisms in polycyclic hydrocarbon carcinogenesis. In: Chemical carcinogenesis (Ts'o, P.O.P., and DiPaolo, J.A., eds.), part A, p. 113–147. New York: Marcel Dekker, Inc. 1974
559. Brookes, P., Baird, W.M., Dipple, A.: Interaction of the carcinogen 7-methylbenz(a)anthracene with DNA of mammalian cells. In: Chemical carcinogenesis (Ts'o, P.O.P., DiPaolo, J.A., eds.), part A, p. 149–157. New York: Marcel Dekker, Inc. 1974
560. Heidelberger, C.: *In vitro* studies on the role of epoxides in carcinogenic hydrocarbon activation. In: Topics in Chemical Carcinogenesis (Proceedings of the 2nd Internat. Symposium of the Princess Takamatsu Cancer Research Fund) (Nakahara, W., Takayama, S., Sugimura, T., and Odashima, S., eds.), p. 371–386. Baltimore: University Park Press 1972
561. Heidelberger, C.: Chemical oncogenesis in culture. In: Advances in cancer research (Klein, G., Weinhouse, S., and Haddow, A., eds.), vol. 18, p. 317–336. New York and London: Academic Press 1973
562. Nebert, D.W., Gielen, J.E.: Genetic regulation of aryl hydrocarbon hydroxylase induction in the mouse. Fed. Proc. **31**, 1315–1325 (1972)
563. Gurtoo, H.L., Bejba, N.: Hepatic microsomal mixed function oxygenase: enzyme multiplicity for the metabolism of carcinogens to DNA-binding metabolites. Biochem. biophys. Res. Commun. **61**, 685–692 (1974)
564. Rasmussen, R.E., Wang, I.Y.: Dependence of specific metabolism of benzo(a)pyrene on the inducer of hydroxylase activity. Cancer Res. **34**, 2290–2295 (1974)
565. Khandwala, A., Kasper, C.B.: Preferential induction of aryl hydroxylase activity in rat liver nuclear envelope by 3-methyl-cholanthrene. Biochem. biophys. Res. Commun. **54**, 1241–1246 (1973)
566. Bleecker, W., Capdevila, J., Agosin, M.: Sequential solubilization of microsomal mixed function oxidases. J. biol. Chem. **248**, 8474–8481 (1973)
567. Abramson, R.K., Hutton, J.J.: Effects of cigarette smoking on aryl hydrocarbon hydroxylase activity in lungs and tissues of inbred mice. Cancer Res. **35**, 23–29 (1975)
568. Weber, R.P., Coon, J.M., Triolo, A.J.: Nicotine inhibition of the metabolism of 3,4-benzopyrene, a carcinogen in tobacco smoke. Science **184**, 1081–1083 (1974)
569. Loub, W.D., Wattenberg, L.W., Davis, D.W.: Aryl hydrocarbon hydroxylase induction in rat tissues by naturally occurring indoles of cruciferous plants. J. nat. Cancer Inst. (in press)
570. Weber, R.P., Coon, J.M., Triolo, A.J.: Effect of the organophosphate insecticide parathion and its active metabolite paraoxon on the metabolism of benzo(a)pyrene in the rat. Cancer Res. **34**, 947–952 (1974)
571. Stoming, T.A., Bresnick, E.: Hepatic epoxide hydrase in neonatal and partially hepatectomized rats. Cancer Res. **34**, 2810–2813 (1974)
572. Jerina, D.M., Daly, J.W.: Arene oxides: a new aspect of drug metabolism. Science **185**, 573–582 (1974)
573. Owens, I.S., Akira, N., Nebert, D.W.: Expression of aryl hydrocarbon hydroxylase induction in liver- and hepatoma-derived cell cultures. In: Gene expression and carcinogenesis in cultured liver (Gerschenson, L.W., and Thompson, E.B., eds.), p. 378–401. New York-San Francisco-London: Academic Press, Inc. 1975
574. Belman, S., Troll, W.: Phorbol-12-myristate-13-acetate effect on cyclic adenosine 3′,5′-monophosphate levels in mouse skin and inhibition of phorbol-myristate-acetate-promoted tumorigenesis by theophylline. Cancer Res. **34**, 3446–3455 (1974)
575. Estensen, R.D., Hadden, J.W., Hadden, E.M., Touraine, F., Touraine, J.L., Haddox, M.K., Goldberg, N.D.: Phorbol myristate acetate: effects of a tumor promoter on intracellular cyclic GMP in mouse fibroblasts and as a mitogen on human lymphocytes. In: Control of proliferation in animal cells (Clarkson, B., and Baserga, R., eds.), p. 627–634. Cold Spring Harbor, N.Y.: Cold Spring Harbor Laboratory 1974
576. Kubinski, H., Strangstalien, M.A., Baird, W.M., Boutwell, R.F.: Interactions of phorbol esters with cellular membranes *in vitro*. Cancer Res. **33**, 3103–3107 (1973)
577. Berwald, Y., Sachs, L.: *In vitro* transformation of normal cells to tumor cells by carcinogenic hydrocarbons. J. nat. Cancer Inst. **35**, 641–661 (1965)
578. DiPaolo, J.A.: Quantitative aspects of *in vitro* chemical carcinogenesis. In: Chemical carcinogenesis (Ts'o, P.O.P., and DiPaolo, J.A., eds.), part B, p. 443–455. New York: Marcel Dekker, Inc. 1974
579. Marx, J.L.: Restriction enzymes: new tools for studying DNA. Science **180**, 482–485 (1973)
580. Commoner, B., Vithayathil, A.J., Henry, J.I.: Detection of metabolic carcinogen intermediates in urine of carcinogen-fed rats by means of bacterial mutagenesis. Nature (Lond.) **249**, 850–852 (1974)
581. Ames, B.N., Lee, F.D., Durston, W.E.: An improved bacterial test for the detection and classification of mutagens and carcinogens. Proc. nat. Acad. Sci. (Wash.) **70**, 782–786 (1973)
582. Kao, F.T.: Cell mutagenesis studies *in vitro* using auxotrophic markers. In: Chemical carcinogenesis (Ts'o, P.O.P. and DiPaolo, J.A., eds.), part B, p. 565–573. New York: Marcel Dekker, Inc. 1974
583. Malling, H.V., Chu, E.H.Y.: Development of mutational model systems for study of carcinogenesis. In: Chemical carcinogenesis (Ts'o, P.O.P. and Di Paolo, J.A., eds.), part B, p. 545–563. New York: Marcel Dekker, Inc. 1974
584. Violo, P.L.: Pathology of vinyl chloride. Med. Lavoro **60**, 174–180 (1970)
585. Smyth, H.F., Jr.: Improved communication—hygiene standards for daily inhalation. Amer. industr. Hyg. Ass. Quart. **17**, 129–185 (1956)
586. Marsteller, H.J., Lelbach, W.K., Müller, R., Jühe, S., Lange, C.E., Rohner, H.G., Veltman, G.: Chronisch-toxische Leberschäden bei Arbeitern in der PVC-Produktion. Dtsch. med. Wschr. **98**, 2311–2314 (1973)
587. Editorial: Vinyl chloride, P.V.C., and cancer. Lancet **1974I**, 1323–1324
588. Creech, J.L., Johnson, M.N.: Angiosarcoma of liver in the manufacture of polyvinyl chloride. J. occup. Med. **16**, 150–151 (1974)
589. Baum, J.K., Holtz, F., Bookstein, J.J., Klein, E.W.: Possible association between benign hepatomas and oral contraceptives. Lancet **1973II**, 926–929
590. Kelso, D.R.: Benign hepatomas and oral contraceptives. Lancet **1974I**, 315–316
591. Rothman, K., Keller, A.: The effect of joint exposure to alcohol and tobacco on risk of cancer of mouth and pharynx. J. chron. Dis. **25**, 711–716 (1972)
592. Dietzman, D., Horta-Barbosa, L.: Slow virus infections. In: Brenneman's practice of pediatrics, vol. 2, chap. 43. New York: Harper & Row, Publishers 1973
593. Field, E.J.: Slow virus infections of the nervous system. Int. Rev. exp. Path. **8**, 129–239 (1969)
594. Johnson, R.T., Johnson, K.P.: Slow and chronic virus infections of the nervous system. In: Recent advances in neurology (Plum, F., ed.), p. 33–78. Philadelphia: F.A. Davis Company 1969
595. Diener, T.O.: Viroids: the smallest known agents of infectious disease. Ann. Rev. Microbiol. **28**, 23–39 (1974)
596. Sambrook, J.: Transformation by polyoma virus and simian virus 40. In: Advances in cancer research (Klein, G., Weinhouse, S., and Haddow, A., eds.), vol. 16, p. 141–180. New York and London: Academic Press 1972
597. Shatkin, A.J.: Animal RNA viruses: genome structure and function. Ann. Rev. Biochem. **43**, 643–665 (1974)
598. Hill, M., Hillova, J.: RNA and DNA forms of the genetic material of C-type viruses and the integrated state of the DNA form in the cellular chromosome. Biochim. biophys. Acta (Amst.) **355**, 7–48 (1974)
599. Mangel, W.F., Delius, H., Duesberg, P.H.: Structure and molecular weight of the 60–70S RNA and the 30–40S RNA of the Rous sarcoma virus. Proc. nat. Acad. Sci. (Wash.) **71**, 4541–4545 (1974)
600. Bauer, H.: Virion and tumor cell antigens of C-type RNA tumor viruses. In: Advances in cancer research (Klein, G., Weinhouse, S., and Haddow, A., eds.), vol. 20, p. 275–341. New York-San Francisco-London: Academic Press 1974
601. Temin, H.M.: The cellular and molecular biology of RNA tumor viruses, especially avian leukosis-sarcoma viruses, and their relatives. In: Advances in cancer research (Klein, G., Weinhouse, S., Haddow, A., eds.), vol. 19, p. 47–104. New York-San Francisco-London: Academic Press 1974
602. Temin, H.M.: On the origin of the genes for neoplasia: G.H.A. Clowes memorial lecture. Cancer Res. **34**, 2835–2841 (1974)
603. Chattopadhyay, S.K., Lowy, D.R., Teich, N.M., Levine, A.S., Rowe, W.P.: Evidence that the AKR murine-leukemia-virus genome is com-

plete in DNA of the high-virus AKR mouse and incomplete in the DNA of the "virus-negative" NIH mouse. Proc. nat. Acad. Sci. **71**, 167–171 (1974)

604. Poiesz, B.J., Seal, G., Loeb, L.A.: Reverse transcriptase: correlation of zinc content with activity. Proc. nat. Acad. Sci. (Wash.) **71**, 4892–4896 (1974)
605. Gibson, W., Verma, I.M.: Studies on the reverse transcriptase of RNA tumor viruses. Structural relatedness of two subunits of avian RNA tumor viruses. Proc. nat. Acad. Sci. (Wash.) **71**, 4991–4994 (1974)
606. Sarin, P.S., Gallo, R.C.: RNA directed DNA polymerase. In: Biochemistry series one (Burton, K., ed.), vol. 6, p. 219–254. London: Butterworths; Baltimore: University Park Press 1974
607. Green, M., Gerard, G.F.: RNA-directed DNA polymerase—properties and functions in oncogenic RNA viruses and cells. In: Progress in nucleic acid research and molecular biology (Cohn, W.E., ed.), vol. 14, p. 187–334. New York and London: Academic Press 1974
608. Balda, B.R., Birkmayer, G.D.: Further evidence for viral etiology of human melanoma. Naturwissenschaften **60**, 304 (1973)
609. Spiegelman, S.: Molecular evidence for viral agents in human cancer and its chemotherapeutic consequences. Cancer Chemother. Rep. **58**, 595–613 (1974)
610. Schlom, J., Spiegelman, S.: Breast cancer: molecular probing for a viral etiology. In: Pathobiology annual (Ioachim, H.L., ed.), vol. 3, p. 269–290. New York: Appleton-Century-Crofts 1973
611. Atkinson, J.N.C., Galton, D.J., Gilbert, C.: Regulatory defect of glycolysis in human lipoma. Brit. med. J. **1974I**, 101–102
612. Hatanaka, M.: Transport of sugars in tumor cell membranes. Biochim. biophys. Acta (Amst.) **355**, 77–104 (1974)
613. Paoletti, C.A., Riou, G.: The mitochondrial DNA of malignant cells. In: Progress in molecular and subcellular biology (Hahn, F.E., ed.), vol. 3, p. 203–248. New York-Heidelberg-Berlin: Springer 1973
614. Storr, J.M., Burton, A.F.: The effects of arginine deficiency on lymphoma cells. Brit. J. Cancer **30**, 50–59 (1974)
615. Terz, J.J., Curutchet, P.: Analysis of the cell kinetics of human solid tumors: results following infusion of 3H thymidine. Presented at the Thirteenth Hanford Biology Symposium, "The Cell Cycle in Malignancy and Immunity," October, 1973
616. Terz, J.J., Curutchet, P., Lawrence, W.: Analysis of the cell kinetics of human solid tumors. Cancer (Philad.) **28**, 1100–1110 (1971)
617. Schumm, D.E., Webb, T.E.: Modified messenger ribonucleic acid release from isolated hepatic nuclei after inhibition of polyadenylate formation. Biochem. J. **139**, 191–196 (1974)
618. Schumm, D.E., Webb, T.E.: Transport of informosomes from isolated nuclei of regenerating rat liver. Biochem. biophys. Res. Commun. 1259–1265 (1972)
619. Cholon, J.J., Studzinski, G.P.: Metabolic differences between normal and neoplastic cells: effects of aminonucleoside on cytoplasmic messenger RNA. Science **18**, 160–161 (1974)
620. Shill, J.P., Neet, K.E.: Allosteric properties and the slow transition of yeast hexokinase. J. biol. Chem. **250**, 2259–2268 (1975)
621. Chakrabarti, U., Kenkare, U.W.: Dimerization of brain hexokinase induced by its regulatory glucose 6-phosphate. J. biol. Chem. **249**, 5984–5988 (1974)
622. Felig, P., Wahren, J.: Protein turnover and amino acid metabolism in the regulation of gluconeogenesis. Fed. Proc. **33**, 1092–1097 (1974)
623. Beneziale, C.M., Lohmar, P.H.: Gluconeogenesis in isolated hepatic parenchymal cells. J. biol. Chem. **248**, 7786–7791 (1973)
624. Magner, L.N., Kim, K.H.: Regulation of rat liver glycogen synthetase. J. biol. Chem. **248**, 2790–2795 (1973)
625. Kirsten, E.S., Watson, J.A.: Regulation of 3-hydroxy-3-methylglutaryl coenzyme A reductase in hepatoma tissue culture cells by serum lipoproteins. J. biol. Chem. **249**, 6104–6109 (1974)
626. Hoogenraad, N.J., Lee, D.C.: Effect of uridine on *de novo* pyrimidine biosynthesis in rat hepatoma cells in culture. J. biol. Chem. **249**, 2763–2768 (1974)
627. Bagnara, A.S., Letter, A.A., Henderson, J.F.: Multiple mechanisms of regulation of purine biosynthesis *de novo* in intact tumor cells. Biochim. biophys. Acta **374**, 259–270 (1974)
628. Green, C.D., Martin, D.W., Jr.: Characterization of a feedback-resistant phosphoribosylpyrophosphate synthetase from cultured, mutagenized hepatoma cells that overproduce purines. Proc. nat. Acad. Sci. (Wash.) **70**, 3698–3702 (1973)
629. Gaja, G., Cajone, F., Ferroro, M.E., Bernelli-Zazzera, A.: Anaerobic glycolysis and patterns of glycolytic intermediates during liver carcinogenesis and in hepatoma. J. nat. Cancer Inst. **44**, 1269–1280 (1970)
630. Gerschenson, L.E.: Hormonal effects on two rat liver cell lines cultured in chemically defined medium. In: Gene expression and carcinogenesis in cultured liver (Gerschenson, L.E. and Thompson, E.B., eds.), p. 220–231. New York-San Francisco-London: Academic Press, Inc. 1975
631. Gerschenson, L.E., Thompson, E.B.: Gene expression and carcinogenesis in cultured liver (Gerschenson, L.E. and Thompson, E.B., eds.), p. 1–491. New York-San Francisco-London: Academic Press, Inc. 1975
632. Pariza, M., Becher, J., Yager, J., Jr., Bonney, R., Potter, V.: Control of differentiation: induction of differentiation enzyme induction in primary cultures of rat liver parenchymal cells. In: Differentiation and control of malignancy of tumor cells (Nakahara, W., Ono, T., Sugimura, T., and Sugano, H., eds.), p. 267–285. Baltimore-London-Tokyo: University Park Press 1973
633. Stein, G.S., Spelsberg, T.C., Kleinsmith, L.J.: Nonhistone chromosomal proteins and gene regulation. Science **183**, 817–824 (1974)
634. Chae, C.B., Carter, D.B.: Degradation of chromosomal proteins during dissociation and reconstitution of chromatin. Biochem. biophys. Res. Commun. **57**, 740–746 (1974)
635. Gilmour, Stewart: The role of acidic proteins in gene regulation. In: Acidic proteins of the nucleus (Cameron, I.L. and Jeter, J.R., Jr., eds.), p. 297–315. New York-San Francisco-London: Academic Press 1974
636. Kleinsmith, L.J.: Acidic nuclear phosphoproteins. In: Acidic proteins of the nucleus (Cameron, I.L. and Jeter, J.R., Jr., eds.), p. 103–135. New York-San Francisco-London: Academic Press 1974
637. Bonner, J.: Molecular events in differentiation and de-differentiation. In: Chemical carcinogenesis (Ts'o, P.O.P. and DiPaolo, J.A., eds.), part p. 531–541. New York: Marcel Dekker, Inc. 1974
638. Silverman, B., Mirsky, A.E.: Addition of histones to histone-depleted nuclei: effect on template activity toward DNA and RNA polymerases. Proc. nat. Acad. Sci. (Wash.) **70**, 2637–2641 (1973)
639. Gourevitch, M., Puigdoménech, P., Cavé, Etienne, G., Méry, J., Parello, J.: Model studies in relation to the molecular structure of chromatin. Biochimie **56**, 967–985 (1974)
640. Van Lancker, J.L., Tomura, T.: Unpublished material
641. Augenlicht, L., Nicolini, C., Baserga, R.: Circular dichroism and thermal denaturation studies of chromatin and DNA from BrdU-treated mouse fibroblasts. Biochem. biophys. Res. Commun. **59**, 920–926 (1974)
642. Stein, G.S., Criss, W.E., Morris, H.P.: Properties of the genome in experimental hepatomas: variations in the composition of chromatin. Life Sci. **14**, 95–105 (1974)
643. Arnold, E.A., Buksas, M.M., Young, K.E.: A comparative study of some properties of chromatin from two "minimal deviation" hepatomas. Cancer Res. **33**, 1169–1176 (1973)
644. Kadohama, N., Turkington, R.W.: Altered populations of acidic chromatin proteins in breast cancer cells. Cancer Res. **33**, 1194–1201 (1973)
645. Davidson, R.L., de la Cruz, F.F.: Somatic cell hybridization (Davidson, R.L. and de la Cruz, F., eds.), p. 1–281. New York: Raven Press 1974
646. Pierce, G.B., Nakane, P., Mazurkiewicz, J.E.: Natural history of malignant stem cells. In: Differentiation and control of malignancy of tumor cells (Nakahara, W., Ono, T., Sugimura, T., and Sugano, H., eds.), p. 453–470. Baltimore-London-Tokyo: University Park Press 1973
647. Prasad, K.N., Sahu, K.C., Kumar, S.: Relationship between cyclic AMP level and differentiation of neuroblastoma cells in culture. In: Differentiation and control of malignancy of tumor cells (Nakahara, W., Ono, T., Sugimura, T., and Sugano, H., eds.), p. 287–310. Baltimore-London-Tokyo: University Park Press 1973
648. Bondy, S.C., Prasad, K.N., Purdy, J.L.: Neuroblastoma: drug-induced differentiation increases proportion of cytoplasmic RNA that contains polyadenylic acid. Science **186**, 359–361 (1974)
649. Gullino, P.M., Cho-Chung, Y.S., Losonczy, I., Grantham, F.H.: Increase of RNA synthesis during mammary tumor regression. Cancer Res. **34**, 751–757 (1974)
650. Hozumi, M., Sugiyama, K., Mura, M., Takizawa, H., Sugimura, T., Matsushima, T., Ichikawa, Y.: Factor(s) stimulating differentiation of mouse myeloid leukemia cells found in ascitic fluid. In: Differentiation and control of malignancy of tumor cells (Nakahara, W., Ono, T., Sugimura, T., and Sugano, H., eds.), p. 471–484. Baltimore-London-Tokyo: University Park Press 1973
651. Ostertag, W., Cole, T., Crozier, T., Gaedicke, G., Kind, J., Kluge, N., Krieg, J.C., Roesler, G., Steinheider, G., Weimann, B.J., Dube, S.K.: Viral involvement in the differentiation of erythroleukemic mouse and human cells. In: Differentiation and control of malignancy of tumor cells (Nakahara, W., Ono, T., Sugimura, T., and Sugano, H., eds.), p. 485–514. Baltimore-London-Tokyo: University Park Press 1973
652. Thompkins, G.: Specific enzyme production in eukaryotic cells. In: Advances in cell biology (Prescott, D., Goldstein, L., McConkey, E., eds.), vol. 2, p. 299–322. New York: Meredith Corporation 1971
653. Cellehrter, T.D.: Regulatory mechanism of enzyme synthesis. In: Enzyme induction (Parke, D.V., ed.), p. 165–199. New York-London: Plenum Press 1975
654. Ord, M.G., Stocken, L.A.: Further studies on phosphorylation and the thiol-disulphide ratio of histones in growth and development. Biochem. J. **112**, 81–89 (1969)
655. Mantal, M., Korenbrot, J.I.: Incorporation of rhodopsin proteolipid into bilayer membranes. Nature (New Biol) **246**, 219–221 (1973)
656. Mason, W.T., Fager, R.S., Abrahamson, E.W.: Ion fluxes in disk membranes of retinal rod outer segments. Nature (New Biol) **247**, 562–563 (1974)
657. Klein, G., Weinhouse, S.: Advances in cancer research (Klein, G., ed.), vol. 20. New York-San Francisco-London: Academic Press 1974
658. Pollack, R.E., Hough, P.V.C.: The cell surface and malignant transformation. In: Annual review of medicine (Creger, W.P., Coggins, C.H., Hancock, E.W., eds.), vol. 25, p. 431–446. California: Annual Reviews Inc. 1974
659. Hakomori, S.: Glycolipids of tumor cell membrane. In: Advances in cancer research (Klein, G., Weinhouse, S., Haddow, A., eds.), p. 265–315. New York-London: Academic Press 1973

660. Critchley, D.R.: Gycolipids and cancer in membrane mediated information. In: Biochemical function (Kent, P.W., ed.), vol. 1, p. 20–47. New York: American Elsevier Publishing Co., Inc. 1973
661. Spiro, R.G.: Glycoproteins: their biochemistry, biology and role in human disease. New Engl. J. Med. **281**, 1043–1056 (1969)
662. Verstraete, M., Vermylen, J., Collen, D.: Intravascular coagulation in liver disease. In: Annual review of medicine (Creger, W.P., Coggins, C.H., Hancock, E.W., eds.), vol. 25, p. 447–455. California: Annual Reviews Inc. 1974
663. Inbar, M., Sachs, L.: Interaction of the carbohydrate-binding protein concanavalin A with normal and transformed cells. Proc. national Acad. Sci. **63**, 1418–1425 (1969)
664. Roberts, E., Simonson, D.G.: Free amino acids and related substances in normal and neoplastic tissues. In: Amino acids, proteins, and cancer biochemistry (Edsall, J.T., ed.), p. 121–145. New York: Academic Press, Inc. 1960
665. Moyer, G.H., Pitot, H.C.: Static and dynamic aspects of amino acid pools in rat liver and Morris hepatomas 9618A and 7800. Cancer Res. **34**, 2647–2653 (1974)
666. Lawson, D., Woon, K.P., Morris, H.P., Weinhouse, S.: Carbamyl phosphate synthetases in rat liver neoplasms. Cancer Res. **35**, 156–163 (1975)
667. Rothschild, K.J., Stanley, H.E.: Model of ionic transport in biological membranes. In: Ninth Annual ASCP Research Symposium on Cell Membranes and Disease; Genes, Viruses, Hormones and the Immune Response. Amer. J. clin. Path. **63**, 695–713 (1975)
668. Rosenthal, P.N., Robinson, H.L., Robinson, W.S., Hanafusa, T., Hanafusa, H.: DNA in uninfected and virus-infected cells complementary to avian tumor virus RNA. Proc. nat. Acad. Sci. **68**, 2336–2340 (1971)
669. Karasaki, S.: Subcellular localization of surface adenosine triphosphatase activity in preneoplastic liver parenchyma. Cancer Res. **32**, 1703–1712 (1972)
670. Zucker, S., Howe, D.M., Weintraub, L.R.: Bone marrow response to erythropoietin in polycythemia vera and chronic granulocytic leukemia. Blood **39**, 341 (1972)
671. Greenblatt, M., Warren, B.A., Kommineni, V.R.: Tumour angiogenesis: ultrastructure of endothelial cells in mitosis. Brit. J. exp. Path. **53**, 216–224 (1972)
672. Hellström, K.E., Hellström, I.: Immunological enhancement as studied by cell culture techniques. Ann. Rev. Microbiol. **24**, 373–398 (1970)
673. Hellström, K.E., Hellström, I.: Some aspects of the immune defense against cancer, I & II. Cancer (Philad.) **28**, 1266–1271 (1971)
674. Baldwin, R.W.: Immunological aspects of chemical carcinogenesis. In: Advances in cancer research (Klein, G., Weinhouse, S., Haddow, A., eds.), vol. 18, p. 1–75. New York-London: Academic Press 1973
675. Rubin, B.A.: Alteration of the homograft response as a determinant of carcinogenicity. In: Progr. exp. tumor res. 14 (Homburger, F., ed.), p. 138–195. Basel: S. Karger 1971
676. Kitagawa, M., Yamamura, Y.: Cancer immunology, surveillance and specific recognition of tumor antigen (Kitagawa, M., Yamamura, Y., eds.), No. 16. Baltimore-London-Tokyo: University Park Press 1974
677. Kopf, A.W.: Host defenses against malignant melanoma. Hosp. Pract. 116–124 (1971)
678. Morton, D.L., Eibler, F.R., Malmgren, R.A., Wood, W.C.: Immunological factors which influence response to immunotherapy in malignant melanoma. Surgery **68**, 158–164 (1970)
679. Smith, J.L., Stehlin, J.S.: Spontaneous regression of primary malignant melanomas with reginal metastases. Cancer (Philad.) **18**, 1399–1415 (1965)
680. Golub, S.H., O'Connell, T.X., Morton, D.L.: Correlation of in vivo and in vitro assays of immunocompetence in cancer patients. Cancer Res. **34**, 1833–1837 (1974)
681. Gross, R.L., Latty, A., William, E.A., Newberne, P.M.: Abnormal spontaneous rosette formation and rosette inhibition in lung carcinoma. New Engl. J. Med. **292**, 439–443 (1975)
682. Jehn, U.W., Nathanson, L., Schwartz, R.S., Skinner, M.: In vitro lymphocyte stimulation by a soluble antigen from malignant melanoma. New Engl. J. Med. **283**, 329–341 (1970)
683. Smith, R.T.: Possibilities and problems of immunologic intervention in cancer. New Engl. J. Med. **287**, 439–450 (1972)
684. Bast, R.C., Zbar, B., Borsos, T., Rapp, H.: BCG and cancer. New Engl. J. Med. **290**, 1413–1420 (1974)
685. Grant, R.M., Cochran, A.J., Hoyle, D., Mackie, R., Murray, E.L., Ross, C.: Results of administering B.C.G. to patients with melanoma. Lancet **1974II**, 1096–1100
686. Kaliss, N.: Immunological enhancement. Int. Rev. exp. Path. **8**, 241–276 (1969)
687. Vaage, J., Doroshow, J.H., DuBois, T.T.: Radiation-induced changes in established tumor immunity. Cancer Res. **34**, 129–134 (1974)
688. Onóe, T., Dempo, K., Kaneko, A., Watabe, H.: Significance of α-fetoprotein appearance in the early stage of azo-dye carcinogenesis. In: Alpha-fetoprotein and hepatoma (Hirai, H., Miyaji, T., eds.), No. 14, p. 233–247. Baltimore-London-Tokyo: Univ. Park Press 1973
689. Kitagawa, T., Yokochi, T., Sugano, H.: α-fetoprotein and hepatocarcinogenesis in rats. In: Alpha-fetoprotein and hepatoma (Hirai, H., Miyaji, T., eds.), No. 14, p. 249–268. Baltimore-London-Tokyo: University Park Press 1973
690. Shikata, T., Skakibara, K.: Relationship between α-fetoprotein and histological patterns of hepatoma, and localization of α-fetoprotein in hepatoma cells using the peroxidase antibody technique. In: Alphafetoprotein and hepatoma (Hirai, H., Miyaji, T., eds.), No. 14, p. 269–277. Baltimore-London-Tokyo: University Park Press 1973
691. Sell, S., Nichols, M., Becker, F.F., Leffert, H.L.: Hepatocyte proliferation and α_1-fetoprotein in pregnant, neonatal, and partially hepatectomized rats. Cancer Res. **34**, 865–871 (1974)
692. Becker, F., Sell, S.: Early elevation of α_1-fetoprotein in N-2-fluorenylacetamide hepatocarcinogenesis. Cancer Res. **34**, 2489–2494 (1974)
693. Banwo, O., Versey, J., Hobbs, J.R.: New oncofetal antigen for human pancreas. Lancet **1974I**, 643–645
694. Gold, P.: Tumor-specific antigen in GI cancer. Hosp. Pract. 79–88 (1972)
695. Eveleigh, J.W.: Heterogeneity of carcinoembryonic antigen. Cancer Res. **34**, 2122–2124 (1974)
696. Dhar, P., Moore, T.L., Zamcheck, N., Kupchik, H.Z.: Carcinoembryonic antigen (CEA) in colonic cancer. J. Amer. med. Ass. **221**, 31–35 (1972)
697. Livingstone, A.S., Hampson, L.G., Shuster, J., Gold, P., Hinchey, E.J.: Carcinoembryonic antigen in the diagnosis and management of colorectal carcinoma: current status. Arch. Surg. **190**, 259–264 (1974)
698. Zamcheck, N., Kupchik, H.Z.: The interdependence of clinical investigations and methodological development in the early evolution of assays for carcinoembryonic antigen. Cancer Res. **34**, 2131–2136 (1974)
699. Zamcheck, N.: Carcinoembryonic antigen: quantitative variations in circulating levels in benign and malignant digestive track diseases. In: Advances in internal medicine (Stollerman, G.H., ed.), vol. 19, p. 413–433. Chicago: Year Book Med. Pub. 1974
700. Holyoke, D., Reynoso, G., Chu, T.M.: Carcinoembryonic antigen (CEA) in patients with carcinoma of the digestive tract. Ann. Surg. **176**, 559–564 (1972)
701. Ravry, M., Moertel, C.G., Schutt, A.J., Go, V.L.W.: Usefulness of serial serum carcinoembryonic antigen (CEA) determinations during anti-cancer therapy or long-term follow-up of gastrointestinal carcinoma. Cancer (Philad.) **34**, 1230–1234 (1974)
702. Burnet, F.M.: The evolution of bodily defence. Med. J. Austr. **1963II**, 817–821
703. Prehn, R.T.: Immunosurveillance, regeneration and oncogenesis. In: Progress in experimental tumor research (Homburger, F., ed.), vol. 14, p. 1–24. Basel: S. Karger 1971
704. Thomas, L.: Discussion, Reaction to homologous tissue antigens. In: Cellular and humoral aspects of the hypersensitive state (Lawrence, H.S., ed.), p. 529–532. New York: Hoeber 1959
705. Coggin, J.H., Ambrose, K.R., Eierlam, P.J., Anderson, N.: Proposed mechanisms by which autochthonous neoplasms escape immune rejection. Cancer Res. **34**, 2092–2101 (1974)
706. Glascow, A.H., Nimberg, R.B., Menzoian, J.O., Saporoschetz, I., Cooperband, S.R., Schmid, K., Mannick, J.A.: Association of anergy with an immunosuppressive peptide fraction in the serum of patients with cancer. New Engl. J. Med. **291**, 1263–1267 (1974)
707. Hyman, R.: Genetic alterations in tumor cells resulting in their escape from the immune response. Cancer Chemother. Repts, Part I, **58**, No. 4, 431–439 (1974)
708. DeLucia, P., Cairns, J.: Isolation of an *E. coli* strain with a mutation affecting DNA polymerase. Nature (Lond.) **224**, 1164–1166 (1969)
709. Gross, J., Gross, M.: Genetic analysis of an *E. coli* strain with a mutation affecting DNA polymerase. Nature (Lond.) **224**, 1166–1168 (1969)

Subject Index

Abetalipoproteinemia II 711
Abscesses I 282
Acatalasia I 163
Accelerated globulin deficiency I 407
Acetaldehyde II 644
Acetamide, Drug induced hemolytic anemia I 170
Acetonuria in galactosemia I 167
Acetylaminofluorene metabolism II 980
Acetyl-CoA carboxylase I 60
Acetoacetyl-CoA I 54
Acetyl-CoA I 54
Acetyl-CoA carboxylase I 278
Acetyl-CoA-ACP transacylase I 62
Acetylcholine I 260
Acetylcholine receptors I 528
Acid base I 570
— Acetic acid I 570
— Hydronium ion, I 571
— Muriatic acid I 570, 571
— Natron I 570
— Potash I 570
— Sulfuric acid I 570
Acid phosphatase II 937
— Gaucher's disease I 193
Acidosis I 574
— Albright's disease I 575
— Lung I 576
— Metabolic I 574
— Proximal tubular I 576
— Tubular I 575
Aconitase I 29
— Mechanism of action I 30
Acrodermatitis enteropathica I 252
2-Acroleyl-3-amino-fumarate I 272
Acromegaly I 426
— Diabetes I 431
— Glucose tolerance I 431
— Gonadal function I 431
— Eosinophilic adenoma I 429
— Lactogenic effect I 431
— Osteoporosis I 432
ACTH I 530
— Corticotropin-releasing factor (CRF) I 475
— Covalent structure I 472
— Humoral feedback I 475
— Metabolic effect I 476
— — Adenosine cyclic phosphate I 476
— — Adenyl cyclase I 476
— — Corticosteroidgenesis I 476
— — Cyclic adenylate I 476
— — Lipogenesis I 476
— — Urea formation I 476
— Properties I 471
— Release I 475
— — Adrenal weight, effect of hypophysis I 475
— Secretion control, median eminence I 475
— — Releasing hormones I 474
— — Hypothalamic nuclei I 474
— — Portal system of the hypophysis I 473
Actinomycin D II 615
Active carcinogens II 982
Adenine I 210
Adenosine triphosphatase, nucleus I 83
Adenyl cyclase I 455, 529, 530
5'-Adenylic phosphatase, nucleus I 83
Addison's disease I 565, 559
— Azotemia I 565
— Electrolyte I 565
— Hyperpigmentation I 565, 566
— Hypertension I 565
— Ketosteroids I 566
Adiposogenital dystrophy I 433
Adrenal adenoma, virilizing I 494
Adrenal carcinoma I 494
Adrenal cortex I 458
— Anatomy I 458
— Embryonic development I 459
— Fascicularis I 459
— Glomerulosa I 459
— Histophysiology I 459
— — x-zone I 460
— Reticularis I 459
— Spongiocytes I 459
— Sympathogonia I 459
Adrenal deficiency I 277
Adrenals I 282
Adrenocortical hormones I 460
— Glucocorticoid I 460
— Mineralocorticoid I 460
Adrenogenital syndrome I 493
— Hyperpigmentation I 493
— Hypertension I 493
— Virilism I 493
Afibrinogenemia I 420
Aflatoxin II 983, 994
Agammaglobulinemia I 159
Aging, cholesteryl esters in arteriosclerosis II 683
Alanine RNA I 110
Alanine tRNA base sequence I 111
Albers-Schönberg disease I 358
Albinism I 178
— Melanin I 178
— Melanocyte I 178
— Tyrosinase I 178
Albumin I 158
Alcohol I 208
— α-aminolevulinic dehydrase II 650
— Congeners II 642
Alcohol and diet II 643
Alcohol and drugs II 650
Alcohol dehydrogenase I 311, II 642
Alcohol metabolism II 642, 646
— Acetaldehyde II 642, 644
— Catalase II 643
— Fatty acid shuttle II 644
— Fatty acid synthesis II 646
— α-glycerophosphate shuttle II 644
— Malate aspartate II 644
— Malate citrate shuttle II 644
— Mitochondria II 642, 646
— Mixed function oxidase II 643
— NADH/NAD ratios II 644
— Neurological adaptation II 643
— Smooth endoplasmic reticulum II 647
— Transhydrogenase II 644
— Triglyceride oxidation II 646
Alcoholism I 266, 382
— Bronchiectasis II 648
— Deterioration II 650
— Fatty cyst II 647
— Intoxication II 650
— Mallory bodies II 647
— Myocardial disease II 649
— Myopathy II 649
— Pulmonary emphysema II 648
— Pulmonary fibrosis II 648
— Vitamin B1 I 266
Aldolase, nucleus I 80
Aldosterone I 554
— ACTH I 557
— Addison's disease I 559
— Atrial receptors I 556
— Blood volume I 555
— Cardiac failure I 555
— Cirrhosis I 555
— Glomerulosa cells I 554
— Mode of action I 559
— Potassium I 555
— Receptor I 560
— Secretion I 555
— Stretch receptor I 556
Aldosteronism I 562
— Baroreceptors I 563
— Blood volume I 564
— Hypernatremia I 563
— Hypertension I 562, 564
— Hypokalemia I 563, 564
— Osmoreceptors I 563
— Primary I 562
— Secondary I 563
Aleutian mink disease II 1009
Alkaline phosphatase I 340; II 937
Alkalosis I 581
— Metabolic I 574
— Respiratory I 582
Alkaptonuria I 177
— Articular cartilages I 178
Allergic encephalitis II 668
Allergic granulomatous, angiitis II 879
Alloisoleucine in maple syrup disease I 181
Allopurinol I 224
Alloxan I 211
— Diabetes I 514

Alloxan, Diabetic rats I 513
Alloxantin I 211
Alpha-Amanitin I 120
Alzheimer cells I 160
Alzheimer's disease II 662
— Neurofibril densification II 662
α-Amanitine II 615
Amino acid I 149, 587
— Concentration in muscle I 283
— Decarboxylation I 300
— Excretion I 546
— Ketogenic I 589
— Metabolism
— — Ammonium acetate administration II 1034
— — Fluoroacetate administration II 1034
— — In hypoglycemia II 1034
— Liver I 585
— — Mitochondrial infarct II 1034
— — Transport I 585
— — — Cystinuria I 585
— — — Hartnup disease I 585
— — — Pyridoxal phosphate I 585
Amino acid acetylation I 587
— Phenylacetylglutamine I 588
Amino acid activation I 107
Amino acid code I 115
— Amber mutation I 118
— Nonsense codon I 118
— Ocre mutation I 118
— Punctuation codons I 118
— Termination codons I 118
— Tobacco mosaic virus I 107
— Tryptophan synthetase I 118
D-Amino acid oxidase I 36
L-Amino acid oxidase I 36
Amino acyl RNA synthetase I 108
δ-amino levulinic acid I 203
δ-amino levulinic acid dehydrase I 203
δ-amino levulinic acid synthetase I 203, 208
— Porphyria I 209
Aminopterin I 227
D-amino oxidation I 301
Aminoaciduria in galactosemia I 167
Aminopeptidase II 937
α-aminolevulinic dehydrase II 650
6-aminopurine I 210
Ammonia I 573
— Glutaminase I 573
— Glutamine I 573
— Secretion I 573
Amiphipatic protein II 1078
Amniocentesis I 241
Amylases I 503
— Calcium I 503
Amyloid fibrils II 660
Amyloidosis II 655
— Diabetes II 659
— Experimental II 659
— — Amyloid fibrils II 659
— — Bacteria II 658, 659
— — Casein diet II 659
— — Chondroitin sulfate II 659
— — γ-globulin II 659
— Heart II 656
— Hodgkin's disease II 659
— Immunoblasts II 660
— Kidney II 656, 657
— Leprosy II 659
— Liver II 656, 658
— Myxedema II 659
— Pathogenesis II 658
— — Plasmocytosis II 659
— Pathological anatomy II 655
— Primary II 655
— Secondary II 655
— Spleen II 656
— TB II 659
Amyotrophic lateral sclerosis II 672
Amytal I 50, 52
Anaphase I 87
Anaphylaxis II 834
Anderson's disease, see Glycogen storage disease I 166
Anemia I 264
— Hemolytic I 391
— Thalassemia I 157
Anephrotensin I 478
Anesthetics I 550
Angina pectoris II 697, 705
Angiotensin, Dipeptidyl carboxypeptidase I 558
Angiotensin II
— Arterioles I 558
— Blood pressure I 559
— Cyclic AMP I 599
— Epinephrine I 558
— Zona glomerulosa I 558
Angiotensinogen I 557
Aniline derivatives II 983
— Naphthylamine II 984
— 2-Naphthylhydroxylamine II 984
Antemortem I 417
Anterior poliomyelitis II 672
Antibodies II 805
— Age II 816
— Antigen-binding sites II 807
— Blood levels II 816
— Constant segment II 807
— C region II 819
— Cytotoxic II 833
— — Membrane II 833
— Cytotropic II 832
— — Bradykinin II 833
— — Cyclic AMP II 833
— — Degranulation II 833
— — Eosinophilia II 833
— — Histamine II 833
— — Pausnitz-Kustner reaction II 832
— — Reagin II 832
— — Serotonin II 833
— Domains II 807
— Fa fraction II 807
— Fc fraction II 807
— Fa fragment II 805
— Fc fragment II 805
— Gamma globulins II 805
— Heavy chain II 806
— Heredity II 816
— Host II 816
— IgA II 805
— IgD II 805
— IgE II 805
— IgG II 805
— IgM II 805
— γ-chain II 806
— j-chain II 819
— K chain II 806
— K type II 806
— L type II 806
— Light chain II 806
— Molecular structure II 807
— Synthesis II 817
— — Somatic mutation II 817
— — Template theory II 817
— Variable segment II 807
— V region II 819
Antigens II 805, 808
— Administration II 817
— Antibody reaction II 812
— — Agglutinins II 812
— — Hemolysins II 812
— — Precipitins II 812
— Determinants II 808
— — Conformational II 809
— — Sequential II 809
— Haptenes II 808
Anoxia I 542
Antimycin I 43
Antimycin A I 40
α_1-Antitrypsin deficiency II 633
— Chronic obstructive lung disease II 633
— Cirrhosis of the liver II 633
Apatite crystals I 336
Apoferritin synthesis I 364
Apoproteins II 688
— ApoA-II II 688
— ApoB II 688
— ApoC II 688
— ApoC-I II 688
— ApoC-III II 688
— Apo HCL II 688
— Chylomicrons II 689
Apotranscarboxylase I 280
Arachidonic acid II 639
Arginase, nucleus I 84
Arthus reaction II 836
— Pathology II 836
— Systemic II 836
Aromatic amino acids I 173
— Intermediary metabolism I 173
— — Pathology I 173
Arteries II 679
— Biochemistry II 679
— — Enzymes II 680
— — Glucose-6-phosphate dehydrogenase II 680
— — Glyolysis II 680
— — Hydrolases II 680
— — Polysaccharide II 680
— Caveolae II 679
— Desmosomes II 679
— Endothelium II 679
— Lathyrism II 679
— Media II 679
— Morphology II 679
— Regeneration II 680
— — Copper deficiency II 681
— — Freezing II 681
— — Thrombi II 681
Arteriosclerosis I 369
— Blood lipids II 701
— — HDL II 701
— — α-lipoprotein II 701
— Cholesterol levels II 697
— Cortisone II 699
— Cushing's syndrome II 699
— Diet II 697
— Disease II 697
— Epidemiology II 697
— Estrogen II 698
— Experimental II 700
— — Irradiation II 701
— Fatty acid essential II 697
— Hemodynamic factors II 702
— Heredity II 697
— Hormones II 697
— Hypothyroidism II 698
— Insulin II 699
— Myocardial infarct II 701
— Nicotinic acid II 698
— Origin of lipids II 702
— Pathogenesis II 697, 709
— Pyridoxine deficiency II 698
— Triac II 699
Articular cartilages in alkaptonuria I 178

Astrocytes II 663
Aschoff body II 869
Ascobic acid I 24, 25, 281
– in Phenylketonuria I 174, 175
Aspartic acid oxidase I 36
Astrocyte II 663
– Blood-brain barrier II 663
– Clasmatodendrosis II 663
– Dendrophagia II 663
– Fibrous II 663
– Protoplasmic II 663
– Sucker feet II 663
Astrocytosis II 663
Astrogliosis II 663
Atherosclerosis I 303, 326; II 679
– Angina pectoris II 705
– Brain infarct II 708
– Cerebral hemorrhage II 708
– Consequences II 705
– Coronary occlusion II 705
– Diabetes II 700
– Edema II 681
– Electrocardiographic findings II 707
– Elementary lesions II 681
– Embolism II 707
– Encephalomalacia II 708
– Endothelial injuries II 682
– Esterification of cholesterol II 704
– Fat metabolism II 685
– Fibrosis II 683
– – Copper deficiency II 683
– Hemodialysis II 700
– Lipid accumulation II 683
– – Free cholesterol II 683
– – Cholesteryl esters II 683
– – Cholesteryl oleate II 683
– – Lecithin II 683
– – Sphingomyelin II 683
– Myocardial infarct II 705
– Myxedema II 700
– Nephrosis II 700
– Polyol metabolism II 682
– Smooth muscle proliferation II 683
– Smoking II 700
– Sphingomyelin II 705
– Stress II 700
– Thrombosis II 684
– Thrombus II 707
ATP-ADP exchange reaction I 52
ATP lyase I 61
ATP-$^{32}P_i$ exchange I 52
ATPase release I 52
Atrial receptor I 556
Autoimmune disease II 870
– Acquired hemophilia II 870
– Allergic granulomatous angiitis II 879
– Fibrinoid necrosis II 879
– Hemolytic anemia II 870
– Hypersensitivity angiitis II 879
– Immunological neutropenia II 870
– Immunological thrombocytic purpura II 870
– Immunologic vasculitis II 878
– Lupus erythematosus II 871
– Polyarteritis nodosa II 878
– Polymyositis II 881
– Rheumatoid arthritis II 875
– Sarcoidosis II 880
– Scleroderma II 881
– Thyroiditis II 870
– – Hashimoto's disease II 870
– Wegener's granulomatosis II 879
Autoimmune thyroiditis, Askanazy cells II 870
Autoimmunity II 671
Autolysis I 610

Avian leukosis viruses II 1010
– Lymphomatosis II 1010
– Rous sarcoma II 1011
Avidin I 278
Azaserine, purine metabolism I 214
Axon II 664
– Degeneration II 668
Axoplasm II 664
Azauracil I 226
Azide I 52
Azo derivatives II 977
– Amination II 977
– Aminoazotoluene II 977
– Amino-4-azobenzene II 977
– Changes in liver cells II 979
– – Basophilia II 979
– – Hyaline bodies II 979
– – Mitochondria II 979
– Demethylation II 978
– Halogenation II 977
– Hydroxylation II 977
– Methylation II 977
– Protein binding II 978
– – H_25S protein II 978
Azobenzene II 977
Azonaphthalene II 977
– α-α-azonaphthalene II 977
– β-β-azonaphthalene II 977

B cells II 824
– Antigen recognition II 825
– Receptors II 825
Bacterial transformation I 94
Bacteriophage I 96; II 997
– Fate I 96
Bacteriostatic agents II 788
– Cationic proteins II 788
– H_2O_2, II 788
– Lactic acid II 788
– Myeloperoxidase II 788
– Phagocytin II 788
Balanced Polymorphism I 149
– Drug induced hemolytic anemia I 170
Barbiturates I 24
Basal cell carcinoma II 1100
Basement membranes II 861, 930
Behinic acid I 195
Benamid I 224
Bence Jones proteins II 806
Benzoquinoacetic acid and methemoglobinemia I 157
Beriberi II 266, 268
– Adenosine-5′-phosphatase I 270
– Cerebellar ataxis I 270
– Clinicopathological aspects I 267
– Demyelination I 267
– Edema I 266
– Hyperoxaluria I 270
– α-ketoglutarate decarboxylase I 270
– Lactic acid I 268
– Oxythiamine I 267
– Pathogenesis I 268
– Polyneuritis I 266
– Pyrithiamine I 267
– Pyruvemia I 269
Pyruvic acid I 268, 269
– Pyruvic decarboxylase I 269, 270
– Thiaminase I 267
– Transketolase I 270
– Vitamin B1 I 266
Bicarbonate absorption I 573
Biguanides I 508
Bilirubin I 385
– Glucuronide I 387
– Glucuronyl transferase I 387

– Direct van den Bergh reaction I 387
– Excretion I 387
– Hemolytic jaundice I 387
– Indirect van den Bergh reaction I 387
– Metabolism I 388
– Transport I 385
– UDP-glucuronic acid I 387
Biocytin I 279
Biotin I 31
– Acetyl CoA carboxylase I 278
– Biocytin I 279
– Biotinidase I 279
– Deficiency I 278
– – Avidin I 278
– – Methylmalonyl I 278
– Mitochondria I 278
– Propionyl CoA I 278
– – Carboxylase I 278
Biotinidase I 279
Bile acids I 596; II 685
– Cholestasis I 596
– Cholecystolithiasis I 596
– Cholic acid formation I 596
– Conjugation, Glycine I 597
– – Taurine I 597
– Disease I 597
– Intestinal bypass I 599
– Metabolism I 598
– Primary I 596
– Secondary I 596
Bile duct I 599
– Cholecystokinin I 599
– Cystic duct I 599
Bile pigment I 385
– Bilirubin I 385
– Hemoglobin breakdown I 385
– Metabolism I 385
– Protoporphyrin breakdown I 386
Bittner virus II 1012, 1017
Bladder cancer II 1100
Blocking antibodies II 1103
Blocking antigens II 1103
Blood brain barrier I 389
Blood coagulation I 396
– Antihemophilic globulin I 399
– Autoprothrombin I-C I 401
– Autoprothrombin III I 401
– Factor V I 401
– Factor VII I 400
– Factor X I 401
– Factor XIII deficiency I 408
– Fibrin I 399, 405
– Fibrinogen I 399, 404
– Fibrinolysis I 413
– Fibrinopenia I 408
– Hageman factor I 400
– – Deficiency I 408
– Idiopathic thrombocytopenia I 412
– Inactive plasma, thromboplastin component I 401
– Plasma-accelerating globulin I 399
– Plasma AC globulin I 399
– Platelets I 409
– – Viscous metamorphosis I 401
– Prothrombin I 401
– – Deficiencies I 408
– Prothromboplastin I 399
– Stuart-Prower factor I 400
– Symptomatic thrombocytopenia purpura I 412
– Theory I 399
– Thrombin I 399, 401, 402
– Thrombocytopenic purpura, neonatal I 413
– Thromboplastin I 399, 400

Blood coagulation, Thromboplastin antecedent I 400
— Thromboplastin component deficiency I 408
— Thromboplastin extrinsic formation I 400
— Thromboplastin intrinsic formation I 400
— Tissue factors I 400
— Vascular factors I 413
— Vitamin K I 399
— — Deficiency I 409
Blood groups II 840
— A group II 841
— ABO system II 841
— B group II 841
— Cancer II 842
— Coombs' reaction II 841
— Globosides II 842
— H gene II 842
— Incompatibility, newborn II 843
— O group II 841
— Rh group II 841
— Rh system II 843
— Transfusion II 842
— Trophoblast II 842
Blood leukocyte, purine metabolism I 216
Blood lipids II 689
Blood pH I 574
— Acidosis I 574
— Alkalosis I 574
— Respiration I 574
Blood platelets, viscous metamorphosis I 401
Blood pressure I 543, 559
Blood volume I 555, 557
Bloom syndrome II 732
Body fluids I 539
— Donnan equilibrium I 539
— Electrolytes I 539
— Extracellular I 539
— Intracellular I 539
Bone atrophy I 351
Bone growth I 307
Bone marrow hyperplasia and thalassemia I 157
Bone marrow, purine metabolism I 216
Bone metabolism I 334
Bone resorption I 352
Bouyant density I 66
Bradykinin I 319; II 771, 833
— Amino acid sequence II 772
— Bradykininogen II 773
— Shock II 773
Bragg's equation I 337
Brain I 514
— Tay-Sachs disease I 186, 187, 188
Branched amino acids in maple syrup disease I 181
Breast cancer II 1012, 1016, 1100
— Cystic hyperplasia II 961
— Dialyzable inhibitor II 1012
— Estrogens II 959, 961
— Menopause II 961
— Methylcholanthrene II 960
— Nursing II 961
— Precancerous lesions II 961
— Prolactin II 960
— Thyroid function II 961
— Tumor inducing factors II 1012
— Tumor inhibiting factors II 1012
Bregen-Moloney virus II 1012
Bronchiectasis II 648
Burkitt's lymphoma II 1100
Burkitt's sarcoma II 1025
Butyryl dehydrogenase I 55
Caffeine I 210
Calcitonin I 356, 562
— Albers-Schönberg disease I 358
— Amino acid sequence I 356
— C cells I 357
— Calcium, intestinal absorption I 358
— Calcium, resorption I 358
— Hypocalcemia I 357
— Osteoporosis I 358
— Receptors I 358
— Thyroid carcinoma I 358
— Thyrocalcitonin I 356
Calcium I 333
— Excretion I 334
— Hormone action I 532
— Intestinal absorption I 343
— Mitochondria I 532
— Resorption I 358
— Serum I 333
— Sources I 333
— — Food I 333
— — Milk I 333
Calcium absorption I, 333 358
— Bile salt I 333
— Carrier protein I 333
Calcium metabolism, skeleton I 333
Cancer II 937
— Adrenals II 964
— — ACTH II 964
— — Gonadotropins II 964
— Ascites II 953
— Bladder II 996
— — Schistosomiasis II 996
— Blood group II 842
— Breast II, 949, 953, 961, 1025
— Carcinogenesis, Human, Kidney II 994
— Carcinoma *in situ* II 952
— Cervix II 962
— — Among Jewish II 962
— — Among poor II 962
— — Among virgins II 962
— — Coitus II, 962
— — Estrogen II 962
— — Herpes virus II 962
— — Pregnancy II 962
— — Smegma II 962
— Chromosomes II 957
— — Heteroploidy II 957–959
— — Philadelphia chromosome II 957
— — Stem line II 959
— Colon II, 950, 951, 1096
— Differentiation II 954, 955
— DNA contents I 94; II 1039
— DNA methylation II 1040
— DNA physical difference II 1040
— DNA synthesis II 1040
— Drugs II 994
— Glycolysis I 9
— — Lipomas II 1029
— — Pasteur effect II 1029
— Growth rate II 1038
— — Chemotherapy II 1038
— Heredity II 955
— — Animals II 955
— — — Breast cancer II 956
— — — Leukemias II 956
— — — Lung cancer II 955, 956
— — — Lymphosarcoma II 956
— — — Mammary cancer II 955
— — Chromosomes II 957
— — Humans II 956
— — — Breast cancer II 956
— — — Identical twins II 957
— — — Medullary thyroid carcinoma II 957
— — — Multiple exostosis II 957
— — — Multiple polyposis II 957
— — — Neurofibromatosis II 957
— — — Nevoid basal cell carcinoma II 957
— — — Retinoblastoma II 957
— — — Xerodermapigmentosum II 957
— — Polyendocrine adenomatosis II 957
— High malignancy II, 1082
— Hormones II 959
— — Adrenal II 964
— — Androgen II 970
— — Autonomous II 968
— — Biochemistry II 967
— — Bladder II 966
— — Blood levels II 969
— — Breast cancer II 959
— — Cervix II 962
— — Dependent II 968
— — Hypophysis II 964
— — 17-Ketosteroids II 969
— — Kidney II 966
— — Liver II 966
— — Lymphatic tissue II 966
— — Ovary II 963
— — Prostate II 965
— — Skin II 966
— — Steroid levels II 969
— — Subcutaneous tissue II 966
— — Testicles II 966
— — Transplacental II 967
— — Urinary estrogens II 969
— — Uterus II 962
— Host II, 1088
— — Stroma II 1089
— — Toxohormone II 1089
— Host reactions II 1088
— Host relationship II 1096
— — Anemia II 1097
— — Angiogenesis II 1098
— — Ectopic hormones II 1096
— — — Bronchial carcinomas II 1097
— — — Cancer pancreas II 1096
— — — Carcinoid II 1096
— — — Colon II 1096
— — — Cushing's syndrome II 1096
— — — Diabetes II 1096
— — — Diabetes insipidis II 1096
— — — Glucose tolerance test II 1096
— — — Gonadotropin elaboration II 1096
— — — Hepatomegaly II 1097
— — — Hypercalcemia II 1096
— — — Hypoglycemia II 1096
— — — Mammary glands II 1096
— — — Oat cell carcinoma II 1096
— — — Ovary II 1096
— — — Parathyroid II, 1096
— — — Pheochromocytomas II 1096
— — — Prostate II 1096
— — — Sympatheticoblastomas II 1096
— — — Thymus II 1096
— — — Thyroid hormone II 1096
— — — TSH secretion II 1096
— — Hyperuricemia II 1098
— — Immunity II 1098
— — Kidney enlargement II 1097
— — Neural degeneration II 1097
— — Nutrition II 1097
— — — Cachexia II 1097
— — — Negative nitrogen balance II 1097
— — — Negative phosphorus balance II 1097
— — — Nitrogen II 1097
— — Uric acid accumulation II 1097
— Hypophysis II 964

— — Adrenocorticotropic II 964
— — Autonomous II 965
— — Dependent II 965
— — Mammotropic II 964
— — Thyrotropic II 964
— Invasion II 951, 1088
— — Cancer en cuirasse II 952
— — Cytotoxic substances II 1088
— — Hydrolytic enzymes II 1088
— — Pressure II 1088
— Isozymes II 1086
— — Carbamyl phosphate synthetase II 1087
— — Serine dehydrase II 1097
— Kidney II 994
— Liver II 994, 996
— — Aflatoxin II 994
— — Schistosomiasis II 996
— Lung II 1096
— Lymph nodes II 952
— Metabolic regulation II 1041
— — Glycolysis II 1042
— Metabolism
— — Amino acids II 1034
— — — Asparaginase II 1035
— — — ATP utilization II 1036
— — — Azaserine II 1035
— — — Hodgkin's disease II 1034
— — — Leukemia II 1034
— — — Oxygen utilization II 1036
— — — Yoshida sarcoma II 1034
— — ATPase II 1033
— — Carrier System II 1030
— — Cytochrome c II 1032
— — Electron transport II 1034
— — Electron transport chain II 1031
— — Glycolysis II 1028, 1030
— — — Hepatomas II 1029
— — — High aerobic II 1028
— — — Pasteur effect II 1028
— — Hepatomas II 1031, 1034
— — Hexose monophosphate shunt II 1030, 1031
— — Krebs cycle II 1030
— — Levels of NAD II 1033
— — Mitochondria II 1033
— — Mitochondrial DNA II 1032
— — Mitochondrial number II 1033
— — Mitochondrial permeability II 1033
— — NADase II 1033
— — Nucleic acid, DNA synthesis, exploitable differences II 1037
— — Nucleic acid synthesis II 1036
— — — *de novo* pathway II 1037
— — — Salvage pathway II 1037
— — Oxidative phosphorylation II 1032, 1033
— — — ATP catabolism II 1032
— — — Number of mitochondria II 1032
— — Oxygen consumption II 1032
— — Oxygen uptake II 1030
— — Respiration II 1032
— — Sugar transport II 1030
— Metastasis II 951, 952, 1088, 1089
— — Adhesiveness II 1090
— — Blood vessels II 1090
— — Cell adhesion II 1094
— — Cell membrane II 1093
— — Contact inhibition II 1094
— — Lymphatic invasion II 1090
— — Macrophages II 1095
— — Retrograde progression II 1092
— — Stroma II 1090,1091
— Minimal deviation hepatomas II 1082
— Ovary II 954, 963, 1096
— — Carcinogen II 963
— — Implantation in spleen II 963
— — X-irradiation II 963
— Pancreas II 1096
— Prostate II 965, 1096
— — Castration II 965
— — Chinese II 965
— — Estrogen II 965
— — Japanese II 965
— — Testosterone II 965
— Radiation II 742
— RNA, Walker tumor II 1041
— RNA base composition II 1041
— RNA metabolism II 1040
— — RNA release II 1041
— Schistosomiasis II 996
— Stomach II 994
— Skin, squamous cells cells carcinoma II 955
— Teratomas II 954
— Testicles II 966
— — Androgen II 966
— — Cryptorchidism II 966
— — Estrogen II 966
— — Progesterone II 966
— — Zinc chloride II 966
— Thyroid II 1096
— Toxohormones II 953
— Transplacental II 967
— — Vagina II 967
— Uterus II 962
— — Endometrial hyperplasia II 962
— — Estrogen II 962
— — Estrus II 962
— — Pregnancy II 962
— — Progesterone II 962
— Vagina II 967
— Virus II 996
— — Antigenic properties II 1017
— — — Bittner virus II 1017
— — — Cross-immunity II 1017
— — — Shope papilloma II 1017
— — Biochemistry II 1018
— — — Polyoma virus II 1018
— — — Rauscher leukemia virus II 1019
— — — Rous sarcoma II 1918
— — Bittner virus II 1012
— — Breast carcinoma II 1025
— — Burkitt's sarcoma II 1025
— — Cervical cancer II 1026
— — Characteristics II 1014
— — — Morphology II 1014
— — — Size II 1014
— — — Type A II 1014
— — — Type B II 1014
— — — Type C II 1014
— — Epstein-Barr virus II 1026
— — Herpes-like agent II 1025
— — Herpes virus II 1025
— — Hodgkin's disease II 1013, 1025
— — Hypothesis II 1027
— — Infectious myxomatosis II 996
— — In humans II 1024
— — Leukemia II 1012, 1025
— — Liposarcomas II 1026
— — Lucke's disease II 1026
— — Melanomas II 1026
— — Modulating factors II 1015
— — — Age II 1016
— — — Carcinogens II 1015, 1016
— — — Helper virus II 1015
— — — Heredity II 1015
— — — Host II 1015
— — — Tissue susceptibility II 1015
— — — X-irradiation II 1016
— — Oncogenic gene theory II 1027
— — Papilloma II 1012, 1026
— — Parotid tumors II 1013
— — Protovirus theory II 1027
— — Rous sarcoma II 996
— — Shope papilloma virus II 1011
— — Transformation II 1023
— — Type D II 1014
— — Viral replication II 1019
— — X-irradiation II 1041
Cancer Cells,
— Electrophoretic mobility II 1095
— — Calcium II 1095
— — Fibroblast transformation II 1095
— — Metastasis II 1095
— — Neuraminidase II 1095
— — Ribonuclease II 1095
— — Sialic acid II 1096
— Gene expression II 1065
Cancer immunity II 1098
— Antigen loss II 1101
— Antigens II 1100
— — Cell surface proteins II 1101
— — Chemistry II 1101
— — Intracellular II 1101
— — Membranes II 1101
— Basal cell carcinoma II 1100
— BCG II 1099
— Blocking antibodies II 1103
— Burkitt's lymphoma II 1100
— Cancer in smokers II 1103
— Cancer in young people II 1103
— Carcinoembryonic antigens II 1101, 1102
— Carcinoma of bladder II 1100
— Carcinoma of breast II 1100
— Carcinoma of colon II 1100
— Carcinoma of esophagus II 1100
— Carcinoma of lung II 1099, 1100
— Carcinoma of pancreas II 1100
— Carcinoma of parathyroid II 1100
— Carcinoma of stomach II 1100
— Carcinoma of thyroid II 1100
— Carcinoma of urinary tract II 1099
— Chemical carcinogens II 1100, 1102
— Circulating antigens II 1103
— Circulating lymphocytes II 1103
— Colony inhibition test II 1102
— α-fetoprotein II 1101
— α_1-fetoprotein II 1101
— Hepatomas II 1100
— Hodgkin's disease II 1099
— Hypernephroma II 1100
— Immune RNA II 1099
— Immunological enhancement II 1102
— Immunosuppression II 1102
— Immunosurveillance II 1103
— In animals II 1100
— — Antigens II 1100
— — Tumor specific antigens II 1100
— — Viral antigens II 1100
— In spontaneous tumors II 1104
— Irradiation II 1099
— Leukemia II 1099, 1100
— Liposarcoma II 1100
— Melanoma II 1100
— Neuroblastoma II 1100
— Osteogenic sarcoma II 1100
— Retinoblastoma II 1100
— Squamous cell carcinoma II 1100
— Transfer factors II 1099
— Wilm's tumor II 1100
CAP factor I 119
Carbamyl aspartic acid synthetase I 226
Carbamyl phosphate I 226
Carbamyl phosphate synthetase II 1087

Carbohydrate metabolism I 163
– Inborn errors I 163
– – Glycogen storage disease I 163
Carbohydrates, sparing effect on proteins I 589
Carbon tetrachloride intoxication II 637
– ATPase II 640
– ATP level II 638
– Chloroform II 639
– Conjugated-dienes II 639
– Endoplasmic reticulum II 638
– Fatty acid II 639
– Free radicals II 639, 640
– Glucose-6-phosphatase II 640
– Heterolytic fission II 639
– Homolytic cleavage II 639
– Lysosomes II 638
– Malonyl dialdehyde II 640
– Mitochondria II 638
Mixed function oxidase II 640
– Peroxidation II 640
– Solvent theory II 638
– Toxic metabolites II 638
Carbonic anhydrase I 554
Carbonic hydrase I 377
– Zinc I 377
Carboxypeptidase I 256
– Procarboxypeptidase I 259
– Zinc I 259
Carcinogens II 970
– Aflatoxin II 983
– Aniline derivatives II 983
– Azo derivatives II 977
– Cycasin II 983
– 1,2,5,6-dibenanthracene II 970
– Electronic structure II 972
– Fluorene derivatives II 979
– K region II 972
– L region II 972
– Mixed-function oxidase II 975
– Polycyclic hydrocarbons II 970
– – 3,4,-benzene pyrene II 971
– – Cholanthrene II 971
– – 1,2,5,6-dibenzanthracene II 970
– – 1,2,7,8-dibenzanthracene II 970
– Epoxide II 973
– Epoxide hydrase II 976
– Hydrogenation II 971
– K region epoxide II 973, 974
– Methylation II 971
– 9,10-methyldibenzanthracene II 971
– Polymers II 984
– – Free radicals II 985
– Protein binding II 972
– Tar II 970
– Urethane II 984
Carcinogenesis II 970
– Chemical II 970
– – DNA repair II 990
– – Humans II 991
– – – Aniline II 992
– – – Asbestos II 992
– – – Chrome II 995
– – – Contraceptives II 992
– – – Creosote II 995
– – – Dyes II 994
– – – Insecticides II 992
– – – Isoniazid II 995
– – – Liver II 994
– – – Marijuana II 993
– – – Nickel II 995
– – – Penicillin G II 994
– – – Petroleum products II 994
– – – Pionolactone II 994
– – – Propylactone II 994
– – – Reserpine II 995
– – – Smoking II 993
– – – Stomach II 995
– – – Talc II 992
– – – Vinyl chloride II 992
– – Lung cancer II 993
– – Mechanism II 985
– – – Activation scheme of AAF II 986
– – – Metabolism of dimethylamino-azobenzene II 986
– – Silicates II 992
– – Transformation II 988
– – – Cyclic AMP II 989
– – – Cyclic GMP II 989
– – Transformation *in vitro* II 988
– Cyclic GMP II 988
– Drugs,
– – Prospective approach II 995
– – Retrospective approach II 995
Mechanism,
– – Activation II 986
– – N-hydroxy derivatives II 985
– Mutation II 990
– Two-stage II 986
– – Croton oil II 987
– – Cyclic AMP II 988
– – Initiator II 987
– – Methylcholanthrene II 987
– – Promotors II 987
– 12-0-tetradecanoylphorbol-13-acetate II 987
– Viral II 1010
– – Avian Leukosis viruses II 1010
Carcinoembryonic antigen II 1101
Carcinoids II 1096
– In phenylketonuria I 174
Cardiac failure I 555
– Angiotensin II I 584
– Renin I 584
– Salt and water retention I 583
Cardiac Hypertrophy II 919
– Cell membrane II 920
– DNA synthesis II 920
– Glucose uptake II 920
– Glucose utilization II 920
– Mitochondria II 920
– Nuclear pores II 920
– Nucleotide pools II 920
– Polyploidy II 920
– Shunt pathway II 920
Carrier mechanism II 1077
Catalase I 41, 272; II 643
Cataracts I 284, 354
Cell adhesion II 1094
– Calcium II 1094
– Hepatoma II 1094
Cell communication II 1094
Cell hybridization II 1061
Cell cultures I 238
– Cell lines I 238
– Diploid cell lines I 238
– Primary I 238
Cell cycle II 752
Cell membrane II 1065, 1093
– Adenylcyclase II 1077
– Adhesion II 1068
– – Ionic milieu II 1068
– – Potential barrier II 1068
– Adhesive substances II 1069
– Aggregation II 1069
– Amphipatic protein II 1078
– Binding to agglutinin II 1079
– Binding to IgG II 1079
– Cancer II 1081
– – Adhesiveness II 1081
– – Agglutination II 1081
– – Charge II 1081
– – Enhanced transport II 1081
– – Glycoproteins II 1081
– – Loss of communication II 1081
– – Loss of contact inhibition II 1081
– – Sialic acid II 1081
– – Tumor antigens II 1081
– Capping II 1079
– Carrier-mediated transport II 1066
– Cell periphery II 1078
– Chemotactism II 1067
– Concavanalin A II 1069
– Contact guidance II 1067
– Contact inhibition II 1067, 1068, 1079
– Cross-link II 1079
– Disaccharidases II 1067
– Disaccharide intolerance II 1067
– Enzymes II 1065, 1074
– – β-glactoside permease II 1074
– – Diglyceride kinase II 1074
– – Neuraminidase II 1079
– – Phosphohydrolases II 1075
– – Sodium-potassium-sensitive ATPase II 1074
– Erythrocyte ghosts II 1072
– – Glycophorin II 1073
– – Protein II 1073
– – Sialic acid II 1073
– Exchange diffusion II 1066
– Facilitated diffusion II 1066
– Feedback mechanism II 1065
– Flip-flop motion II 1078
– Free diffusion II 1066
– Genome II 1065
– Glycolipid II 1069
– Glycoprotein II 1080
– Glycosidic linkage II 1080
– Hormones II 1078
– Hydrolases II 1079
– Microfibrils II 1067
– Microtubules II 1079
– Molecular composition II 1072
– – Erythrocyte ghosts II 1072
– Molecular organization II 1075
– – Carrier mechanism II 1077
– – Cytochrome b_5 II 1076
– – Danielli model II 1075
– – Gramicidin A II 1077
– – Iceberg model II 1076
– – Lipid layers II 1075
– – Mitochondria II 1075
– – Rhodopsin II 1076
– – Subunit theory II 1075
– – Valinomycin II 1077
– Movements II 1065, 1067
– Pinocytosis II 1066
– Plasminogen II 1079
– Pores II 1066
– Potassium sodium ATPase II 1078
– Proteins II 1078
– Receptors II 1066, 1079
– Ruffled edge II 1067
– Sodium potassium ATPase II 1067
– Synthesis II 1078
– Transport II 1065
– Virus II 1078
Cell periphery,
– Actin-like microfilaments II 1078
– Microtubules II 1078
β Cells I 497
– Fibrosis I 497
– Hyalinization I 497
Cellular communication II 1070
– Calcium II 1070
– Colicine II 1071

– Desmosomes II 1070
– Electric current II 1070
– Electric organ II 1070
– Gap junction II 1070
– Permeases II 1071
– Potassium concentration II 1071
– Regenerating liver II 1071
– Sodium pump II 1071
– Tight junction II 1070
Cellular death I 470, 607; II 613
– Actinomycin D II 614
– Aging red cell II 619
– α_1-antitrypsin deficiency II 633
– Biology I 607
– Cloudy swelling II 627
– Conclusion II 634
– Cyclic AMP II 630
– D-galactosamine II 629
– DNA synthesis II 613
– Ethionine II 616
– Hydrolases II 620
– Ischemia II 616, 628
– Membrane lesions II 617
– – Irreversibility II 618
– – Ischemia II 618
– – Lysosome II 618
– – Mitochondria II 618
– – Osmotic shock II 618
– – Phalloidine II 619
– Membrane permeability II 617
– Mitomycin II 614
– Oxidative phosphorylation II 616, 617
– Phosphatidylcholine level II 619
– Point of no return II 627
– Provoked II 629
– Red cell I 608
– Rifamycin II 614
– Sodium pumping II 617
– Source of energy II 616
– Spherocytosis II 619
– Spontaneous II 629
– Tannic acid II 716
– Trypsin I 630
– – Pancreatitis II 630
– UTP depletion II 614
Cellular life span I 607
Centromere I 234
Ceramides I 188
– Biosynthesis I 188
Cerebellar ataxia I 270
Cerebrosides I 193
– Biosynthesis I 193
Ceroids I 315
Ceruloplasmin I 159
Cervical cancer II 1026
CFU I 373
Chalone II 916
– Epidermal II 916
– Erythrocytes II 916
– Fibroblasts II 916
– Granulocyte II 916
– Lymphocytes II 916
– Rat liver II 916
Chondroitin sulfates II 934
Charcot-Marie-Tooth disease II 668
Chelate I 376
– Hemoglobin I 379
– Peroxidase I 379
Chemiosmotic coupling I 53
Chemoreceptor I 579
– Aortic I 579
– Carotid bodies I 579
– Low levels of oxygen I 580
– Partial pressure oxygen I 580
Chemotactism II 1067
Chemotaxis II 779
– Actin filament II 782
– Acute glomerulonephritis II 781
– Bacteria II 781
– Calcium II 782
– Glycolysis II 782
– Hodgkin's disease II 781
– Immunological vasculitis II 781
– Magnesium II 782
– Membrane II 781
– Microtubules II 782
– Mononuclears II 782
– Plants II 781
Chemotherapy II 1005
Chloride metabolism I 570
– Alkalosis I 570
Chlorosis I 363
Chlorpromazine I 52
Cholestasis I 601
– Pathogenesis I 602
Cholate synthesis I 587
Cholycystokinin I 262
Cholesterol I 271
– Cholestyramine I 599
– Formula II 692
Cholesterol esterification II 704
Cholesterol metabolism II 692
– Control II 1050
– – Absorption II 1051
– – HMG-CoA reductase II 1052
– – – Posttranscriptional control II 1052
– – HMG-CoA synthesis II 1051
– – Sterol biosynthesis II 1052
– Endogenous II 693
– Esterification II 692
– Exogenous II 692
– Mevalonic acid formation II 693
– Regulation II 696
– – Cyclic AMP II 696
– – Squalene sterol carrier protein II 696
– Sitosterol II 692
– Squalene formation II 694
Chromatin II 1056
Chromosomal anomalies I 233
– Acetylaminofluorene I 240
– Acquired I 238
– – Viruses I 238
– Autosomal transmission I 233
– Cold shocks I 239
– DDT I 240
– Dominant transmission I 233
– Hexachlorophene I 240
– Ionizing radiation I 239
– Magnetic fields I 239
– Mosaicism I 236
– Nondisjunction I 236
– Recessive transmission I 233
– Ring chromosome I 239
– Sound waves I 239
– Teratogens I 238
– Thalidomide I 240
– Translocation I 236, 240
– Trisomy I 234
– Ultraviolet light I 239
Chromosomal trisomies I 235
Chromosomes I 104
– Breaks I 241
– Centromere I 234
– Chemistry I 88
– Chromatid I 234
– Color Blindness I 85
– Crossing over I 86
– Dicentric I 239
– DNA I 104
– Genetics I 84
– Hemophilia I 85
– Histones I 89
– Linkage I 86
– Morphology I 84
– Nucleic acid I 88
– Nuclein I 88
– Protamines I 88
– Protein I 88
– Ring I 239
– Ultrastructure I 104
Chronic renal disease I 592
Chvostek's sign I 354
Chymotrypsin I 256, 403
Chymotrypsinogen I 257
– Activation I 258
Cirrhosis I 321, 555
– Gross findings II 648
– Portal gross findings II 648
– Postnecrotic II 648
Citrate synthetase II 1048
Citric acid I 54
Clathrate I 550
Clefts of Schmidt-Lanterman II 664
Cloudy swelling II 627
– Diphtheria toxin II 627, 628
– Protein synthesis I 628
Cll-cis-retinol I 305
Coenzyme A I 277
– Biosynthesis I 277
– Ovaries I 277
Coenzyme Q I 43, 317
– Reductase I 44
Colchicine I 106, 224; II 1064
Collagen I 279, 281, 550; II 924
– Basement membranes II 926
– Biosynthesis II 931
– – Cross-linking II 931
– – Cytochalasin B II 932
– – Galactose II 932
– – Glucosylgalactose II 932
– – Glycine tRNA II 931
– – Peptidyl galactosyl hydroxylysine transferase II 932
– – Peptidyl glucosyl galactosyl hydroxylysine transferase II 932
– – Peptidyl lysine hydroxylase II 932
– – Peptidyl proline hydroxylase II 932
– – Polysomes II 931
– – Pro α chains II 931
– – Procollagen II 931
– – Proline tRNA II 931
– – Tropocollagen II 931
– – Tubular system II 932
– Breakdown II 932
– – Collagenase II 932
– α_1 Chain II 925
– Cross-links II 927, 928
– – Allysine II 929
– – β-mercaptoethylamine II 929
– – Copper II 929
– – Dehydrohydroxylysinorleucine II 929
– – Hydroxylysinorleucine II 929
– – Hydroxylysine II 929
– – δ-hydroxylysinorleucine II 929
– – Lysinorleucine II 929
– – Penicillamine II 929
– – Pyridoxal deficiency II 929
– Disease II 932
– – Decreased proline hydroxylase activity II 934
– – Decreased soluble collagen II 934
– – Dermatosparaxis II 933
– – Ehlers-Danlos syndrome II 934
– – Hydroxylysine deficiency II 933

Collagen, Disease, Increased glycosyl transferases II 934
— — Increased proline hydroxylase activity II 934
— — Lysine oxidase II 933
— — Osteogenesis imperfecta II 933
— Molecule II 924
— — Models II 925
— — Sequences II 925
— — — Apolar II 925
— — — Polar II 925
— — Soluble II 934
— — Suprahelix II 926
— — Tripeptide II 925
— — Triple helical structure II 926
Collagenase II 932
Colon carcinoma II 1100
Colony inhibition test II 1102
Color blindness I 85, 86
Compensatory polycythemia in methemoglobinemia I 155
Complement II 813
— Activation II 813
— — binding of $C4_b$ II 814
— — $C3_b$ peptidase II 815
— — splitting of C3
— Activation of C1 II 813
— Activation of C2 II 814
Complex ion I 376
Concavanalin A I 521; II 1069
Condroitin II 934
Cones I 310
Conformational coupling I 53
Congenital anomalies I 276, 308
Contact guidance II 1067
Contact inhibition II 1068, 1094
Convulsion I 354
Coombs' reaction II 841
Copper I 42, 159
— Tyrosinase I 174
Copper metabolism I 160
— Ceruloplasmin I 162
— Copper and blood I 162
— Copper bound I 162
— Erythrocuprein I 162
— Polypeptides I 162
Coproporphyrinogen I I 205
Cordycepin II 615
Coronary occlusion II 705
Corticoid hormones I 467
— Metabolic effects I 467
— — ATP synthesis I 468
— — Eosinophilia I 471
— — Erythropoiesis I 471
— — Gluconeogenesis I 468
— — Glycogen synthesis I 468
— — Lipid metabolism I 469
— — Lipogenesis I 469
— — Lymphopoietic tissue I 469
— — Mitochondrial swelling I 468
— — Monocytes I 471
— — Nitrogen balance I 467
— — Nucleic acids I 470
— — Protein metabolism I 467
— — Protein synthesis I 470
— — Pyruvate carboxylase I 469
— — Receptors I 471
Corticosteroid hormones I 491
— Adrenogenital syndrome I 492
— — Androgens I 493
— Inborn errors I 491
— — Adrenogenital syndrome I 492
— — Cryptorchidism I 492
— — 21-hydroxylase deficiency I 492
— — 3β-hydroxysteroid dehydrogenase deficiency I 492
— Inborn errors of metabolism I 491
— — 11β-hydroxylase deficiency I 493
— — 17α-hydroxylase deficiency I 493
— — Hypospadias I 492
Councilman bodies II 1003
Countercurrent exchange I 545
Coupling factors I 51
Coupling mechanisms I 47
Covalent bond, coordinated I 376
Crabtree effect II 1044, 1045
Cretinism I 457
— Abnormal peroxidase I 458
— Iodine deficiency I 458
— Iodine pumping mechanism I 458
— TRH deficiency I 458
Creutzfeldt-Jakob disease II 1009
Cri-du-chat syndrome I 237
Crohn's disease II 885
Cross-links II 927, 928
— β Aminopropionitrile II 931
— Lathyrism II 930
— Soluble collagen II 931
Crotonase I 55
— Reactions I 56
Croton oil II 987
Cryptorchidism II 966
Crypt of Lieberkühn, Alkaline phosphatase I 322
— Hexose monophosphate shunt I 323
— Proliferation I 323
Cushing's syndrome I 477; II 1096
— Adenocarcinoma I 477
— Adenoma I 477
— Anephrotensin I 478
— Adrenal hyperplasia I 477
— Basophilic adenoma I 477
— Cortisol levels I 478
— Diabetes I 479
— Hypertension I 478
— 17-hydroxycorticosteroid I 478
— Moon-faced I 478
— Nitrogen balance I 478
— Obesity I 478
— Osteoporosis I 478
— Skin I 479
Cyanosis and methemoglobinemia I 155
Cycasin II 983
Cyclic AMP I 455, 529, 559; II 988, 989, 1022, 1048, 1088
— ACTH I 530
— Adenyl cyclase I 529
— Cell division I 532
— Enzyme turnover I 531
— Epinephrine I 530
— Glucagon I 530
— GTP I 530
— Histones I 530
— Insulin I 530
— Metabolism I 530
— Phosphodiesterase I 529, 530
— Phosphofructokinase I 531
— Phosphoprotein phosphatase I 531
— Protein kinase I 530, 531
— Psoriasis I 532
— Receptor I 531
— Steroid metabolism I 531
— Translation I 530
Cyclic GMP I 531; II 988, 989
— Guanylate cyclase I 531
Cyanide I 42
Cyclohexamide I 66
Cystathioninuria I 232
Cystine I 229
Cystinosis I 231
Cystinuria I 229, 594
— Arginine I 229
— Cystine stone I 230
— Lysine I 229
— Ornithine I 229
Cystic fibrosis I 241, 320
— Atelectasis I 321
— Cirrhosis I 321
— Fatty liver I 321
— Mucus secretion I 321
— Pathogenesis I 321
— Portal hypertension I 321
Cytochrome I 37, 40
Cytochrome b_5 I 36; II 1076
Cytochrome c I 36, 37; II 1032
— Amino acid sequence I 38
Cytochrome oxidase I 41
— Nucleus I 84
Cytochrome p_{450} I 41
Cytolysis II 840
Cytomegalovirus I 1003
Cytoplasmic alteration, viruses II 1001

Deamido NAD I 274
Debye units I 547
Decarboxylase in maple syrup disease I 181
Defective leukocytic response II 791
— Chediak-Higashi's disease II 791
— Erythroleukemia II 791
— Granulocytopenia II 791
— Hodgkin's disease II 791
— Lazy leukocyte syndrome II 791
— Leukemia II 791
— Leukotactic defects II 791
— Polycythemia II 791
Dehydration I 546, 584
— Hyposmolarity I 584
Deiodination I 422
— Tetra- and triiodo-derivatives I 443
Dementia I 271
Demyelination I 267; II 668
— Allergic encephalitis II 668
— Axon degeneration II 668
— Electron microscopy II 668
— Multiple sclerosis II 669
De novo pathway II 1037
De novo synthesis with isotopes I 82
Dermatosparaxis II 933
Dexamethasone receptor I 528
Diabetes I 247, 272, 277, 326, 479, 495; II 700, 1047
— Alloxan I 513, 514
— Anti-insulin I 497
— Fatty acid synthesis I 523
— Growth hormones I 507
— Insipidus I 437; II 1096
— Ketosis I 522
— Pathogenesis I 524
— Pathology, β cells I 496
— Phosphopyruvic carboxylase I 525
— Clinicopathological correlation I 496
— — By increased diuresis I 496
— — Dehydration I 496
— — Electrolytes I 496
— — Fatty acid metabolism I 496
— — Glucosuria I 496
— — Hyperglycemia I 496
— — Ketone bodies I 496
— — Polydypsia I 496
— — Protein I 496
— — Urine nitrogen I 496
— Complications I 498
— — Abnormal delivery I 498
— — Amyotrophies I 501
— — Arteriosclerosis I 498
— — Cataracts I 498, 501
— — Glomerular nephrosclerosis I 498

— — Infections I 498, 501
— — Neuropathy I 501
— — Osteopathies I 501
— — Polyneuritis I 498
— — Pseudoerythroblastosis I 501
— — Retinitis I 498
— — Xanthelasmas I 498
— Glomerulonephrosclerosis I 499, 500
— — Glycoproteins I 499
— — Kimmelstiel and Wilson disease I 499
— Onset I 495
— — Diseases I 496
— — Dietary habits I 496
— — Hemochromatosis I 496
— — Lithiasis I 496
— — Pancreas carcinoma I 496
— — Pancreatectomy I 496
— — Pancreatitis I 496
— — Stress I 496
Dialysis disequilibrium syndrome I 566
Diamine oxidase I 301
Diatomic molecule I 376
Dicumarol I 42
Dihydrouridine I 110
1,25-dihydroxycholecalciferol I 343
Dihydroxyphenylalanine in phenylketunoria I 174
Diiodothyronine, deiodination I 442
Diiodotyrosine, Deiodination I 442
Dimers, function II 731
Diphosphopyridine nucleotide (NAD) I 33
Diphtheria toxin II 1008
— Electron transport II 1009
— Iron II 1009
— Protein synthesis II 1009
Dipole moment I 547
Direction of reading message I 128
Disaccharidases II 1067
Disaccharide intolerance II 1067
Disseminated coagulation I 419, 420
— Afibrinogenemia I 420
— Azotemia I 421
— Cor pulmonale I 420
— Dypsnea I 420
— Ecchymosis I 420
— Endocarditis I 421
— Hemorrhagic diathesis I 420
— Ischemia I 420
— Necrosis I 420
— Oliguria I 421
— Pathogenesis I 421
— Petechiae I 420
— Shock I 420
DNA I 93
— Base composition I 98
— Base pairing I 99
— Bouyant density I 98
— Cancer I 94
— Chemistry I 97
— Content and nucleus I 93
— Erythroblasts I 94
— Guanine-cytosine I 98
— Histones I 91
— Intestinal polyps I 94
— Megaloblast I 94
— Nearest neighbor bases I 101
— Okazaki fragments I 102
— Unwinding protein I 102
— Watson-Crick model I 99
DNA methylase I 114
— S-Adenosyl methionine I 114
DNA Polymerase I 101
— Nucleus I 83
DNA repair II 727, 990
— Aging II 732
— Bloom syndrome II 732
— Chemical carcinogenesis II 990
— Disease II 731
— Excision repair II 728
— Fanconi syndrome II 732
— Hitchinson-Gilford syndrome II 733
— Postreplication repair II 730
— Progeria II 733
— Thymine dimers II 728
DNA Replication I 100
— Enzymic mechanism I 100
— Semiconservative I 100
DNA synthesis II 1064
Donnan body fluids I 539
Donnan law I 568
Dopa decarboxylase I 174
— Phenylketonuria I 174
Dopamine-β-hydroxylase I 225
Down's syndrome I 236, 237
— Nondisjunction I 236
Drosophila I 85
— Chromosomes I 85
— Red eye I 85
— White eye I 85
Drug induced hemolytic anemia I 170
— Balanced polymorphism I 170
— Glutathione peroxidase I 171
— Glyoxalase I 171
— Heinz bodies I 170
— Hyperbilirubinemia I 170
— Jaundice I 170
— Lifa span of the red cell I 171
— Malaria I 170
— Naphthalene I 170
— Primaquine I 171
— One gene, one enzyme theory I 171
— Sulfanilamide I 170
— Vitamin K I 170
dsRNA I 121
Duane equation II 717
Dumping syndrome,
— Bradykinin I 319
— Pathogenesis I 319
Duodenal ulcers I 276, 314
Dwarfism I 432
— Achondroplasia I 433
— Hereditary I 433
— Malnutrition I 433
— Pituitary, acquired I 433
Dwarf mice I 433

Edema I 546, 582
— Central nervous system lesions I 582
— Cyclic idiopathic I 584
— Pulmonary I 582
— — Anoxemia I 482
— — Lymphatic obstruction I 582
— — Pathogenesis I 582
— Salt and water retention I 583
— Systemic I 583
— — Pathogenesis I 583
Effect of thyroid hormone I 445
— Calcium I 446
— Chloride I 446
— Diabetes I 446
— Electrolytes I 446
— Electron transport I 446
— Gluconeogenesis I 446
— Glucose metabolism I 446
— α-glycerophosphate shuttle I 448
— Iron I 446
— Magnesium I446
— Mitochondria I 447
— NADPH concentration I 447
— Nitrogen metabolism I 445
— Oxygen consumption I 448
— Oxygen uptake I 446
— Potassium I 446
— Sodium I 446
— Transhydrogenase I 448
Ehlers-Danlos syndrome II 934
Einstein-Planck equation II 717
Elastase I 256
Elastin II 929
— Cross-links II 929
— Desmosine II 929
— Fibroblasts II 930
— Smooth muscle cells II 930
Electric organ II 1070
Electron transport I 317; II 1034
— Antimycin I 44
— Chain I 44; II 1009, 1031
— Oxidative phosphorylation I 45
— Mitochondrion I 45
Electrolytes I 539
Electrodialysis I 376
Electrophilic reagent I 50
Electron II 717
Emboli I 415, 418
Endochondral ossification I 279
Endoplasmic reticulum I 133, 587; II 646
— DNA content I 135
— Morphology I 133
— Nuclear membrane I 75
— Origin I 135
— Role in protein synthesis I 134
— Rough I 135
— Smooth I 135
Enolase, nucleus I 80
Enzyme, nucleus I 83
Enzyme turnover I 531
Eosiniphilic adenoma I 429, 430
Eosinophils II 788
— Cortisone II 788
— Granules II 788
Epinephrine I 530
— Receptors I 528
Epinine in phenylketonuria I 174
Epitheliomesenchymal interactions II 938
— Mammary gland II 938
— Pig epithelium II 938
— Salivary glands II 938
Erb's sign I 354
Ergot preparation I 208
Erythroblast, DNA content I 94
Erythroblastosis fetalis II 844
— Host-versus-graft reaction II 845
Erythrocuprein I 162
Erythrocyte ghosts II 1072
— Lipids II 1072
— Plasmalogens II 1072
Erythron I 371
Erythropoiesis I 372
— Colony forming units, CFU I 373
— Erythropoietin I 373
— Polycythemia I 373
— Porphyrin I 373
Erythropoietin I 373, 557
Esophagus cancer II 110
Essential amino acids I 265
Estrogen I 247
— Cancer II 962, 966
— Leiomyoma II 963
— Ovaries I 480
Exophthalmia I 452
Eye in Gaucher's disease I 191

Fabry's disease I 233
— Pathogenesis I 198
— Telangectases I 198
Factor XIII deficiency I 408
Factor M I 119

Factor T I 119
Familial iminoglycinuria I 232
Fanconi syndrome II 732
Farnesoate II 694
Farnesyl pyrophosphate II 694
Fat absorption,
— Bile acid II 685
— Chylomicrons II 686
— Heparin II 686
— Lipoprotein lipase II 686
— Pinocytosis II 686
Fat metabolism, fat absorption II 685
Fatty acid II 1048
— a-Oxidation I 59
— Acetyl-CoA-ACP transacylase I 62
— Acyl dehydrogenase I 55
— ATP lyase I 61
— Avidin I 61
— B-hydroxyacyl-ACP dehydrase I 62
— B-Ketoacyl-ACP-reductase I 62
— B-Oxidation pathway I 54, 55
— Biotin I 61
— Branched oxidation I 57
— Butyryl dehydrogenase I 55
— Citrate I 61
— Crotonase I 55
— Cyanide I 55
— Hydroxyacyl dehydrogenase I 56
— Intracellular distribution I 57
— Ketoacyl thiolase I 57
— Ketosis I 55
— Malonyl CoA-ACP transacylase I 62
— Maple syrup disease I 57
— Methylglutaconase I 57
— Minimal deviation hepatomas I 61
— Mitochondria I 55
— Oligomycin I 55
— Palmitaldehyde dehydrogenase I 55
— 4′-phosphopantothenic acid I 62
— Shuttle II 644
— Synthesis I 60; II 646
— — in Mitochondria I 60
— Synthetase I 61, 62
— Thiokinase I 55
— w-Oxidation I 59
Fatty Acid Oxidation I 54
— Acetoacetyl-CoA I 54
— Acetyl-CoA I 54
— Citric acid I 54
— Thiokinase I 54
Fatty liver I 264, 321
Ferritin I 363
— Apoferritin I 364
— Biosynthesis I 363
— Structure I 363
Ferrochetalase I 206
Fetal liver I 175
Fetus II 830
— Bioenergetic pathway I 248
— Blastocyst II 830
— Carbohydrate oxidation I 248
— Decidua II 830
— Fat I 249
— Fat Oxidation I 248
— Glucose oxidation I 248
— Glucose-6-phosphatase I 249
— Hexokinase I 249
— Lactic dehydrogenase I 249
— Oxygen consumption I 248
— Phosphofructokinase I 249
— Phosphorylase I 249
— Protein synthesis I 250
— Trophoblast I 830
— Tryptophan pyrrolase I 248
Fibers of Remak II 664
Fibrin I 399
— Cross-linking I 405
— Factor LLF I 406
— Factor XIII I 406
— Fibrinase I 405
— Hyperfibrinogenemia I 415
— Polymerization I 405
Fibrinase I 405
Fibrinogen I 158, 399, 403
— Amino acid sequence I 403
— Conversion to fibrin I 404
— Fibrin or peptides I 404
— Sialidase I 403
Fibrinoid necrosis II 660, 116, 879
Fibrinolysis I 413
— Fibrinogenase I 413
— Nicotinic acid I 414
Plasma, hyperproteolytic activity I 415
— Plasmin I 413, 414
— Plasminogen I 414
— Pseudomembranes I 414
— Streptokinase I 414
— Urokinase I 415
Fibrinopenia, Blood coagulation I 408
Fibroadenoma II 948
Fibroblasts I 279
Flavin adenine dinucleotide pyrophosphorylase I 35
Flavokinase I 35
Fluorapatite I 336
Fluoride, inhibition of initiation I 129
Fluorocytes I 206
Fluorene derivatives II 980
— Acetylaminofluorene II 980
— Active carcinogens II 982
— Chelates I 983
— Effect of diet II 981
— Hormones I 981
— Metabolism II 982
— — Deacylation II 982
— — Hydroxylation II 982
— N-hydroxy-2-acetylaminofluorene II 980
— N-hydroxyl metabolites II 982
— Other carcinogens II 981
— Substitution II 980
— — Acetamide II 980
— — Halogen II 980
— — Hydroxyl II 980
— — Sulfur group II 980
Fluorene derivatives II 979
— Hyperplastic nodules II 983
— Liver changes II 983
Foam cells II 711
Focal cytoplasmic degradation II 624
Folic acid I 294
— Aminopterin I 294
— Anhydride of hydroxymethyl THFA I 294
— Citrovorum factor I 294
— Deficiency I 297
— — Megaloblast I 297
— — Methotrexate I 297
— Deoxycytidylate hydroxymethylase I 296
— Dihydrofolic acid reductase I 294
— Folic acid reductase I 294
— Formyltetrahydrofolate synthetase I 294
— Formiminotetrahydrofolic acid cyclodeaminase I 296
— Formininotransferase I 295
— L-serine hydroxymethyltransferase I 296
— Metabolism I 295
— N-formyl, 5,6,7,8-tetrahydrofolic acid I 294
— N^5-formyltetrahydrofolate isomerase (cyclodehydrolase) I 295
— N^5, N^{10}-methyltetrahydrofolate cyclohydrolase I 294
— Pteroylglutamic acid I 294
— Serine hydroxymethyltransferase I 296
Forbes' disease (see glycogen storage disease) I 165
Formyl methionyl tRNA I 129
N-formyltetrahydrofolic acid I 294
Free radicals II 639, 640, 985
Friend virus II 1013
Fröhlich's syndrome I 432
Fructoaldolase I 170
Fructokinase I 170
Fructose diphosphatase II 1046
Fructosuria I 169
— Fructoaldolase I 170
— Fructokinase I 170
— Phosphoglucomutase I 170
FSH I 487
Fumarase I 30

Galactosemia I 167
— Acetonuria I 167
— Aminoaciduria I 167
— Bilirubin I 168
— Cataracts I 169
— Cerbrosides I 168
— Fatty Liver I 168
— Galactosuria I 167
— Hepatomegaly I 167
— Mental Deficiency I 168
— Pathogenesis I 168, 169
— Pathology I 167
— Phosphoglucomutase I 168
— Polyuria I 167
— Transferase Deficiency I 169
Galactose metabolism, Regulation I 169
Galactose synthesis I 168
Gallbladder I 599
Gallstones I 599
— Pathogenesis I 600
Gammaglobulinopathies II 882
— Heavy-chain disease II 882
— Light-chain disease II 882
Gammopathies, Polyclonal II 885
Ganglioside and ceramides I 188
— Breakdown I 185
— Sialic acid I 186
— Sphingosine I 186
— Structure I 189
— Unsaturated fatty acid I 185
Ganglioside structure and metabolism I 185
Ganglioside tissue fractionation I 188
Gastrectomy I 286
Gastric glands I 255
Gastric juice I 255
Gastrin I 260
— Amino acid sequence I 261
Gastrin secretion I 260
— Acetylcholine I 260
— Gastrin I 260
— Gastrones I 261
Gastric section, Control I 259
Gastrones I 261
Gaucher's disease I 191
— Acid phosphatase I 193
— Cerebrosides I 192, 193
— Eye I 191
— Galactolipids I 192
— Globoside I 193
— Glucosidase I 193
— Liver cells I 191, 192
— Pathogenesis I 198

– Pigmentation I 191
Genes I 130
Gene expression II 1052
– Activator II 1059
– Cancer cell, Reversion II 1065
– Cell differentiation II 1053
– – Pancreas II 1053
– – Predifferentiation stage II 1054
– Cell division II 1062
– Cell hybridization II 1061
– Chromatin II 1056, 1059
– Chromosomal RNA II 1058
– Colchicine II 1062, 1064
– Corticoid receptors II 1061
– Cyclic AMP II 1056, 1058
– Differentiated stage II 1054
– DNA II 1059
– – Reassociation II 1059
– – Synthesis II 1053, 1064
– Enzyme induction, Tyrosine aminotransferase II 1054
– Gene batteries II 1060
– Generation cycle II 1062
– Hepatomas II 1055, 1059
– Histones II 1059
– Integrator gene II 1059
– Isolated hepatocytes II 1056
– Liver regeneration II 1063
– Messenger RNA II 1060
– Nonhistone chromosomal protein II 1057, 1059
– Nuclear transplantation II 1061
– Pancreas regeneration II 1063
– Polyribosome II 1064
– Prodifferentiation stage II 1054
– Producer gene II 1059
– Protein kinase II 1058
– Receptors II 1055
– Receptor gene II 1059
– Redundant DNA II 1060
– Regulatory protein II 1060
– Repetitive sequences II 1060
– Repressor II 1056
– Sensor gene II 1058, 1059
– Sodium II 1064
– Spindle II 1064
– Structural gene II 1060
– Structural messenger II 1060
– Transcription regulation II 1060
– Translation II 1060
– Translation control II 1060
– tRNA II 1061
– Vinblastine II 1062
Generalized gangliosidosis I 190
Germinal gland, histogenesis I 479
Gigantism I 430
Gilbert's disease I 393
Gliadin I 323
Globin I 145
Globoid lipoidosis (see Krabbe's disease) I 196
Globoside, Gaucher's disease I 193
Globulin I 158
Glomerular filtration, Autoregulation I 543
Glomerulonephritis II 781
– Acute streptococcal II 865
– Antigen-antibody complex II 861
– Anti-glomerular membrane II 861
– Chronic II 865, 866
– Diffuse II 865
– Focal II 865
– Goodpasture II 863
– Goodpasture's syndrome II 862, 866
– Human II 861
– Malignant progressive II 865
– Renal transplant II 863
– Streptococcal II 862
– Subacute II 866
Glomerulosa cells I 554
Glucagon I 326, 506, 513, 530; II 1048
– Ketosis I 507
– Receptors I 528
Gluconeogenesis I 504, 514; II 1045
– ADP II 1046
– ADP/ATP ratio II 1048
– AMP II 1046
– ATP II 1046
– Biotin II 1046
– Citrate synthetase II 1048
– Cyclic AMP II 1048
– Diabetes II 1047
– Diphosphatase II 1046
– Fatty acids II 1048
– Fatty acyl CoA II 1048
– Fructose diphosphatase II 1046
– Glucagon II 1048
– Glucose II 1047, 1049
– Glucose administration II 1049
– Glucose-6-phosphatase II 1046
– Glutamate oxaloacetate transaminase II 1048
– Hepatocytes II 1049
– Hexokinase II 1046
– Malic enzyme II 1047
– Mitochondria II 1048
– NADH/NAD ratio II 1048
– Oxaloacetate II 1046
– Phosphocarboxykinase II 1046
– Phosphofructokinase II 1046
– Pyrophosphate II 1047
– Pyruvic carboxylase II 1046, 1047
– Pyruvic kinase II 1046, 1047
– Regulation in vivo, Pyruvic carboxylase II 1047
Glucoreceptors I 326
Glucosekinase II 1084
Glucose I 545
– Carrier I 545
– Reabsorption I 545
Glucose metabolism, Hormonal control I 505
Glucose-6-phosphatase II 640, 1042, 1046
– Fetus I 249
– Infancy I 250
Glucose-6-phosphate dehydrogenase, Pentose phosphate pathway I 21
Glucose tolerance I 283; II 1096
Glucose transport I 545
Glucose uptake I 514
Glucose uptake in brain I 514
Glucose uptake in lens I 514
Glucose uptake in tumor cells I 514
Glucosidase, Gaucher's disease I 193
Glucosuria, Renal I 545
Glucuronic acid cycle I 24
Glucoronic pathway I 282
– Intracellular distribution I 25
β-glucuronidase II 626, 937
Glutamic aspartic transaminase I 300
Glutamine I 588
Glutamine synthetase I 588
Glutathione reductase I 369
Glutathione synthesis I 588
Glutathione transferase II 976
Glycerokinase I 519
α-Glycerophosphate shuttle II 644
Glycine Oxidase I 36
Glycogen metabolism I 164
– Control II 1049
– – 5′-AMP II 1049
– – Anoxemia II 1050
– – Calcium II 1050
– – Glucose-6-phosphate increase II 1050
– – Glycogen synthetase II 1049, 1050
– – Kinase-activating factor II 1049
– – Phosphorylase II 1049
– – Trypsin II 1050
– – UDP-glycogen glycosyl transferase II 1049
– – Von Gierke's disease II 1050
– Glycogen synthetase, Phosphorylation II 1050
Glycogen storage disease I 163
– Anderson's disease I 166
– Branching enzymes I 166
– Convulsions I 164
– Forbes' disease I 165
– Glucose-6-phosphatase I 164
– 1,6-glucosidase I 165
– Glycogen in liver I 165
– Hers' disease I 166
– Hyperlipidemia I 164
– Ketosis I 164
– McArdle's disease I 166
– Pathogenesis I 166
– Phosphorylase I 166
– Phosphorylase kinase I 166
– Portocaval transposition I 165
– Types I 167
– Van Gierke's disease I 164
Glycogen synthesis, Control, Glycogen synthetase II 1050
– Active II 1050
– Calcium II 1050
– Inactive II 1050
– Phosphorylation II 1050
– Trypsin II 1050
Glycolipid II 1069
Glycolysis I 514; II 1045
– Control II 1042
– – Allosteric regulation II 1043
– – Crossover II 1042
– – Cyclic AMP II 1043
– – Fluoroacetate II 1043
– – Glucose II 1042
– – Glucose phosphatase II 1042
– – Phosphoenolpyruvic carboxykinase II 1042
– – Phosphofructokinase, Polymerization II 1042, 1043
– – Pyruvic carboxylase II 1042
– – Pyruvic kinase II 1042
– Nucleus I 80
Glycoproteins II 1080
– Biosynthesis, Transferases II 1080
– Receptors II 1080
– Regulation of growth II 1080
– Sialyl transferase II 1080
Glycosyl transferase II 934
Golgi apparatus I 135
– ATP sulfurylase I 136
– Galactosyl transferase I 136
– Glycoprotein biosynthesis I 136
– Lysosomal enzymes I 136
– Sulfation I 136
– Sulfatransferase I 136
Gonadotropin, elaboration II 1096
Gout I 218, 546, 594
– Allopurinol I 224
– Benamide I 224
– Colchicine I 224
– Feedback inhibition I 223
– Glutaminase I 223
– Glutamine PRPP Amidotransferase I 223
– Glutamine synthetase I 223

Gout, Indomethacin I 224
— Methylguanine I 218
— 1-methylguanine I 218
— 7-methylguanine I 218
— methyl-8-hydroxyguanine I 218
— 1-methylhypoxanthine I 218
— N, 2-methylguanine I 218
— Pathogenesis I 221
— Phenylbutazone I 224
— Phosphoribosyl transferase I 223
— Therapy I 224
— Tophi I 219
— Urate crystals I 220
Graffi virus II 1012
Graft-versus-host reaction II 840
— Cytolysis II 840
— Secondary disease II 840
— Wasting disease II 840
Gramicidin II 1077
Granulocytes II 1088
Graves' disease I 451
— Diarrhea I 452
— Excitability I 452
— Exophthalmia I 452
— Increased basal metabolism I 452
— Iodine I 452
— Muscle wasting I 452
— Pathogenesis I 455
— — LATS I 456
— — Receptors I 456
— Pathology I 451
— Protein bound iodine I 451
— Symptoms I 451
— Tachycardia I 452
— Thymicolymphatic state I 453
— Thyroid bound globulin I 451
— Thyroid bound proalbumin I 451
— Thyroxine I 452
— Vomiting I 452
Griseofulvin I 106
Gross virus II 1012
Ground substance II 934
— Biosynthesis II 936
— Chondroitin II 934
— Chondroitin sulfates II 934
— Heparin sulfate II 934
— Hyaluronic acid II 934
— Keratinosulfates II 935
— Keratosulfate II 934
— Marfan's syndrome II 934
— Polysaccharide II 936
— PPL fraction II 935
— Protein-polysaccharide complexes II 935
Growth factors II 914
— Epidermal growth II 914
— Erythropoietin II 914
— Fetuin II 915
— Lymphocytic proliferation II 914
— Nerve II 914
— — Microfilaments II 915
— — Microtubules II 915
— Receptors II 914
— Submaxillary gland II 914
— Zeatin II 915
Growth Hormone I 425, 507
— Amino acid sequence I 426
— Insulin effect I 427
— Metabolic effect I 427
— — Amino acid and protein synthesis I 428
— — Anti-insulinic effect I 427
— — Calcium I 429
— — Carbohydrate metabolism I 427
— — Electrolytes I 429
— — Fatty acid synthesis I 428
— — Glucose uptake I 427
— — Glucose uptake in muscles I 427
— — Hexose monophosphate shunt I 428
— — Insulin effect I 427
— — Ketosis I 428
— — Lipid metabolism I 427
— — Lipid mobilization I 428
— — Nitrogen balance I 428
— — Phosphorus I 429
— — Potassium I 429
— — Sodium I 429
— Receptors I 429
— Releasing factor I 429
— Sulfating factor I 431
Growth regulation II 1080
GTP, Purine metabolism I 214
Guanine I 210
Guanine hypoxanthine phosphoribosyl transferase I 225
Guanylate cyclase I 531
Guarnieri's bodies II 1003
Gulonolactone oxidase I 25

$H_2{}^{18}O$-ATP Exchange reaction I 52
$H_2{}^{18}O$-P_i Exchange reaction I 52
$H_2$5S protein II 978
Hageman factor deficiency I 407
Hand-Shüller-Christian disease I 438
Haptenes II 837
Havers canal I 335
HCG I 487
Heart diaphorase I 36
Heinz bodies I 158
— Drug induced hemolytic anemia I 170
Heinz bodies in thalassemia I 158
Hematopoietic, Erythroblast I 366
Hematopoietic system I 366
— Angioblast I 366
— Erythron I 366
— Hematopoiesis I 366
— Megaloblast I 366
— Megalocytes I 366
— Red cells I 366
Heme I 145, 158
— Iron I 206
— Myoglobin I 153
— Porphyria I 209
Heme in Thalassemia I 158
Heme synthesis I 302
Hemochromatosis I 383
— Pancreatitis I 383
— Xanthine oxidase I 383
Hemodialysis II 700
Hemoglobin I 145, 369
— A I 146
— C I 146
— D I 146
— Disease, clinical molecular correlation I 154
— D punjab I 147
— E I 147
— Electrophoretic mobility I 147
— F I 146
— Fetal I 145
— G I 146
— G Honolulu I 147
— G San Jose I 147
— Georgetown I 147
— Lepore I 146
— M Boston I 147, 156
— M Milwaukee I 147
— M Saskatoon I 147, 156
— Nomenclature I 145
— Norfolk I 147
— O Arabis I 147
— Reabsorption I 546
— S I 146, 147
— S tactoids I 147
— Structure I 153
Hemolytic anemia I 175, 391
— Bone marrow I 391
— Hemosiderin I 391
— Urobilinogen I 391
Hemolytic Jaundice I 387
Hemophilia I 406
— Transfusion I 407
— Von Willebrand's disease I 406
Hemosiderosis I 379, 380, 381
— Alcoholism I 382
— Marchiafava-Micheli syndrome I 381
Hemosiderosis in Thalassemia I 157
Heparin II 686
Heparin sulfate II 934
Hepatic lobules I 601
Hepatitis II 650
— A II 651
— B II 651
— Chronic II 652
— Clinical manifestation, Jaundice II 651
— Drugs II 652
— Viral II 650
— — Epidemic II 651
— — Experimental II 652
— — — Heredity II 653
— — — Immune reaction II 653
— — — Kupffer cell II 653
— — — Lysosomes II 653
— — — Toxic II 654
— — Fulminant II 651
— — Serum hepatitis II 651
Hepatomas II 1031, 1059, 1082, 1100
— Minimal deviation II 1031, 1082
— — Allosteric inhibition II 1085
— — Amino acid pool II 1085
— — Cholesterol biosynthesis II 1085
— — Enzyme induction II 1085
— — — Tryptophan pyrrolase II 1086
— — — Tyrosine glutaryl transaminase II 1086
— — Glycolysis II 1084
— — — Glucosekinase II 1084
— — — Hexokinase II 1084
— — — Ketone bodies II 1084
— — — Velocity of growth II 1084
— — — Histology II 1083
— — Isozymes, 5′-nucleotidase II 1087
— — Receptors II 1087
Hepatomegaly in galactosemia I 167
Hepatomegaly in thalassemia I 157
Hereditary angioneurotic edema II 858
Hereditary disease, Sickle cell anemia I 145
Hermaphroditism I 491
— Mosaicism I 491
— Ovotestis I 491
— Sex chromosomes I 491
Herpes virus II 1025
— Cancer II 962
Herpetic infection II 1008
Hers' disease (see Glycogen storage disease) I 166
Heterogeneous RNA I 121
— Cordycepin I 121
— dsRNA I 121
— snRNA I 121
Heterolytic fission II 639
Hexachlorobenzene, Porphyria I 209
Hexokinase II 1044, 1046, 1084
— Conformation II 1045
— Dimerization II 1045
— Fetus I 249

— Regulation II 1044
— — Conformation II 1045
— — Crabtree effect II 1045
— — Dimerization II 1045
— — Glucose-6-phosphate II 1044, 1045
— — Glycolysis II 1045
— — Lens II 1045
— — Muscle II 1045
— — Orthophosphate II 1044
Hexosaminidase in Tay-Sachs disease I 190
Hexose monophosphate shunt II 1030, 1031
Hippuric acid synthesis I 587
Histamine II 768
— Degranulation II 833
— Metabolism II 768, 770
— — Diamino oxidase II 768
— — Histaminase II 768
— — Histamine AD II 769
— — Histidine decarboxylase II 768
— — Methylation II 769
— — Xanthine oxidase II 769
— Release II 769
— — Cyclic AMP II 770
— — Degranulation II 769
— — Mast cells II 769
— — Phospholipase II 770
Histidase in histidinemia II 179
Histidine deaminase I 179
Histidine decarboxylase II 768
Histidine degradation I 180
Histidine pathogenesis I 181
Histidine pyruvic transaminase in histidinemia I 179
Histidinemia I 179
— Histidase I 179
— Histidine pyruvic transaminase I 179
— Imidazolone propionate hydrolase I 179
— Urocanase I 179
— Urocanic acid I 179
Histocompatibility II 845
— Genes II 839, 845
— Major II 845
— Minor II 845
Histones I 89; II 919, 1056
— After partial hepatectomy I 91
— Amino acid sequence I 90
— And DNA I 91
— Lysine I 90
— In simulated lymphocytes I 90
— Nomenclature I 92
— Phosphokinase I 91
— Role and metabolism I 90
HL-A system II 846
— Celiac disease II 848
— Cross-reactions II 847
— Disease II 847
— Mixed-lymphocyte culture II 848
— Transplantation II 847
HMG-CoA reductase II 1052
Hodgkin's disease II 781, 1025
Holotranscarboxylase I 280
Homocystinuria I 231
Homolytic cleavage II 639
Homoserine dehydrase I 301
Host-versus-graft reaction II 845
Houssay preparation I 60
Hunger I 326
Hunter's syndrome II 938
Hurler's syndrome II 938
Hyalinization II 660
Hyaluronic acid II 934
Hydrocephalus I 308
Hydrogen bonds I 152, 547
Hydrolases II 620
— Experimental necrosis II 623
— Insect metamorphosis II 623
— Necrobiosis II 622
— — Breast tissue II 623
— — Mullerian ducts II 622
— — Tadpoles II 622
— Nucleus I 83
— Shock II 624
— X-irradiation II 624
Hydrolases in autolysis II 621
Hydrolysine deficiency II 933
Hydronium iron I 571
Hydroxyacyl dehydrogenase I 56
B-Hydroxyacyl-ACP dehydrase I 62
Hydroxyanthranilic acids I 274
3-hydroxyanthranilic acid I 272
3-hydroxyanthranilic oxidase I 272
25-hydroxycholecalciferol, formula I 343
17-hydroxycorticosteroid I 283
Hydroxyproline I 284
Hydroxylation of proline I 285
5-Hydroxymethylcytosine I 96
Hydroxyphenylpyruvic hydroxylase I 283
Hydroxyprolinemia I 231
5-Hydroxytryptamine, Hypertension II 771
Hyper β-alaninemia I 231
Hyperbilirubinemia I 393
— Pernicious anemia I 393
— Drug induced hemolytic anemia I 170
Hypercalcemia I 351; II 1096
Hypercholesterolemia I 277
Hyperfibrinogenemia I 415
Hyperglobulinemia II 881
— Monoclonic II 882
— Polyclonic II 882
Hyperkalemia I 569
— Heart failure I 569
— Muscular dystrophy I 569
— Myasthenia I 569
Hyperlipidemia II 710, 712
— Abetalipoproteinemia II 711
— Familial II 710
— Foam cells II 711
— Lipemic retinitis II 711
— Pancreatitis II 711
— Tangier disease II 711
— Xanthoma II 710
— Xanthomatosis tuberosa II 711
Hyperlysemia I 231
Hyperoxaluria I 270
Hyperparathyroidism I 350, 592, 594
— Adenoma I 350
— Bone atrophy I 351
— Bone resorption I 352, 354
— Carcinoma I 350, 351
— Chief cell hyperplasia I 350
— Hypercalcemia I 351
— Hypertension I 352
— Muscle excitability I 352
— Nephrolithiasis I 351, 352
— Nerve excitability I 352
— Pancreatitis I 352
— Peptic ulcer I 352
— Primary I 350
— Secondary I 350, 352, 592
— — Acidosis I 353
— — Bone I 352
— — Chronic nephritis I 352
— — Congenital malformation I 352
— — Hypocalcemia I 353
— — Osteoclasts I 352
— — Phosphorus I 353
— Thrombosis I 352
— Uremic osteodystrophy I 352
— Von Recklinghausen's disease I 352
— Wasserhelle cell hyperplasia I 350
Hyperplasia II 898
Hypersarcosinemia I 231
Hypersensitivity II 836, 837
— Antigens II 837
— Antigen-antibody complexes II 836
— Cell-mediated II 837
— Haptenes II 837
— Macrophage inhibitory factor II 837
Hypersensitivity angiitis II 879
Hypertrophy II 898
Hyperuricemia I 218
— Heredity I 218
— Primary I 218
— Secondary I 218
Hypertension I 326, 352, 478, 493
Hypoadrenocorticism, Pituitary I 433
Hypocalcemia I 357
Hypoglycemia I 526; II 1096
— Alcohol I 527
— Classification I 525
— Clinicopathological correlation I 526
— Gluconeogenesis I 527
— In fetus I 527
— In newborns I 527
— Leucine I 527
— 5-methoxyindole-2-carboxylic acid I 527
— Nonpancreatic tumors I 526
— Pancreatic tumors I 526
— Propranolol I 527
— Quinaldinic acid I 527
Hypogonadism, Pituitary I 433
Hypoparathyroidism I 354
— Cataracts I 354
— Chvostek's sign I 354
— Convulsion I 354
— Erb's sign I 354
— Renal clearance I 354
— Serum calcium I 354
— Teeth I 354
— Tetany I 354
— Trousseau's sign I 354
Hypophysis I 425
— Anterior lobe I 425
— Basophilic cells I 425
— Cancer I 964
— Chromophobe cells I 425
— Eosinophilic cells I 425
— Organogenesis I 425
— Pars intermedia I 425
— Pars nervosa I 425
— Pars tuberalis I 425
— Pathology I 438
— Posterior lobe I 434
— — Oxytocin I 434
— — Vasopressin I 434
Hypopituitarism I 432
— Frohlich's syndrome I 432
— Idiopathic I 433
— Laurence-Moon-Biedl syndrome I 432
— Simmonds' cachexia I 432
Hypothalamic nuclei I 435
Hypothyroidism I 456
— Anemia I 457
— Carotenemia I 457
— Cholesterol levels I 457
— Cretinism I 456
— Facies I 457
— Fatty acid metabolism I 457
— Hexose monophosphate shunt I 457
— Mucopolysaccharide infiltration I 457
— Mucopolysaccharides I 457
— Myxedema I 456
— Skin I 457
— Steroid hormones I 457

Hypoxanthine guanine phosphoribosyl transferase I 224
Hypoxemia I 375
Hypoxia I 551

Imidazolone propionate hydrolase
– Histidinemia I 179
Iminoglycinuria I 232
Immunity
– Cellular II 820
– Graft-versus-host reponse II 828
– Hemangioblasts II 825
– Lymphatic system II 820
– Lymphocytes II 820, 825
– Macrophages II 825, 827
– Plasmoblasts II 825
– T and B cell interactions II 828
– Tolerance II 830
– – Capping II 832
– – Fetus II 830
– – High-zone II 832
– – Low-zone II 832
Immunodeficiency disease II 850, 851, 852
– Agammaglobulinemia II 853
– Third and fourth pharyngeal pouch syndrome II 853
Immunological disease II 854
– Allergens II 854
– Allergy II 854
– Atopic II 854
– Atopic eczema II 858
– – Benzylpenicillin II 855
– – Bronchial asthma II 856
– – Contact dermatitis II 858
– – Hereditary angioneurotic edema II 858
– – Pollen II 855
– – Reagins II 854
– – Rhinitis II 855
– – Urticaria II 857
– Glomerulonephritis II 860
– – Antigen-antibody complex II 860
– – Anti-basal membrane, II 860
– Immune reaction to drugs II 859
– – Acetophenetidin II 859
– – Aminosalicylic acid II 859
– – Aspirin II 859
– – Hydantoin II 859
– – Methyldopa II 859
– – Quinidine II 859
Immunological enhancement II 1102
Immunological response to bacteria II 848
– Receptors II 849
Immunological response II 848
– Parasites II 848
– Tuberculosis II 848
– Viruses II 848
– Urticaria pigmentosa II 858
– – Choriomeningitis virus II 849
Immunosuppression II 840
Immunosurveillance II 1103
Inborn errors of metabolism
– – Amino acid I 172
– – – Albinism I 178
– – – Arginase I 233
– – – Argininuria I 233
– – Aromatic amino acid I 172
– – – Alkaptonuria I 177
– – – Phenylketonuria I 172
– – – Tyrosinosis I 177
– – Carbohydrate metabolism I 163
– – – Drug induced hemolytic anemia I 170
– – – Fructosuria I 169
– – – Galactosemia I 167
– – – Hereditary hemolytic anemia I 231
– – – Therapy I 232
Inclusion bodies II 663, 1002
– Bilirubin II 663
– Ferrugination II 663
– Hematin II 663
– Lafora bodies II 663
– Lewy bodies II 663
– Negri bodies II 1003
– Rabies II 1003
Indomethacin I 224
Infancy I 250
– Glucose-6-phosphatase I 250
– Iron I 250
– Phenylalanine hydroxylase I 250
– Protein intake I 250
– Tyrosine transaminase I 250
– Tryptophan pyrrolase I 251
Infantile Amaurotic Familia Idiocy (scc Tay-Sachs-Disease) I 184
Inflammation
– Abscess II 795
– Acute II 791
– Angioneurotic edema II 774
– Appendicitis II 793
– Axon reflex II 766
– Bacteriostatic agents II 788
– Bradykinogen II 773
– Capillary dilation II 766
– Capillary permeability II 767, 771
– – Bradykinin II 771
– – Cement II 767
– – Exudine II 771
– – GF II 771
– – Kaleidin II 771
– – Leukotaxine II 771
– – Plasmin II 771
– – Pores II 768
– Caseation II 797
– Catarrhal II 792
– Cellular changes II 778
– – Leukocytic migration II 778
– Chemical mediators II 768
– – Histamine II 768
– Chemotaxis II 779
– Defective leukocytic response II 791
– Diapedesis II 779
– Eosinophils II 788, 789
– Epitheloid cells II 796
– Fibrinous II 792
– Fibrosis II 795
– Giant cells II 796
– Granulomas II 795
– Granulation tissue II 765
– Gross appearance II 792
– Hemorrhagic II 792
– Hemorrhage II 765
– 5-Hydroxytryptamine II 771
– Kallidin II 773
– Kallikreins II 773
– Leprosy II 799
– Lymphocytes II 789
– Macrophages II 789
– Necrosis II 765, 795
– Phagocytosis II 782
– Plasmocytes II 789
– Phlegmon II 795
– PMN migration II 765
– Process as a whole II 765
– Prostaglandin II 775
– Purulent II 792
– Pus formation II 765
– Pustules II 793
– Repair II 765
– Serous II 792
– Syphilis II 797
– Tuberculosis II 796
– Vascular reaction II 766
– Vasodilation II 765
Initiation Factors I 130
– M_2A I 130
– M_2B I 130
– M_3 I 130
– R I 130
– S I 130
– TR I 130
Initiation of translation
– Eukaryotes I 129
Initiator II 987
– Factors I 129
– – F_1 I 129
– – F_2 I 129
Inosine I 110
Insulin I 283, 495, 530
– Adenylate cyclase I 521
– Antibodies I 502
– Binding I 520
– – Adipose tissue I 521
– Binding
– – Diaphragm I 521
– Deficiency I 502
– Diabetes and glucagon I 506
– Effect on adipose tissue I 519
– – Glycerokinase I 519
– – Lipogenesis I 519
– Glutathione-insulin transhydrogenase I 502
– Guanylate cyclase I 521
– Insulinase I 502
– Metabolic effect I 510
– – Liver I 512
– – Muscle I 510
– – – Glycogen synthesis I 511
– – – Oxidation of pyruvate I 511
– Mode of action
– – ATP synthesis I 518
– – Carrier I 516
– – Effect on adipose tissue I 519
– – Gluconeogenesis I 513
– – Glucose-6-phosphatase I 513
– – Glucose output I 513
– Mode of action (con'd)
– – Glycogen synthesis I 513
– – Hexokinase theory I 516
– – Protein synthesis I 518
– – – Transcription I 519
– – – Translation I 519
– – Transport theory I 515
– Receptors I 521, 528
– Secretion I 506
– – Islets of Langerhans I 506
– – Regulation I 520
– Sinalbumin I 502
– Structure I 508
– Transport I 510
Interferon
– Inducers II 1007
– – Polyanionic macromolecules II 1007
– Induction II 1006
– Picronavirus II 1007
– RNA-dependent RNA polymerase II 1006
– Thymidine kinase II 1006
Intermediates in oxidative phosphorylation I 47
Interphase I 87
Intestinal, bypass I 599
– Bypass I 599
Intestinal flora I 323
Intestinal polyps II 948

— DNA contents I 94
Intestinal secretion I 262
— Aminopeptidase I 262
— Amylase I 262
— Enterokinase I 262
— Exopeptidase I 262
— Invertase I 262
— Lactase I 262
— Lipase I 262
— Maltase I 262
Intestine, Irradiation I 607
Intracellular Distribution I 7
— Fatty acids I 57
— Glucuronic pathway I 25
— Krebs Cycle I 31
— Pentose pathway I 25
Intrinsic factor I 286
— Antibodies I 287
— Assay I 287
— Gastrectomy I 286
Invertase I 503
Iodide Oxidation I 440
Iodinated tyrosine I 440
Iodine I 439
— metabolism I 440
— — Thiocyanate I 440
— Oxidation I 439
— Pump I 439
— Release I 439
— Storage I 439
— Trapping I 439
Ionizing radiation II 733, 746
— Biological effects II 733
— Effect on gastrointestinal tract II 736
— Effect on gonads II 735
— Effect on hematopoietic organs II 735
— Effect on mammary glands II 735
— Effect on ovaries II 735
— Effect on skin II 733
— Types of exposure II 733
Iron II 1009
— Absorption I 363
— Atom I 377
— Catalase I 379
— Cytochromes I 378
— Deficiency I 383, 384
— — Dysphagia I 383
— — Incidence I 363
— — Pathogenesis I 385
— — Plummer-Vinson syndrome I 383
— Ferrochetalase I 206
— Heme I 206
— Hemoproteins I 378
— Incorporation in red cells I 371
— — Kinetics I 371
— Metabolism I 363, 375
— — Chlorosis I 363
— — Control I 373
— — Hemolytic anemia I 375
— — Hypoxemia I 375
— Orbitals I 378
— Release I 364
— Requirement I 363
— Role in hematopoietic system I 366
— Secretion I 365
— Tissue distribution I 365
— Transport, Intestinal I 363
— Uptake in red cells I 371
— Xanthine oxidase I 364
Irridation II 701, 1099
— Beer-Lambert law II 721
— Ionization II 720
Isobutyryl CoA I 58
— Pathway I 58
Isocitric dehydrogenase I 30
Isolated hepatocytes II 1056
Isoleucine, Maple syrup disease I 181
Isopentenyl pyrophophate II 694
Isotope I 82
— Uptake I 82
Isovaleric CoA I 58
— Pathway I 58

Jaundice I 389
— Bilirubin I 385
— — Diglucuronide I 389
— — Monoglucuronide I 389
— Blood brain barrier I 389
— Drug induced hemolytic anemia I 170
— Gilbert's disease I 393
— Hemolytic pathogenesis I 393
— Hepatic I 392
— Kernicterus I 389, 390
— Neonatal I 389
— — UDPGA transferase I 389
— Nonhemolytic I 389
— — Congenital familial I 390
— — — Enzymes I 391
— — — Glucuronyl transferase I 390
— — — Kernicterus I 391
— — Pathogenesis I 394
— Obstructive I 392
— Pathogenesis I 389
J-chain II 819
Juxtaglomerular apparatus I 557
— Blood volume I 557
— Erythropoietin I 557
— Lace cells I 557
— Renin I 557

Kallidin II 773
Karyolysis I 610
Karyorrhexis II 611
Karyotype I 234
— Giemsa banding I 235
Kaschin-Beck disease I 379
Keratinization I 307
Keratinosulfates II 935
Keratosulfate II 934
Kernicterus I 389, 390
Ketoacyl thiolase I 57
B-Ketoacyl-ACP-Reductase I 62
α-Ketoglutarate decarboxylase I 30, 270
Ketosis I 55, 58
— Acetoacetic acid I 522
— Acetoacetyl CoA deacylase I 522
— β-hydroxybutyric acid I 522
— Diabetes I 522
— Gluconeogenesis I 525
— Malnutrition I 253
— — Mechanism I 523
Kidney I 539
— Amino acid excretion I 546
— Anatomy I 539
— Arteriolae rectae I 540
— Glucose reabsorption I 545
— Gout I 546
— Hemoglobin reabsorption I 546
— Hypernephroma II 1100
— Lithiasis I 546
— Mutarotase I 545
— Phlorhizin I 545
— Renal artery I 540
— Renal glucosuria I 545
— Renal tubles I 540
— Sodium reabsorption I 553
— Transplant II 839
— Uric acid reabsorption I 545
Kinins in disease II 774
— Anaphylactic shock II 774
— Angioneurotic edema II 774
— Carcinoid II 774
— Carcinoma of lung II 774
— Carcinoma of thyroid II 774
— Flushing II 774
— Retroperitoneal neuroblastoma II 774
Krabbe's disease I 196, 197
— Brain I 197
Krebs cycle I 27, 1030
— Aconitase I 29
— Citric Acid synthesis I 28
— Distribution in tissues I 31
— Fate of Succinyl-CoA I 28
— Fumarase I 30
Isocitric dehydrogenase I 30
— α-Ketoglutarate decarboxylase I 30
— Lipoic acid I 30
— Pyruvate metabolism I 31
— Succinic dehydrogenase I 30
— Thiamine pyrophosphate I 30
— Three-point attachment theory I 28
Kuru II 1009
Kwashiorkor I 262
— Anemia I 264
— Brain I 264
— Edema I 265
— Essential amino acids I 265
— Fatty liver I 264
— Glucose I 265
— Mental retardation I 264
— Pancreas I 265
— Pathogenesis I 263, 266
— Pathology I 263
— Potassium I 262, 265
— Protein I 262
— Protein turnover I 265
— Water retention I 265
Kynurenase I 272
Kynurenic acid I 274
Kynurenine formamidase I 272
Kynurenine-3-hydroxylase I 272
Kynurenine transaminase I 273

Lactases I 503
Lactase intolerance I 231
Lactic dehydrogenase,
— Fetus I 249
— Nucleus I 80
Lactonase I 21, 25
Lafora bodies II 663
Laurence-moon-biedl syndrome I 432, 433
Lectins I 521
Leiomyoma II 963
— Estrogen II 963
Lens I 514
Leprosy,
— Lepromatous cell II 799
Lesch-Nyhan syndrome I 216, 224
— Dopamine-β-hydroxylase I 225
— Hypoxanthine guanine phosphoribosyl transferase I 224
Leucine in maple syrup disease I 181
Leukemia II 743, 1100
— Viruses II 1012
— — Bregen-Moloney virus II 1012
— — Erythroleukemia II 1013
— — Friend virus II 1013
— — Graffi virus II 1012
— — Gross virus II 1012
— — Horizontal transfer II 1012
— — Lymphatic leukemia II 1013
— — Moloney virus II 1012
— — Myeloid leukemia II 1013
— — Rauscher virus II 1013
— — Schwartz virus II 1012
— — Thymus II 1013
— — Vertical transmission II 1012
— — X-irradiation II 1012

Leukocytic migration II 778
— Leukocytic margination II 778
— Membranes II 778
— Stickiness II 778
Leukocyte movement II 1095
Leukodystrophies I 196
— Globoid lipoidosis I 196
— Krabbe's Disease I 196
— Metachromatic I 197
— Sulfatides I 196
— Sulfatase I 196
— Sulfatide synthetase I 196
Lewy bodies II 663
L-glyceric aciduria I 232
Ligands I 376
Linoleic acid II 639
Linolenic acid II 639
Lipemia I 271
Lipemic Retinitis II 711
Lipids
Blood II 689
— — Cerebrosides II 685
— — Cholesterol II 689
— — Cholesterol esters II 689
— — Diabetes II 690
— — Esterified fatty acids II 689
— — Neutral fats II 689
— — Nonesterified fatty acids II 689
— — Phospholipids II 689
— — Principal sources II 690
— — α-triglycerides II 689
— — β-triglycerides II 689
— — Origin II 690
— — — ApoC II 690
— — — Chylomicrons II 690, 691
— — — Fatty acids II 691
— — — HDL II 690
— — — LDL II 690
— — — Protein lipase II 691
— — — Triglycerides II 691
— — — VLDL II 690
Lipogenesis I 519
Lipoic acid I 283
— Fat infiltration I 26
Lipoic Dehydrogenase I 26
Lipoidosis I 184
— Metachromatic leukodystrophy I 197
— Tay-Sachs disease I 184
Lipoprotein,
— Blood II 687
— — Apoproteins II 688
— — Cholesterol II 688
— — Density-gradient centrifugation II 687
— — Flotation II 687
— — Low-density II 687
— — Micellar II 687
— — Mobility II 688
— — Pseudomolecular II 687
— — Sf value II 687
— — Solubility II 688
— — Very high-density II 687
— — Very low-density II 687
Lipoprotein lipase II 686
Liposarcomas II 1026, 1100
Lithiasis I 302, 546, 592
— Renal calculi I 593
Liver Disease I 277, 278
— Endoplasmic reticulum I 587
— Hepatic artery I 585
— Hepatic cells I 585
— Hepatic lobule I 585
— Kiernan's spaces I 585
— Kupffer's cells I 585
— Microbodies I 587
— Proteases I 587
— Steroid hormones I 494
— Protein turnover I 586
— — Arginase I 586
— — Starvation I 586
Liver regeneration II 1063
Liver steatosis II 635
— Alcohol II 642
— Carbon tetrachloride intoxication II 638
— Cardiac insufficiency II 640
— Diabetes II 640
— Endoplasmic reticulum II 637
— Ethionine II 640
— Galactosemia II 640
— Lipophanerosis II 637
— Liposomes II 636
— Microscopy II 635
— Mitochondria II 637
— Phosphorus II 640
— Puromycin II 640
— Starvation II 640
— Triton X-100 II 637
— Ultrastructure II 635
LSH, I 487
Lung, I 577
— Alveolar wall, I 577
— Cancer, II 993, 1100
— Fetus, I 577
— Function,
— — Gas exchange, I 576, 577
— Passive congestion, I 577
— Pneumonia, I 577
— Septae, I 577
Lupus erythematosus, II 871
— Afferent limb theory, II 872, 875
— Am antigen, II 873
— DNA antibodies, II 872
— Efferent limb theory, II 875
— Endocarditis of Libman-Sacks, II 873
— Forbidden clones, II 872
— Natural history, II 871
— Onion skin arteriolar sclerosis, II 873
— Vasculitis, II 873
Lymphangioma II 948
Lymphocytes II 821
— B cells, II 823
— — Bursa, II 823
— Life span II 821
— Lymphokinins, II 829
— Null cells, II 826
— Proliferation, II 918
— — DNA synthesis, II 918
— — Histones, II 919
— Recirculation, II 821
— T cells, II 822
— — Thymus, II 823
Lymphocytes B, II 824
— Factors, II 829
— Histones, I 91
— Interaction with T cells, II 825
Lymphokinins, II 829
— Blastogenic factors, II 830
— Growth inhibitory factor, II 830
— Migration inhibitory factor, II 829
— Mitogenic factor, II 830
— Transfer factor, II 829
Lymphotoxic factors, II 829
Lyon's hypothesis, I 491
Lysine oxidase, II 933
Lysogeny, II 1008
Lysosomal disease, I 199
Lysosomes, I 316, 620, 653
— Enzymes, II 627
— — A form, II 627
— — B form, II 627
— Physiological role, II 621
— Pinocytic theory, II 621

Macroglobulinemia, Waldenstrom's disease, II 882, 883
Macrophage inhibitory factor, II 837
Macrophage movement, II 1095
Macrophages, II 789, 827
— Phagocytosis, II 790
— — Acid hydrolases, II 790
— — Electron transport, II 790
— — Respiratory activity, II 790
— Promonocyte, II 790
Malaria, I 149
Malaria in drug induced hemolytic anemia, I 170
Malate aspartate shuttle, II 644
Malate citrate shuttle, II 644
Malatonin, I 106
Male sex hormones, leydig cells, I 483
Malnutrition, I 159
— Body size, I 252
— Diabetes, I 247
— Fetus, I 248
— General, I 247
— Glucose alanine cycle, I 253
— Growing child, I 252
— Growth retardation, I 252
— Ketosis, I 253
— Lactation, I 247
— Osteoporosis, I 253
— Placenta, I 247
— Pregnancy, I 247
— Protein deficiency, I 253
— Steroid hormones, I 248
Malnutrition in disease, I 318
— Disaccharidases, I 318
— Dumping syndrome, I 318
— Steatorrhea, I 318
Malonyl CoA-ACP transacylase, I 62
Maltases, I 503
Mammary cancer, II 1096
Mammary tumors, B particles, II 1014
Maple syrup disease, I 57
— Alloisoleucine, I 181
— Branched amino acids, I 181
— Decarboxylase, I 181
— Isoleucine, I 181
— Leucine, I 181
— Pyridoxal phosphate, I 181
— Transaminase, I 181
— Valine, I 181
Maple syrup urine disease, I 179
Marchiafava-Micheli syndrome, I 381
— Transferrin, I 381
— Transferrinemia, I 381
Marfan's syndrome, II 934
Mast cells, II 769, 770
McArdle's disease (see glycogen storage disease), I 166
Megaloblast, DNA content, I 94
Megaloblastic anemia, orotic aciduria, I 229
Meiosis, I 489
— Chiasmata, I 489
— Chromatids, I 489
— Crossover, I 489
— Pachytene, I 489
— Zygotene, I 489
Melanin in albinism, I 178
Melanin in phenylketonuria, I 174
Melanocyte in albinism, I 178
Melanocyte-stimulating hormones, I 472
Melanoma, II 1100
Membranes, I 542, 550
— Nuclear, I 73

Mental retardation, I 264
Messenger RNA, II 1021, 1060
— Binding to ribosomes, I 126
— Polycistronic, I 133
Metabolic acidosis, I 580
Metachromatic leukodystrophy, I 197
— Brain, I 198
— Pathogenesis, I 198
Metaphase, I 87
Metastasis, II 1089
— Liver, II 951
Methemoglobinemia, I 155
— Benzoquinoacetic acid, I 157
— Compensatory polycythemia, I 155
— Cyanosis, I 155
— Diaphorase, I 156
— Hemoglobin M, I 156
— Methemoglobin reductase, I 155
— NADPH-dependent methemoglobin reductase, I 156
Methotrexate, I 297
Methoxytyramine in phenylketonuria, I 174
Methylcholanthrene, II 987
β-methylcrotonyl CoA carboxylase, I 279
— Mode of action, I 280
Methylglutaconase, I 57
1-methylhistidine, I 160
3-methylhistidine, I 160
2-methylhydronaphthoquinone, I 36
Methylmalonate CoA-isomerase, I 59
Methylmalonic aciduria, I 232
Methyl purine, I 110
Mevalonic acid, II 693, 694
Mevalonic kinase, II 694
M factor, I 119
Michaelis-Menten theory, I 503
Microbodies, I 137, 587
— D amino oxidase, I 137
— Half life, I 137
— Isocitrate dehydrogenase, I 137
— L-hydroxy acid oxidase, I 137
— Nucleoids, I 137
Microglia, II 664
Microsomes, I 316
Microtubules, I 105
Milk, II 1014
— B particles, II 1014
— Composition, I 251
Mineralization, I 339
— Alkaline phosphatase, I 340
— Fluorine, I 340
— Helmholtz double layer, I 338
— Sodium, I 340
— Strontium, I 340
— Surface ions, I 338
Minimal deviation, II 1030
Mitochondria, I 55, 60, 316; II 646, 1033, 1048
— DNA, I 66
— Gene expression, I 67
— Ribosomes, I 67
— RNA, I 67
— RNA polymerase, I 67
— Transfer RNA, I 67
Mitochondrial DNA, II 1032
Mitochondrion, I 45, 63
— Cardiolipin, I 65
— Chloramphenicol, I 66
— Cristae, I 63
— Membranes, I 65
— Movements, I 65
— Origin, I 65
— Particles, I 45
— — Antimycin, I 46
Mitomycin, II 615
Mitosis, I 87
— Anaphase, I 87
— Aster, I 87
— Centromere, I 87
— Centrosome, I 87
— Interphase, I 87
— Nuclear membrane, I 87
— Nucleoli, I 87
— Prophase, I 87
— Spindle, I 87
— Telophase, I 87
— X-radiation, I 87
Mitotic apparatus, I 105
— And colchicine, I 106
— And griseofulvin, I 106
— And melatonin, I 106
— And podophyllotoxin, I 106
— And UV light, I 106
— And vinblastine, I 106
Mixed-function oxidase, I 60; II 640, 643, 975
— Benzoflavone, II 976
— Cigarette smoking, II 976
— Indole-3-acetonitrite, II 976
— Induction, II 975
— Nicotine, II 976
— Parathion, II 976
Polycyclic hydrocarbons, glutathione transferase, II 976
Mixed-lymphocyte culture, II 848
Molecular orbital, I 376
Moloney virus, II 1012
Molybdenum, I 161
Mongoloid facies and thalassemia, I 157
Monotyrosine, deiodination, I 442
Mosaicism, I 489, 491
Mucopolysaccharide, ^{35}S-incorporation, I 284
Mucopolysaccharidosis, I 241; II 938
— Corrective factors, II 939
— β-galactosidase, II 939
— Hunter's syndrome, II 938
— Hurler's syndrome, II 938
— Sanfilippo syndrome, II 938
— Syndrome S, II 938
Multiple sclerosis, II 669
— Astrocytosis, II 670
— Autoimmunity, II 671
— Charcot's triad, II 669
— Demyelinization, II 670
— Geography, II 669
— Gliosis, II 670
— Intention tremor, II 669
— Lead, II 669
— Measle viruses, II 672
— Microglial infiltration, II 670
— Nystagmus, II 669
— Parasthesia, II 671
— Pathology, II 670
— Plaque, II 670
— Scrapie, II 672
— Slurred speech, II 669
— Spastic paraplegia, II 671
— Thrombi, II 671
— Transient blindness, II 671
— Virus, II 669, 672
Muscular dystrophy, I 569; II 672
Muscular injuries, I 315
Mushroom toxins, II 654
— *Amanita muscaria,* II 654
— *Amanita phalloides,* II 654
— Amanitine, II 654
— Muscarine II 654
— Phallin, II 654
— Phalloidine, II 654
— RNA polymerase, II 654
Mutagens, I 94
Mutation, II 990
— Carcinogenesis, II 990
— Operator 0 mutants, I 131
— Polarity, I 131, 133
Mutarotase, I 545
Myasthenia gravis, II 824
Myelin, II 665
— Birefringent, II 665
— Histochemistry, II 666
— Lipid, II 666
— Protein, II 666
— — Amino acid sequence, II 667
— Proteolipids, II 667
— Schmidt-Lanterman clefts, II 665
— Schwann cell, II 665
— X-ray diffraction, II 665
Myelination, II 667, 668
— Charcot-marie-tooth disease, II 668
Myeloma,
— Clasmatosis, II 883
— Flame cell, II 884
— Multiple, II 883
— Russell's bodies, II 884
— Thesaurocytes, II 884
Myeloperoxidase, deficiency, II 788
Myocardial disease, II 649
Myocardial infarct, II 697, 701, 705
— Electrocardiographic findings, II 707
— Norepinephrine, II 707
Myoglobin, I 152
— Heme, I 153
— Structure, I 152
Myopathy, II 649
Myxedema, I 433, 456; II 700
— Primary, I 456
— Secondary, I 456

NADase, I 34
NADH coenzyme Q reductase, I 43
NADH/NAD ratio, II 644
NAD metabolism, I 275
NAD synthetase, I 274
NADP-L-hexonate dehydrogenase, I 25
Naphthalene, drug induced hemolytic anemia, I 170
Natriuretic hormone, I 560, 561
Necrocytosis, dynamic changes, II 611
Necrosis, I 608
— Coagulation, I 608
— Fat I 609
— Liquefaction I 608
— Microscopic I 609
— Type I 608
Negri bodies II 1003
Neonatal jaundice I 389
— Placental barrier I 390
— UDPG dehydrogenase I 389
Neo-oncogene II 1104
Nephrolithiasis I 351, 352
Nephrosis II 700
Nernst equation I 568
Nernst potential I 569
Nerolidol pyrophosphate, II 695
Nerve cells, II 661
— Acetylcholine, II 662
— Astrocytes, II 663
— Axon flow, II 662
— Betz cells, II 661
— Cylindraxile, II 661
— Dendrite, II 661
— Inclusion bodies, II 663
— Injury, nissl substance, II 662
— Neurofibril injury, II 662
— Neurofibrillar structure, II 661
— Nissl substance, II 661

Nervous fibers, II 664
— Axon, II 664
— Axoplasm, II 664
— Clefts of Schmidt-Lanterman, II 664
— Fibers of Remak, II 664
— Myelin, II 665
— Nodes of Ranvier, II 664
— Schwann cell, II 664
Nervous system, II 661
Neuroblastoma, II 1100
Neurofibril, II 661
— Densification, II 662
— Disintegration, II 662
— Fibrolysis, II 662
— Swelling, II 662
Neurofisin, I 436
Neurons, purine metabolism, I 216
Neurophysins, I 437
N^{10}-formyltetrahydrofolic acid, I 294
Niacin, I 271
Niacinogen, I 271
Nicotinic acid, I 272, 414
— Deficiency, I 271
— — Cholesterol, I 271
— — Lipemia, I 271
— Metabolism, I 271, 272
— — Deamido NAD, I 274
— — NAD synthetase, I 274
— — Niacin, I 271
— — Niacinogen, I 271
— — Tryptophan, I 274
— — Xanthurenic acid, I 272
— Ribonucleotide, I 273
— Tryptophan metabolism I 272
Niemann-Pick disease I 193
— Behinic acid I 195
— Brain I 194
— Liver I 194
— Pathogenesis I 196
— Sphingomyelin I 195
— Spingomyelinase I 196
— Spleen I 194
Nissl substance II 661
— Chromatolysis II 662
— Densification II 662
Nitrogen balance I 478
Node of Ranvier II 664, 666
Nodules of Minet II 869
Nonenzymic transanimation, Schiff base I 300
Nontropical sprue
— Celiac disease I 324
— Gliadin I 324
Norepinephrine in phenylketonuria I 174
Nuclear inclusion II 1003
Nuclear injuries, viruses II 1001
Nuclear membrane
— And endoplasmic reticulum I 75
— Annuli I 74
— Permeability I 74
Nuclear transplantation II 1061
Nucleic acid I 88
Nuclein I 88
Nucleolus I 75, 120
— Chromosomes I 79
— Liver regeneration I 77
— Regenerating liver I 78
— Ribosomal RNA I 79
— Starvation I 77, 78
— Thioacetamide I 78
— Ultraviolet light I 77
— X-irradiation (nucleolus) I 77
Nucleophilic reagent I 50
Nucleoside diphosphokinase I 31
Nucleotide I 24
Nucleotide pyrophosphatase I 34
Nucleus
— Adenosine triphosphatase I 83
— 5′-adenylic phosphatase I 83
— Aldolase I 80
— Arginase I 84
— Cytochrome oxidase I 84
— DNA content I 93
— DNA polymerase I 83
— Enzymes I 83
— Glycolysis I 80
— Hexokinase I 80
— Hydrolytic enzymes I 83
— Ionizing radiation I 81
— Lactic dehydrogenase I 80
— Membrane, pores I 73
— Oxidative phosphorylation I 81
— Protein synthesis I 82
— Sources of energy I 80
— Triose phosphate dehydrogenase I 80
— Urea-forming system I 84
Nutrition, infancy I 250

Obesity I 325, 326
— Atherosclerosis I 326
— Glucagon I 326
— Glucoreceptors I 326
— Hunger I 326
— Hypertension I 326
— Ketogenesis I 327
— Metabolic regulation I 326
— Psychological factors I 327
— Satiety center I 326
Ocre mutation I 118
Odontoblasts I 279
Okazaki fragments I 102
Oligodendrocytes II 663
— Satellitosis II 664
— Sensitivity II 664
Oligomycin I 50, 52
One gene-one enzyme theory in drug induced hemolytic anemia I 171
Operator genes I 130
Operon theory I 130
— Histidine I 130
— Lactose I 130
— Polarity I 131
Opsin I 306
Optical isomerism I 56
Orotic aciduria I 225, 228
— Aspartic transcarbamylase I 229
— Megaloblastic anemia I 229
— Ureidosuccinic acid I 229
Ossification I 334
— Cancellous bone I 335
— Compact bone I 335
— Havers canal I 335
— Osteoblast I 334
— Osteoclast I 335
— Osteocyte I 334
Osmotic pressure I 540
— Anoxia I 542
— Membrane I 542
— Selective solvation I 542
Osteoblasts I 279, 334
Osteoclast I 335
Osteogenesis imperfecta II 933
Osteogenic sarcoma II 1100
Osteoid I 279
Osteoporosis I 355, 358, 478
— Aged I 356
— Calcium/PO ration I 355
— Immobilization I 356
— Pathogenesis I 355
— Schmorl's nodules I 356
Oxalic acid metabolism I 183
Oxaluria I 182, 594
— 2,3-diketo-L-gulonic acid I 182
— Glyoxylic acid I 182
— Glyoxylic acid dehydrogenase I 182
— N-glyoxylglutamic acid I 182
— Lithiasis I 182
— Oxalic acid metabolism I 183
α-Oxidation I 59
β-Oxidation pathway of fatty acids I 54, 55
ω-Oxidation I 59
Oxidative phosphorylation I 46
— Alcohol dehydrogenase I 49
— Amytal I 47, 50, 52
— ATP-ADP exchange reaction I 52
— ATPase release I 52
— ATP-^{32}P; exchange I 52
— Azide I 52
— Chemiosmotic coupling I 53
— Chlorpromazine I 52
— Conformational coupling I 53
— Coupling factor I 51
— Coupling mechanisms I 47
— Cyanide I 47
— $H_2{}^{18}O$-ATP exchange reaction I 52
— $H_2{}^{18}O$-P_i exchange reaction I 52
— Intermediates I 47, 48
— Oligomycin I 50, 52
— Sites of phosphorylation I 47
— Uncoupling agents I 47
Oxythiamine I 267

Palmitaldehyde dehydrogenase I 55
Pancreas cancer II 1100
Pancreas regeneration II 1063
Pancreatic secretion I 261
— Cholecystokinin I 262
— Hormones I 262
— Pancreozymin I 262
— Secretinase I 262
— Secretin I 262
Pancreatitis I 352; II 630, 711
— Amylase II 632
— Chronic II 631
— Fatty necrosis II 631
— Hypocalcemia II 632
— Lipase II 632
— Pancreozymin I 532
— Pathogenesis II 632
— Secretin II 632
— Trypsin II 632
— Trypsinogen II 631
Pancreozymin I 262
Pantothenic acid deficiency I 275
— Diabetes I 277
— Hypercholesterolemia I 277
— Coenzyme A I 276
— Congenital anomalies I 276
— Duodenal ulcer I 276
— Liver disease I 277, 278
— Renal deficiency I 277
Papillomas II 1026
Paraaminoazobenzene II 977
Paraglobulinemia II 881
Paramonomethylaminoazo-benzene II 977
Parathormone I 346
— Aconitase I 348
— Adenylcyclase I 349
— Amino acid sequence I 347
— Bone resorption I 348
— Citric acid I 348
— Collagenolytic effect I 349
— Condensing enzyme I 348
— Control of secretion I 347
— Cyclic AMP I 349
— DNA metabolism I 349
— Effect I 348

– Effect on bone I 348
– Glomerular filtration of phosphate I 349
– Isocitric dehydrogenase I 348
– Lactate I 348
– Mitochondrial I 349
– Phosphaturic action I 349
– Protein synthesis I 349
– Purification I 347
– RNA metabolism I 349
Parathyroid, cancer II 1100
Parathyroid glands, oxyphilic cells I 346
Partial hepatectomy, histones I 91
Partial pressures of CO_2 I 580
Passive congestion I 577
Pasteur effects II 1028, 1029, 1043
– ADP II 1043
– Inorganic phosphate II 1043
– NADH II 1044
– Phosphofructokinase II 1044
Pathogenesis of nontropical sprue I 324
Pathogenesis of vitamin C deficiency I 285
Pathological calcification I 358
– Microincineration I 358
– Von Kossa staining I 358
Pellagra I 271
– Black tongue I 271
– Clinicopathology I 271
– Dementia I 271
– Dermatitis I 271
– Diarrhea I 271
– Nicotinic acid I 271
– Pathogenesis I 274
Penicillin G II 994
Pentose pathway I 21
– Intracellular distribution I 25
– Transaldolase I 22
Pentose phosphate pathway I 21
– Distribution I 24
– Glucose-6-phosphate dehydrogenase I 21
– Goal in metabolism I 22
– Metabolic sequence I 23
– Phosphogluconate dehydrogenase I 21
Pentosuria I 24, 232
Pepsin I 256
– Inhibitor I 257
– Phosphoserine I 257
Pepsinogen I 256
Peptic ulcer I 352
Peptide bonds, polyglycine I 151
Peptide bond synthesis I 126
Peptidyl transferase I 127
Periodic paralysis I 564
Periodic table I 375
Pernicious anemia I 284, 289
– Anisocytosis I 289
– Bone marrow I 289
– Demyelination I 289
– Gastric smears I 289
– Hematological changes I 289
– Heredity I 288
– Megaloblast I 289
– Nucleated red cells I 289
– Neurological degeneration I 289
– Normoblast I 289
– Pathogenesis I 293
– Polymorphonuclears I 289
– Thrombocytes I 289
– Tongue I 289
– Vitamin B12 I 286
Peroxisomes (see Microbodies) I 137; II 643
– Petroleum products II 994
pH I 571
– Acidosis I 571
– Alkalosis I 571
– Bicarbonate absorption I 573
– Blood I 571
– Carbonic anhydrase I 573
– Cell I 572
λ Phage II 1008
Phagocytin II 788
– Deficiency II 788
Phagocytosis I 24; II 782, 1000
– Choline II 784
– Ehrlich ascites cells II 788
– Glucose II 784
– Glycogen II 785
– Glycolysis II 785
– Histamine II 784
– Macrophages II 790
– Membrane II 784
– Opsonin II 783
– Opsonization II 784
– Phospholipids II 785
– Phagosome II 784
– Polymorphonuclear II 786
– Respiration II 785
– Salt II 784
Phenylalanine hydroxylase infancy I 250
Phenylbutazone I 224
Phenylketonuria I 108, 172
– Ascorbic acid I 174, 175
– Biosynthesis of melanin I 174
– Carcinoids I 174
– Copper I 175
– Dihydropteridine I 172
– 3,4-dihydroxyphenylalanine I 174
– Dopa decarboxylase I 174
– Epinine I 174
– Fetal liver I 175
– Glutamic acid decarboxylase I 176
– Hydroxytryptophan decarboxylase I 176
– Metabolic alterations I 175
– Methoxytyramine I 174
– M-tyramine I 174
– Neurological lesions I 176
– Norepinephrine I 174
– Pathogenesis I 175, 177
– Pathogenesis of neurological lesions I 176
– Phenylalanine hydroxylase I 172
– Phenyltryptamine I 176
– Pyridoxal phosphate I 174
– S-adenosylmethionine transferase I 174
– Serotonin I 174
– Tetrahydropteridine I 172
– Tyrosinase I 174
– Tyrosine transaminase I 174
Pheochromocytomas II 964, 1096
Phlorhizin I 545
Phorbol II 987
Phosphocarboxykinase II 1046
Phosphodiesterase I 529
Phosphoenolpyruvate kinase I 31
Phosphoenolpyruvic carboxykinase II 1042
Phosphofructokinase I 531; II 1043, 1046
– Fetus I 249
Phosphoglucomutase I 170
– Galactosemia I 168
6-Phosphogluconate dehydrogenase I 21
Phosphoprotein phosphatase I 531
Phosphoribosyl pyrophosphate I 211
Phosphorylase I 301; II 1049
– Conversion from active to inactive I 166
– Fetus I 249
– Nucleus I 83
Photochemistry II 723
– Free radical II 723
– Nucleic acid II 723
Photosensitivity I 206
Pionolactone II 994
Picolinic acid I 273
Pigmentation in Gaucher's disease I 191
Placenta I 247
– Glutamic dehydrogenase I 248
– 17-B-hydroxysteroid dehydrogenase I 248
– Steroid hormones I 248
Placental barrier I 390
Plasma proteins I 158
– Inborn errors
– – Actalasia I 159
– – Agammaglobulinemia I 159
– – Wilson's disease I 159
Plasmin I 413–414
Plasminogen I 414
Platelets
– Agglutination I 411
– Aggregation I 410
– Collagen I 410, 411
– Enzyme I 409
– Histamine I 409
– Megakaryocytes I 409
– Romanofsky staining I 409
– Serotonin I 409
– Thromboplastin I 401
– Thrombosthenin I 410
Plummer-Vinson syndrome I 383
Podophyllotoxin I 106
Polyarteritis nodosa II 878
– Prodromic factor II 878
Polycythemia I 373
Polyglycine I 151
Polyhedroses II 1003
Polyoma virus II 1013
Polyp II 951
Polymorphonuclear II 786
– Granules II 786
– – Streptolysin A II 787
Polypeptide bonds I 149
– Hormones, Extended I 510
Polypeptide chains I 123
– Elaboration I 123
Polyribosomes I 123, 135; II 1064
Polyuria in galactosemia I 167
Polyunsaturated fatty acids II 639
Pompe's disease I 199
Pores I 73
Porphobilinogen I 202, 203
Porphyria I 200
– Acquired I 209
– δ-amino levulinic acid synthetase I 209
– Coproporphyrins I 209
– Cutanea tarda I 209
– Erythropoietica I 206
– Fluorocytes I 206
– Heme I 209
– Hepatica I 207–209
– – Alcohol I 208
– – δ-amino levulinic synthetase I 208
– – Barbiturates I 208
– – Ergot preparation I 208
– – Sulfonal I 208
– Hexachlorobenzene I 209
– Isomerase I 207
– Photosensitivity I 206
– Ultaviolet light I 209
– Uroporphyrins I 209
Porphyrinogens, Conversions I 205
Porphyrins I 37, 200, 201, 373
– δ-amino levulinic acid I 203
– – Dehydrogenase I 203
– – Synthetase I 203
– Biosynthesis I 202

Porphyrins, Chemistry I 200–201
– Copper porphyrin I 201
– Heme I 205
– Porphobilinogen I 202
– Pyridoxal I 203
– Side chain I 201
– Succinate-glycine cycle I 203
– Uroporphyrins I 201
– – Biosynthesis I 204
Portocaval transposition in glycogen storage disease I 165
Posttranscriptional regulation I 1052
Potassium I 567
– Acidosis I 567
– Alkalosis I 567
– Body fluids I 567
– Carbonic anhydrase I 567
– Donnan's law I 568
– Cellular metabolism I 569
– – Acetyl kinase I 569
– – Fructose-1,6-diphosphate I 569
– – Fructose-1-phosphate I 569
– – Hyperkalemia I 569
– – Pyruvic kinase I 569
– Membrane I 567
– Metabolism I 567
– Nernst equation I 568
– Structural water I 567
Prausnitz-Kustner reaction II 834
Prematurity I 250
Primaquine, Drug induced hemolytic anemia I 171
Progesterone I 247
– Cancer II 962
– Ovaries I 480
Proinsulin covalent structure I 509
Proline I 284
– Hydroxylase I 284; II 934
Promonocyte I 790
Promotor II 987
PRPP synthetase I 211
Prophage II 1008
Prophase I 87
Propionic acid I 59
– Metabolism I 59
Propionyl CoA carboxylase I 278
Propylactone II 994
Prostaglandin II 775, 833
– A_3 II 775
– E_1 II 775
– E_3 II 775
– Biosynthesis II 776
– Function II 777
– – Aspirin II 777, 778
– – Carcinoma of thyroid II 777
– – Cholera II 777
– – Electrolyte transport II 777
– – Fertility II 777
– – Hyperemia II 777
– – Hypertension II 778
– – Inflammation II 777
– – Menstrual fluid II 777
– – Parturition II 777
– – Synaptic transmission II 777
– – Transport of water II 777
– Metabolism II 775
– – Degradation II 777
– – Hormones II 776
– – Lung II 776
– – Phospholipase II 775
– – Prostaglandin dehydrogenase II 775
– – Prostaglandin reductase I 775
– – Prostaglandin synthetase II 775
– – Synthesis II 775
– Structure II 776
Protamines I 88
Protein deficiency I 253
– Amino acid imbalance I 254
– Menstruation I 254
– Nitrogen balance I 253
Protein digestion I 255
– α-amylase I 255
– Carboxypeptidase I 256
– Chymotrypsin I 256
– Elastase I 256
– Gastric juice I 255
– Kallikrein I 255
– Lysozyme I 255
– Pepsin I 256
– Salivary glands I 255
– Trypsin I 256
– Zymogens I 256
Proteins I 149
– Amino acids I 151
– – Sequence I 149
– Configuration I 151
– – Cysteine I 151
– – Histidine I 151
– – Proline I 151
– – Serine I 151
– Hydrogen bonds I 152
– Inborn errors I 158
– Kinase I 531
– Metabolism, Liver I 585
– Peptide bonds I 151
– Polypeptide bonds I 149
– Sparing effect of carbohydrates I 589
– Structure I 149
– Synthesis I 106, 124; II 1009
– – Amino acid activation I 107
– – Amino acyl RNA synthetase I 108
– – Fetus I 250
– – *In vitro* I 107
– – *In vivo* I 106
– – Mitochondria I 449
– – Nucleus I 82
– – Phenylketonuria I 108
– Tertiary structure I 152
– Turnover I 265
Prothrombin, Deficiency® I 401
– Vitamin K I 408
Proton transfer I 550
Protoporphyrin breakdown I 386
Provirus II 1021
Proximal tubule I 594
Pseudohermaphroditism I 491
Pseudohypoparathyroidism I 354
Pseudouridine I 110
Psi factor I 119
Pulmonary acidosis I 581
– Emphysema I 581
– Pleuritis I 581
– Pneumonia I 581
– Pulmonary edema I 581
Pulmonary emphysema II 648
Pulmonary fibrosis II 648
Punctation codons I 118
Purine biosynthesis I 212, 213
– Control II 1052
– – Amidophosphoribosyltransferase II 1052
– – PRPP II 1052
– Inborn errors of metabolism I 209
Purine metabolism I 210
– Adenosinic kinase I 216
– Adenylosuccinase I 214
– AMP pyrophosphorylase I 215
– 5-amino-4-imidazole N-succinocarboxamide ribotide I 213
– 5-amino-4-imidazole carboxamide ribotide I 213
– N^5, N^{10}anhydroformyltetrahydrofolic acid I 212
– Azaserine [212, 214
– Deaminase I 217
– Formylglycinamide ribotide 212
– 5-formamido-4-imidazole carboxamide ribotide I 213
– N^{10}-for-myltetrahydrofolic acid I 213
– Guanase I 217
– Glutamine I 211
– Glycinamide ribonucleotide synthetase I 212
– Glycinamide ribotide I 212
– GTP I 214
– Isonicase I 213
– Nucleoside Hydrolases I 217
– Nucleoside phosphorylase I 215, 217
– Nucleotidases I 216
– 5′-nucleotidase I 216
– Nucleotide interconversion I 215
– Origin of various atoms of purine ring I 214
– Phosphatases I 216
– Phosphoribosyl pyrophosphate I 211
– PRPP synthetase I 211
– Purine nucleotide after conversion I 214
– Ribosylamine pyrophosphorylase I 211
– Salvage pathway I 216
– Transferases I 216
– Xanthine oxidase I 217
– Xanthosine-5-phosphate I 214
Pygmies I 433
Pyknosis I 610, 612
Pyridine nucleotides I 33
Pyridoxal I 297
– Phosphate I 60
– Maple syrup disease I 181
– Phenylketonuria I 174
Pyridoxamine I 297
Pyrimidine I 225
– Cytosine I 225
– 5-hydroxymethylcytosine I 225
– Inborn errors of metabolism I 209
– 5-methylcytosine I 225
– Pseudouracil I 225
– Thymine I 225
– Uracil I 225
– Biosynthesis I 227
Pyrimidine metabolism I 225
– Aspartic acid synthetase I 226
– Azauracil I 226
– Carbamyl phosphate I 226
– Control II 1052
– – Carbamyl phosphate II 1052
– – UTP II 1052
– Cytosine deaminases I 228
– Dehydropyrimidine dehydrogenase I 228
– 6-diazo-5oxo-L-norleucine I 227
– Dihydroorotic acid dehydrogenase I 226
– Dihydrothymine hydrolase I 228
– Dihydrouracil hydrolase I 228
– Hypoxanthine guanine phosphoribosyl transferase I 216
– 5′-nucleotidases I 228
– Orotidylic pyrophosphorylase I 226
– 5′-orotidylic acid I 226
– Orotidine-5′-phosphate decarboxylase I 226
– Phosphatases I 228
– Phosphodiesterases I 228
– Phosphoribosyl pyrophosphate I 226
– Phosphotransferases I 228

– Thymidylate synthetase I 227
– Ureidoisobutyric acid I 228
– Ureidopropionic acid I 228
Pyridoxine I 297
– Amino acid decarboxylation I 300
– Cow's milk I 298
– Cystathione I 301
– D-amino oxidation I 301
– D-amino acid racemization I 301
– Dehydrases I 301
– Deoxypyridoxine I 297
– Diamine oxidase I 301
– Glutamic aspartic transaminase I 300
– Heme synthesis I 302
– Homoserine dehydrase I 301
– Phosphorylase I 301
– Pyridoxamine phosphate I 297
– 4-pyridoxic acid I 297
– Pyridoxine phosphate oxidase I 297
– Schiff base I 299
– Serine hydroxymethyl transferase I 302
– Transamination I 299
– Urocanase I 301
– Vitamin B_6 I 297
Pyridoxine deficiency I 298
– Arteriosclerosis I 298
– Clinicopathological correlations I 298
– Convulsions I 298
– Dental caries I 298
– Lithiasis I 298, 302
– Magnesium I 298
Pyrithiamine I 267
Pyruvate decarboxylase I 270
Pyruvate metabolism I 31
– Nucleoside diphosphokinase I 31
– Phosphoenolpyruvate kinase I 31
Pyruvemia I 269
Pyruvic acid I 269
Pyruvic acid decarboxylation I 26, 27
Pyruvic carboxylase II 1042, 1046, 1047
Pyruvic decarboxylase I 269
Pyruvic kinase II 1042, 1046, 1047

Quinolinic acid I 272, 273
Quinolinic-2-carboxylic acid I 272

Rabies II 997, 1005
Radiation I 391
– Biochemical effects II 746
– – Acetic acid biosynthesis II 748
– – CO_2 elimination II 748
– – Cytoplasmic radiosensitivity II 746
– – DNA II 746
– – Enzymes II 746
– – – Amino acid oxidase II 746
– – – ATPase II 747
– – – Catalase II 746
– – – Carboxypeptidase II 746
– – – Chymotrypsinogen II 747
– – – DNase II 746
– – – Hexokinase II 747
– – – Hydrolases II 747
– – – Phosphoglyceraldehyde dehydrogenase II 747
– – – Polyphenol oxidase II 746
– – – Ribonuclease II 747
– – – Succinoxidase II 747
– – – Trypsin II 747
– – Fructose-1,6-diphosphate II 748
– – Nuclear radiosensitivity II 746
– – Oxygen consumption II 748
– Biological effect II 733
– – Delayed necrosis II 737
– – Duodenum II 737
– – Enzymes II 746
– – Jejunum II 737
– – Lung II 737
– – Nephritis II 737
– – Parotid II 737
– – Stomach II 737
– Cancer II 742
– Cause of death II 737
– Effect on antibody formation II 751
– Effect on cell population kinetics II 752
– Effects on DNA synthesis II 749, 751
– Effect on DNA synthesis, Regenerating liver II 749
– Effect on mitosis II 751
– Effects on ribosomes II 750
– Leukemia II 743, 745, 746
Radiation carcinogenesis II 742
– Xeroderma pigmentosum II 742
Rauscher virus II 1013
Receptors I 288, 437, 488, 527, 528, 531, 533, 560; II 1061, 1066, 1080
– Acetylcholine I 528
– Clustering II 1079
– Dexamethasone I 528
– Epinephrine I 528
– Glucagon I 528
– Insulin I 528
– Virus II 1000
Red cells I 566, 608
– Aging II 619
– Embden-Meyerhof pathway I 369
– Enucleation I 608
– Fate I 370
– Glutathione I 369
– Glutathione reductase I 369
– Hemoglobin I 369
– Hexose monophosphate shunt I 369
– Sodium leakage I 566
– Spherocytosis II 619
– Stromatin I 369
Red cells life span, Drug induced hemolytic anemia I 148, 171
Refsum disease I 59
Regenerating liver II 898
– Chalone II 916
– Nucleolus I 78
Regeneration II 895
– Adrenal II 920
– Blood vessels II 920
– Bone marrow II 920
– Gonads II 920
– Intestinal mucosa II 920
– Kidney II 916
– – DNA synthesis II 917
– – Mitosis II 917
– Lens II 897
– Limb II 896
– Miscellaneous II 920
– Pancreas II 917
– – Amylase II 917
– – DNA synthesis II 917
– – Ethionine II 917
– – Methionine II 918
– – Pancreatectomy II 918
– – Zymogen granules II 918
– Skin II 920
– Spleen II 920
– Tail II 895
– Liver II 898
– – Amino acid content II 900
– – Cephalin synthesis II 899
– – Cofactors II 914
– – Deoxyribonucleotides origin II 905
– – DNA synthesis II 907
– – – Regulation II 911
– – Enzyme activities II 901
– – Fatty acid synthesis II 899
– – Glycogen metabolism II 899
– – Hypertrophy II 908
– – Hypophysectomy II 914
– – Lecithin synthesis II 899
– – Lipid content II 899
– – Mitochondria II 899
– – Mitosis II 914
– – Nucleotide pools II 904
– – – Orotidylic pyrophosphorylase II 904
– – – UMP kinase II 904
– – Ornithine II 914
– – Ornithine decarboxylase II 913
– – Plasma protein II 900
– – Polyamines II 913
– – Protein synthesis II 899
– – Putrescine II 913
– – Regulation of gene expression II 908
– – RNA synthesis II 901, 902
– – – Regulation II 910
– – Spermidine II 913
– – Triggering II 914
– – Urea cycle II 914
– – Urea formation II 900
Regulator genes I 130
Releasing factor I 488, 533
Releasing hormones I 455
– LRF, CRF, GRF, PRF, MRF I 455
Renal calculi I 594
– Cysteinuria I 594
– Gout I 593, 594
– Hyperparathyroidism I 594
– Oxaluria I 594
– Phosphatic calculosis I 595
– Proximal tubule I 594
– Silicon I 595
– Tams protein I 595
– Urinary protein I 594
– Uromucoids I 595
– Vitamin A I 594
Renin I 256, 557
Renin-angiotensin system I 558
Renin-angiotensin I I 558
Renin-angiotensin II I 558
Repressor I 132
Respiratory center I 578
– Expiration I 578
– Inspiration I 578
– Pneumotaxic center I 578
– Receptor I 579
– – Chemorecepter I 579
– – Pressure receptor I 579
– – Stretch receptor I 579
Respiratory chain I 32
– Actimycin I 43
– Coenzyme Q I 43
– Cytochrome c I 43
– NADH coenzyme Q reductase I 43
– Pyridine nucleotides I 33
– Succinic coenzyme Q reductase I 43
– Ubiquinone I 42
– Vitamin E I 42
– Vitamin K I 42
Respiratory quotient I 33
Retina I 309
Retinene i I 311
Retinoblastoma II 1100
Retinol, All trans I 305
Reverse transcriptase II 1021
Reye's syndrome II 654
– Mitochondria II 654
– Ornithine-transcarbamylase deficiency II 654

Reye's syndrome, Viruses I 654
Rh System II 843
— Anti-C antibody II 843
— Anti-E antibody II 843
— D antigen II 843
— Fisher-Race theory II 843
— Weiner's theory II 844
Rheumatic fever II 866
Rheumatic heart disease II 866
— Angina pectoris II 869
— Aortic stenosis II 868
— Aschoff body II 869
— Hypostatic pneumonia II 868
— Mitral stenosis II 867
— Nodules of Minet II 869
— Verruca II 867
Rheumatoid arthritis II 875
— Amyloidosis II 877
— Clinical symptoms II 876
— Granulation tissue II 877
— Incidence II 876
— Lysosomes II 878
— Membrane II 878
— Pathogenesis II 876
— Pathology II 877
— Rheumatoid factor II 876
— Subcutaneous nodules II 877
Rhodopsin II 1076
— Vision I 312
Riboflavin I 35, 302
— Atherosclerosis I 303
— Burns I 302
— Deficiency I 303
— — Cheilitis I 303
— — Glossitis I 303
— Formula I 303
— Glycogen synthesis I 302
— Requirements I 302
Ribosomal RNA, Nucleolus I 79
Ribosomes I 123
— Proteins I 126
— — Acetylation I 125
— — Phosphorylation I 125
— RNA I 125
Ribosome binding I 126
— EF-T factor I 127
— EF-T_s factor I 127
— EF-T_u factor I 127
— Messenger RNA I 127
— Transfer RNA I 126
Ribosome in mitochondria I 67
Ribosylamine pyrophosphorylase I 211
Ribulose-5-phosphate I 21
Rickets I 341, 345
— Calcium resorption in bone I 345
— Intestinal absorption of calcium I 345
— Reabsorption of phosphate in kidney I 345
Rifampicin I 102
Rifampin II 615
dsRNA I 121
RNA methylases I 114
— S-adenosly methionine I 114
— Tumors I 115
RNA polymerase I 118; II 1020
— CAP factor I 119
— Initiation I 119
— Y factor I 119
— M factor I 119
— Mammalian I 119
— — α-amanitin I 120
— — Nucleolar I 120
— Mitochondria I 67
— Mitochondrial RNA I 449
— Nucleoplasmic I 120
— T factor I 119
— T4 phage I 119
— Units I 119
RNA release, Regenerating liver II 1041
RNA replicase II 1020
RNA synthetase II 1020
RNA transfer I 122
— Nuclear membrane I 122
— Nuclear pores I 122
Rods I 310
Rous sarcoma II 1016
— Virus II 1011

Saccharase I 503
Saccharase intolerance I 231
S-Adenosyl Methionine I 114
S-Adenosylmethionine Transferase in Phenylketonuria I 174
Salivary Gland
— DNA synthesis II 919
— Proliferation II 919
Salmonellosis and Sickle Cell Anemia I 149
Salvage pathway II 1037
Sanfilippo syndrome II 938
S antigen II 1022
Scarlatinal toxin II 1009
Sarcoidosis, Schaumann's bodies II 880
Satellite DNA I 79
Satiety center I 326
Schiff base I 300
Schwann cell II 664, 665
Schwartz virus II 1012
Scurvy II 279
— Abscesses I 282
— Adrenals I 282
— Amino acid Concentration I 283
— Cataracts I 284
— Clinicopathology I 279
— Collagen I 279, 281
— Dentin I 279
— Endochondral Ossification I 279
— Fibroblasts I 279
— Glucose tolerance I 283
— Glucuronic pathway I 282
— 17-Hydroxycorticosteroid I 283
— Hydroxyphenylpyruvic hydroxylase I 283
— Insulin I 283
— Lipoic acid I 283
— Mucopolysaccharide I 284
— Odontoblasts I 279
— Osteoblasts I 279
— Osteoid I 279
— Proline hydroxylase I 284
— Stress I 282
— Subperiosteal hemorrhage I 281
— Trummerfeld zone I 281
— Wound healing I 281
— X-irradiation I 283
Seborrheic dermatitis I 278
Secretinase I 262
Secretin I 262
Selenium I 317
Serine hydroxymethyl transferase I 302
Serotonin II 833
Serotonin in Phenylketonuria I 174
Serum calcium I 354
Sex chromatin I 241
Sex chromosomes I 85, 489
— Anomalies I 490
— — Amenorrhea I 490
— — Deletion I 490
— — Ring X I 490
— — Sterility I 490
— Lyon's hypothesis I 491
Sex glands
— Hereditary disease I 489
— — Klinefelter's syndrome I 489
— — Turner's syndrome I 490
Sex hormones I 479
— Breast I 482
— Cervical gland I 482
— Effect of hypophysis I 486
— Effect of male sex hormones I 482
— Feedback regulation I 487
— Fertilization I 482
— Hypophysis FSH I 486
— Hypophysis ICSH I 487
— Hypophysis LSH I 486
— Menstrual cycle I 481
— Placenta I 482
— Receptor I 488
— Stein-Levanthal syndrome I 494
— Vaginal epithelium I 482
Shope papilloma II 1017
Shope papilloma virus II 1011
— Carcinogens II 1011
— Hormones II 1011
Sialic acid biosynthesis I 189
Sialic acid synthesis I 185
Sialyl transferase II 1080
Sickle cell anemia I 145
— Aspirin I 155
— Balanced polymorphism I 149
— Bone marrow pathology I 149
— Cyanate I 154
— Malaria I 149
— Pathogenesis I 148
— Pathology I 147
— Radiological Picture I 149
— Red cell life span I 148
— Salmonellosis I 149
— Urea I 154
Sickle cell trait I 149
Siderosis I 379
— Cytosiderosis I 379
— Kashin-Beck disease I 379
— Lungs I 379
— Nerves I 379
Sigma unit I 119
Simmonds' cachexia I 432
Sinalbumin I 502
Sites of phosphorylation I 47
Skin cancer II 950
Slow virus diseases II 1009
— Aleutian mink disease II 1009
— Creutzfeldt-Jakob disease II 1009
— Heredity II 1009
— Kuru II 1009
Smallpox II 1005
Smegma cancer II 962
Smoking II 700
Smooth endoplasmic reticulum II 647
snRNA I 121
Sodium II 1064
Sodium balance I 555
Sodium inhibition of initiation I 129
Sodium leakage, glycolysis I 566
Sodium leakage, red cells I 566
Sodium load I 560
Sodium losses I 560
Sodium metabolism I 551
— Sodium chloride I 551
— Sodium pool I 551
— Sodium potassium dependent ATPase I 552
— Sodium pump I 551
Sodium potassium ATPase II 1967
Sodium potassium dependent/ATPase I 552
— Membranes I 552

Sodium pump I 551
– Hypoxia I 551
Sodium reabsorption I 553
– Carbonic anhydrase I 554
– Congestive heart failure I 554
– Regulation I 554
– – Aldosterone I 554
Somatomedin A I 429
Somatostasin I 429
Spherocytosis II 619
Sphingolipids metabolism I 199
Spindle II 1064
Spingosine biosynthesis I 186
Splenomegaly in thalassemia I 157
Sprue I 320, 322
– Crypts of lieberkuht I 322
– Gliadin I 323
– Idiopathic steatorrhea I 322
– Intestinal flora I 323
Squalene conversion II 695, 696
– Squalene oxidocyclase II 696
Squalene formation II 695
– Farnesoate II 694
– Farnesyl pyrophosphate II 694
– 48–47 Isomerases II 696
– Isopentenyl pyrophosphate II 694
– Mevalonic kinase II 694
– Nerolidol pyrophosphate II 695
Squamous cell carcinoma II 1100
Staphylococcal toxin II 1009
Starvation I 77, 252
Steatorrhea I 319, 343
– Cystic fibrosis I 320
– Sprue I 320
Steatosis II 647
– Alcoholism II 647
Stein-Leventhal syndrome I 494
– Amenorrhea I 494
– Block of 3-β-oldehydrogenase I 494
– Flushes I 494
– Hirsutism I 494
– Obesity I 494
– Polycystic ovary I 494
Steroid hormone biosynthesis I 460
– ACTH I 461
– Adrenodixin reductase I 463
– Aldosterone I 465
– Androstendione I 463
– Cholesterol I 460
– Conversion of cholesterol to pregenolone I 461
– Desmolase I 463
– 17-estradioldehydrogenase I 465
– Estrogen I 465
– Formation of cortisol I 462
– Formation of progresterone I 462
– 20-hydroxycholesterol I 460
– 22-hydroxycholesterol I 460
– 11-hydroxylase I 463
– Isomerase I 463
– Pathway for estrogen I 466
– Pathway for testosterone I 465
– Pregnanediol I 460
– Sex hormone synthesis I 464
– Sex hormone testosterone I 465
Steroids I 21, 24
Steroid hormone inactivation I 466
– Aryl sulfate I 466
– Cirrhosis I 466
– Conjugation I 466
– Dehydrogenase I 467
– Glucuronidase I 466
– Glucuronides I 466
– Hydroxysteroid dehydrogenase I 467
– Hypothyroidism I 466
– 4-reductase I 466
– Reductases I 467
Steroid hormones I 494
– Amino acid uptake I 483
– Aryl sulfatase I 466
– Glucose-6-phosphate dehydrogenase I 483
– Glutamic dehydrogenase I 483
– Hormone gene theory I 485
– Liver disease I 494
– Mechanisms of action I 483
– Protein biosynthesis I 484
– Receptors I 486
– RNA synthesis I 485
– Transhydrogenase I 483
– Uptake of α-aminoisobutyric acid I 483
Steroid metabolism I 531
Stillbirth I 250
Stomach cancer II 1100
Streptococcal toxin II 1009
Stress I 282
Stretch receptor I 556
Stromatin I 369
Structural genes I 130
Structured water II 725
Succinate-glycine cycle I 203
Succinic coenzyme Q reductase I 43
Succinic dehydrogenase I 30, 36
Sucrase I 503
Sugar absorption I 504
– Carrier I 504
– Energy I 504
– Sodium I 504
Sulfanilamide drug induced hemolytic anemia I 170
Sulfatase I 196
Sulfatides I 196
Sulfatide synthetase I 196
Sulfating factor I 431
Sulfonal I 208
Sympatheticoblastomas II 1096
Syphilis II 797
– Gumma II 797
Syndrome S II 938
Syringomyelia II 672

T Factor I 119
Taka-diastase I 34
T antigen II 1022
Tangier disease II 711
Tay-Sachs disease I 184
– Brain I 186, 187, 188
– Gangliosides I 185
– Hexosaminidase I 190
– Pathogenesis I 190
– Retina I 184
T cells II 822
– Antigen recognition II 825
– Helper substance II 826
– Receptor II 825
– Rosette formation II 826
Telophase I 87
Teratomas II 954
Termination codons I 118
12-O-tetradecanoyl-phorbol-13-acetate II 987
Thalassemia I 157
– Anemia I 157
– Bone marrow hyperplasia I 157
– Hair on end I 157
– Heme I 158
– Hemosiderosis I 157
– Heinz bodies I 158
– Hepatomegaly I 157
– Mongoloid facies I 157
– Spenomegaly I 157
– Vicarious liver erythropoiesis I 157
Throphylline I 210
Thiamine hydroxyethylthiamine I 269
Thiamine pyrophosphate I 22
Thiamine pyrophosphokinase I 268
Thioacetamide I 78
Thiokinase I 54, 55
Thiouracil I 441
Thiouridine I 110
Thrombi I 415, 416, 671
– Platelets I 416
– Postmortem I 417
– Red I 417
Thrombin I 401, 403
Thromblastin component deficiency I 407
Thromblastin deficiency christmas disease I 407
Thrombocytopenia I 412
Thrombosis I 352
Thrombocytopenic purpura I 412
– Neonatal I 413
Thromboplastin I 402
Thrombosthenin I 410
Thrombus I 415
– Mural I 417
– Opthalmotonometry II 708
– Steps in formation I 418
– Vegetation I 417
Thymidine methylation I 227
– Aminopterin I 227
Thymidylate synthetase I 227
Thymine dimers II 725
Thymopoietin II 824
Thymopoietin II II 824
Thymus II 824
– Products II 824
– Myasthenia gravis II 824
Thymus tumors II 1096
Thyroglobulin I 441
Thyroglobulin synthesis I 441
Thyroid disease I 439
Thyroid adenoma hyperthyroidism I 451
Thyroid cancer II 1100
Thyroid carcinoma I 358
Thyroid hormone I 441, 444
– Binding I 443
– Effect on mitochondrial RNA I 449
– Effect on protein synthesis in mitochondria I 449
– Effect on RNA polymerase I 449
– Liver disease I 444
– Metabolism I 445
– Respiratory and metabolic acidosis I 444
Thyroid hormone in blood I 443
Thyroid hormone metabolism I 442
– Nicotinic acid I 446
– Riboflavin I 446
– Thiamine I 446
– Vitamin A I 446
Thyroid pathology I 450
– Heterotrope factor (HTF) I 453
– Long acting thyroid stimulus (LATS) I 453
– Short acting thyroid stimulus (SATS) I 453
– Thyrotropin I 453
– TSH I 453
Thyroid hormone secretion control I 453
Thyroxine I 306
– Crystallization I 444
– Free I 444
Thyroxine metabolism I 442
Tissue graft II 838
– Allograft II 838

Tissue graft, Autograft II 838
— Histocompatibility genes II 839
— Isograft II 838
— Transplantation antigens II 839
— Xenograft II 838
Tobacco mosaic virus, amino acid code I 117
Tobacco mosaic virus, organization II 998
Tolbutamide I 508
Tophi I 219
Tower skull and sickle cell anemia I 149
Toyocamycin II 615
Transaminase in maple syrup disease I 181
Transamination, nonenzymic I 299
Transcription I 122
— Nucleoli I 122
Transfer factors II 1099
Transfer RNA binding to ribosomes I 126
Transfer RNA in mitochondria I 67
Transferrin I 365, 381
Transferrinemia I 381
Transformation II 1023
— Hybridization II 1024
— Morphology II 1023
— Partial transcription II 1023
— Phenotypic changes II 1023
— Reserve transcriptase II 1024
— Viral genome II 1023
Transformation in vitro II 988
Transformylase activity I 129
Transhydrogenase I 34; II 644
Transketolase I 21, 270
Translation inhibitors II 616
Transmethylation I 589
Transplantation antigens II 839
TRH structure I 455
tRNA I 109; II 1061
— Alanine RNA I 110
— Configuration I 112
— Dihydrouridine I 110
— Inosine I 110
— Methyl purines I 110
— Pseudouridine I 110
— Sequence I 110
— Synthesis tRNA I 109
TSH secretion II 1096
TSTA antigen II 1022
Tricarboxylic acid I 26
— Pyruvic acid decarboxylation I 26
— Thiamine pyrophosphate I 26
Triglycerides biosynthesis II 692
3,5′,3′-Triiodothyronine I 444
Triphosphopyridine nucleotide (NADP) I 33
Triose phosphate dehydrogenase nucleus I 80
Trisomy I 489
— X I 489
— XX I 490
— XXY I 489
— XYY I 490
Tropocollagen II 926, 927
Tropoelastin II 929
Trousseau's sign I 354
Trummerfeld zone I 281
Trypsin I 256
Trypsinogen I 257
— Amino acid sequence I 258
Tryptophan I 274
Tryptophan metabolism I 272, 273
— 2-Acroleyl-3-amino-fumarate I 272
— Catalase I 272
— Diabetes I 273
— 3-hydroxyanthranilic acid I 272, 274
— 3-hydroxyanthranilic oxidase I 272
— Kynurenase I 272, 274
— Kynurenine formamidase I 272
— Kynurenine-3-hydroxylase I 272
— Kynurenine transaminase I 273
— Nicotinic acid I 272
— Nicotinic ribonucleotide I 273
— Picolinic acid I 273
— Quinolinic acid I 272, 273
— Quinolonic-2-carboxylic acid I 272
— Tryptophan pyrrolase I 272
— Xanthurenic acid I 272
Traptophan pyrrolase I 272
TSH secretion I 454, 455
— Control hypothalamus I 454
— Control neurohormone (TRH) I 454
— Receptors I 454
— Releasing hormones I 455
Tuberculosis II 796
— Caseation II 797
— Macrophages II 848
— Miliary II 798
— Prostate II 799
Tumors II 947
— Benign II 947
— — Acquired I 947
— — Congenital II 947
— Cystic II 947
— Malignant II 947, 948
— — Cytoplasmic abnormalities II 949
— — Nuclear changes II 949
Tumor cells I 514
Tumors RNA methylase I 115
Turner's syndrome I 490
— Amenorrhea I 490
— Breast I 490
— Gonadotropins I 490
— Ovaries I 490
— Sterility I 490
Turnover, endoplasmic reticulum I 587
— microbodies I 587
— proteases I 587
M-tyramine in phenylketonuria I 174
Tyrosinase in albinism I 179
— phenylketonuria I 174
Tyrosine aminotransferase II 1054
— transaminase, infancy I 250
— — phenylketonuria I 174, 175
Tyrosinosis I 177

Ubiquinone I 42
UDP-glucuronide pyrophosphatase I 24
UDP-transglucuronylase I 24
Ulcerative colitis II 885
Ultraviolet light porphyria I 209
Ultraviolet radiation in albinism I 178
Unsaturated fatty acid I 185
Unwinding protein I 102
Urea I 226
Urea cycle I 589
— Arginine synthetase I 590
— Carbamyl phosphate synthetase I 590
— Inborn errors I 588, 591
— Ornithine carbamyl transferase I 590
— Rate-limiting step I 590
Urea-forming system nucleus I 84
Urea metabolism I 585
Urea synthesis I 589
Uremia I 591
— Chronic renal disease I 592
— Erythropoietin I 591
— Glucose tolerance I 591, 592
— Pericarditis I 591
— Secondary hyperparathyroidism I 592
— Toxin I 591, 592
Urethane II 984
— N-hydroxy derivative II 984
Uric acid I 210
— Reabsorption I 545
Uric acid degradation I 211
Uric acid metabolism I 217
— Uricase I 217
Uricase I 217
Uridine diphosphoglucose dehydrogenase I 24
Urine formation I 542
— Antidiuretic hormones I 545
— Autoregulation of glomerular filtration I 543
— Blood pressure I 543
— Convoluted tubules I 544
— Countercurrent exchanges I 545
— Glomerular filtration I 543
— Loop of Henle I 544
Urobilinogens I 388
— Enterohepatic cycle I 388
— Stercobilin I 388
Urocanase I 301
— Histidinemia I 179
Urocanic acid in histidinemia I 179
Uroporphyrinogen I I 204, 205
— Uroporphyrinogen III I 204, 205
Uroporphyrin I I 204
— Uroporphyrin III I 204
Uterus II 962
— Deciduomas II 963
— Endometrial moles II 963
— Polyps II 963
UV irradiation II 724
— Base alteration II 724
— Biological effects II 717, 724
— Effect on skin II 726
— Structured water II 725
— Thymine dimers II 725
UV light I 106

Vagina, cancer II 967
Valine in maple syrup disease I 181
Valinomycin II 1077
van den Bergh reaction I 387
— Direct I 387
— Indirect I 387
Vasopressin I 434
— Acenyl cyclase I 437
— Alteration in functional activity I 434
— Amino acid sequence I 434
— Cyclic AMP I 437
— Microtubules I 437
— Receptors I 437
— Secretion I 435
— — Baroreceptors I 436
— — Epinephrine I 436
— — Prostaglandin E I 436
— — Volume receptor I 436
— Synthesis I 434
Vicarious liver erythropoiesis in thalassemia I 157
Vinblastine I 106
Viral replication II 1019
— Catabolism II 1022
— Changes in cell membrane II 1022
— Cyclic AMP II 1022
— DNA synthesis II 1021
— Enzyme induction II 1021
— Minus strand II 1020
— Murine leukosis virus II 1021
— Plus strand II 1020
— Provirus II 1021
— Reverse transcriptase II 1021
— RNA polymerase II 1020
— RNA replicase II 1020
— RNA synthetase II 1020
— RNA virus II 1019
— S antigen II 1022

— T antigen II 1022
— TSTA antigen II 1022
— Vaccinia II 1019
— Viral messenger RNA II 1021
Viroids II 1010
Viruses II 996
— Affectiveness of RNA II 998
— Bacteriophage II 997
— Capsid II 999
— Chemotherapy II 1005
— — Halogenated pyrimidines II 1005
— — N′,N′-Anhydrobis (β-hydroxyethyl) biguanide hydrochloride II 1005
— — N-Methylisatin 3-thiosemicarbazone II 1005
— Cytoplasmic alterations I 1001
— Hepatitis II 650
— Inclusion, viral II 1002
— — Cytomegalovirus II 1003
— — Nuclear II 1003
— — Polyhedroses II 1003
— Inclusion bodies II 1002
— — Councilman bodies II 1003
— — Guarnieri's bodies II 1003
— Injuries II 1000
— Interferons II 1006
— Lysogeny II 1008
— — Diptheria toxin II 1008
— — Herpetic infection II 1008
— — λ phage II 1008
— — Prophage II 1008
— Molecular biology II 997
— *Molluscum contagiosum* II 1003
— Morphopoietic factors II 1000
— Morphopoietic genes II 1000
— Myxoviruses II 998
— Nuclear injuries II 1001
— Phagocytosis II 1000
— Polykaryocytosis II 1004
— Properties II 998
— — DNA II 998
— — RNA II 998
— — Shapes II 998
— — Size II 998
— Protein II 997
— Rabies II 997
— Receptors II 1000
— RNA II 997
— Rod shape II 998
— Self-assembly II 999
— — Of tobacco mosaic virus II 999
— Spherical II 998
— — Icosahedral II 999
— — Octahedral II 999
— Structural organization II 998
— Temperate II 1007
— Tetrahedral II 999
— Tobacco mosaic II 997, 998
— Toxins II 1007
— — Diphtheria II 1007
— Turnip yellow mosaic II 999
— Ultrastructural changes II 1002
— Vaccinia II 998
— Vaccination II 1004
— — Rabies II 1005
— — Smallpox II 1005
— Virulent II 1007
Viscous metamorphosis, Product I I 401
Viscous metamorphosis, Product II I 401
Vision, molecular events I 312
Vitamin A (C11-cis-Retinol) I 305
— Carotene I 306
— Geometric isomers I 304
— Kupffer cells I 306
— Opsin I 306
— Retinol I 305
— Retinol binding protein I 306
— Sources I 305
— Storage I 306
Vitamin A deficiency I 304
— Aureomycin I 306
— Bone growth I 307
— Clinical pathological correlation I 307
— Hemeralopia I 304
— Hydrocephalus I 308
— Keratinization I 307
— Keratomalacia I 304
— Nyctalopia I 307
— Steatorrhea I 305
— Thyroxine I 306
— Xerophthalmia I 304, 307
Vitamin A metabolism I 308
— Alcohol dehydrogenase I 311
— Chondroitin sulfate I 308
— Differentiation I 309
— DNA synthesis I 309
— Glycolysis I 308
— Keratinization I 308
— Lysosomes I 309
— Mucous synthesis I 308
— Protein synthesis I 309
— Retina I 309
— Retinene 1 I 311
— Rhodopsin I 312
— Rods and cones I 310
— Vision I 312
Vitamin B_1 I 266
— Alcoholism I 266
Vitamin B_6 I 297
Vitamin B_{12} I 59, 286
— Absorption I 286
— Acetate synthesis I 291
— Aminomutases I 290
— Cancer I 292
— Cobamide I 289
— Corrin ring I 290
— Cyanocobalamin I 290
— Dehydrase I 291
— DNA synthesis I 292
— Ethanolamine deaminase I 291
— Intrinsic factor I 286
— Megaloblast I 292
— Methionine synthesis I 292
— Methotrexate I 292
— Methylaspartate I 290
— Methyl transfer I 291
— Methylitaconate I 290
— Methylmalonic aciduria I 291
— Methylmalonyl CoA I 290
— Receptors I 288
— Releasing factor I 288
— Ribose to deoxyribose conversion I 291
— RNA synthesis I 292
— Thioredoxin I 291
— Thymidylate synthetase I 292
— Werner's theory I 286
Vitamin D I 341
— Absorption I 343
— Calciferol I 342
— Calcium binding to protein I 344
— Calcium sensitive ATPase I 344
— Chemistry I 341
— 1,25-dihydroxycholecalciferol I 343
— Ergosterol I 342
— Esterification I 343
— Formula I 342
— Formula of calciferol I 341
— 25-Hydroxycholecalciferol I 343
— Intestinal absorption of calcium I 343
— Lumisterol I 342
— Precalciferol I 342
— Provitamin D I 342
— Steatorrhea I 343
— Tachysterol I 342
Vitamin D metabolism I 343, 344
Vitamin deficiency I 266, 284
— Ascorbic acid deficiency I 279
— Beriberi I 266
— Biotin deficiency I 278
— Nicotinic acid I 271
— Pantothenic acid deficiency I 276
— Pellagra I 271
— Scurvy I 279
— Seborrheic dermatitis I 278
— Thiamine deficiency I 266
Vitamin E I 42
— Antioxidant I 316
— Dimers I 315
— Electron transport I 317
— α-Ketopheronic acid I 315
— Lysosomes I 316
— Microsomes I 316
— Mitochondria I 316
— Organic degradation I 313
— Organic synthesis I 314
— Tocopherols, formulas I 313
— α-Tocopherol hydroquinone conjugate I 315
— α-Tocopheronolactone conjugate I 315
— Trimers I 315
Vitamin E deficiency I 313
— Ceroid accumulation I 315
— Duodenal ulcers I 314
— Muscular injury I 315
— Pregnancy I 315
— Spermatogenesis I 315
— Zenker degeneration I 315
Vitamin E metabolism I 315
— Coenzyme Q I 317
— Creatine phosphokinase I 317
— Hydrolases I 317
— Selenium I 317
Vitamin K I 42, 408
— Drug induced hemolytic anemia I 170
Von Gierke's disease I 164, 199
Von Recklinghausen's disease I 352
Von Willebrand's disease I 406

Water metabolism I 546
— Bound water I 549
— Dehydration I 546
— Edema I 546
— Thirst I 546
— Water reabsorption I 546
Water molecule I 547
— Debye units I 547
— Dipole moment I 547
— Flickering iceberg I 548
— Hydrogen bond I 547
— Ice crystals I 548
— Polarity I 547
— Water cage I 548
— Water clusters I 548
Water retention I 265
Water structure I 547
— Anesthetics I 550
— Clathrate I 550
— Collagen I 550
— Membranes I 550
— Proteins I 550
— Proton transfer I 549, 550
— Water molecule I 547
Watson-Crick model of DNA I 99
Weber-Fechner law I 311
Wegener's granulomatosis II 879
Werner's theory I 286
Wilm's tumor II 1100

Wilson's disease I 159
— Aciduria I 160
— Alzheimer cells I 160
— Amino aciduria I 163
— Ceruloplasmin I 159, 160
— Cirrhosis I 159, 160
— Copper I 159
— Hepatolenticular degeneration I 159
— 1-Methylhistidine I 160
— 3-Methylhistidine I 160
— Pathogenesis I 162
Wound healing I 281; II 920
— β-Aminopropionitrile II 937
— Amphibians II 921
— Ascorbic acid deficiency II 937
— Biochemistry II 924, 937
— — Acid phosphatase II 937
— — Alkaline phosphatase II 937
— — Aminopeptidase II 937
— — Cell proliferation II 924
— — Collagen formation II 924
— — β-Glucuronidase II 937
— Causes II 920
— Epitheliomesenchymal interactions II 938
— First intention II 921
— Homeostasis II 921
— Inflammation II 921
— Low-protein diet II 937
— Mammals II 922
— — Collagen II 923
— — — Tensile properties II 923
— — Contact inhibition II 922
— — Chalones II 922
— — Desmosomes II 922
— — Fibroblasts II 922
— — Fibrogenesis II 922
— — Mitosis II 922
— — Scar tissue II 923
— Penicillin II 937
— Purposes II 920
— Second intention II 920
— X-irradiation effects II 937

Xanthine I 210
Xanthine oxidase I 217
Xanthinuria I 217, 232
Xanthoma II 710
Xanthomatosis tuberosa II 711
Xanthurenic acid I 272, 274
X-irradiation I 283
— Absorption II 717
— Biological effects II 717
— Carcinogenesis II 1041
— Compton effect II 718, 719
— Cross-linking II 726
— DNA repair II 756
— Double-strand breaks II 756
— Effect on chromosomes II 753
— Effect on DNA *in vitro* II 753
— Effect on DNA *in vivo* II 755
— Effect on mitosis II 755
— Excitation II 720
— Free radicals II 753
— G value II 723
— Hydrated electron II 722
— Photoelectric effects II 718
— Radiation holes II 723
— Radiolysis II 722
— Repair, cycloheximide II 756
— Single-strand breaks II 754, 755
— — 3'hydroxyl 5' phosphoryl bond, II 755
— Thomson effect II 718
— Thymine products II 753
— Thymine radiolysis II 754
— Xeroderma pigmentosum II 756
X-Radiation, mitosis I 87
X-ray, nucleolus I 79
X-ray carcinogenesis II 742

Zinc I 376
Zymogen granules I 52
Zymogens I 256

Related Titles

T.E. Barman

Enzyme Handbook

2 Volumes, not sold separately

The Enzyme Handbook, the first compilation of its kind, provides in a concise and orderly manner molecular data on 800 enzymes.

Cyclic AMP, Cell Growth, and the Immune Response

Proceedings of the Symposium Held at Marco Island, Florida, January 8–10, 1973. Editors: W. Braun, L.M. Lichtenstein, C.W. Parker

This book is an attempt to define what is known about the pathogenesis of the complex events that underlie the immune response, with particular reference to the possible role of cyclic AMP as a modulating agent.

T. Kawai

Clinical Aspects of the Plasma Proteins

What is currently known about plasma proteins is reviewed clearly and with great thoroughness. The author first explains the physico-chemical and pathophysiological basis of plasma proteins and then calls upon his own extensive experience in discussing their clinical importance.

Lipids and Lipidoses

Editor: G. Schettler

Contributors: R.M. Burton, D.G. Cornwell, W. Fuhrmann, W. Kahlke, L.W. Kinsell, D. Kritchevsky, R.J. Rossiter, G. Schettler, G. Schlierf, B. Shapiro, W. Stoffel, H. Wagener

Springer-Verlag
Berlin Heidelberg New York

Metabolic Changes Induced by Alcohol

Editors: G.A. Martini, C. Bode

With contributions by numerous experts

Metabolic Interconversion of Enzymes 1973

3rd International Symposium held in Seattle, June 5–8, 1973. Organized by E.H. Fischer, E.G. Krebs, H. Neurath, E.R. Stadtman

This report continues the series of published proceedings on one of the most urgent themes of current biochemical research, begun in 1971 with the appearance of the report of the Sixth Scientific Conference of the Gesellschaft Deutscher Naturforscher und Ärzte.

Proteinase Inhibitors

Proceedings of the 2nd International Research Conference on Proteinase Inhibitors held at Grosse Ledder near Cologne, Germany, October 16–20, 1973. Editors: H. Fritz, H. Tschesche, L.J. Greene, E. Truscheit. (Bayer-Symposium 5)

This collection of original papers and reviews conveys a good overall impression of the present state of knowledge and research on proteinase inhibitors. The various classes – from animal sera, organs and secretions, as well as from plants and bacteria – are discussed together with their chemical, physiochemical, and molecular characteristics, and their importance in physiology and pathophysiology.

D.F.H. Wallach, R.J. Winzler

Evolving Strategies and Tactics in Membrane Research

Research on the structure and function of biological membranes constitutes one of the most important areas of experimental medicine and biology. This up-to-date, critical, interdisciplinary overview deals with the techniques and methods used in research.

Related Titles

The Dynamic Structure of Cell Membranes

Editors: D.F. Hölzl Wallach, H. Fischer
(22. Colloquium der Gesellschaft für Biologische Chemie, 15.–17. April 1971 in Mosbach/Baden)

This book comprises tutorial reviews of the most exciting areas of membrane biology by noted worldwide authorities. Its diverse, interdisciplinary material is knit together in a comprehensive round-table discussion.

Protein-Calorie Malnutrition

A Nestlé Foundation Symposium. Editor: A.v. Muralt

The symposium on protein-calorie malnutrition, which gathered experts from 12 countries, discussed, among other subjects mainly the possibility of a biochemical assessment of human adaptation to a low protein intake. It became clear that there is no single and unique method, but that the approach has to be made with a "battery" of biochemical methods. A new trend developed at this symposium: the introduction of highly refined biochemical methods in the study of world problems of nutrition.

Connective Tissues

Biochemistry and Pathophysiology. Editors: R. Fricke, F. Hartmann. Editorial Board: E. Buddecke, R. Fricke, F. Hartmann, H. Muir, K. Kühn

These symposium proceedings present current research on connective tissues and cover the latest information on metabolism and catabolism in their various components, including the findings of biochemists, immunobiologists, and pathophysiologists. Each chapter is virtually a self-contained review of one particular area of the field.

Journals

Berichte Biochemie und Biologie

Biochemistry – Biology

Referierendes Organ der Deutschen Botanischen Gesellschaft und der Zoologischen Gesellschaft
Managing Editors: G. Czihak, R. Lehmann, G. Schoser, E. Schwartz, J. Schwoerbel, L. Träger, M. Wiedemann, I. Ziegler

Berichte Physiologie, physiologische Chemie und Pharmakologie

Physiology – Physiological Chemistry – Pharmacology

Edited by K. Lang
Managing Editors: K. Lang in cooperation with A. Fricker

European Journal of Biochemistry

Published on behalf of the Federation of European Biochemical Societies (FEBS)

Editor-in-Chief: C. Liébecq

Histochemistry

Managing Editor: T.H. Schiebler

Molecular and General Genetics

An International Journal

Managing Editors: G. Melchers, H. Stube

Springer-Verlag
Berlin Heidelberg New York

7633731
3 1378 00763 3731